FELINE GASTROENTEROLOGY

Fabio Procoli
Karin Allenspach
Silke Salavati Schmitz

FELINE GASTROENTEROLOGY

edra

Feline Gastroenterology
Fabio Procoli, Karin Allenspach, Silke Salavati Schmitz

ISBN: 978-88-214-5233-8
eISBN: 978-88-214-5234-5

Book Publishing Manager: Costanza Smeraldi
Paper, Printing and Binding Manager: Paolo Ficicchia

Cover and Layout: Grupo Asís Biomedia S.L., Zaragoza, Spain
Copyediting: Grupo Asís Biomedia S.L., Zaragoza, Spain
Scientific consultant: Enrico Febbo

Edra S.p.A.
Via G. Spadolini 7, 20141 Milano (Italy)
Tel. 02 881841
www.edizioniedra.it

Printed by "Printer Trento" S.r.l., Trento (Italy), October 2021

(*) Edra S.p.A. is part of LSWR GROUP

Editors

FABIO PROCOLI

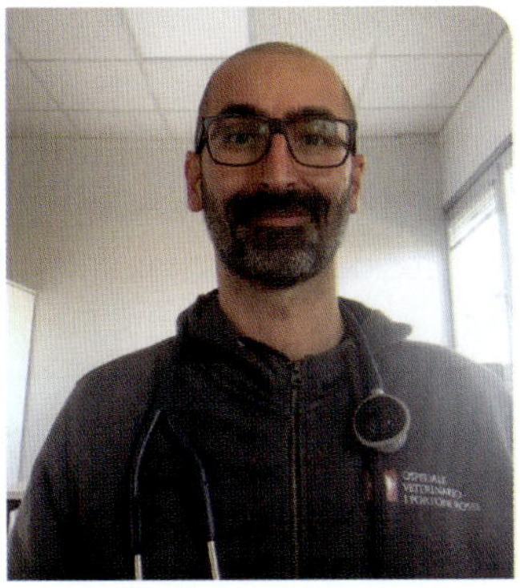

DMV, MVetMed, DipACVIM, DipECVIM-CA, MRCVS

Fabio Procoli graduated from the University of Bari (Italy) in 2003. After moving to the UK, he worked in small animal general practice for 5 years. He then did an internship in small animal medicine and surgery at The Royal (Dick) School of Veterinary Studies in Edinburgh, followed by a residency in small animal internal medicine at the Royal Veterinary College in London. He is a diplomate of the American College of Veterinary Internal Medicine and the European College of Veterinary Internal Medicine. Fabio worked as an internal medicine and gastroenterology consultant in a private referral hospital in Hampshire (UK) for 3 years before returning to Italy to lead the Internal Medicine Department at Ospedale Veterinario I Portoni Rossi, a private small animal referral hospital in Bologna.

Besides consulting in gastroenterology cases, Fabio is responsible for the training of aspiring ECVIM Diploma candidates. Fabio is member of the Exam Committee of the ECVIM. He has published in peer-reviewed journals on small animal gastroenterology and is actively involved in postgraduate continuing education courses aimed at general practitioners with an interest in small animal gastroenterology.

KARIN ALLENSPACH

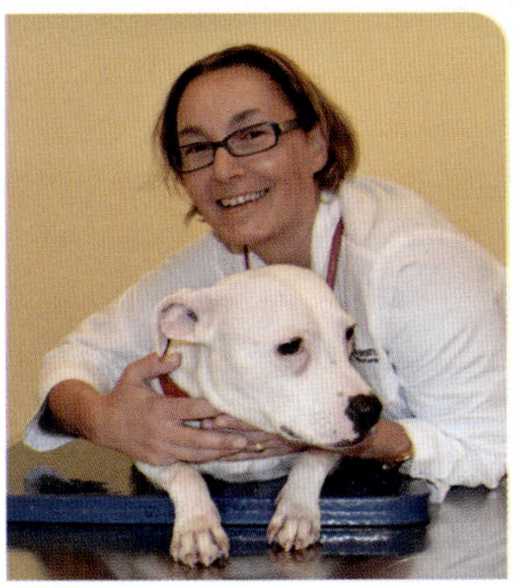

DVM, PhD, DipECVIM-CA

Karin Allenspach graduated from the University of Zurich (Switzerland). She did an internship in small animal emergency medicine and critical care at Tufts University (USA) and a residency in small animal internal medicine at the University of Pennsylvania (USA). Karin is a diplomate of the European College of Veterinary Internal Medicine. She was awarded a PhD in veterinary immunology from the University of Bern (Switzerland) for her work on canine chronic enteropathies. Karin is currently employed as Professor in Internal Medicine and Translational Health at Iowa State University, Ames (USA), where she also supervises the SMART Comparative Medicine Laboratory.

Karin is passionate about gastrointestinal diseases in dogs and cats and about using spontaneous animal diseases in clinical trials as models for human disease. She has published over 100 peer-reviewed articles and over 20 book chapters and was named a Fellow of the American Gastroenterology Association in 2018.

SILKE SALAVATI SCHMITZ

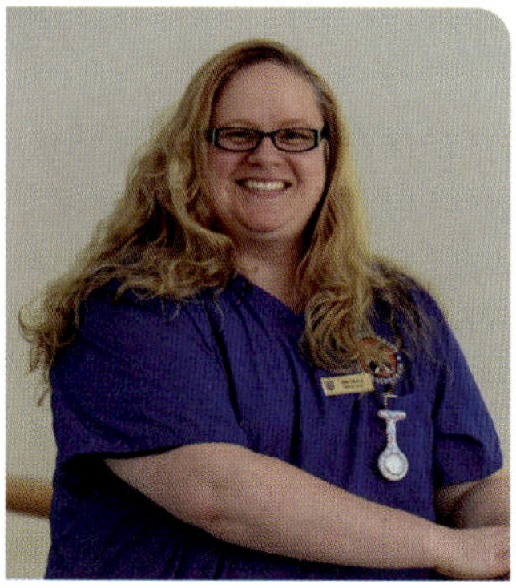

DrMedVet, PhD, DipECVIM-CA, FHEA, MRCVS

Silke Salavati Schmitz graduated from the Justus-Liebig University in Giessen (Germany), where she subsequently completed her first doctoral thesis (DrMedVet) in canine gastroenterology. She did a rotating internship and a residency in small animal internal medicine at the same university. Apart from being a diplomate of the European College of Veterinary Internal Medicine, she has also been actively involved with the ECVIM in different roles (e.g. exam and education committee member; ESCG president). She was awarded a PhD from the Royal Veterinary College, London, for her research on the clinical and immunological effects of a single-strain probiotic in canine IBD. She is currently a Senior Lecturer in Small Animal Internal Medicine at The Royal (Dick) School of Veterinary Studies in Edinburgh.

Silke continues to have a great interest in canine and feline gastroenterology and has over 30 publications around these topics and several book chapters in relevant textbooks. She has presented her work in numerous conferences throughout the years and held a large number of CPD events in various countries. She is equally passionate about teaching and mentoring future veterinarians and small animal specialists and holds a postgraduate certificate in academic practice (PGAP) as well as a Fellowship of the Higher Education Academy (FHEA).

Contributors

Mark Ackermann, DVM, PhD, DipACVP
Oregon State University, USA

David J. Argyle, BVMS, PhD, DipECVIM-CA, FRSE, FRSA, FRCVS
University of Edinburgh, UK

Davide Berlato, DipECVIM-CA, MSc(Clin Onc), PhD, MRCVS
AniCura Animal Oncology and Imaging Center, Hünenberg, Switzerland

Kelly L. Bowlt Blacklock, BVM&S, DipECVS, SFHEA, PGCert, PhD, MRCVS
University of Edinburgh, UK

Craig Breheny, BVM&S, DipECVIM-CA, MRCVS
University of Edinburgh, UK

Daniel L. Chan, DVM, DipACVECC, DipECVECC, DipACVN
University of London, UK

Fiona Da Riz, DVM
École nationale vétérinaire d'Alfort, France

Julien R. S. Dandrieux, BSc, DrMedVet, PhD, DipACVIM
University of Melbourne, Australia

Georgia Diakoudi, PhD
University of Bari Aldo Moro, Italy

Alessia Diana, DVM, PhD
University of Bologna, Italy

Valérie Freiche, DVM, PhD, DESV (Internal Medicine)
École nationale vétérinaire d'Alfort, France

Frédéric P. Gaschen, DrMedVet, DipACVIM, DipECVIM-CA
Louisiana State University, USA

Emily N. Gould, DVM, MS, DipACVIM
Texas A&M University, USA

Adam G. Gow, BVM&S, PhD, DSAM, DipECVIM-CA, FHEA, FRCVS
University of Edinburgh, UK

Christine Griebsch, DrMedVet, DipECVIM-CA
University of Sydney, Australia

Thomas Grönthal, DVM, PhD, Specialist in Veterinary Medicine (Infectious Animal Diseases)
University of Helsinki, Finland

Danièlle Gunn-Moore, BSc(Hons), BVM&S, PhD, MANZCVS, FHEA, FRSB, FRCVS
University of Edinburgh, UK

Romy M. Heilmann, DrMedVet, DipACVIM, DipECVIM-CA, MANZCVS(Small Animal Medicine), PhD
University of Leipzig, Germany

Chelsea Iennarella-Servantez, BSc, MSc
Iowa State University, USA

Albert E. Jergens, DVM, PhD, DipACVIM, AGAF
Iowa State University, USA

Aarti Kathrani, BVetMed(Hons), PhD, DipACVIM, DipACVN, FHEA, MRCVS
University of London, UK

Susanne Kilpinen, DVM, PhD, Specialist in Veterinary Medicine (Small Animal Diseases)
University of Helsinki, Finland

Lauren Lacorcia, BVSc(Hons), MVSc, GCertUniTeach, GDipClinEd, MANZCVS, DipACVIM
University of Melbourne, Australia

Karla C. L. Lee, MA, VetMB, PhD, CertSAS, DipECVS, PGCAP, FHEA, MRCVS
Veterinary Specialists Scotland, Livingston, UK

Jonathan A. Lidbury, BVMS, PhD, MRCVS, DipACVIM, DipECVIM-CA
Texas A&M University, USA

Michael Linton, BVSc, FANZCVS, MANZCVS(Med)
Sydney Veterinary Emergency and Specialists, Rosebery, Australia

Vicky J. Lipscomb, MA, VetMB, CertSAS, DipECVS, MRCVS
University of London, UK

Vito Martella, DVM, PhD
University of Bari Aldo Moro, Italy

Brenda Mulherin, DVM, DipAVDC
Iowa State University, USA

Reto Neiger, DrMedVet, PhD, DipECVIM-CA, DipACVIM
IVC Evidensia DACH, Munich, Germany

Conor O'Halloran, BVSc, MSc, PhD, MRCVS
University of Edinburgh, UK

Pascaline Pey, DVM, PhD, DipECVDI
Ospedale Veterinario I Portoni Rossi, Bologna, Italy
Antech Imaging Services, Irvine, USA

Nathalie Rademacher, DrMedVet, DipACVR, DipECVDI
Louisiana State University, USA

Thomas Spillmann, DipMedVet, DrMedVet, DipECVIM-CA
University of Helsinki, Finland

Joerg M. Steiner, MedVet, DrMedVet, PhD, DipACVIM, DipECVIM-CA, AGAF
Texas A&M University, USA

Christiane Stengel, DrMedVet, DipECVIM-CA
www.zweitmeinung-tierarzt.de, Germany

Jan Suchodolski, MedVet, DrMedVet, PhD, AGAF, DipACVM
Texas A&M University, USA

Mickey S. Tivers, BVSc, PhD, CertSAS, DipECVS, MRCVS
Paragon Veterinary Referrals, Wakefield, UK

M. Katherine Tolbert, DVM, PhD, DipACVIM
Texas A&M University, USA

Chiara Valtolina, DVM, PhD, DipACVECC, DipECVECC
Utrecht University, Netherlands

Kassandra Wilson, DVM
Louisiana State University, USA

Panagiotis G. Xenoulis, DVM, DrMedVet, PhD
University of Thessaly, Greece
Texas A&M University, USA

Preface

We are delighted to present the first edition of a dedicated feline gastroenterology book to you. It has been a great journey, and we are happy and proud to see the final product.

The aim of this book is to focus on problems unique to the feline alimentary tract in comparison to dogs—for example, feline gastrointestinal eosinophilic sclerosing fibroplasia—and to discuss them in detail, but also to highlight areas where knowledge is lacking or can only be derived from comparison with other companion animal species or humans. Instead of being a comprehensive work of "all things GI" in the cat, this book aims to shine a light on topics that are novel—such as the microbiome or probiotics—and might not have been covered by other standard textbooks.

As all three of us editors are internal medicine specialist, this book focuses on "a medic's perspective" on feline alimentary tract health, which starts with considering differential diagnoses in a structured way based on the most common clinical signs. It also includes the invaluable input from other specialties we so often draw on in clinical practice, namely laboratory diagnostics, diagnostic imaging, clinical pathology and histopathology, and nutrition, which—as we all know—can be a particular challenge in cats. It also covers feline-specific infectious and neoplastic diseases. Appropriate methods for retrieving adequate samples from organs of the alimentary tract in cats are discussed, and a particular focus on the challenges of differentiating inflammation from neoplasia is present in several chapters.

All authors have contributed their unique viewpoint on their specific topic by highlighting evidence-based approaches to common feline clinical problems and conditions, but also by drawing on their own invaluable experience as experts in their field. We are therefore very grateful to all authors for taking the time to contribute to this unique book and sharing their expertise.

We hope you enjoy the book as much as we enjoyed being part of the editing journey. Particular thanks go to our colleagues and families who had to put up with us being preoccupied with this work while juggling other commitments—halfway through a pandemic no less! We would also like to thank Jorge and Costanza from Edra publishing for being patient with us and to create the wonderful layout and final finish of this book.

Fabio Procoli, Karin Allenspach, Silke Salavati Schmitz

Abbreviations

5-HT 5-hydroxytryptamine (serotonin)
α_1PI alpha$_1$-proteinase inhibitor
AA amyloid A
AAFCO Association of American Feed Control Officials
AC ameroid constrictor
ACh acetylcholine
AChR acetylcholine receptor
ACTH adrenocorticotropic hormone
ACVIM American College of Veterinary Internal Medicine
AEEC attaching and effacing *Escherichia coli*
AFO acid-fast organism
AFR adverse food reaction
AGA American Gastroenterology Association
AGP alpha-1-acid glycoprotein
AIEC adherent–invasive *Escherichia coli*
AKI acute kidney injury
ALP alkaline phosphatase
ALT alanine aminotransferase
ANS autonomic nervous system
APC antigen presenting cell
APHA Animal and Plant Health Agency
APO apolipoproteins
aPTT activated partial thromboplastin time
APUD amine precursor uptake and decarboxylation
ARE antibiotic-responsive enteropathy
ASBT apical sodium-dependent bile acid transporter
AST aspartate aminotransferase
AstV astrovirus
ATP adenosine triphosphate
AUC area under the curve
AVDC American Veterinary Dental College
BA bile acid
BCS body condition score
BIPS barium-impregnated polyethylene spheres
BP blood pressure
BUN blood urea nitrogen
CB_1 cannabinoid type 1
CBC complete blood count
CBD common bile duct
CBuV canine bufavirus
CCD charge-coupled device
CCHC cholangitis/cholangiohepatitis complex
CCoV canine coronavirus
C. diff *Clostridioides* (*Clostridium*) *difficile*
CE chronic enteropathy
CEUS contrast-enhanced ultrasonography
CFU colony-forming unit
CGS Comparative Gastroenterology Society
CHOP cyclophosphamide, doxorubicin, vincristine, prednisolone
CK creatine kinase
CKD chronic kidney disease
CLO *Campylobacter*-like organism
CM contrast medium
C_{max} maximum plasma concentration
CMPA caudal mediastinal paraoesophageal abscesses
CNS central nervous system
COP cyclophosphamide, vincristine, prednisolone
COX-2 cyclooxygenase 2
CPE *Clostridium perfringens* enterotoxin
cPLI canine pancreatic lipase immunoreactivity
CPSS congenital portosystemic shunt
CPT1 carnitine palmitoyltransferase 1
CPV-2 canine parvovirus type 2
CRESS circular replication-associated protein-encoding single-stranded
CRI constant-rate infusion
CRP C-reactive protein
CRTZ chemoreceptor trigger zone
C&S culture and sensitivity
CT computed tomography
CTA computed tomography angiography
cTLI canine trypsin-like immunoreactivity
CYP450 cytochrome P450
DEC diarrhoeagenic *Escherichia coli*
DGGE denaturing gradient gel electrophoresis
DGGR 1,2-o-dilauryl-rac-glycero-3-glutaric acid-(6'-methylresorufin) ester
DIC disseminated intravascular coagulation
DKA diabetic ketoacidosis

DM diabetes mellitus
DSS dioctyl sodium succinate
EAEC enteroaggregative *Escherichia coli*
EATL enteropathy-associated T-cell lymphoma
EF *Enterococcus faecium*
EFA essential fatty acid
EGC eosinophilic granuloma complex
EGFR epidermal growth factor receptor
EHBDO extrahepatic bile duct obstruction
EHEC enterohaemorrhagic *Escherichia coli*
EIEC enteroinvasive *Escherichia coli*
EPEC enteropathogenic *Escherichia coli*
EPI exocrine pancreatic insufficiency
ERCP endoscopic retrograde cholangiopancreatography
ESBL extended-spectrum beta-lactamase
ESPEN European Society for Clinical Nutrition and Metabolism
ETEC enterotoxigenic *Escherichia coli*
EUS endoscopic ultrasound
fα_1PI feline alpha$_1$-proteinase inhibitor
FA fatty acid
FAO Food and Agriculture Organization
FAST focused assessment with sonography for trauma
FAstV feline astrovirus
FBoV feline bocavirus
FcaGHV1 Felis catus gammaherpesvirus 1
FCE feline chronic enteropathy
FCEAI feline chronic enteropathy activity index
FCGS feline chronic gingivostomatitis
FCoV feline coronavirus
FCV feline calicivirus
FDA Food and Drug Administration
FECAVA Federation of European Companion Animal Veterinary Associations
FECV feline enteric coronavirus
FeKoV feline kobuvirus
FeLV feline leukaemia virus
FePV feline picornavirus
FeSCV feline stool-associated circular DNA virus
FFA free fatty acid
FGESF feline gastrointestinal eosinophilic sclerosing fibroplasia
FHL feline hepatic lipidosis
FHV-1 feline herpesvirus 1
FIP feline infectious peritonitis
FIPV feline infectious peritonitis virus
FISH fluorescence in situ hybridisation
FIV feline immunodeficiency virus
FMT faecal microbiota transplantation
FNA fine needle aspiration
FOS fructooligosaccharides
FOSCC feline oral squamous cell carcinoma
fPL feline pancreatic lipase
fPLI feline pancreatic lipase immunoreactivity
FPV feline parvovirus
FRE food-responsive enteropathy
fTLI feline trypsin-like immunoreactivity
GALT gut-associated lymphoid tissue
GC glucocorticoid
GGT gamma-glutamyltransferase
GI gastrointestinal
GIL gastrointestinal lymphoma
GIST gastrointestinal stromal tumour
GLP-1 glucagon-like peptide 1
GM-CSF granulocyte–macrophage colony-stimulating factor
GMS Grocott–Gomori's methenamine silver
GO gastrooesophageal
GOS galactooligosaccharides
H_2RA histamine type 2 receptor antagonist
HAVM hepatic arteriovenous malformation
HE hepatic encephalopathy
HGIL high-grade intestinal lymphoma
HGMS histology-guided mass spectrometry
HIV human immunodeficiency virus
HNSCC head and neck squamous cell carcinoma
HPA hypothalamic–pituitary–adrenal
HPC hepatic progenitor cell
HPF high-power field
HPLC high-performance liquid chromatography
HU Hounsfield unit
IAPP islet amyloid polypeptide

IBD inflammatory bowel disease
ICC interstitial cell of Cajal
ICCJ ileocaecocolic junction
ICTV International Committee on Taxonomy of Viruses
ICU intensive care unit
IEC intestinal epithelial cell
IEL intraepithelial lymphocyte
IF intrinsic factor
IFA immunofluorescence assay
IFN interferon
Ig immunoglobulin
IGF-2 insulin-like growth factor 2
IGH immunoglobulin heavy chain
IGIL intermediate-grade intestinal lymphoma
IGRA interferon gamma release assay
IHC immunohistochemistry
IL interleukin
IM intramuscular
IMHA immune-mediated haemolytic anaemia
IOMP intraoperative mesenteric portovenography
IRE immunosuppressant-responsive enteropathy
IV intravenous
JAK Janus kinase
J-tube jejunostomy tube
LAB lactic acid bacteria
LBTT large bowel transit time
L-CHOP L-asparaginase, cyclophosphamide, doxorubicin, vincristine, prednisolone
L-COP L-asparaginase, cyclophosphamide, vincristine, prednisolone
LCPUFA long-chain polyunsaturated fatty acid
LDA linear discriminate analysis
LDH lactate dehydrogenase
LGITL low-grade intestinal T-cell lymphoma
LGL large granular lymphocyte
LGLL large granular lymphocyte lymphoma
LIPyV Lyon-IARC polyomavirus
LOS lower oesophageal sphincter
LPD lymphoproliferative disorder
LPE lymphoplasmacytic enteropathy
MAC *Mycobacterium avium–intracellulare* complex
MALDI-TOF-MS matrix-assisted laser desorption/ionisation time-of-flight mass spectrometry
MALT mucosa-associated lymphoid tissue
MAPK mitogen-activated protein kinase
MAS multiple acquired shunts
MBP major basic protein
M cell microfold cell
MCT mast cell tumour
MCV mean corpuscular volume
MDB minimum database
ME metabolisable energy
MEITL monomorphic epitheliotropic intestinal T-cell lymphoma
MER maintenance energy requirement
MG myasthenia gravis
MIC minimum inhibitory concentration
MMA methylmalonic acid
MMF mycophenolate mofetil
MPA mycophenolic acid
MPAG mycophenolic acid glucuronide
MRCP magnetic resonance cholangiopancreatography
MRI magnetic resonance imaging
MRSP/A methicillin-resistant *Staphylococcus pseudintermedius/aureus*
MSC mesenchymal stem cell
MST median survival time
MTBC *Mycobacterium tuberculosis* complex
NAC N-acetylcysteine
NDMA N-nitrosodimethylamine
NEFA nonesterified fatty acid
NF-κB nuclear factor kappa B
NG tube nasogastric tube
NK natural killer
NK_1 neurokinin-1
NLR neutrophil:lymphocyte ratio
NMDA N-methyl-D-aspartate
NMH N-methylhistamine
NOD nucleotide-binding oligomerisation domain
NO tube nasooesophageal tube
NoV norovirus
NSAID nonsteroidal anti-inflammatory drug

NTC normal-transit constipation
NTEC necrotoxigenic *Escherichia coli*
NTM nontuberculous mycobacteria
ORF open reading frame
PANS post-attenuation neurological signs
PARR PCR for antigen receptor rearrangements
PAS periodic acid–Schiff
PCoA principal coordinate analysis
PCV packed cell volume
pE1 pancreatic elastase-1
PEG percutaneous endoscopic gastrostomy
PH portal hypertension
phospho-STAT phosphorylated signal transducer and activator of transcription
PIVKA proteins induced by vitamin K antagonism
PLE protein-losing enteropathy
PLN protein-losing nephropathy
PN parenteral nutrition
PO per os
PPI proton pump inhibitor
PPVH primary portal vein hypoplasia
PRAA persistent right aortic arch
PSS portosystemic shunt
PT prothrombin time
PU/PD polyuria and polydipsia
qPCR quantitative polymerase chain reaction
RER resting energy requirement
rFeIFN-ω recombinant feline interferon omega
RI reference interval
RPLAA reverse passive latex agglutination assay
RT-PCR reverse transcriptase polymerase chain reaction
RT-qPCR reverse transcriptase quantitative polymerase chain reaction
RVA rotavirus A
SAA serum amyloid A
SAMe S-adenosylmethionine
SARS-CoV severe acute respiratory syndrome coronavirus
SC subcutaneous
SCC squamous cell carcinoma
SCFA short-chain fatty acid
SCL small-cell lymphoma
SEGRAM selective glucocorticoid receptor agonist and modulator
SIADH syndrome of inappropriate antidiuretic hormone secretion
SIRS systemic inflammatory response syndrome
SM sphingomyelin
SNP single nucleotide polymorphism
SR1 Sulphur River 1
SRE steroid-responsive enteropathy
SST somatostatin
STAT signal transducer and activator of transcription
STC slow-transit constipation
STT Schirmer tear test
TCR T-cell receptor
TDF total dietary fibre
TDM therapeutic drug monitoring
TFB thin film band
TG triglyceride
TGEV transmissible gastroenteritis virus
TGF transforming growth factor
THC tetrahydrocannabinol
Th cell T-helper cell
TK tyrosine kinase
TLI trypsin-like immunoreactivity
TLR toll-like receptor
TMAO trimethylamine N-oxide
TNF tumour necrosis factor
TPMT thiopurine methyltransferase
Treg cell regulatory T cell
tsp teaspoon
TT_4 total thyroxine
UOS upper oesophageal sphincter
UPC urine protein:creatinine
VLDL very-low-density lipoprotein
VSD virulent systemic disease
WBC white blood cell count
WHO World Health Organization
WSAVA World Small Animal Veterinary Association

Table of contents

Oesophageal diseases

Gastric diseases

Infectious diseases of the gastrointestinal tract

Intestinal inflammation

Neoplasia

Motility disorders

SECTION III Diseases of the pancreas and hepatobiliary system

SECTION IV Management strategies for diseases of the gastrointestinal and hepatobiliary tract

Pharmacological approach to gastrointestinal and hepatobiliary disorders

Novel and alternative treatment options of gastrointestinal disorders

Nutritional strategies for gastrointestinal and hepatobiliary disorders

CHAPTER 1

Differential diagnoses for clinical signs of the gastrointestinal tract

Karin Allenspach, Silke Salavati Schmitz, Fabio Procoli

Gastrointestinal (GI) disease is complex in all animal species, and the domestic cat is no exception. Clinical signs can be vague and nonspecific, or pronounced, but differential diagnoses always overlap with conditions of other organ systems. A systematic problem-oriented workup is best suited to determine a precise diagnosis, which itself allows targeted treatment. In this chapter, the authors elaborate the most pertinent aspects of differential diagnoses for common clinical signs of the GI tract, with the aim of highlighting where deviations from general thought concepts are indicated due to conditions specific to the domestic cat.

ANOREXIA AND WEIGHT LOSS

Anorexia is defined as absolute lack of food intake or appetite. This is usually differentiated from inappetence (reduced food intake) or pseudoanorexia (inability to pick up or swallow food; see Chapters 10 and 11). Mechanistically, anorexia can be divided into primary anorexia, which involves changes within higher centres for hunger and satiety of the central nervous system or sensory input (lack of sense of smell—anosmia), and secondary anorexia, where the cause is outside the central nervous system. Secondary anorexia is much more common in small animals.

Weight loss is defined as a loss of body mass due to a negative energy balance, while cachexia describes very low body condition with severe loss of muscle mass, weakness, and lethargy. Physiological reasons for reduced appetite and loss of body/muscle mass include pregnancy or lactation, and—particularly in cats—old age.

As anorexia and weight loss are very common but unspecific presenting complaints in cats, involvement of any organ system or systemic disease has to be considered (Box 1.1). Often, careful exploration of the history and a thorough physical examination give additional hints for potential causes.

Broad categories of differential diagnoses for anorexia involve toxic insults, inflammatory or infectious conditions, metabolic or endocrine diseases, pain (generalised or of musculoskeletal origin as well as local abdominal pain), and neoplasia. For anorexia without an immediately identifiable cause, differential diagnoses are identical to the ones for weight loss. These range from insufficient quality, composition, or availability of food; maldigestion (e.g. exocrine pancreatic insufficiency; see Chapter 25); malabsorption (e.g. inflammatory bowel disease [IBD]; see Chapters 17 and 18; intestinal lymphoma; see Chapter 20); malassimilation (e.g. hepatopathy; see Chapters 26, 27, 30, and 31); loss of nutrients (e.g. diabetes mellitus, proteinuria, protein-losing enteropathy [PLE]; see below), and pathologically increased metabolic turnover (e.g. hyperthyroidism, systemic inflammatory and infectious conditions, neoplasia, congestive heart failure).

Based on the wide variety of causes, diagnostic workup and treatment is variable but often includes laboratory tests (see Chapters 3 and 4) and diagnostic imaging procedures (see Chapters 5 and 6). If extraintestinal/systemic causes are ruled out and initial diagnostics do not reveal a potential cause, appropriate measures for tissue sampling can be considered (see Chapters 7–9).

Appetite stimulants like cyproheptadine or mirtazapine can be very effective in cats but should only be used for

Box 1.1. Causes of reduced appetite or anorexia in cats.

Inability to eat
- Facial/mandibular fractures
- Temporomandibular disease
- Cranial nerve neuropathy (e.g. bilateral trigeminal neuropathy)
- Dental disease
- Oral ulceration/stomatitis

Nausea
- Primary gastrointestinal disease (e.g. chronic enteropathy)
- Parasitic disease
- Gastrointestinal foreign bodies
- Alimentary neoplasia
- Gastrointestinal irritation/inflammation
- Ileus

Extragastrointestinal causes
- Pancreatitis
- Hepatic disease
- Central disease (e.g. forebrain neoplasm)
- Vestibular disease
- Acute kidney injury
- Chronic kidney disease
- Congestive heart failure

Medications
- Chemotherapeutics
- Nonsteroidal anti-inflammatories
- Steroids
- Cyclosporin
- Mycophenolate mofetil
- Opioids

Behavioural/others
- Anxiety
- Fear
- Cervical arthritis preventing ventroflexion to food bowl
- Osteoarthritis preventing access to food bowls

a short period of time, especially if the underlying cause of anorexia and weight loss is unclear (see Chapters 39 and 40). Due to cats' tendency to develop hepatic lipidosis (see Chapter 27), nutritional support should be considered early in the course of any disease (see Chapters 38–40), and tube feeding should be started early (see Chapter 40). Care must be taken not to initiate too aggressive nutrition, as cats can develop severe complications due to refeeding syndrome (see Chapter 29).

VOMITING

Vomiting (emesis) is an active reflex with the purpose of retrograde evacuation of the proximal GI tract contents. It involves contractions of the stomach, diaphragm, and abdominal wall muscles while relaxing upper and lower oesophageal sphincters and positional changes of the larynx and epiglottis to protect the airways. As such, this active process has to be differentiated from the more passive expulsion during regurgitation (indicating oesophageal disease; see Chapter 11), which is rare in cats.

Even though vomiting is a common presenting complaint, there is some debate if and when occasional vomiting can be physiological or accepted as "normal" in cats. Long-haired cats in particular might bring up trichobezoars relatively frequently due to grooming. Grass-eating behaviour with subsequent vomiting is also often considered a normal occurrence in cats.

Causes for pathological vomiting can be divided into central (endogenous and exogenous substances stimulating the vomiting centre via breaching the blood–brain barrier in the chemoreceptor trigger zone) and peripheral (irritating stimuli within the GI tract). However, differentiation into GI vs. extra-GI causes might be more helpful. Differential diagnoses for vomiting are plentiful (Table 1.1) and can—besides gastric, intestinal, hepatobiliary, pancreatic, or dietetic causes—include toxic, metabolic, renal, infectious as well as neurological conditions.

Information from history, physical examination, and initial laboratory and diagnostic imaging tests (see Chapters 3–6) should be aimed at identifying a serious or potentially life-threatening situation that requires immediate action. Single episodes of vomiting in an otherwise well animal can prompt short-term symptomatic treatment (see Chapter 35). In recurrent or more chronic episodes that are either mild or where investigations have ruled out serious or extra-GI causes, a dietary change is often recommended (see Chapters 18 and 39). Probiotics can be considered as adjunctive treatments in both acute and chronic uncomplicated cases (see Chapter 36).

Further diagnostic steps should be initiated for both chronic GI (e.g. endoscopy with mucosal biopsies; see Chapter 7) and hepatobiliary diseases (e.g. surgical or laparoscopic biopsies; see Chapter 8) before empirical or definitive treatment is initiated (e.g. with antimicrobials; see Chapter 34; or anti-inflammatories; see Chapter 35). This is particularly important to differentiate inflammatory causes (see Chapters 18 and 19) from neoplastic (see Chapters 20, 21, and 32) or infectious conditions (see Chapters 30 and 31).

Table 1.1. Causes of vomiting in cats.

Category	Location/type	Cause	Comment
Gastrointestinal	Stomach	Gastritis	Mostly unspecific or as part of inflammation of the entire upper gastrointestinal tract (CE)
		Erosion, ulceration	Often NSAIDs; less often neoplasia
		Obstruction • Foreign body • Pyloric stenosis/hypertrophy • Mass, diffuse neoplasia	 See Chapter 12 See Chapters 20 and 21
		Parasites: *Ollulanus tricuspis*	Rarely causes clinical signs
	Small intestine	Steroid-responsive CE/IBD	Most common form of CE
		Dysbiosis, antibiotic-responsive CE	See Chapters 16 and 18
		Obstruction	As for stomach
		Ileus, intestinal hypomotility	See Chapter 22
		Intestinal parasites	See Chapter 15
		Infections • Panleucopenia • Enteric coronavirus or FIP • FeLV	See Chapter 13
		Neoplasia (e.g. lymphoma)	See Chapters 20 and 21
	Large intestine	Colitis	See Chapter 18
		Constipation, obstipation	Vomiting can be a reflectory response of colonic overdistension; see Chapter 23
	Dietetic	Spoilt food, foreign material	Rare
		Abrupt dietary change	
		Food hypersensitivity/allergy/intolerance (food-responsive CE)	See Chapter 18
Extragastrointestinal	Metabolic	Acute kidney injury, chronic kidney disease (azotaemia, uraemia)	
		Hepatobiliary disease	See Chapters 26–31
		Pancreatitis (chronic >> acute)	See Chapter 24
		Electrolyte and acid–base disturbances	
	Endocrine	Diabetic ketosis/ketoacidosis	
		Hyperthyroidism	
	Intoxications	Ethylene glycol	
		Herbicides, heavy metals, bleach	
	Drugs	NSAIDs	
		Cytotoxic drugs	
		Xylazine, medetomidine	
		Glycosides	
		Glucocorticoids	
		Antibiotics	e.g. erythromycin, penicillins, tetracycline
	Intra-abdominal disease	Peritonitis (septic or FIP)	
		Pyelonephritis	
		Neoplasia	
	Neurological	Vestibular disease	
		Traumatic head injury	
		Seizures	

CE, chronic enteropathy; FeLV, feline leukaemia virus; FIP, feline infectious peritonitis; IBD, inflammatory bowel disease; NSAID, nonsteroidal anti-inflammatory drug.

SMALL INTESTINAL DIARRHOEA

Diarrhoea is defined as production of faeces with a higher than normal water content. History reveals if diarrhoea is acute (<1-week duration), chronic (>3 weeks), or recurrent. It can be classified as mainly of large or small intestinal origin (Table 1.2), even though in a lot of cases components can be mixed.

Acute diarrhoea is most commonly idiopathic, but both dietary causes and infectious diseases (see Chapters 13–15) have to be considered as major differential diagnoses.

Chronic diarrhoea has potentially many causes that can be classified as intra- or extraintestinal and further divided into infectious, noninfectious, organ-specific, and systemic conditions (Fig. 1.1).

Diagnostic approach and treatment of diarrhoea are very similar to those described above for vomiting (see Chapters 3–9). Acute and/or uncomplicated cases can be treated symptomatically and/or with a dietary change. In more serious conditions, more extensive testing is required, particularly to rule out either the need for emergency measures (e.g. intestinal obstruction) or common extra-GI causes (e.g. hyperthyroidism, chronic kidney disease). If specific conditions are identified, treatment should address the underlying cause. Detection of low serum albumin in a diarrhoeic cat might prompt considering PLE as a differential. However, in comparison to dogs, this is a rare condition in cats, and other causes of low albumin (e.g. hepatopathy, protein-losing nephropathy, infectious conditions) should be thoroughly ruled out before considering PLE as a diagnosis. Serum cobalamin determination is of particular importance in cats, as body stores of cobalamin in cats deplete faster than in dogs. Also, as the intrinsic factor necessary for cobalamin absorption is only produced in the pancreas in felines, both diffuse small intestinal disease and exocrine pancreatic insufficiency make them prone to the development of hypocobalaminaemia (see Chapters 3 and 25).

Specific infectious and noninfectious GI diseases (see Chapters 13–23 and 31) and pancreatic (see Chapters 24, 25, and 32) and hepatobiliary disorders (see Chapters 26, 27, and 30–32) relevant to the cat are discussed in detail in other parts of this book. The nutritional approach to GI, pancreatic, and hepatobiliary conditions that can cause diarrhoea is detailed in Chapters 38–41.

LARGE INTESTINAL DIARRHOEA

In cats, large intestinal diarrhoea is most frequently a sign of colitis (see Chapter 18). However, straining or dyschezia due to colitis can be difficult to differentiate from constipation (see below and Chapter 23) or urinary straining, especially in female cats. Differential diagnosis and associated workup usually focus on ruling out infectious diseases (see Section II, Subsection D), particularly tritrichomoniasis. Especially in young pedigree cats, in which this condition is often suspected but sometimes difficult to definitively prove, differential diagnoses include food-responsive chronic enteropathy, antibiotic-responsive chronic enteropathy (see Chapter 18), and dysbiosis (see Chapter 16). Because of this, alternative treatment options are increasingly explored for "idiopathic" colitis in cats (see Chapters 36 and 37).

Table 1.2. Differentiating characteristics of small intestinal vs. large intestinal diarrhoea.

Characteristic	Small intestinal diarrhoea	Large intestinal diarrhoea
Volume/weight	Increased	Normal to decreased
Frequency	Mildly increased	Severely increased
Consistency	Watery	Cow patty to normal
Melaena	Possible	Not present
Haematochezia	Not present	Possible
Mixed or coated with mucus	Not present	Typically present
Steatorrhoea	Possible	Not present
Weight loss	Common	Rare
Inappetence and/or systemic unwellness	Common	Rare

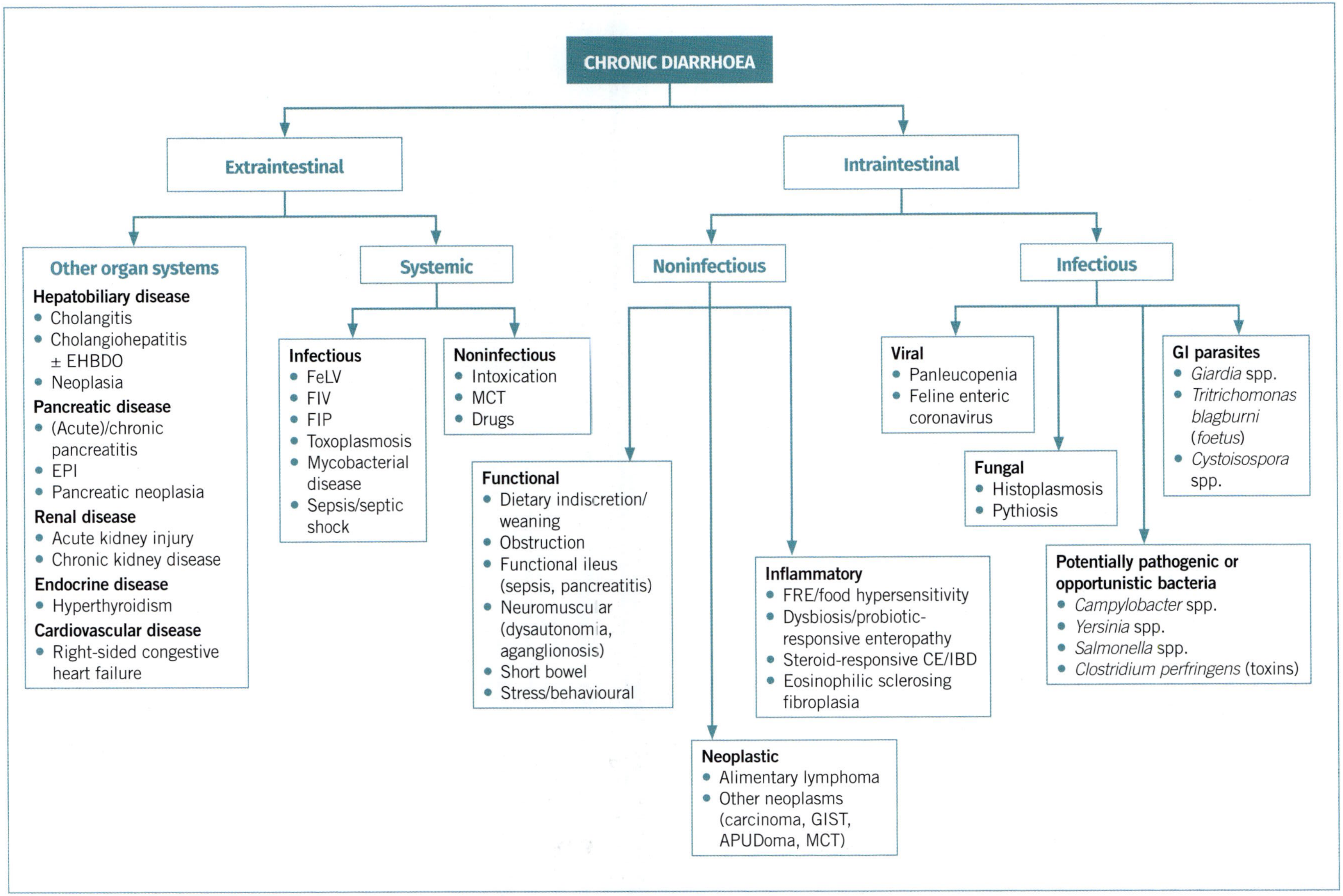

Figure 1.1. Causes of chronic diarrhoea in cats. APUD, amine precursor uptake and decarboxylation; CE, chronic enteropathy; EHBDO, extrahepatic bile duct obstruction; EPI, exocrine pancreatic insufficiency; FeLV, feline leukaemia virus; FIP, feline infectious peritonitis; FIV, feline immunodeficiency virus; FRE, food-responsive enteropathy; GI, gastrointestinal; GIST, gastrointestinal stromal tumour; IBD, inflammatory bowel disease; MCT, mast cell tumour.

Steroid-responsive chronic enteropathy or IBD manifest rarely in large intestinal diarrhoea only in cats. However, if this is suspected, endoscopy with mucosal biopsies for histological assessment is indicated (see Chapters 7 and 9), as it will also help to rule out large intestinal lymphoma or colorectal masses (rare in cats). Haematochezia should prompt assessment of a systemic coagulopathy, but this is rarer in cats than in dogs.

CONSTIPATION AND OBSTIPATION

Constipation is defined as infrequent, difficult, or painful evacuation of faeces without permanent loss of function, while obstipation is defined as complete inability to pass faeces, often indicating permanent functional impairment. Generalised dilation with hypomotility of the colon is termed (idiopathic) megacolon.

Causes for constipation can be within the large intestine (extramural, mural, or luminal) or external (e.g. neuromuscular, endocrine, or metabolic), as well as idiopathic (see Chapter 23). In neonates, congenital abnormalities like hypoganglionosis, aganglionosis (Hirschsprung's disease), or *atresia ani* have to be considered. Outdoor cats could suffer from asymmetrical fusion of a pelvic fracture, while neoplasia is more likely in elderly animals. A breed-specific condition associated with constipation is sacral malformations in Manx cats.

The diagnostic approach to patients with constipation will vary depending on the findings from signalment, history, and physical examination. Treatment of constipation is also guided by the underlying cause. Alleviating constipation or treating obstipation is warranted, in addition, in most cases. The specifics of this depend on the severity of constipation (see Chapter 23).

Take-home messages

- Clinical signs of gastrointestinal disease in cats are very similar to those in dogs and give an indication of the part of the gastrointestinal tract affected.
- Differential diagnostics of gastrointestinal disease should be approached systematically (e.g. gastrointestinal vs. extragastrointestinal).
- In cats, causes of gastrointestinal disease are more often infectious than in dogs for both small and large intestinal diarrhoea.
- Constipation is more common in cats than in dogs and can have several causes, but megacolon as a diagnosis of exclusion is unique to the cat.

CHAPTER 2

Differential diagnoses for clinical signs of the pancreas and hepatobiliary system

Silke Salavati Schmitz, Fabio Procoli, Karin Allenspach

Clinical signs of the pancreas and hepatobiliary system are often indistinguishable from signs associated with primary gastrointestinal (GI) disease. In contrast to dogs, in cats they are often vague and unspecific (anorexia, lethargy, resentment of abdominal palpation). Even though more specific clinical signs or findings on physical examination can be present (e.g. vomiting, icterus, palpable cranial abdominal mass), overall telltale signs considered to be somewhat pathognomonic in dogs (e.g. the combination of acute vomiting, severe cranial abdominal pain, or even a "prayer position" in acute pancreatitis; or ascites as a sign of end-stage hepatic disease and/or portal hypertension) are hardly ever present in cats. Even signs of hepatic encephalopathy are more difficult to recognise in cats compared to dogs, as they include signs such as pyrexia, hypersalivation, blindness, or seizures (see Chapters 26 and 28) which would be considered atypical in dogs. Hence, differential diagnoses always overlap with conditions of other organ systems. In addition, infectious diseases are overall more common in cats compared to dogs and thus have to be considered a more likely differential diagnosis (e.g. feline infectious peritonitis [FIP], toxoplasmosis). A systematic problem-oriented workup based on the predominant clinical sign(s) is best suited to determine a precise diagnosis but can involve a considerable number of laboratory tests (see Chapter 4) and diagnostic imaging procedures (see Chapter 6). In this chapter, the authors elaborate the most pertinent aspects of differential diagnoses for specific clinical signs of the pancreas and hepatobiliary system in cats. Differential diagnoses for unspecific signs like anorexia, weight loss, vomiting, and diarrhoea have already been covered in Chapter 1.

CLINICAL SIGNS AND DIFFERENTIAL DIAGNOSES OF PANCREATIC DISEASE

Feline pancreatic diseases are extensively covered in Chapters 24, 25, and 32. As a brief summary, acute pancreatitis is rare in cats, but if present (or experimentally induced), signs are nonspecific and ill-defined (anorexia, lethargy, weight loss). Acute deterioration with hypovolaemic shock, dehydration, and hypovolaemia can follow, whilst abdominal mass effects, vomiting, or diarrhoea are rare. Chronic pancreatitis is much more common in cats and often associated with cholangitis and inflammatory bowel disease (IBD) (triaditis; see Chapter 30), where clinical signs again are either unspecific or predominantly associated with the other organ systems affected (e.g. vomiting and diarrhoea in IBD, icterus and pyrexia in cholangitis).

The hallmark signs of exocrine pancreatic insufficiency are diarrhoea and weight loss (see Chapters 1 and 25), so a number of differential diagnoses within and outside the GI tract have to be considered (see Chapter 1).

CLINICAL SIGNS AND DIFFERENTIAL DIAGNOSES OF HEPATOBILIARY DISEASE

Hepatobiliary disease (detailed in Chapters 26, 27, 30, and 31, including neoplasia in Chapter 32) can be primary or secondary (with hepatic lipidosis being the most common and most significant secondary liver disease in cats; see Chapter 27) and can manifest in a plethora of clinical signs (Table 2.1), even though most of these are seen more frequently in dogs compared to cats. Similar to pancreatic disease, signs in cats are often unspecific (e.g. lethargy, inappetence or anorexia, vomiting, diarrhoea, recent weight loss), and a number of tests are necessary to answer critical clinical questions, narrow down the type of hepatic disease (hepatocellular damage, functional impairment, or cholestasis), and confirm a diagnosis (Fig. 2.2).

Differential diagnoses of icterus (Fig. 2.1) are equally not limited to hepatobiliary diseases but should firstly be divided into prehepatic (haemolytic), hepatic (hepatocellular), and posthepatic (biliary or obstructive) causes (Box 2.1). Once haemolysis is excluded, hepatic causes (e.g. hepatic lipidosis, see Chapter 27; or neoplasia, see Chapter 32) have to be differentiated from posthepatic causes. The latter can be involving the intrahepatic biliary canaliculi (e.g. cholangitis/cholangiohepatitis; see Chapter 30) or the extrahepatic bile duct (e.g. extrahepatic bile duct obstruction) and gallbladder (see Chapter 31). Pancreatitis (see Chapter 24) or triaditis (see Chapter 30) should also be considered common differential diagnoses of posthepatic icterus in cats.

A number of systemic infections have to be considered as a cause of icterus and appropriately ruled out. The suspicion for FIP should be high in either young (kittens) or geriatric cats with pyrexia, icterus, or ascites and appropriate supportive findings on routine laboratory work (hyperglobulinaemia, albumin:globulin ratio from serum or ascites <0.3). In cases with ascites, reverse transcriptase quantitative polymerase chain reaction (RT-qPCR) for feline coronavirus from the peritoneal fluid is the best diagnostic tool available. Ultimately, the final diagnosis, especially in cases of dry FIP or for the differentiation from lymphocytic cholangitis or hepatic small-cell lymphoma, can only be achieved by histopathological assessment of hepatic biopsies. Toxoplasmosis can be diagnosed based on IgG and IgM titres or on finding tachyzoites in hepatic (or other tissue) biopsies or bile samples.

Overall, likely differential diagnoses need to be adapted based on history, signalment, and initial findings, even

Table 2.1. Common clinical signs associated with hepatobiliary disease in cats. Significance and differences with dogs are outlined.

Clinical signs associated with hepatobiliary disease in cats	Significance/mechanism	Frequency in the context of hepatobiliary disease	Common differential diagnoses
Anorexia/inappetence	Unspecific	Common	Many
Acholic faeces	Suggests complete blockage of common bile duct (e.g. EHBDO; see Chapter 31)	Rare	None
Bleeding/coagulopathy	Reduced or absent synthesis and activation of coagulation factors by the liver	Rare as main presenting complaint but often observed clinically (e.g. after venepuncture)	Thrombocytopenia, thrombocytopathia, rodenticide intoxication, DIC, factor XII deficiency
Blindness/loss of vision	Often a sign of HE	Overall rare, but can be seen more often in cats with PSS than in dogs	Ocular disease (chorioretinitis, toxoplasmosis); inflammatory, infectious, or neoplastic CNS disease (cortical blindness); systemic hypertension
Diarrhoea	Usually small bowel diarrhoea, result of GI ulceration, malabsorption, toxin production, osmotic	Uncommon in comparison to dogs	Many primary GI diseases (infectious, inflammatory, neoplastic), pancreatitis, EPI, CKD, hyperthyroidism
Dysuria	Due to urolithiasis Ammonium urate crystals or stones do not typically develop in cats with hepatic functional failure/PSS; the cause of most urate urolithiasis cases in cats is unknown	Very rare	Urolithiasis of nonhepatic cause (calcium oxalate, struvite), urinary tract infection, feline idiopathic cystitis

though several tiers of investigation are often necessary to find a final diagnosis (see Fig. 2.2 and Chapters 4, 6, 8, and 9). Treatment needs to be directed at the underlying cause (see Section III for specific diseases) but can include antimicrobials (see Chapter 34), anti-inflammatories, or immunosuppressants (see Chapter 35) as well as symptomatic treatment (see Chapter 33). Antioxidants and hepatoprotective agents are also often administered. Appropriate nutritional measures have to be considered in addition, either as adjunctive treatment (see Chapters 39–41) or as causative intervention (e.g. in hepatic lipidosis; see Chapter 27).

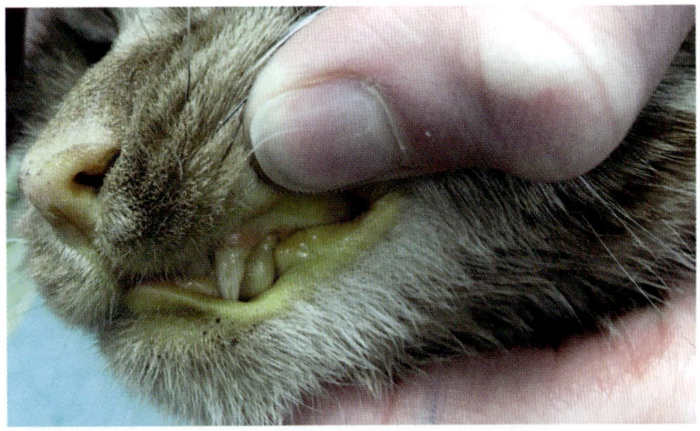

Figure 2.1. A cat with visible icterus of the skin and oral mucosa. Image courtesy of Glynn Woods, The Royal (Dick) School of Veterinary Studies, University of Edinburgh, UK.

Clinical signs associated with hepatobiliary disease in cats	Significance/mechanism	Frequency in the context of hepatobiliary disease	Common differential diagnoses
Enlarged abdomen	Hepatomegaly or hepatobiliary mass; free peritoneal fluid	Uncommon	Other organ enlargement or mass, intra-abdominal fat Differentials for peritoneal fluid to be determined by type of fluid: transudate (hypoalbuminaemia, cardiac disease [also if chyle]), modified transudate (inflammatory, infectious, neoplastic, uroabdomen), exudate (FIP, biliary rupture, septic peritonitis)
Hyperthermia/fever	True infectious cause (systemic or local) or lack of clearance of endotoxins by portal circulation	Overall uncommon, but seen in PSS or FIP	Any other inflammatory or infectious cause (organs or systemic), based on predominant signs and initial findings
Icterus	To be differentiated into prehepatic, hepatic, and posthepatic	Common	See Box 2.1
Pale mucous membranes	Anaemia or suboptimal perfusion (shock)	Uncommon	Haemolysis, GI bleeding (acute or iron deficiency), bone marrow disorder, shock (hypovolaemic, distributive/anaphylactic, cardiogenic, neurogenic)
Polyuria/polydipsia	Medullary washout (reduced urea production), psychogenic	Rare	CKD, hyperthyroidism, hypercalcaemia, diabetes mellitus (insipidus rare), drug-induced
Ptyalism/hypersalivation	Often a sign of HE	Common in PSS or with other causes of HE	Salivary gland disease, oral/dental disease, neurological condition (trigeminal nerve), dysphagia/odynophagia, drug reaction
Seizures (and other CNS signs like stupor, coma, circling, head pressing, ataxia)	Often a sign of HE	Seizures overall rare, but more common in cats with PSS than in dogs Other CNS signs rarely observed	Infectious, inflammatory, or neoplastic CNS diseases; idiopathic (epileptic) seizures; ear disease; intoxication To be differentiated from syncope
Vomiting	Pathogenesis often unclear, but likely combination of central vomiting due to endogenous toxin accumulation and possible GI mucosa injury	Less common than in dogs	Idiopathic, infectious GI disease, foreign body/GI obstruction, hyperthyroidism, DKA, AKI or CKD, intoxication, drug-induced
Weight loss	Unspecific, secondary to anorexia, catabolic state	Common	Many

AKI, acute kidney injury; CKD, chronic kidney disease; CNS, central nervous system; DIC, disseminated intravascular coagulation; DKA, diabetic ketoacidosis; EHBDO, extrahepatic bile duct obstruction; EPI, exocrine pancreatic insufficiency; FIP, feline infectious peritonitis; GI, gastrointestinal; HE, hepatic encephalopathy; PSS, portosystemic shunt.

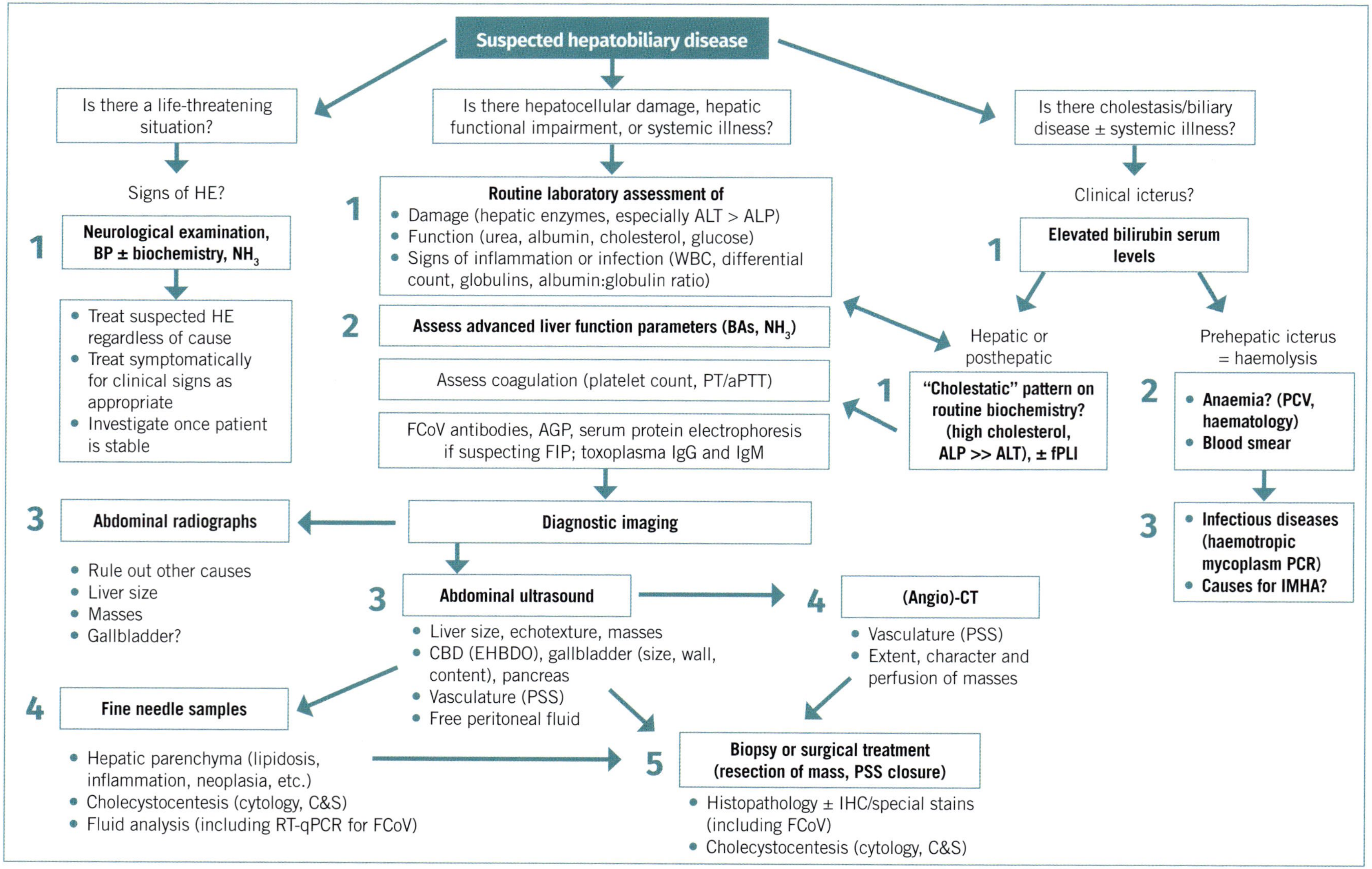

Figure 2.2. Algorithm for clinical scenarios of hepatobiliary disease and their respective workup. Numbers indicate layer/order of investigations. AGP, alpha-1-acid glycoprotein; ALP, alkaline phosphatase; ALT, alanine aminotransferase; aPTT, activated partial thromboplastin time; BA, bile acids; BP, blood pressure; CBD, common bile duct; C&S, culture and sensitivity; CT, computed tomography; EHBDO, extrahepatic bile duct obstruction; FCoV, feline coronavirus; FIP, feline infectious peritonitis; fPLI, feline pancreatic lipase immunoreactivity; HE, hepatic encephalopathy; IHC, immunohistochemistry; IMHA, immune-mediated haemolytic anaemia; NH_3, ammonia; PCV, packed cell volume; PSS, portosystemic shunt; PT, prothrombin time; RT-qPCR, reverse transcriptase quantitative polymerase chain reaction; WBC, white blood cell count.

Box 2.1. Differential diagnoses for icterus and hyperbilirubinaemia.

Prehepatic (haemolytic) icterus
- Immune-mediated (primary and secondary) haemolytic anaemia
- RBC infections:
  - *Babesia* spp.
  - Haemotropic *Mycoplasma* spp.
  - *Cytoauxzoon felis*
- RBC oxidative injury (Heinz body anaemia):
  - Acetaminophen/paracetamol
  - Onion, garlic
  - Zinc
  - Vitamin K
  - Benzocaine and other local anaesthetics
  - Propylene glycol
  - Naphthalene (moth balls)
- Envenomation (spiders, snakes, bees):
- Hypophosphataemia:
  - Insulin therapy in diabetes or DKA
  - Refeeding syndrome (see Chapter 29)
- Hereditary RBC defects:
  - Pyruvate kinase deficiency
  - Phosphofructokinase deficiency
  - Stomatocytosis
- Microangiopathic RBC fragmentation:
  - DIC
  - Vasculitis
  - Haemangiosarcoma
  - Heatstroke
  - Heartworm infection
- Incompatible blood transfusion
- Neonatal isoerythrolysis

Hepatic (hepatocellular) icterus
- Adverse drug reaction (many)
- Hepatotoxins (many)
- Infectious hepatitis or multi-organ/systemic infection:
  - FIP
  - Toxoplasmosis
  - Atypical feline calicivirus infection
  - Ascending infection from biliary tract
- Cholangitis/cholangiohepatitis (see Chapter 30)
- Neutrophilic/suppurative
- Lymphocytic
- Feline hepatic lipidosis (see Chapter 27)
- Hepatic neoplasia (primary or metastatic; see Chapter 32)
- Cholestasis of sepsis

Posthepatic (biliary or obstructive) icterus
- Cholelithiasis, choledocholithiasis
- Choledocal cyst
- Bile duct inflammation (granulomatous), stricture, or cyst
- Biliary fluke infestation (*Platynosomum concinnum, Amphimerus pseudofelineus*)
- Biliary neoplasia (see Chapter 32)
- Cholecystitis
- Pancreatic disease (pancreatitis, see Chapter 24; pancreatic neoplasia, see Chapter 32)
- Triaditis (see Chapter 30)
- Bile duct or gallbladder rupture (bile peritonitis)

Adapted from Washbau RJ, Day MJ, editors. *Canine and Feline Gastroenterology*. St Louis, Saunders Elsevier, 2012.
DIC, disseminated intravascular coagulation; DKA, diabetic ketoacidosis; FIP, feline infectious peritonitis; RBC, red blood cell.

Take-home messages

- Clinical signs of hepatobiliary disease are commonly nonspecific or associated with the gastrointestinal tract.
- Even more specific clinical signs (e.g. icterus, bleeding) have a plethora of differential diagnoses that need to be ruled out.
- It seems prudent to initially assess if a life-threatening situation is present (e.g. hepatic encephalopathy, biliary peritonitis) and to diagnose and treat this appropriately.
- Routine laboratory assessments usually allow the differentiation between hepatocellular injury, hepatic functional impairment, and cholestasis.
- Diagnostic imaging is essential in many cases to establish a final diagnosis and can also aid in sampling (e.g. hepatic fine needle aspiration, cholecystocentesis, Tru-Cut biopsies).
- A number of common feline hepatobiliary conditions can only be diagnosed by fine needle or biopsy samples with associated tests (e.g. bile culture, special stains on histopathology).

CHAPTER 3

Laboratory approach to gastrointestinal disorders

Romy M. Heilmann

Gastrointestinal (GI) disorders are a common reason for cats to be presented to the veterinary practice. The diagnostic and therapeutic approach to these cases varies depending upon the chronicity and severity of the disease. Still, patient and environmental factors will also determine the best individual diagnostic strategy. Common clinical signs in cats with GI disease are weight loss, reduced appetite (hyporexia) or anorexia, diarrhoea, and vomiting. Compared to dogs, abdominal pain and borborygmus are infrequently seen in cats. The clinical picture of some GI diseases in cats can also include tenesmus, increased faecal volume, steatorrhoea, salivation, and regurgitation. The diagnostic workup of cats with GI disorders usually requires a sequential evaluation that includes laboratory tests, diagnostic imaging, and—in some cats—also more invasive diagnostics.

Acute GI signs might be self-limiting or respond to symptomatic treatment of the cat without needing further diagnostics, mainly if the clinical signs are mild. However, cats that are presented with either moderate to severe acute GI signs or with an acute episode of a seemingly more chronic disease process and cats with chronic persistent clinical signs generally require further diagnostics after stabilisation of the patient.

Particularly, chronic GI signs are one of the most common reasons for a feline patient to be presented to a veterinary surgeon. For suspicion of a chronic disease process such as a chronic enteropathy (CE), clinical signs are either persistently or intermittently shown for at least 3 weeks.[1] Because many differential diagnoses have to be considered, the diagnostic workup of some cats with chronic GI signs can be time-consuming and also cost-intensive. Noninvasive diagnostic tests should always precede more invasive diagnostics. Client education about the necessity, the time required, and the associated costs for the diagnostic workup will result in a better understanding of particularly chronic inflammatory (but also neoplastic) GI diseases. It can also increase owner compliance.

A detailed medical history and a thorough physical examination are fundamental prerequisites for the diagnostic evaluation of any feline patient that is presented with clinical signs of acute or chronic GI disease. In the presence of persistent GI signs, a distinction should be attempted between small intestinal, large intestinal, and mixed small and large intestinal signs to initiate more targeted diagnostics based on pertinent differential diagnoses for the presumed or predominant location of the disease (distal vs. proximal GI tract).

A clinical scoring system, the feline chronic enteropathy activity index (FCEAI), has been developed for assessing the severity of clinical signs of cats with chronic GI disease.[2] For the FCEAI, five clinical parameters (attitude/activity, appetite, vomiting, diarrhoea, and weight loss) are evaluated on a scale from 0 (normal) to 3 (severely abnormal), and one endoscopic parameter (presence of endoscopic lesions) and three clinicopathologic parameters (serum total protein concentration, alanine aminotransferase [ALT]/alkaline phosphatase [ALP] activity, and serum phosphorus concentration) are assessed as dichotomised variables (0 = normal, 1 = abnormal).[2] The sum of all individual scores results in the cumulative FCEAI score, which is directly proportional to the severity of clinical signs. The FCEAI system can be used to semiobjectively assess the severity of the cat's clinical signs at the time of diagnosis and also at follow-up evaluations during treatment to monitor for patient improvement.

A minimum database (MDB) in cats with GI signs should include routine haematology, serum biochemistry profile (including a total thyroxine [TT_4] measurement in cats ≥7 years of age and/or with a palpable thyroid gland [thyroid slip] during physical examination), feline retrovirus (feline leukaemia virus [FeLV] and feline immunodeficiency virus [FIV]) status, and a urinalysis with urine sediment examination (and, if needed, bacterial culture and antimicrobial susceptibility testing). In addition to these clinicopathologic parameters, a faecal examination and diagnostic imaging (thoracic and/or abdominal radiographs, abdominal ultrasonography with doppler or contrast-enhanced ultrasonography if needed, and in some cases also advanced imaging techniques including computed tomography or magnetic resonance imaging) are essential tools for assessment of the overall health status of the patient. These diagnostics can also help to diagnose GI diseases (e.g. solitary masses or marked coprostasis with underlying megacolon) and exclude or diagnose extra-GI aetiologies (that can clinically or clinicopathologically mimic GI disorders). These modalities are also useful to rule out differentials that require surgical intervention (e.g. intestinal intussusception, obstructive neoplasia, perforation of the GI wall, or GI foreign body). Immunological or molecular-based diagnostic tests can further help to evaluate the patient for specific GI disease processes, to further characterise the disease, to determine the best course of treatment, and also, in some cases, to determine the individual prognosis. In some cats, more invasive diagnostics (GI endoscopy, laparoscopy, or laparotomy to obtain GI tissue biopsies) might be needed to characterise the disease process better and arrive at a definitive diagnosis. The diagnosis of CE is a diagnosis of exclusion. Thus, other GI and also extra-GI causes need to be ruled out first.

LABORATORY DIAGNOSTIC APPROACH IN CATS WITH ACUTE OR CHRONIC GASTROINTESTINAL SIGNS

Routine laboratory diagnostic tests

The MDB in a cat with GI signs (Fig. 3.1) should include routine haematology (with a differential blood cell count if needed) and serum biochemistry (including measurement of serum TT_4 concentration) as well as a urinalysis. Typically, there are nonspecific findings in the complete blood count (CBC). In some cases, a mild leucocytosis with neutrophilia reflecting typical changes of an inflammatory leucogram and/or a stress leucogram can be found. Lymphopenia is also part of the stress leucogram but can also be seen with viral infections affecting rapidly dividing tissues (e.g. parvovirus infection, also known as feline panleucopenia). Lymphocytosis can be a benign finding resulting from an infectious disease (e.g. viral or vector-borne diseases) or routine vaccination. Still, it can also reflect a malignant disease process (e.g. lymphoma or lymphocytic leukaemia). The diagnostic or prognostic value of the neutrophil:lymphocyte ratio (NLR) has not been reported in cats with GI disease. A mild nonregenerative, normocytic normochromic anaemia (anaemia of inflammation or anaemia of chronic disease) is often detected in cats with chronic GI disease. Nonregenerative, microcytic anaemia (and decreased reticulocyte haemoglobin concentration or erythrocyte hypochromia) is consistent with an iron-deficiency anaemia, and more subtle changes (particularly a decreased reticulocyte haemoglobin concentration) suggest iron-limited erythropoiesis. Together with a mild to moderate thrombocytosis and an increased blood urea nitrogen (BUN) concentration, this finding might indicate the presence of chronic GI bleeding. Peripheral eosinophilia can be seen in cats with eosinophilic gastroenteritis, fungal enteritis, endoparasite infections, or alimentary lymphoma or mast cell tumour. However, it should be emphasised that a normal CBC does not rule out the presence of a significant disease process.

Blood biochemistry tests should also be included in the MDB in cats with acute or chronic GI disease. These tests allow for the detection of either acute or chronic renal and hepatic diseases, which can also be associated

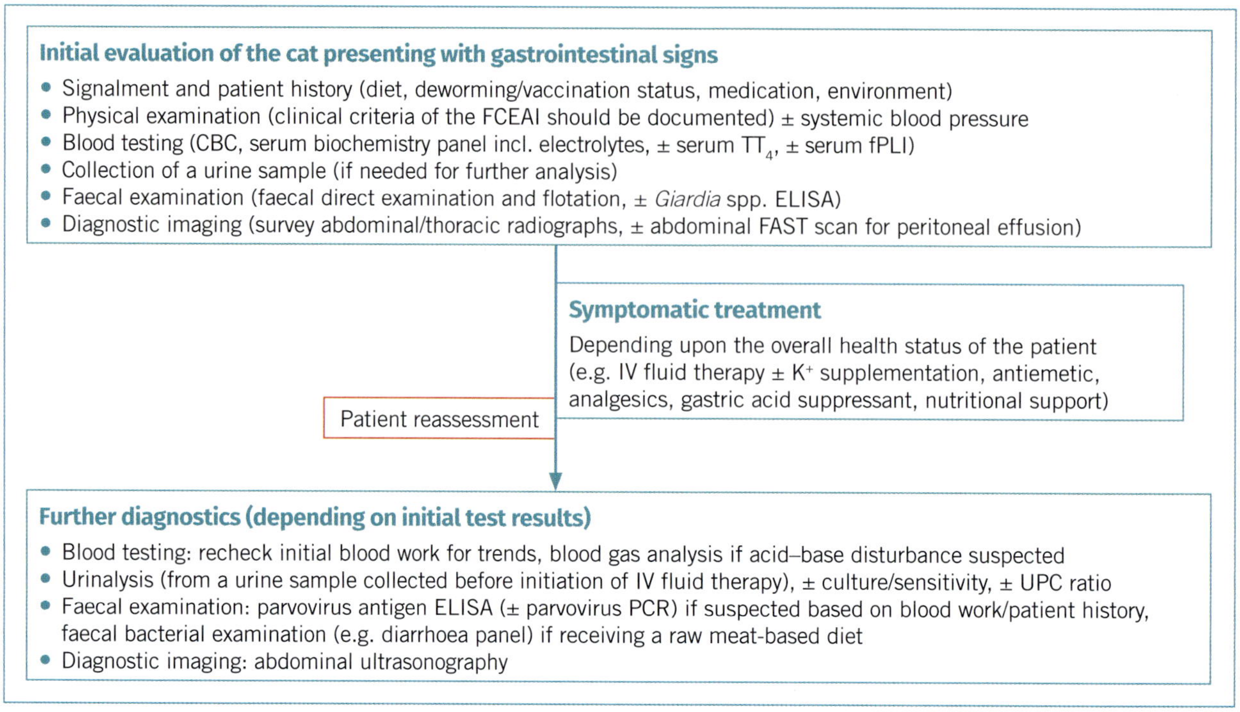

Figure 3.1. General algorithm for laboratory diagnostics in cats with clinical signs of moderate to severe acute or chronic gastrointestinal disease. CBC, complete blood count; FAST, focused assessment with sonography for trauma; FCEAI, feline chronic enteropathy activity index; fPLI, feline pancreatic lipase immunoreactivity; IV, intravenous; TT_4, total thyroxine; UPC, urine protein:creatinine.

with GI signs. Occasionally, a mild to moderate increase in serum liver enzyme activities (mainly ALP and ALT activity) can be observed in the absence of primary disease of the liver in cats with chronic intestinal disease, and this finding is often the result of a reactive hepatopathy.[2] However, similar degrees of increases in serum liver enzyme activities could also signal a concurrent cholangiohepatopathy (e.g. lymphocytic or neutrophilic cholangitis) or hepatic parenchymal (e.g. hepatic lipidosis) or vascular disease (e.g. portosystemic shunt). Evaluation of the liver substrates (i.e. the pseudofunction markers serum BUN, albumin, bilirubin, glucose, and cholesterol concentrations) and a bile acid stimulation test to assess the excretory function of the liver can also be helpful. Hypophosphataemia is reported in 48% of cats with CE,[3] and BUN is higher in cats with intestinal lymphoma compared to cats with chronic inflammatory enteropathy. Hypoalbuminaemia is a rare finding in cats with GI disease. Still, severe infiltrative GI disorders (e.g. large-cell lymphoma or fungal enteritis) can be associated with GI protein loss and hypoalbuminaemia, carrying a worse prognosis (see Chapter 20). Hyperglobulinaemia (leading to hyperproteinaemia) can be detected with chronic inflammatory enteropathy, fungal enteritis, granulomatous feline infectious peritonitis (FIP), or alimentary lymphoma. Extra-GI primary or secondary inflammatory diseases are also important differential diagnoses for this finding. Serum or plasma electrolytes (sodium, potassium, and chloride) should also be measured in cats with either acute or chronic vomiting or diarrhoea, or both, as significant electrolyte abnormalities can be present (e.g. hypokalaemia, hyponatraemia) that need to be considered in the cat's initial treatment plan. Detecting acid–base disturbances also requires a blood gas analysis to be performed. The most common abnormality is metabolic acidosis.

Urinalysis with sediment analysis (and if needed, bacterial culture of urine with antimicrobial susceptibility testing and/or interpretation of the urine protein:creatinine ratio) should also be performed to evaluate the cat for chronic renal or lower urinary tract pathologies.

A diagnostic abdominocentesis for fluid analysis should be attempted in any cat with ultrasonographic evidence of peritoneal effusion. The fluid sample obtained should be macroscopically evaluated, followed by routine laboratory evaluation of the fluid for further characterisation. These tests include the measurement of fluid specific gravity, protein concentration, and total and nucleated cell counts. Also, cytological examination of the fluid sample (as a direct smear and/or after centrifugation) and microbiological culture followed by antimicrobial susceptibility testing of any isolated organisms should be performed if a septic exudate is suspected (that requires surgical intervention). Further molecular diagnostics might be needed to diagnose or rule out other differential diagnoses (e.g. FIP or lymphoma).

The feline pancreatic lipase immunoreactivity (fPLI) concentration in serum should be determined to evaluate cats with compatible clinical signs (anorexia, vomiting, diarrhoea) and/or diagnostic imaging findings (e.g. enlarged hypoechoic pancreas with peripancreatic hyperechogenicity or hyperechoic pancreas with or without nodular lesions) for acute, chronic, or acute-on-chronic pancreatitis (see Chapter 24). The serum Spec fPL test (concentration ≥5.4 µg/l) currently has the highest sensitivity (47%–100%, depending upon disease severity) and specificity (63%–100%) for diagnosing cats with pancreatitis and should be measured in samples collected after 8–12 hours of fasting the cat. The SNAP fPL test is a rapid, semiquantitative fPLI test available for point-of-care analysis. With a moderate to high sensitivity (81%) and specificity (82%) of the SNAP fPL test,[4] a positive result should prompt measurement of fPLI (by Spec fPL) to verify the diagnosis of pancreatitis and to obtain a baseline concentration for future disease monitoring. A negative SNAP fPL rules out pancreatitis with approximately 80% certainty.[4] Also, chronic renal failure or glucocorticoid administration do not appear to have a clinically relevant effect on serum fPLI concentrations in cats. However, severe hyperbilirubinaemia can cause slightly lower fPLI levels. The Spec fPL and SNAP fPL tests have been optimised for diagnosing feline pancreatitis and cannot be used to establish or rule out a diagnosis of exocrine pancreatic insufficiency (EPI) in cats.

As an alternative to serum fPLI measurement by Spec fPL, serum lipase activity can be a sensitive (37%–100%, depending upon disease severity) and specific (63%–100%) laboratory test for diagnosing pancreatitis in cats, if measured by the 1,2-o-dilauryl-rac-glycero-3-glutaric acid-(6'-methylresorufin) ester (DGGR) lipase activity assay and following a proper preanalytic and clinical validation of the test.[5] Because of a high false-positive and also false-negative rate, the measurement of serum amylase activity alone or in combination with serum lipase activity (measured by standard 1,2-diglyceride assay) is not suitable for diagnosing pancreatitis in cats. It is important to recognise that cats with chronic GI (chronic inflammatory enteropathy) and/or hepatobiliary inflammation (cholangitis; see Chapter 30) can have concurrent pancreatitis—the combination of these comorbidities is referred to as feline triaditis (see Chapter 30). The exact aetiology of feline triaditis remains unclear, but host inflammatory and exaggerated immune responses, as well as the intestinal microbiota, appear to play a central role. In contrast to dogs, increased pancreatic lipase concentrations do not appear to affect the outcome or to potentially impact the individual prognosis in cats with CE. Whether a diagnosis of exocrine pancreatic neoplasia (e.g. pancreatic adenocarcinoma or lymphoma) is associated with increased fPLI concentrations (measured by Spec fPL test) or DGGR lipase activities is currently unknown.

Cats with weight loss, diarrhoea, anorexia or polyphagia, vomiting, lethargy, and an unkempt haircoat should also be evaluated for EPI (see Chapter 25). It is important to recognise that this disease often produces a different clinical picture of maldigestion than in dogs. Also, EPI can be challenging to recognise due to the high rate of comorbidities in cats. The test of choice for diagnosing cats with EPI is the measurement of feline trypsin-like immunoreactivity (fTLI) in serum, which reflects the amount of functional pancreatic tissue present. This test (serum fTLI concentration ≤8.0 µg/l is consistent with a diagnosis of EPI) has the highest sensitivity and specificity for the diagnosis of EPI. Still, the correct interpretation of the test requires that the serum sample is collected after an 8- to 12-hour period of fasting. It is unknown whether equivocal serum fTLI concentrations (i.e. serum fTLI concentrations of 8.0–12.0 µg/l) can be detected in cats developing EPI and whether low–normal or even normal serum fTLI concentrations can be seen in cats with EPI secondary to chronic pancreatitis and in the face of an acute exacerbation of inflammation in the residual pancreatic tissue. Thus, equivocal serum fTLI concentrations should best be followed-up by retesting the cat 3–4 weeks later. Because fTLI reflects the functional glandular mass of the pancreas, dietary enzyme replacement therapy does not affect serum fTLI concentrations. Serum fTLI levels can be increased in cats with pancreatitis. Still, both sensitivity (33%–86%) and specificity (56%–90%) of the serum fTLI test for the diagnosis of feline pancreatitis are inferior to those of Spec fPL, and serum fTLI levels can also be increased in cats with renal failure. Measurement of the digestive protease pancreatic elastase-1 (pE1) concentration in faeces is not available for samples from cats, and also is no longer recommended for diagnosing EPI in dogs.

Atypical hypoadrenocorticism as a cause of waxing and waning GI signs has not been reported in cats, and hypoadrenocorticism, in general, is a very rare disease in this species. Thus, measurement of serum cortisol concentration (unstimulated or as ACTH stimulation test) is not warranted in cats with signs of GI disease.

Hypovitaminosis D occurs commonly in cats with chronic GI inflammation or small-cell intestinal lymphoma. However, more research and confirmatory data is needed before routine measurement of serum 25-hydroxyvitamin D concentrations in cats with chronic intestinal disease can be recommended.

Routine coagulation testing is currently also not performed or recommended as there is minimal evidence for coagulopathy in cats with chronic GI inflammation. Two studies support a potential hypovitaminosis K–associated hypocoagulability, but hepatobiliary diseases could not be completely ruled out in the cases reported.[6,7] Another study suggests a hypercoagulable state in feline chronic inflammatory enteropathy due to the incidence of pulmonary thromboembolism diagnosed post-mortem. Still, the contribution of treatment (e.g. glucocorticoids) could not be completely ruled out in these cases.[8] Thus, more research is needed to determine the coagulation (primary and secondary haemostasis) and fibrinolysis status (e.g. by thromboelastography) and the potential need for intervention (e.g. vitamin K supplementation, thromboprophylaxis) in cats with chronic intestinal inflammation.

Faecal examination

Faecal consistency can vary substantially in cats with GI disease and should be assessed using the individual criteria and characteristics of the standard faecal scoring system. This semiobjective grading system allows the veterinary surgeon and also the owner to determine the degree of abnormal faecal consistency and its progression during treatment. The faecal consistency score must be assigned based on the evaluation of a faecal sample immediately after defecation.

Routine parasitological examination of faecal samples collected from three consecutive days for helminth infections with nematodes or cestodes (by faecal sedimentation and flotation techniques or individual coproantigen ELISAs) and protozoa (e.g. *Giardia* spp., *Tritrichomonas blagburni*, *Cryptosporidium* spp.) is an integral part of the initial evaluation of cats with clinical signs of GI disease (Table 3.1), particularly in cats with vomiting or diarrhoea, or both. Also, empirical deworming with fenbendazole for 3 days (or administration of metronidazole for *Giardia* spp.) is usually recommended in cats with chronic diarrhoea before pursuing more invasive diagnostics. For further details, see Chapter 15.

Table 3.1. Parasites that can cause gastrointestinal signs in cats.

Common parasites	Less common parasites
Nematodes *Toxocara cati*	**Nematodes** *Toxascaris leonina* *Trichuris felis* *Physaloptera* spp. *Ollulanus tricuspis*
Cestodes *Ancylostoma* spp. *Taenia* spp. *Dipylidium* spp.	**Cestodes** *Mesocestoides* spp.
Protozoa *Cystoisospora* spp. *Giardia* spp.	**Protozoa** *Tritrichomonas blagburni* *Cryptosporidium* spp. *Sarcocystis* spp. *Hammondia hammondi*
Trematodes *Alaria* spp.	**Trematodes** *Platynosomum fastosum*

Trophozoites of *Giardia* spp. can be detected by microscopic examination (at ×100 magnification) of a fresh faecal smear or faecal wet mount by its characteristic smooth "falling leaf" pattern of motility. The addition of methylene blue or Lugol's solution to the faecal wet mount can aid in better visualising *Giardia* spp. trophozoites. *Giardia* spp. cysts are more resistant, which makes them microscopically detectable in fresh faecal material after $ZnSO_4$ or (less preferred) sugar centrifugal flotation at low speed for 5 minutes (which lyses the more labile *Giardia* spp. trophozoites). Examination of three consecutive faecal samples collected within 5 days can help to maximise the sensitivity of this test to more than 90%.[9] Visualisation of *Giardia* spp. cysts via direct immunofluorescence assay (IFA) using monoclonal antibodies is currently considered as the reference gold standard diagnostic test to detect *Giardia* spp. The sensitivity and specificity of the IFA are reported to be both approximately 100%, and the assay is unlikely to produce false-positive results as it is based on an immunodetection technique that is combined with the evaluation of pathogen morphology. However, this test is costly and cumbersome for routine diagnostics. Detection of faecal *Giardia* spp. antigen by ELISA is also a sensitive diagnostic test but should only be used in cats with clinical signs of small intestinal diarrhoea. Analysis of three faecal samples collected within 5 days can help to maximise the sensitivity of commonly used ELISA kits to approximately 70%–80% (range 50%–100%).[9] The patient-side *Giardia* spp. ELISA has a high agreement with the IFA and a low false-positive and false-negative rate (2%). Faecal PCR for *Giardia* spp. DNA is less sensitive (40%) than ELISA or IFA,[9] and is thus not recommended as a routine test. The current consensus recommendation for routine diagnostics is to use a combination of centrifugal flotation and *Giardia* spp. antigen ELISA for the detection of *Giardia* spp. in cats.[9] *Giardia* spp. isolates (assemblages) are host-specific. Cats carry predominantly assemblages A and F, which are of little zoonotic importance—except for immunocompromised people. The prevalence of *Giardia* spp. in cats in the United States of America is similar (2%–14%, higher prevalence in younger animals) in health and disease, suggesting that *Giardia* spp. should not per se be seen as a primary pathogen. However, clinical giardiasis might be more likely in immunocompromised cats or cats with either coinfections (e.g. *T. blagburni*; see below) or an underlying chronic GI disease (e.g. chronic inflammatory enteropathy or lymphoma).

Particularly young cats (<2 years of age) with a history of chronic or recurrent (often malodorous) large intestinal diarrhoea should also be evaluated for *T. blagburni* (formerly known as *Tritrichomonas foetus*) infection. *T. blagburni* is an anaerobic protozoan species, and feline isolates are biologically, genetically, and pathologically different from *T. foetus* isolates in cattle.[10] The prevalence of *T. blagburni* infection in purebred cats in the United States of America is approximately 30% and ranges from 2% to 59% in other countries (Europe and Australasia).[10] Diagnosis of *T. blagburni* is ideally made by PCR analysis of a faecal sample (collected immediately following natural defecation or via rectal loop technique), which has the highest sensitivity and specificity for detecting *T. blagburni* in faecal samples from cats.[10] Trophozoites of *T. blagburni* can also be detected during direct microscopic examination of a faecal smear or faecal wet mount preparation with saline solution (×100 magnification) based on their rather jerky and rapid pattern of anterior motility. However, this test has the lowest sensitivity (14%) to detect *T. blagburni*, and motile flagellates of *T. blagburni* can be either misdiagnosed as *Giardia* spp. trophozoites or difficult to distinguish from apathogenic *Pentatrichomonas hominis*. Detection of *T. blagburni* by the culture of a fresh faecal sample (e.g. by using the InPouch TF system) has a moderate sensitivity (55%), but the final result of this test might take between 2 and 12 days, and the test is also not specific for *T. blagburni*.

Cryptosporidium spp. (*C. parvum* and *C. felis*) oocysts are best detected by direct IFA using a monoclonal antibody following centrifugal flotation. This test is currently considered as the reference gold standard for the detection of *Cryptosporidium* spp. in feline patients. Because the prevalence of *Cryptosporidium* spp. in cats is generally very low (<1%), test sensitivity is crucial. Molecular analysis by PCR amplification of *Cryptosporidium* spp. is also a sensitive and specific diagnostic tool. Immunoassays have only a moderate sensitivity for *Cryptosporidium* spp., and traditional Ziehl–Neelsen staining is even less sensitive.

Infection with the trematode *Heterobilharzia americana*, endemic in the coastal areas of the Gulf of Mexico and the southern Atlantic, has only been reported in dogs but can also occur in other mammals, including cats. Diagnosis is made by demonstrating *H. americana* eggs on faecal sedimentation and/or fine needle aspirate cytology or histopathology (tissue samples from the liver and/or intestines).

Feline panleucopenia is a highly contagious disease caused in cats primarily by feline parvovirus (FPV) but also by the closely related canine parvovirus type 2 (CPV-2) antigenic variants CPV-2a, CPV-2b, and CPV-2c.[11] Feline panleucopenia should be evaluated as a differential diagnosis in cats with anorexia, lethargy, fever, and marked leucopenia/neutropenia (see Chapter 13). Some affected cats (3%–15%) also show vomiting and haemorrhagic diarrhoea, and other clinicopathologic changes include anaemia and thrombocytopenia, (prerenal) azotaemia, hypokalaemia, and less frequently hypoalbuminaemia.[11] Hypoglycaemia is not typically seen in cats. Abortion can be a sign in pregnant queens. The diagnosis is usually made by a positive faecal parvovirus antigen ELISA result, and the availability of a point-of-care test format developed for CPV-2 detection allows for rapid and reliable detection of FPV. The ELISA has a high specificity and a moderate sensitivity, but false-positive test results can occur within 2 weeks of vaccination with a modified-live vaccine against FPV. False-negative outcomes that are not associated with the sensitivity of the ELISA can occur approximately 2 weeks past the initial parvovirus infection as a result of decreased virus shedding, but this has no clinical relevance. Faecal FPV PCR analysis has the highest sensitivity and specificity for the detection of FPV, but this test is less practical than the point-of-care ELISA test. The FPV PCR cannot per se differentiate between FPV infection and vaccine strain, and the test will also detect CPV-2a–c.

The diagnostic value of a bacteriological faecal examination has remained a matter of debate, particularly in cats with chronic GI signs (see comments on antimicrobial use in Chapter 34). The most common pathogens cultured from faeces in cats are *Salmonella* spp., *Clostridium perfringens*, *Campylobacter* spp., and *Clostridioides* (*Clostridium*) *difficile* (*C. diff*).[12] However, interpretation of the findings can be challenging because these bacteria can also be isolated at reasonably high rates (up to approximately 60%) in healthy nondiarrhoeic cats, and shedding can be transient.[12] It often also remains unknown whether the bacteria are the cause of diarrhoea or the result of intestinal bacterial dysbiosis due to an underlying GI disease. Further, the majority of affected cats showing clinical signs will have acute, uncomplicated, self-limiting (occasionally haemorrhagic) diarrhoea that resolves with supportive therapy alone. However, faecal bacterial testing might be warranted in specific situations, such as the implications of a zoonotic concern.[12]

Salmonella spp. can be shed in healthy cats, especially stray or shelter cats, and also cats fed a raw meat-based diet (Table 3.2), and similar prevalences exist in healthy (up to approximately 14%) and diarrhoeic cats (up to about 9%).[12] All *Salmonella* spp. express virulence genes, but merely the isolation of *Salmonella* spp. from faeces in a diarrhoeic cat does not prove a diagnosis of *Salmonella* spp.–induced enteritis. However, feline salmonellosis has zoonotic relevance and should be considered as an important differential diagnosis when the organism is isolated by culture or PCR amplification in a cat with compatible acute or chronic clinical signs and potential risk factors are present (e.g. environment, prior antibiotic use, feeding of a raw meat-based diet).[12]

Table 3.2. Presence of potential pathogens that can be associated with feeding of a raw meat-based diet in small animals.

Bacteria	**Parasites**
• *Campylobacter* spp.	Protozoa
• *Clostridioides difficile*	• *Cryptosporidium* spp.
• *Clostridium perfringens*	• *Toxoplasma gondii*
• *Clostridium botulinum*	• *Sarcocystis* spp.
• *Escherichia coli* (EHEC)	Cestodes
• *Listeria* spp.	• *Echinococcus* spp.
• *Mycobacterium bovis*	• *Diphyllobothrium latum*
• *Salmonella* spp.	Nematodes
• *Yersinia enterocolitica*	• *Trichinella spiralis*

C. perfringens is a commensal organism with a prevalence in healthy cats that is lower (up to 63%) than in healthy dogs (approximately 80%).[12] *C. perfringens* enterotoxin (CPE) might be associated with acute (haemorrhagic) diarrhoea (4%), especially when present at a high concentration. Still, a 2% prevalence of CPE has also been reported in nondiarrhoeic cats.[12] Thus, *C. perfringens*–associated diarrhoea more likely occurs as a result of a disruption in the intestinal microenvironment. Diagnosis requires real-time faecal PCR for enterotoxigenic (CPE-producing) *C. perfringens* strains together with the immunodetection of faecal CPE by coproantigen ELISA. An association of *C. perfringens* NetE and NetF toxins with acute or chronic diarrhoea has not been reported in cats.

Campylobacter spp. (particularly *C. upsaliensis* and *C. helveticus*, but also *C. jejuni*), isolated by culture or quantitative PCR, show similar isolation rates in health and disease in cats. *Campylobacter* spp. are more likely to be associated with clinical disease (i.e. diarrhoea) in younger animals (<3 years of age) and with specific environmental conditions (e.g. crowding in shelters or kennels) and feeding practices (e.g. raw meat-based diets).

The incidence rate of *C. diff* infection is low in cats, and colonisation rates in cats are generally lower (0%–21%) than in dogs but can be higher in hospitalised cats (9%–38%).[12] Detection of *C. diff* infection requires detection of the organism by real-time PCR and detection of the two main toxins—toxin A (TcdA) and toxin B (TcdB)—by ELISA.

Escherichia coli is a commensal microorganism in cats but also has the potential to be pathogenic with certain virulence factors and an impaired immunity of the host. The role of different *E. coli* pathotypes in cats is currently unclear. Still, adherent–invasive *E. coli* (AIEC) strains can cause granulomatous colitis (formerly known as histiocytic ulcerative colitis) in cats. Diagnosis is made, similar to the disease in dogs, by demonstrating the typical histopathological features in colonic tissue biopsies (periodic acid–Schiff staining-positive macrophages, loss of goblet cells, and mucosal ulceration) and confirmation of AIEC within macrophages by fluorescence in situ hybridisation (FISH) technique followed by AIEC isolation and antimicrobial susceptibility testing. Merely the isolation of *E. coli* from faecal samples in cats with chronic large intestinal diarrhoea does not prove a diagnosis of granulomatous or *E. coli*-induced colitis.

Care should be taken to not indiscriminately perform faecal bacterial testing on every cat with GI signs (mainly if these are chronic) because this practice can lead to misinterpretation of the results and potentially also the administration of unnecessary treatment (particularly antimicrobial drugs). Also, proper handling of the fresh faecal material for bacterial culture is essential. Samples should be processed within 2 hours of collection (if processed at an on-site laboratory) or be placed in a transport medium (e.g. Amies gel) and shipped at 4°C–10°C (if samples are sent to an outside laboratory).

Infection with the fungal organism *Histoplasma capsulatum* should be considered as a (common) differential diagnosis in cats from the southern United States of America if presenting with acute or chronic small, large, or mixed small and large intestinal signs. The diagnosis of GI or disseminated histoplasmosis is typically made by cytology (e.g. fine needle aspiration from a lymph node or rectal scrape) or histopathology (intestinal tissue biopsies obtained via endoscopy, laparoscopy, or laparotomy). The detection and quantification of *H. capsulatum* antigen in serum and/or urine can aid in the diagnosis and also in monitoring cats for the response to antifungal treatment.[13] *Pythium insidiosum* infection should be considered as a (rare) differential diagnosis in cats from the southeastern United States of America (states lining the Gulf of Mexico) if presenting with small, mixed, or large intestinal signs and the suspicion of an abdominal mass based on palpation and/or abdominal ultrasonography. Diagnosis of feline pythiosis is confirmed—similar to the disease in dogs—by histopathology (haematoxylin/eosin and Gomori methenamine silver stain, *P. insidiosum* immunohistochemistry) and isolation by culture or PCR amplification. Also, *P. insidiosum* antigen ELISA serology can help with the diagnosis and disease monitoring.

FURTHER DIAGNOSTIC EVALUATION OF CATS SUSPECTED TO HAVE A CHRONIC ENTEROPATHY

In cats, CE is a broad term that comprises different disease entities: food-responsive enteropathy (FRE), steroid- or immunosuppressant-responsive enteropathy (SRE/IRE, typically referred to as idiopathic inflammatory bowel disease or IBD), and gastrointestinal lymphoma (GIL). The first two forms of the disease are histologically indistinguishable and are generally classified retrospectively based on the cat's response (or lack thereof) to sequential treatment trials. GIL is further subclassified as either small- (lymphocytic) or large-cell (lymphoblastic) lymphoma.

FRE is a common diagnosis, particularly in younger cats. The diagnosis (Fig. 3.2) requires a clinical response within 2–4 weeks of implementing a strict elimination diet trial using a novel antigen or hydrolysed protein diet. A provocation trial to confirm the diagnosis of FRE is very rarely performed in clinical practice. Unfortunately, there is currently no biomarker that can help predict the response to treatment (FRE vs. SRE) in cats with CE. SRE/IRE is a diagnosis of exclusion, and the disease is characterised by an inflammatory infiltrate of the

GI mucosa.[1] Treatment is multimodal by giving anti-inflammatory and/or immunosuppressive medication (e.g. glucocorticoids, chlorambucil) together with at least the initial feeding of an elimination diet. From a therapeutic aspect—and potentially also from a prognostic point of view—the importance of differentiating SRE/IRE from particularly small-cell alimentary (intestinal) lymphoma is currently a matter of debate. Cats diagnosed with SRE/IRE or small-cell intestinal lymphoma generally respond more favourably to medical treatment, whereas cats with large-cell intestinal lymphoma have a poor prognosis. A protein-losing enteropathy as a result of primary intestinal lymphangiectasia (as described in dogs) has not been reported in cats.

The gut microbiome of cats with SRE/IRE or intestinal lymphoma is significantly different from that in healthy cats, pointing to an intestinal dysbiosis. Antimicrobial treatment (e.g. metronidazole or tylosin for 2–4 weeks) can modify the intestinal microbiome in cats and, also, has an immunomodulatory effect, but typically these positive effects of treatment are short-lived, and clinical signs return after discontinuing the antimicrobial medication. Thus, there is currently no convincing evidence to support the existence of an antibiotic-responsive enteropathy in cats. An exception to this concept is granulomatous colitis associated with AIEC, typical histological lesions, and durable response to treatment with a fluoroquinolone antibiotic.

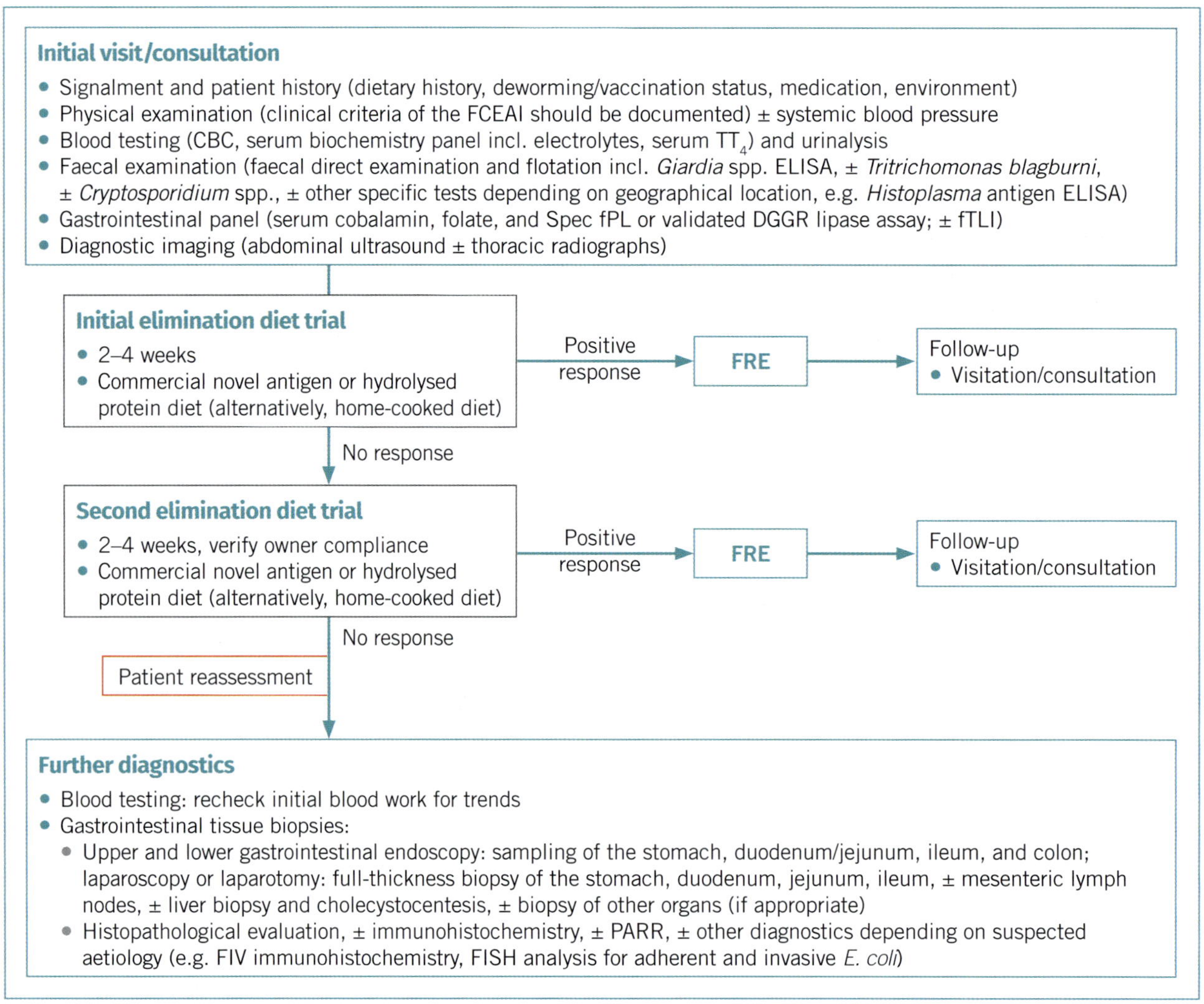

Figure 3.2. Diagnostic algorithm in cats with a suspicion of a diagnosis of chronic enteropathy. CBC, complete blood count; DGGR, 1,2-o-dilauryl-rac-glycero-3-glutaric acid-(6'-methylresorufin) ester; FCEAI, feline chronic enteropathy activity index; FISH, fluorescence in situ hybridisation; FIV, feline immunodeficiency virus; fPL, feline pancreatic lipase; FRE, food-responsive enteropathy; fTLI, feline trypsin-like immunoreactivity; PARR, PCR for antigen receptor rearrangements; TT_4, total thyroxine.

Food antigen testing

Semiquantitative determination of food-specific IgG and IgE titres in serum is not a reliable test to diagnose FRE.[14] Increased IgG and IgE titres reflect a response to individual food ingredients. Still, they do not prove an antigenic effect, and healthy cats can also have increased serum IgG and IgE titres simply as a result of exposure. Also, IgE titres can be affected by many variables, and immune cross-reactions are known to occur. If at all, these tests can potentially identify food antigens that the cat has not been exposed to in the past. A lymphocyte proliferation test appears to be more reliable to detect allergenic food components in cats,[14] but this test is currently not routinely available.

Functional markers of gastrointestinal disease

Determining the serum vitamin B_{12} (cobalamin) status in cats with chronic GI signs is of diagnostic and therapeutic importance. The water-soluble vitamin B_{12} is usually abundant in food, and once complexed with intrinsic factor—which in cats originates exclusively (>99%) from the exocrine pancreas—it is absorbed via specific cobalamin–intrinsic factor receptors located in the distal small intestine (ileum). The current consensus is that a serum cobalamin concentration below 400–500 ng/l can reflect a suboptimal serum cobalamin status that warrants either oral or parenteral supplementation of cobalamin[15] to replete cobalamin stores and aid with the regeneration of the GI mucosa. Hypocobalaminaemia or a low–normal serum cobalamin concentration can be seen in the presence of EPI (prevalence >80%),[16] chronic inflammatory enteropathy (FRE or SRE/IRE), and neoplastic infiltration of the intestinal wall (intestinal small-cell lymphoma). Similar to dogs, the exact aetiology of a suboptimal serum cobalamin status or hypocobalaminaemia in cats with CE is currently unknown. Possible causes include a decreased expression or intraepithelial translocation of the ileal cobalamin–intrinsic factor receptor as a result of inflammation or neoplastic cell infiltration, the development of secondary small intestinal dysbiosis, a decreased half-life of cobalamin, or alterations in the cobalamin transport proteins. The prevalence of hypocobalaminaemia ranges from 17% in cats with chronic inflammatory enteropathy (lower prevalence with FRE compared to SRE/IRE) to 78% in cats with intestinal lymphoma.[3,17,18] Serum cobalamin concentrations are also generally lower in cats with intestinal lymphoma compared to those cats diagnosed with SRE/IRE.[17] However, the concentration of cobalamin in serum does not allow to differentiate between these two aetiologies, nor does a suboptimal cobalamin status allow any inferences or conclusions about the involvement of other segments of the GI tract. It is important to recognise that normocobalaminaemia does not rule out the diagnosis of a CE, as the cat's cobalamin stores may not have been exhausted at the time of serum cobalamin measurement despite ongoing cobalamin malabsorption. Furthermore, hypercobalaminaemia (without prior cobalamin supplementation) has also been documented in cats with CE.[18] Hence, the decision for or against further diagnostics (e.g. GI endoscopy with tissue biopsy specimen collection and the decision to perform both an upper and lower GI endoscopy) should not be based solely on the cat's serum cobalamin status. Hypocobalaminaemia with concurrent hyperfolataemia may reflect secondary small intestinal dysbiosis (e.g. with SRE/IRE or EPI), whereas concurrent hypofolataemia could indicate a diffuse chronic small intestinal disease. Cats with untreated hyperthyroidism can also be hypocobalaminaemic (with a rate of up to 41%). Still, in the absence of concurrent GI disease, this appears to be a transient finding resolving with the control of hyperthyroidism and not requiring cobalamin supplementation. There are no cases of a primary hereditary cobalamin deficiency (Imerslund–Gräsbeck syndrome) in cats in the literature. Also, nutritional cobalamin deficiency has not been reported in cats and should be very unlikely or rare with a balanced feline diet.

Because cobalamin is an essential cofactor of various intracellular enzymes, an increase in the concentrations of substrates of cobalamin-dependent enzymes or alternative metabolic pathways can occur as a result of cellular cobalamin deficiency. Decreased activity of the cobalamin-dependent enzyme methylmalonyl-CoA mutase leads to an accumulation of methylmalonic acid (MMA). This metabolite can be measured in serum or urine to evaluate the cellular cobalamin status for early evidence of a suboptimal intracellular cobalamin supply. Serum (or urine) MMA concentration is routinely determined in human medicine, but the MMA test is not routinely available yet in small animal medicine.

Folic acid (vitamin B_9) is also abundant in commercial pet foods, and a diet-related deficiency is very uncommon. Following the enzymatic digestion of dietary folate polyglutamate, folate is absorbed in its monoglutamate form by carrier-mediated endocytosis in the proximal small intestine. A serum folate deficiency state can, therefore, point to a chronic proximal small intestinal disease (reported prevalence of up to about 40%).[3] Oral supplementation of approximately 200–400 µg folic acid daily for 5–7 days is recommended if serum folate concentration is moderate to markedly decreased. Because certain intraluminal intestinal bacteria are capable of producing folic acid, increased serum folate concentrations might signal an intestinal dysbiosis (e.g. secondary to a chronic inflammatory enteropathy or EPI).[16] Because folic acid is also an essential cofactor in some cobalamin-dependent intracellular pathways, folic acid can accumulate in cobalamin deficiency states and lead to falsely higher serum folate levels. Thus, careful interpretation of alterations in serum cobalamin and folate concentrations is advised.

Alpha$_1$-proteinase inhibitor (α_1PI) is a proteolysis-resistant protein that has a similar molecular weight to albumin. Thus, with intestinal protein loss, the rate of α_1PI being lost into the intestinal lumen is expected to be comparable to that of albumin. In contrast to albumin, however, α_1PI is not enzymatically digested during the intestinal passage, allowing for a quantitative assessment of feline (f)α_1PI in faecal samples by use of a species-specific immunoassay. Concentrations of fα_1PI in faeces (samples collected from 3 consecutive days) are increased in cats with chronic intestinal inflammation (SRE/IRE) and are highest in cats with severe SRE or GIL. This faecal biomarker can also indicate intestinal protein loss in cats without noticeable serum biochemical changes (i.e. hypoalbuminaemia). This test is currently not routinely available to veterinary surgeons.

Investigation of the faecal microbiome in cats with CE indicates the presence of dysbiosis that also might be associated with the progression of GI neoplasia. However, a clinically applicable dysbiosis index, similar to that established and validated in dogs, is currently not available for the evaluation of intestinal dysbiosis in cats. Metabolomic derangements have been identified in cats with CE,[19] but further studies into the feline metabolome, specifically the metabolomic signature of feline CEs, are needed and are currently underway to determine its use as a biomarker in feline gastroenterology.

The deficiency of several essential plasma amino acid (especially taurine but also arginine, histidine, lysine, methionine, phenylalanine, and tryptophan) and non-essential plasma amino acid (asparagine, aspartic acid, glutamic acid, glycine, hydroxyproline, proline, and serine) concentrations in cats with CEs[19] might be a sensitive nutritional marker. However, further study is required to determine the clinical utility of plasma amino acid concentrations as a biomarker in cats with chronic GI disease. Increased serum D-lactate levels have also been reported in cats with GI disease.[20]

The GI absorptive function can be evaluated by determining the absorption of ^{51}Cr-EDTA or iohexol, and GI permeability testing can be assessed by using simple sugar probes. Determination of urine sucrose after oral administration can evaluate gastric permeability, whereas intestinal permeability can be determined by the serum or urine lactulose:rhamnose ratio or the xylose:methylglucose ratio. However, these functional tests are impractical and not used routinely in feline patients.

Gastric emptying time can be noninvasively assessed by the ^{13}C-octanoic acid breath test, but this test is also impractical (particularly in cats), and with the advent of newer modalities, this test is no longer used in small animal clinical practice.

Biomarkers of gastrointestinal inflammation

Serum amyloid A (SAA) and alpha-1-acid glycoprotein (AGP) are major acute-phase proteins in cats that can be measured by immunoassays. Serial SAA measurement might be useful to monitor the response to treatment in cats with pancreatitis. Still, neither SAA nor AGP has been evaluated for their potential as biomarkers of chronic GI or hepatobiliary inflammation in cats.

C-reactive protein (CRP) is a positive acute-phase protein that is produced by hepatocytes as a result of various inflammatory reactions. Measurement of serum CRP concentration might be a useful biomarker for response to treatment in dogs with SRE. However, there is currently no CRP assay available for use with serum samples from cats.

Calprotectin (S100A8/A9 protein complex) and S100A12 are calcium-binding proteins that are mainly secreted by neutrophilic granulocytes and activated macrophages. Calprotectin indicates mononuclear inflammatory processes and can be a useful biomarker to distinguish dogs with SRE from those with FRE. Also, faecal canine calprotectin concentrations correlate with the severity of clinical signs and also the severity of inflammatory lesions in the duodenum and ileum. S100A12 is another biomarker for mononuclear inflammation and, if measured in faecal samples, is specific for the GI tract. Faecal canine S100A12 concentrations correlate with the severity of clinical signs and small intestinal endoscopic lesions, and a failure to respond to treatment in dogs with SRE was associated with higher faecal S100A12 concentrations. Canine calprotectin and S100A12 immunoassays show sufficient cross-reactivity and have been successfully validated for use with feline samples,[21] but clinical validation of these tests in cats is currently still underway. Measurement of calprotectin and S100A12 in faeces is presently only possible at the Texas A&M University Gastrointestinal Laboratory, United States of America. A calprotectin assay that is commercially available in Europe is also currently being validated for feline samples.

N-methylhistamine (NMH) is a stable metabolite of histamine, an important inflammatory mediator that is released proportionally to the activation of mast cells but has a short half-life. NMH can be measured in faeces or urine, and increased NMH concentrations suggest a mast cell component of the intestinal inflammatory process in some dogs with CE. NMH has not been studied in cats with CE, but the test is not species-specific and should be suitable for use with samples from cats. A stable product of the eosinophilic enzyme peroxidase and noninvasive indicator of eosinophilic inflammation, 3-bromotyrosin, has potential as a biomarker in dogs with CE. However, serum 3-bromotyrosine concentrations have not been reported in cats with CE, particularly those cats with eosinophilic gastroenteritis.

Faecal microRNAs hold promise as diagnostic markers for GI disease in cats, but further research is needed in this area of novel biomarker discovery in feline gastroenterology.

Histopathological diagnosis and differentiation markers

If FRE has been ruled out, more invasive diagnostics need to be pursued to arrive at a definitive diagnosis and to further characterise the disease (i.e. quality, severity, and distribution of inflammation, differentiation of inflammation from a neoplastic condition). Tissue samples can be procured via endoscopy, which is minimally invasive and allows the collection of multiple tissue biopsy samples from each site (stomach, duodenum/proximal jejunum, ileum, and colon) under direct visualisation of the mucosa. Full-thickness GI tissue biopsies, collected laparoscopically or via laparotomy, allow for the evaluation of all GI wall layers, but the procedure carries a risk of suture dehiscence, leads to a treatment delay (for the administration of immunosuppressive drugs or chemotherapy), and colonic samples cannot be collected due to the high risk of dehiscence after a colonic surgical biopsy. It is imperative to avoid (if necessary, taper and/or discontinue) pretreatment with glucocorticoids, which can compromise postsurgical wound healing and accurate diagnosis (e.g. masking GIL and leading to an incorrect final diagnosis).

Histopathological examination of GI tissue biopsies should be performed using the histopathological standards established by the World Small Animal Veterinary Association (WSAVA) Gastrointestinal Standardisation Group (see Chapter 9).[1] This guideline aims at the semiobjective assessment of GI tissue biopsies by an individual grading of several structural and inflammatory criteria.[1] In some cats, concurrent tissue biopsy sampling of the liver (for histopathological examination, bacterial culture, and quantification of copper) and the GI tract is essential to distinguish a reactive hepatopathy from a primary disease of the liver parenchyma or the biliary tract. A pancreatic biopsy is seldom performed (e.g. if suspicion of pancreatic neoplasia) and also would be very unlikely to change the treatment plan in a cat suspected to have pancreatitis in addition to the risk of potential postsurgical complications.

The most common histopathological finding in cats with chronic inflammatory enteropathy is lymphoplasmacellular enteritis.[1] The inflammatory infiltrates can also have a minor eosinophilic and/or neutrophilic component in some cats, whereas a marked degree of eosinophilic infiltration (feline eosinophilic enteritis) is infrequently seen. Granulomatous inflammation is very rare in cats and should prompt further investigation for an underlying noneffusive form of FIP (by immunohistochemistry), vector-borne disease (e.g. *Bartonella* spp. by PCR analysis), fungal enteritides (by special stains, fungal culture, and typing, or antigen ELISA), and—if localised to the colon—granulomatous colitis (by FISH analysis followed by bacterial isolation and antimicrobial susceptibility testing). The histopathological finding of a marked lymphoplasmacellular infiltrate might indicate an intestinal small-cell lymphoma,[17] which can be difficult to distinguish from an inflammatory enteropathy based on histopathological examination alone. Intestinal lymphoblastic (large-cell) and large granular lymphocyte lymphoma typically have more obvious diagnostic features on histopathology. Immunohistochemical evaluation of B cell (by immunodetection of CD20 or CD79a) and T cell markers (by immunodetection of CD3) can further help to differentiate lymphoplasmacytic inflammation (mixed infiltrate of B and T cells) from an intestinal small-cell lymphoma (clonal expansion of T or B cells). PCR for antigen receptor rearrangements (PARR) to determine the clonality of the infiltrative lymphocytes in tissue biopsies (performed on stained or unstained microscopy slides) or flow cytometric analysis (performed on a tissue biopsy sample or fine needle aspirate placed in EDTA solution) to assess for clonal expansion of lymphocytes can further help to distinguish mixed lymphocytic inflammation from a small-cell intestinal lymphoma. Still, these tests have to be appropriately analytically and clinically validated. Histology-guided mass spectrometry (HGMS), performed on formalin-fixed, paraffin-embedded tissue biopsy samples, appears to be a very sensitive and specific technique to differentiate a diagnosis of lymphocytic inflammation from a small-cell lymphoma. Still, more research is needed to validate the clinical utility of the assay, and the test is currently only available through a single laboratory in the United States of America.

SUMMARY

The laboratory approach to cats with clinical signs of GI disease should be based on the severity and chronicity of the clinical picture of the individual feline patient. Using a systematic sequential approach is recommended. A detailed patient history, together with a thorough physical examination of the cat, should precede any diagnostic test. Noninvasive diagnostics such as routine blood (haematology, serum biochemistry, and—if appropriate—also additional laboratory tests such as a serum TT_4 or Spec fPL analysis), urine, and faecal examinations as well as diagnostic imaging should present the first steps in the diagnostic evaluation of a cat with GI signs. Routine laboratory tests might reveal or point to the final diagnosis in some cats. In other cats, these tests will be more important for obtaining a good overall impression of the cat's health status and to rule out some differentials. Still, then a more costly and time-consuming diagnostic evaluation will need to follow. Particularly the diagnosis and subclassification of a CE requires the exclusion of several other differential diagnoses and, eventually, more invasive diagnostics. Exclusively feeding at least one elimination diet is an integral part of the diagnostic workup in a clinically stable cat suspected to have CE. If that diagnostic step is adequately done but fails twice (i.e. with two different elimination diets), a diagnosis of FRE can be excluded, and tissue biopsy samples of the GI tract for histopathology (and if needed, further molecular-based tests) are required to document the final diagnosis. Compared to dogs, only a few biomarkers have been studied in cats with chronic GI disease, and even fewer biomarkers are available for routine diagnostics in feline patients with GI disease, highlighting the need for further biomarker research in feline gastroenterology.

Take-home messages

- The laboratory approach to cats with clinical signs of gastrointestinal disease should be based on the severity and chronicity of the clinical signs.
- A systematic and sequential approach to laboratory diagnostics is recommended in cats with signs of chronic gastrointestinal disease.
- Noninvasive and routine diagnostic tests should be performed before proceeding to more invasive diagnostics in these cases.
- Only few functional or biochemical markers of gastrointestinal disease are available for routine diagnostics in cats, and further biomarker research is needed in feline gastroenterology.

REFERENCES

[1] WASHABAU RJ et al. Endoscopic, biopsy, and histopathologic guidelines for the evaluation of gastrointestinal inflammation in companion animals. *J Vet Intern Med* 24:10, 2010.

[2] JERGENS AE et al. A clinical index for disease activity in cats with chronic enteropathy. *J Vet Intern Med* 24:1027, 2010.

[3] REED N et al. Cobalamin, folate and inorganic phosphate abnormalities in ill cats. *J Feline Med Surg* 9:278, 2007.

[4] SCHNAUSS F et al. Diagnosis of feline pancreatitis with SNAP fPL and Spec fPL. *J Feline Med Surg* 21:700, 2019.

[5] OPPLIGER S et al. Glycero-3-glutaric acid-(6'-methylresorufin) ester assay in 60 cats using standardized assessment of pancreatic histology. *J Vet Intern Med* 30:764, 2016.

[6] EDWARDS DF et al. Probable vitamin K-deficient bleeding in two cats with malabsorption syndrome secondary to lymphocytic-plasmacytic enteritis. *J Vet Intern Med* 1:97, 1987.

[7] CENTER SA et al. Proteins invoked by vitamin K absence and clotting times in clinically ill cats. *J Vet Intern Med* 14:292, 2000.

[8] NORRIS CR et al. Pulmonary thromboembolism in cats: 29 cases (1987–1997). *J Am Vet Med Assoc* 215:1650, 1999.

[9] UCHÔA FFM et al. Assessment of the diagnostic performance of four methods for the detection of *Giardia duodenalis* in fecal samples from human, canine and feline carriers. *J Microbiol Methods* 145:73, 2018.

[10] GOOKIN JL et al. The conundrum of feline tritrichomonosis. *J Feline Med Surg* 19:261, 2017.

[11] BARRS VR. Feline panleukopenia: a re-emergent disease. *Vet Clin North Am Small Anim Pract* 49:651, 2019.

[12] MARKS SL et al. Enteropathogenic bacteria in dogs and cats: diagnosis, epidemiology, treatment, and control. *J Vet Intern Med* 25:1195, 2011.

[13] HANZLICEK AS et al. Antigen concentrations as an indicator of clinical remission and disease relapse in cats with histoplasmosis. *J Vet Intern Med* 30:1065, 2016.

[14] MUELLER RS et al. Critically appraised topic on adverse food reactions of companion animals (4): can we diagnose adverse food reactions in dogs and cats with in vivo or in vitro tests? *BMC Vet Res* 13:275, 2017.

[15] TORESSON L et al. Oral cobalamin supplementation in cats with hypocobalaminemia: a retrospective study. *J Feline Med Surg* 19:1302, 2017.

[16] XENOULIS PG et al. Feline exocrine pancreatic insufficiency: a retrospective study of 150 cases. *J Vet Intern Med* 30:1790, 2016.

[17] KISELOW MA et al. Outcome of cats with low-grade lymphocytic lymphoma: 41 cases (1995–2005). *J Am Vet Med Assoc* 232:405, 2008.

[18] KATHER S et al. Prevalence and clinical relevance of hypercobalaminaemia in dogs and cats. *Vet J* 265:105547, 2020.

[19] SAKAI K et al. Decreased plasma amino acid concentrations in cats with chronic gastrointestinal diseases and their possible contribution in the inflammatory response. *Vet Immunol Immunopathol* 195:1, 2018.

[20] PACKER RA et al. Serum D-lactate concentrations in cats with gastrointestinal disease. *J Vet Intern Med* 26:905, 2012.

[21] HEILMANN RM et al. Preanalytical validation of an in-house radioimmunoassay for measuring calprotectin in feline specimens. *Vet Clin Pathol* 47:100, 2018.

CHAPTER 4

Laboratory approach to exocrine pancreatic and hepatobiliary disorders

Emily N. Gould, Joerg M. Steiner

Feline pancreatic and hepatobiliary disorders have become recognised with increasing frequency and also better characterised over the last decade. This is in part due to both improved understanding of pathophysiology and advances in the development and appropriate utilisation of diagnostics. As most differential diagnoses discussed in Chapter 2 are associated with nonspecific clinical signs, clinicians must use a combination of history, physical examination, and minimum database (i.e. complete blood count [CBC], biochemistry panel, urinalysis) results to guide the need for organ-specific testing (e.g. plasma ammonia, bile acids [BAs], species-specific pancreatic enzymes) and/or diagnostic imaging. It is also paramount to remember that abnormalities in clinicopathologic parameters are based on reference intervals (RIs) established from clinically healthy individuals, assuming that a small percentage of healthy animals (approximately 5%) will have values that fall outside these RIs. Similarly, some values that fall on the low or high end of the RI are actually abnormal for that animal and can provide clues to the clinician as to what the underlying disorder is. For these reasons, examining the trends for clinicopathologic parameters over time is important in reaching a definitive diagnosis and monitoring disease progression.

A minimum database is indicated in nearly every cat with suspected hepatobiliary or exocrine pancreatic disease, with the need for organ-specific testing determined on a case by case basis. Appropriate interpretation of laboratory abnormalities depends on accompanying clinical signs, diagnostic imaging findings, and, in the case of liver enzymes, consideration of species-specific serum or plasma half-lives. This chapter is designed to provide a practical approach to the application and interpretation of laboratory tests for commonly occurring feline exocrine pancreatic and hepatobiliary disorders.

DIFFERENTIAL DIAGNOSES FOR EXOCRINE PANCREATIC AND HEPATOBILIARY DISORDERS IN CATS

The most common exocrine pancreatic disorders in the cat are pancreatitis, both chronic and acute, and exocrine pancreatic insufficiency (EPI). Hepatobiliary diseases frequently seen in cats include a variety of inflammatory disorders (e.g. infectious or sterile inflammatory cholangitis), primary or secondary feline hepatic lipidosis (FHL), less commonly vascular anomalies (e.g. portosystemic shunt [PSS] and primary portal vein hypoplasia [PPVH]), and rarely copper storage hepatopathies. Cholangitis can be seen in isolation or, potentially more commonly, as a comorbidity with chronic pancreatitis and/or chronic enteropathy. The combination of all three disease processes is referred to as triaditis. Tables 4.1 and 4.2 summarise the main differential diagnoses for specific clinicopathologic abnormalities most commonly seen on the CBC and biochemistry panel, respectively, in cats affected by these disorders. See Chapter 2 for a complete list of differential diagnoses and clinical signs associated with these conditions.

EVALUATION OF THE COMPLETE BLOOD COUNT

It is common for cats with hepatobiliary and exocrine pancreatic disease to have an unremarkable CBC, and neither the presence nor absence of abnormalities are sensitive or specific for identifying individual disorders. If abnormalities are present, a spectrum of changes to both the leucogram and haemogram are possible (Table 4.1). The presence of a leucocytosis, with or without bands, anaemia, altered erythrocyte morphology, and hyperproteinaemia (often secondary to dehydration or hyperglobulinaemia) should all be noted. These changes often provide the clinician with important information about the primary disease process or comorbidities.

Although only approximately half of cats with cholangitis have leucogram abnormalities, a neutrophilia with or without left shift is most commonly noted.[1,2] Those with neutrophilic cholangitis more commonly have a leucocytosis with a left shift compared to those with other hepatobiliary diseases.[1,3] This more frequently occurs if the cat is also febrile. Cats with pancreatitis can range from having a completely normal leucogram to a significant leucocytosis with a left shift and even degenerate neutrophils. Multiple studies have shown that pancreatitis with concurrent leucopenia carries a worse prognosis.[4,5] This might directly reflect severity of pancreatic inflammation or result from a comorbidity predisposing to or exacerbating inflammation. Cats with lymphocytic cholangitis and FHL often exhibit no alterations of the leucogram, unless the FHL is secondary to an underlying inflammatory process.

If an anaemia is present, it must be appropriately classified and the severity noted and closely monitored. Poikilocytosis (Fig. 4.1), that is, any abnormally shaped erythrocyte, and microcytosis are two of the more commonly encountered abnormalities in cats with hepatobiliary disorders.

Erythrocyte abnormalities are seen most frequently with FHL,[6,7] varying types of cholangitis,[1,3] and PSS.[8,9] One of the largest retrospective studies of FHL showed that of 77 cats, 31% had a moderate anaemia and up to 53% had poikilocytes.[7] Heinz body formation,[6] as well as ovalocytes (i.e. elliptocytes)[10] and acanthocytes,[11] have also been documented in lipidotic cats. It is unknown if this is directly related to FHL or the sequela of an underlying disease process that is associated with lipidosis.[6] Because many of the erythrocyte abnormalities noted in cats with FHL do not fit into one category, the term poikilocytosis is often used to encompass all changes.[11] Most cats with a PSS and microcytosis are anaemic, but up to one-third of cats with vascular anomalies might be presented with a normal haematocrit.[8] While the pathophysiology of microcytosis with hepatic disease is not fully understood, the most likely explanation is a disruption of iron transport and/or storage.

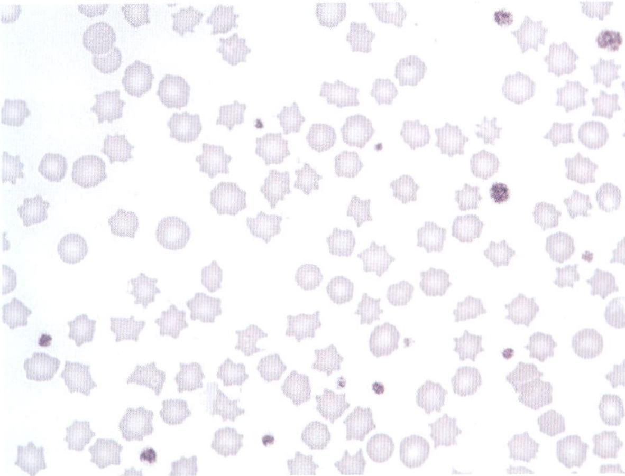

Figure 4.1. Poikilocytosis in a cat with a marked cholestatic hepatopathy and hyperbilirubinaemia. The abnormal erythrocyte shapes are characterised by predominantly echinocytes and rare acanthocytes. Modified Wright's stain, ×100. Image courtesy of Dr Candice Pei-Hua Chu, Texas A&M University, USA.

Hyperglobulinaemia, causing an increase in total protein, is a nonspecific finding and is most often indicative of systemic inflammation or, if markedly elevated, a neoplastic process. This can be seen in cats with cholangitis and pancreatitis, but it also might reflect systemic disorders, namely feline infectious peritonitis or toxoplasmosis.

Alterations of platelet counts are uncommon for cats with hepatobiliary or exocrine pancreatic disease,[12] but thrombocytopenia can develop secondary to a concurrent consumptive process or disseminated intravascular coagulation. Most cats documented to have developed disseminated intravascular coagulation and subsequent thrombocytopenia had developed hepatic dysfunction due to acute liver failure rather than a more commonly seen hepatobiliary disorder. Thrombocytopenia in general is more commonly reported in dogs than cats, but this might simply reflect a lack of literature regarding the effects of hepatic dysfunction on platelet counts in cats.

Table 4.1. The most common abnormalities seen on the complete blood count of cats with hepatobiliary and pancreatic disease, along with corresponding rule outs.

Abnormality	Primary hepatobiliary and pancreatic causes	Extrahepatobiliary and extrapancreatic causes
Leucocytosis (+/– left shift)	Cholangitis (neutrophilic more common)* FHL (secondary)* Pancreatitis EHBDO	Any systemic inflammatory disease (sterile or infectious)
Leucopenia	Pancreatitis (associated with worse prognosis)* Bacterial cholangitis	Septicaemia* Viral (FeLV, FIV)* Primary bone marrow disorders
Anaemia (more commonly nonregenerative)	Anaemia of inflammatory disease (with pancreatitis, cholangitis)* PSS disease* Any hepatic dysfunction	Any systemic inflammatory disease Primary bone marrow disorder Haemorrhage (usually regenerative) Haemolysis (usually regenerative)
Poikilocytosis (abnormal erythrocyte shape)	FHL (primary and secondary, acanthocytes and elliptocytes overrepresented)* PSS disease* Cholangitis Pancreatitis	DIC Heartworm disease
Microcytosis	PSS disease (overrepresented)* Any primary hepatic disease	Gastrointestinal bleeding* Preanalytic factors (e.g. underfilling of collection tube with resulting increased ratio of EDTA) Young age of patient Breed related (i.e. Abyssinian cats have normally low MCV)

DIC, disseminated intravascular coagulation; EHBDO, extrahepatic bile duct obstruction; FeLV, feline leukaemia virus; FHL, feline hepatic lipidosis; FIV, feline immunodeficiency virus; MCV, mean corpuscular volume; PSS, portosystemic shunt.
*Differential diagnoses overrepresented to develop that specific biochemical change.

EVALUATION OF THE BIOCHEMISTRY PANEL

A biochemistry panel is nearly always indicated in cats with suspected hepatobiliary and/or exocrine pancreatic disease. Key aspects of a chemistry panel to evaluate include:

- pattern of liver enzyme activity increases
- markers of hepatic synthetic capacity
- additional analytes that might provide clues for correct identification of the primary disorder or comorbidities.

Examples of this would be a hyperglobulinaemia, resulting from underlying systemic inflammation or concurrent hypercholesterolaemia signifying to the clinician that a cholestatic process is most likely.

Increases in liver enzyme activities can be differentiated as either hepatocellular or cholestatic in nature, depending on where the liver enzyme originates from, and, importantly, do not reflect hepatic function. While a marked hepatocellular hepatopathy alerts the clinician that there has been more significant damage to the hepatocytes than an injury resulting in mild increases, severity of enzyme activity increase is not necessarily prognostic. It also does not differentiate reversible from nonreversible hepatic injury.[13] Instead, enzyme activities are important for prioritising which disease processes are most likely as well as for monitoring disease progression and/or response to therapy. It is important to be aware that while there are usually increases in liver enzyme activities prior to hepatic failure, enzyme activities do decline with progression of disease as the liver loses functional hepatocytes.

While patterns of liver enzyme activity increase alone are by no means diagnostic for specific aetiologies, a hepatopathy of some sort is usually present with nearly any hepatobiliary and/or exocrine pancreatic disorder. Exceptions to this might include certain hepatic or biliary neoplasms, vascular anomalies (i.e. PSS, PPVH), or end-stage liver disease, resulting in depletion of functional hepatocytes. If present, the hepatopathy can be any combination of cholestatic, hepatocellular, or mixed pattern. Hepatopathies can also fluctuate significantly in severity. Because previously established guidelines for liver enzyme activity increases were developed with multiple species in mind, some of these cutoff values are not appropriate for cats. This is due to differences in their enzyme half-lives compared to other species. In a cat, 2- to 5-fold increases should probably be considered moderate instead of mild, and greater than 5-fold increases classified as severe.

Hepatocellular hepatopathy

Alterations in hepatocellular enzyme activities include increases in the intracellularly located enzymes alanine aminotransferase (ALT) and aspartate aminotransferase (AST). ALT is a predominantly cytosolic enzyme, while AST is found in high amounts in both the cytosol and the mitochondria. The most severe increases in hepatocellular enzyme activities usually result from inflammatory or necrotising processes. In the authors' opinion, 2- to 5-fold increases in hepatocellular enzyme activities in cats require a complete diagnostic investigation, and greater than a 5-fold increase necessitates an immediate workup as well as therapeutic intervention. Any increase in ALT or AST activity in a cat should be taken seriously and investigated.

Alanine aminotransferase activity

Although the liver contains the largest amount of ALT, other isoenzymes are found in the kidneys, heart, muscle, and—in some species—erythrocytes.[10] Because feline erythrocytes do contain ALT, haemolysis can also cause serum/plasma enzyme activity increases. This means that while damage to hepatocytes is often the main cause of an elevated ALT activity, it is imperative to remember that any active muscle damage and potentially haemolysis can contribute to increases and should not be overlooked. Lipaemia can also falsely elevate serum/plasma ALT activities.[10]

Peak serum/plasma activities of ALT occur 12–28 hours following hepatocyte injury and, in the absence of an ongoing insult, are expected to decrease fairly rapidly due to a short half-life. Of note, ALT has a markedly shorter half-life (approximately 3.5–6 hours) in cats[10,14] compared to dogs (approximately 2–3 days). This is significant because even a mild increase in ALT activity in a cat implies an active process whereas in a dog might simply indicate residual hepatocellular damage that occurred days before the blood sample was collected.

Increases in serum/plasma ALT activity can be seen secondary to any type of hepatobiliary disease or pancreatitis, and the degree of increase can fluctuate on a case by case basis. Increases in ALT activities are most sensitive (inability to exclude the disease if elevated) for extrahepatic bile duct obstruction (EHBDO) and cholangitis in the cat, with sensitivities of 80%–100%.[13] It is very rare for cats with EHBDO to have a normal ALT activity, making this differential diagnosis much less likely if the enzyme activity is within the RI. While most cats with cholangitis have increases in ALT activity, some animals with neutrophilic cholangitis have been documented to have liver enzymes within the RI.[15] Also, a recent study found that ALT activity in conjunction with bilirubin concentration were the two most likely parameters to be increased in cats with copper storage hepatopathy.[16] The presence or magnitude of the ALT activity increase was not useful to differentiate these cats from those with other common hepatobiliary diseases (i.e. cholangitis, EHBDO). Because copper storage hepatopathy is rare in cats, there is still a lack of understanding about the most common biochemical abnormalities seen in cats with this hepatopathy.

Severe, acute increases in serum/plasma ALT activity should alert the clinician that hepatotoxicosis must be a top differential diagnosis until proven otherwise. Both generic and brand-name oral diazepam have been reported to cause an idiosyncratic hepatotoxicity characterised by dramatic increases in ALT activity.[17] The same has not been reported with injectable diazepam. Though acetaminophen administration can cause hepatotoxicity in cats, it is more common for this species to develop methaemoglobinaemia and haematologic abnormalities. Close monitoring of ALT activity is necessary in cats that have recently been started on either oral or transdermal methimazole for treatment of hyperthyroidism, especially because many of these cats already have an increased ALT activity as a result of uncontrolled hyperthyroidism prior to initiation of methimazole therapy. Hepatotoxicity secondary to methimazole is idiosyncratic and can cause either an exclusively hepatocellular or cholestatic hepatopathy, with or without accompanying hyperbilirubinaemia. Approximately 1%–2% of cats receiving methimazole will develop hepatotoxicity within the first month of therapy.[18] It is usually reversible, if detected early, with immediate discontinuation of the medication.

Even though ALT is the most specific enzyme for hepatocellular injury, hyperthyroidism and myopathies should be ruled out prior to pursuing further diagnostics, especially if the remainder of the liver enzyme activities are within the RI. Muscle damage will usually cause increases in both ALT and AST activities, with AST increases exceeding those of ALT (Fig. 4.2).

Aspartate aminotransferase activity

Because AST is located predominantly in the mitochondria of hepatocytes, as opposed to the cytosol, greater cellular damage must occur in order to liberate the enzyme into circulation.[10] In contrast to ALT, where the largest amount of the enzyme is stored in the liver, significant amounts of AST are found in skeletal muscle and cardiac tissue. A smaller amount is also found in erythrocytes, and AST can thus be released with severe haemolysis. Similar to ALT, AST has a very short half-life in the cat (1.5 hours).[10] For these reasons, AST is usually a less specific marker of hepatocellular injury compared to ALT.

Despite this, it is important to recognise that exceptions do occur. In some cats diagnosed with hepatic necrosis, cholangitis, hepatic lymphoma, or chronic bile duct obstruction, AST activity was the only liver enzyme that was increased.[13]

If AST activity is increased in the absence of an increase in ALT activity, it is recommended that creatine kinase (CK) activity, haematocrit, and potentially bilirubin be evaluated (Fig. 4.2). If CK is significantly increased, there is a high likelihood that muscle, rather than the liver, is the cause of the increase. Haemolysis is usually easily ruled in or out by the presence of a regenerative anaemia with or without hyperbilirubinaemia. A very recent haemolytic process (<3–5 days) might lack evidence of regeneration (i.e. reticulocytosis) if the bone marrow has not had time to mount an appropriate response.

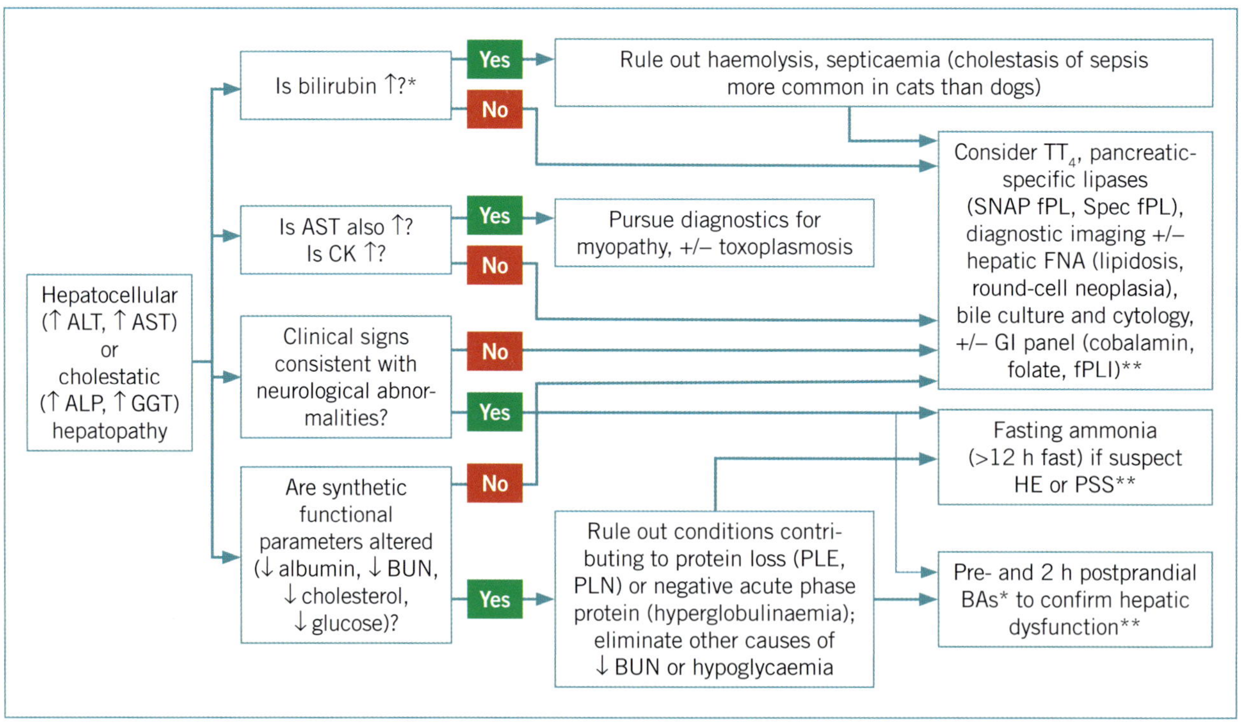

Figure 4.2. Flow chart illustrating an appropriate diagnostic tree for cholestatic and hepatocellular hepatopathies in cats. A single asterisk (*) denotes that bile acids (BAs) are contraindicated if the bilirubin is already elevated. A double asterisk (**) denotes that these are also appropriate times to assess for coagulation defects (e.g. platelet count, prothrombin time, activated partial thromboplastin time), especially if any sampling of the liver such as fine needle aspiration (FNA) or liver biopsy are pursued. ALP, alkaline phosphatase; ALT, alanine aminotransferase; AST, aspartate aminotransferase; BUN, blood urea nitrogen; CK, creatine kinase; fPL, feline pancreatic lipase; fPLI, feline pancreatic lipase immunoreactivity; GGT, gamma-glutamyltransferase; GI, gastrointestinal; HE, hepatic encephalopathy; PLE, protein-losing enteropathy; PLN, protein-losing nephropathy; PSS, portosystemic shunt; TT_4, total thyroxine.

If the serum/plasma globulins and CK are both elevated, toxoplasmosis must be ruled out, as these protozoa target both the liver and muscle.

Cholestatic hepatopathy

A cholestatic hepatopathy refers to a disease that is associated with an increase in serum/plasma activities of membrane-bound alkaline phosphatase (ALP) or gamma-glutamyltransferase (GGT), often in conjunction with increased concentrations of cholesterol and/or total bilirubin. While the latter two are not enzymes, concurrent increase of either can help the clinician more confidently attribute the changes observed to a disease process causing intra- or extrahepatic cholestasis.

Alkaline phosphatase activity

Increased serum/plasma activities of ALP in the cat arise due to a variety of cholestatic processes as well as non-hepatobiliary disorders (Table 4.2). In contrast to ALT and AST, which are found within the cell, the hepatic iso-

Table 4.2. The most common abnormalities seen on the biochemistry panel of cats with hepatobiliary and pancreatic disease, along with corresponding rule outs.

Abnormality	Primary hepatobiliary and pancreatic causes	Extrahepatobiliary and extrapancreatic causes
↑ ALT	Cholangitis* EHBDO* Hepatotoxicity (diazepam, methimazole >> acetaminophen)* Pancreatitis* FHL (primary or secondary) Neoplasia (hepatic, hepatobiliary) PSS disease Toxoplasmosis FIP	Hyperthyroidism* Hypoxia (e.g. congestive heart failure, hypotension, seizures)* CE Preanalytic factors (i.e. lipaemia, haemolysis [species-specific, occurs in cats])
↑ AST	Hepatotoxicity* Cholangitis* EHBDO* Pancreatitis* FHL (primary or secondary) Neoplasia (infiltrative hepatic lymphoma) Chronic bile duct obstruction Hepatotoxicity (methimazole) Toxoplasmosis FIP	Muscle damage* Haemolysis*
↑ ALP	FHL (usually significantly ↑ in primary, but also seen with secondary)* Pancreatitis* Cholangitis* Infiltrative round-cell neoplasms (lymphoma > MCT)* EHBDO (from neoplasia or severe inflammation)* Hepatotoxicity (methimazole)	Diabetes mellitus* Hyperthyroidism* Primary bone tumours Duodenal foreign body causing EHBDO
↑ GGT	Cholangitis EHBDO Biliary hyperplasia Neoplasia (primary or secondary) FHL (secondary >>> primary)	Preanalytic factors (e.g. underfilling of collection tube), otherwise very specific for biliary tract disorders
Mixed hepatopathy (↑ in equal magnitude of hepatocellular and cholestatic enzymes)	Pancreatitis (acute and chronic)* FHL (secondary >> primary)* Cholangitis Neoplasia Toxoplasmosis FIP	CE* Hyperthyroidism

CE, chronic enteropathy; EHBDO; extrahepatic bile duct obstruction; FHL, feline hepatic lipidosis; FIP, feline infectious peritonitis; MCT, mast cell tumour; PSS, portosystemic shunt.
*Differential diagnoses overrepresented to develop that specific biochemical change.

enzyme of ALP is located on the hepatocyte membrane of cells lining sinusoids and bile canaliculi.[10] Cats have less hepatic ALP than dogs, and while they also possess intestinal, bone, and renal isoenzymes, a consensus has not been reached on which type contributes the most to circulating ALP activity in cats.[13] It is currently believed that the intestinal and hepatic isoenzymes of ALP are the biggest contributors to increased serum/plasma ALP activities in cats, but this has not been definitively proven. However, cats lack corticosteroid-induced ALP, which is of note because increases in ALP activity cannot be attributed to endogenous or exogenous steroids in the cat as it can in dogs. The half-life of hepatic ALP is shorter in the cat (approximately 6 hours) compared to the dog, and it is also actively excreted by the kidneys.[10] These two characteristics about feline ALP might make it an inferior marker for cholestatic disease compared to its cholestatic counterpart, GGT.

Because cats lack the steroid-induced enzyme, it is rare to see isolated increases in serum/plasma ALP activity in the absence of other increases in liver enzyme activities. When this does occur, the most common causes are intra- or posthepatic cholestatic processes that lack significant inflammation, as is the case with primary FHL. A defining feature of primary FHL is that affected cats show marked increases in serum/plasma ALP activity, with only mild to moderate increases in other enzyme activities, and often no increase in GGT activity. However, this does not hold true if there is an underlying infectious or inflammatory disorder (e.g. cholangitis, neoplasia) acting as the inciting cause of the lipidosis.[7,13] Some cats with hyperthyroidism develop increases in ALP activity from increases in both liver and bone isoenzymes, which most likely is due to the effect of thyroid hormone on bone turnover. However, it is also possible that hyperthyroidism leads to hepatic pathology, an area of further research interest. While, in general, hepatotoxicities do not commonly manifest themselves as being cholestatic in nature, methimazole toxicity can cause an exclusively cholestatic or mixed hepatopathy.

Gamma-glutamyltransferase activity

Another enzyme found in large quantities in feline hepatocytes and biliary epithelium is GGT. It is very uncommon for cholestatic processes to lack an increase in GGT, and most diseases causing increases in ALP activity will similarly increase GGT activity (Table 4.2).[19] Biliary ducts contain large amounts of this enzyme, which might explain why GGT activity is almost always increased in cats with inflammatory, necrotic, or neoplastic processes of the biliary tree.[13,20] GGT also has a longer half-life than ALP in the cat, making it a more sensitive indicator of cholestatic disease in this species.[19] The one exception to this appears to be primary FHL, where ALP activity is nearly always increased, while that of GGT is not. Furthermore, if GGT activity is increased in a cat with primary FHL, it often is increased to a much lesser magnitude compared to ALP activity.[7,13,19] If a cat is definitively diagnosed with FHL but has increases in ALP and GGT activities of approximately the same magnitudes, this should pique the clinician's interest enough to search for an underlying disorder acting as a trigger for the lipidosis. Finally, while GGT activity increases following administration of oral steroids or anticonvulsants in dogs, this has not been reported to occur in cats.

Mixed hepatopathy

A mixed hepatopathy refers to conditions that lead to increases of both hepatocellular and cholestatic liver enzyme activities of equal magnitude. This pattern is nonspecific and can be seen with primary hepatic, biliary, or exocrine pancreatic disease in the cat. Cats with both acute[4,21] and chronic[21] pancreatitis will often have increases in ALT and ALP activities of equal magnitude, along with secondary FHL. Mixed hepatopathies are also common in cats with cholangitis but are less commonly seen with primary FHL or EHBDO.

Hepatic synthetic function parameters and specific testing

Markers of hepatic synthetic function that are routinely assessed include albumin, blood urea nitrogen (BUN), cholesterol, coagulation factors, and glucose. Naturally, the liver synthesises a large number of other molecules, such as acute phase reactants and fibrinolytic factors, amongst many others. However, none of these are routinely measured, and thus they cannot be employed to assess hepatic function. A loss of more than 70% of liver function is necessary to cause alterations in most of these parameters, and they are rather insensitive markers for hepatic disease. Therefore, results of these parameters within the RI do not confidently rule out hepatic dysfunction. Importantly, each product of hepatic synthesis has a different minimal residual hepatic function to maintain homoeostasis. Maintaining serum albumin, BUN, and cholesterol concentrations within the RI will require the most residual function, with glucose and coagulation factors requiring the least residual function. This can be very helpful in assessing the degree of hepatic dysfunction in a cat with hepatic failure. Additionally, all of these markers are not specific to the liver and can be influenced by other disease processes. Thus, careful attention to the pattern of alterations in functional parameters, as well as elimination of extrahepatic diseases and/or preanalytic conditions that can cause alterations in these markers, is important (Box 4.1). If hepatic dysfunction seems most likely, additional testing such as measurement of serum BAs and/or ammonia is often necessary (see section "Additional tests of hepatic function" in this chapter).

Blood urea nitrogen

BUN refers to a nitrogenous waste product that is produced in the liver and excreted in the kidneys. While BUN decreases with decreasing liver function, it is necessary to remember that a plethora of other systemic conditions may also lower the BUN. Examples of this would include overhydration, polyuria and polydipsia, and syndrome of inappropriate antidiuretic hormone secretion (SIADH). Although BUN is one of the earliest functional markers to decrease with hepatic dysfunction, it is nonspecific for discriminating between various disease processes. Cats with PSS more commonly have a low BUN than hypoalbuminaemia or alterations in other synthetic hepatic functional parameters.[22,23] This is in contrast to canine PSS disease, in which albumin is one of the most common synthetic parameters to be altered.

Albumin

Albumin is produced exclusively by the liver and can be decreased either due to increased loss (e.g. protein-losing enteropathy [PLE], protein-losing nephropathy [PLN], haemorrhage, exudative processes associated with vasculitis), as a negative acute phase protein, or as a result of primary liver disease and inadequate hepatic synthesis. PLE occurs less commonly in cats compared to dogs and, if present, is usually secondary to gastrointestinal (GI) lymphoma or severe inflammatory enteropathy. While concurrent hypoalbuminaemia and hypocholesterolaemia is most often due to hepatic dysfunction or PLE, the concurrent presence of hypoalbuminaemia and hypoglobulinaemia would suggest a loss through the GI tract or the skin and should steer the clinician away from a problem solely with the liver. In general, hypoalbuminaemia is seen far more commonly in dogs than in cats, which also holds true for cats with PSS.[22,23] There is a shortage of published literature specifically looking at hypoalbuminaemia and hepatobiliary disease in cats, but it is not recognised as commonly as it has been reported in dogs with hepatic dysfunction.

Cholesterol

Similar to albumin, cholesterol is also produced in the liver and decreases with hepatic dysfunction. However, because cholesterol is also excreted in the bile, it is often increased in cats with diseases that lead to impaired biliary transport (i.e. cholestasis). Cholesterol concentrations can be variable in cats with hepatobiliary disorders, but hypercholesterolaemia is one of the most commonly reported abnormalities on the biochemistry profile of cats with pancreatitis, with almost 75% of cats presenting with elevated serum cholesterol concentrations in multiple studies.[4,5,21] This finding is not specific for pancreatitis, as any disease causing intra- or posthepatic cholestasis will also usually result in hypercholesterolaemia.

Coagulation function

Although clinical evidence of a coagulopathy is rarely observed in cats with hepatobiliary and pancreatic disease, studies investigating coagulation function in feline hepatobiliary disease have shown that 45%–73% of these patients display alterations in haemostasis.[7,12] Mechanisms that are thought to contribute to coagulopathies in this population are multifactorial. While hepatic insufficiency can cause both hyper- and hypocoagulability, most coagulopathies documented in the literature describe hypocoagulability secondary to impaired clotting factors. Not only does the liver produce all of the clotting factors except a subset of factor VIII, but cholestatic disease also interferes with vitamin K–dependent factors in multiple ways. Firstly, because successful absorption of vitamin K requires normal flow of bile and subsequent delivery of BAs to the small intestine, malabsorption of vitamin K increases with worsening cholestasis. Secondly, resident bacteria in the small intestine also produce vitamin K, leading to potentially decreased vitamin K concentrations in cats that receive antimicrobial therapy for a suspected infectious cholangitis. For these reasons, altered function of vitamin K–dependent clotting factors is thought to be the most significant problem leading to hypocoagulability seen in cats with hepatobiliary disease.

The fact that BA homoeostasis is important for vitamin K homoeostasis explains why cats with cholestatic disorders (e.g. cholangitis, FHL, EHBDO) are overrepresented[3,7,12,24] and more frequently have a coagulopathy when compared to cats with strictly hepatocellular disease. In a large retrospective study of cats with both primary and secondary FHL, a coagulopathy was identified in almost half of the population despite no evidence of clinical bleeding.[7] Similarly, up to 50% of cats with EHBDO have been identified as having a prolongation in prothrombin time (PT) and activated partial thromboplastin time (aPTT).[25] In cases for which surgical correction of the EHBDO was pursued, nearly half still required blood products despite administration of injectable vitamin K perioperatively.

Box 4.1. Important extrahepatic diseases, conditions, and preanalytic factors to take into consideration when interpreting abnormal synthetic functional parameters. All conditions listed cause decreases in functional parameters, with the exception of total bilirubin, which elevates.

BUN
- Overhydration
- SIADH
- Any disease causing PU/PD

Albumin
- PLE, especially if panhypoproteinaemia (↓ globulins, cholesterol)
- PLN as long as no concurrent ↓ in globulins, cholesterol
- Haemorrhage, especially if concurrent anaemia
- Vasculitis
- Severe burns

Cholesterol
- PLE
- Severe malnutrition

Glucose
- Spurious (e.g. sample sitting prior to processing)
- Septicaemia
- Overdose of exogenous or endogenous insulin (i.e. insulinoma)
- Paraneoplastic (e.g. intestinal leiomyoma, leiomyosarcoma, hepatic and renal tumours)
- Glycogen storage disorders

Total bilirubin
- Haemolysis
- ↑ CK
- Septicaemia
- Cytauxzoonosis
- FIP

BUN, blood urea nitrogen; CK, creatine kinase; FIP, feline infectious peritonitis; PLE, protein-losing enteropathy; PLN, protein-losing nephropathy; PU/PD, polyuria and polydipsia; SIADH, syndrome of inappropriate antidiuretic hormone secretion.

While coagulopathies are well described in dogs with PSS, the literature on feline PSS is sparse and disturbances in haemostasis in these populations remain poorly understood. In one of the few studies evaluating coagulation abnormalities in cats with intra- and extrahepatic PSS, up to 88% and 69% of cats had prolongations in PT and aPTT, respectively.[9] In contrast to what has been documented in cats with EHBDO, none of these cats developed significant intraoperative bleeding requiring blood products during surgical correction of their PSS. Vitamin K–responsive coagulopathy has been reported in two cats diagnosed with EPI,[26] but this is an uncommon sequela in cats with this condition.

There is very little literature documenting altered coagulability in cats with hepatic disease. One report has documented portal vein thrombosis in six cats with hepatobiliary disease.[27] All cats had either FHL, cholangitis, or hepatic neoplasia, and 50% of these cats had a PSS identified. A pilot study evaluating 18 cats with cholestatic disease identified nearly half of these cats to be hypercoagulable and only approximately one-quarter as hypocoagulable based on thromboelastography.[28] Similarly to previous literature on FHL, lipidotic cats in this study were more likely to be hypocoagulable and have greater increases in ALP activity. While larger studies are necessary to better characterise altered coagulability in feline hepatobiliary disorders, clinicians should know that both exaggerated and diminished coagulation are possible.

It is important to note that while most cats do not exhibit spontaneous bleeding, those with significant hepatobiliary disease often have prolonged bleeding following routine venepuncture or placement of an intravenous catheter. Also, cats with FHL are more prone to bleed following fine needle aspiration of the liver or gallbladder despite a normal platelet count, PT, aPTT, and hepatic synthetic functional parameters. Clinicians should be aware that normal clotting times do not exclude the possibility of significant haemorrhage. Thus, cats should be supplemented with vitamin K periprocedurally, and blood products should be available during the procedure.

Glucose

Glucose is produced (via gluconeogenesis) and stored in the liver in the form of glycogen. Because glucose is essential for normal function of vital organs (i.e. brain, heart, kidneys), the functional capacity of the liver is very high, and serum glucose concentration is the last of the hepatic synthetic parameters to decrease. A loss of at least 75% of liver function is necessary for hypoglycaemia to result solely from liver failure.[10] There is a lack of literature specifically evaluating feline hepatic dysfunction, and much of what we know has been extrapolated from dogs. As with dogs, hypoglycaemia in the absence of other decreased synthetic functional parameters should raise suspicion for an extrahepatic process leading to a low blood glucose concentration (e.g. spurious hypoglycaemia due to delayed analysis, insulin overdose, septicaemia).

Other biochemical parameters and diagnostics of importance

Depending on the magnitude of the increase and concurrent pattern of liver enzyme increases, hyperglobulinaemia should prompt the clinician to consider ascending bacterial cholangitis, other infectious aetiologies (e.g. feline infectious peritonitis, toxoplasmosis, fungal disease—histoplasmosis), and/or neoplasia as top differential diagnoses. As many cats with neutrophilic cholangitis and pancreatitis are believed to also have a chronic enteropathy (i.e. triaditis) contributing to inflammation and ascending infection,[15] testing to rule in or rule out intestinal disease is warranted in cats with either chronic or waxing and waning hepatopathies. These diagnostics include, but are not limited to, the measurement of serum concentrations of cobalamin (vitamin B_{12}), folate, feline trypsin-like immunoreactivity (fTLI), and feline pancreatic lipase immunoreactivity (fPLI), also referred to as a GI panel, as well as a dietary trial. Decreases in either cobalamin and/or folate are supportive of a small intestinal malabsorptive process. A blood sample for a GI panel should be collected after withholding food for 8–12 hours. However, a shorter period of withholding food is acceptable for diabetic patients.

Lipidotic cats usually lack both hyperglobulinaemia and significant increases in GGT activity (as mentioned in section "Cholestatic hepatopathy" of this chapter), unless the lipidosis is secondary to an underlying inflammatory process of the biliary tract. Hypokalaemia is frequently seen with both primary or secondary FHL and is associated with a worse prognosis.[7] Cats with FHL are also often hyperglycaemic, and it is imperative that the clinician distinguishes diabetes mellitus (DM) from transient increases in blood glucose given that uncontrolled DM can cause FHL.[7] Because glycosuria is often not sufficient to differentiate between stress hyperglycaemia and DM in cats, serum fructosamine is a useful diagnostic marker to differentiate between the two. See Chapter 27 for further discussion of FHL.

For cats with pancreatitis, careful attention should be given to abnormalities such as hyperglycaemia, hyperbilirubinaemia, hypoalbuminaemia, ionised hypocalcaemia, and/or concurrent DM and azotaemia (prerenal and, less commonly, renal).[4,21,29] These findings suggest advanced severity of disease or comorbidities that warrant a more aggressive therapeutic approach and might carry a more guarded prognosis. Hyperglycaemia and hyperbilirubinaemia are commonly observed in cats with severe pancreatitis, likely because this disease causes both insulin resistance and cholestasis. These parameters should be vigilantly monitored, along with potential electrolyte derangements.[30] It is not uncommon for cats with pancreatitis to require electrolyte supplementation. Although decreases in serum total calcium concentrations can occur secondary to hypoalbuminaemia, ionised calcium should be assessed in any cat with total hypocalcaemia. The presence of ionised hypocalcaemia should alert the clinician to the possibility of a necrotising process requiring aggressive therapy.[29,31] See Chapter 24 for further discussion of feline pancreatitis.

TOTAL BILIRUBIN

Quantification of total bilirubin in the bloodstream is the end result of the degradation of haemoglobin from senescent erythrocytes, transport of conjugated bilirubin through the liver, and excretion of total bilirubin as a component of bile. Thus, any process leading to excessive haemolysis and/or disruption to the normal flow of bile will result in hyperbilirubinaemia.

Differential diagnoses for hyperbilirubinaemia can be classified into three distinct categories depending on the underlying pathophysiological process: prehepatic (i.e. haemolysis), primary hepatic (i.e. any process causing intrahepatic cholestasis), and posthepatic (i.e. any process causing posthepatic cholestasis or biliary obstruction). Figure 4.3 provides an algorithm of differential diagnoses for hyperbilirubinaemia. When faced with hyperbilirubinaemia, the clinician must first eliminate haemolysis as a cause or contributing factor before considering hepatic or posthepatic aetiologies. Haemolysis can often either be ruled in or out based on the presence of a concurrent, often regenerative, anaemia with normal total solids. Since an acute haemolytic process will lack an accompanying reticulocytosis, it is important to not exclude haemolysis based solely on absence of regeneration. The presence of spherocytes might point towards an immune-mediated aetiology for haemolysis, though spherocytes are seen much more commonly in dogs than in cats. Once a haemolytic aetiology has been confidently excluded, the severity of hyperbilirubinaemia is neither sensitive nor specific for further differentiating between diseases of the liver, biliary tract, or exocrine pancreas. Therefore, the clinician must use a combination of concurrent clinicopathologic and often ultrasonographic abnormalities to further localise the primary disease process.

The most common hepatobiliary diseases causing disruptions in bilirubin transport in the cat are cholangitis, FHL, and EHBDO. While cats with cholangitis might lack a true hepatopathy, up to 66% of them display hyperbilirubinaemia.[1] However, total bilirubin can range from being completely normal to, more commonly, moderately to markedly increased in cats with primary or secondary

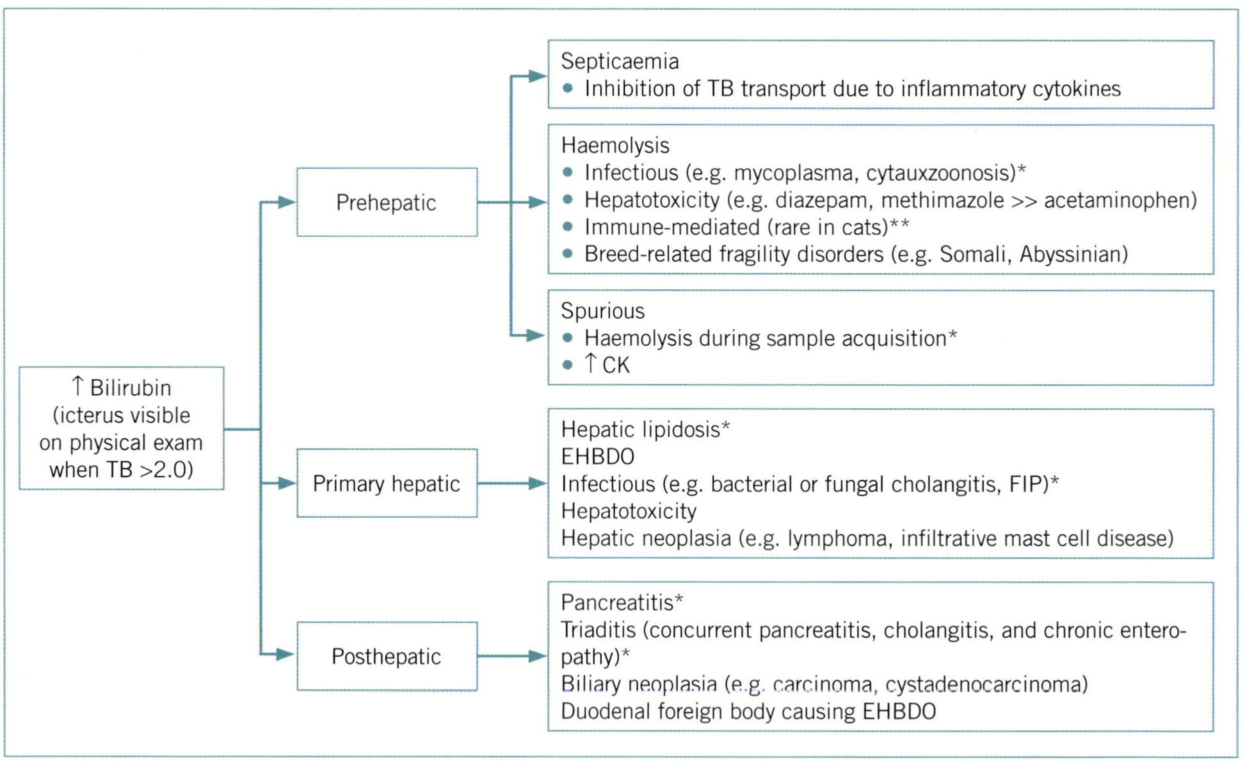

Figure 4.3. Flow chart illustrating an appropriate algorithm for causes of hyperbilirubinaemia in the cat. A single asterisk (*) indicates commonly seen aetiologies. A double asterisk (**) denotes that immune-mediated diseases are difficult to identify in cats, as their erythrocytes lack the central pallor of dogs, making spherocytes much harder to detect. Posthepatic causes are often accompanied by a cholestatic hepatopathy, leading to increases in alkaline phosphatase (ALP) or gamma-glutamyltransferase (GGT) activities and/or cholesterol concentrations. CK, creatine kinase; EHBDO, extrahepatic bile duct obstruction; FIP, feline infectious peritonitis; TB, total bilirubin.

FHL.[7] Up to 95% of lipidotic cats reported in the veterinary literature were hyperbilirubinaemic at presentation,[6] which makes FHL one of the most important rule-outs for increases in total bilirubin in a cat. Most cases of hyperbilirubinaemia that are due to primary hepatobiliary or pancreatic disease will also be associated with a hepatopathy. Cats with hepatotoxicity will usually have accompanying increases in hepatocellular enzymes,[10] while those with cholestasis usually also display elevated ALP and GGT activities and/or cholesterol concentrations.

A variety of diseases can also cause hyperbilirubinaemia in the absence of hepatobiliary disease, most notably feline cytauxzoonosis or septicaemia. Septic patients can develop hyperbilirubinaemia in the absence of hepatobiliary disease because inflammatory cytokines can inhibit the expression of bilirubin transporters in the liver. Hepatic vascular anomalies do not typically alter serum bilirubin concentrations unless there is a concurrent active cholestatic or hepatotoxic process.

Because bilirubin can become irreversibly bound to albumin during transport in the liver, increases in total bilirubin commonly persist for longer periods even if the inciting cause has already resolved. This is why the disappearance of clinically detectable icterus often lags improvement in clinical signs and laboratory abnormalities.

URINALYSIS

Abnormalities that can be observed on the urinalysis of cats with pancreatic or hepatobiliary disease include bilirubinuria, ammonium biurate crystalluria, and alterations in urine specific gravity. Urine specific gravity can reflect either overly concentrated urine (indicating dehydration) or reduced urine concentrating ability (if synthetic hepatic function is compromised resulting in low BUN followed by medullary washout). Because cats have a much higher renal threshold for bilirubin than dogs and do not have renal tubules that actively excrete bilirubin, any amount of bilirubinuria is significant in the cat and warrants investigation. See section "Hepatic synthetic function parameters and specific testing" in this chapter for more details on hyperbilirubinaemia. Although PSS is less commonly reported in cats, 15%–42% of confirmed cases have been identified to have ammonium biurate crystalluria.[32–34] Figure 4.4 shows urate crystals from a cat. Cats with FHL have been reported to have lipiduria, which can be seen as refractile fat globules on urine sediment examination;[6] however, this only occurs uncommonly.

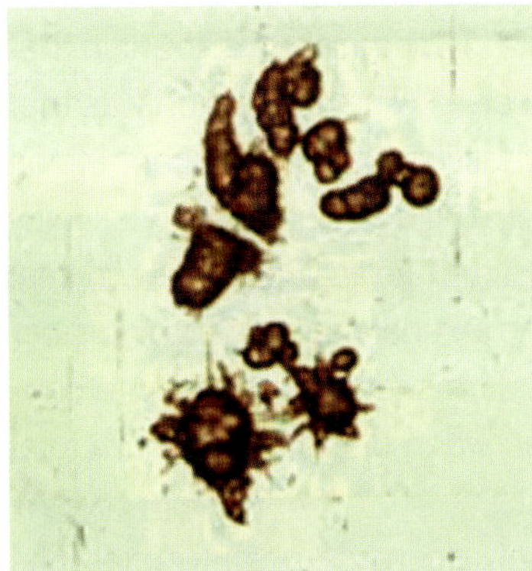

Figure 4.4. Ammonium urate crystals recovered from the urine sediment of a cat with hepatic dysfunction. Image courtesy of Dr Joe Bartges, University of Georgia, USA.

ADDITIONAL TESTS OF HEPATIC FUNCTION

Serum total bile acid concentration

BAs, with cholic acid being the predominant primary BA in both the cat and dog, are synthesised from cholesterol in the liver, excreted in the bile, and reabsorbed in the ileum. Normal hepatic perfusion, biliary flow, and a healthy ileum are all requirements for normal BA homoeostasis. Because measurable concentrations of BAs are altered to variable degrees during hepatic dysfunction, they are often measured in cases where dysfunction is suspected based on clinical signs and biochemistry results. An example of this would be decreases in synthetic functional parameters in which extrahepatic diseases have already been ruled out as contributing factors.

It is important to note that conditions other than liver failure can also cause increases in total BAs, namely vascular anomalies (i.e. PSS or PPVH), hepatic parenchymal diseases, or disorders leading to cholestasis.[35] BAs are felt to be particularly helpful in screening for vascular anomalies, such as PSS, with high sensitivity (>90%) for an increased postprandial BA in both cats and dogs. Limited studies have looked at the utility of fasted and 2-hour postprandial BAs specifically for the diagnosis of PSS in cats.[35,36] One study found that a lower cutoff threshold for fasting BAs in the cat (34 µmol/l) compared to that which is used for the dog (58 µmol/l) resulted in zero false-negative results for diagnosis of a shunt in that particular population of cats.[36] The conclusion was that cats with PSS had lower fasting total BA concentrations compared to what is commonly seen in dogs. These findings would suggest that using cutoff values for serum total BAs for dogs would lead to an unacceptably high number of false-negative results. This should be taken into consideration by the clinician when interpreting serum total BA concentrations in cats.

Factors that can falsely decrease postprandial BAs are ileal resection, as this reduces normal reabsorption of BAs, haemolysis, and feeding a meal that is deficient in fat or protein. Fat and protein reaching the small intestinal lumen are two factors that initiate gallbladder contraction under the hormonal influence of cholecystokinin. False increases in BAs can occur if the sample is lipaemic or the patient is already hyperbilirubinaemic. Intestinal disease and alterations in GI motility can both falsely increase or decrease BAs, and results in cats with these conditions should be interpreted with caution. A preprandial, fasted measurement exceeding that of the postprandial sample can occur due to spontaneous gallbladder contraction and should not be misinterpreted as liver dysfunction. Patients that have undergone cholecystectomy or ileal resection might have altered BA results independent of hepatic dysfunction. These limitations must be considered when interpreting results from cats with these demographics.

Urine BAs have been studied in cats given that they can be measured minimally invasively and might provide a sensitive and specific test for hepatic dysfunction. One study evaluated the utility of urine BAs (both sulphated and nonsulphated) for differentiating cats with hepatobiliary disease from those with nonhepatobiliary systemic illness and healthy controls.[37] Unfortunately, study limitations were that some cats were already hyperbilirubinaemic and not all cats had routine assessment of serum BAs. In addition, at the moment, the measurement of urine BAs is not routinely offered by a commercial laboratory. Therefore, urine BAs are not currently recommended for assessment of hepatic dysfunction in cats.

Plasma ammonia

Ammonia is produced by microbes in the GI tract from the breakdown of nitrogenous compounds, is carried via the portal circulation to the liver, and then metabolised as urea nitrogenous waste in the urea cycle. This nitrogenous waste can then be excreted by the kidneys. In cases of hepatic dysfunction or PSS, ammonia is no longer efficiently converted to urea and the end result is hyperammonaemia in the bloodstream. That being said, because the liver has a high reserve capacity for ammonia breakdown, significant function must be lost before clinical evidence of hyperammonaemia is apparent. Therefore, ammonia is a less sensitive indicator of early hepatic dysfunction in comparison to serum BA concentrations. The most useful reasons for assessing ammonia would be if the patient is hyperbilirubinaemic and serum BAs cannot reliably be interpreted or if the clinician is suspicious of hepatic encephalopathy (HE) or a PSS, as both dogs and cats with PSS often have elevated plasma ammonia concentrations. Chapter 28 discusses feline HE in more detail.

Because ammonia is extremely labile, the blood needs to be placed into a chilled EDTA tube and the tube must be placed on ice and then analysed within 30 minutes of collection. Failure to do so might result in false increases.[38] Haemolysis also falsely increases ammonia concentrations due to the release of ammonia from erythrocytes.[38] While such studies were only performed in dogs, it is reasonable to extrapolate this to cats, as studies refuting these findings have not been performed.

Controlled studies investigating the utility of ammonia for diagnosis of hepatobiliary disease in cats are limited. The same study evaluating serum BAs for the diagnosis of PSS in cats also investigated fasted plasma ammonia concentrations. This study concluded that hyperammonaemia is less specific for the diagnosis of PSS in cats when the same cutoff established for dogs is used,[36] failing to exclude a shunt in unaffected cats. In other words, cats without a PSS had higher plasma ammonia concentrations compared to dogs; therefore, a higher cutoff value signifying a "positive" result should be used in cats being screened for PSS disease to reduce false-positive results. One possible reason for this species-specific difference maybe that cats tend to develop arginine deficiency, which can result in falsely elevated ammonia concentrations, whereas dogs do not. The prevalence of vascular anomalies is also significantly higher in dogs than in cats, which might impede the establishment of a valid cutoff value for the diagnosis of PSS in cats.

An ammonia tolerance test refers to a diagnostic procedure that can be performed if an initial plasma ammonia concentration is within the RI but hepatic dysfunction is still being suspected. The premise behind an ammonia tolerance test is to administer ammonia rectally via a red rubber catheter and then quantify the ammonia in blood after a set amount of time. Ammonia is quantified at baseline, 20 minutes, and 40 minutes after administration. Patients with normal hepatic function should have results within the RI for all three time points, whereas those with hepatic dysfunction will have elevated plasma ammonia concentrations at the two time points after ammonia challenge. Because the ammonia tolerance test is contraindicated for patients with HE, and clinical signs of HE are not always clinically apparent, this test is no longer considered appropriate in the United States of America but is still used in parts of Europe.

ASSAYS FOR ASSESSMENT OF EXOCRINE PANCREATIC FUNCTION AND DISEASE

Pancreatitis, both acute and chronic, and EPI are the most commonly encountered exocrine pancreatic diseases seen in the cat. Both types of disease can present with a wide array of clinical signs and clinicopathologic changes. Because of this, measurement of pancreatic-specific enzymes is nearly always a crucial part of the diagnostic puzzle required in order to obtain a definitive diagnosis (Fig. 4.2). When interpreting any pancreatic enzyme assay, it is important to consider how specific the assay is for detecting enzymes of strictly pancreatic origin. The measurement of serum amylase and lipase activity is not helpful in establishing a diagnosis because these assays lack both sensitivity and specificity for pancreatitis in cats.[4,39] The poor performance of these assays is likely due to a lack of a substrate that is specific for pancreatic lipase, leading to other lipases as well as other molecules being detected by these tests. This results in an unacceptably high number of false-positive results.

For these reasons, it was necessary that tests be developed that would only quantify pancreatic lipases and not measure lipases released from other organs. The premise behind measuring fPLI specifically is that this enzyme is only released following direct damage to pancreatic acini, improving both sensitivity and specificity for detection of pancreatic inflammation.

Conversely, cats with EPI lack certain enzymes, and documentation of low to often undetectable concentrations of trypsinogen is necessary in order to reach a definitive diagnosis. Analytically validated assays for the measurement of fPLI (as measured by Spec fPL) and fTLI are commercially available and considered to be the gold standard for diagnosis of pancreatitis and EPI in cats, respectively. These tests are discussed briefly below but are reviewed more comprehensively in Chapters 24 and 25.

Feline pancreatic lipase immunoreactivity

Several studies have reported the sensitivity and specificity of fPLI measured by Spec fPL for the diagnosis of feline pancreatitis. An in-clinic, patient-side assay known as the SNAP fPL was created to provide clinicians with a rapid means of ruling out pancreatitis prior to submission of a Spec fPL or pursuing diagnostic imaging. The Spec fPL is currently considered the best serum test available to aid in a definitive diagnosis.[39]

As mentioned above, the SNAP fPL is a patient-side modification of the Spec fPL. It has been shown to have good agreement with the Spec fPL based on both published clinical studies[30] and unpublished data acquired from the manufacturer.[40] Agreement reported by the manufacturer shows 89%–100% agreement between assays depending on whether the results are within the RI or whether they are abnormal.[40] The current recommended use for the SNAP fPL is to rule out pancreatitis if the result is normal, not to definitively diagnose it. Because the sensitivity of this test is so high, false-negative results are extremely unlikely. While a positive result indicates that there is an increased amount of pancreatic-specific lipase in circulation, increases in this enzyme may not be due to primary pancreatitis, as they can also be caused by secondary pancreatic inflammation or pancreatic hypoxia (e.g. acute kidney injury, severe gastroenteritis, intestinal foreign body), especially in cats with results in the "grey zone". Therefore, the authors recommend this test be used to screen cats in which pancreatitis is a likely differential diagnosis. If the test is negative, pancreatitis can most likely be ruled out. If the test is positive, submitting a quantitative Spec fPL is recommended.

Although the Spec fPL is the best serum test currently available to help diagnose pancreatitis in cats, it is not a perfect test and should not be used in isolation to reach a definitive diagnosis, as both false-positive and false-negative results are possible. The clinician must always consider clinical signs, clinicopathologic findings, and diagnostic imaging findings in conjunction with a serum fPLI concentration in order to reach a diagnosis of pancreatitis. Data is lacking to confidently conclude if the degree of Spec fPL increase is useful for prognosticating outcome, but it has been used for monitoring disease progression and recovery.[41]

Other lipase assays

Over the last few years, two other lipase tests, the triolein substrate–based v-LIP-P slide and the 1,2-o-dilauryl-rac-glycero-3-glutaric acid-(6'-methylresorufin) ester (DGGR) assay, have received considerable attention for the diagnosis of feline pancreatitis.

Multiple studies have looked at agreement of the DGGR lipase assay with the Spec fPL for diagnosis of feline pancreatitis and found good agreement between the tests in one study,[42] despite limited to poor agreement of both tests with pancreatic histology in another.[43] However, such correlation studies are insufficient to conclude that these tests can be used interchangeably. Instead, various studies in humans, dogs, and cats have shown that DGGR is not specific for the measurement of pancreatic lipase and also can serve as a substrate for other lipases, such as hepatic or lipoprotein lipase, pancreatic lipase-related protein 2, and even esterases. It should be noted that measurement of serum lipase activity in people is not considered as a definitive diagnostic test for pancreatitis but merely used to suggest further workup regarding the possibility of pancreatitis.

Feline trypsin-like immunoreactivity

The fTLI is the diagnostic test of choice for diagnosing feline EPI. A serum concentration of fTLI less than 8.0 µg/l

Table 4.3. Indications for and limitations of tests used to assess for hepatic dysfunction and species-specific pancreatic enzymes.

Test	Indications	Limitations
BAs	Strong suspicion of vascular anomaly (PSS) Concern for hepatic dysfunction in absence of hyperbilirubinaemia	False (+) if hyperbilirubinaemia or lipaemia present False (–) if fat or protein content of food fed between samples too low, or an inadequate amount is consumed Falsely decreased postprandial BAs with severe ileal disease or ileal resection
Ammonia	Suspicion of hepatic encephalopathy Suspicion of hepatic dysfunction but hyperbilirubinaemia precludes BA measurement BAs not elevated but still suspect hepatic dysfunction	Labile, must be put on ice immediately and processed within 30 minutes of collection Can be elevated from high-protein meal, gastrointestinal bleeding, haemolysis, excess exercise, urea cycle deficiencies (e.g. arginine deficiency in the cat) Ideally, sample should be fasted
Total lipase (DGGR, triolein based)	Evaluation of total lipase is not recommended to rule in or out pancreatitis	Not specific for pancreatic lipases (detects lipases of gastric and intestinal origin) False (+) for triolein-based assay with haemolysis, lipaemia, icterus Not recommended for ruling in or out pancreatitis Further studies required to establish appropriate cutoff values for DGGR-based assays in cats
SNAP fPL	To rule out pancreatitis (if SNAP [–]) in patients with clinical signs	Not a stand-alone test for diagnosis of pancreatitis Must be followed up by Spec fPL if "grey zone" or strong (+)
Spec fPL	To quantify species-specific lipase in cats suspicious of pancreatitis that are SNAP (+)	Some abdominal and systemic conditions are associated with acinar cell damage, which may lead to increases in serum fPLI concentrations
fTLI	To definitively diagnose or rule out EPI	Not useful for diagnosing or ruling out pancreatitis Not specific for pancreatitis if elevated (increases in fTLI with feline chronic enteropathy) "Grey zone" values might represent early EPI

BA, bile acid; DGGR, 1,2-o-dilauryl-rac-glycero-3-glutaric acid-(6'-methylresorufin) ester; EPI, exocrine pancreatic insufficiency; fPL, feline pancreatic lipase; fPLI, feline pancreatic lipase immunoreactivity; fTLI, feline trypsin-like immunoreactivity; PSS, portosystemic shunt.

is considered diagnostic for EPI, and many cats have serum fTLI concentrations well below this cutoff value.[44] It should also be noted that serum trypsin-like immunoreactivity (TLI) assays are exquisitely species-specific, and assays developed for use in other species (e.g. dogs, humans) cannot be used in cats.

Serial monitoring of the TLI following supplementation with pancreatic enzymes is of no value given that the fTLI only detects the feline enzyme and cats with EPI are supplemented with porcine or, rarely, bovine or game pancreas. For this reason, there is no benefit to monitoring serial fTLIs following diagnosis because the result is not expected to increase with supplementation therapy. The TLI has poor sensitivity and specificity for both acute and chronic pancreatitis and should only be used for the diagnosis of EPI.[5] Importantly, all cats diagnosed with EPI should also have serum cobalamin (vitamin B_{12}) concentration measured. Because successful cobalamin absorption (Fig. 4.5) relies on binding of cobalamin to intrinsic factor for absorption and the pancreas is the sole site of production of intrinsic factor in the cat, many cats with EPI require lifelong supplementation of vitamin B_{12}. While it is recommended that all animals with cobalamin concentrations below 400 ng/l be supplemented, this test is not an accurate reflection of total body tissue cobalamin. For this reason, cats with normal cobalamin concentrations might still have a total body deficiency of cobalamin, and supplementation is recommended if cats are experiencing clinical signs (i.e. weight loss and poor haircoat despite pancreatic enzyme replacement therapy) regardless of a normal serum cobalamin concentration.

Table 4.3 summarises the indications and limitations of tests for assessment of hepatic and exocrine pancreatic function.

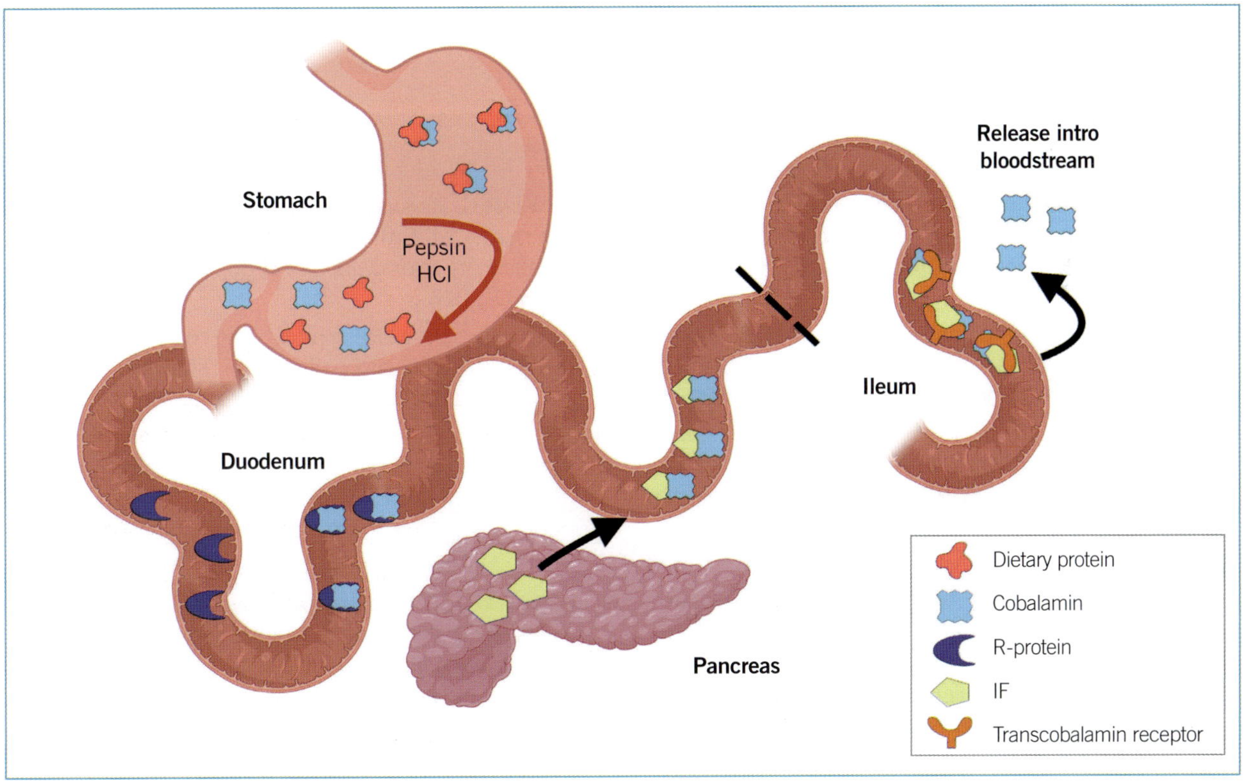

Figure 4.5. Diagram depicting the process of cobalamin absorption in the human gastrointestinal tract, which is similar to that in the cat. Cobalamin (vitamin B_{12}) is ingested tightly bound to dietary protein and subsequently liberated from said proteins in the stomach by pepsin and HCl. It is then complexed with R-protein, which is released by both salivary glands and gastric parietal cells, and transported to the duodenum. Pancreatic proteases cleave the R-protein in the proximal duodenum, after which cobalamin is free to complex with intrinsic factor (IF) secreted by the pancreas. The pancreas is the sole site of IF production in the cat, whereas the dog and human have extra-pancreatic production. Complexed cobalamin–IF then travels to the distal ileum, where it is absorbed via cobalamin receptors. Following absorption, cobalamin binds to transcobalamin II, which transports cobalamin to the liver and other tissues. Image courtesy of Travis Burdick (Gastrointestinal Laboratory, Texas A&M University, USA), created with BioRender.com.

Take-home messages

- Unlike dogs, cats lack a corticosteroid-induced isoenzyme of alkaline phosphatase (ALP). Thus, if an elevated serum/plasma ALP activity is identified in a feline patient, a primary hepatobiliary disease is likely.
- The half-lives of nearly all hepatic enzymes are shorter in cats than in dogs. This means that increases of even mild magnitude should not be ignored and necessitate a diagnostic workup with serial monitoring.
- ALP activity is elevated to a much greater magnitude than gamma-glutamyltransferase (GGT) activity in nearly all cats with primary hepatic lipidosis. If both GGT and ALP activities are elevated to the same magnitude, an underlying disease process of hepatic lipidosis is most likely.
- Species-specific cutoff values are necessary when interpreting serum bile acids and ammonia concentrations in cats, as they differ from those in dogs. Failure to do so will result in an unacceptable amount of false-positive and false-negative results when evaluating cats for possible portosystemic shunts or hepatic encephalopathy.
- Alterations in vitamin K–dependent clotting factors (with associated prolongations of prothrombin time and/or activated partial thromboplastin time) is the most common coagulopathy seen in cats with cholestatic hepatobiliary disease. These cats are at high risk for haemorrhage periprocedurally.
- Measurement of serum feline pancreatic lipase immunoreactivity (fPLI) is the most sensitive and specific diagnostic test currently available for the diagnosis of pancreatitis in cats.
- A negative SNAP fPL test can be used to exclude pancreatitis as a differential diagnosis. An abnormal (i.e. positive) result necessitates confirmation of the diagnosis by Spec fPL, which will also provide a baseline value for monitoring of disease progression.

REFERENCES

[1] Forman MA. Feline inflammatory/infectious hepatic disease. In: Ettinger SJ, Feldman EC, Côte E, editors. *Textbook of Veterinary Internal Medicine*, 8th ed. St Louis, Elsevier: 1633, 2017.

[2] Brain PH et al. Feline cholecystitis and acute neutrophilic cholangitis: clinical findings, bacterial isolates and response to treatment in six cases. *J Feline Med Surg* 8:91, 2006.

[3] Gagne JM et al. Clinical features of inflammatory liver disease in cats: 41 cases (1983–1993). *J Am Vet Med Assoc* 214:513, 1999.

[4] Hill RC, Van Winkle TJ. Acute necrotizing pancreatitis and acute suppurative pancreatitis in the cat. A retrospective study of 40 cases (1976–1989). *J Vet Intern Med* 7:25, 1993.

[5] Swift NC et al. Evaluation of serum feline trypsin-like immunoreactivity for the diagnosis of pancreatitis in cats. *J Am Vet Med Assoc* 217:37, 2000.

[6] Center SA. Feline hepatic lipidosis. *Vet Clin North Am Small Anim Pract* 35:225, 2005.

[7] Center SA et al. A retrospective study of 77 cats with severe hepatic lipidosis: 1975–1990. *J Vet Intern Med* 7:349, 1993.

[8] Weisse C, Berent AC. Hepatic vascular anomalies. In: Ettinger SJ, Feldman EC, Côte E, editors. *Textbook of Veterinary Internal Medicine*, 8th ed. St Louis, Elsevier: 1639, 2017.

[9] Tzounos CE et al. Haematology and coagulation profiles in cats with congenital portosystemic shunts. *J Feline Med Surg* 19:1290, 2017.

[10] Chapman SE, Hostutler RA. A laboratory diagnostic approach to hepatobiliary disease in small animals. *Clin Lab Med* 35:503, 2015.

[11] Christopher MM, Lee SE. Red cell morphologic alterations in cats with hepatic disease. *Vet Clin Pathol* 23:7, 1994.

[12] Lisciandro SC, Hohenhaus A, Brooks M. Coagulation abnormalities in 22 cats with naturally occurring liver disease. *J Vet Intern Med* 12:71, 1998.

[13] Center SA. Interpretation of liver enzymes. *Vet Clin North Am Small Anim Pract* 37:297, 2007.

[14] Zinkl JG et al. Comparative studies on plasma and tissue sorbitol, glutamic, lactic and hydroxybutyric dehydrogenase and transaminase activities in the dog. *Res Vet Sci* 12:211, 1971.

[15] Callahan Clark JE et al. Feline cholangitis: a necropsy study of 44 cats (1986–2008). *J Feline Med Surg* 13:570, 2011.

[16] Hurwitz BM et al. Presumed primary and secondary hepatic copper accumulation in cats. *J Am Vet Med Assoc* 244:68, 2014.

[17] Center SA et al. Fulminant hepatic failure associated with oral administration of diazepam in 11 cats. *J Am Vet Med Assoc* 209:618, 1996.

[18] Peterson ME, Kintzer PP, Hurvitz AI. Methimazole treatment of 262 cats with hyperthyroidism. *J Vet Intern Med* 2:150, 1988.

[19] Center SA et al. Diagnostic value of serum gamma-glutamyl transferase and alkaline phosphatase activities in hepatobiliary disease in the cat. *J Am Vet Med Assoc* 188:507, 1986.

[20] Fahie MA, Martin RA. Extrahepatic biliary tract obstruction: a retrospective study of 45 cases (1983–1993). *J Am Anim Hosp Assoc* 31:478, 1995.

[21] Ferreri JA et al. Clinical differentiation of acute necrotizing from chronic nonsuppurative pancreatitis in cats: 63 cases (1996–2001). *J Am Vet Med Assoc* 223:469, 2003.

[22] Hunt GB. Effect of breed on anatomy of portosystemic shunts resulting from congenital diseases in dogs and cats: a review of 242 cases. *Aust Vet J* 82:746, 2004.

[23] Havig M, Tobias KM. Outcome of ameroid constrictor occlusion of single congenital extrahepatic portosystemic shunts in cats: 12 cases (1993–2000). *J Am Vet Med Assoc* 220:337, 2002.

[24] Webster CR. Hemostatic disorders associated with hepatobiliary disease. *Vet Clin North Am Small Anim Pract* 47:601, 2017.

[25] Kavanagh C, Shaw S, Webster CR. Coagulation in hepatobiliary disease. *J Vet Emerg Crit Care (San Antonio)* 21:589, 2011.

[26] Perry LA et al. Exocrine pancreatic insufficiency with associated coagulopathy in a cat. *J Am Anim Hosp Assoc* 27:109, 1991.

[27] Rogers CL et al. Portal vein thrombosis in cats: 6 cases (2001–2006). *J Vet Intern Med* 22:282, 2008.

[28] Kakar N et al. Thromboelastography in cats with cholestatic liver disease. *J Feline Med Surg* 23:160, 2021.

[29] Kimmel SE, Washabau RJ, Drobatz KJ. Incidence and prognostic value of low plasma ionized calcium concentration in cats with acute pancreatitis: 46 cases (1996–1998). *J Am Vet Med Assoc* 219:1105, 2001.

[30] Schnauss F, Hanisch F, Burgener IA. Diagnosis of feline pancreatitis with SNAP fPL and Spec fPL. *J Feline Med Surg* 21:700, 2019.

[31] Dias C, Carreira LM. Serum ionised calcium as a prognostic risk factor in the clinical course of pancreatitis in cats. *J Feline Med Surg* 17:984, 2015.

[32] Center SA, Magne ML. Historical, physical examination, and clinicopathologic features of portosystemic vascular anomalies in the dog and cat. *Semin Vet Med Surg Small Anim* 5:83, 1990.

[33] VanGundy TE, Boothe HW, Wolf A. Results of surgical management of feline portosystemic shunts. *J Am Anim Hosp Assoc* 26:55, 1990.

[34] Dear JD et al. Feline urate urolithiasis: a retrospective study of 159 cases. *J Feline Med Surg* 13:725, 2011.

[35] Center SA, Erb HN, Joseph SA. Measurement of serum bile acids concentrations for diagnosis of hepatobiliary disease in cats. *J Am Vet Med Assoc* 207:1048, 1995.

[36] Ruland K, Fischer A, Hartmann K. Sensitivity and specificity of fasting ammonia and serum bile acids in the diagnosis of portosystemic shunts in dogs and cats. *Vet Clin Pathol* 39:57, 2010.

[37] Trainor D et al. Urine sulfated and nonsulfated bile acids as a diagnostic test for liver disease in cats. *J Vet Intern Med* 17:145, 2003.

[38] Hitt ME, Jones BD. Effects of storage temperature and time on canine plasma ammonia concentrations. *Am J Vet Res* 47:363, 1986.

[39] Xenoulis PG. Diagnosis of pancreatitis in dogs and cats. *J Small Anim Pract* 56:13, 2015.

[40] Xenoulis PG, Steiner JM. SNAP tests for pancreatitis in dogs and cats: SNAP canine pancreatic lipase and SNAP feline pancreatic lipase. *Top Companion Anim Med* 31:134, 2016.

[41] Stockhaus C et al. Serial serum feline pancreatic lipase immunoreactivity concentrations and prognostic variables in 33 cats with pancreatitis. *J Am Vet Med Assoc* 243:1713, 2013.

[42] Oppliger S et al. Agreement of the serum Spec fPL™ and 1,2-o-dilauryl-rac-glycero-3-glutaric acid-(6'-methylresorufin) ester lipase assay for the determination of serum lipase in cats with suspicion of pancreatitis. *J Vet Intern Med* 27:1077, 2013.

[43] Oppliger S et al. Comparison of serum Spec fPL™ and 1,2-o-dilauryl-rac-glycero-3-glutaric acid-(6'-methylresorufin) ester assay in 60 cats using standardized assessment of pancreatic histology. *J Vet Intern Med* 30:764, 2016.

[44] Xenoulis PG et al. Feline exocrine pancreatic insufficiency: a retrospective study of 150 cases. *J Vet Intern Med* 30:1790, 2016.

CHAPTER 5

Diagnostic imaging of the gastrointestinal tract

Pascaline Pey, Alessia Diana

Diagnostic imaging represents a crucial part of the diagnostic workup of gastrointestinal (GI) disorders in cats. The aim of diagnostic imaging is to localise the pathology within the GI tract, to identify its origin, to determine its extent, and to describe how it will affect GI motility. This information guides the clinician in choosing the next diagnostic step, such as ultrasound-guided fine needle aspiration (FNA), endoscopy-guided mucosal biopsy, or full-thickness surgical biopsy. The main advantage of diagnostic imaging is that it provides a general overview of the GI tract and adjacent organs and complements other modalities, such as endoscopy, that provide only endoluminal information. In this chapter, a detailed overview of the main diagnostic imaging modalities (ultrasound, contrast ultrasound, radiology, contrast study, and computed tomography [CT]) of the entire GI tract are presented. See Online Supplement 5.1 for detailed information on techniques, patient preparation, and preprocedural considerations.

Magnetic resonance imaging and scintigraphy are not discussed in this chapter, as, to date, there is no evidence of their utility or superiority when imaging the feline GI tract.

Online Supplement 5.1. Imaging of the gastrointestinal tract. Techniques, patient preparation, and preprocedural considerations.

NORMAL ANATOMY AND APPEARANCE OF THE GASTROINTESTINAL TRACT

Oral cavity and oropharynx

Radiography

Evaluation of dental and skull radiographs is complex and requires the reader to be familiar with the anatomy and interpretation paradigm. The dental formula of the adult cat is 2× (3/3I, 1/1C, 3/2P, 1/1M). The use of the modified Triadan dental numbering system should be preferred to describe a tooth or a lesion referring to a tooth.

As the quality of the study dramatically affects the interpretation, perfect positioning of the patient is fundamental. The teeth are anchored in alveoli within the mandible or maxilla. The root is embedded in bone, whereas the crown is within the oral cavity. Radiopaque components of the tooth include the dentin, enamel, and lamina dura that surround each tooth root. Soft tissue structures of the tooth include the pulp cavity and periodontal membrane. The pharynx corresponds to the space located between the base of the tongue and the retropharyngeal wall. It is composed of the nasopharynx and oropharynx, and the soft palate separates them. A laterolateral projection of the pharynx provides important information on the presence or absence of a space-occupying lesion that would create a mass effect on adjacent structures. The soft palate should be seen as a thin, smoothly outlined soft tissue band running horizontal and extending from the hard palate to the level of the epiglottis. Dorsally to the soft palate, the nasopharynx can be seen as an air-filled space, which should be completely radiolucent from the nasopharyngeal meatus to the pharyngeal sphincter. The presence of an endotracheal tube may alter the position of the soft palate and reduce the lumen of the nasopharynx. Any displacement of the soft palate, reduction of the lumen of the nasopharynx, or thickening of the soft palate should be interpreted as pathological.

Contrast radiography

An oropharyngeal contrast study involves taking a series of radiographs during a swallow and after the swallow is completed. The normal appearance of the oropharyngeal region after a swallow of contrast medium (CM) shows coating of the mucosa. A small amount of CM may occasionally remain in the cervical oesophageal lumen. No CM should be seen or persist in the piriform recesses, nasopharynx, larynx, or trachea. A dynamic study with fluoroscopy should be preferred when available and is indicated to explore functional abnormalities, although pharyngeal and oesophageal dysmotility are rare in cats.[6] As in dogs, the swallowing process in cats is composed of three phases: oropharyngeal, oesophageal, and gastrooesophageal. The oropharyngeal phase is characterised by food prehension and bolus formation (oral stage), reflex pharyngeal peristalsis (pharyngeal stage), and reflex upper oesophageal sphincter (UOS) relaxation (cricopharyngeal stage). Several quantitative parameters may be evaluated with a dedicated software. Quantitative assessment of the swallowing reflex (pharyngeal constriction ratio 0.17 ± 0.09; time to maximum pharyngeal contraction 0.13 ± 0.02 s; time to UOS opening 0.07 ± 0.02 s; time to UOS closed 0.23 ± 0.05 s; time to opening of the epiglottis 0.27 ± 0.04 s) is similar to the quantitative swallowing parameters previously reported in healthy dogs.[6]

Computed tomography

Thin-slice bone algorithm CT images offer excellent visualisation of the dental and periodontal tissues. Due to the shape of the teeth and their peculiar alignment, the use of multiplanar reformatted images along the axis of the maxilla or mandible is essential. Increasing the window width (7000–10000) of the standard bone window improves visualisation of dental tissues such as the pulp cavity, dentine layer, enamel layer of the crown, periodontal ligament surrounding the tooth root apex, hyperdense lamina dura, and the alveolar crest demarcating the top of the alveolar socket. Prognathism is frequently observed in brachycephalic cats.

CT allows a 3D visualisation of the pharynx removing all the composite images due to superimposition and border effacement between fluid and soft tissue structures. All the adjacent structures that may lead to oropharyngeal diseases can be observed, including the tongue, soft palate, auditory (Eustachian) tube, larynx, tonsils, thyroid, salivary glands, and regional lymph nodes. Any asymmetry, convex margins, bulging, increased size, abnormal position, alterations in contours, or heterogeneous enhancement of one of the aforementioned structures should be carefully evaluated.

Ultrasonography

Ultrasonography may be used to evaluate the oropharynx and the glands of the cranial neck that may induce oropharyngeal diseases. The tongue is hyperechoic to the supporting musculature (mylohyoid and geniohyoid muscles). The mandibular salivary glands are easily observed caudal to the ramus of each mandible. They are well-defined, large, pyramidal in shape, and hypoechoic with a well-defined hyperechoic capsule and a central hyperechoic hilum. The parotid salivary glands appear as ill-defined, heterogeneous, and poorly marginated structures located laterally and caudally to the external ear canals. The entire larynx can also be imaged, but this is beyond the scope of this chapter. The medial retropharyngeal lymph nodes are located medially to the mandibular salivary glands and dorsally to the pharynx. They are fusiform in shape and measure $20.7 \times 12.4 \times 3.7$ mm in cats. The mandibular lymph nodes are located ventrally to the mandibular salivary glands and very superficial. There are generally two mandibular lymph nodes, one on each side of each linguofacial vein. Lymph nodes should be homogeneous and overall hypoechoic relative to adjacent tissue. Perinodal adipose tissue should be isoechoic relative to adipose tissue located in the neck.

Oesophagus

The oesophagus is a musculomembranous tubular organ extending from a cranial sphincter (upper, cricopharyngeal, or proximal) to a caudal sphincter (lower, cardiac, or distal). It is composed of four layers: the mucosa, a keratinised stratified squamous epithelium; the submucosa, composed of fibrous connective tissue, smooth muscle, and mucous glands (the glands are present solely in the cranial cervical half); the muscularis, which in cats is composed of striated muscle in the cranial two-thirds and exclusively of smooth muscle in the caudal third; and the outer adventitia. In its course, the distal oesophagus is narrowed at the level of the diaphragm and becomes progressively wider towards the cardia.

Radiography and contrast radiography

The oesophagus is located dorsally in the mediastinum, slightly to the left of the midline. It is rarely visible on survey radiographs. The caudal third may occasionally be visible on the left lateral projection as an ill-defined soft tissue band running dorsally and parallel to the caudal vena cava. A small amount of oesophageal air may be observed due to stress-related aerophagia. Normal survey thoracic radiographs do not preclude the presence of oesophageal diseases. Indirect signs of oesophageal disease, such as tracheal displacement, pneumomediastinum, tracheal stripe sign, or aspiration pneumonia, should be searched. The tracheal stripe sign corresponds to the border effacement of both the dorsal tracheal wall and the ventral wall of the oesophagus. It suggests the presence of oesophageal luminal gas. It should not be confused with pneumomediastinum.

Redundant oesophagus may be incidentally observed in cats with brachycephalic conformation, but it is usually not clinically relevant.

The muscular anatomy and conformation of the feline oesophagus give a very peculiar appearance following oral CM administration (see Fig. 5.2 in Online Supplement 5.1). As the muscularis is exclusively composed of smooth muscle in the caudal third, with the corresponding mucosa thrown into obliquely directed folds, a characteristic herringbone pattern is seen in the feline species on contrast radiography. This pattern may be observed from the cranial to the caudal mediastinum, as smooth muscular fibres are already present—although in a lesser number—in the muscularis layer from the cranial mediastinum. CM usually proceeds rapidly through the oesophagus. The oesophageal phase is characterised by primary peristalsis, initiated by the oropharyngeal phase, and secondary peristalsis, which occurs in response to mechanical stimulation by a food bolus in the oesophagus. A postperistaltic refractory period exists during which new peristalsis cannot occur. Repeated rapid swallowing can, therefore, result in accumulation of ingesta in the oesophagus. The gastrooesophageal phase occurs when a bolus passes through the gastrooesophageal junction, an area which functions as the lower oesophageal sphincter. Transit time is longer in cats compared to dogs.

Computed tomography

The four soft tissue layers of the oesophageal wall are not distinguishable on CT. In its cervical portion, the oesophagus runs dorsal and to the left of the trachea. It crosses over the tracheobronchial bifurcation dorsally and then remains in the midline until it reaches the diaphragm, with the aortic arch on its left. Its shape in cross section is variable: rounded to ovoid in the neck and cranial and middle mediastinum, and triangular in the caudal mediastinum. Its degree of gaseous distension is also variable, and this is mainly related to sedation or anaesthesia. An oesophageal probe may help identifying its position. Gas inflation may also be considered to visualise the intraluminal surface; sufficient gaseous distension should be employed to avoid mistaking smaller nodules for oesophageal folds.

Ultrasonography

The cervical oesophagus runs parallel to the trachea, but its position compared to the trachea varies depending on the swallowing phase. It is mainly located dorsal and to the left of the trachea. Gas and mucus pattern can be observed in the oesophageal lumen. The oesophageal wall displays a typical intestinal layering (see section "Duodenum, jejunum, and ileum" in this chapter). Five layers can be identified in normal caudal oesophageal and cardial walls. The inner oesophageal layer is echogenic, corresponding to the cornified mucosa and glandular portion of the submucosa. The cardia is characterised by a thick muscularis and a transitional zone between the echogenic oesophageal mucosal layer and the hypoechoic gastric mucosal layer (see Fig. 5.1a in Online Supplement 5.1).

Stomach, cardia, and pylorus

Ultrasonography and contrast-enhanced ultrasonography

The feline stomach is mainly located to the left of the midline, nearly parallel to the spine. In the near field, the stomach wall is thin, layered, and curvilinear. Rugal folds are identified as small invaginations of the wall into the lumen (see Fig. 5.1b in Online Supplement 5.1). Optimising the exam (i.e. performing a stress-free exam of the patient) is particularly important in cats, as they easily develop stress-related aerophagia. When a large amount of gas is present in the gastric lumen, acoustic shadowing and reverberation artefacts can obscure the view of deeper portions of the stomach. A fluid-filled stomach or sonolucent ingesta may allow evaluation of a larger portion of the deeper parts.

The ultrasonographic image of the stomach is characterised by concentric tissue layers which create a pattern of alternating hyperechoic and hypoechoic layers. The lumen may be represented by an anechoic layer if fluid filled. When empty, it displays an echogenic appearance due to the interface with the inner margins of the mucosa and the lumen content (admixture of gas and fluid). The mucosal layer is thick and hypoechoic, the submucosal layer is thin and hyperechoic, the muscularis layer is thin and hypoechoic, and the outer serosal surface is thin and hyperechoic.

The empty stomach in cats demonstrates a typical spoke-wheel, or wagon-wheel, pattern; the striated pattern is created by the rugal folds and crypts. It is more conspicuous in cats in good body condition due to a presumed higher amount of adipose tissue in the submucosa layer.

The pyloric antral region is located in the midline; this differs from dogs, in which the pylorus is located to the right of the midline. It corresponds to a progressive decrease of the lumen size. The stomach gently curves cranially from the gastric body to the pyloric antrum. The pyloric outflow tract leading into the duodenum is visualised as a transition from the muscular portion of the pylorus to the duodenum, which has the typical layered appearance of the small intestine.

Gastric peristalsis varies between four and six contractions per minute—a gastric contraction should be observed every 12 seconds. The normal ranges used to evaluate the gastric wall thickness are shown in Table 5.1. A 2 mm interrugal thickness and a 4.4 mm rugal fold thickness have also been reported. Normal reference ranges for the measurement of the lymph nodes draining the stomach are shown in Table 5.2.

The enhancement of the gastric wall during contrast-enhanced ultrasonography (CEUS) has not yet been reported. However, in the authors' experience, the gastric wall demonstrates an enhancement similar to that observed in the intestinal wall (see section "Duodenum, jejunum, and ileum" in this chapter for more details).

Radiography

The stomach is located caudal and slightly dorsal to the liver (see Fig. 5.3 in Online Supplement 5.1). The fundus and the body are located in the left cranial abdominal quadrant. In cats, the stomach demonstrates a "J" shape, and the pyloric antrum remains on the left side with the pylorus being superimposed to the midline and thoracolumbar spine (see Fig. 5.4 in Online Supplement 5.1). The gastric volume depends on the prandial phase of the cat. The stomach tends to empty faster in cats compared to dogs and hence to be smaller and to contain very little gas. Sometimes it can even be rather difficult to differentiate it from the liver. With stress, feline patients tend to accumulate gas in the GI tract due to aerophagia.

Table 5.1. Published wall thickness of the different gastrointestinal segments of the cat.

	Wall thickness (mm) Mean (range)						
	Gastric fundus	Gastric body	Pylorus	Duodenum	Jejunum	Ileum	Colon
Winter et al. 2014[9]	1.8 (1.6–2.0)	2.2 (1.9–2.6)	2.1 (1.7–2.7)	2.4 (2.2–2.7)	2.3 (2.0–2.5)	2.8 (2.3–3.2)	1.2 (1.1–1.3)
Di Donato et al. 2014[8]	—	—	—	2.78 (2.3–3.2)	2.36 (2–2.82)	3.01 (2.44–3.57)	—
Goggin et al. 2000[22]	2–4		—	2.2	2.2	2.8	1.5

Table 5.2. Width and length measurements of the abdominal lymph nodes draining the feline gastrointestinal tract obtained by ultrasonography and computed tomography.

Lymph node	Ultrasonography		Computed tomography	
	Width (mm) Mean (range)	Length (mm) Mean (range)	Width (mm) Mean (range)	Length (mm) Mean (range)
Hepatic	2.9 (2.5–3.6)	7.6 (5.9–9.5)	3 (1–7)	7 (2–23)
Splenic	3.2 (1.9–4.8)	8.4 (5.0–11.2)	3 (1–8)	5 (1–8)
Gastric	1.9 (1.9–1.9)	5.1 (4.6–6.4)	3 (1–5)	6 (2–19)
Pancreaticoduodenal	4.6 (3.6–6.2)	8.4 (6.6–13.0)	4 (2–8)	7 (2–14)
Jejunal	5.0 (2.8–7.2)	20.1 (11.4–39.0)	5 (2–10)	17 (3–48)
Ileocaecal	4.1 (2.7–4.8)	11.8 (6.7–23.2)	4 (4–7)	6 (2–13)
Colic	3.1 (1.9–5.2)	9.0 (4.6–12.1)	4 (2–8)	7 (2–20)
Caudal mesenteric	2.1 (2.1–2.1)	6.0 (6.0–6.0)	4 (1–10)	8 (1–20)

The gastric gas follows the nondependent portion of the gastric lumen according to the recumbency of the patient. In right lateral recumbency, the gas is located in the fundus and body; in left lateral recumbency, the gas is located in the pyloric antrum; in dorsal recumbency, the gas is located in the fundus; and in ventral recumbency, the gas is located in the pyloric antrum and body. The pattern of distribution of the gas within the gastric lumen can be used to localise lesions.

The gastric wall cannot be evaluated for its thickness on radiographs. The typical spoke-wheel pattern observed on ultrasound is also observed on radiographs, especially when fat accumulates in the gastric wall.[7] In geriatric cats, the gastric fundus is frequently observed sliding in the caudodorsal thorax, representing an intermittent paraoesophageal sliding hiatal hernia which is generally not clinically significant.

Contrast study

In cats, the stomach should immediately start emptying after CM administration, with a maximal delay of 15 minutes that may be attributable to stress. It should completely empty within 15–60 minutes, with a maximum upper limit of gastric emptying of 3 hours. Beyond 3 hours, it should be considered pathological. The interface between the CM and the gastric mucosa should be evaluated for its contours. The presence of filling defects should be evaluated. The thickness of the gastric wall can be assessed (3–5 mm) during contrast gastrography.

Computed tomography

A hydro-CT should be performed to allow sufficient distension of the stomach and good visualisation of the enhancing wall. A collapsed gastric wall may lead to mistakes in overlooking or overinterpreting disease. On CT, an intramural hypoattenuating layer is seen and corresponds to the fat deposition in the gastric submucosa. To date, there is no description in the literature regarding the normal aspect and enhancement of the gastric wall on CT. Normal reference ranges for the measurement of the lymph nodes draining the stomach are shown in Table 5.2.

Duodenum, jejunum, and ileum

Ultrasonography and contrast-enhanced ultrasonography

Generally, the small intestine should be assessed for uniformity in diameter, wall thickness, wall layering, luminal contents, and peristalsis. The ultrasonographic image of the small intestine is characterised by concentric tissue layers which create a pattern of alternating hyperechoic and hypoechoic layers (see Figs. 5.1c and 5.1d in Online Supplement 5.1). The lumen may be represented by an anechoic layer if fluid filled. When empty, it displays an echogenic appearance due to the interface with the inner margins of the mucosa and the lumen content (admixture of gas and fluid). In addition, reverberation artefacts and acoustic shadowing may also be observed depending on the nature of the lumen content. The mucosal layer is thick and hypoechoic, the submucosal layer is thin and hyperechoic, the muscularis layer is thin and hypoechoic, and the outer serosal surface is thin and hyperechoic.

A summary of the published reference values for the thickness of the intestine in cats is shown in Table 5.1.[8,9,22] The major duodenal papilla is also systematically observed in cats, and it measures 2.9–5.5 mm in thickness in transverse section (Figs. 5.5a and 5.5b). The distal portion of the common bile and pancreatic ducts ends at this level.

The thickness of the duodenum in cats, unlike in dogs, is similar to that of the jejunum. In these two segments, the mucosa is the thickest layer. The ileum is easy to distinguish from the duodenum and the jejunum, as it displays a prominent hyperechoic submucosal layer and a prominent hypoechoic muscularis layer (see Fig. 5.1e in Online Supplement 5.1). The ileum demonstrates a wagon-wheel appearance in transverse section. It is the thickest intestinal segment and has a sphincter-like role to avoid colic content moving back into the small intestine.

Mucosal indentations along the antimesenteric border may also be observed and correspond to Peyer's patches (Fig. 5.5c). To the eyes of the unexperienced sonographer, Peyer's patches can be misinterpreted as transmural lesions. Unlike in dogs, Peyer's patches are not identified in the duodenum of cats but only further in the jejunum and ileum.

Normal reference ranges for the measurement of the lymph nodes draining the small intestine are shown in Table 5.2.

Evaluation of the perfusion of the intestinal wall is possible with CEUS.[2] In normal cats, a rapid intense enhancement of the serosal and submucosal layers followed by gradual enhancement of the entire wall section during the early phase is observed. At peak enhancement, a loss of demarcation between the intestinal wall layers is seen. In the late phase, there is a gradual wash-

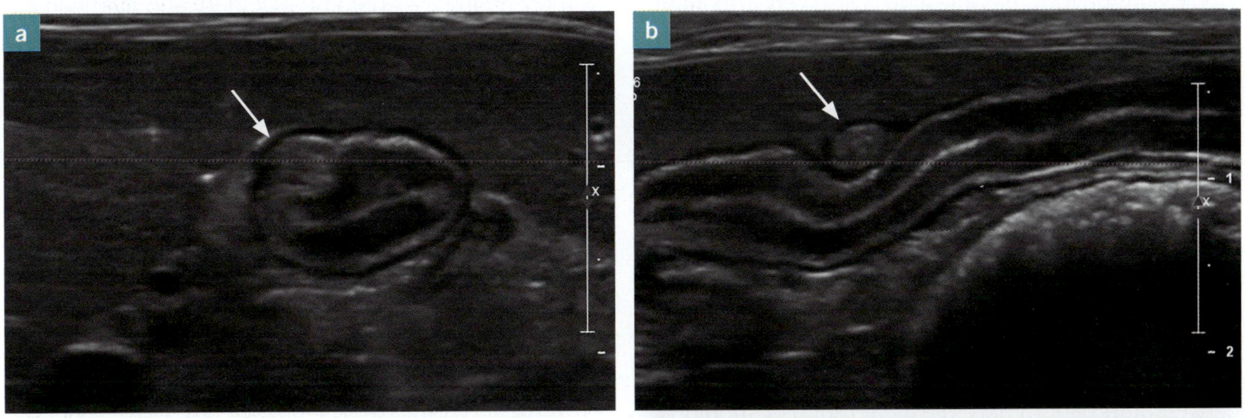

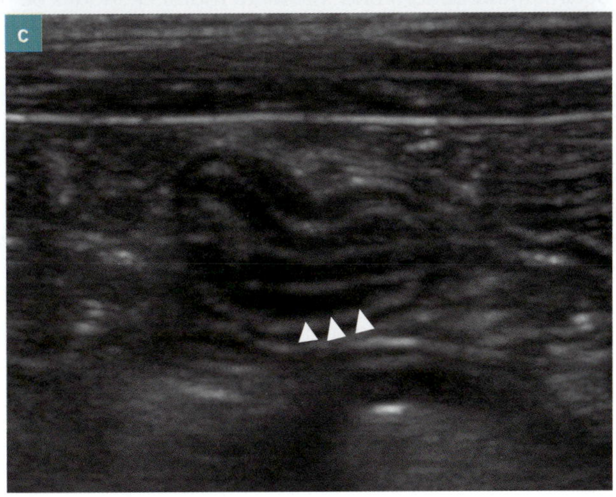

Figure 5.5. Ultrasonographic views of different segments of the feline intestine. Transverse (a) and longitudinal (b) sections of the proximal portion of the descending duodenum of an adult cat. The major duodenal papilla appears as an echogenic ring-like structure (arrow) on the transverse view and as an ovoidal structure on the longitudinal plane. Transverse section of a jejunal loop of a young cat (c). An asymmetrically positioned hypoechoic extra layer is evident within the deeper submucosal layer of the jejunal wall (arrowheads). This feature is histologically related to an asymmetrically positioned normal lymphatic tissue (Peyer's patch) in the lamina propria and submucosa.

out of signal from the intestinal wall with the submucosal washout occurring last. This is a characteristic radial enhancement pattern.[2]

Radiography

The small intestine is in the central portion of the abdomen and generally more on the right side, especially in cats with abundant mesenteric fat (see Figs. 5.4d and 5.4e in Online Supplement 5.1) The small intestine is extremely mobile, and its position can easily be modified by the increase in size of any other abdominal organ. The duodenum is the only portion of the small intestine with a fixed location that also makes it more recognisable. In cats, it is located immediately on the right side of the lumbar spine and midline. As for the stomach, the thickness of the intestinal wall cannot be assessed on survey radiographs, as intraluminal fluid may mimic parietal thickening. The small intestine generally contains a small amount of gas and liquid. The diameter of the small intestine in cats should not exceed 12 mm. Evaluating gas distribution inside the small intestine is also very important. Gas should have a tubular, smoothly outlined distribution without abrupt interruption. It is normal to observe a small variation in diameter and gas distribution, which are due to normal peristalsis. In cats, the normal peristalsis may demonstrate a characteristic string-of-pearls appearance (see Fig. 5.4d in Online Supplement 5.1).

Contrast radiography

An intestinal transit time longer than 3 hours should be considered pathological in cats. In addition, the interface between the barium and intestinal mucosa should be studied for the presence of a filling defect. The intestinal wall can also be evaluated for thickness. It should not be thicker than 1–2 mm and should be homogeneous. The characteristic string-of-pearls appearance may be observed, probably more frequently on contrast radiographs compared to survey radiographs (see Fig. 5.4e in Online Supplement 5.1). Prominent circular muscle contractions cause almost complete obliteration of the duodenal lumen during segmental peristalsis. A linear filling defect may also be seen in between the "pearls"; this is attributed to a longitudinal fold of mucosa in the incompletely distended intestine (so-called pseudostring sign) and should not be interpreted as a linear foreign body. Unlike in dogs, pseudoulcers are not identified in the duodenum in cats but only further in the jejunum and ileum.

Computed tomography

To date there is no study published on the normal CT appearance of the small intestine in cats. Therefore, there is no evidence of the superiority of CT over ultrasound for the evaluation of the GI tract in small animals, and this is particularly true in the feline species. In the authors' experience and opinion, ultrasound is far superior to CT for evaluating the GI tract in cats, either in case of diffuse GI disease or multifocal or focal lesions. Extrapolating the scarce published data from dogs, mucosal villi and intestinal wall layering cannot be observed on CT. The intestinal thickness can be evaluated on CT, and the reference values extrapolated from ultrasonography can be applied to CT interpretation. On postcontrast CT, the normal intestinal wall shows marked homogeneous contrast enhancement, with the mucosa and submucosa demonstrating a higher enhancement and attenuation.

Normal CT reference ranges for the measurement of the lymph nodes draining the small intestine are shown in Table 5.2.

Caecum and ileocaecocolic junction

Ultrasonography

The caecum is a blind diverticulum of the colon located at the transition between the colon and the ileum in the right hemiabdomen. It is divided in a proximal (close to the colon) and distal part (end of the cul-de-sac). Both proximal and distal parts of the caecum have distinct layering: the interface with the luminal content (hyperechoic line), a thick layer of multiple hypoechoic coalescent nodular areas, a thin hyperechoic band with scalloped borders, a thin hypoechoic layer, and a thin hyperechoic even layer (Fig. 5.6).[10] As the hypoechoic nodular inner layer corresponds on histology to the coalescence of multiple lymphoid follicles originating from the submucosa and protruding in the mucosa, hampering the distinction of the two layers, the combined mucosal and submucosal layers may be called the "follicular layer".[10] A recent study demonstrated that a subclinical mild caecal inflammation (detected on histopathology) can be seen in asymptomatic cats and would correspond on ultrasound to a slightly increased thickness of the follicular layer at the entrance of the caecum. An ultrasonographically normal caecum is characterised by a proximal follicular layer diameter of up to 2.0 mm.[10] The ileocaecocolic junction (ICCJ) is almost always visible in cats, unlike in dogs, because the caecum is rarely filled with gas which could hamper its recognition. Normal reference ranges for the dimensions of the lymph nodes draining the caecum and ICCJ are shown in Table 5.2.

Radiography

In cats, the caecum and ICCJ are generally not visible on radiographs. If the caecum contains gas or faecal material, it appears as a small comma-shaped structure on the right side of the central abdomen, at the height of L1–L3, on the ventrodorsal and dorsoventral views.

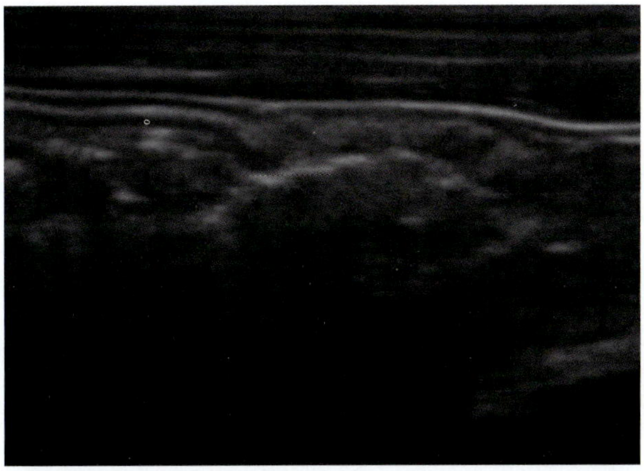

Figure 5.6. Longitudinal section of the caecum of an asymptomatic cat. Multiple hypoechoic coalescent nodules surrounded by a thin hyperechoic band with scalloped borders are evident in the mucosal and submucosal layers. This ultrasonographic finding is defined as "follicular layer".

Contrast radiography

The caecum, being in direct continuity with the ascending colon, may be visualised during colonography or pneumocolonography. See section "Colon and rectum" in this chapter for further details on the appearance of the ICCJ.

Computed tomography

There is no description in the literature of the normal CT appearance of the caecum and the ICCJ in cats. Generally, it should be assessed for position, uniformity in diameter, wall thickness, and luminal contents. Normal reference ranges for the measurement of the lymph nodes draining the caecum and ICCJ are shown in Table 5.2.

Colon and rectum

Ultrasonography

The ascending colon is medial and ventral to the right kidney, the transverse colon is caudal to the stomach and the left lobe of the pancreas, and the descending colon is in the left lateral abdomen, lateral and then, at the pelvic inlet, dorsal to the urinary bladder. It has a thin wall, and its content is commonly represented by acoustic shadowing due to dense faecal material (see Fig. 5.1f in Online Supplement 5.1). The layering remains always visible, but it is less conspicuous when the degree of distension of the large intestine increases. Normal reference ranges for the measurement of the wall thickness of the large intestine and of the lymph nodes draining the large intestine are shown in Table 5.1 and Table 5.2, respectively. The ultrasound image of an empty colon may be difficult to recognise. As for the caecum, hypoechoic micronodular well-defined areas may be seen in the submucosa of the colic wall and correspond to reactive intraparietal lymphoid follicles. Their clinical importance is uncertain, as they are regularly seen with a linear transducer in asymptomatic cats.

Radiography

The localisation of the colon and rectum is relatively constant, and their appearance depends mainly on the size, quantity, consistence, and content of the faecal material in addition to the amount of colic and rectal gas. The colon generally has a question-mark shape on the ventrodorsal and dorsoventral views. It generally remains within the central abdomen on the lateral view, extending from the anal sphincter/rectum to the greater curvature of the stomach in a horizontal axis. This course may be displaced ventrally if a large amount of faecal matter is present.

A study established that the ratio of maximal diameter of the colon to the length of the vertebral body of L5 is an accurate and repeatable method to evaluate the normal or acceptable degree of distension of the large intestine. A ratio below 1.28 is a strong indicator of a normal colon (sensitivity 96%, specificity 87%).[11]

Contrast radiography

As for the other contrast studies of the GI tract, the contours of the barium–mucosa interface, spasm of the bowel lumen, filling defect, and position of the large intestine should be carefully examined. When distended with barium, the normal colon has a smooth CM–mucosa interface and a uniform diameter. After evacuation of the CM, longitudinal mucosal folds are visible as radiopaque longitudinal lines. Images difficult to interpret are related to adherence of barium to mucus, colic spasm if the CM has not been warmed up prior to administration, clumping and flocculation, and filling defects of faeces. The caecum and the colon of cats have lymphoid follicles in the mucosa which appear as spicules on barium study.

Computed tomography

There is no available data in the literature regarding the normal CT appearance of the colon and rectum in cats. Generally, the large intestine should be assessed for position, uniformity in diameter, wall thickness, and luminal contents. Normal reference ranges for the measurement of the lymph nodes draining the large intestine are shown in Table 5.2.

PATHOLOGICAL APPEARANCE OF THE OROPHARYNX AND OESOPHAGUS

Oropharyngeal pathologies

Ultrasonography and contrast-enhanced ultrasonography

Ultrasound of the cranial neck may allow identification of cranial oesophageal or pharyngeal masses or para-oesophageal lesions in cats with dysphagia. Ultrasound of pathological salivary and thyroid glands and larynx is beyond the scope of this chapter. Lymphoma and squamous cell carcinoma can appear as masses in the pharyngeal wall and may also distort and obliterate the normal pharyngeal structures. Both can have a well-circumscribed appearance, hypoechoic or with mixed echogenicity, arising from the pharyngeal or oesophageal wall. Squamous cell carcinoma may demonstrate a more aggressive pattern and irregular margins. Laryngeal cysts originating from the epiglottis have been rarely reported in cats and are seen as anechoic masses distorting the rima glottidis.

Radiography

Although radiography provides little information about gingival tissues, it provides important information on bony structures, particularly the teeth. Typical radiographic signs associated with stomatitis on dental radiographs include:

- radiolucent halo in the alveolar bone and periodontal membrane surrounding the tooth root suggesting potential periodontal abscess formation, external or internal resorption, root resorption, or destruction of the periodontal attachment apparatus (i.e. gingiva, cementum, periodontal ligaments, and alveolar bone);
- exposure of the furcation of one or several teeth;
- carious lesions within the furcation of one or several teeth;
- dense pinpoint shape opacity in the furcation between the roots of a single tooth.

Oropharyngeal and cranial oesophageal foreign bodies such as sewing needles are regularly seen in cats. Oropharyngeal radiographs are particularly indicated when signs of mechanical ileus due to a linear foreign body are identified on abdominal radiographs. The metallic needle-like opacity might be seen at the base of the tongue or UOS.

Contrast radiography and fluoroscopy

Oropharyngeal swallowing disorders are uncommon in cats. To the authors' knowledge, there are no case reports in the literature of cricopharyngeal achalasia or dyssynchrony in cats. As in dogs, a delay in the time to opening and closure of the UOS can be expected in cats with cricopharyngeal achalasia. A dyssynchrony between the closure of the larynx and the opening of the UOS, failing to close the laryngeal/tracheal opening during the expulsion of the oropharyngeal bolus into the pharynx and consequently aspiration, can be expected in cats with dyssynchrony.

Computed tomography

The same interpretative paradigm used for dental radiographs (see above) is applied for the interpretation of head CT studies of cats with suspected stomatitis. Squamous cell carcinoma is the most frequent oropharyngeal neoplasia in cats; it generally originates from the tonsils but may also be seen in the gingiva. On contrast-enhanced images of the head, a small to large, intensely enhancing mass in the soft palate and tonsillar region can be observed. When located in the gingiva, a diffuse soft tissue swelling of the gingiva associated with polyostotic mottled lysis of adjacent bones including the mandible, maxilla, and temporal bone is generally observed. The mandibular and medial retropharyngeal lymph nodes are generally markedly enlarged and heterogeneously contrast enhancing. Fluid can also be visible in the tympanic bulla secondary to soft palate thickening. A normal CT appearance of the tonsils does not preclude their neoplastic infiltration. On the contrary, a classical CT presentation includes a normal aspect of the tonsils and soft palate but a massive medial retropharyngeal lymphadenopathy.

Oesophageal pathologies

Ultrasonography and contrast-enhanced ultrasonography

Ultrasound may be used to confirm the adequate placement of an oesophageal feeding tube. It has also been reported being useful in confirming the presence of a megaoesophagus. Oesophageal or paraoesophageal masses located within the cervical or intra-abdominal oesophagus can be evaluated with ultrasonography and CEUS (Fig. 5.7). Squamous cell carcinoma is the most common neoplasia, but its incidence is low. Similar imaging findings to those observed in the small intestine are generally seen (see section "Neoplastic diseases" in this chapter). Ultrasound may be useful in confirming the presence of an oesophageal foreign body using a transdiaphragmatic window. In case of suspected vascular ring anomaly, the advantage of ultrasound is to evaluate the heart for potential concomitant congenital cardiac defects such as patent ductus arteriosus. *Spirocerca* spp. infection in cats is seldom reported. It can be associated with the presence of granulomas within the caudal oesophageal wall, which may undergo neoplastic transformation to fibrosarcoma or osteosarcoma. Their ultrasonographic appearance has not yet been reported.

Radiography and contrast radiography

The most common findings in dysphagic cats are hiatal hernias, oesophageal strictures, and oesophageal dysmotility. Oesophageal dysmotility may occur alone or together with other oesophageal disorders, and on videofluoroscopy it appears as a high proportion of unproductive swallows from which no peristaltic waves are produced.

Congenital megaoesophagus in cats is rare, but Siamese cats may be predisposed. Radiographs show generalised oesophageal gaseous distension visible as two thin converging soft tissue lines representing the oesophageal wall, tracheal stripe sign, well-defined interface between the oesophagus and the longissimus colli muscle, rightward and ventral displacement of the trachea, and may create a mass effect over the cardiac silhouette, which will appear smaller.

Contrast studies are required only if the oesophagus is not identified on plain radiographs or to rule out a vascular ring anomaly. Radiographic findings of a vascular ring anomaly include oesophageal dilation cranial to an abrupt tapering at approximately the level of the fourth intercostal space, just cranially to the heart base; a ventral deviation of the trachea; and a marked focal leftward kink of the trachea on the dorsoventral and ventrodorsal views, close to the heart base (Fig. 5.8). The latter is a pathognomonic sign of a vascular ring anomaly, and when observed there is no need to further perform a contrast study. A narrowing of the lumen of the trachea may be seen in case of a double aortic arch. A contrast study will confirm the location of the oesophageal obstruction and severity of oesophageal distension. The right lateral view generally demonstrates a curved filling defect associated with a persistent right aortic arch.

In cases of oesophagitis, a contrast study might show generalised or focal oesophageal dilation, a thickened oesophageal wall, irregularities of the oesophageal mucosa, prominent mucosal striation, delayed oesophageal emptying, a crater-like filling defect consistent with ulceration, perforation with mediastinal leakage, and strictures. Videofluoroscopy might be necessary to demonstrate the presence of gastrooesophageal reflux that may be the cause of the oesophagitis.

Strictures are seen as persistent luminal narrowing on sequential radiographs or videofluoroscopy (Fig. 5.9). Strictures are generally due to inflammation or injury to

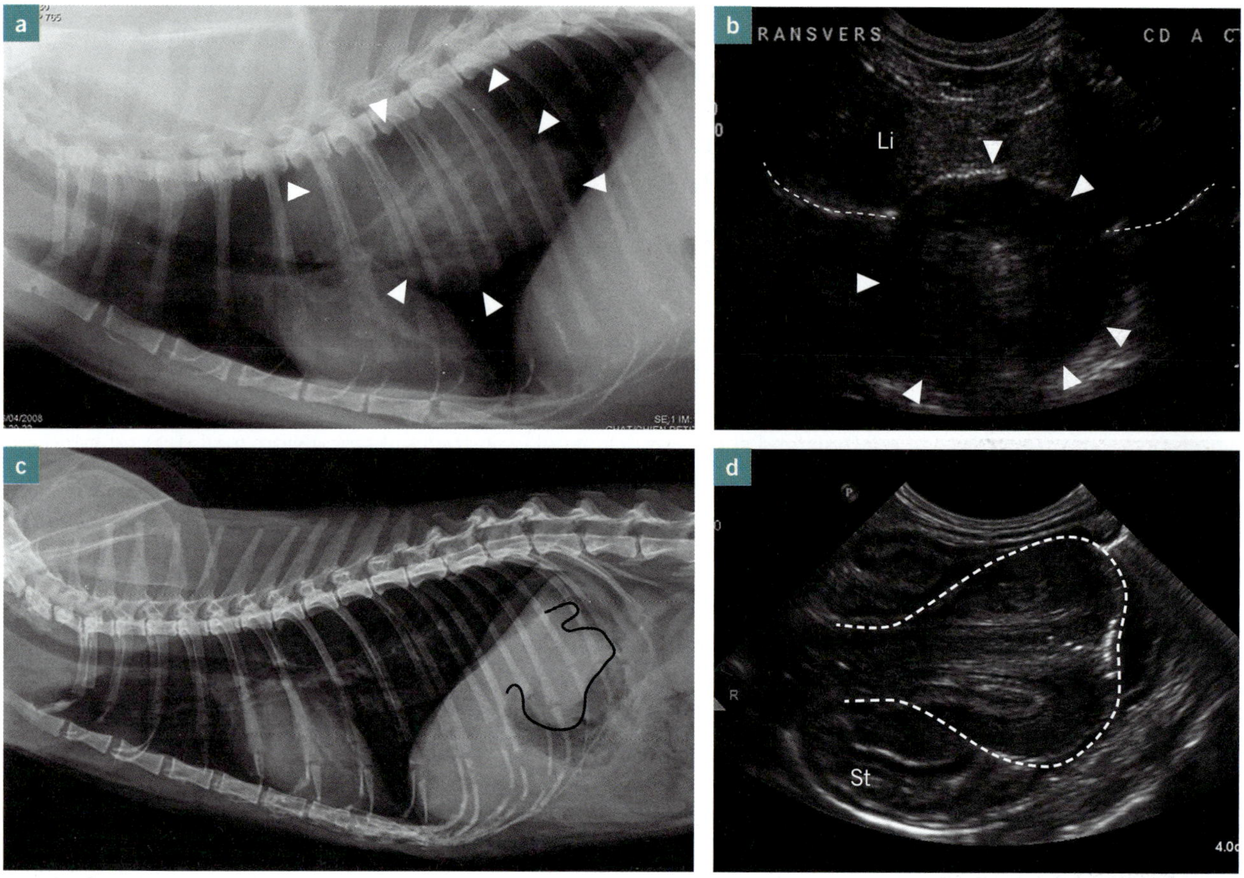

Figure 5.7. Imaging of caudal oesophageal and gastrooesophageal masses in two senior cats presented with a history of regurgitation. In the first cat, the left lateral thoracic radiograph (a) shows a large homogeneous soft-tissue opacity (arrowheads) in the caudodorsal mediastinum which displaces the caudal portion of the trachea, the carina, and the main left bronchus ventrally. In the corresponding ultrasonographic image obtained with a ventral transhepatic approach (transverse plane) at the level of the oesophageal hiatus (b), the mass (arrowheads) appears as a more rounded echogenic parenchymal structure. The dashed lines show the lung–diaphragm interface. The histological diagnosis was squamous cell carcinoma. In the second cat, the left lateral thoracic radiograph (c) shows a soft-tissue opacity (solid line) in the stomach at the level of the cardia. The mass is clearly visible due to the spontaneous contrast provided by gas. The corresponding ultrasonographic image obtained with a transhepatic approach at the level of the cardia (d) shows a severe transmural thickening of the wall of the cardia (dashed line), with loss of normal layering. Endoscopic biopsy confirmed the diagnosis of squamous cell carcinoma. Li, liver; St, stomach.

the oesophageal/intestinal wall, but they may also be due to extraluminal mass lesions (e.g. rib osteoma, mediastinal cryptococcal granuloma), as rarely reported in the literature.

A hiatal hernia can be seen on radiographs as an ovoid soft tissue opacity in the caudodorsal thorax with effacement of the borders of the diaphragm between the aorta and caudal vena cava on the lateral view, and as a central, slightly left-sided, opacity on the dorsoventral and ventrodorsal views (Fig. 5.10). Gas present in the herniated stomach may allow recognition of the rugal folds. Radiographic signs may be absent due to the sliding nature of the hernia. Gastric rugal folds may be highlighted with the presence of CM, visible both in the caudal mediastinum and cranial abdomen and separated by a marked narrowing at the level of the oesophageal hiatus.

Oesophageal neoplasms are generally seen as a focal soft tissue oesophageal dilation, a perioesophageal lesion displacing the oesophagus, a soft tissue stripe between the descending aorta and the caudal vena cava, or a midline soft tissue opacity with convex margins on the dorsoventral or ventrodorsal views. A contrast study allows the visualisation of an intraluminal mass or a filling defect obstructing completely or partially the oesophagus. The oesophagus is generally distended orally, with pooling of the CM.

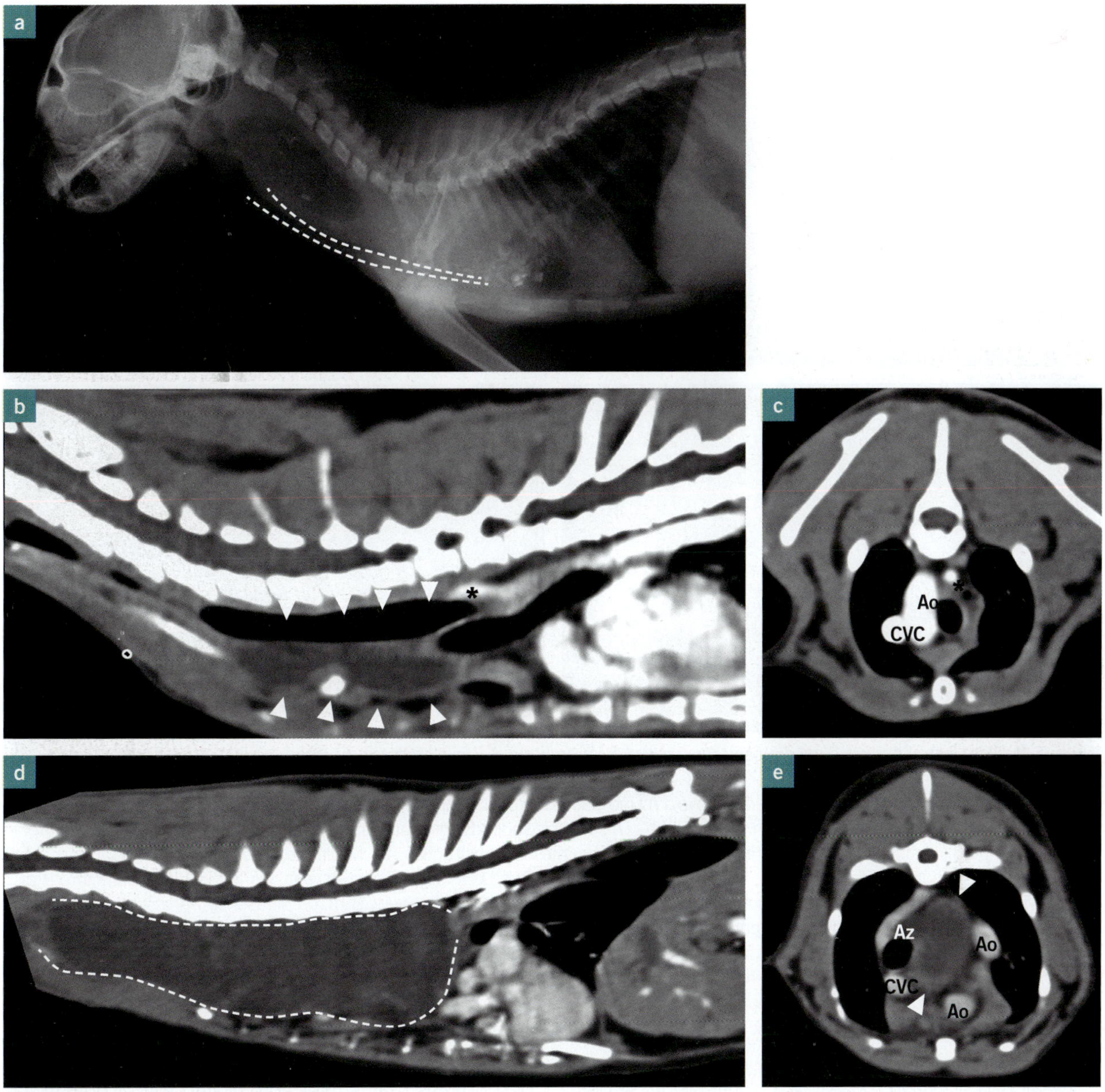

Figure 5.8. Marked oesophageal distension in three different kittens affected by a vascular ring anomaly (a–c) and an oesophageal duplication cyst (d,e). Left lateral radiograph of the neck and thorax (a) showing a marked dilation of the cervical and cranial thoracic oesophagus, with fluid, gas, and mineralised ingesta, which causes ventral displacement of the trachea (dashed lines). The oesophageal lumen abruptly ends at the level of the heart base, approximately at the fourth and fifth intercostal spaces. The caudal aspect of the oesophagus is not identified. Sagittal (b) and transverse (c) multiplanar reformatted postcontrast computed tomographic images of the thorax of a 4-month-old Ragdoll kitten with a persistent right aortic arch (Ao) and an aberrant left subclavian artery (asterisk). The cervical and cranial thoracic oesophagus (delineated by arrowheads) is markedly distended with gas and fluid, and its lumen abruptly ends at the level of the heart base. On the transverse image, the aortic arch is seen on the right side of the trachea displacing the cranial vena cava (CVC) to the right. Note that the left subclavian artery (asterisk) is passing dorsally to the oesophagus, contributing to the vascular ring and oesophageal constriction. Sagittal (d) and transverse (e) multiplanar reformatted postcontrast computed tomographic images of the thorax of a kitten presenting with an oesophageal duplication cyst. The cyst (dashed lines) is seen as a voluminous fluid-filled pouch running along the wall of the cervical and cranial thoracic oesophagus, creating a mass effect on the oesophageal lumen and hampering its clear distinction. The cyst was initially misinterpreted as the oesophageal lumen; however, as homogeneous fluid content is not commonly seen in oesophageal diverticula, a cyst was considered most likely. On the transverse image, the duplication cyst (between arrowheads) is visible between the cranial vena cava (CVC) and aorta (Ao). The aortic arch is normally positioned on the left side of the trachea. Note the distension of the azygous (Az) vein, most likely due to mass effect and compression on the cranial vena cava. Images b and c courtesy of Lumbry Park Veterinary Specialists, Alton, UK; d and e courtesy of the Clinique Vétérinaire Alliance, Bordeaux, France.

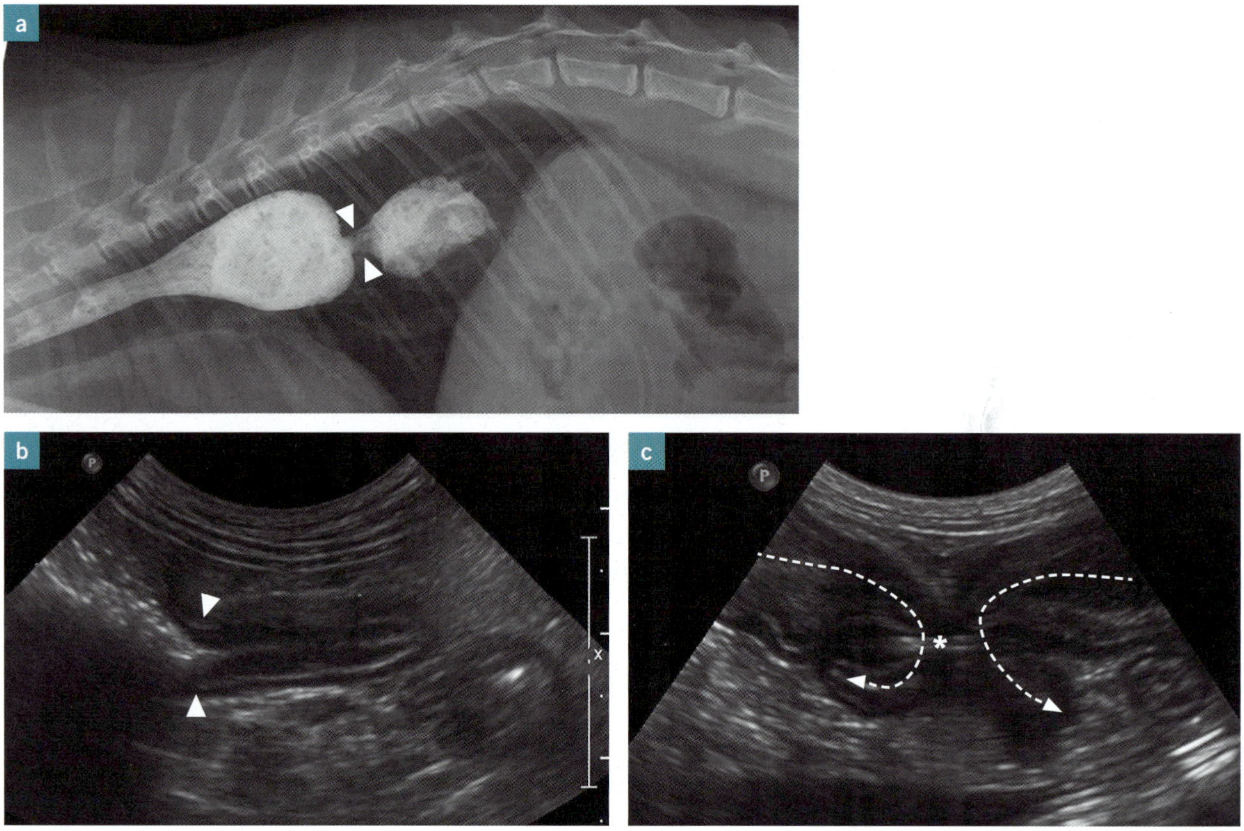

Figure 5.9. Right lateral barium sulphate oesophagram of a 10-month-old Bengal cat with an oesophageal stricture after doxycycline administration and a hiatal hernia (a). Focal oesophageal dilation cranial to the stricture (arrowheads), with abrupt tapering at the level of the caudal thoracic oesophagus, is identified. An ovoid mixed soft tissue/barium opacity is also observed, just caudal to the stricture, with gas and a rugal fold pattern consistent with the stomach. This finding supports the diagnosis of hiatal hernia. B-mode ultrasonographic image showing an intestinal stricture in an adult cat with chronic intestinal obstruction (b). Moderate distension of the jejunum is noted proximal to the stricture site (arrowheads). Mild wall thickening associated with slightly altered wall layering within the stricture is also evident. The fibrostenotic nature of the stricture was histologically diagnosed after surgery. B-mode ultrasonographic image showing an intestinal strangulation in an adult cat with chronic vomiting (c). Two different jejunal loops (dashed arrows) are hooked by a hyperechoic stripe (asterisk) causing mild focal distension of both loops proximal to the stricture. Surgery was required to resect adherences, resolve intestinal entrapment, and suture the mesenteric defect. Image a courtesy of the Centre Hospitalier Universitaire Vétérinaire de Saint-Hyacinthe, Université de Montréal, Canada.

Oesophageal foreign bodies, particularly sewing needles in cats, are generally seen on radiographs due their metallic opacity. For radiolucent foreign bodies, a contrast study may be necessary to reveal a filling defect and oesophageal dilation orally to the obstruction. It is important to use nonionic iodinated CM due to the risk of oesophageal perforation and leakage of CM into the thoracic cavity.

Computed tomography

Vascular ring anomalies can be further evaluated using CT, although the diagnosis is generally achieved with survey or contrast radiography. In case of persistence of the right aortic arch, thoracic CT shows a cranial thoracic oesophagus that is markedly dilated with fluid and gas and an aortic arch located to the right of the trachea, causing tracheal displacement and luminal narrowing (Figs. 5.8d and 5.8e). The ligamentum arteriosum is not directly identified. The position of the subclavian arteries should also be carefully evaluated, as they may contribute to oesophageal compression. Cases of vascular ring anomaly due to an aberrant right subclavian artery with or without Kommerell diverticulum have been reported. Kommerell diverticulum is a dilation of the proximal portion of an aberrant subclavian artery near its origin from the aorta, thought to represent a remnant of the left fourth aortic arch.

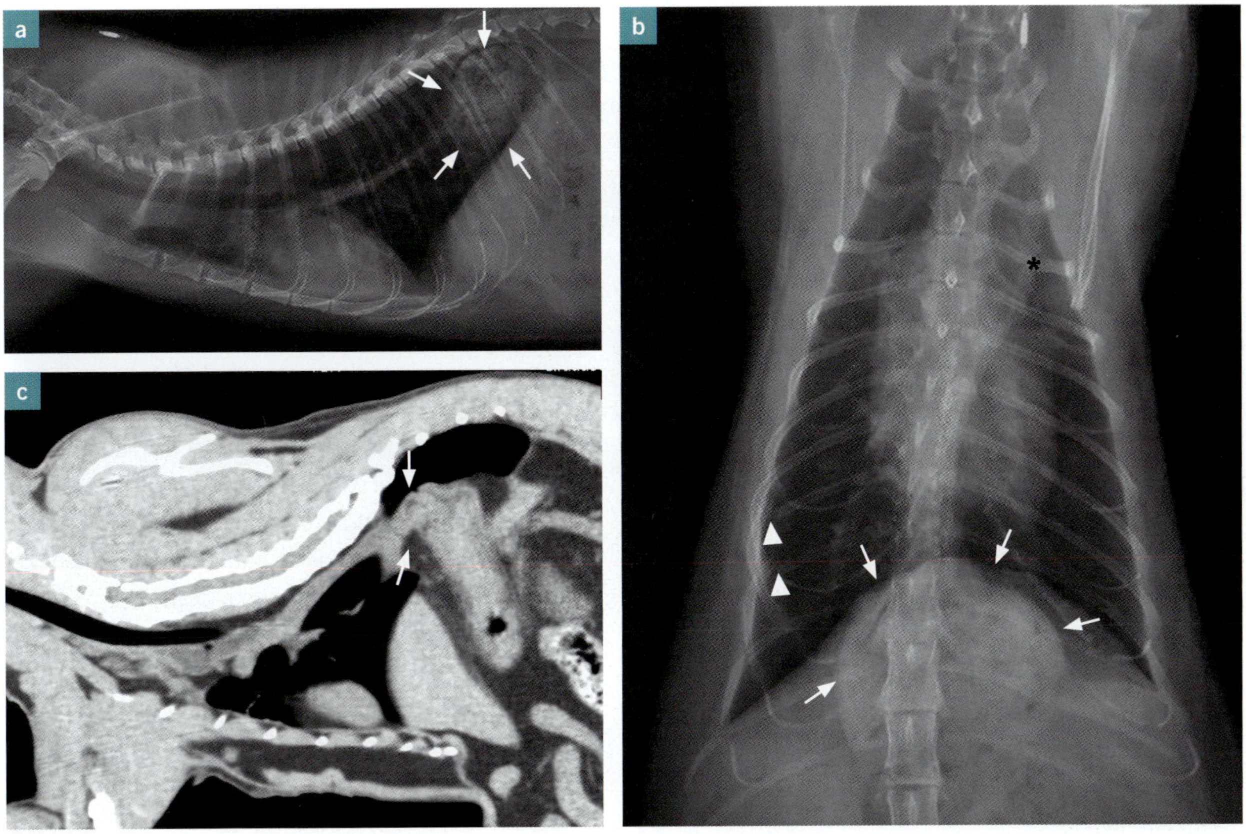

Figure 5.10. Lateral (a) and ventrodorsal (b) thoracic radiographs of a 9-year-old Singapura cat with chronic coughing due to chronic bronchitis. A mild bronchial pattern associated with soft tissue opacity nodules (tree-in-bud pattern) (asterisk) in the left cranial lung lobe is present. Multiple spontaneous fractures of the caudal ribs on the right side (arrowheads) are also evident. A mixed granular soft tissue/gas opacity in the caudodorsal thorax (arrows) with effacement of the borders of the diaphragm was detected on the lateral projection, between the aorta and caudal vena cava. On the ventrodorsal view, the same opacity was recognised at the level of diaphragmatic cupola, supporting the diagnosis of hiatal hernia. The hiatal hernia was thought to be secondary to chronically increased respiratory effort. Sagittal multiplanar reformatted postcontrast computed tomographic image of the thorax of the same cat (c), confirming the continuity of the stomach with the intrathoracic gas/soft tissue structure and the presence of the gastric fundus in the thorax. Images courtesy of the École nationale vétérinaire d'Alfort, France.

Paraoesophageal abscesses may be evaluated using CT. They are generally well-delineated, fluid-filled, spheroid to ellipsoid masses arising in the mediastinum. On transverse CT images, the oesophagus appears as a thin soft tissue–attenuating ring associated with part of the abscess margin. Abscesses are fluid attenuating in their centre and demonstrate peripheral contrast enhancement. The flattened oesophageal mucosa has a characteristic curvilinear pattern of contrast enhancement conforming to the curvature of the abscess.

An intraluminal mass creating complete or partial obstruction with heterogeneous, moderate contrast enhancement and irregular, ill-defined margins seems the most common feature of intraluminal abscesses.

A rare condition of oesophageal duplication cyst has been reported in the literature, and it was recently observed by the authors. CT imaging demonstrated a well-defined space-occupying lesion within the cranial mediastinum. The lesion was fluid attenuating (mean 10 HU), circumscribed by a thin enhancing wall. The lesion compressed the trachea and cranial vena cava. The oesophagus, in the authors' case, could not be clearly identified as empty. The duplication cyst was initially misinterpreted as a diverticulum, with no vascular ring anomaly identified that could explain its focal dilation up to the heart base. However, the complete fluid attenuating pattern in the absence of a fluid level and a gas interface, which is generally seen in a distended oesophagus, made the second interpretation more consistent with a cystic lesion.

PATHOLOGICAL APPEARANCE OF THE GASTROINTESTINAL TRACT

Hernia, intussusception, volvulus, and ischaemia

Radiography and contrast radiography

Sliding hiatal hernias are the most common occurrence in cats, and its radiographic appearance is detailed elsewhere in this chapter (see section "Oesophageal pathologies" in this chapter). Peritoneopericardial diaphragmatic hernias are frequent congenital defects in cats, but there are very few situations in which the GI tract is herniated in the pericardial sac. Radiographic signs include an enlarged cardiac silhouette that merges with the diaphragmatic outline ventrally ("remnant line"). The visualisation of different soft tissue opacities with the presence of a gas pattern or, better, the use of CM may allow identification of herniated GI segments.

Diaphragmatic or abdominal wall rupture due to trauma may result in "herniation" of the GI tract, but this is not considered a true hernia as no hernial sac is present. Common sites of rupture include the diaphragm, paracostal abdominal wall, and inguinal region. When a GI segment is displaced in the thorax, subcutaneous tissues, or inguinal region, strangulation and vascular compromise may happen and lead to ischaemia and mechanical ileus. Radiographic identification of the wall rupture and displaced GI segments is crucial. If doubt exists about the presence of a herniated GI segment, a contrast study should be performed.

Intussusception occurs when one part of the intestine (the intussusceptum) is invaginated into the lumen of the adjacent intestinal segment (the intussuscipiens). Any portion of the intestine may be affected, but the most common intussusceptions in cats are jejunojejunal and enterocolic. On survey radiographs, the intussusception may be seen as an elongated, sausage-shaped soft tissue opacity. Ileocolic intussusceptions are located in the midabdomen, caudal to the stomach, and displace the small intestine caudally. In this type of intussusception, a gas opacity may outline the crescentic end of the intussusceptum. An upper GI contrast study can help confirm the suspicion of intussusception. A sharply demarcated narrowing of the intestinal lumen is generally seen. When the CM enters the space between the intussusceptum and the intussuscipiens, a typical corkscrew or coiled-spring pattern is observed.

Gastric dilatation–volvulus in cats is a rare event and might occur in combination with a traumatic diaphragmatic hernia or, less commonly, spontaneously. Similar radiographic signs to those reported in dogs are seen, including gaseous distension of the stomach associated with compartmentalisation and dorsal displacement of the pylorus. Intestinal volvulus or mesenteric torsion has also been rarely reported in cats. Abdominal radiographic findings are rather nonspecific and include marked distension of gas-filled, small intestinal loops.

Ultrasonography and contrast-enhanced ultrasonography

Ultrasound is very useful to confirm or exclude the presence of a herniated GI segment, identify abdominal wall rupture, and evaluate the size of the defect. In addition, it provides information regarding the GI wall integrity, permeability, and vascularisation. The classic ultrasonographic appearance of intussusception is a circular target-like lesion in the transverse plane (bull's-eye appearance) due to the presence of several concentric rings reflecting the various layers inside the intussuscipiens and the adjacent intussusceptum walls (Fig. 5.11). The appearance in the longitudinal plane is similar. Hyperechoic tissue can be seen in the centre of the lesion, representing mesenteric fat pulled together with the intussusceptum into the intussuscipiens. Dilated lymphatic and blood vessels are seen as anechoic areas inside the hyperechoic centre.

In chronic cases, the outer intussuscipiens may become thicker and hypoechoic, and individual wall layers may become less discernible due to oedema and impairment to blood flow.

Since the condition in older cats has been reported to occur in association with inflammatory bowel disease (IBD), intestinal neoplasia, caecal inversion, and caecal polyps, the intestine should always be carefully assessed to determine whether additional conditions may be present.

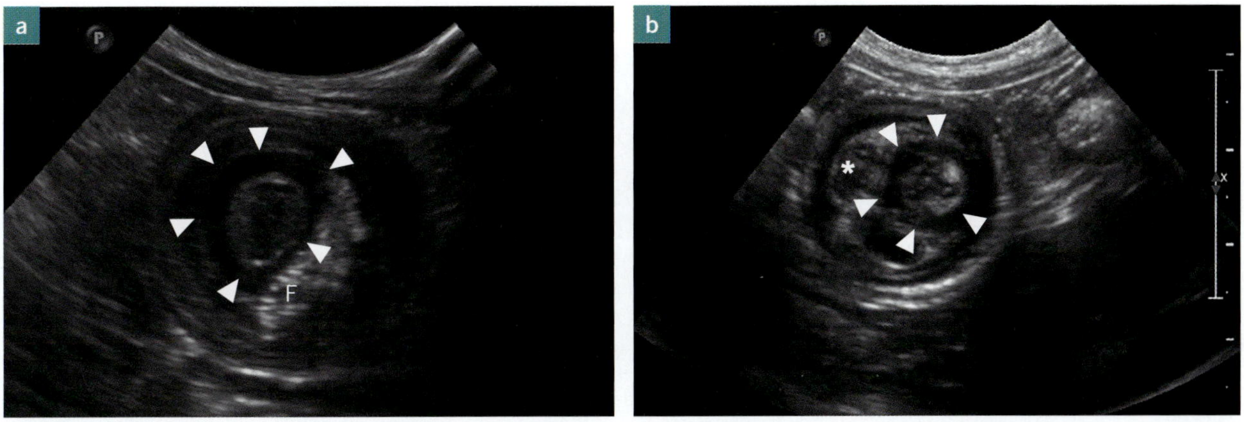

Figure 5.11. Transverse ultrasonographic images of a jejunojejunal (a) and an ileocolic (b) intussusception in two adult cats. The multilayered appearance of the wall represents the superimposed wall layers of the intussusceptum and intussuscipiens. The arrowheads are depicting the invaginated intestine. Hyperechoic mesenteric fat (F) and a hypoechoic lymph node (asterisk) are invaginated within the intussuscipiens.

The ultrasonographic appearance of an intestinal volvulus or mesenteric torsion consists in two distinct populations of intestinal loops: one population of distended intestinal loops displaying focal wall thickening (layering maintained), loss of intestinal peristalsis, and absence of intraluminal or intramural obstruction, and another population of normal looking intestinal loops. Doppler ultrasonography may be performed to confirm loss of intestinal perfusion. In the authors' experience, CEUS is the technique of choice following B-mode ultrasound to confirm volvulus and ischaemia. Absence of enhancement of the twisted segment is confirmatory.

A very recent study has described the use of CEUS in four cats with intestinal ischaemia.[3] The diagnoses included a perforating duodenal ulcer, jejunal necrotising enteritis, secondary necrosis due to jejunojejunal intussusception, and iatrogenic damage to jejunal arteries. On B-mode ultrasound, all intestinal lesions were characterised by nonspecific findings such as focal hypoechoic thickening of the wall with loss of normal layering associated with a hyperechoic mesentery. CEUS displayed a diminished or absent enhancement of the intestinal lesions compared to the adjacent perfused wall (Video 5.2). CEUS is therefore indicated to diagnose this life-threatening condition.

Video 5.2. Ultrasound study of a 12-year-old domestic shorthair cat presented with anorexia and acute vomiting and diagnosed with intestinal ischaemia due to necrotising enteritis. The B-mode ultrasound demonstrates generalised ileus characterised by fluid-filled distended intestinal loops and decreased peristalsis. The small intestine has a diffusely thickened muscularis layer. A focal transmural asymmetrical eccentric hypoechoic thickening of the wall with loss of layering is observed in one segment (blue arrow). After intravenous administration of contrast medium, no enhancement is observed in the lesion, whereas adjacent small intestinal loops demonstrate normal enhancement. This was highly suggestive of ischaemia of the intestinal wall. The final diagnosis was obtained on necropsy following euthanasia, as the owner declined surgery due to the critical status of the patient.

Computed tomography

CT may be useful in cases of trauma for a more rapid and precise visualisation of the wall defect, size and location of the rupture, and displaced GI segment. Vascular compromise may be seen as absence of enhancement of the herniated loop. CT is particularly interesting in case of intestinal volvulus or mesenteric torsion, as it allows the visualisation of a whirl sign corresponding to the looping of the mesenteric root and vessels. Multiplanar reformatted images are useful in visualising the whirl sign: small and large intestinal loops and nearby mesenteric vessels form a spiral. The cranial and caudal mesenteric veins and their tributaries may also be dilated and tortuous. The mesenteric fat may show multiple lines of increased attenuation consistent with focal oedema, steatitis, and/or peritoneal fluid accumulation.

Foreign bodies

Radiography and contrast radiography

Foreign bodies most commonly ingested by cats include sewing needles, Christmas ornaments, and shoelaces. Sewing needles are easily recognised due to their metallic opacity and shape (Fig. 5.12a). Shoelaces are generally seen as a soft tissue linear band and tend to accumulate in the stomach (Fig. 5.12b). Christmas ornaments are challenging to identify, as they may be radiolucent or of soft tissue opacity. They are commonly associated with a linear mechanical ileus obstruction type (Figs. 5.12d and 5.12f). Indigestible material such as trichobezoars is frequently encountered in long-haired cats. When chronic, it tends to mineralise and displays a characteristic radiographic appearance of an amorphous mixed mineral/soft tissue opacity within the stomach. Obstructive gastric foreign bodies are generally more easily seen on the left lateral view, as the gas can be seen surrounding the foreign body in the pyloric antrum. If the stomach is empty of gas because the patient has just vomited, a contrast study may be considered. The absence of gastric emptying, the visualisation of a filling defect, or the persistence of CM within the gastric foreign material is suggestive of pyloric outflow obstruction due to foreign or indigestible material. In the small intestine, an obstruction due to a foreign body is suspected when two populations of small intestinal loops of different diameter are seen, one of which being larger than 12 mm. An upper GI contrast study may be considered to confirm the obstruction and highlight the contours and shape of the cause of the obstruction. An abrupt filling defect is seen in case of foreign body. Linear foreign bodies are generally suspected when intestinal plication is seen, with multiple small intestinal loops bunched together in an accordion-like aspect. Teardrop-shaped, crescent-shaped, or geometric/triangular gas bubbles are commonly seen in the plicated loops. Loss of serosal detail is generally observed. An upper GI contrast study highlights the bunching of the small intestinal loops.

Figure 5.12. Imaging of gastrointestinal foreign bodies.

Ultrasonography

Mechanical ileus due to a linear foreign body generally occurs when part of the foreign material is anchored at the pylorus or around the tongue base, while the remaining material progresses distally into the small intestine. Peristaltic contractions unsuccessfully try to move the foreign body aborally, ultimately resulting in intestinal plication (Fig. 5.12c). Evidence of intestinal plication is highly indicative of the existence of a linear foreign object. All layers of the intestinal wall are involved within an affected segment of the intestine, including the serosa; this differs from simple corrugation, which describes normal, symmetrical undulations of the intestinal wall in the presence of a straight serosa. The precise visualisation of the linear foreign body depends on the degree to which the object transmits or attenuates the ultrasound beams. Since linear foreign bodies typically cause only partial intestinal obstruction, the resulting intestinal dilation is often mild or absent.

Roundworms or grass can potentially resemble linear foreign material, as they appear as paired parallel hyperechoic lines within the intestinal lumen. They are easily distinguished from linear foreign bodies because they do not cause bowel plication or acoustic shadowing, and movement of live worms can often be observed. Occasionally, nonlinear foreign bodies can be identified by the appearance of an intraluminal structure with a highly echogenic interface associated with variable acoustic shadowing and edge enhancement. The typical ultrasonographic appearance of trichobezoars is that of a cylindrical or spherical mixed-echogenicity mass associated with variable acoustic shadowing (Figs. 5.12e and 5.12g).

Computed tomography

The same rules for interpretation may be used to look for GI foreign bodies. To date there are no scientific reports evaluating the CT appearance and technique to find GI foreign bodies. In the authors' experience, a bone or lung window may facilitate the visualisation of abnormal GI content when evaluating the abdomen. A distended loop may be easily detected on an abdominal window of a postcontrast CT study, but abnormal content may easily be overlooked due to gaseous distension or ingesta.

Inflammatory diseases

Infectious inflammatory diseases

Ultrasonography and contrast-enhanced ultrasonography

Pyogranulomas due to feline infectious peritonitis (FIP) may be seen in the GI tract. They have been reported to occur in the jejunum, ICCJ, and colon. In an old study, 26 out of 156 cats with a histological diagnosis of FIP had apparently solitary mural intestinal lesions. All 26 cats had a mass, believed to be a neoplasm, in the colon or ICCJ. Affected intestines were markedly thickened, nodular, and associated with enlarged lymph nodes, making the distinction with neoplasia impossible.

In a recent report regarding GI ultrasonographic findings in cats infected with feline panleucopenia virus, the most frequent signs included decreased motility of the GI tract with fluid accumulation, decreased total wall thickness of the duodenum and jejunum, decreased thickness of the mucosal layer, thickening of the muscular layer, hyperechogenicity of the mucosa, and a nonspecific hyperechoic mucosal band paralleling the submucosa.

Histoplasmosis has also been documented to cause selective thickening of the small intestine muscularis in cats. Other reported findings in cases with histoplasmosis are thickening of a jejunal loop with loss of layering and peritoneal effusion. In parasitic infections, a nonspecific submucosal thickening can be seen. Gas dissemination within the intestinal wall (pneumatosis) can be seen in the entire GI tract on ultrasound, radiographs, and CT, but its clinical importance is unclear. Reported ultrasonographic findings include diffuse wall thickening, loss of or indistinct wall layering, and the presence of one or more strong echogenic intramural interfaces within the GI wall associated with reverberation artefacts. On radiographs and CT, a thin radiolucent or gas-attenuating line is seen within the wall of the GI tract. This may be due to proliferation of gas-producing bacteria such as *Clostridium* spp. and *Escherichia coli.*

A case of gastric pseudotumour due to *Actinomyces hordeovulneris* has been reported. The lesion is called a pseudotumour in human medicine because the chronic inflammatory process is able to induce granulomatous lesions that mimic a malignant tumour on clinical, ultrasonographic, and gross examination. *Actinomyces* species are gram-positive, branching, filamentous bacteria that are common inhabitants of the feline oral cavity and GI tract. Abdominal ultrasound showed a hypoechoic transmural thickening (approximately 9 mm) at the gastric body, associated with loss of normal wall layering and hyperechoic speckles possibly consistent with focal fibrosis. Gastric and hepatic lymph nodes were mildly enlarged and hypoechoic, but normal in shape.

CEUS may be useful for diagnosis, as it may show a benign behaviour of the nonneoplastic mass and guide for FNA in order to avoid necrotic, poorly cellular, or richly vascularised areas.

Radiography and contrast radiography

Infectious GI diseases are generally associated with a nonspecific radiographic appearance of gastroenteritis (i.e. small amount of gas in the GI tract, several loops being corrugated). Only in case of intraluminal granuloma of fungal or parasitic origin, or when FIP-related, mechanical obstruction may occur. Functional ileus may also be seen in case of feline panleucopenia.

Noninfectious inflammatory diseases

Ultrasonography and contrast-enhanced ultrasonography

Generally speaking, inflammatory enteropathies are accompanied by intestinal wall changes on ultrasound.[12] These changes include mild diffuse and symmetrical thickening of the intestinal wall with maintenance of the layering or diffuse thickening of individual layers of the wall (Fig. 5.13). Eventually, inflammatory conditions of the feline GI tract can sometimes be associated with a normal appearance of the intestine on ultrasound. Although no significant changes may be seen, an occult nonultrasonographically visible alteration of the intestinal wall is still possible. A decision tree is proposed to help the veterinary surgeon evaluate the type of pathology depending on the ultrasonographic alterations of the intestinal wall (Fig. 5.14).

In cats, a thin hyperechoic mucosal band, which correspond to mucosal fibrosis on histopathology, may be seen parallel to the submucosa.[13] However, as it is identified in cats with and without clinical signs of GI disease, the clinical significance of this finding is still unknown. It was hypothesised that prior intestinal wall inflammation or insult may be at the origin of the fibrosis or that it

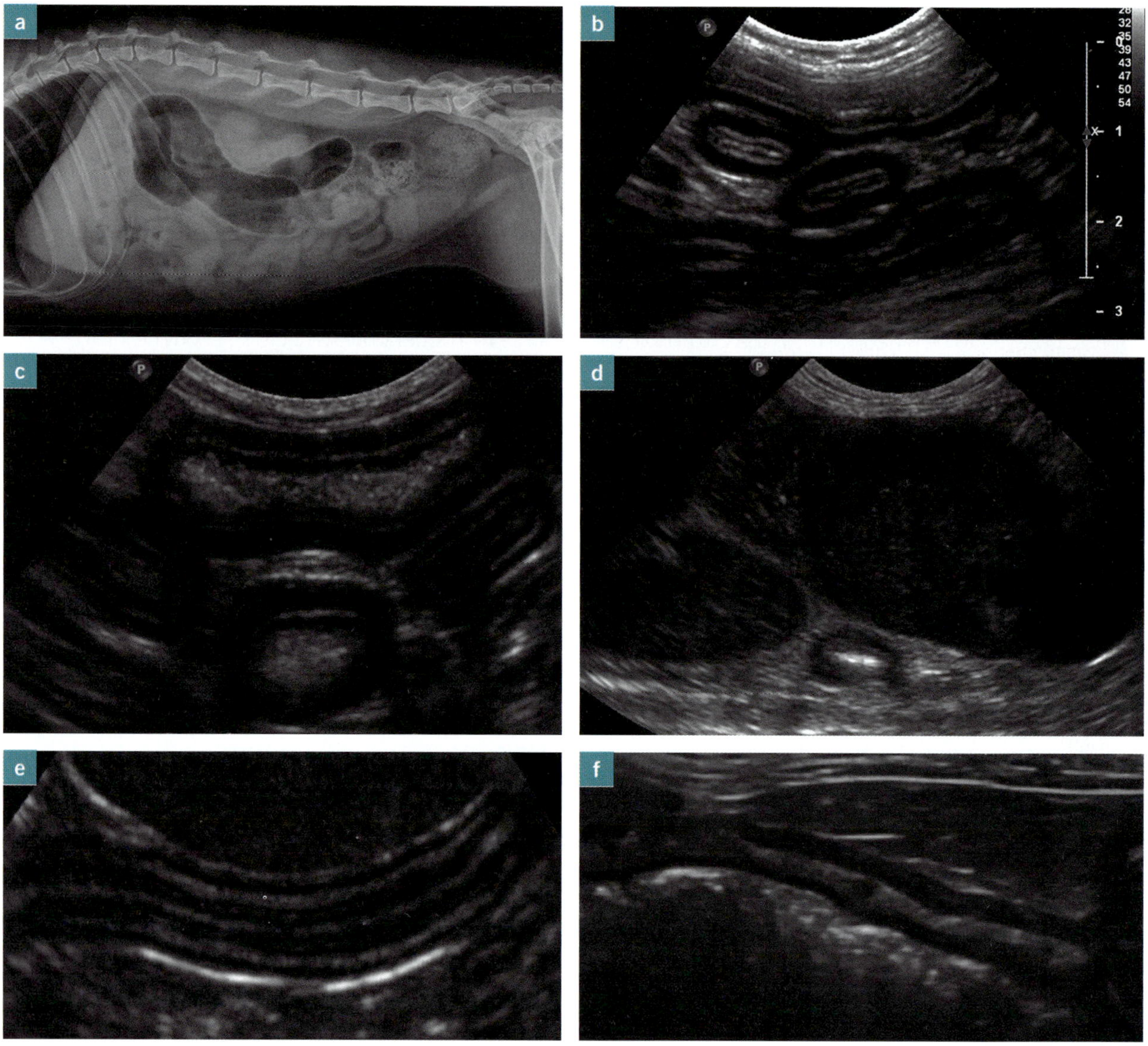

Figure 5.13. Imaging of diffuse thickening of the intestinal wall. Lateral radiograph of the abdomen of a cat with chronic diarrhoea (a). Jejunal loops are mildly distended with a fluid-filled pattern. Ultrasonographic images of two adult cats displaying thickening of the muscularis layer of the small intestine (b,c). The intestinal wall is moderately thickened. Final histopathological diagnosis was lymphocytic enteritis (b) and low-grade (small-cell) lymphoma (c). Ultrasonographic image showing markedly enlarged, rounded and hypoechoic jejunal lymph nodes associated with intestinal wall alterations in a cat with alimentary lymphoma (d). Longitudinal ultrasonographic image of a jejunal loop in a cat with chronic diarrhoea (e). Mild thickening of the wall associated with prominence of the submucosal layer is evident. A thin hyperechoic line within the mucosa paralleling the lumen is seen (likely representing fibrosis). Final histopathological diagnosis was lymphocytic enteritis. Longitudinal ultrasonographic image of the colon of a cat with acute diarrhoea (f) showing moderate thickening of the wall of the descending colon with visualisation of small submucosal hypoechoic nodules. This finding is histopathologically related to intraparietal reactive lymphoid follicles.

may represent visible lymphatic vessels. In severe cases of inflammation of the intestinal wall, a loss of layering may occasionally be seen, although this is much less common. Very rarely, intestinal thickening may be seen with colic or intestinal wall infarction. In the latter case, a thickening of the mucosa and submucosa may be observed, accompanied by a complete loss of layering in the advanced stages. Corrugation of the small intestine may also be observed ("angry" appearance). Regular and symmetrical undulations of the wall are generally seen but are not specific of inflammatory diseases of the GI tract, as they may also be observed in case of peritonitis. Unlike

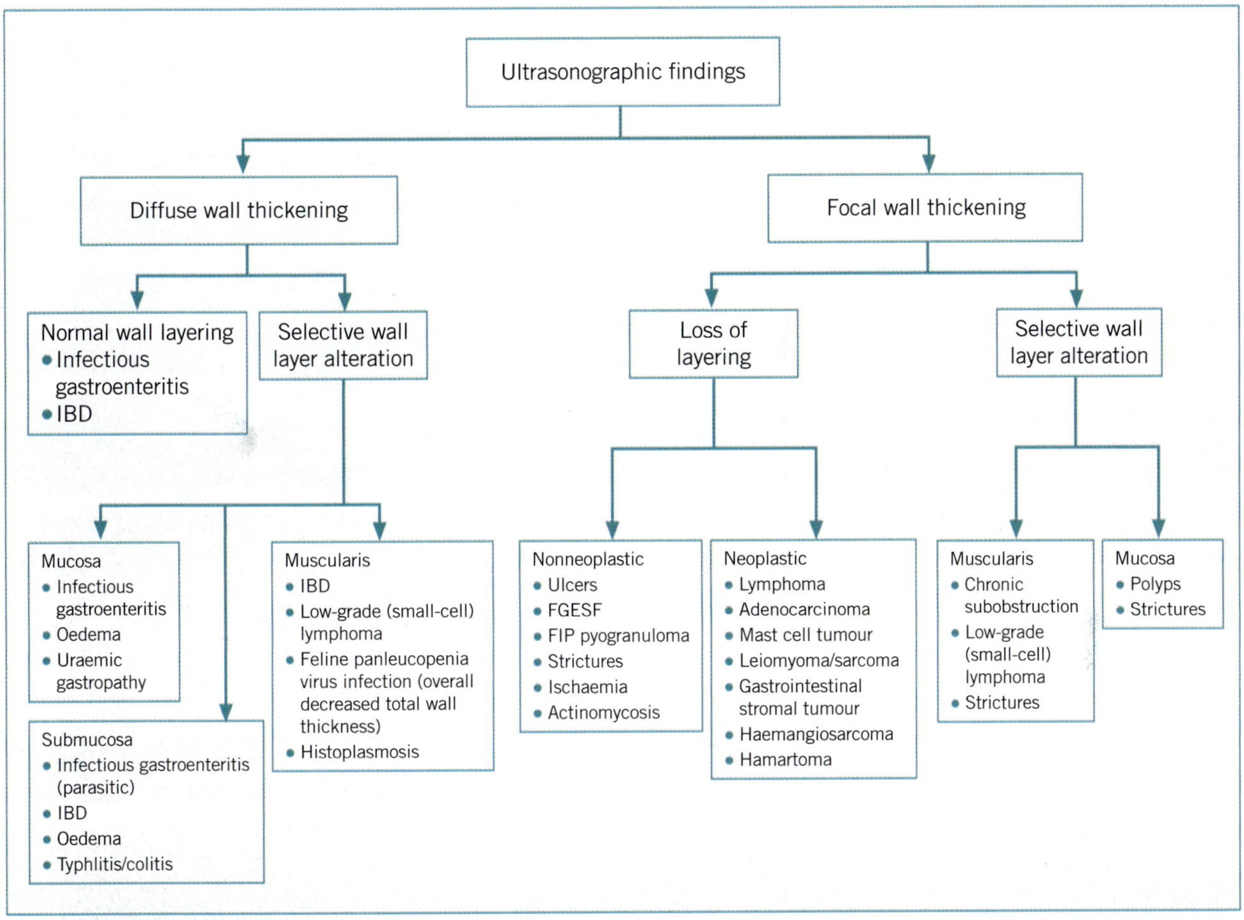

Figure 5.14. Decision tree to guide the veterinary surgeon in the interpretation of ultrasonographic abnormalities in the feline intestinal wall. FGESF, feline gastrointestinal eosinophilic sclerosing fibroplasia; FIP, feline infectious peritonitis; IBD, inflammatory bowel disease.

intestinal plication in the presence of an intraluminal linear foreign body, the serosal layer remains relatively linear in case of corrugation.

In case of gastritis (Fig. 5.15a), diffuse or focal wall thickening associated with a decreased motility may be observed. A concomitant increased echogenicity or decreased visualisation of the wall layers is consistent with severe gastritis. Gastric wall oedema is routinely seen with inflammatory gastric diseases (Fig. 5.15b). On ultrasound, it appears as a diffuse moderate to severe thickening of the gastric wall associated with an altered layering. The mucosa is generally hyperechoic and very swollen. Gastric ulcers (Fig. 5.15c) are typically associated with the image of a crater or a single discrete mucosal defect, depending on severity and extent. Hyperechoic microbubbles accumulating in the crater or being trapped in the gastric wall associated with hyperechoic speckles and comet tails artefacts are also very suggestive of an ulcer. In addition, the stomach is fluid filled and hypomotile when ulcers are present. The adjacent wall is generally thickened with a loss of layering, making the distinction between a benign and a malignant origin almost impossible. In cats with chronic uraemia, uraemic gastropathy may develop (Fig. 5.15d). It is characterised by ultrasonographic features of gastric oedema associated with a hyperechoic line at the mucosal–luminal interface due to mineralisation of the mucosa.

Cats with eosinophilic and lymphocytic enteritis commonly have diffuse circumferential thickening of the muscularis layer of the small intestine with maintenance of the wall layering.[12] This ultrasonographic feature may also be encountered with low-grade (small-cell) lymphoma (see section "Neoplastic diseases" in this chapter).[14] Thickening of the muscularis layer that exceeds half the

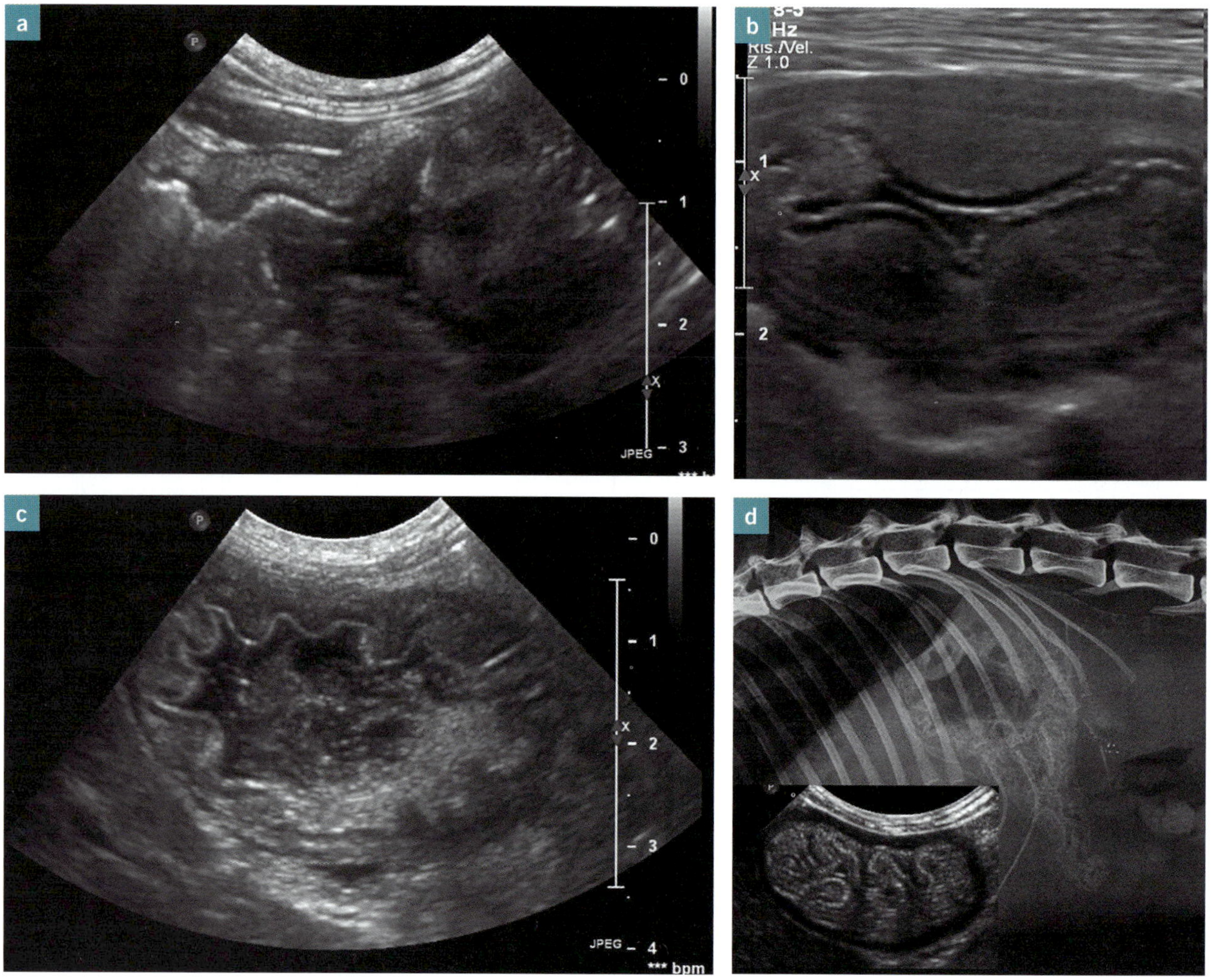

Figure 5.15. Imaging of gastritis. Ultrasonographic image of the stomach of an adult cat presenting with acute vomiting (a). The stomach is mildly dilated with fluid and shows a moderately thickened hyperechoic wall. Ultrasonographic image of the stomach of a young cat (b) showing an extensive and severe thickening with altered layering. The thin inner mucosal anechoic layer borders the remaining hyperechoic wall. This feature is consistent with gastric oedema. Ultrasonographic image of the stomach of an old cat with chronic ulcerative gastritis (c). The stomach is moderately distended with echogenic fluid, and the gastric wall is thickened and hyperechoic. Lateral radiograph of an old cat with gastric mineralisation secondary to chronic kidney disease (d). Thin, curvilinear, mineralised opacities that parallel the rugal folds of the stomach are caused by gastric calcification. The corresponding ultrasonographic image is characterised by a moderately thickened gastric wall with prominent rugal folds and a hyperechoic line at the mucosal–luminal interface secondary to mineralisation of the mucosa.

thickness of the submucosal layer was reported in cases of IBD as a specific feature. However, subsequent work on the ultrasonographic appearance of the feline normal GI tract found the muscularis layer to be normally equal to or thicker than the width of the submucosal layer in the stomach, duodenum, jejunum, and ileum. Lymphadenopathy may occur with both IBD and lymphoma. However, the changes are generally more severe in case of lymphoma compared to enteritis. Therefore, as the appearance of both diseases on ultrasound can significantly overlap, further diagnostic workup, including full-thickness surgical biopsy, might be required to achieve a diagnosis.[14]

Colonic inflammatory changes are generally discrete, characterised by a subtle thickening of the wall. Prominence of the folds associated with diffuse wall thickening despite normal wall layering may be seen with colonic wall oedema. In the large intestine and caecum, the visualisation of 1–3 mm diameter hypoechoic nodules in the follicular layer and submucosa of either the caecum or colonic wall, respectively, are thought to represent reactive intraparietal lymphoid follicles and may indicate the presence of caecal and colonic inflammatory disease. However, they may also be seen in asymptomatic cats, making their clinical relevance equivocal. Typhlitis is probably underestimated in cats due to the variety and lack of specificity of clinical signs. Associated ultrasonographic abnormalities include prominence of the follicular layer, diffuse wall thickening of the proximal and distal part of the caecum, and loss of caecal wall layering.[15] Although not correlated to the severity of the inflammation, loss of layering in the caecum seems to be a marker of caecal inflammation. Cats with typhlitis generally tend to also have colitis. Selective muscularis thickening of the intestine proximal to a stenosis caused by a foreign intestinal body has also been reported in cats, with smooth muscle hypertrophy thought to be the reason due to chronic subobstruction.

Although less common, intestinal masses can also be caused by benign or nonneoplastic lesions.

Feline gastrointestinal eosinophilic sclerosing fibroplasia (FGESF) is an inflammatory condition that mainly affects middle-aged cats, and it has been suggested that Ragdoll cats may be overrepresented. FGESF is a major differential diagnosis in a cat with an intestinal mass and may be a primary step towards a neoplastic transformation.[16] See Chapter 19 for further details.

Adenomatous polyps are another type of benign intestinal mass that may be seen in cats.[17] Their ultrasonographic aspect has been recently described at the pyloroduodenal junction of six cats. They typically appear as a thin, echogenic homogeneous nodule projecting into the lumen of either the proximal duodenum or the pyloroduodenal junction. They can easily be mistaken for ingesta. Although benign, they may cause luminal obstruction, GI bleeding, and biliary tract obstruction if located in the proximity of the duodenal papilla.

Intramural small intestinal obstruction caused by a benign stricture should be considered in the differential diagnosis for chronic progressive GI disease, especially in younger, debilitated cats.[18] On ultrasound, a moderate to marked fluid gastric distension and moderate to marked distension of the small intestine oral to the stenotic segment may be observed. The stricture can be located in the duodenum, mid- to distal jejunum, or proximal ileum. Two types of strictures have been identified: annular strictures (napkin-ring appearance, length <15 mm, abrupt transition between dilated intestine oral and non-dilated intestine aboral to stricture) and long-segment strictures (uniform diameter and cylindrical in shape, length >15 mm, more gradual transition). The wall of the stenotic segment can be mildly to moderately thickened (3–6 mm), and layering is usually abnormal.

Radiography and contrast radiography

Noninfectious inflammatory GI diseases are generally associated with a nonspecific radiographic appearance of gastroenteritis with a small amount of gas within the GI tract and several corrugated loops. Only in case of intraluminal granuloma or polyp, or fibrotic intestinal strictures, mechanical obstruction may occur. In this situation, nonspecific signs of mechanical ileus will be seen.

Computed tomography

To date no specific CT features have been described for noninfectious inflammatory intestinal diseases. Nonspecific signs of enteritis are expected to be observed. Granulomas and polyps are expected to display features of benign lesions on CT such as the presence of an intraluminal mass with smooth margins, homogeneous enhancement or peripheral rim enhancement, and normal adjacent wall thickness.

Neoplastic diseases

Ultrasonography and contrast-enhanced ultrasonography

A decision tree is proposed to help the veterinary surgeon evaluate the type of pathology depending on the ultrasonographic alterations of the intestinal wall (Fig. 5.14).

Focal GI masses are generally neoplastic, although there may be exceptions. Lymphoma is the most common intestinal tumour, and adenocarcinoma is the most common nonlymphoid tumour, followed by mast cell tumour (Fig. 5.16).

Figure 5.16. Imaging of focal thickening of the gastrointestinal wall.

The Siamese breed and increasing age (particularly cats aged 10–14 years) are associated with an increased risk of carcinoma. Lymphoma is the most common tumour of the feline stomach; compared to dogs, gastric adenocarcinoma is very rare in cats. Lymphoma can present with a variety of ultrasonographic features.[19] The most frequently observed are solitary or multiple intestinal masses or a diffuse thickening of the small intestinal muscular layer with otherwise normal layering of the wall. When it takes the appearance of a mass, it is more likely to be intermediate or high in grade. The ultrasonographic features are generally transmural, hypoechoic, circumferential thickening of the GI wall associated with loss of normal wall layering and decreased motility of the affected intestinal segment (Video 5.3).[19] The mass can be symmetrical or asymmetrical, and ulceration may or may not occur. Ultrasonographic evidence of regional lymphadenopathy is common and often corresponds to a mass palpated during physical examination. Mesenteric involvement due to direct extension from a lymphomatous mass, which results in the presence of small hypoechoic nodules within the adjacent mesenteric fat, has also been described. Gastric and intestinal lymphomas show a radiating or sun-rising vascular pattern on both colour Doppler interrogation and CEUS due to the presence and prominence of large vessels running perpendicular to the lumen and serosa.

Similarly, the ultrasound appearance of feline GI adenocarcinomas has been reported. Adenocarcinomas are typically present as solitary intestinal masses. Circumferential segmental wall thickening characterised by transmural loss of normal wall layering is a feature described in cats with GI adenocarcinoma. These tumours may be symmetrical or asymmetrical and may have a similar appearance to GI lymphoma. One reported difference is that intestinal adenocarcinoma is more likely to present a mixed echogenicity, whereas lymphoma is more commonly associated with a uniformly hypoechoic intestinal wall, although the definitive diagnosis must be based on histopathological examination of tissue samples. Intestinal tumours, particularly adenocarcinomas, may cause intestinal obstruction, and fluid may accumulate within the loops proximal to the lesion due to mechanical ileus. In the authors' experience, GI adenocarcinoma shows a mixed heterogeneous vascular pattern on both colour Doppler interrogation and CEUS, with early washout on CEUS, consistent with a malignant behaviour.

Video 5.3. Ultrasound study of a 13-year-old Siberian cat presented with chronic vomiting. The B-mode ultrasound shows a massive transmural asymmetrical hypoechoic circumferential thickening of the wall of the pyloric antrum and a normal aspect of the gastric fundus and body. On colour Doppler, multiple intralesional vessels running perpendicular to the lumen are seen. On contrast-enhanced ultrasound, a homogeneous intense "radiating" washing is observed followed by a homogeneous progressive slow washout. Ultrasound-guided fine needle aspiration of the lesion was then performed using a 22-gauge needle and capillary technique, avoiding the lumen of the stomach. Cytological examination was consistent with high-grade lymphoma.

Mast cell tumours have been reported to occur in cats as focal masses in the duodenum, jejunum, ICCJ, and colon or, more rarely, as diffuse intestinal wall thickening.[20] They have also been documented to cause selective thickening of the small intestine muscularis in cats. Mast cell tumours are most commonly identified as a focal hypoechoic thickening of the intestinal wall associated with loss of normal layering and may be either noncircumferential and eccentric or circumferential, asymmetrical, and eccentric. Cats with low-grade lymphoma display a diffuse selective thickening of the muscularis layer.[14] Average wall thickness is usually within the normal range in cats with lymphoma, and wall layering is generally preserved. In one study of cats with low-grade lymphoma, the mean wall thickness was 4.3 mm (median 4.5 mm, range 3.4–5 mm). Mesenteric lymphadenopathy is also frequent. Another study reported a diffuse intestinal wall thickening in 22/27 (81%) cats with low-grade lymphoma. Focal intestinal mass formation, intussusception, and decreased mucosal echogenicity were also found occasionally in cats with low-grade lymphoma. However, normal intestinal wall thickness and the absence of changes in the mesenteric lymph node do not rule out low-grade lymphoma.

Carcinoma and lymphoma are commonly encountered tumours of the caecum and colon in cats. Carcinomas cause annular thickening with obstruction, which is rarely seen in cases of colic lymphoma. Other tumours such as leiomyoma and leiomyosarcoma of the caecum and colon also occur but are rare. No ultrasonographic description of their aspect in the large intestine of cats is available in the literature. In the authors' experience, they demonstrate similar features to those described in the small intestine. Mast cell tumours have been described in the ICCJ and colon in cats. Haemangiosarcomas have been reported in the ICCJ, colon, and rectum in cats and cause luminal narrowing and obstruction.

Radiography and contrast radiography

Although survey radiographs may be suggestive of gastric or intestinal wall thickening, a normal intestinal wall associated with intraluminal fluid cannot be differentiated from true wall thickening, as soft tissue and fluids have similar radiographic opacities. Therefore, in many cases, survey radiographs will be unremarkable. If focal thickening is severe enough to cause a chronic partial obstruction, a gravel sign may be observed (Fig. 5.17). Granular soft tissue and mineral material accumulate in a distended intestinal segment orally to the obstruction site. If focal thickening is severe enough, a "rigid" appearance of an intestinal loop may be seen, and this image will be persistent on subsequent radiographs. Small intestinal masses are usually visible in the central abdomen, with peripheral displacement of the other small intestinal loops. Neoplastic infiltration may cause perforation, and pneumoabdomen and loss of serosal details may be seen.

For subtle or moderate wall thickening, an upper GI study or barium enema are necessary for an accurate assessment of the intestinal or rectocolic wall diameter and better define the intraluminal lesion, its point of attachment to the intestinal or colonic wall, and its symmetry in the wall. If a mass lesion is visible, it typically appears either as an irregular filling defect originating from one side of the intestinal wall, as an annular constriction with luminal narrowing, as pedunculated, or as mural eccentric. These findings are nonspecific, and ultrasound is necessary to further evaluate the wall thickening and layering. CM adherence to the mucosa is indicative of mucosal ulceration.

Computed tomography

In a recent study on the use of hydro-CT to evaluate gastric lesions, three cats had gastric lymphoma in different locations such as cardia/fundus, lesser curvature, and fundus/body. All cats had moderate to severe gastric wall thickening at that level, with moderate heterogeneous contrast enhancement of the lesion. One cat also had a hiatal hernia. Lymphoma in the intestine is often circumferential, with moderate heterogeneous contrast enhancement and a hyperattenuating mucosa. Increased tortuous arteries may be seen supplying the affected portion of the stomach. Gastric adenocarcinomas appear as a focal wall thickening without discrete wall layering. Contrast enhancement is heterogeneous with a hyperattenuating mucosa. In the intestine, adenocarcinomas appear as a circumferential wall thickening with heterogeneous contrast enhancement. Leiomyomas or leiomyosarcomas are generally an eccentric, homogeneously (leiomyoma)

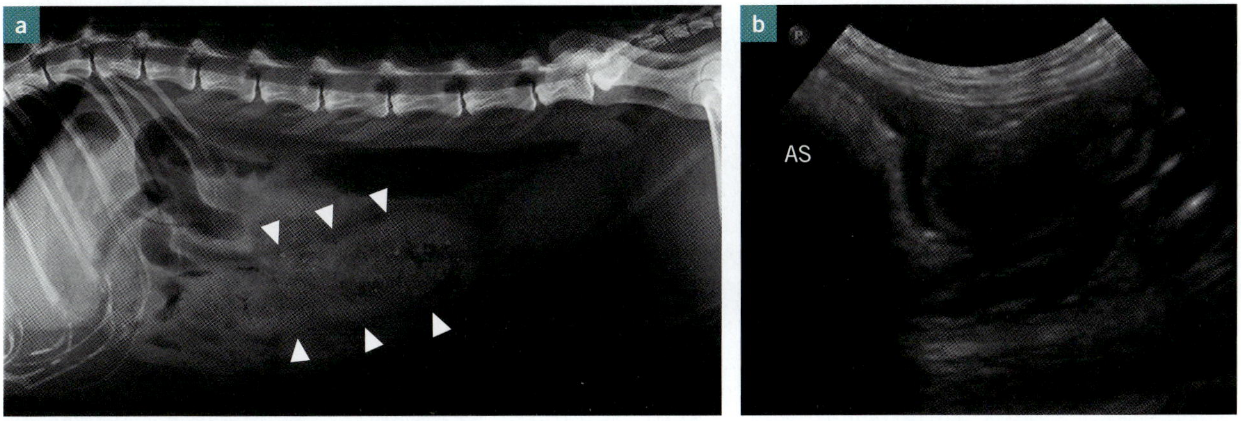

Figure 5.17. Lateral radiograph (a) and ultrasonographic image (b) of a cat presenting with a chronic subobstruction due to a jejunal adenocarcinoma. Note the gravel sign in the central abdomen due to the presence of heterogeneous mixed soft tissue and mineral material in a markedly distended small intestinal loop (arrowheads). This material casts a strong acoustic shadow (AS) on ultrasound, aboral to the asymmetrical hypoechoic mass that distorts the jejunal wall and lumen.

or heterogeneously (leiomyosarcoma) contrast-enhancing mass originating from the intestinal or colonic wall. The mass may obstruct the intestinal or colonic lumen. Colic adenocarcinomas may present central mineral foci on unenhanced CT images. They are generally seen as an eccentric heterogeneously and peripherally contrast-enhancing mass arising from the wall of the colon, and the colonic lumen may be obstructed by the mass.

Postoperative follow-up and complications

Enterotomy and enterectomy sites are generally well identified on ultrasound; the suture can be seen as bright foci in the intestinal wall. Focal thickening of the intestine with loss of layering is generally observed. This should resolve completely or partially with time. Normal peristalsis should be observed in the next hours following surgery. Postoperative dehiscence is challenging to diagnose, as free fluid and free gas may be normally seen postoperatively. However, collection of fluid close to the surgical site, thinning of wall, and trapped gas bubbles inside and outside the intestinal wall are strongly suggestive of dehiscence. A fluid sample cytological examination result consistent with septic fluid further supports the diagnosis of dehiscence. Adjacent mesentery may also be hyperechoic, but this is also routinely observed on normal postoperative ultrasound. In case of intestinal wall perforation, hyperechoic mesentery due to focal peritonitis or steatitis is generally seen near the perforation site as a consequence of spontaneous omentalisation. The affected wall is generally thickened and hypoechoic with loss of layering in case of perforation secondary to foreign body migration, deep ulceration, or postoperative dehiscence. A hyperechoic tract due to the presence of the perforating foreign body or migration tract filled with gas bubbles can be seen crossing the wall, with accumulation of a pocket of anechoic or cellular-free fluid at the same level.

Congenital disorders

Congenital abnormalities of the anus and/or rectum associated with urogenital malformations originate from abnormal embryonic development of the cloacal region. Rectovaginal fistulae and *atresia ani* have been reported in cats. They are correlated with a failure of the urorectal septum to completely divide the cloaca into the vestibulo-vesical and rectal segments and a failure of the anal membrane to perforate after anal formation. As shown by the literature and the authors' experience, type II *atresia ani* may be the most common form encountered

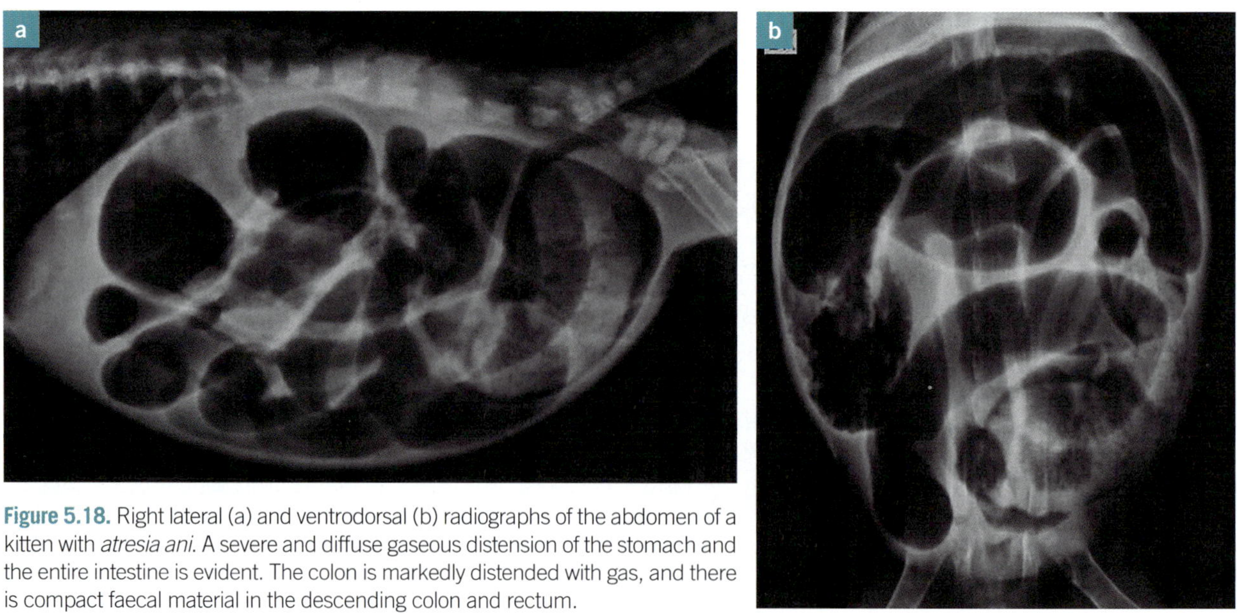

Figure 5.18. Right lateral (a) and ventrodorsal (b) radiographs of the abdomen of a kitten with *atresia ani*. A severe and diffuse gaseous distension of the stomach and the entire intestine is evident. The colon is markedly distended with gas, and there is compact faecal material in the descending colon and rectum.

in cats. Megacolon or severe gaseous distension of the large intestine is generally present on plain radiographs (Fig. 5.18). A vaginogram (intravaginal administration of 2 ml iohexol using a 22-gauge catheter) is generally performed to illustrate a connection between the vagina and the rectum. As the anus is not perforated or is absent, a barium enema cannot be performed. The CM is seen entering the faeces-filled colon from the vagina through a small fistula, indicating a rectovaginal communication.

Duplication cysts have been reported in cats as a cause of oesophageal compression (see section "Oesophageal pathologies" in this chapter). Enteric duplication cysts are unusual congenital malformations that may result from small or large, single or multiple duplications of the oesophagus, duodenum, jejunum, ileum, colon, or rectum. In general, affected cats are young (<2 years). Three main features characterise intestinal duplication cysts: an established relationship with the GI tract, a well-developed smooth muscle layer, and an epithelial lining that may differ from that of the adjacent intestinal section.

Ultrasonographically, they are fluid-filled spherical or tubular cysts containing sterile fluid. They typically do not communicate with the intestinal lumen. The presence of a distinct hypoechoic layer of smooth muscle inside the cyst wall has been recently identified as a "muscular rim sign" and is usually continuous to the adjacent intestinal segment of smooth muscle. The cyst wall contains an inner hyperechoic surface (the mucosa) surrounded by an outer hypoechoic layer (muscular layer), an appearance considered unique to this disorder. A case of malignant transformation of a duodenal duplication cyst has been described in a 15-year-old domestic shorthair cat. Therefore, surgical excision is recommended. Duplication cysts have also been reported in different species in conjunction with vertebral abnormalities; therefore, radiography should be considered in affected cats.

Motility disorders

Common causes of megacolon include chronic constipation and nutritional, metabolic, or mechanical disorders. Chronic renal disease and the associated subclinical dehydration are also commonly associated with megacolon. In addition, idiopathic cases of megacolon can occur, more commonly in cats. Neurological diseases associated with megacolon include spinal cord diseases such as cauda equina syndrome (most common cause in cats is traumatic sacrococcygeal luxation), sacrococcygeal agenesis in Manx cats, dysautonomia, and Hirschsprung's disease. Radiography is the technique of choice to confirm megacolon; to assess the degree of distension of the colon, the shape and density of the faecal material, and the width of the pelvic canal for mechanical causes of obstruction; and to monitor the efficacy of enemas (Fig. 5.19). Ultrasound is indicated to find a primary cause of megacolon not identified on radiographs. Radiographically, it is difficult to differentiate constipation and obstipation from megacolon. Several studies have attempted to define some rules to assist with this differentiation: megacolon is suspected when the colon is three times larger than the small intestines or greater than the length of the vertebral body of L7 or more than 1.4 times the length of the vertebral body of L5.[11] The opacity of the faeces depends on the duration of the obstipation. The longer the faecal material remains in the colon, the more desiccated and opaquer it becomes.

Short colon syndrome has been sporadically described in cats. Its main radiographic features include the lack of visualisation of the ascending and transverse colon and subjective colonic shortening. On ultrasound, the ascending and transverse colon cannot be identified, and the ICCJ is displaced towards the left side of the abdomen, close to the left kidney and immediately cranial to the apex of the urinary bladder. Thickening of the wall is also observed, with severe irregular submucosal and muscularis layer thickening. The layering is generally maintained.

Feline dysautonomia is characterised by general degeneration of the autonomic nervous system, resulting in distension and/or impairment of the oesophagus, distension and hypomotility of the stomach and intestine, distension of the urinary bladder, and pupillary impairment. Radiographic anomalies suggesting feline dysautonomia include megaoesophagus, dilated stomach, severe diffuse functional ileus, aspiration pneumonia, and distended urinary bladder (Fig. 5.20). Delayed transit of CM may be seen on an upper GI contrast study.

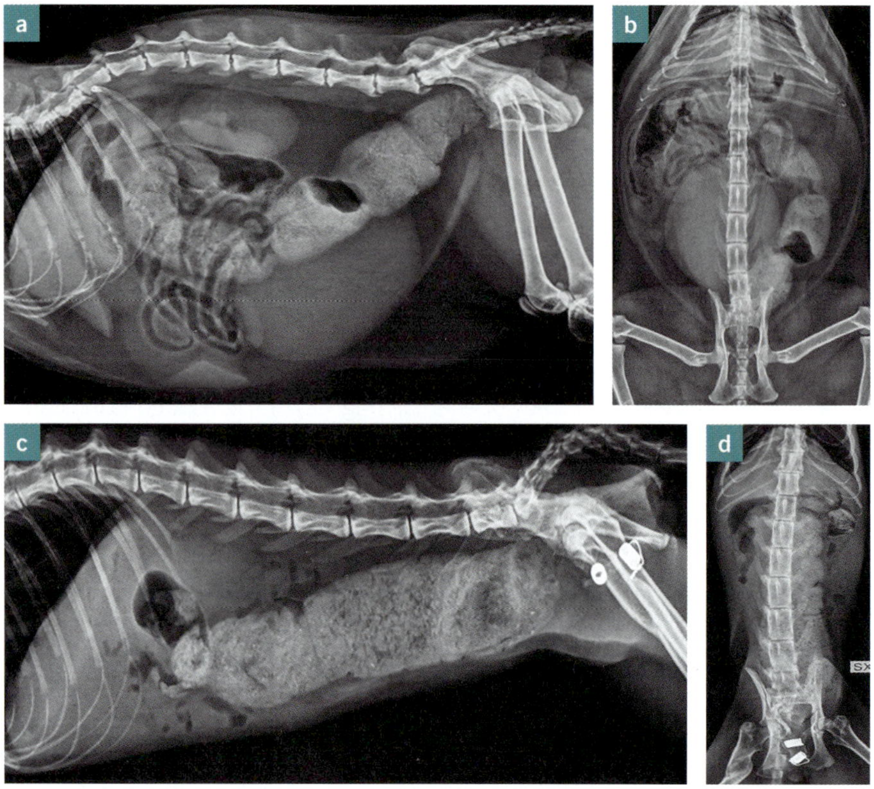

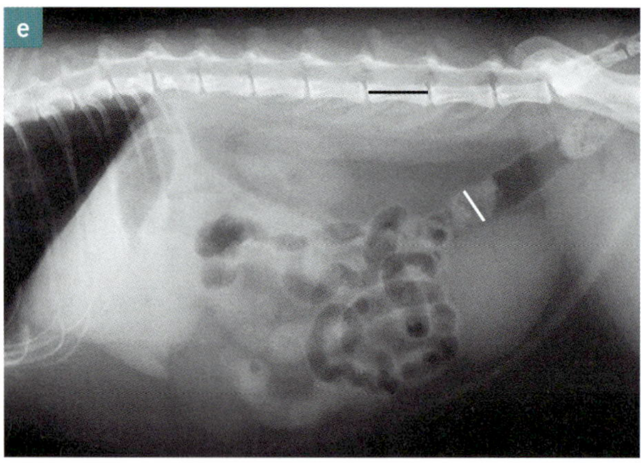

Figure 5.19. Imaging of motility disorders of the colon. Lateral (a) and ventrodorsal (b) radiographs of the abdomen of a senior cat with megacolon due to the narrowing of the pelvic canal, most likely due to prior nutritional hyperparathyroidism (documented in the cat's history). Lateral (c) and ventrodorsal (d) radiographs of the abdomen of a cat affected by megacolon due to multiple pelvic fractures. Note the increased opacity of the faecal material due to desiccation. Lateral radiograph of the abdomen of a clinically healthy adult cat (e) showing the normal course of the descending colon, which contains a combination of gas and formed faecal material. In cats without gastrointestinal disease, a ratio of maximal colonic diameter (white line) to L5 vertebral body length (black line) below 1.28 is consistent with a normal colon.

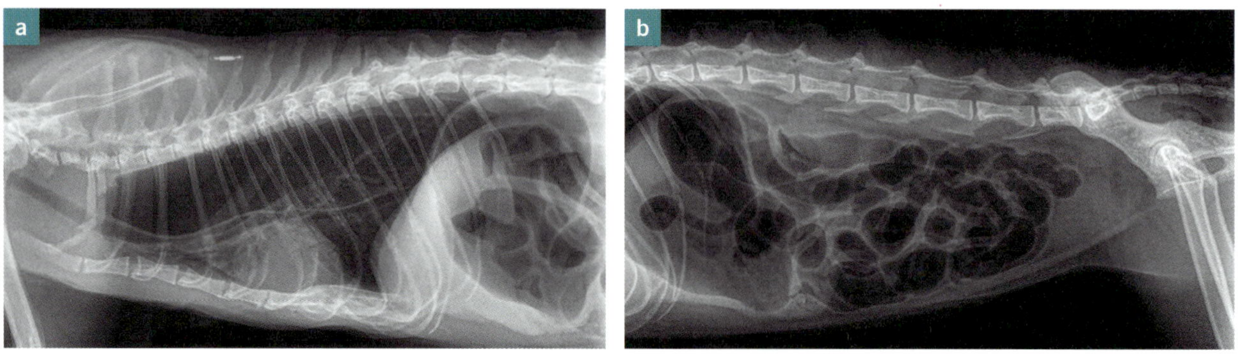

Figure 5.20. Lateral radiographs of the thorax (a) and the abdomen (b) of a cat with dysautonomia. A severe and diffuse gaseous dilation of the oesophagus (megaoesophagus), stomach, and small intestine (functional ileus) can be seen.

IMAGE-GUIDED INTERVENTIONAL PROCEDURES OF THE GASTROINTESTINAL TRACT

Percutaneous ultrasound-guided FNA and biopsy are useful and safe procedures for the diagnostic workup of GI lesions.[21] Depending on the location of the lesion, these procedures may be alternative to endoscopic or surgical biopsy. They are generally performed when lesions are not accessible with endoscopy, particularly when lesions are located in the small intestine or in the deeper portion of the GI wall (muscularis and serosal layers). They may also be considered when surgery is not a viable option (e.g. unstable patient, declined by owners as too invasive).

The most important principle is to avoid the lumen, as sampling could lead to perforation of the GI wall and septic peritonitis. Therefore, the thickness of the lesion should be sufficient to limit the risk of passing through the lumen. The main limitation of the techniques is the thickness of the lesion itself, its position with regard to the lumen, and the limited size of the sample. Even with ultrasound-guided biopsy, the sample will never be as large as the one obtained with surgery and will never provide a full-thickness visualisation of the intestine, thereby offering a limited aspect of the disease.

FNA is generally performed using either a 22- or 20-gauge needle or a spinal needle. Capillary, aspiration, or a mixed technique may be used depending on the lesion (the authors personally adapt the technique depending on the specimen obtained on the first FNA). Some lesions such as carcinoma may not easily exfoliate; therefore, aspiration may be required to obtain an adequate number of cells. FNA or biopsy of the adjacent lymph nodes are also strongly advised by the authors, as they usually complete or provide the cytological or histopathological diagnosis of the GI lesion. Semiautomatic or automatic biopsy using a 16- or 18-gauge Tru-Cut needle is generally performed to obtain ultrasound-guided biopsy samples from GI lesions. Care should be taken when a mast cell tumour is considered in the differential diagnosis, as they may degranulate during the procedure.

Take-home messages

- Ultrasound is the technique of choice to evaluate the feline gastrointestinal tract due to the dimensions of the patient and recently advanced technologies. It cannot be replaced by cross-sectional modalities due to their lower spatial resolution and their lack of dynamic and real-time evaluation of the gastrointestinal tract.
- The main limitation of ultrasound is the impossibility of distinguishing low-grade lymphoma from inflammatory bowel disease.
- Ultrasound is a fundamental step in the diagnostic workup of a gastrointestinal lesion, as it guides the clinician in choosing the next diagnostic step; for instance, deciding between ultrasound-guided fine needle aspiration, endoscopic-guided biopsy, and surgical full-thickness wall biopsy.
- Radiography is the first step to exclude mechanical ileus and obstruction.
- Radiography and computed tomography are useful for evaluating the intrathoracic oesophagus and intrapelvic colon and rectum.
- Diagnostic imaging is very useful to diagnose many emergent/newly recognised diseases (e.g. feline gastrointestinal eosinophilic sclerosing fibroplasia, mast cell tumour, strictures, ischaemic, ileocaecocolic junction disease).

REFERENCES

[1] Couturier L et al. Ultrasonographic characterization of the feline cardia and pylorus in 34 healthy cats and three abnormal cats. *Vet Radiol Ultrasound* 53:342, 2012.

[2] Diana A et al. Contrast-enhanced ultrasonography of the small bowel in healthy cats. *Vet Radiol Ultrasound* 52:555, 2011.

[3] Linta N et al. Two-dimensional and contrast-enhanced ultrasound of intestinal ischaemia in cats: four cases. *J Feline Med Surg* 22:384, 2020.

[4] Chandler ML, Guilford G, Lawoko CR. Radiopaque markers to evaluate gastric emptying and small intestinal transit time in healthy cats. *J Vet Intern Med* 11:361, 1997.

[5] Terragni R et al. Stomach wall evaluation using helical hydro-computed tomography. *Vet Radiol Ultrasound* 53:402, 2012.

[6] Levine JS, Pollard RE, Marks SL. Contrast videofluoroscopic assessment of dysphagic cats. *Vet Radiol Ultrasound* 55:465, 2014.

[7] Heng HG et al. Fat is responsible for an intramural radiolucent band in the feline stomach wall. *Vet Radiol Ultrasound* 46:54, 2005.

[8] Di Donato P et al. Ultrasonographic measurement of the relative thickness of intestinal wall layers in clinically healthy cats. *J Feline Med Surg* 16:333, 2014.

[9] Winter MD et al. Ultrasonographic evaluation of relative gastrointestinal layer thickness in cats without clinical evidence of gastrointestinal tract disease. *J Feline Med Surg* 16:118, 2014.

[10] Hahn H et al. Ultrasonographic, endoscopic and histological appearance of the caecum in clinically healthy cats. *J Feline Med Surg* 19:85, 2017.

[11] Trevail T et al. Radiographic diameter of the colon in normal and constipated cats and in cats with megacolon. *Vet Radiol Ultrasound* 52:516, 2011.

[12] Tucker S et al. Clinicopathological and ultrasonographic features of cats with eosinophilic enteritis. *J Feline Med Surg* 16:950, 2014.

[13] Penninck DG, Webster CR, Keating JH. The sonographic appearance of intestinal mucosal fibrosis in cats. *Vet Radiol Ultrasound* 51:458, 2010.

[14] Zwingenberger AL et al. Ultrasonographic evaluation of the muscularis propria in cats with diffuse small intestinal lymphoma or inflammatory bowel disease. *J Vet Intern Med* 24:289, 2010.

[15] Taeymans O et al. Ultrasonographic characterization of feline ileocecocolic abnormalities. *Vet Radiol Ultrasound* 52:335, 2011.

[16] Weissman A et al. Ultrasonographic and clinicopathological features of feline gastrointestinal eosinophilic sclerosing fibroplasia in four cats. *J Feline Med Surg* 15:148, 2013.

[17] Daure E et al. Ultrasonographic and clinicopathological features of pyloroduodenal adenomatous polyps in cats. *J Feline Med Surg* 19:141, 2017.

[18] Holloway A, Pivetta M, Rasotto R. Ultrasonographic and histopathological features in 8 cats with fibrotic small intestinal stricture. *Vet Radiol Ultrasound* 60:423, 2019.

[19] Penninck DG et al. Ultrasonography of alimentary lymphosarcoma in the cat. *Vet Radiol Ultrasound* 35:299, 1994.

[20] Laurenson MP et al. Ultrasonography of intestinal mast cell tumors in the cat. *Vet Radiol Ultrasound* 52:330, 2011.

[21] Penninck DG et al. The technique of percutaneous ultrasound guided fine-needle aspiration biopsy and automated microcore biopsy in small animal gastrointestinal diseases. *Vet Radiol Ultrasound* 34:433, 1993.

[22] Goggin JM et al. Ultrasonographic measurement of gastrointestinal wall thickness and the ultrasonographic appearance of the ileocolic region in healthy cats. *J Am Anim Hosp Assoc* 36:224, 2000.

CHAPTER 6

Diagnostic imaging of the biliary system and pancreas

Nathalie Rademacher, Kassandra Wilson

The biliary tree and gallbladder constitute the biliary system, and its evaluation in cats relies heavily on diagnostic imaging. Main clinical indications for performing diagnostic imaging of the biliary tract and pancreas are suspected cholecystitis, pancreatitis, pancreatic or biliary neoplasia, or to rule out extrahepatic biliary obstruction.

RADIOGRAPHIC EVALUATION OF THE BILIARY TRACT AND PANCREAS

While radiographs are a common first line of diagnostic imaging, they are neither sensitive nor specific for diagnosing biliary or pancreatic disease. Mineralised densities involving the biliary tree can reflect stasis of bile flow or dystrophic mineralisation associated with congenital malformations, acquired duct "sacculation", chronic duct inflammation, or cholelithiasis. Some choleliths contain enough calcium bilirubinate to be radiographically visible (Fig. 6.1). In cats, especially those with obesity, the pancreas can sometimes be visualised on the ventrodorsal view between the spleen and the caudal stomach as a wispy to triangular soft tissue opacity. A mass effect in the right cranial quadrant in suspected extrahepatic bile duct obstruction (EHBDO) may represent an engorged gallbladder, pancreatitis, neoplasia, or focal bile peritonitis. Radiographic suspicion of abdominal effusion (poor abdominal detail) may prompt early diagnosis of bile peritonitis or pancreatitis. Gas within biliary structures

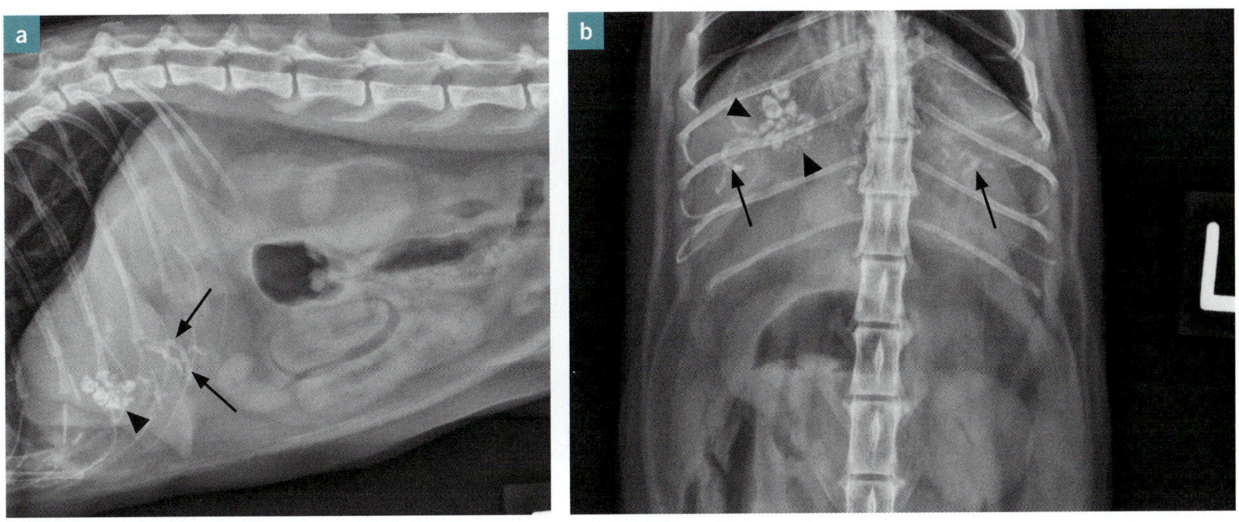

Figure 6.1. Lateral (a) and ventrodorsal (b) radiographs of the abdomen of a 17-year-old spayed female Burmese cat with intrahepatic bile duct mineralisation (arrows) seen as linear tubular mineralisation and cholelithiasis (arrowheads) superimposed with the right cranioventral liver. The findings were incidental.

or the liver might indicate an emphysematous process (e.g. cholecystitis, choledochitis, infected biliary cyst, hepatic abscess, necrotic tumour mass). Anticipated radiographic changes for feline pancreatitis include a mass effect in the region of the pancreas, loss of serosal detail due to peripancreatic effusion, and the presence of dilated bowel loops due to ileus.[1]

ULTRASONOGRAPHIC EVALUATION OF THE BILIARY TRACT AND PANCREAS

Ultrasound is superior to radiography in the evaluation of the biliary tract and pancreas, particularly in cats with poor body condition or those that have abdominal effusion, both of which decrease serosal detail and reduce the clinician's ability to assess the pancreas and biliary system radiographically. In veterinary medicine, B-mode ultrasound imaging is used frequently but has proven to be unsatisfactory in many patients. Ultrasonography has low sensitivity and specificity to cholangitis and pancreatitis and correlates poorly with histopathological diagnosis, although advanced stages of disease can be detected.

Normal ultrasonographic appearance

The gallbladder is located to the right of the midline between the two parts of the right medial liver lobe. The gallbladder wall may or may not be visible with ultrasound. When seen, it forms an echogenic line less than 1 mm in thickness.[2,3] On average, over 12% of cats have some form of accessory gallbladder, and most represent incidental findings during ultrasound, surgery, or at necropsy and cause no clinical signs. In some individuals, the gallbladder is bilobed, which represents a congenital anomaly that arises during embryonic development.[4] Two different types of bilobed gallbladder have been described. In the first type, the gallbladder lumen is partially divided by an internal longitudinal septum (Fig. 6.2). The two resulting chambers communicate at their proximal extent by a single shared cystic duct, and the external appearance of the gallbladder is normal. In the second type, the fundus of the gallbladder is completely divided, and the two cavities fuse only at the neck, resulting in a "V" or valentine heart shape when viewed externally.[4] Duplex gallbladders, which have rarely been reported in the cat, involve two entirely separate cavities, each supplied by their own cystic duct.[4] Gallbladder volume and contractility can be assessed during ultrasound, and a wide range in gallbladder volume of 0.84–4.5 ml (mean volume 2.41 ml), with no correlation to body weight, has been reported.[5] Mean pre- and postprandial (2 hours after eating) volumes of 2.47 ± 1.16 ml and 0.88 ± 0.13 ml, respectively, have been reported in the normal cat.[6]

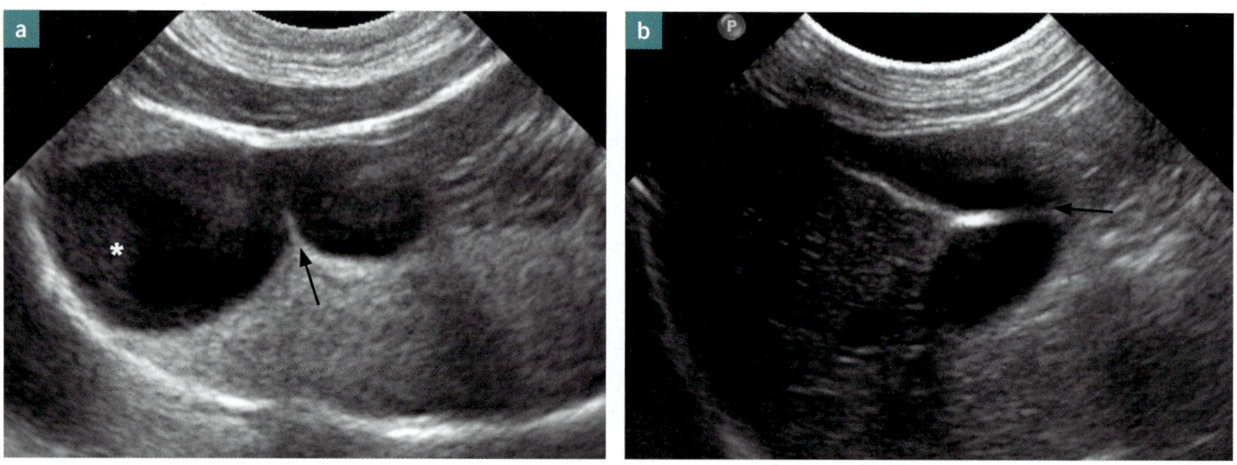

Figure 6.2. Ultrasonographic appearance of a bilobed gallbladder in two different cats. In the first cat (a), an incomplete septum (arrow) is present in addition to a mild amount of gravity-dependent hyperechoic gallbladder sludge (asterisk). In the other cat (b), a longitudinal ultrasound image shows a bilobed gallbladder, with the septum present (arrow).

The feline common bile duct (CBD) is long and tortuous compared with its canine counterpart (Fig. 6.3a) and can be routinely identified on ultrasound as a tubular anechoic structure with echogenic walls located ventral to the portal vein at the porta hepatis using either a subcostal approach or a right cranial intercostal window.[7] The normal CBD may be differentiated from blood vessels by its thicker walls, tortuosity, and absence of flow signal when examined with colour Doppler ultrasound (Fig. 6.3b). It can usually be followed caudally without too much difficulty to the junction where it merges with the major pancreatic duct prior to its entry into the duodenum via the major duodenal papilla (Figs. 6.3c and 6.3d).[7] Only 20% of cats are estimated to have an accessory pancreatic duct with its own separate opening into the duodenum. The normal CBD should measure no greater than 4 mm in diameter, and the wall of the duct should be less than 1 mm in thickness. Intra- and extrahepatic ducts are not normally visible unless pathologically dilated. The pancreatic duct can be visualised as an anechoic tubular structure with highly echogenic walls and is very prominent in the feline pancreas (Fig. 6.4a). The pancreatic duct diameter ranges from 0.7 to 2.5 mm, with a mean of about 1.0 mm. There is a slight increase in pancreatic duct diameter with increasing age (Fig. 6.4b).[7]

The feline pancreas is a well-defined organ when imaged with a good-quality ultrasound machine and a high-frequency transducer, although it can initially appear somewhat inconspicuous to the untrained eye. The pancreas can be visualised in most cats, and anatomic landmarks are essential in defining the pancreatic area. Ultrasound imaging is very sensitive at identifying biliary and pancreatic abnormalities but often lacks specificity, and therefore cytology or histopathology are required for

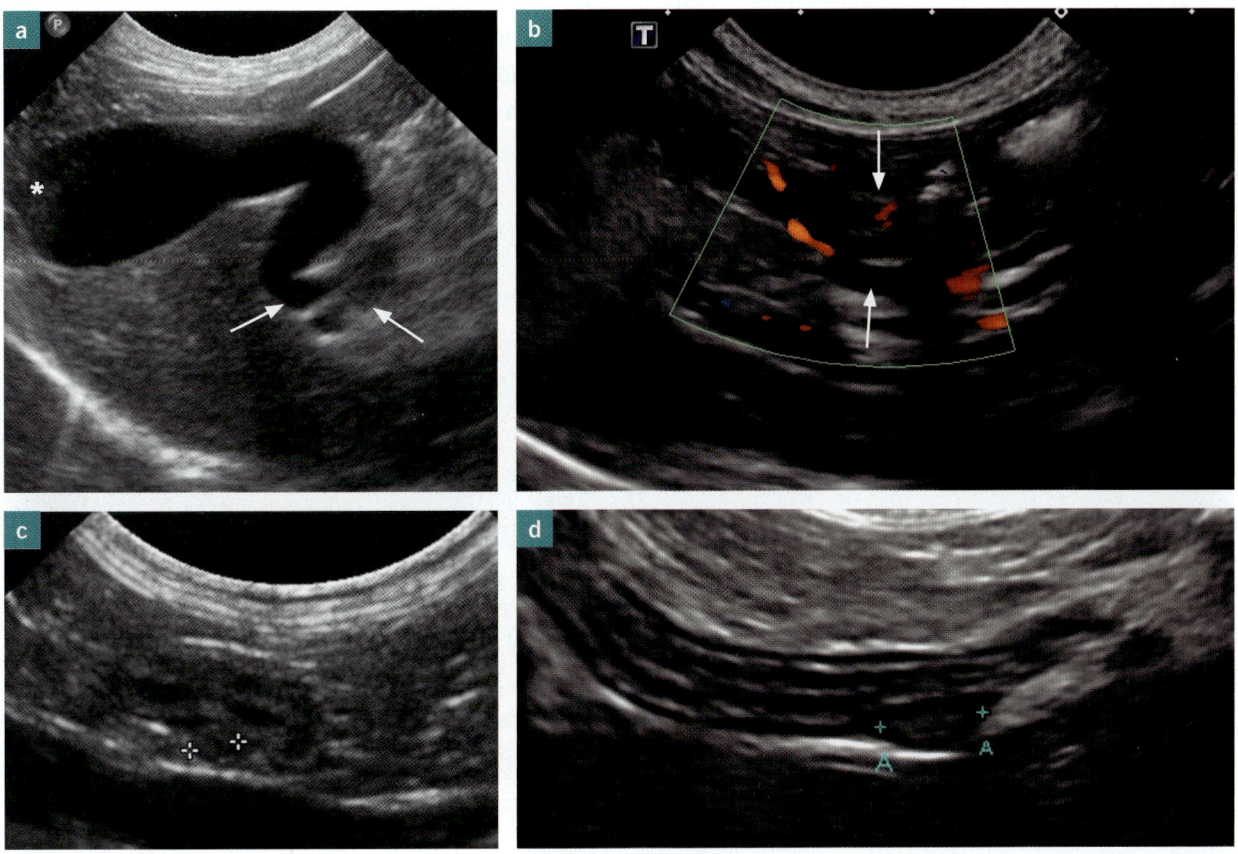

Figure 6.3. Longitudinal ultrasound image of the gallbladder of a cat (a) showing a mild amount of gravity-dependent hyperechoic gallbladder sludge (asterisk). Note the long and tortuous common bile duct (arrows), which is a normal finding in the cat. With power Doppler ultrasound (b), the common bile duct (arrows) can be differentiated from a blood vessel by the lack of flow signal. Transverse (c) and longitudinal (d) ultrasonographic images of the duodenum of a cat showing the major duodenal papilla (callipers), where the common bile duct merges with the pancreatic duct in 80% of cats.

definitive diagnosis. Ultrasound is the modality of choice because of the advantages that awake or sedated patients can be examined, the ability to use nonionising sound waves, and the ability to evaluate the size, echogenicity, and echotexture of the pancreas. Furthermore, simultaneous evaluation of the peripancreatic fat and regional lymph nodes can be performed during the assessment of the pancreas. However, it is generally accepted that false-positive and false-negative results can occur.[2,7] Understanding what constitutes a normal biliary and pancreatic appearance on ultrasound is essential to recognise any abnormalities.

The pancreas is composed of the left lobe, the body, and the right lobe. The body and left limb of the pancreas are most easily identified in the cat. The left limb of the pancreas is much easier to visualise in the cat and lies dorsal and caudal to the greater curvature of the stomach, cranial to the transverse colon along the left abdomen, and is oriented towards the left kidney (Figs. 6.4a and 6.4b). The right limb of the pancreas is located along the descending duodenum and extends caudally towards the right kidney (Fig. 6.4c). The pancreatic body lies immediately caudal and dorsal to the pyloroduodenal junction, ventral to the portal vein, and medial to the proximal duodenum.[7] The pancreas is isoechoic or slightly hypoechoic to the surrounding mesentery and the liver, with the pancreatic parenchyma having a uniform, homogeneous appearance.[7] Normal ranges for the feline pancreatic body and left limb width are 0.3–1.0 cm, with a mean of approximately 5.0 mm. The right limb is smaller, at 0.3–0.6 cm.[2] The pancreaticoduodenal vein extends through the right limb, coursing caudally in an undulating fashion, parallel to the descending duodenum, and creates a helpful landmark to identify the right pancreas in the dog but is less conspicuous in the cat.[7]

Appearance of biliary system disease

In cats, diseases of the gallbladder and bile ducts are more common than diseases of the liver parenchyma.[8] However, a lack of pathological changes does not rule out the possibility of disease.

Gallbladder sludge and mucocele

Gallbladder sludge (Figs. 6.2a, 6.3a, and 6.5) is an accumulation of mixed particulate solids that have precipitated from bile and is an uncommon ultrasonographic finding

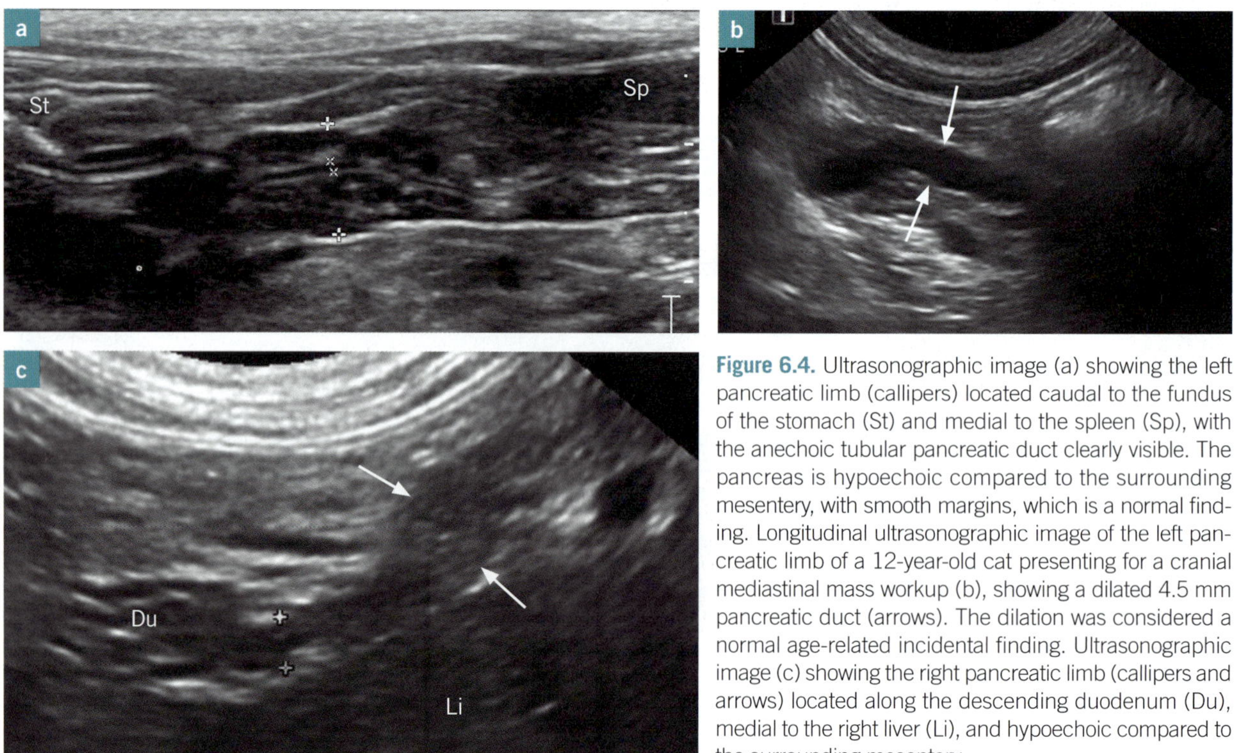

Figure 6.4. Ultrasonographic image (a) showing the left pancreatic limb (callipers) located caudal to the fundus of the stomach (St) and medial to the spleen (Sp), with the anechoic tubular pancreatic duct clearly visible. The pancreas is hypoechoic compared to the surrounding mesentery, with smooth margins, which is a normal finding. Longitudinal ultrasonographic image of the left pancreatic limb of a 12-year-old cat presenting for a cranial mediastinal mass workup (b), showing a dilated 4.5 mm pancreatic duct (arrows). The dilation was considered a normal age-related incidental finding. Ultrasonographic image (c) showing the right pancreatic limb (callipers and arrows) located along the descending duodenum (Du), medial to the right liver (Li), and hypoechoic compared to the surrounding mesentery.

in cats. An association has been identified between the presence of sludge and hepatobiliary or gastrointestinal disorders and extrahepatic biliary obstruction, and therefore cholestasis seems to be a significant factor.[9,10]

Gallbladder sludge must be differentiated from a mucocele. Cats have fewer mucous glands in the gallbladder than dogs, which may explain why mucoceles have been reported less frequently in cats than in dogs.[4,11,12] Gallbladder mucoceles result from cystic mucinous hyperplasia, which causes an abnormal increase in mucin production and consequently gallbladder distension that can ultimately lead to wall necrosis and rupture.[12] Mucinous plugs associated with the mucocele can enter and travel along the CBD and may result in EHBDO.[11] Descriptions for gallbladder mucoceles in the cat differ from the classically reported hyperechoic stellate or kiwi fruit–like pattern reported in the dog. In two cats with mucoceles diagnosed at necropsy or during surgery, the gallbladder content was described as echoic and organised,[11,12] while a third report documented no ultrasonographically visible changes and the diagnosis was made via histopathology.[4]

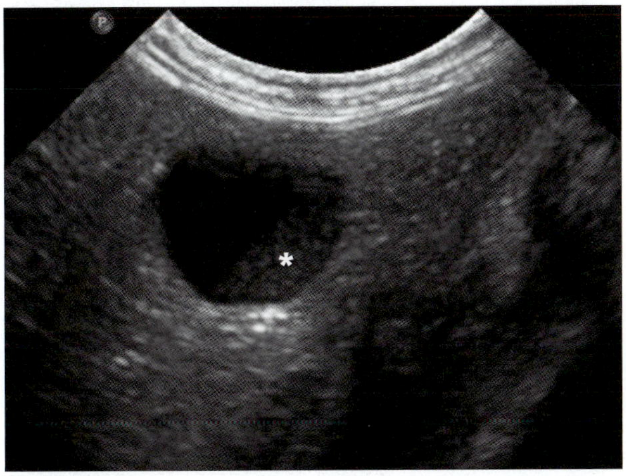

Figure 6.5. Transverse ultrasonographic image of the gallbladder of a cat showing moderate amount of hyperechoic gravity-dependent sludge (asterisk).

Gallbladder wall thickening

A gallbladder wall thickness greater than 1 mm is reported to be an accurate predictor of gallbladder disease in cats, although a thickness less than 1 mm does not rule out mild or chronic inflammation.[2] Diffuse gallbladder wall thickening is considered to be a nonspecific finding and can occur as a result of inflammation (cholecystitis, cholangitis, cholangiohepatitis), oedema (especially due to biliary obstruction), or mucosal gland hyperplasia.[13,14] Pseudothickening of the gallbladder wall due to peritoneal effusion has also been described and is believed to be the result of the acoustic interface between the peritoneal fluid and the wall of the gallbladder (Fig. 6.6).[2]

Inflammation of the biliary tree

Cholangitis is a common inflammatory disorder of the biliary system in cats. The World Small Animal Veterinary Association Liver Standardization Group[8] recognises three forms of feline cholangitis: neutrophilic,

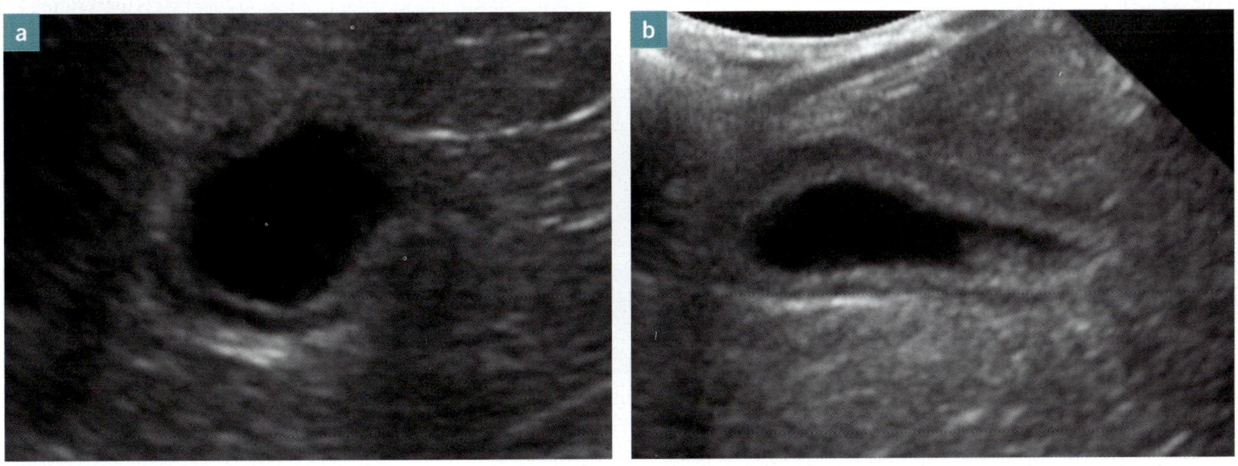

Figure 6.6. Transverse (a) and longitudinal (b) ultrasonographic images of a thickened gallbladder wall secondary to abdominal effusion in an 11-year-old spayed female Persian cat. A small amount of gallbladder sludge is present.

lymphocytic, and chronic, the latter associated with liver flukes.[13,15] Since concurrent involvement of the liver parenchyma is common, the term cholangitis/cholangiohepatitis complex (CCHC) is sometimes used. In many cases, the ultrasound examination of the liver and biliary tree is unremarkable.[13] Still, ultrasound is considered a fairly accurate diagnostic test for cholangitis in cats, with a sensitivity and a specificity reported at 87% and 90%, respectively.[16] When abnormalities are present, they can include gallbladder and/or CBD wall thickening (Fig. 6.7a); hyperechoic gallbladder contents, possibly due to either gallbladder dysfunction or biliary stasis; choleliths and/or choledocholiths; and dilation of the CBD (Fig. 6.7a) and a heterogeneous hyperechoic liver surrounding portal vessels.[13,17,18] Changes in the appearance of the gallbladder in cats with neutrophilic cholangitis may be the result of concurrent bacterial cholecystitis. *Platynosomum* species (liver flukes) are cat-specific parasitic trematodes that parasitise the biliary ducts and gallbladder and have been linked to chronic cholangitis.[15] Choledocholiths may be mineralised or nonmineralised and can be both a cause and consequence of biliary obstruction; if obstruction is complete, regardless of the underlying cause, rupture of the gallbladder or CBD can occur. Mineralised choleliths (Fig. 6.7b) and choledocholiths (Fig. 6.7c) are easily recognisable on ultrasound examination due to their hyperechoic interface and associated distal acoustic shadowing. Gallbladder choleliths are often an incidental finding; however, they can cause biliary obstruction if they migrate from the gallbladder into the CBD.

Extrahepatic bile duct obstruction

EHBDO results in a retrograde dilation of the biliary system and can often be diagnosed with ultrasound. In normal cats, intra- and extrahepatic ducts are not visible; thus, any duct visible on ultrasonography is considered dilated.[11] The diameter of the CBD is a useful parameter in diagnosing EHBDO since it is greater than 5 mm in 97% of affected cats; the upper limit for healthy cats has been established at 4 mm. In contrast, gallbladder dilation was noted in only 43% and thus is not a reliable indicator of obstruction.[11,19] In dogs with complete obstruction, the gallbladder and cystic duct start to distend within 24 hours after obstruction, with progressive dilation of the CBD within 48 hours. Further dilation of the CBD and hepatic ducts occurs during the next 3–4 days, with additional dilation of lobar and interlobar ducts seen by 7 days. Multiple tortuous, irregularly branching anechoic tracks (without Doppler signal) can be seen (Fig. 6.8a).[19] Obstruction of the CBD in cats frequently occurs close to or at the level of the duodenal papilla and can arise as a result of mural thickening, extraluminal compression, or obstruction of the lumen. Specific causes include cholangitis, acute necrotising pancreatitis, extra- or intraluminal masses (Figs. 6.8b and 6.8c), choledocholithiasis (Fig. 6.7c), and congenital abnormalities of the biliary tract (Fig. 6.8d).[11] Sludge accumulation within the bile duct associated with cholangiohepatitis and causing extrahepatic biliary obstruction is not easily differentiated from a neoplastic mass in the bile duct (Fig. 6.8b). It is important to note that incomplete or early obstruction may not cause visible biliary dilation.

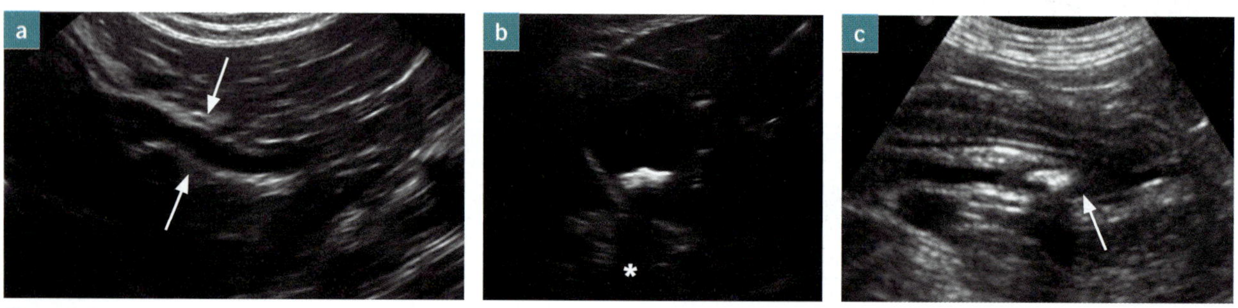

Figure 6.7. Ultrasonographic images of a cat with icterus. The common bile duct is dilated, measuring 4 mm in diameter, and has a thickened hyperechoic wall (arrows), and the surrounding mesentery is hyperechoic (a). These findings are consistent with cholangitis and choledochocystitis. The gallbladder contains a moderate amount of hyperechoic gravity-dependent material, with distal acoustic shadowing (asterisk), consistent with cholelithiasis (b). A longitudinal ultrasonographic image of the descending duodenum shows a dilated common bile duct that contains a hyperechoic shadowing choledocholith (arrow) adjacent to the major duodenal papilla (c).

In addition, the CBD in the cat can remain distended after the obstruction is relieved because of inflammation and prolonged distension resulting in a reduction of the elasticity of the duct.

Biliary cysts

Biliary cysts are classified according to whether or not they communicate with the biliary tree. Cysts that communicate with the biliary tree are known as choledochal cysts and are defined as segmental cystic dilations of extrahepatic and/or intrahepatic biliary ducts. Segmental dilation of the CBD of up to 5 mm on ultrasound with concurrent tubular to saccular intra- and extrahepatic bile duct dilation, accumulation of echogenic debris within the biliary tree, and hepatomegaly has been reported. Some cats might have ultrasonographic evidence of bile duct obstruction. However, because the maximum diameter of the dilated CBD segment may exceed 5 mm, this can easily lead to a misdiagnosis of EHBDO. It is not clear whether choledochal cysts represent congenital or acquired biliary malformations. Biliary cysts can become so large that they occupy a significant portion of the abdominal cavity, causing mechanical compression and displacement of adjacent structures such as the stomach and liver.[2,20] Multiple uni- or multilocular hepatic cysts have also been reported in association with pancreatic and renal cysts in a large proportion of cats with polycystic kidney disease.[21]

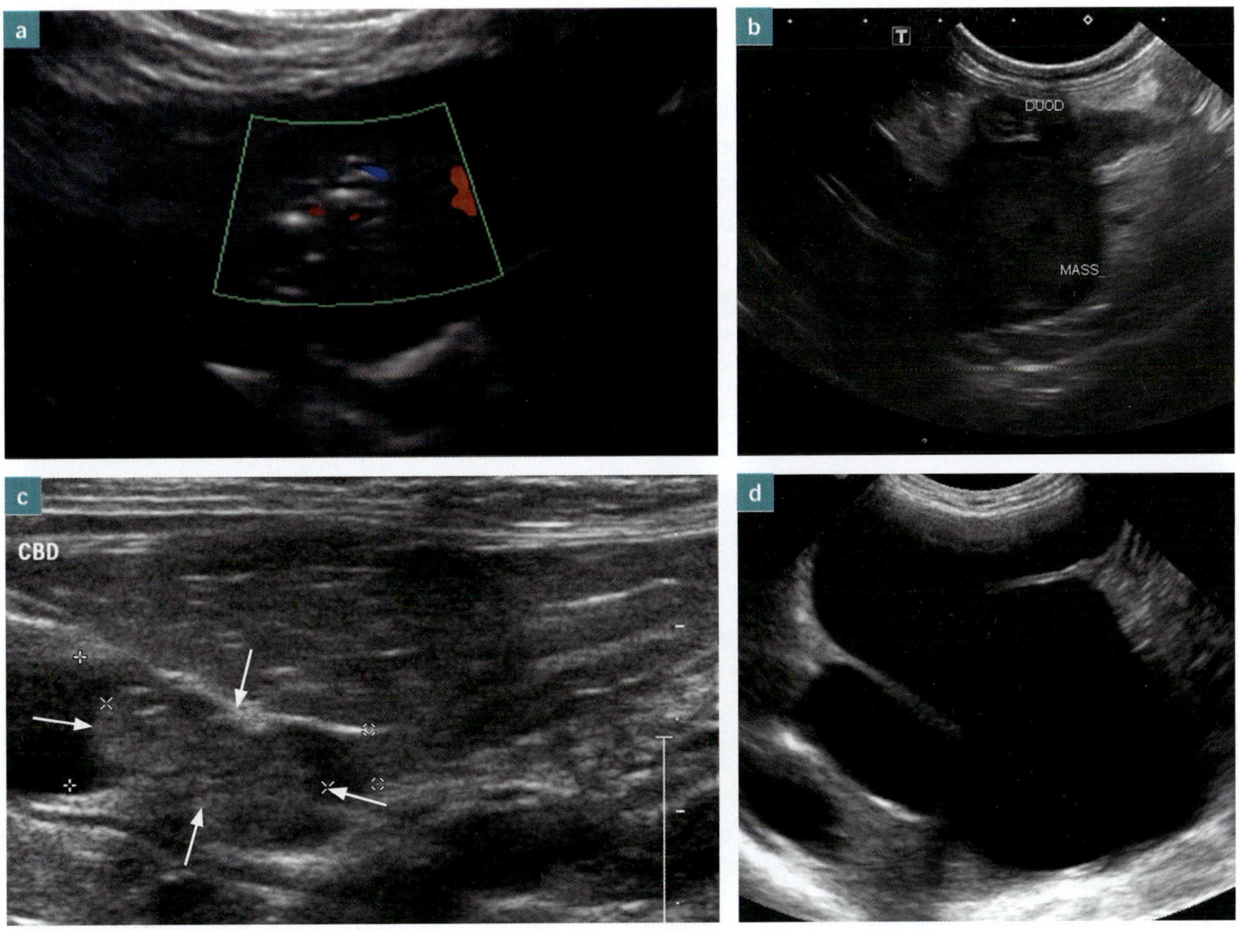

Figure 6.8. Longitudinal Doppler ultrasonographic image of the liver of a cat (a) showing intrahepatic bile duct dilation seen as anechoic tubular structures without Doppler signal parallel to portal veins. A large hypoechoic pancreatic carcinoma with secondary obstruction of the common bile duct is noted (b), with dilation of the cystic duct and incorporation of the major duodenal papilla and descending duodenum. In another cat (c), extrahepatic bile duct obstruction was present due to a well-defined hyperechoic mass (arrows) in the distal common bile duct, close to the major duodenal papilla. The common bile duct measures 7 mm in diameter. Differential diagnoses for the intraluminal mass include biliary sludge and infiltrative disease such as biliary adenoma or adenocarcinoma. Severe dilation of the common bile duct is present in this cat (d), without a specific cause identified in this case.

Biliary neoplasia

Neoplasms of the biliary system occur more frequently than neoplasms of hepatic cell origin, with the most common histotype being bile duct adenoma (45.4%), also referred to as biliary adenomas or biliary cystadenomas, followed by bile duct carcinomas (36.3%) with metastasis commonly detected.[22,23] Biliary cystadenomas (Fig. 6.9) of cats are benign liver tumours that most often appear as focal or multifocal thin-walled cystic lesions, varying in size from several millimetres to more than 10 cm, in animals that are usually 10 years of age or older.[23] Acoustic enhancement may be seen distal to some of these masses. Lesions with very small-diameter cysts may appear hyperechoic because of the increased number of acoustic interfaces. Cystadenomas may also appear as hyperechoic lesions or have mixed echogenicity. This is possibly due to the variable size and number of cystic components within the tumour and the amount of fibrous tissue stroma present.[2] Few neoplastic lesions have specific ultrasonographic features. There is poor correlation between the ultrasound appearance and cytology and histopathology, and due to overlapping features on ultrasound, even with contrast-enhanced ultrasound, differentiation of histotypes is ultrasonographically not possible.[23] Additionally, cholangitis may be involved in the aetiology of biliary tumours and can be present concurrently in cats with biliary tumours. Feline neuroendocrine epithelial tumours have been reported, possibly the result of a malignant transformation of hepatic stem cells, and can be intrahepatic or extrahepatic involving the bile duct but rarely involve the gallbladder.[24] Neoplasia arising from the gallbladder epithelium is very rare in the cat. A case of a primary gallbladder lymphoma has been described ultrasonographically in a 15-year-old cat as severe generalised mural thickening (up to 14 mm), which almost completely obliterated the gallbladder lumen.[25] Multiple sessile hyperechoic nodules protruding from the wall into the lumen were described in a second cat with gallbladder lymphoma.[26]

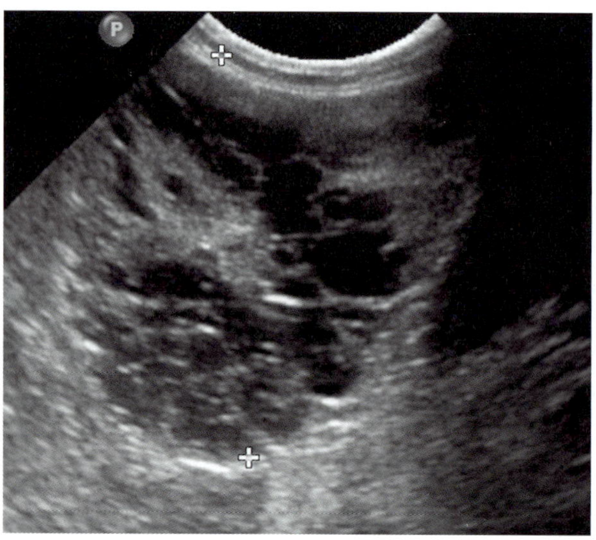

Figure 6.9. Ultrasonographic image of the liver of a 15-year-old cat showing right-sided very small-diameter anechoic cysts and mixed echogenicity consistent with a feline biliary cystadenoma.

Appearance of pancreatic disease

The diagnosis of pancreatic disease is based on a combination of imaging and clinicopathologic findings. The ultrasound appearance of various pancreatic diseases overlaps. In some cases, no changes are visible despite histological pancreatic disease. Histopathology of the pancreas is considered the gold standard but is not feasible in most patients. Multiple pancreatic samples are required for a reliable diagnosis because of the potential presence of very localised disease. The differential diagnoses for mass lesions of the pancreas include pancreatitis, asymptomatic nodular hyperplasia, benign pseudocysts, adenomas, exocrine pancreatic tumours, metastatic tumours, and rare endocrine tumours such as beta cell tumours, gastrinomas, or multiple endocrine neoplasia.[27] Ultrasound imaging of the feline pancreas lacks the specificity to differentiate chronic and acute forms of the disease. In many cases, feline chronic pancreatitis is not associated with any ultrasound changes at all, or the changes are so subtle that they cannot be identified.[7] Due to the link between pancreatitis and inflammatory bowel disease and hepatic disease (i.e. triaditis), the liver and gastrointestinal tract should be evaluated ultrasonographically at the same time as the pancreas.

Acute pancreatitis

Pancreatitis is the most common disorder of the feline exocrine pancreas. When ultrasonographic abnormalities suggestive of acute pancreatitis are identified, they are often more subtle than those seen in the dog. Furthermore, the absence of changes on ultrasound is not sufficient to rule out pancreatitis. The sensitivity of ultrasound for the detection of pancreatitis in the cat has traditionally been regarded as relatively low, with reported values of 11%–35%.[2,7] Due to continued and significant advances in ultrasound technology and markedly improved radiologist skill levels, sensitivities up to 84% and specificities of up to 75% in cats with moderate to severe pancreatitis have been reported more recently.[28] However, in a recent study, elevated serum feline pancreatic lipase immunoreactivity (fPLI) was used as the standard for diagnosis of pancreatitis, which has been shown to have only fair agreement with ultrasonography in cats with a suspicion of pancreatitis.[29] It should also be noted that all of these studies were conducted at university teaching hospitals, and most ultrasound examinations would have been performed by board-certified radiologists using high-end equipment. Hence, it is reasonable to assume that sensitivity is likely to be reduced when scans are performed by clinicians that are less experienced in ultrasound and using lower-quality equipment. Pancreatitis in cats is frequently accompanied by diseases in other organs, including hepatic lipidosis, inflammatory liver disease, bile duct obstruction, inflammatory bowel disease, and diabetes mellitus. Pancreatitis (based on serum markers and ultrasound changes) seems to be common in cats at the time of diagnosis of diabetes mellitus, and a subset of diabetic cats develop pancreatitis within 6 months of being diagnosed with diabetes mellitus. Pancreatitis in these cats was reported to be subclinical. It is important to perform a complete ultrasound examination in any cat suspected of having pancreatitis. High fPLI concentrations can indicate acute or chronic active purulent pancreatitis, but underlying pancreatic neoplasia needs to be considered as well.[30] For a more in-depth description of the clinical diagnosis of pancreatitis, including the interpretation of fPLI values, see Chapter 24.

Ultrasonographically reported abnormalities consistent with pancreatitis include an enlarged, hypoechoic or mixed echoic pancreas (Fig. 6.10a) with irregular or scalloped margins, a surrounding hyperechoic mesentery because of focal steatitis, fluid accumulation secondary to focal peritonitis, and dilation of the CBD and pancreatic duct (Fig. 6.7a).[2] Hyperechoic peripancreatic fat may be one of the most sensitive indicators of pancreatitis; it was identified in 68% of cats (n = 35) that had elevated serum fPLI in one study[28] and was the most frequently identified ultrasonographic abnormality in 55% of cats with raised fPLI in another study.[18] Accordingly, this would suggest that there is a moderate likelihood of cats having pancreatitis when such abnormalities are found on ultrasonographic examination, although it is important to note that the authors of these studies do not differentiate between cats with acute and chronic pancreatitis. The authors of the former of these two studies report that, in addition to hyperechoic pancreatic fat, the presence of a thick left pancreatic limb and severely irregular pancreatic margins in cats with appropriate clinical signs and raised serum fPLI concentrations can be highly supportive of pancreatitis.[28] When inflammation of peripancreatic fat is severe, the fat can become hazy in appearance and pancreatic margins may appear ill-defined. In cases in which the ultrasonographic appearance of the pancreas is unremarkable, but there is a high clinical suspicion of pancreatitis, ultrasound can be repeated after 2–4 days,

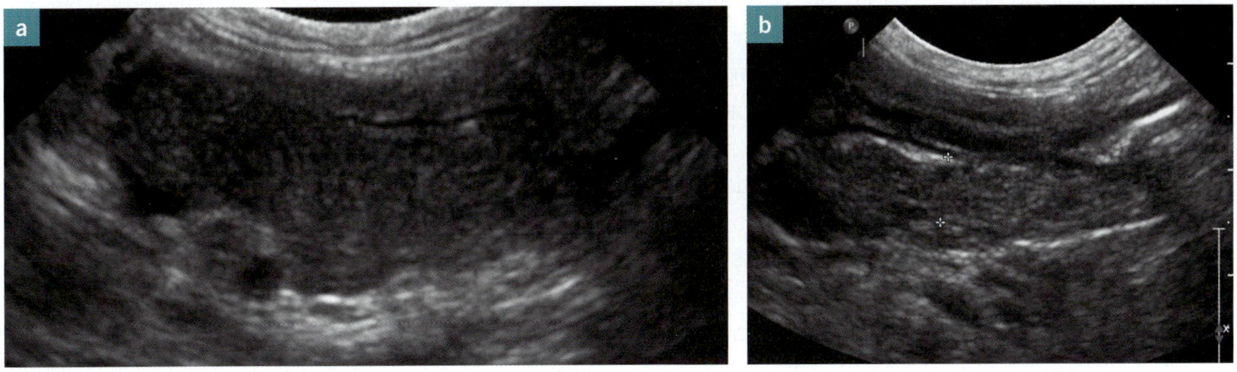

Figure 6.10. Ultrasonographic image of a 15-year-old cat (a) showing an enlarged left pancreatic limb, with irregular margins and surrounding hyperechoic mesentery, consistent with a suspected acute pancreatitis. Ultrasonographic image of a different cat (b) showing a mildly enlarged, irregular right pancreatic limb with heterogeneous parenchyma, consistent with chronic pancreatitis.

which may allow sufficient time for ultrasonographic changes to appear.[7]

Pancreatic rupture resulting in severe pancreatitis and peripancreatitis has been described in cats with high-rise syndrome in 0.6%–1% of cats that have fallen out of windows, with a higher prevalence of pancreatic rupture when falling from greater heights and a mean height of 4.9 stories. Without the correct diagnosis, the condition can lead to multi-organ failure and death. On ultrasound, the pancreas in four affected cats appeared hyperechoic and was surrounded by hyperechoic peripancreatic mesenteric fat, with the left pancreatic lobe considered to be more vulnerable to rupture.[31] Additional findings in all affected cats included abdominal effusion and hypomotility of the gastrointestinal tract. Traumatic pancreatitis has also been reported in association with high-rise syndrome. Abdominal ultrasonography of affected cats may reveal any combination of pancreatic enlargement, decreased or heterogeneous pancreatic echogenicity, hyperechoic mesentery, and peritoneal effusion.[32]

Chronic pancreatitis

Recurrent episodes of inflammation over months or years can lead to the development of chronic pancreatitis. Ultrasonographic changes observed in cats with chronic pancreatitis tend to vary between individuals since the disease processes present may not be sufficient to induce an alteration in the appearance of the pancreas on ultrasound. In addition, a normal ultrasound does not exclude the possibility of chronic pancreatitis. Whereas acute pancreatitis is typically associated with neutrophilic inflammation, necrosis, and oedema, chronic pancreatitis eventually leads to irreversible acinar loss and fibrosis and resembles the process seen in humans, where fibrosis is more pronounced than inflammation. The condition is often mild and asymptomatic and has a high prevalence in apparently healthy cats, causing some to question its clinical significance. Histological evidence of chronic pancreatitis was identified in 67 out of 115 cats undergoing necropsy in one study; in comparison, 18 cats showed histological evidence of acute pancreatitis.[33] Despite this, there is relatively little evidence in the literature regarding the ultrasonographic appearance of feline chronic pancreatitis. Abnormal pancreatic thickness, an irregular pancreatic margin, nodularity and hypoechogenicity of the pancreas, an hyperechoic mesentery, and abdominal effusion have all been reported in cats with chronic pancreatitis confirmed by histopathology (Fig. 6.10b).[7] Thus, it appears that there is a degree of overlap in the ultrasonographic appearance of acute and chronic pancreatitis in the cat. As with acute pancreatitis, dilation of the CBD may also be recognised, and if adhesions occur secondary to chronic inflammation, the duodenum and/or part of the stomach can become displaced from their normal position within the abdomen. However, a further separate study found no correlation between pancreatic duct width and clinically significant pancreatic disease. Furthermore, since dilation of the pancreatic duct can occur as a normal ageing change, it should not be used as the sole indicator of pancreatitis in the geriatric cat.[34] Causes of pancreatic duct dilation in feline pancreatitis are postulated to be secondary to progressive atrophy of both endocrine and exocrine tissues, ductal inflammation, partial to complete ductal obstruction secondary to intraluminal mucoprotein accumulation or pancreatolith, epithelial metaplasia, and/or ductal mucinous hyperplasia.[33] The authors of the study theorised that dilation of the pancreatic duct may first be identified in the body of the pancreas in cats with pancreatitis due to its close proximity to the major duodenal papilla and potential functional or mechanical obstruction to flow. A pancreatolith was not identified in any of the cats in this study and appears to be an uncommon finding, even on histopathology.[33] In view of the fact that an ultrasonographic diagnosis of chronic pancreatitis is not always straightforward, attempts have been made to discover alternative means of obtaining a more definitive diagnosis using ultrasound in combination with secretin. In healthy individuals, secretin stimulates the pancreas to secrete bicarbonate, resulting in dilation of the pancreatic duct. Mean pancreatic duct diameter increased from 0.77 ± 0.33 mm to 1.42 ± 0.40 mm following secretin administration, and the mean percentage increase in pancreatic duct diameter over basal diameter up to 15 minutes after secretin administration was $101.9 \pm 58.8\%$.[35] To date, the relationship between secretin administration and ductal diameter in the diseased feline pancreas has not been evaluated, and therefore the ability of this diagnostic procedure to identify cats with chronic pancreatitis has yet to be determined.

Pancreatic oedema

Pancreatic oedema results in pancreatic enlargement and fluid accumulation within the interlobular septae. This gives rise to multiple hypoechoic striations dispersed throughout the parenchyma—the so-called tiger stripe appearance (Fig. 6.11).[2] Oedema often occurs with pancreatitis but can also occur secondary to nonpancreatic disease, such as hypoalbuminaemia and portal hypertension, and hence it is not considered to be pathognomonic for inflammation.

Pancreatic pseudocysts and abscesses

Pancreatic pseudocysts are focal collections of pancreatic enzymes, blood, and products of tissue digestion contained within a nonepithelialised fibrous sac and are a potential sequela to pancreatitis in both dogs and cats. Pseudocysts appear generally hypoechoic or anechoic, may have acoustic enhancement, usually contain echogenic debris, and may be surrounded by a thick wall. It is difficult to differentiate a pancreatic pseudocyst from a pancreatic abscess or neoplastic mass on ultrasound examination alone (Fig. 6.12).

Pancreatic abscesses are uncommon in cats but may develop as a consequence of pancreatitis or an infected pseudocyst.[2] Abscesses are collections of purulent material and necrotic tissue within the pancreas or extending into adjacent tissues. Pancreatic abscesses develop from secondary infection of necrotic pancreatic tissue and are a serious and often fatal complication of acute pancreatitis. Abscesses may appear as ill-defined mass lesions within the pancreas, containing both hypoechoic and hyperechoic areas. Echogenic foci with distal shadowing indicating gas may be present within the lumen. A thick or poorly defined wall may surround the abscess. Abscesses can be highly variable in appearance but usually present as thick-walled cavitary lesions with hyperechoic or flocculent contents. Occasionally, gas is also present and recognised on ultrasound by the presence of hyperechoic foci associated with a reverberation artefact.

Pancreatic nodular hyperplasia

Nodular hyperplasia of the pancreas seems to be common in older cats and is likely not clinically significant. Hypoechoic small nodules (3–10 mm in cats) distributed diffusely within normal pancreatic parenchyma may be seen as an incidental finding on ultrasound examination (Fig. 6.13). However, nodular hyperplasia cannot be reliably differentiated from malignant pancreatic neoplasia, and a biopsy is needed for a definitive diagnosis.[2] There is significant overlap in the ultrasonographic appearance of pancreatic neoplasia, nodular hyperplasia, and pancreatitis, and therefore examination of tissue samples obtained via either biopsy or fine needle aspiration is usually required to make a definitive diagnosis.

Pancreatic neoplasia

Pancreatic neoplasia is rare in cats and represents a differential diagnosis for any mass lesion within the pancreas. Ancillary findings in cases of pancreatic neoplasia include evidence of pancreatic mineralisation, invasion of the duodenal wall, free abdominal fluid, hyperechogenicity of peripancreatic fat, lymphadenopathy, and obstruction of the CBD. Ultrasound examination cannot reliably differentiate neoplasia from pancreatitis, pseudocysts, abscesses, or nodular hyperplasia. A focal solid

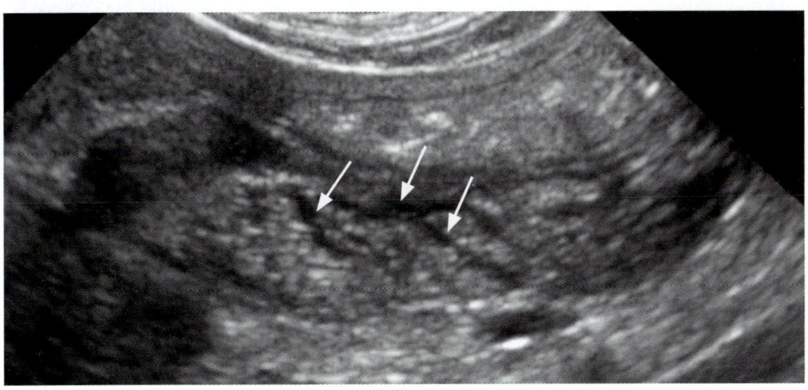

Figure 6.11. Ultrasonographic image of a 2-year-old neutered male domestic shorthair cat presenting with acute kidney injury. The left limb of the pancreas is enlarged, with fluid accumulation within the interlobular septae seen as multiple hypoechoic striations (arrows) dispersed throughout the parenchyma, also known as the "tiger stripe" sign.

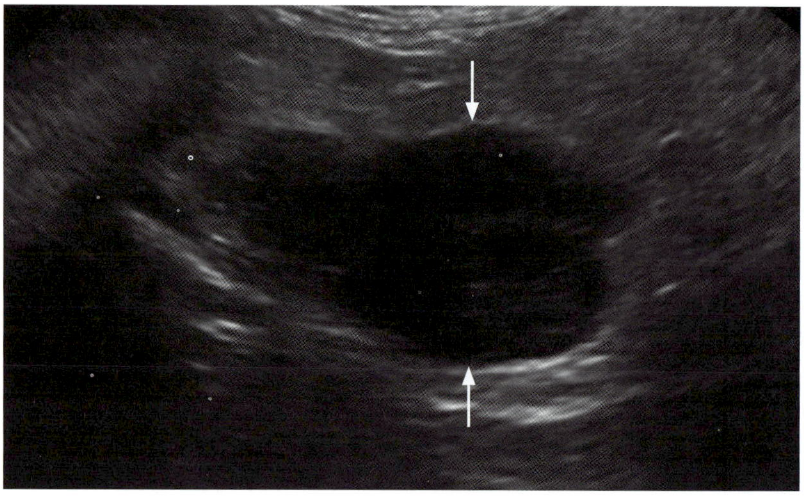

Figure 6.12. Ultrasonographic image of a 1-year-old cat with an enlarged right hypoechoic pancreatic limb, which expands into a hypoechoic, fluid-filled structure (arrows) surrounded by hyperechoic mesentery, consistent with a pancreatic abscess, a pseudocyst, or focal pancreatitis and focal peritonitis.

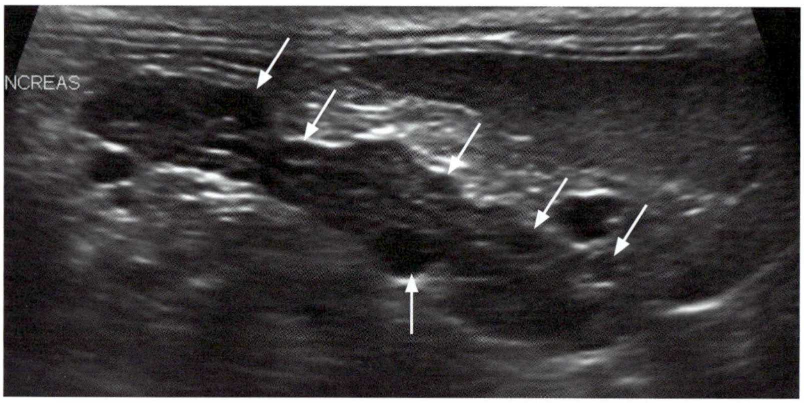

Figure 6.13. Ultrasonographic image of the left pancreatic limb of a cat. Hypoechoic small nodules (arrows) of about 5 mm in diameter and slightly irregular margins are distributed diffusely within the pancreatic parenchyma. These findings are consistent with nodular hyperplasia.

mass is the most common ultrasound appearance for malignant neoplasia. The only ultrasound feature unique to malignant pancreatic neoplasia vs. nodular hyperplasia in cats is the presence of a single mass greater than 2.0 cm in at least one dimension (Fig. 6.14a). In one study, feline pancreatic neoplasms tended to have a single larger mass lesion, whereas nodular hyperplasia tended to have multiple smaller nodules. Carcinoma is the most common tumour type reported,[36] but adenomas, sarcomas, lymphomas, mast cell tumours, unclassified tumours, and metastatic neoplasms have also been described.[37] Cystic pancreatic neoplasms occur in 35% of cats, with the majority (60%) being benign, while solid tumours are typically malignant. Pancreatic tumours, especially carcinomas, usually affect older cats, with a mean age of 12 years;[27] however, one study reported that young cats between 2 and 7 years of age can also be affected.[36] Additionally, pancreatic neoplasms may be accompanied by inflammation, and histopathological investigation is required to differentiate pancreatitis from an inflamed pancreatic neoplasm.[7] The presence or absence of abdominal effusion can also be used as a prognostic indicator. In one report of 34 cats with pancreatic adenocarcinoma, the median survival of those cats with abdominal effusion at the time of diagnosis (16 in total) was 30 days compared with 165 days for cats with no effusion.[27] Unfortunately, feline pancreatic adenocarcinoma has a poor prognosis and has often already metastasised by the time of diagnosis, particularly to the liver, lung, and small intestine (Fig. 6.14b).

Lymphoma of the pancreas is also recognised in the cat but may represent pancreatic involvement in multicentric disease rather than being a primary tumour of the pancreas.[37] Lymphoma in the pancreas has been reported to result in irregular margination, diffuse enlargement, and hypoechogenicity of the pancreas.

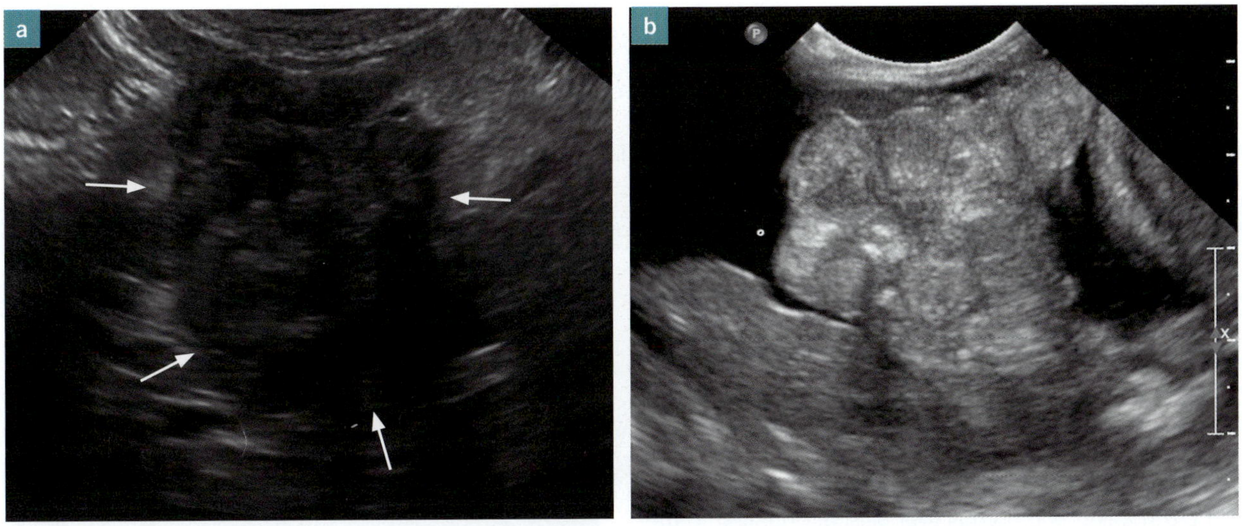

Figure 6.14. Ultrasonographic image of a cat (a) showing a large, well-defined, irregular, hypoechoic mass (arrows) in the right limb of the pancreas. Examination of fine needle aspiration samples revealed pancreatic carcinoma as definitive diagnosis. Abdominal effusion is present in this different cat with carcinomatosis (b), which is noted as multiple hypoechoic, ill-defined confluent masses in the mesentery.

Pancreatic endocrine tumours are extremely rare in cats. Insulinomas have been most commonly reported affecting older cats, with a total of nine cases, and a good prognosis has been reported following surgical removal.[38]

Metastatic spread of pancreatic neoplasia to the mesentery (carcinomatosis) can occur, resulting in a nodular-appearing omentum and peritoneal effusion (Fig. 6.14b). Metastatic lesions in adjacent lymph nodes or liver may be more reliably imaged. There are only occasional reports of metastatic disease occurring within the pancreas in cats. Pancreatic metastases were identified in 2 out of 26 cats with visceral haemangiosarcoma in one study.[39]

Contrast-enhanced ultrasonography

Contrast-enhanced ultrasound has been evaluated in the diagnosis of hepatobiliary neoplasms[23] and pancreatic disease in the cat. A study evaluating 44 cats with primary hepatobiliary neoplasms showed overlapping contrast enhancement pattern and was therefore not useful in differentiating the subtypes.[23] Contrast enhancement of the pancreas correlates with perfusion and can be used to evaluate areas of inflammation (more intensely enhancing) and necrosis (nonenhancing).[40] These initial results are promising, and further large-scale studies of cats with spontaneously occurring pancreatic disease are warranted.

Endosonography

Endoscopic ultrasound (EUS) has been used to evaluate cats with pancreatitis.[41] Although there was no difference in the ability to detect changes associated with pancreatitis between EUS and abdominal ultrasound, pancreatic margins and parenchymal detail were better visualised on EUS. Disadvantages of EUS include the necessity for specialised equipment, general anaesthesia, and the expertise and experience needed for this procedure.

ADVANCED IMAGING

With the increased availability of computed tomography (CT) and magnetic resonance imaging (MRI) scanners in veterinary hospitals, these imaging modalities are more readily available for diagnosis of abdominal diseases in cats. The ability to image veterinary patients without superimposition of other organs or bowel gas and to perform a complete assessment of the biliary tree and pancreas offers distinct advantages over current imaging methods. With the advent and increased availability of multislice CT scanners, the speed at which CT studies can be performed has increased, and sedating rather than anaesthetising animals for some studies is now a possibility. Both CT and MRI use intravenous contrast to better evaluate the blood flow to organs and adjacent tissues. Nevertheless, while no imaging modality is poised to replace abdominal ultrasound for the routine evaluation of the feline pancreas and biliary system, some other modalities have potential for this purpose.

Computed tomography

This imaging technique provides excellent contrast resolution of soft tissues and bones. With the ability to perform multiplanar reconstructions, the biliary tract and pancreas can be evaluated in dorsal and sagittal imaging planes in unlimited angles for thorough assessment. Disadvantages of CT imaging include the use of ionising radiation, added expense, need for anaesthesia or sedation, and decreased availability compared with ultrasound. On CT imaging, the normal liver is isoattenuating to the spleen, with a hypoattenuating gallbladder due to storage of bile. The bile should be hypoattenuating, with no evidence of internal contents such as debris or calculi. The normal CBD can be seen consistently in normal cats (Fig. 6.15) and cats with elevated fPLI[42] on CT. A protocol for cholangiography was described in normal cats that provided only moderate enhancement of the biliary tract, with optimal imaging time 65 minutes after injection of the contrast agent.[43] Another study evaluated a drip infusion protocol for CT for the visualisation of the bile duct in healthy cats and cats with EHBDO due to cholelithiasis.[44] A triple-phase CT protocol has been established in 15 healthy sedated cats, and the normal appearance of the pancreas was described as hypo- to isoattenuating to both the liver and spleen in all phases in the majority of cats, with a homogeneous enhancement pattern noted in all 15 cats (Fig. 6.16).[45] Mean pancreatic attenuation was 48, 79, 166, and 126 HU respectively on precontrast, arterial, portal, and delayed-phase images. In addition, mean height, length, and width of the left lobe of the pancreas were larger than those of the right lobe in all 15 cats. There were no associations between volume and volume:body weight ratio with age ($P = 0.6518$, $P = 0.6968$) or sex ($P = 0.7013$, $P = 0.2043$). This baseline information may be beneficial for use in future studies characterising pancreatic disease in cats as well as in future research studies evaluating pancreatic endocrine function. The results of an early study evaluating the accuracy of CT for the diagnosis of feline pancreatitis were not encouraging, as only 2 out of 10 cats had CT changes consistent with pancreatitis.[46]

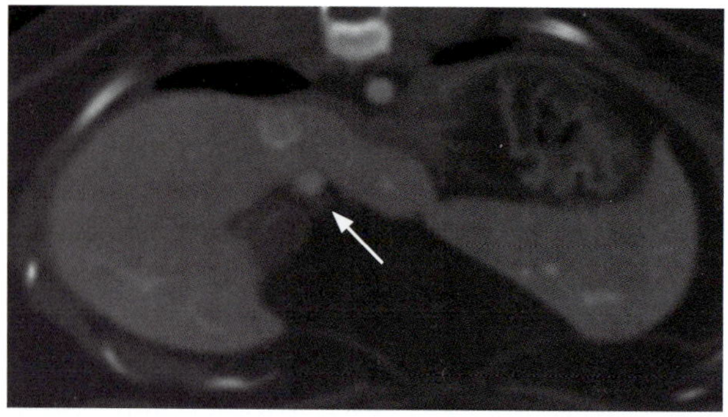

Figure 6.15. Postcontrast CT scan in a bone window of the abdomen at the level of the porta hepatis. The hypodense common bile duct (arrow) can be seen medioventral to the portal vein.

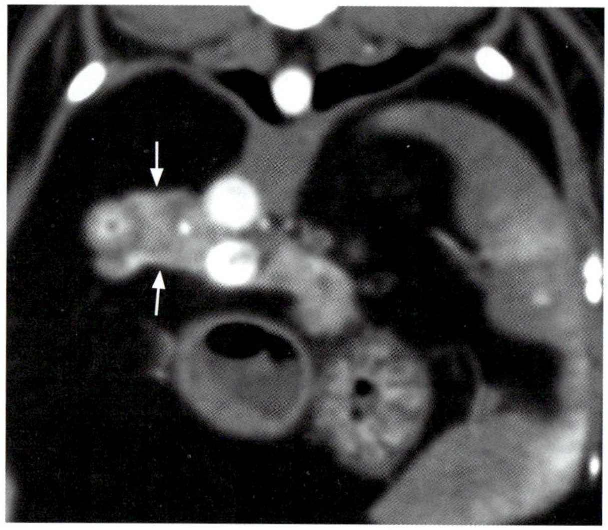

Figure 6.16. Postcontrast CT scan in a soft tissue window of the abdomen depicting the right pancreatic limb (arrows) medial to the descending duodenum.

Further large-scale studies are needed to determine the accuracy of CT for the diagnosis of pancreatic disease in both dogs and cats.

Magnetic resonance imaging

This imaging technique offers excellent contrast resolution of the soft tissues and provides multiple anatomic planes to visualise organs in the abdomen. Disadvantages of MRI are the need for general anaesthesia, added expense, and decreased availability compared with ultrasound and CT. A protocol for MRI incorporating cholangiopancreatography sequences (magnetic resonance cholangiopancreatography [MRCP]) and secretin stimulation has been developed in healthy cats and provided high-quality images of the normal liver, biliary ductal system, pancreas, and pancreatic duct without the use of ionising radiation or intravenous contrast.[43] In a study of 10 cats with suspected pancreatitis and/or cholangitis, pancreatic changes were identified in 9 cats, including gallbladder wall thickening, moderate contrast enhancement of the gallbladder wall, and/or gallbladder debris. The pancreatic parenchyma was characterised as T1 precontrast hypointense and T2 hyperintense, but the findings were nonspecific. The authors of the study concluded that MRI/MRCP provided excellent comprehensive visualisation of the pancreatic and hepatobiliary systems.[47] These findings suggest that MRI may be a feasible and useful imaging modality for the assessment of cholangitis and other biliary tract disorders in cats.

Take-home messages

- Ultrasound is the most common modality used to initially evaluate the pancreas and biliary system in cats due to its wide availability.
- An unremarkable ultrasound examination does not rule out biliary or pancreatic disease.
- Due to overlap in imaging features of inflammation and neoplastic disease, histopathology or cytology are required for a definitive diagnosis in most cases.
- Advanced imaging is becoming more and more common for evaluating biliary and pancreatic disease in cats. However, it requires anaesthesia and is associated with higher costs.

REFERENCES

[1] Larson MM. Liver and spleen. In: Thrall DE, editor. *Textbook of Veterinary Diagnostic Radiology*, 7th ed. St Louis, Elsevier: 792, 2018.

[2] Nyland TG, Mattoon JS, editors. *Small Animal Diagnostic Ultrasound*, 3rd ed. St Louis, Elsevier, 2015.

[3] Griffin S. Feline abdominal ultrasonography: what's normal? what's abnormal? The biliary tree. *J Feline Med Surg* 21:429, 2019.

[4] Woods KS et al. Congenital duplex gallbladder and biliary mucocele associated with partial hepatic cholestasis and cholelithiasis in a cat. *Can Vet J* 53:269, 2012.

[5] Penninck DG, Brisson JO, Webster CR. Sonographic assessment of gallbladder volume in normal cats. *Vet Radiol Ultrasound* 51:665, 2010.

[6] Diana A et al. Ultrasonographic evaluation of preprandial and postprandial gallbladder volume in healthy cats. *Am J Vet Res* 73:1583, 2012.

[7] Griffin S. Feline abdominal ultrasonography: what's normal? what's abnormal? The pancreas. *J Feline Med Surg* 22:241, 2020.

[8] van den Ingh TSGAM et al. Morphological classification of biliary disorders of the canine and feline liver. In: Rothuizen J et al., editors. *WSAVA Standards for Clinical and Histological Diagnosis of Canine and Feline Liver Diseases.* Edinburgh, WB Saunders: 61, 2006.

[9] Harran N et al. Gallbladder sludge on ultrasound is predictive of increased liver enzymes and total bilirubin in cats. *Can Vet J* 52:999, 2011.

[10] Policelli Smith R et al. Association between gallbladder ultrasound findings and bacterial culture of bile in 70 cats and 202 dogs. *J Vet Intern Med* 31:1451, 2017.

[11] Gaillot HA et al. Ultrasonographic features of extrahepatic biliary obstruction in 30 cats. *Vet Radiol Ultrasound* 48:439, 2007.

[12] Bennett SL et al. Gallbladder mucocoele and concurrent hepatic lipidosis in a cat. *Aust Vet J* 85:397, 2007.

[13] Marolf AJ et al. Ultrasonographic findings of feline cholangitis. *J Am Anim Hosp Assoc* 48:36, 2012.

[14] Mayhew PD et al. Pathogenesis and outcome of extrahepatic biliary obstruction in cats. *J Small Anim Pract* 43:247, 2002.

[15] Köster L et al. Percutaneous ultrasound-guided cholecystocentesis and bile analysis for the detection of *Platynosomum* spp.–induced cholangitis in cats. *J Vet Intern Med* 30:787, 2016.

[16] Newell SM et al. Correlations between ultrasonographic findings and specific hepatic diseases in cats: 72 cases (1985–1997). *J Am Vet Med Assoc* 213:94, 1998.

[17] Brain PH et al. Feline cholecystitis and acute neutrophilic cholangitis: clinical findings, bacterial isolates and

response to treatment in six cases. *J Feline Med Surg* 8:91, 2006.

[18] Moser K et al. Prognostische Bedeutung sonographischer Parameter der Pankreatitis der Katze [Evaluation of sonographic parameters as prognostic risk factors in cats with pancreatitis—a retrospective study in 42 cats]. *Tierarztl Prax Ausg K Kleintiere Heimtiere* 46:386, 2018.

[19] Nyland TG, Gillett NA. Sonographic evaluation of experimental bile duct ligation in the dog. *Vet Radiol* 23:252, 1982.

[20] Best EJ, Bush DJ, Dye C. Suspected choledochal cyst in a domestic shorthair cat. *J Feline Med Surg* 12:814, 2010.

[21] Grand JG et al. Cyst of the common bile duct in a cat. *Aust Vet J* 88:268, 2010.

[22] Balkman C. Hepatobiliary neoplasia in dogs and cats. *Vet Clin North Am Small Anim Pract* 39:617, 2009.

[23] Banzato T et al. Contrast-enhanced ultrasonography features of hepatobiliary neoplasms in cats. *Vet Rec* 186:320, 2020.

[24] Patnaik AK et al. Hepatobiliary neuroendocrine carcinoma in cats: a clinicopathologic, immunohistochemical, and ultrastructural study of 17 cases. *Vet Pathol* 42:331, 2005.

[25] Geigy CA et al. Extranodal B-cell lymphoma in the urinary bladder with cytological evidence of concurrent involvement of the gall bladder in a cat. *J Small Anim Pract* 51:280, 2010.

[26] Baxter KJ et al. Gastrointestinal small-cell lymphoma with gall bladder involvement in a cat. *J Feline Med Surg* 14:267, 2012.

[27] Linderman MJ et al. Feline exocrine pancreatic carcinoma: a retrospective study of 34 cases. *Vet Comp Oncol* 11:208, 2013.

[28] Williams JM et al. Ultrasonographic findings of the pancreas in cats with elevated serum pancreatic lipase immunoreactivity. *J Vet Intern Med* 27:913, 2013.

[29] Oppliger S et al. Agreement of serum feline pancreas-specific lipase and colorimetric lipase assays with pancreatic ultrasonographic findings in cats with suspicion of pancreatitis: 161 cases (2008–2012). *J Am Vet Med Assoc* 244:1060, 2014.

[30] Törner K et al. Histopathology and feline pancreatic lipase immunoreactivity in inflammatory, hyperplastic and neoplastic pancreatic diseases in cats. *J Comp Pathol* 174:63, 2020.

[31] Liehmann LM et al. Pancreatic rupture in four cats with high-rise syndrome. *J Feline Med Surg* 14:131, 2012.

[32] Zimmermann E et al. Serum feline-specific pancreatic lipase immunoreactivity concentrations and abdominal ultrasonographic findings in cats with trauma resulting from high-rise syndrome. *J Am Vet Med Assoc* 242:1238, 2013.

[33] De Cock HE et al. Prevalence and histopathologic characteristics of pancreatitis in cats. *Vet Pathol* 44:39, 2007.

[34] Hecht S et al. Relationship of pancreatic duct dilation to age and clinical findings in cats. *Vet Radiol Ultrasound* 47:287, 2006.

[35] Baron ML et al. Ultrasonographic observation of secretin-induced pancreatic duct dilation in healthy cats. *Vet Radiol Ultrasound* 51:86, 2010.

[36] Törner K et al. Primary solid and cystic tumours of the exocrine pancreas in cats. *J Comp Pathol* 169:5, 2019.

[37] Törner K et al. Clinical and pathological data of 17 non-epithelial pancreatic tumors in cats. *Vet Sci* 7:55, 2020.

[38] Cervone M et al. Use of contrast-enhanced ultrasonography for the detection of a feline insulinoma. *JFMS Open Rep* 5:2055116919876140, 2019.

[39] Culp WT et al. Feline visceral hemangiosarcoma. *J Vet Intern Med* 22:148, 2008.

[40] Rademacher N et al. Contrast-enhanced power and color Doppler ultrasonography of the pancreas in healthy and diseased cats. *J Vet Intern Med* 22:1310, 2008.

[41] Schweighauser A et al. Evaluation of endosonography as a new diagnostic tool for feline pancreatitis. *J Feline Med Surg* 11:492, 2009.

[42] Park JY et al. Feline pancreatic ducts are consistently identified on CT and more likely to be dilated in the body of pancreas in cats with elevated feline pancreatic lipase immunoreactivity. *Vet Radiol Ultrasound* 61:255, 2020.

[43] Marolf AJ. Computed tomography and MRI of the hepatobiliary system and pancreas. *Vet Clin North Am Small Anim Pract* 46:481, 2016.

[44] Tanaka T et al. Drip infusion cholangiography with CT in cats. *J Feline Med Surg* 20:1173, 2018.

[45] Secrest S, Sharma A, Bugbee A. Triple phase computed tomography of the pancreas in healthy cats. *Vet Radiol Ultrasound* 59:163, 2018.

[46] Forman MA et al. Evaluation of serum feline pancreatic lipase immunoreactivity and helical computed tomography versus conventional testing for the diagnosis of feline pancreatitis. *J Vet Intern Med* 18:807, 2004.

[47] Marolf AJ et al. Magnetic resonance (MR) imaging and MR cholangiopancreatography findings in cats with cholangitis and pancreatitis. *J Feline Med Surg* 15:285, 2013.

CHAPTER 7

Endoscopy of the feline gastrointestinal tract

Christiane Stengel, Reto Neiger

Flexible endoscopy is an integral part in the diagnostic workup of cats with gastrointestinal (GI) signs such as retching, regurgitation, vomiting, or diarrhoea. It is minimally invasive and almost atraumatic, with a low risk of procedure-related morbidity and mortality. It should be used after noninvasive investigations (see Chapters 3 and 4 for laboratory assessment and Chapters 5 and 6 for other diagnostic imaging modalities) and when trial therapy failed to provide a diagnosis or resolution of clinical signs (see Chapters 1 and 2 for differential diagnoses). Haematology, biochemistry, and potentially other laboratory investigations such as complete faecal analysis (including *Giardia* spp. antigen testing, *Tritrichomonas blagburni* PCR, coronavirus PCR), plasma thyroxin concentrations, trypsin-like immunoreactivity (TLI) and vitamin B_{12} concentrations, and, as in all sick cats, feline leukaemia virus (FeLV) or feline immunodeficiency virus (FIV) testing should be done initially (see Chapters 3, 4, and 15) together with appropriate diagnostic imaging such as plain or possibly contrast radiographs and—most importantly—abdominal ultrasound (see Chapters 5 and 6). Like other diagnostic modalities, endoscopy has limitations for the investigation of GI problems. Motility abnormalities, functional diseases (dietary hypersensitivity, pancreatic insufficiency, etc.), lesions outside the GI tract (liver, pancreas, etc.), or pathological processes restricted to the intestinal submucosal or muscularis layers cannot be visualised endoscopically. It is not possible to investigate the entire GI tract with a standard flexible endoscope as available today. Endoscopy also has therapeutic intent, such as for foreign body retrieval, polyp removal, stricture dilation, or feeding tube placement (percutaneous endoscopic gastrostomy [PEG] or jejunostomy tube; see Chapter 40). The main reason to perform endoscopy lies in obtaining biopsy samples for histopathological investigation (see Chapter 9). Endoscopy should only be performed when indicated and not because the equipment is available and has to be used. If the indications are well chosen, the equipment is appropriate for the cat, and the clinician is experienced in the procedure, endoscopy can not only help to diagnose many diseases in the oesophagus, stomach, and intestine but may even help to treat some problems with minimal invasiveness. In comparison to exploratory laparotomy, which might be the only alternative in some cats but poses several risks itself, flexible GI endoscopy has the major advantage that multiple biopsy samples can be taken exactly at the area of greatest abnormality. Furthermore, there is no problem with wound healing and possible dehiscence, and thus animals can be treated with immunosuppressive drugs, especially steroids, immediately after taking biopsy samples.

The risks and possible benefits to an individual cat must be considered, and the likelihood of gaining a diagnosis through endoscopy has to be counterweighted against the anaesthetic risk and the risks posed by the procedure itself. It is paramount that endoscopists are well versed in these procedures in order to yield appropriate results. Careful recording of all findings, normal and abnormal, should be done immediately after the procedure. There are pro forma standardised GI endoscopy reporting forms available from the World Small Animal Veterinary Association (WSAVA) website.* Besides photographic recording (if possible), the clinician must report the entire procedure in detailed writing.

*https://wsava.org/global-guidelines/gastrointestinal-guidelines/

Endoscopy of the GI tract includes examination of the mouth, oesophagus, stomach, proximal small intestine, ileum, colon, and rectum. The mouth, oesophagus, and also the rectum and descending colon might be examined with a rigid endoscope, but the preferred instrument is a flexible endoscope, which is essential for the complete visualisation of the stomach and intubation of the small and proximal large intestine. Part of minimising the procedure-related risks is to use adequate and fully functioning equipment. The veterinary surgeon performing endoscopy should have a high level of proficiency, as GI endoscopy in cats is more demanding in skill than in dogs due to the small size of the animal and the decreased tolerance to anaesthesia. It takes patience and much practice to perform upper and lower GI endoscopy effectively; one should best start training in a comprehensive endoscopy course including lectures and wet labs before attempting this procedure in sick cats.

In cats, GI endoscopy can safely and adequately be performed only under general anaesthesia. Therefore, a competent anaesthetist or assistant proficient in maintaining and supervising anaesthesia needs to be present throughout the whole intervention to allow the endoscopist to concentrate on the procedure. This anaesthetist should understand endoscopy and the inherent risks to anticipate possible complications (e.g. overinflation of the stomach, stretching of oesophageal sphincters and colon).

EQUIPMENT

Endoscopy equipment consists of the endoscope, imaging system (camera, camera head, and monitor), and illumination system (light source and cable). The selection of the endoscopic equipment in veterinary practice often depends on its expense and therefore on the versatility of application, durability, and ease of guidance of the endoscope. One single flexible endoscope might be used for a variety of procedures in the GI tract (and also respiratory tract in dogs). The versatility of an endoscope depends on its length, diameter of insertion tube, diameter of the working channel, and tip deflection capabilities; its ease of guidance only depends on length and outer diameter. Another important factor to be considered before purchasing the endoscopic equipment is the optical and imaging system.

A flexible endoscope suitable for upper and lower GI endoscopy in cats is typically 90–120 cm long and should have four-way tip deflection. Careful thought should be given to the insertion tube, particularly to its diameter. To be able to pass the endoscope through the feline pylorus into the duodenum and through the ileocolic junction into the ileum, the outer diameter should not exceed 9 mm (preferably <8 mm). Length is not as important unless large felids (tiger, lion, cheetah) are examined. If the same endoscope is also to be used in dogs, a length greater than 130 cm is recommended.

To obtain adequately sized biopsy samples, the instrumentation channel should be at least 2.2 mm (preferably ≥2.5 mm). Simply stated, the ideal endoscope is thin but has a large instrumentation channel. One videoendoscope model specifically designed for use in cats is 110 cm long, with an outer diameter of 5.9 mm and an instrumentation channel of 2.0 mm (Feline Videoendoscope, Karl Storz SE & Co. KG) (Fig. 7.1a).

The two basic types of flexible endoscopes used in veterinary medicine are fibre-optic endoscopes (fibrescopes) and videoendoscopes. They differ in the method of sensing and transmitting the image. In the fibrescope, the image is carried from the tip to the eyepiece via bundles of optical glass fibres. The image can then be viewed directly through the eyepiece or indirectly by attaching an endoscopic charge-coupled device (CCD) video camera. The picture can be transferred via the imaging system onto a monitor. Videoendoscopes need to be connected to a monitor, as they have no eyepiece. The image in a videoendoscope is sensed directly by a CCD chip located at the tip of the endoscope and transmitted electronically. The image quality of videoendoscopes is far superior to that of fibre-optic endoscopes, but they are also more expensive. If a good-quality fibre-optic endoscope is combined with a high-intensity light source and a good-quality video camera, the resulting image is in most instances sufficient for adequate visualisation.

For both types of endoscopes, an imaging system offers distinct advantages, not only comfort for the operator but also for documentation, client information, and teaching purposes. Taking and recording images and video sequences helps owners to understand the procedure and condition of their pet. Imaging systems differ in quality, as standard definition is typically 768 pixels wide

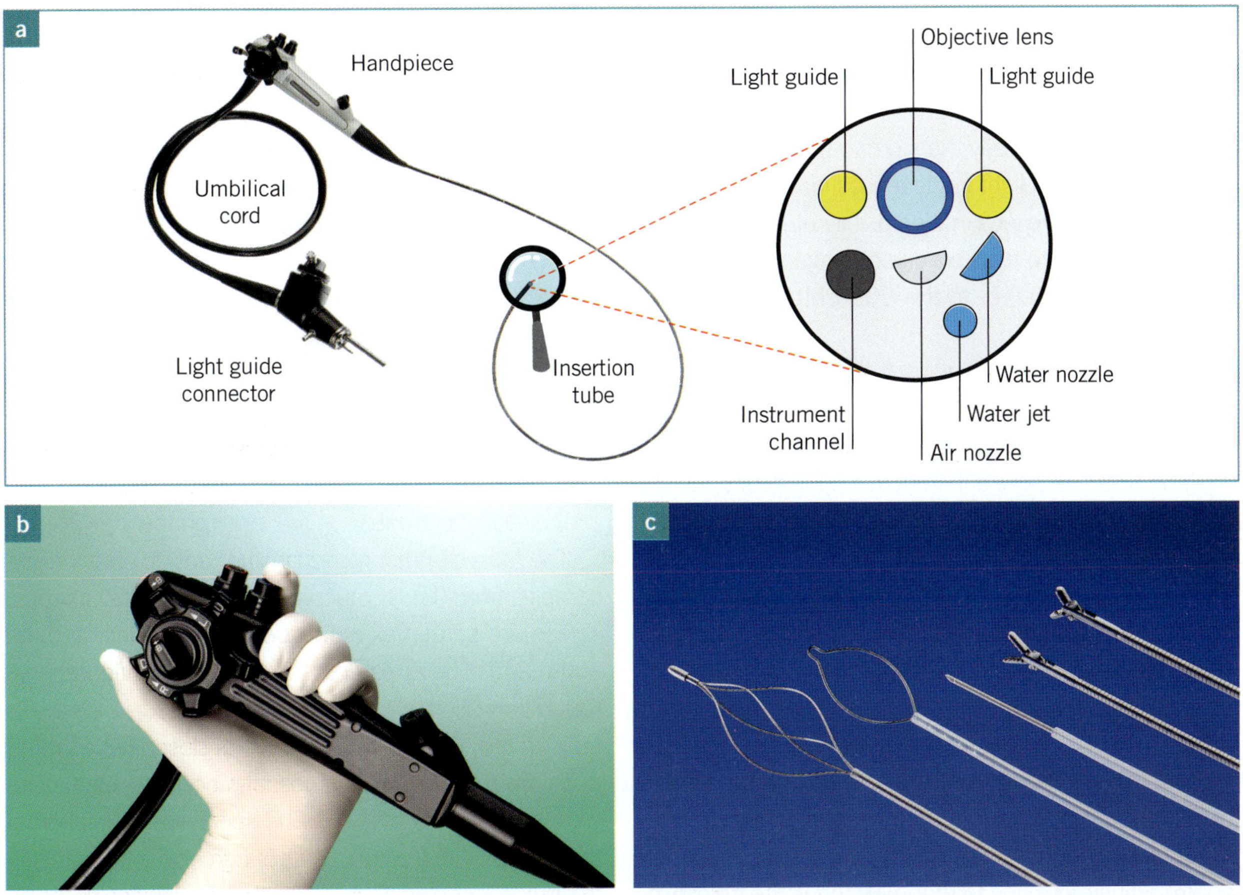

Figure 7.1. Equipment needed for flexible endoscopy of the gastrointestinal tract in a cat. Silverline Video Gastroscope (Karl Storz SE & Co. KG) with 110 mm length, 5.9 mm outer diameter, and 2.0 mm working channel, specifically designed for feline gastrointestinal endoscopy (a). A diagram of the endoscopic tip is shown on the right, with the various end points for light source, working channel, and water/air nozzle. Handpiece of a flexible endoscope held in the left hand, with the thumb on the inner deflection knob (up/down) and the index finger controlling the air/water valve (b). Commonly used accessory instruments for flexible gastrointestinal endoscopy (c): from left to right, four-wire basket retrieval instrument, snare, injection needle, alligator grasper, and nonfenestrated biopsy forceps without central spike. Images a left, b, and c courtesy of Karl Storz SE & Co. KG.

by 576 pixels high, while high definition is most commonly available in 720p, 1080i, and 1080p resolutions.

Flexible endoscopes

Flexible endoscopes consist of three major parts: the insertion tube, handpiece, and umbilical cord (Figs. 7.1a and 7.1b). The insertion tube is the most complex part because it contains fibre-optic bundles for light transmission and image transmission (fibrescope); channels for insufflation, irrigation, and suction/instrumentation; deflection cables (two or four); and several layers of protective sheathing along its entire length. The last several centimetres of the endoscopic tip are called the bending section. In this portion, the insertion tube can be deflected in one or two planes (up and down, left and right). This movement is controlled by the deflection cables, which are connected to the deflection knobs on the handpiece of the endoscope. Smaller diameter endoscopes can only deflect the tip in one plane (one- or two-way tip deflection: up and down); however, endoscopes designed for GI use (gastro-, duodeno-, colonoscopes) are equipped with four-way tip deflection. In most flexible endoscopes, the up deflection is at least 180°, while deflection in the other three directions is about 90°. The tip deflection enables the endoscopist to guide the endoscope in almost any forward direction by coordinated movement of up/down, right/left, and twisting of the whole insertion tube and handpiece around its longitudinal axis.

Fibre-optic light transmission bundles terminate at the distal tip in one or two light guide lenses close to the objective lens. As a strong light is needed for illumination of the GI tract, especially the stomach, GI endoscopes usually contain two light guide lenses located on either side of the objective lens in the tip. The objective lens is either connected to the fibre-optic image transmission bundles (fibrescope) or to the CCD chip (videoendoscope).

The irrigation channel ends at the irrigation nozzle, which is located on the endoscope tip close to the objective lens. The water jet exiting this nozzle is directed over the objective lens to remove adherent mucus or debris, which might obscure the view. Room air is used to insufflate and hence distend the GI tract, enabling a clear view of the mucosa for complete and thorough examination. The instrumentation/suction or accessory/working channel is used for insertion of accessory flexible instruments and for suction of fluids and air. The handpiece also contains the deflection knobs with the deflection locks (Fig. 7.1b), the opening of the instrumentation channel, and the valves for insufflation/irrigation and suction. In a fibrescope, the handpiece ends with the eyepiece and also contains a dioptre adjustment ring to manually focus the objective lens. The handpiece of some videoendoscopes also hold programmable buttons for control of various functions (e.g. light gain, magnification, image freeze).

The light guide connector connects the umbilical cord to the light source and includes fittings for insufflation and irrigation. Most light sources used for GI endoscopy contain an integral air pump for insufflation, which also provides the positive pressure that forces the irrigation water from an attached bottle though the irrigation channel. A separate suction pump can be attached to the suction connector on the light guide connector. Located on the light guide connector is also the pressure compensation port used for leakage testing with a manometer-type pressure tester and to prevent damage from external pressure changes (gas sterilisation, shipping by air) by attaching the pressure compensation cap to this valve. In videoendoscopes, the connection for the video cable is integrated into the light guide connector, combined with an air and water tight fitting cap, which needs to be tightly screwed on the connector whenever the endoscope is cleaned and is left there when not in use.

The endoscope has to be cleaned and disinfected between uses. An unclean endoscope should never be used in another animal. Each type of endoscope is cleaned and disinfected individually, and information about the cleaning procedure and approved disinfectants needs to be obtained from the manufacturer.

Accessory instruments

A variety of accessory instrumentation is available for use with endoscopes. The most widely used in cats are biopsy forceps and foreign body grasping instruments (Fig. 7.1c). Other potentially useful instruments include injection/aspiration needles, polypectomy snares, and coagulation electrodes.

The most commonly used instruments to obtain tissue samples from the GI mucosa are pinch biopsy forceps. These are small flexible forceps with opposing cups at the end. The cups come in different configurations: round or oval, with a smooth or serrated edge, closed or fenestrated, with or without central spike. Fenestrated cups are reported to produce larger biopsy specimens with less crush artefacts.[1] The spike aids in anchoring the forceps into the mucosa but can lead to artefacts in the tissue samples. Personally, the authors prefer to use nonspiked cups because, with proper technique, a spike is not needed and causes crushing of the samples.

The most important feature of flexible instruments is their appropriate size and handling. To not damage the instrumentation channel and the endoscope itself, their diameter should never exceed the instrument diameter recommended by the manufacturer. To avoid damage to the endoscope, the instrument is never to be forced through the instrumentation channel.

Rigid endoscopes for gastrointestinal endoscopy

For evaluation of the oral cavity, oesophagus, and distal large intestine (descending colon and rectum), rigid endoscopes can be used. Rigid endoscopes are composed of a telescope used in conjunction with a sheath or cannula. The telescope is a metal tube containing high-quality optical glass lenses (rod-lens system) and light bundles. The outer diameter of a rod-lens telescope ranges from 1.9 to 10 mm, the length from 10 to 40 cm. Smaller telescopes are more versatile, but illumination and image size are superior in larger-diameter optics. Rigid endoscopes have a fixed viewing angle which is important to consider, as the viewing angle affects orientation and visual access. For GI endoscopy, 0° to 30° angled telescopes are used. With forward (0°) angle, orientation is quite simple, while view is limited. An angled optical instrument allows the endoscopist a larger viewing area just by rotating the endoscope around its axis, but spatial orientation is more challenging. For GI endoscopy, an operating sheath is locked onto the telescope. It serves to protect the telescope and prevents injury to the cat but also facilitates the ingress and egress of fluids or gases through the two side ports and the introduction of diagnostic and surgical accessory instrumentation through the working channel port. In rigid endoscopes, light is transmitted from a remote light source via a fibre-optic light cable, which is connected to a port near the eyepiece. The endoscopist can look directly through the eyepiece, but the procedure is easier with a connected CCD camera that allows viewing of the projected image on a monitor.

Rigid endoscopes used for oesophagoscopy and proctoscopy in humans use a blunt-tip obturator that fits inside the endoscope to facilitate insertion of the instrument into the oesophageal or rectal lumen. These endoscopes also come with an attachable light source and an air insufflation mechanism, mostly in form of a bulb insufflator. The diameter varies between adult (18–25 mm) and paediatric (9–12 mm), and their length is usually 25 cm. The paediatric size is most suited for feline patients. In oesophagoscopy, rigid endoscopes are mostly used for foreign body removal or balloon dilation of strictures. Examination of the large intestine with rigid endoscopes is limited to the rectum and descending colon, whereas the ileum, caecum, and ascending and transverse colon cannot be visualised. However, in inflammatory disorders which involve the whole colon diffusely, biopsy samples obtained from the distal part are often diagnostic. Large intestinal tumours and polyps are most often located in the distal colon and rectum and can therefore be adequately evaluated, biopsied, or even removed with rigid instruments. Biopsy forceps with an angulated tip might be used parallel to the endoscope in rigid oesophagoscopy and colonoscopy, as with these, the endoscopist is able to place the cups perpendicular to the mucosa, which is essential to obtain adequate biopsy samples. However, visualisation of mucosal detail and the use and handling of biopsy forceps are superior and more targeted with flexible endoscopes.

TECHNIQUES

Handling the endoscope

Flexible endoscopy should not be performed in a sitting position, as this constrains the movement of the arm and upper body of the endoscopist. Therefore, the endoscopist is always standing in front of (for upper GI endoscopy) or behind (for lower GI endoscopy) the cat. The handpiece of the flexible gastroscope is designed to be held in the left hand (Fig. 7.1b).

The thumb of the left hand controls the larger inner deflection knob (up/down), while the index finger controls the valves. The upper valve allows suction when being depressed fully. The insufflation/irrigation valve (lower valve) is controlled either with the index finger as well or with the middle finger. Obstructing this valve with the fingertip (without depressing it) results in air insufflation, while complete depression allows irrigation.

Bending the wrist of the left hand in (supination) and out (pronation) provides rotational torque of the whole insertion tube without causing damage (Video 7.1) The right hand is used to advance or retreat the insertion tube and to insert any accessory instruments into the working channel. The left/right (outer, smaller) deflection knob is either worked by the thumb of the left hand or by the right hand.

During rigid endoscopy, it is recommended for the endoscopist to be in a sitting position, while the endoscope can be held either with the right or left hand. The light guide cable and the cable of the camera head are hanging downwards. The hand holding the endoscope advances and retracts the rigid part of the endoscope and also rotates the endoscope around its axis as needed.

Video 7.1. Correct way of holding a flexible endoscope, and demonstration of endoscope tip flexion by using deflection controls and achieving insertion tube torque by left arm and wrist movement.

The index or middle finger of the hand holding the endoscope controls the opening and closing of the side ports. The other hand can be used to hold the animal in a correct position while the endoscope is advanced. In rigid colonoscopy, the hand not controlling the endoscope needs to be used to pinch the anus closed to allow air insufflation without leakage, or this can be done by an assistant. This hand also introduces and retracts any accessory instrumentation through the working port of the sheath. The air insufflation line is attached to one side port, and the assistant insufflates air into the lumen of the examined organ with a bulb insufflator or another device (e.g. air insufflation pump, pressure bag, syringe).

Handling accessory instruments

Accessory instruments are advanced through the instrumentation channel by the endoscopist. The upper opening of the instrumentation channel is covered by a rubber instrumentation channel cap, which closes the channel to prevent leakage of insufflated air. The lid of this cap can either be opened to introduce the accessory instrument or the instrument is passed through a minute opening in the rubber lid which seals around the instrument. It is paramount to never use force when pushing any instrument through the channel, especially when resistance is met. When the instrument is passed through the deflectable part of the tip, it is advisable to straighten the tip somewhat, advance the instrument until it can be seen in the field of view, and then deflect the tip again as needed. Foreign objects should never be retracted/pulled back into or through the instrumentation channel. Instead, the foreign body is grasped tightly with an accessory instrument (e.g. a grasping forceps, sling/snare, or basket) and pulled close up to the tip of the endoscope, followed by removal of the entire endoscope, instrument, and foreign material. The only material that is allowed to be retrieved through the instrumentation channel are endoscopic biopsy samples inside the biopsy forceps.

In certain circumstances (e.g. when foreign material is retrieved from the oesophagus or stomach but cannot be reached or grasped sufficiently with any of the instruments that can be inserted through the working channel), a separate rigid foreign body grasper can be used by inserting it alongside the endoscope. In cats, this device has to be small enough to fit into the oesophagus together with the endoscope. It often has to be manoeuvred with the help of an assistant, who should take care not to inadvertently grab hold of the endoscope, as this can cause serious damage to the insertion tube. In these circumstances, and once the foreign material is secured, it can be helpful to retract the endoscope completely before attempting to remove the additional grasping instrument. The authors prefer to hold both instruments without help, as this prevents the potential risk of miscommunication. In some cats, it is necessary to deflate the cuff of the endotracheal tube or even extubate in order to pass the foreign body within the grasping instrument through the pharyngeal area. Some rigid endoscopes can be used in conjunction with a sheath that has an integrated foreign body forceps, which is bigger than an accessory instrument used through the working channel.

Obtaining mucosal biopsy samples

The quality of endoscopically obtained biopsy samples greatly influences the likelihood for an accurate histopathological diagnosis of a specific mucosal lesion. In general, at least six to eight (histologically) adequate samples need to be collected of each section of the feline gastric and duodenal mucosa to reliably detect abnormalities.[2,3] An adequate sample should consist of full-thickness mucosa and at least three or four intact, if possible contiguous, villi. Samples containing submucosa are preferred. These requirements can be challenging to meet in the feline intestine due to the small intestinal diameter and therefore limited feasibility to direct the forceps tip into the mucosa at a suitable (preferably perpendicular) angle and depth.

Various techniques for sampling the GI mucosa with flexible forceps are used. Each endoscopist has a preferred method, and any technique that yields adequate tissue specimens without damaging the intestinal wall integrity is acceptable. Taking biopsy samples can be done by the endoscopist alone, but having an assistant to operate the forceps is beneficial. The best samples are obtained if the forceps are advanced perpendicular into the desired area.

If the tip of the endoscope is positioned perpendicular in front of the mucosa, the biopsy instrument is passed through the operating channel until the tip and the hinges of the cups are visible. The jaws are opened and advanced into the mucosa with some pressure. Adequate forward pressure displaces the mucosa away from the endoscope and leads to gentle bowing of the instrument shaft. The jaws are closed, and the forceps are retracted through the working channel, thereby tearing the tissue out of the mucosa (Video 7.2). Except for gastric mucosa in the area of the pylorus, it is not necessary to forcefully tug or jerk the forceps back. To avoid damage to the working channel, it is generally advisable to straighten the endoscope tip as much as possible or at least to let go of the deflecting knobs before retracting the biopsy forceps. This is clearly mandatory if a forceful jerk is deemed necessary. This procedure might not be feasible in cats with a small-diameter intestinal lumen. In this case, the forceps are advanced into the intestinal lumen and then opened and retracted almost against the tip of the endoscope. The tip is then deflected obliquely into the mucosa as much as possible to attain as perpendicular an orientation as possible. During this manoeuvre, it is often impossible to see the mucosa (red-out). The tissue samples are then obtained by gentle pressuring the jaws of the forceps into the mucosa without turning the tip of the instrument away again (happens if too much pressure is applied).

Video 7.2. Obtaining biopsy samples in the small intestine.

Video 7.3. Transferring a mucosal biopsy sample from the endoscopy forceps to a sample pot using the "free floating biopsy" approach. Several samples from one site can be combined like this. The liquid can be saline which is later decanted and replaced by formalin.

In general, larger forceps yield tissue specimens of better quality,[1] but since the intestinal mucosa is relatively thin in the feline patient, adequate samples may be obtained with smaller instruments (working channel 2.0 mm).

After obtaining the specimen, the biopsy forceps are removed from the endoscope, and the tissue sample is carefully removed from the jaws. There are several ways this can be done. The authors prefer placing the jaws containing the sample into a container filled with isotonic saline and then "washing off" the sample by shaking the tip of the forceps; this helps to avoid damaging the edges of the cups (Video 7.3).

Similarly, the tissue sample can be rinsed from the cup with a stream of isotonic saline instead of fiddling it out with a needle. If saline solution is used to remove the tissue from the cup, the container with both sample and saline needs to be carefully decanted to remove as much saline as possible, and then formalin is added to get a liquid:tissue ratio of 10:1. Another technique described by some authors is placing the specimen on a special sponge or prepared cucumber slice in the correct orientation and embedding it directly into the appropriate cups. Prying the specimens from the cups with a hypodermic needle, as often done, might result in crush artefacts and dulling of the biopsy forceps. Irrespective of which technique is used to submit biopsy tissue samples to the histopathology laboratory, discussing it with the pathologist and getting good input will often be helpful to get meaningful results. Specimens should be sent in the fixative to the pathology laboratory as quickly as possible for histopathological examination. Submission of a complete history and macroscopic evaluation report to the pathologist is crucial to obtain the best results. Furthermore, tissue samples can be used for other laboratory investigation (e.g. culture, PCR) or to create touch imprints for cytological evaluation.

Anaesthesia

General anaesthesia is required for GI endoscopy, and intubation with a cuffed endotracheal tube is mandatory because of the risk of gastrooesophageal reflux. The safest anaesthetic regime is one the operator is familiar with, but inhalation anaesthesia is preferable. Even if injection anaesthesia is used throughout the procedure, the animal has to be intubated and the cuff inflated at all times. A non-spring-loaded mouth gag (e.g. cutoff syringe or needle cap) must always be inserted in upper GI endoscopy to prevent damage to the endoscope. Spring-loaded mouth gags should never be used in cats, as they might result in postprocedural blindness due to occlusion of the regional artery.[4,5]

Some anaesthetic agents affect intestinal motility and sphincter function, making the passage of the cardia and pylorus potentially more difficult. Atropine and other anticholinergic drugs should not be used unless necessary to increase heart rate, as these drugs may alter gastric motility patterns and increase pyloric tone. Pure opioid agonists may also increase pyloric tone and should be avoided. Fluid support should be given during anaesthesia; dehydrated animals need to be rehydrated before anaesthesia unless endoscopy needs to be performed as an emergency procedure. In hypoproteinaemic cats, colloid administration should be considered to ensure reasonable oncotic pressure.

Anaesthesia monitoring during upper GI endoscopy includes, at minimum, assessment of heart rate, respiration, and pulse oximetry. Air insufflation is essential in upper GI endoscopy to open the lumen and move the mucosa away from the endoscopic tip. Overinflation of the stomach can cause cardiorespiratory compromise, and both endoscopist and assistant should monitor the degree and possible effects of distension of the GI tract.

Patient preparation

Food should be withheld 12 hours before endoscopy of the upper GI tract, as many animals requiring GI endoscopy are likely to have some delayed gastric emptying. In lower GI tract endoscopy, food should be withheld for at least 24 hours to ensure no further passage of ingesta from the small into the large intestine. If the owner is unable to withhold food (e.g. multiple-cat household, cat complaining severely, outdoor cat), it is advisable to hospitalise the cat prior to the procedure to ensure proper fasting. Normally the feline stomach empties within 8–12 hours; therefore, finding retained food in the stomach of a properly fasted animal may give useful information about a possible anatomical or mechanical outflow obstruction or gastric motility disorder. In these cases, a significant amount of gastric or duodenal ingesta may compromise the endoscopic examination since the entire mucosa cannot be visualised, and lesions or even foreign bodies might be missed. If necessary, fluid can be aspirated through the working channel, or if too much food is present, it can be aspirated through a separate gastric tube alongside the endoscope. In some instances, it is sufficient to gently turn the animal around the endoscope to visualise the entire mucosa of the stomach.

If a barium contrast study has been performed, upper GI endoscopy should be postponed for at least 24 hours to allow complete clearing of the barium from the mucosal surface. Any residual barium should never be aspirated through the instrumentation channel, as this might adhere to the channel's inner lining and clog the lumen.

For lower GI endoscopy, removal of all faeces from the descending colon is required. While in dogs administration of enemas or giving commercial GI lavage solutions based on polyethylene glycol and electrolyte salts is often performed, this is not commonly done in cats, even though recently the use of polyethylene glycol solutions given via nasogastric tube the day before the colonoscopy is advocated by some specialists. The authors empty the colon after the cat has been anaesthetised for the endoscopic procedure. A well-lubricated rubber tube is passed gently into the colon not further than the length up to the last rib, and warm water is slowly injected into the colonic lumen. Care should be taken not to overdistend the colon, as this might lead to vomiting, thus it is imperative that the animal is intubated and the cuff inflated. With adequate massage, almost all faecal material can be removed from the colon allowing a good view of the mucosa.

For flexible GI endoscopy, the cat should be placed in left lateral recumbency. This positions the gastric antrum and pylorus uppermost, which significantly facilitates air insufflation of these structures and hence their intubation with the endoscope (Fig. 7.2). If rigid endoscopy is performed, the cat is in sternal recumbency for oesphagoscopy and in sternal or right lateral recumbency for proctoscopy and colonoscopy. In an animal lying in right lateral recumbency, it is much more difficult to clearly identify all parts of the stomach or pass into the antrum and through the pylorus. The only exception to this positioning is the placement of a PEG feeding tube (see Chapter 40), which is placed through the left flank in an animal lying in right lateral recumbency. For flexible colonoscopy the cat is also placed in left lateral recumbency, so the descending colon lies downward while the transverse and ascending colon are facing up. This position is helpful to properly distend the lumen of the proximal colon by air insufflation.

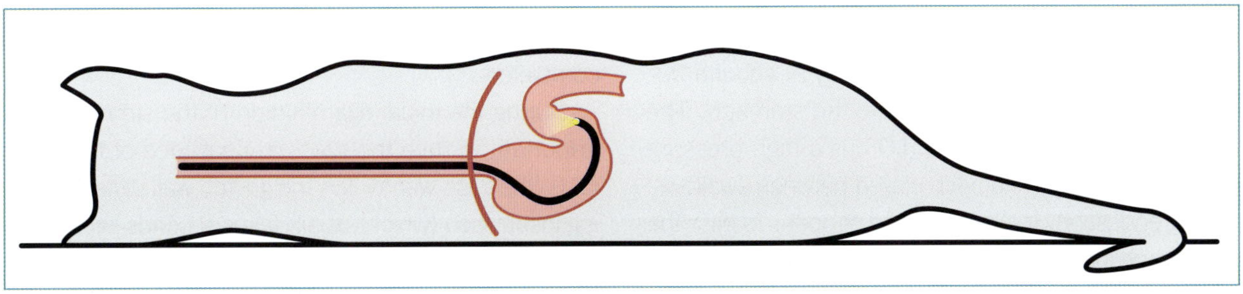

Figure 7.2. Schematic drawing showing positioning of the feline patient in left lateral recumbency for endoscopy of the gastrointestinal tract. The normal orientation of the stomach and correct location of the endoscope entering the gastric antrum are shown.

ENDOSCOPIC PROCEDURES

Oesophagoscopy

Usually only a quick inspection of the oesophagus and stomach is performed on the way to the duodenum, so that apparent lesions are not confused with artefacts caused by the endoscope. After extending the cat's head and neck, the insertion tube is passed carefully along the midline of the hard palate through the oropharynx and guided dorsal to the endotracheal tube until the upper oesophageal sphincter (UOS) comes into view (Fig. 7.3a, Video 7.4). It appears as a star-shaped area of folded mucosa dorsal to the larynx, but often it cannot be sufficiently insufflated with air and is passed blindly (even though visual guidance as much as possible is preferred). As the UOS is a low-resistance sphincter, the tip of the endoscope can be passed easily by applying insufflation, while hardly any pressure is needed. If a rigid endoscope is used, it is passed through the oral cavity under strict visual supervision, as rigid instruments can easily damage the mucosa.

The cervical oesophagus is normally collapsed, so visibility is briefly obscured (red-out). Insufflation is continued once the UOS is passed, but forward motion is halted until the oesophageal lumen is visible as a straight tube with a slight bend at the thoracic inlet. The tip is adjusted into the centre of the lumen, and the endoscope is advanced through the oesophagus in a slow continuous movement with no or very minor resistance. To keep the lumen from collapsing, intermittent or continuous air flow is applied as needed, but overinsufflation should be avoided. In rare instances, slight manual compression of the upper oesophagus is needed to prevent escape of the insufflated air.

Extension of the thoracic oesophagus generally needs minimal insufflation. While passing the endoscope through the length of the oesophagus, the entire mucosal circumference is inspected for colour, texture, and possible pathological lesions. Normal oesophageal mucosa in the cat is smooth, glistening, and pale pink, and superficial mucosal vessels can be seen. As the feline oesophagus is composed of striated muscle in the proximal two thirds and smooth muscle in the distal third, the distal part has the appearance of circular, wavelike ripples (Fig. 7.3b). Over the base of the heart, the pulsation of the aorta can be seen.

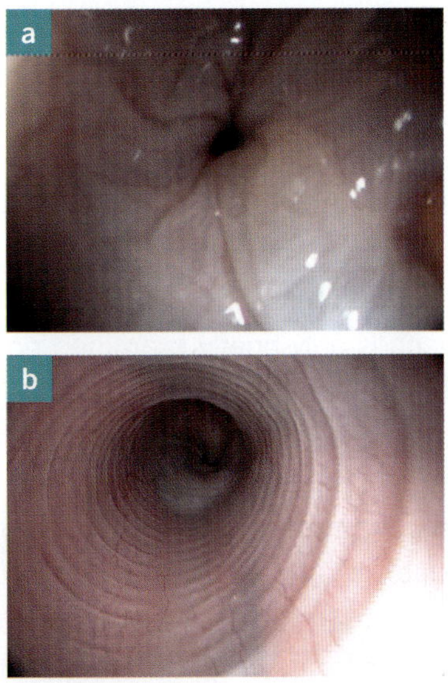

Figure 7.3. Oesophagoscopic views in a cat. Endoscopic appearance of the upper oesophageal sphincter (a). Endoscopic view of the lower third of oesophagus showing typical circular, wavelike ripples—herringbone pattern (b).

Video 7.4. Oesophagoscopy showing the endoscopic passage through the upper oesophageal sphincter.

At the gastrooesophageal junction, the oesophagus is a slit-like opening that passes obliquely at about a 30° angle through the diaphragm into the stomach. The lower oesophageal sphincter (LOS) is a high-pressure zone that keeps the stomach closed between swallows. During endoscopy it may be closed or open. To pass the endoscope into the stomach, the tip is deflected slightly left and upward and the endoscope is advanced under direct visual inspection with slight pressure and variable air insufflation until the gastric lumen is reached. A short red-out may be seen when passing. Little resistance should be encountered. If forward motion is impeded when entering the stomach, it is usually because the tip has missed the LOS. The endoscope should be withdrawn and redirected prior to repeat intubation.

Oesophageal biopsy samples are rarely obtained, as the mucosa is very thin and relatively tough, making perpendicular angling of the endoscope tip challenging. In addition, it results inevitably in very small biopsy specimens. However, oesophageal masses should always be biopsied.

Gastroduodenoscopy

A full examination of all areas of the stomach should be performed in every patient, and all landmarks have to be identified properly. Therefore, the endoscopist has to be familiar with the gastric anatomy to successfully manoeuvre the endoscope through the stomach, obtain retroflexed views of the fundus and cardia, advance around the lesser curvature/incisura angularis (Fig. 7.4a) into the antrum, and traverse the pyloric canal into the duodenum. The stomach is only briefly examined on the way in so as to note the gross appearance, while a full examination and biopsy procedure is performed after duodenoscopy and duodenal biopsies have been completed.

During the initial examination of the stomach, it is important to note the gross appearance of the rugal folds, the ease with which the gastric wall distends during insufflation (which usually takes seconds in cats due to their small gastric volume), and if any fluid or ingesta are present. The mucosa of the stomach is smooth, pale pink, and glistening, and the rugal folds should separate and stretch easily (Figs. 7.4b and 7.4c).

In cats, after insufflating air into the oesophagus, the stomach is usually already filled with air and its mucosa is visible. The degree of gastric distension is judged by increased flattening of the folds, with a completely smooth mucosa seen at maximal insufflation (Fig. 7.4c). However, only moderate distension should be necessary to pass the endoscope through the stomach. This allows orientation and identification of gross lesions (ulcers, foreign bodies, masses) while avoiding overdistension, which might be detrimental to the movement of the diaphragm and lead to serious cardiopulmonary compromise. Providing prior fasting time is appropriate, the stomach in most cats is expected to be completely empty, although the presence of a small amount of intragastric fluid is not considered abnormal. Large amounts of fluid, especially bilious fluids, may suggest reflux of intestinal fluid into the stomach. This could be iatrogenic (in cats that received large-volume enemas) or indicate abnormal motility (gastric emptying disorder, duodenogastric reflux, intestinal obstruction). As bile is an irritant, the gastric mucosa may appear reddened in case of significant biliary reflux.

Insufficient insufflation of the stomach is most commonly due to technical issues with the equipment

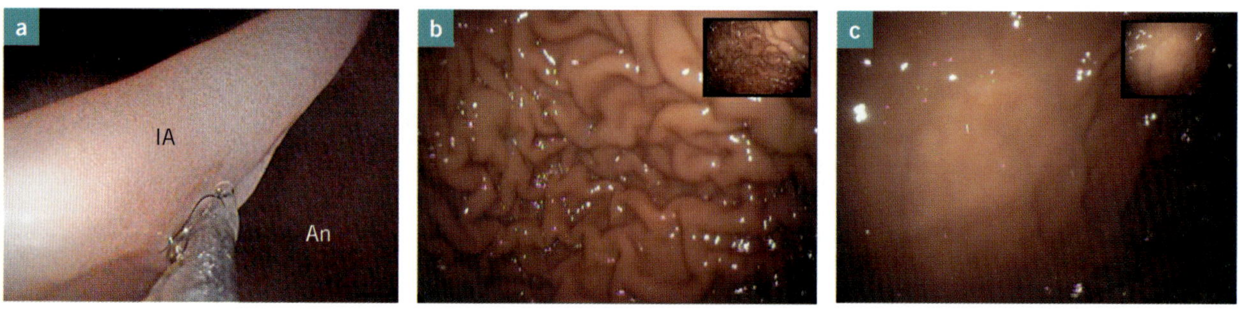

Figure 7.4. Gastroscopic views in a cat. Incisura angularis (IA), with the antrum (An) leading towards the pylorus. A biopsy forceps can be seen at the bottom of the image (a). Rugal folds are clearly visible in the stomach with minimal air insufflation (b). Rugal folds are flattened with increased amounts of insufflated air (c). Image a courtesy of Silke Salavati Schmitz, University of Edinburgh, UK.

(e.g. a blocked air/water channel port, faulty connection of the air pump) or air escaping through the oesophagus, rather than reduced compliance of the gastric wall due to disease that truly prevents distension. With orientation achieved, the endoscope is advanced along the greater curvature by lifting the tip upward and pushing it gently forward using rotational torque if necessary. With the patient in left lateral recumbency and the endoscope held in the conventional manner, the view is predictable. In order to reach the antrum, an important landmark is the incisura angularis (Fig. 7.4a).

By lifting the tip and advancing the endoscope, the incisura comes into view almost automatically. Sometimes the tip has to be deflected down again slightly. The antrum is below the incisura, while the cardia is above it and can be viewed by increased retroflexion of the tip. Once this landmark is reached, the endoscope is advanced through the antrum and pylorus into the duodenum.

Complete assessment of the stomach is performed (after duodenoscopy) by inspecting the antrum and the greater curvature up to the incisura, and then inspecting the cardia and fundus by retroflexion (J-manoeuvre) (Fig. 7.5a). In cats, the J-manoeuvre is started when the endoscope is at the middle part of the gastric body opposite the incisura angularis. The tip is lifted up (counterclockwise deflection of inner control knob) and the endoscope is advanced further, allowing direct visualisation of the incisura first (sometimes this cannot be achieved in cats due to their small size and reduced working space). By deflecting the tip up almost completely—often accompanied by a twist of the left wrist—the cardia comes into view, including the insertion tube of the endoscope itself (Fig. 7.5b).

Sometimes this manoeuvre extends the LOS and air leaks into the oesophagus, so further air insufflation is needed. For a close-up view of the cardia, the endoscopist's right hand retracts the insertion tube, thereby pulling the tip towards the mucosa. By rotational movement of the insertion tube (with the left wrist) and turning the outer deflection knob for a more lateral view, a nearly 360° examination of the proximal stomach can be accomplished. Leaving the endoscope tip in the proximal stomach and turning the deflection controls back into a neutral position allows visualisation of the gastric body. Alternatively, advancing the endoscope while the tip is still deflected provides an additional view of the proximal stomach. Once the incisura angularis is reached, the tip is straightened back into the antrum.

In some cats, the angle of the lesser curvature might be very acute, so a "slide-by" technique might be necessary to pass into the antrum. In this technique, the deflected endoscope tip impinges on the outer lining of the gastric/intestinal bend, and a red-out is seen. If this red-out seems to be moving, it is generally safe to advance until the next straight part, in this case the antrum, can be visualised. However, this manoeuvre can cause some mucosal damage and lead to linear streaks of hyperaemia or mucosal haemorrhage. These artefacts can be avoided by deflecting the endoscope tip within the body of the stomach before advancing into the antrum.

The pylorus has a variety of appearances and can be closed or open to variable degrees (Fig. 7.6). Occasional duodenogastric reflux can be observed. The location can sometimes be difficult to identify because of peristaltic waves, antral masses, or fluid obscuring the view. Pyloric folds are extremely rare in cats.

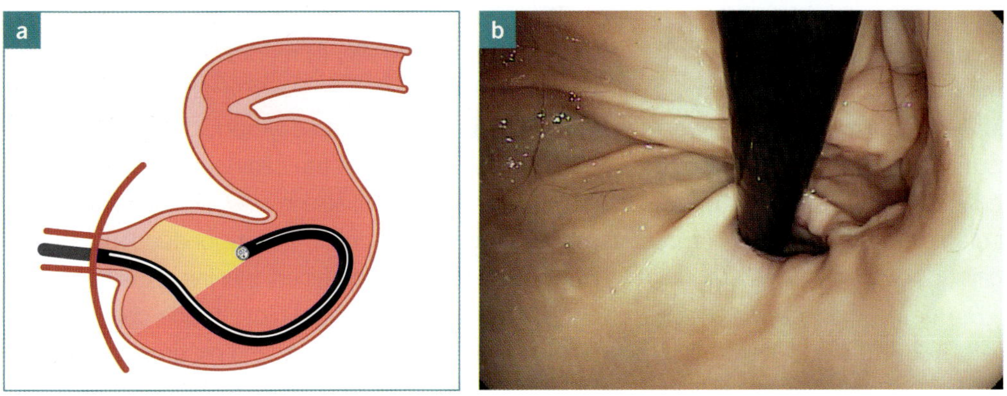

Figure 7.5. J-manoeuvre during gastroscopy. Schematic overview of the J-manoeuvre, with the tip of the endoscope pointing back at the cardia (a). Endoscopic view of a cat's gastric cardia and fundus (and the endoscopic shaft) during the J-manoeuvre (b).

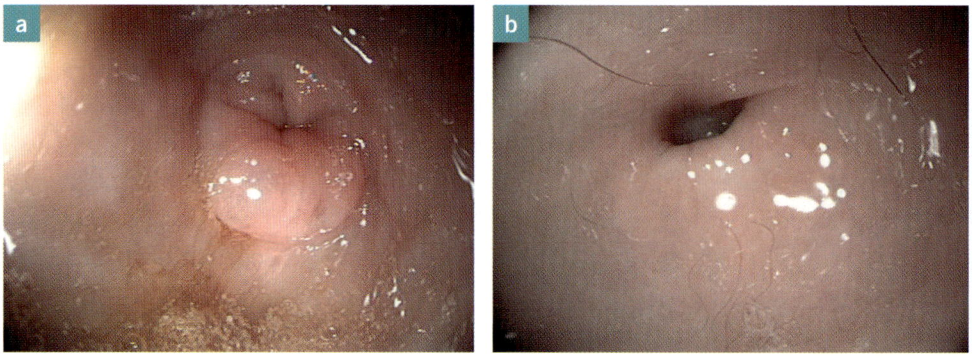

Figure 7.6. Endoscopic views of the feline pylorus. The pylorus has a rosette appearance when firmly closed (a). During opening, the pylorus has a flat appearance (b).

In some cases, the pylorus might be open, and passage can be achieved quite easily; in other cases, the pylorus may be closed tight and offer significant resistance. To intubate the pyloric canal, the pylorus needs to be kept permanently in the centre of the endoscopic field of view. As the pyloric position changes with respiratory movement and peristalsis, small adjustments by up/down deflection and insertion tube rotation might be necessary. The aim is to continually move forward whilst readjusting the centring. Overdistension of the stomach must be avoided during this process, as with increased intraluminal pressure the stomach assumes a round shape while the antral opening is flattened. In addition, antral contractions will be stimulated. However, as pyloric intubation is aided by air insufflation, a constant balance between intermittent insufflation and suction to avoid overdistension has to be found. Despite air insufflation, red-out and image blurring frequently occur when passing the pylorus, in which case, it is often easiest to aim at the blackest area of the field of view. Turning the endoscope tip slightly left and up (both knobs in counterclockwise direction) while advancing forward gradually and gently can help. Vision is blurred inside the pyloric canal, as the pyloric wall closes around the tip. Turning both deflection control knobs clockwise turns the tip into the direction of the proximal duodenum immediately beyond the pylorus. However, excessive turning or advancing against resistance should be avoided, especially during a red-out.

The amount of pressure one dares to use is a matter of experience and judgement. An endoscope less than or equal to 9 mm in outer diameter can be passed in most cats. However, in small cats (<2.5 kg) or cats with a narrow pyloric canal (Siamese, Burmese, Tonkinese), a smaller endoscope (outer diameter <8 mm) is preferred.[6]

As the pylorus of the cat is narrow and offers high constant resistance, it is crucial to carefully monitor the cat's heart and respiratory rates when passing the pylorus appears difficult and the pyloroduodenal junction and proximal duodenum might be stretched and distorted. Transient bradycardia secondary to an increase in vagal tone and/or respiratory depression may occur. If the endoscopic procedure results in significant cardiopulmonary compromise, the endoscope should be withdrawn, the stomach emptied of air, and the patient stabilised before another attempt is made.

Once the junction of the pylorus to the duodenum is reached, the mucosal colour changes from pale pink to pinkish red. If the lumen is still not clearly visible at this point, insufflation might be necessary to distend the intestinal lumen. Further gentle advance usually provides a view into the descending duodenum, seen as a straight tunnel (Fig. 7.7a). In some cases, minor forward or backward adjustments are needed to free the tip from the mucosa. If these manoeuvres do not provide a clear view of the intestinal lumen, the endoscope is retracted under constant insufflation until the view can be obtained. No forward movement should be attempted without clear visualisation, and no force should be used.

The colour of the normal feline duodenal and jejunal mucosa is cream to slightly reddish pink, and the presence of the villi gives it a velvety to villous appearance. Peyer's patches (aggregated lymphoid nodules), which can routinely be seen in the canine duodenal mucosa, are not as readily identifiable in cats, although aggregated lymphoid nodules do occur. The major duodenal papilla, which represents the combined opening of the pancreatic and biliary ducts, is located close to the convex curve formed by the antrum, pylorus, and proximal duodenum.

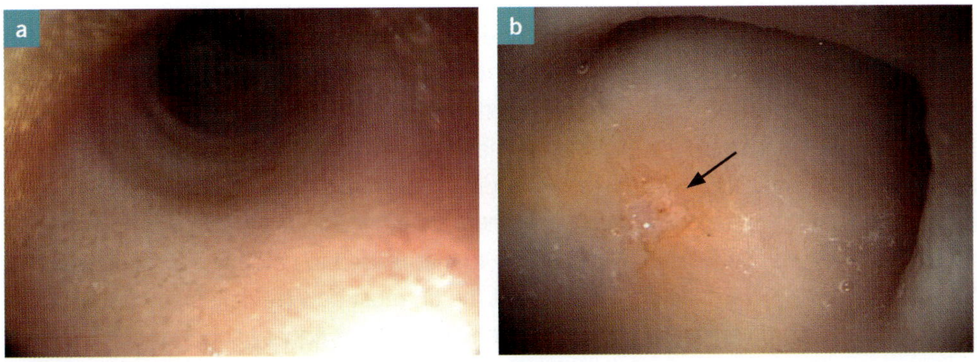

Figure 7.7. Endoscopic views of the feline duodenum. Normal duodenum (a). Duodenal papilla (arrow) (b).

It is a round to oval disc of 1.5–2 mm in diameter that appears almost white against the surrounding reddish mucosa (Fig. 7.7b).

The endoscope can usually be advanced easily through the descending duodenum to the caudal duodenal flexure and almost always up the ascending duodenum and into the proximal jejunum. Variable degrees of insufflation are required to maintain luminal distension and clear view of the mucosa. As there is already a bend in the endoscope insertion tube in the stomach, forward movement in the descending duodenum can, in some cases, be facilitated by withdrawing the endoscope slightly, thereby stretching the loop in the stomach. Forward movement is sometimes accelerated at this point, and great care has to be taken not to move the tip against the mucosal surface. While the insertion tube is slowly advanced, the intestine is closely examined for mucosal surface appearance and obvious lesions. To obtain circumferential views, the insertion tube can be rotated around its longitudinal axis.

After reaching the pelvic flexure of the duodenum, it ascends a short distance before reaching a ventrally directed bend (i.e. the juncture between the duodenum and jejunum). Gradual advance of the endoscope can be continued as long as the lumen can be clearly viewed and no resistance is met. Because the curves of the intestine move easily, only minor adjustments in tip deflection are required. In some cats, the loop in the stomach cannot be straightened and pyloric resistance remains high, which prevents further advancement up to the pelvic flexure of the duodenum. Sometimes massaging the intestinal loops transabdominally relaxes intestinal musculature and may help to facilitate further examination. As soon as resistance is met, the endoscope should be retracted. At this point the mucosa is closely examined, and biopsy samples are taken while slowly retracting.

As the endoscope is retracted through the proximal duodenum and pyloric canal, these areas are closely inspected again, as this has often not been done on the way in. Pyloric ulcers or tumours are frequently only discovered during this second examination.

After completion of gastroduodenoscopy with mucosal biopsy, the stomach is completely deflated. If there is gastric content (bile, fluid, food) in the oesophagus, it needs to be aspirated or washed to prevent aspiration during recovery from anaesthesia and to prevent oesophagitis and possible stricture formation at a later date. The cat has to be supervised closely during recovery and the endotracheal tube removed as late as possible.

Proctoscopy and colonoileoscopy

Before insertion of the endoscope, a digital rectal examination should be performed to assess obvious rectal masses or stricture that could otherwise be missed, especially if very caudal. The endoscope is well lubricated up to a length of about 20 cm and inserted 1–2 cm into the rectum. Air insufflation is started while an assistant closes the perianal tissue tightly around the insertion tube to prevent air leakage. Enough air is insufflated to extend the rectal and colonic lumen, so that the colon is seen as a tunnel and the colonic mucosal folds straighten (Fig. 7.8a). An inability to distend the lumen may indicate severe fibrosis with chronic inflammation, the presence of a stricture, or inadequate manual closure of the anal canal. With intermittent or constant air insufflation (as needed), the endoscope is slowly advanced as far as possible up the colon. The tip of the endoscope is kept in the centre of the lumen by turning the inner angulation knob and rotational torque of the endoscope. No or only minor resistance should be encountered. If the centre of the lumen cannot be visualised, the endoscope is slowly withdrawn while more air is insufflated until the mucosa is visible again. A partial fold separates the rectum from the descending colon but straightens almost completely with air insufflation. The colonic mucosa is pale pink, smooth, and glistening, and submucosal blood vessels can usually be seen throughout the entire colon (Fig. 7.8b). Lymphoid follicles with a diameter of 2–3 mm and an umbilicated centre are visible in the colonic mucosa (Fig. 7.8c).

Hyperaemia should be interpreted carefully, as it can occur secondary to warm-water enema, trauma from the rubber tube and endoscope, or a primary pathological process (e.g. mucosal inflammation). As the endoscope is advanced through the descending colon, the mucosa is inspected and lesions noted. The flexure at the junction of the descending colon to the transverse colon represents an approximate 90° change in direction upward (from left to right) but may be less distinct and less than 90° in some cats. To enter the transverse colon, the tip of the insertion tube is advanced almost against the mucosa of the flexure's outer curve. Air is insufflated and the tip deflected gradually up while the endoscope is advanced until the 90° bend is achieved. Visualisation might be lost for a brief moment until the transverse colon is entered and distended by insufflation. In most cats, insufflation of the descending colon leads to distension of the complete large intestine. Once the endoscope is in the transverse colon, the tip is straightened and centred in the lumen. It is then advanced slowly up to the flexure marking the beginning of the ascending colon. The endoscope should slide easily along the mucosa; however, as the feline intestinal tract is very pliant, manual support of the endoscope insertion tube from the outside might be needed in some instances. If the lumen of the transverse colon is not visible, slight rotational torque and angulation of the outer deflection knob will often help to obtain tunnel vision. The transverse colon of the cat is very short (2–4 cm), and the flexure to the ascending colon may be less distinct than in the dog. Advancement around this flexure is achieved with a similar technique to that utilised to navigate into the transverse colon, but the tip must now be deflected caudally. The feline ascending colon is equally short (about 1–2 cm), and at the end the ileocolic sphincter enters in a slit-like opening adjacent to the caecocolic junction (Fig. 7.9). Due to the small ileal diameter, ileal intubation is rarely possible in cats. If it is attempted, extreme caution is warranted to prevent colonic rupture.[7] If endoscopic intubation is not possible, blind biopsy samples can be collected from the ileum. The caecocolic junction is usually completely or partially open in cats, and, as the caecum is short (1–3 cm), it can be entirely inspected without entering its lumen.

Biopsy samples are again taken on the way out. A perpendicular orientation of the forceps to the mucosa can only be achieved at the flexures, in the caecum, and from luminal masses. Care has to be taken not to cause a caecal inversion when samples are taken. Most areas of the feline colon must be sampled tangentially to the mucosa. The risk of biopsy-related colonic perforation is increased with rigid colonoscopes and the use of angulated-tip forceps parallel to the endoscope.

At the end of the procedure, the endoscope is completely withdrawn; evacuation of the air in the colon is achieved by cessation of anal compression. Insufflation of the large intestine can result in distension of the small intestine and ultimately of the stomach, leading to potential respiratory distress. If overdistension of the stomach has occurred, it can be relieved by passing a tube into the

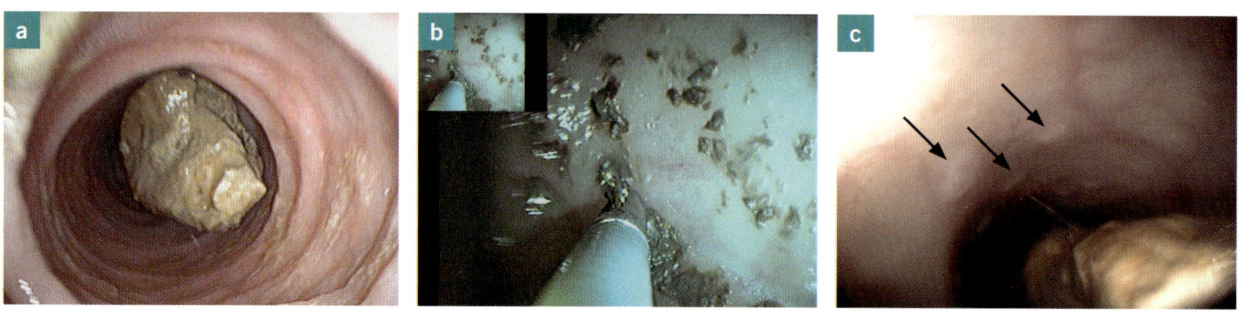

Figure 7.8. Endoscopic views of the feline colon. Normal mucosa of the colon. Residual faecal material is present in the lumen (a). Submucosal blood vessels in the colonic mucosa. Open biopsy forceps can be seen (b). Lymphoid follicles in the colonic mucosa (arrows) (c). Images courtesy of Silke Salavati Schmitz, University of Edinburgh, UK.

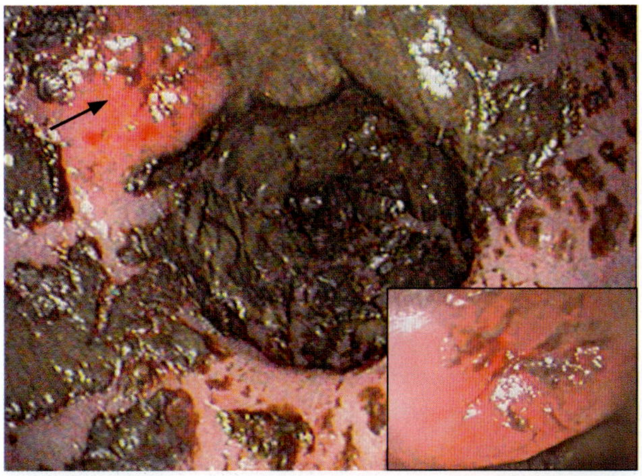

Figure 7.9. Endoscopic view of the feline ileocolic junction, with the caecum (centre of image) and ileocolic sphincter (arrow; close-up in insert). Images courtesy of Silke Salavati Schmitz, University of Edinburgh, UK.

stomach and either evacuating passively or attaching the tube to a suction pump. During recovery from anaesthesia, the cat has to be supervised closely and extubated as late as possible, as some animals tend to vomit. Gastric evacuation makes vomiting much less likely.

PATHOLOGICAL FINDINGS

Endoscopic pathology of the oesophagus

Overall, oesophageal diseases are uncommon in cats and represent about 0.05%–1% of all admissions in a referral situation. Common clinical signs which might necessitate an oesophagoscopy are retching, dysphagia, regurgitation, and possibly unexplained ptyalism. Plain radiographs of the thorax should be performed initially. Radiographs after oral administration of liquid contrast (iodine based or barium) or contrast mixed with food might be indicated in some cats. A swallow study (fluoroscopy) is needed to diagnose functional oesophageal motility problems (see Chapter 22). Endoscopy might still be indicated if the problem cannot be diagnosed sufficiently and it is the only modality to diagnose oesophagitis. Possible abnormalities found during oesophagoscopy are summarised in Box 7.1. Exact localisation of an oesophageal lesion is difficult unless it is directly over the base of the heart (aortic pulsation). To record abnormal findings, the distance from the upper incisors should be guesstimated based on the length markings on the endoscope.

Box 7.1. Possible abnormalities found during oesophagoscopy in cats.

- Oesophagitis (due to drugs [doxycycline, clindamycin], chemical ingestion, reflux, foreign body)
- Eosinophilic oesophagitis
- Stricture
- Foreign body (bezoar, fishhook, toy, bone, others)
- Tumour (squamous cell carcinoma, lymphoma, undifferentiated sarcoma, others)
- Vascular ring anomaly
- Gastrooesophageal intussusception
- Megaoesophagus*

*Megaoesophagus is difficult to diagnose by endoscopy due to air insufflation, and diagnosis should not be attempted by endoscopy.

Oesophagitis is characterised by mucosal erythema, irregularity, erosion, and/or ulceration (Fig. 7.10a). An oesophageal stricture is defined as circumferential narrowing, with a residual opening of varying diameter commonly in the exact centre of the lumen (Fig. 7.10b). It is important not to confuse oesophageal strictures with difficulties to pass the cardia, which might be a problem in some cats. Tumours of the feline oesophagus are rare. They mostly present as intramural masses (Fig. 7.10c) and tend to be ulcerated and friable. Sometimes oesophageal lymphoma may appear simply as a very irregular mucosa with cobblestone appearance. Foreign bodies are readily diagnosed and can often be removed endoscopically (see section "Therapeutic endoscopy" in this chapter). Vascular ring anomalies (e.g. persistent right aortic arch) are not often diagnosed by oesophagoscopy but will display a typical intraluminal band crossing the oesophagus with a diverticulum oral to that (Fig. 7.10d). Protrusion of gastric rugal folds into the oesophagus is the hallmark of a gastrooesophageal intussusception (very rare in cats). Megaoesophagus (generalised dilation of the entire oesophagus) is a rare finding in cats, and oesophagoscopy is infrequently indicated (better diagnosed on radiographs) or might even be contraindicated (risk of aspiration pneumonia during anaesthetic induction or recovery). Furthermore, a dilated oesophagus due to air insufflation and the effects of anaesthesia is difficult to differentiate from true megaoesophagus. Froth, fluid, and fermenting food might be seen in a primary oesophageal dilation or diverticula together with signs of oesophagitis. In some instances, it might even be difficult to reach the LOS because the endoscope keeps being diverted into blind endings.

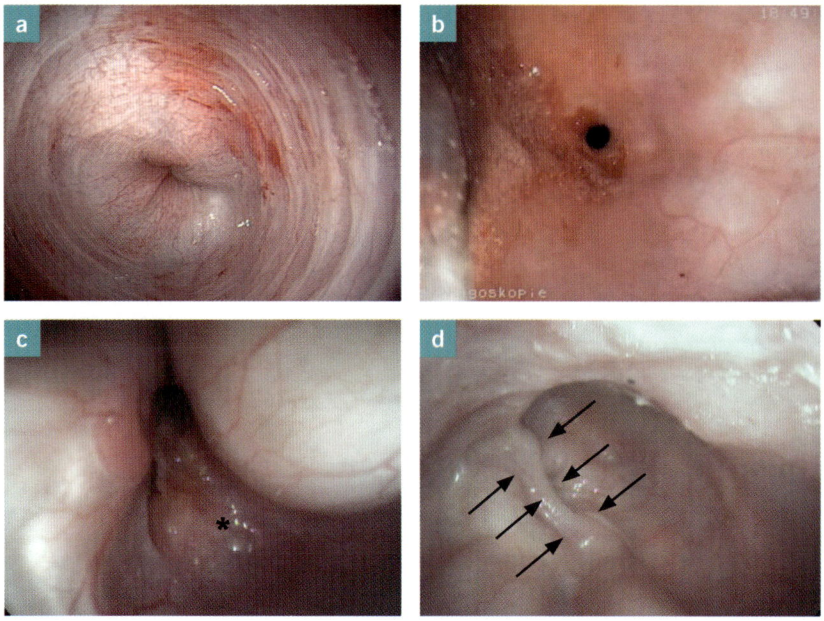

Figure 7.10. Abnormal findings during oesophagoscopy in cats. Oesophagitis with erythema in the lower third of the oesophagus of a 11-year-old cat with chronic vomiting and pretreatment with dexamethasone (a). Oesophageal stricture in a 1-year-old cat 4 weeks after receiving clindamycin tablets (b). Adenocarcinoma (asterisk) in the lower oesophagus of a 6-year-old cat with a 3-week history of regurgitation (c). Oesophagus of a 1-year-old cat with persistent right aortic arch (d). A band compressing the lumen from the outside can be seen (delimited by arrows).

Endoscopic pathology of the stomach

The most common indication for gastroscopy is chronic vomiting for which extra-GI causes have already been excluded (often via laboratory tests; see Chapters 1 and 3) or if the GI tract has been implicated as a likely cause (e.g. via diagnostic imaging procedures; see Chapters 1 and 5). Acute vomiting is rarely an indication unless a foreign body is suspected or diagnosed. Haematemesis—regardless if acute or chronic in nature—is also an indication, especially if there is significant blood loss (anaemia), the cause is not immediately obvious (e.g. historic administration of nonsteroidal anti-inflammatory drugs [NSAIDs]), or it is unresponsive to medical management. Other indications in cats can be unexplained weight loss, anorexia, nausea/ptyalism, or melaena.

Abnormalities seen during gastroscopy can include retention of food longer than 12 hours after feeding (gastric dysmotility), foreign bodies (including trichobezoars) (Fig. 7.11), signs of inflammation in the form of irregular mucosa (friable, cobblestone appearance) (Fig. 7.12a), ulcers (Fig. 7.12b), erosions, or petechial haemorrhage (Fig. 7.12c).

Chronic gastritis is much less well studied in cats than in dogs and is most commonly part of the inflammatory bowel disease (IBD) complex. The mucosa often looks normal but may appear irregular, friable, or show petechiation or larger areas of haemorrhage. For this reason, taking endoscopic biopsy samples of both normal and abnormal areas of the stomach for histopathological examination is mandatory for all animals undergoing diagnostic gastroscopy (see Chapter 9). While gastric

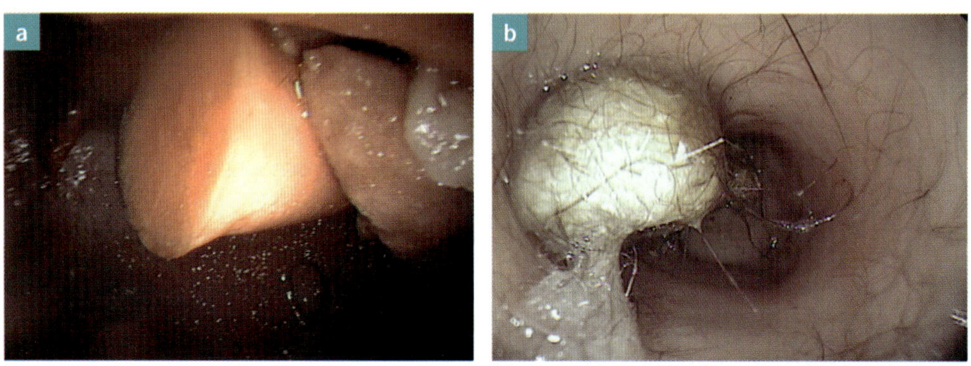

Figure 7.11. Endoscopic views of gastric foreign bodies. Ear plug in a 2-year-old Maine Coon cat (a). Trichobezoar in the gastric antrum of a 15-year-old cat (b).

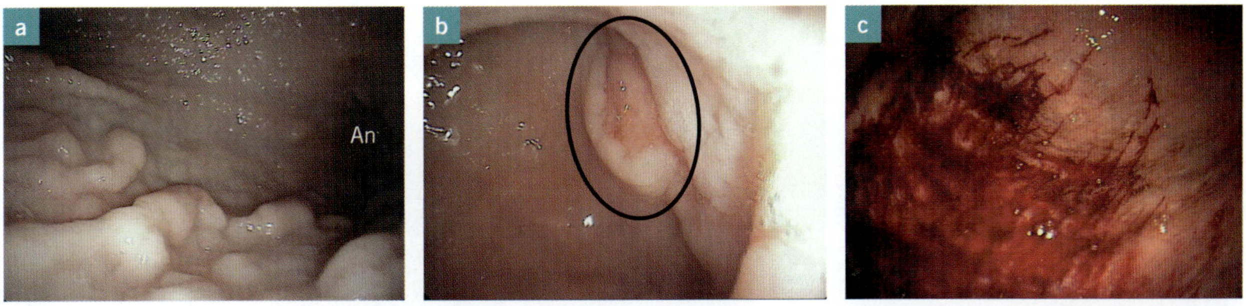

Figure 7.12. Abnormal findings during gastroscopy in cats. Irregular mucosa with cobblestone appearance in the greater curvature of a 10-year-old domestic shorthair cat, histologically confirmed as marked lymphoplasmacytic gastritis (a). In the background, the entrance to the antrum (An) is visible. Gastric ulcer with typical centre and rim (circle) at the entrance to the antrum, histologically confirmed as lymphoma (b). Acute gastritis with severe bleeding in a 12-year-old domestic shorthair cat with vomiting and an invasive gastric adenocarcinoma (c).

samples are sometimes evaluated for *Helicobacter* (*Campylobacter*-like organism [CLO] test, impression smear, etc.), it is most likely that spiral organisms do not play a pathogenic role in cats.

Peptic ulcers in the stomach of cats have rarely been reported; however, the most common causes appear to be tumours and NSAID ingestion. When biopsy samples are taken, it is important to get them from the rim of the ulcer, not from the centre. Taking samples from the centre has the inherent risk of perforating the stomach, and normally histology would only show necrosis and may fail to reveal underlying neoplasia.

Masses in the stomach can either be benign, such as polyps, or malignant (most commonly lymphoma). While the former are generally smooth and small, or occasionally broad-based (Fig. 7.13a), the latter can present as irregular masses (Fig. 7.13b), or potentially ulcerated mucosa (Fig. 7.13c), and can be of variable size. The ultimate differentiation between inflammation and neoplasia can only be made by histopathology (see Chapter 9).

While uncommon, depending on demographics, gastric parasites might be seen (e.g. *Ollulanus tricuspis*, gastric cylicospirurosis, *Physaloptera rara*).

Endoscopic pathology of the duodenum and ileum

Duodenoscopy is mostly performed as part of an upper GI endoscopy (oesophagogastroduodenoscopy). Besides those indications already mentioned earlier, chronic diarrhoea, weight loss, abdominal pain, and thickened bowel loops on physical examination or abdominal ultrasound are common indications for duodenoscopy. Like all endoscopic procedures, duodenoscopy should only be performed if other diagnostic tests or potential empirical treatment trials have not provided a diagnosis or improvement of clinical signs.

Most commonly, the duodenum shows subtle abnormalities or signs of inflammation (increased friability, granularity, areas of focal bleeding) (Fig. 7.14a), while duodenal masses (Fig. 7.14b), foreign bodies, ulcers, intussusception, and parasites are less frequent.

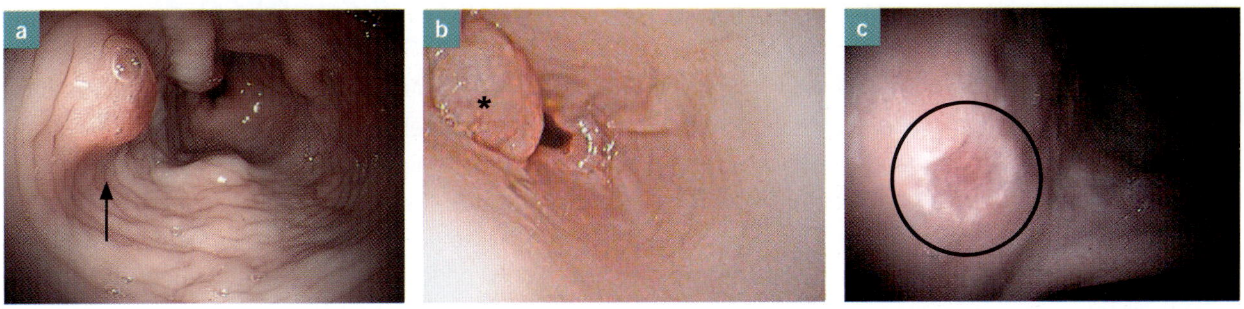

Figure 7.13. Endoscopic views of gastric tumours in cats. Gastric polyp (arrow) in the antrum of a 6-year-old domestic shorthair cat with chronic vomiting (a). Mass (asterisk) in the gastric antrum of a 7-year-old cat with chronic diarrhoea (no vomiting), histologically confirmed as an inflammatory lesion (b). Central ulcer of an adenocarcinoma (circle) in a 10-year-old domestic shorthair cat (c). Image b courtesy of Silke Salavati Schmitz, University of Edinburgh, UK.

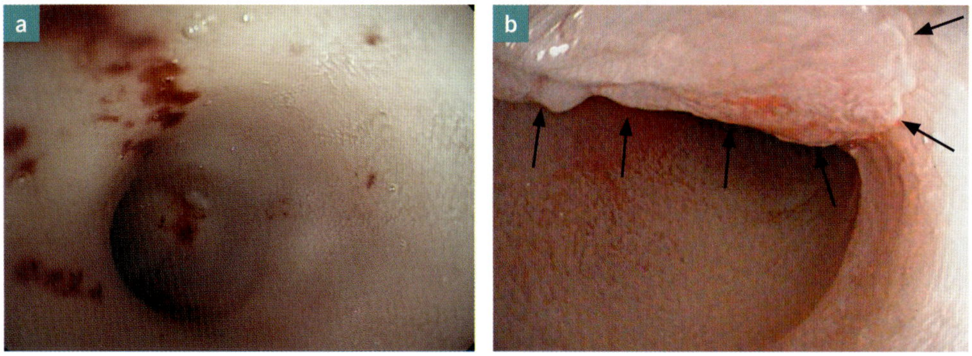

Figure 7.14. Abnormal findings during duodenoscopy in cats. Petechial bleedings (a). Irregular duodenal mass (delimited by arrows), histologically confirmed to be lymphoma (b). Image b courtesy of Silke Salavati Schmitz, University of Edinburgh, UK.

There is often a big discrepancy between macroscopic appearance and final histological diagnosis, emphasising the absolute importance of collecting biopsy samples during all endoscopic examinations. Differentiation between lymphoplasmacytic IBD and small-cell lymphoma is challenging in cats and should be confirmed by immunohistochemistry and/or PCR for antigen receptor rearrangements (PARR). However, recently, PARR has been shown to be less reliable in separating lymphoma from inflammation in cats.[8] For more details on histopathology and intestinal lymphoma, see Chapters 9 and 20.

Intestinal parasites should not be detected by endoscopy, as appropriate investigations and anthelmintic treatment prior to undergoing endoscopic examination should have been performed. Despite this, both roundworms and tapeworms can occasionally be encountered.

Endoscopy of the ileum is commonly performed to obtain ileal biopsy samples, as there might be a discrepancy between duodenal and ileal histological results.[9] If the endoscope cannot be advanced into the ileum due to a closed ileocolic sphincter, obtaining blind samples is recommended.

Endoscopic pathology of the colon and rectum

Indications for lower GI endoscopy include large bowel diarrhoea (including haematochezia) or some cases of constipation. Vomiting is not an uncommon complaint in cats with large bowel disease (see Chapter 1). As mentioned for investigations of the upper GI tract, a thorough investigation for systemic or infectious diseases (especially *Tritrichomonas blagburni*; see Chapters 1, 3, and 15) is warranted prior to endoscopy (see Chapters 3 and 5). Noninfectious inflammation can be limited to the colon (colitis) or be part of generalised IBD.

None of the most common aetiologies for constipation in cats (idiopathic megacolon, pelvic canal stenosis, and neuropathies) requires colonoscopy to establish a diagnosis.

Similar to the small intestine, the macroscopic appearance of the large intestine can range from fairly normal to markedly irregular with friable, thickened mucosa and lymphoid hyperplasia (Fig. 7.15a). Again, neoplasia is the major differential diagnosis, and especially lymphoma can appear identical to colitis; hence, histopathological differentiation and often immunohistochemistry or PARR is required for definitive diagnosis. Other large intestinal tumours in cats include adenocarcinoma and leiomyosarcoma, both of which are more focal, have an irregular proliferative appearance, and often invade the lumen (Fig. 7.15b). Obtaining diagnostic biopsy samples of rectal or colonic masses can be difficult, as samples are often superficial and will hence only reveal inflammation.

Other rare findings in cats include ileocolic or ileocaecal intussusception (often diagnosed via ultrasound prior to endoscopy), caecal neoplasia, or rectal stricture.

THERAPEUTIC ENDOSCOPY

Besides diagnostic purposes, endoscopy can also be used for therapeutic intervention and management. This includes mainly removal of foreign bodies from the oesophagus and stomach, feeding tube placement, and stricture dilation. Endoscopic placement of stents has rarely been performed in the GI tract but might become more important when adequate biodegradable stents become available.

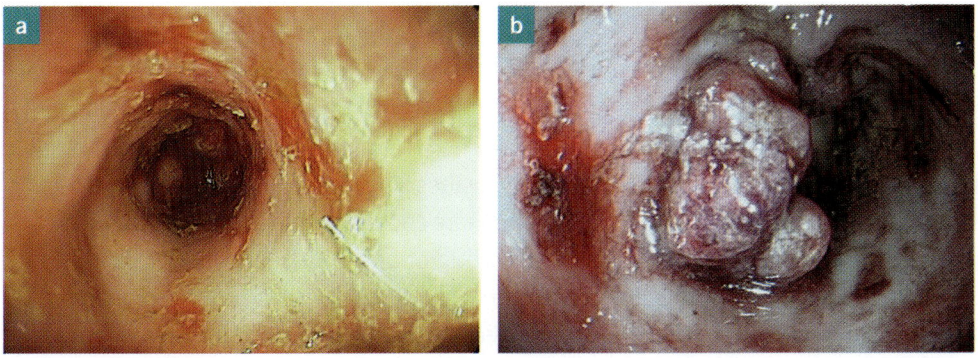

Figure 7.15. Abnormal findings during colonoscopy in cats. Bleeding colon in a 10-year-old domestic shorthair cat with signs of large bowel diarrhoea, histologically confirmed as moderate lymphoplasmacytic infiltration (a). Irregular mass in the colon of a 13-year-old Abyssinian cat with haematochezia, histologically confirmed as adenocarcinoma (b).

Foreign body removal

Due to the fastidious eating behaviour of cats, GI foreign bodies are much less common in cats compared to dogs. Nevertheless, a variety of objects can be found in the oesophagus, stomach, and intestine. Endoscopy for foreign body removal from the oesophagus and stomach is performed identically to diagnostic endoscopy. Before the procedure is initiated, however, the endoscopist must evaluate if the procedure can be performed successfully by assessing the type (sharp-ended object, needle, ball) and size of the foreign object and the available retrieval instruments as well as the own experience. Foreign bodies which can rarely be removed endoscopically include large/wide hairballs, rubber objects that have been in the stomach for a prolonged period of time, large round objects (stone), or fishhooks with three barbed hooks. Foreign bodies in the intestine are not removable via endoscopy, including thread or cloth fully or partially passing the pylorus, both of which pose a major risk of intestinal plication during removal attempts. It is clinically unwise to attempt to retrieve an object for prolonged periods of time if the object could be removed via exploratory surgery (potentially even without opening the stomach) in a fraction of the time.

Endoscopic foreign body removal is, in general, much quicker than surgery in the hands of an experienced clinician, requiring normally less than 30 minutes after anaesthesia has been induced. Another advantage of endoscopy over surgery is minimal invasiveness, resulting in rapid discharge. However, owners must be made aware of potential complications of the endoscopic procedure (unsuccessful procedure, GI tract perforation) and thus should provide consent for surgical intervention during the same anaesthesia if necessary. While severe oesophagitis after foreign body removal is rare in cats, placing a temporary gastrostomy feeding tube might be indicated and should ideally be discussed with the owner prior to performing the procedure.

Foreign body removal instruments can either pass through the working channel or be pushed alongside the endoscope. Rat-tooth, alligator-jaw, multipronged forceps, basket forceps, and snares are available for 2.8 mm working channels and some also for smaller working channels. It is not necessary to have all of these available, and many objects can be successfully grasped and removed with one type of prong and one type of grasper. The choice of the instrument lies mainly in the hands of the endoscopist, and sometimes different instruments will need to be tried to grasp the object satisfactorily. Foreign body prongs used alongside the endoscope, which is only used to visualise the object, have a much better gripping strength.

Oesophageal foreign body removal

Since needles and fishhooks may still have a thread or line attached, careful sublingual inspection should be performed during clinical examination. The thread or line should never be cut until the foreign body has been removed, irrespective of the technique. Thoracic radiographs must be carefully inspected for pneumomediastinum and/or fluid accumulation indicating potential oesophageal perforation.

The procedure is similar to diagnostic oesophagoscopy with the cat lying in left lateral recumbency, so the oesophagus is situated above the aorta. Careful inspection of the mucosa for potential foreign body–related injury is done during air insufflation. In case of perforated oesophagus, respiratory compromise may occur and should be anticipated. Once the foreign body has been visualised, it should be gripped firmly with a foreign body grasper or forceps. Pointed objects are initially pushed aborally to dislodge them from the mucosa, and then the pointed tip is grabbed and pulled towards the endoscope. While some traction is needed, it must be remembered never to use force to remove a foreign object. In case of bony objects, careful rotational torque may help to dislodge them. If a foreign body grasper is used alongside the endoscope, the endoscope should be withdrawn first. Rarely, the foreign object is lost just before passing the UOS; in these cases, it is best to remove the object with a long, curved grasping forceps under laryngoscopic control. After removal, the oesophagus should be inspected for mucosal damage due to both the lodgement of the object and its removal.

Gastric foreign body removal

Not all visible gastric foreign bodies cause clinical signs; they are sometimes seen incidentally during diagnostic imaging. Foreign objects in the stomach of cats are uncommon and normally need removal. Immediately after induction of anaesthesia and just before endoscopy, a control abdominal radiograph should be taken to ascertain that the object has not moved into the small intestine.

While endoscopy for gastric foreign body removal is started in left lateral recumbency, it may be necessary to rotate the cat to dorsal or even right lateral recumbency should visualisation or grabbing of the object be difficult. This is commonly the case when the object lies in the fundus directly adjacent to the cardia.

The object dictates the type of removal instrument. For sharp objects, a rubber tubing sleeve over the endoscope can assist with retrieval and protect the mucosa of the stomach and oesophagus from lacerations. Stones or rubber objects (both rare in cats) can be grabbed with a basket or pronged forceps. Pulling them through the cardia may be difficult. It is easiest to have the object as close to the endoscope as possible. Pulling both as a single unit, slowly and with intermittent/simultaneous insufflation, will eventually assist in object removal.

Stricture dilation

If transmural oesophagitis is present, healing may result in fibrosis and subsequent stricture formation. The most common reasons for severe oesophagitis are the administration of ulcerogenic drug formulations and their retention within the oesophagus (e.g. doxycycline, clindamycin) or foreign body trauma (e.g. trichobezoar).[10] Reflux during anaesthesia or voluntary ingestion of caustic substances are rare causes of oesophageal strictures in cats.

While bougienage has been described to dilate oesophageal strictures, it has largely been replaced by balloon dilation, where a balloon causes radial stretching and blunt tearing of the stricture, a procedure that is considered safe and quick.[11,12] Reused cardiac or other high-pressure balloon catheters (tolerating in general >8 bar) are cheap and very effective. The required length in cats is commonly 4 cm, the diameter 1.0–1.2 cm. Under endoscopic control, first a guide wire is passed through the stricture, and then the balloon catheter is placed over the wire along the endoscope into the stricture. There are balloon catheters available that can be used through the working channel of the endoscope; however, these are expensive and single-use only. Once within the stricture, the endoscope is withdrawn a few centimetres and the balloon is inflated with water (better than air) via a screw of the gun-type insufflation device to the pressure permitted for the balloon, kept in place for 1–2 minutes, and then deflated. Using only a syringe will not allow to increase the pressure sufficiently. Endoscopic visual inspection after the procedure should show some tears and bleeding.[13] If this is not the case, the dilation was probably not wide enough or the balloon has slipped, and the procedure must be repeated. If available, fluoroscopy will help to locate the correct location and will demonstrate the tearing of the mucosa.

To prevent restricture formation, the procedure should ideally be repeated twice weekly until there is no significant stricture visible endoscopically.[13] The median number of dilation sessions required is variable between cats but is, in general, two to five. Redilation when regurgitation reoccurs is another approach, albeit often less successful in the long run. After balloon dilation, treatment for severe oesophagitis (oral liquid sucralfate, a proton pump inhibitor, an antiemetic drug, and soft food) is initiated. There are no studies showing that oral prednisolone helps to prevent stricture formation. In severe cases, endoscopically guided intralesional injection of triamcinolone (4–6 mg/cat in 0.5 ml aliquots per quadrant), with a sclerotherapy injection needle, into the cranial edge of the stricture until a bleb forms, is probably more justified. In cats with significant tears of the oesophagus, placement of a PEG feeding tube might be considered. Life-threatening major tears are a rare occurrence (2%–9%) but will result in serious complications like mediastinitis, pneumomediastinum, or potential tension pneumothorax. Surgical repair is needed but carries a risk of further stricture formation (see Chapter 11).

Percutaneous endoscopic gastrostomy tube placement

Assessment of nutritional requirements in sick and debilitated cats and options for nutritional support are discussed in Chapters 38–41. Advantages and relative disadvantages of different types of tubes are discussed in more detail in Chapter 40. PEG tubes should not be placed when short-term usage is anticipated (<7 days) or in unstable patients that cannot tolerate general anaesthesia, are coagulopathic, or in which problems with wound healing are anticipated. The major drawback of PEG tubes is the cost associated with the needed material (especially commercial kits) and with the endoscopic placement procedure.

There are two types of PEG tubes available: commercial kits (from human medicine), which contain all material for quick placement, and homemade kits, which are cheaper but more cumbersome. With both, the placement procedure is similar: under endoscopic visual control, a needle is pushed through the abdominal and gastric wall into the gastric lumen and used to insert a guide wire, which is grabbed endoscopically and pulled out via the oesophagus through the mouth. The actual PEG tube is then attached to this suture and pulled back into the stomach and through the gastric and abdominal wall. A button, mushroom, or T-piece flange on the luminal side secures the PEG tube in place while allowing the stomach wall to be pulled closely towards the abdominal wall, which prevents the stomach from slipping. The external parts of the tube are attached in a way that a secure stoma is formed.

Commercial PEG tubes are made of either silicone or polyurethane and can withstand gastric acidity for the animal's lifetime. In cats, 16–20 Fr size tubes are used. The inner flange varies between different brands, but all are suitable for cats. Commercial kits contain—besides the feeding tube with conical end—the following material, which is also needed in homemade kits: large over-the-needle catheter (16 gauge), strong double-looped suture material (70–100 cm), scalpel, material to fix the feeding tube on the outside (clips or suture), and adaptor for feeding syringe (Fig. 7.16).

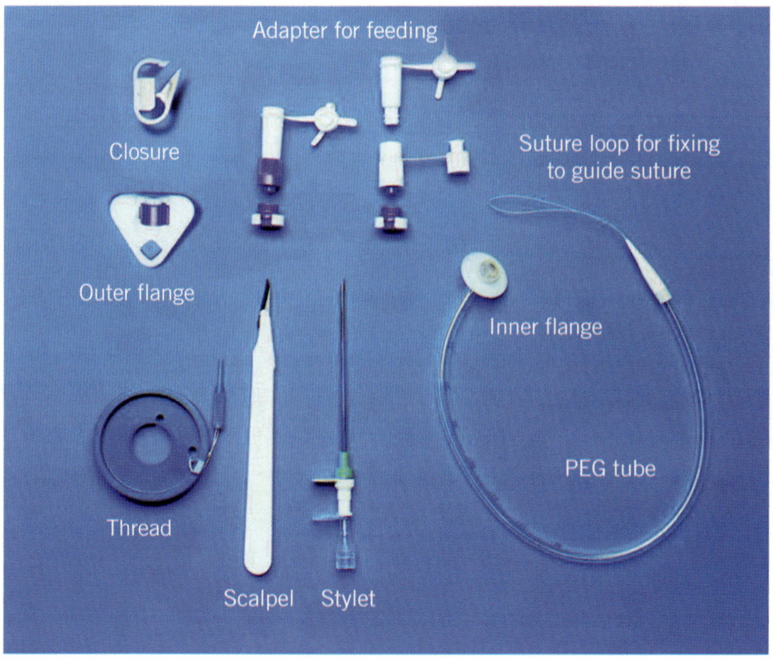

Figure 7.16. Components of a commercial human percutaneous endoscopic gastrostomy (PEG) tube set (Freka, Fresenius Kabi Ltd), 15 Fr size, which is commonly used by the authors in cats.

Endoscopy for PEG tube placement is similar to diagnostic gastroscopy, but the cat lies in right lateral recumbency (see Chapter 40). The left flank caudal to the ribs is clipped generously and surgically prepared. After introducing the endoscope into the stomach, sufficient air is insufflated to push the gastric wall against the abdominal wall and displace abdominal organs (spleen, intestine)—in cats, not too much air must be given. If biopsy samples are needed, they should be taken before PEG tube placement. Next, the site of the tube placement is chosen both by seeing the transillumination of the endoscopic light through the body wall and by gently pushing the sterile sheath of the over-the-needle catheter into the prepared site on the flank in the right direction, which will endoscopically show as an indentation in the stomach. The best place is at the junction between body and antrum. From the outside, this normally translates in cats into 2 cm caudal to the last rib and 5 cm ventral to the vertebral column. Next, the endoscope is withdrawn just to the cardia in order to prevent its accidental puncture. The needle with the over-the-needle catheter is pushed though the abdominal and gastric walls at an approximate angle of 45° forward. As soon as the needle/catheter can be seen endoscopically, the stylet is removed (preventing air leakage by occluding the catheter with a finger temporarily if needed), and the suture material is fed into the stomach and grabbed with an endoscopic grasper (not a biopsy forceps). The suture material is not pulled into the working channel but pulled back towards the oral cavity by holding it with the grasping device. The tip of the PEG tube is then attached to this suture. In commercial kits, this is facilitated by prefabricated loops of suture on both the guide suture and the PEG tube tip, which can then be threaded over each other without knotting. The suture material is now pulled back, taking the attached feeding tube with it. The conical end will eventually appear at the puncture site in the flank, where a very small (1–2 mm) incision of the skin is performed to pull the tube out and into place. The inner flange ensures snug (but not too tight) adherence of gastric and abdominal walls. This is important because if there is too much distance between them, there is potential for the gastric content to seep into the abdominal cavity and cause peritonitis. However, if there is too much pressure or pull on the gastric and abdominal walls, pressure necrosis of the mucosa could develop. Most commercial PEG tube kits contain specific outer flanges to fix the tube to the outer skin with or without suturing. The conical end of the tube is cut off at the desired tube length, and the remainder of the fittings, including a closure clip and a syringe adaptor port, is attached according to manufacturer instructions.

Feeding can be begun 24 hours after placement, initially with half of the daily calorie requirements. In the first few days, feeding should be split into five or six daily meals but can be reduced to three meals per day soon after.

PEG tubes can stay in place for many months, even lifelong. Replacement with low-profile devices (buttons) can be considered. It is important, however, to leave a new PEG tube in place for a minimum of 7 days, or even longer (up to 21 days) in animals with wound healing, to allow for proper stoma formation. Removal in cats should always occur endoscopically, as the inside flange of commercial kits is too big to pass naturally when the tube is cut on the outside.

Take-home messages

- While gastrointestinal endoscopy is an additional tool in the veterinary surgeon's armamentarium, it should only be implemented after a careful workup has been done, including laboratory tests and diagnostic imaging.
- An endoscope of adequate size for gastrointestinal endoscopy in cats should be less than 9 mm in outer diameter (with a working channel of 2.2 mm or bigger) and at least 1 m in length.
- The main purpose of gastrointestinal endoscopy is to obtain gastric and intestinal biopsy samples for histopathological and molecular analysis—it is thus paramount to pass the pylorus and investigate the duodenum.
- The main therapeutic indications of gastrointestinal endoscopy is placement of feeding tubes in the stomach (percutaneous endoscopic gastrostomy tubes), removal of oesophageal or gastric foreign bodies, and dilation of strictures in the oesophagus.

REFERENCES

[1] Goutal-Landry CM et al. Effect of endoscopic forceps on quality of duodenal mucosal biopsy in healthy dogs. *J Vet Intern Med* 27:456, 2013.

[2] Willard MD et al. Effect of sample quality on the sensitivity of endoscopic biopsy for detecting gastric and duodenal lesions in dogs and cats. *J Vet Intern Med* 22:1084, 2008.

[3] Jergens AE, Willard MD, Allenspach K. Maximizing the diagnostic utility of endoscopic biopsy in dogs and cats with gastrointestinal disease. *Vet J* 214:50, 2016.

[4] Stiles J et al. Post-anesthetic cortical blindness in cats: twenty cases. *Vet J* 193:367, 2012.

[5] Barton-Lamb AL et al. Evaluation of maxillary arterial blood flow in anesthetized cats with the mouth closed and open. *Vet J* 196:325, 2013.

[6] Tams TR. Gastroscopy. In: Tams TR, Rawlings CA, editors. *Small Animal Endoscopy*, 3rd ed. St Louis, Elsevier Mosby: 97–172, 2011.

[7] Irom S et al. Gastrointestinal perforation associated with endoscopy in cats and dogs. *J Am Anim Hosp Assoc* 50:322, 2014.

[8] Marsilio S et al. Results of histopathology, immunohistochemistry, and molecular clonality testing of small intestinal biopsy specimens from clinically healthy client-owned cats. *J Vet Intern Med* 33:551, 2019.

[9] Scott KD et al. Utility of endoscopic biopsies of the duodenum and ileum for diagnosis of inflammatory bowel disease and small cell lymphoma in cats. *J Vet Intern Med* 25:1253, 2011.

[10] Bissett SA et al. Risk factors and outcome of bougienage for treatment of benign esophageal strictures in dogs and cats: 28 cases (1995–2004). *J Am Vet Med Assoc* 235:844, 2009.

[11] Leib MS et al. Endoscopic balloon dilation of benign esophageal strictures in dogs and cats. *J Vet Intern Med* 15:547, 2001.

[12] Adamama-Moraitou KK et al. Benign esophageal stricture in the dog and cat: a retrospective study of 20 cases. *Can J Vet Res* 66:55, 2002.

[13] Palma DA, Berent A. Esophageal obstruction: strictures/tumors—balloon, bougie, injections, stent. In: Weisse C, Berent A, editors. *Veterinary Image-Guided Interventions*. Ames, Wiley Blackwell: 130–144, 2015.

CHAPTER 8

Surgical and laparoscopic biopsies of the gastrointestinal tract, pancreas, and hepatobiliary system

Kelly L. Bowlt Blacklock

A biopsy is the removal of cells or tissues for examination by a pathologist.[1] The most common types of biopsy include:

- needle biopsy (fine needle aspiration, FNA)
- incisional biopsy
- excisional biopsy.

Investigation of any abnormal lesion using FNA is an excellent starting point: this is minimally invasive, does not require anaesthesia, and may be particularly useful in identifying lesions with readily exfoliative cells (e.g. lymphoma). Results of FNA may significantly influence case management and prognosis. Disadvantages can include poor cell yield (e.g. spindle cell tumours) or difficulty in interpreting cells in the presence of severe inflammation. Most UK veterinary practitioners perform FNA using a 21- or 23-gauge needle and apply suction using a 2 or 5 ml syringe, which has been shown to be a robust method.[2,3] If neoplasia is suspected, the clinician should not compromise the potential for curative intent surgery and the needle tract should be chosen such that it can be included in any subsequent resection.

If FNA results are unhelpful, surgical biopsy can be performed, which may be incisional or excisional (Table 8.1). If the lesion may be neoplastic, the biopsy tract must be included in the subsequent excision and clinicians should therefore plan the biopsy approach carefully. Potential options for incisional biopsy include a surgical approach (wedge biopsy), needle core (Tru-Cut), or punch biopsy.

Table 8.1. Surgical biopsy techniques.

	Advantages	Disadvantages	Example
Incisional biopsy	Less invasive than excisional biopsy	Requires second anaesthetic if definitive surgery is pursued	Diffuse gastrointestinal disease necessitating full-thickness biopsies Note: biopsy should ideally include a neighbouring margin of normal tissue
Excisional biopsy	Biopsy and gross disease removal are completed in a single surgery and anaesthetic episode	If the surgeon does not know the identity of the lesion, excision may be inadequate or unnecessary If neoplasia is identified, a second, larger resection of the site may be required	Solitary peripheral liver lobe mass

PREPARATION FOR SURGERY

For every surgical procedure, informed client consent should be acquired following a full and frank discussion about the diagnosis, potential complications of surgery/treatment, likely outcomes, additional/alternative treatment options, and estimated costs involved. For the procedures described in this chapter, potential complications include those associated with anaesthesia, surgery of the abdominal cavity (e.g. herniation, infection, haemorrhage, pain), and biopsy of the organ (gastrointestinal [GI] tract: septic peritonitis, ileus; liver: haemorrhage; pancreas: pancreatitis, which may be severe and life-threatening).

Surgical complications occur in every hospital and to every surgeon, leading to increased patient morbidity/mortality, increased cost, and increased stress for the entire clinical and nonclinical team. Complications can arise due to clinician errors or unforeseen circumstances; the former can be addressed by the use of guidelines to improve surgical safety—the author would strongly encourage clinicians to familiarise themselves with the World Health Organization (WHO) "Safe Surgery Saves Lives" campaign* and the current literature on reducing surgical complications.[4-8] Compliance with a surgical checklist significantly decreases the frequency and severity of postoperative complications in veterinary hospitals.[9] In the author's institution, a modified surgical safety checklist is used for every patient undergoing any procedure in theatre, which causes minimum additional workload and reduces harm in the perioperative setting. Additionally, the author would recommend the standardised use of a pain scoring system for postoperative pain management and would encourage the generous provision of multimodal analgesia for all surgical patients. Several validated and reliable tools for acute pain assessment in cats are freely available.[10,11]

This chapter assumes that the surgeon is competent at the ventral midline approach to the abdomen. The reader is directed to a suitable illustrated text if additional information is required.[12,13]

Recent studies have indicated that placing a quilting suture pattern in the subcutaneous tissues after laparotomy significantly reduces seroma and pain levels in cats.[14] The author routinely uses this technique during abdominal closure.

GASTROINTESTINAL BIOPSY

The increasing availability of flexible endoscopes has revolutionised veterinary medicine and, quite rightly, banished surgeons to the sidelines of the GI investigation. However, on occasion, they are required to emerge from the shadows and wield a scalpel. For example, exploratory laparotomy may be indicated if corrective surgery is required alongside biopsy acquisition (e.g. foreign body or intussusception) or if the small size of endoscopic biopsy samples has precluded diagnosis and recourse to full-thickness biopsy sampling is required.

Preoperative considerations

Full-thickness surgical biopsy of the GI tract is not a surgery to undertake lightly, and alternatives (e.g. endoscopic biopsies) should be explored in the first instance. In one recent study of 172 cats undergoing full-thickness GI biopsy at 12 tertiary referral centres, 3.5% were reported to suffer from enteric wound dehiscence, and patients with hypoalbuminaemia were significantly more likely to develop this complication.[15] Septic peritonitis has a mortality rate of up to 50%, even with prompt surgical intervention and high-quality intensive care.[16,17]

The collection of full-thickness GI biopsies is a clean–contaminated procedure. Prophylactic antibiotics are generally indicated and should be provided intravenously 30–60 minutes before surgery to ensure optimal tissue concentration at the time of surgery. Antibiotics should be readministered every 1–2 elimination half-lives during the procedure and discontinued after wound closure (assuming no gross contamination or spillage has occurred). In the author's institution, 20 mg/kg cefazolin IV (serum half-life 70 minutes) is used, but other institutions may preferentially use amoxicillin–clavulanic acid.

*https://www.who.int/patientsafety/safesurgery/en/

Biopsy technique

The GI tract can be biopsied during ultrasonography, endoscopy, laparoscopy, or laparotomy (Table 8.2).

Laparotomy and enterotomy

Following a midline laparotomy, the selected portion of stomach/intestine should be exteriorised and packed off from the remainder of the abdomen using moistened laparotomy pads. Close attention should be paid to minimising contamination by isolating the GI tract to be biopsied (using stay sutures, Doyen bowel clamps, or fingers) and changing kit and gloves following completion of the biopsy and before closure of the abdomen (especially if neoplasia is suspected). The wall of the stomach and intestines has four layers: mucosa, submucosa, muscularis, and serosa. The submucosa is the collagen-containing, strength-holding layer of the GI tract and must be engaged during closure.

Stomach

Biopsy of the stomach is illustrated in Figure 8.1.

Small and large intestine

The small intestine comprises the duodenum, jejunum, and ileum, extending from the pylorus to the ileocolic junction (Fig. 8.2). The large intestine comprises the caecum, colon (ascending, transverse, and descending), and rectum (Fig. 8.2).

The technique recommended to achieve a full-thickness biopsy of the small intestine is illustrated in Figure 8.3. It is imperative that due care and attention is paid to achieving a watertight, appositional closure of the enterotomy site. If the integrity of the repair or the intestines is questionable, it is preferable to resect the site, which may necessitate a sutured/stabled anastomosis. However, on occasion this is not possible. For example, the intimate association of the duodenum with the pancreas means that some regions of the proximal duodenum cannot be readily excised. In such circumstances, use of a serosal patch may be useful to encourage formation of a fibrin seal, and provide increased blood supply and resistance to leakage (Figs. 8.4 and 8.5). Usually, the jejunum is used to create the serosal patch, taking care to avoid stretching, kinking, or twisting the intestine and mesenteric vessels.

Table 8.2. Methods for obtaining gastrointestinal biopsy specimens.

	Advantages	Disadvantages
Ultrasonographic biopsy	Applicable to the entire gastrointestinal tract Safe and quick Specific if neoplasia or fungal disease is present	Insensitive in detecting mucosal lesions Easy to miss focal lesions May be less useful for diagnosis of inflammatory lesions
Endoscopic biopsy	Minimally invasive Allows visualisation of the mucosa Allows collection of multiple biopsies	Specialised equipment and training required Cannot obtain full-thickness biopsies Biopsies are small and readily damaged Usually not possible to examine the entire length of the gastrointestinal tract (particularly the jejunum)
Laparoscopic biopsy	Less invasive than laparotomy Can also obtain hepatic and pancreatic biopsies Can obtain full-thickness biopsies	Specialised equipment and training required Cannot readily biopsy the duodenum or ileum Cannot examine the entire abdomen as thoroughly as with laparotomy Potential risks include septic peritonitis Can miss focal mucosal lesions
Laparotomy	Allows access to entire gastrointestinal tract and abdomen Can biopsy other organs (e.g. liver and pancreas) Can procure full-thickness gastrointestinal biopsies No specialised equipment required	Most invasive approach Can miss focal mucosal lesions Potential risks include septic peritonitis

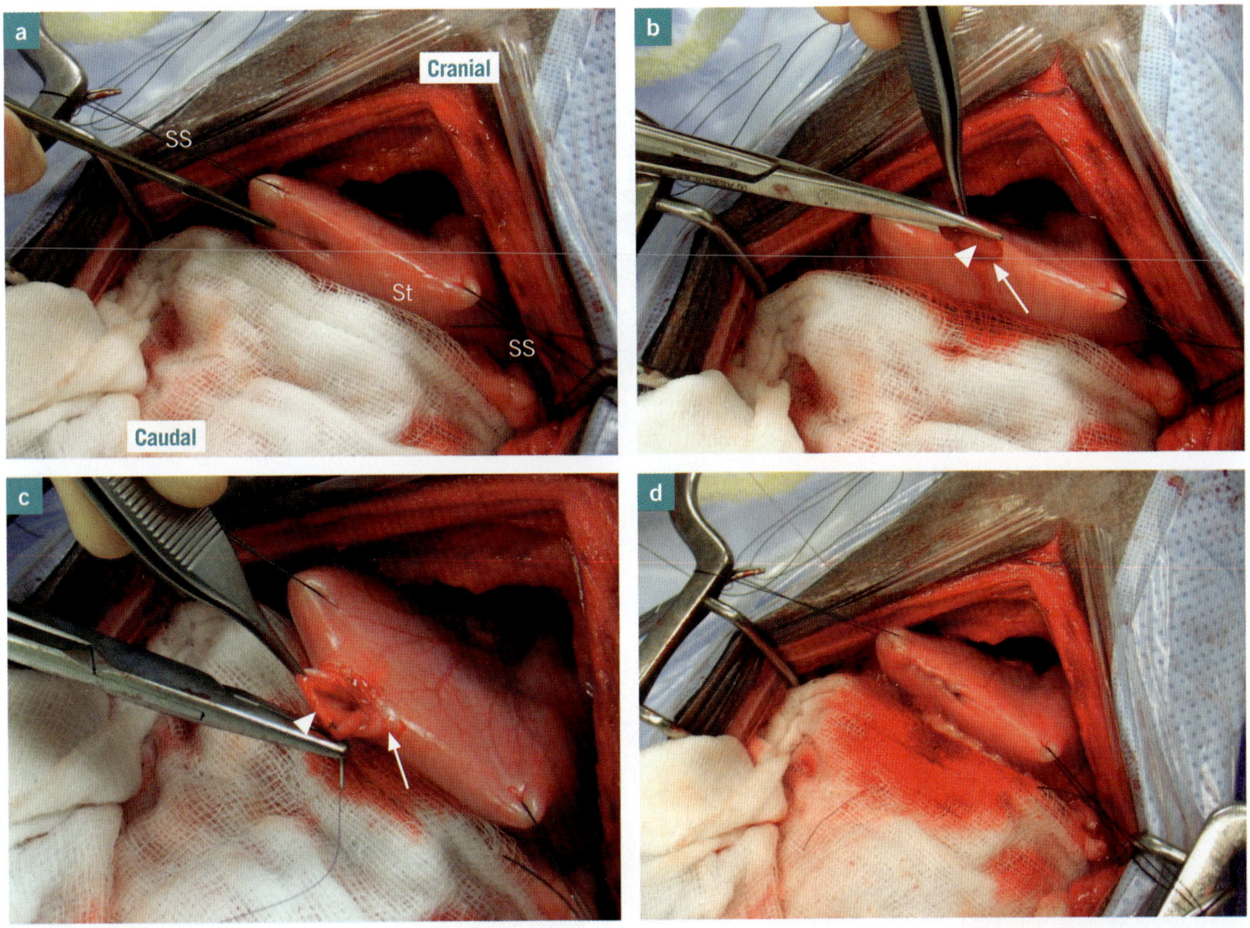

Figure 8.1. Full-thickness biopsy of the stomach. Following midline laparotomy, the stomach (St) is packed off from the remainder of the abdomen using a moist laparotomy pad. The cranially located falciform fat may be removed if it interferes with a complete exploration of the abdominal cavity—there is a vessel sited cranially which should be ligated or sealed. In figure a, the falciform fat has been removed. Monofilament nonabsorbable suture (e.g. monofilament nylon) is used to place full-thickness stay sutures (SS) in a relatively avascular area of the ventral stomach. This will facilitate exteriorisation and stabilisation and reduce spillage of stomach contents. A full-thickness stab incision is made into the stomach using a #11 scalpel blade. The incision is enlarged with Metzenbaum scissors, and a full-thickness biopsy of the stomach wall is taken (b). Note that the stomach separates readily into two distinct, thick layers: the mucosa/submucosal layer (arrowhead) and the seromuscular layer (arrow). The biopsy must comprise both of these layers. The gastric wall can be closed in one or two layers. The volume of the stomach lumen and thickness of each stomach wall layer means that a two-layered closure is technically very easy. Closure is performed with a monofilament absorbable suture material (e.g. poliglecaprone 25) on a swaged, taper-cut needle (c). An appositional pattern is used in the mucosa and seromuscular layers—the author prefers a simple continuous pattern because it is more likely to achieve a watertight seal. An appositional or inverting pattern (e.g. Cushing or Lembert pattern) is used in the seromuscular layer, with the same suture material (d). The suture line should be omentalised, laparotomy pads removed, kit/gloves changed, and the abdominal cavity lavaged and closed in three layers.

The large bowel contains high numbers of intraluminal bacteria, and the risk of infection after colorectal surgery is high. The surgical principles for large intestinal surgery are the same as those for small intestinal surgery, however the risk of dehiscence is greater. It is for these reasons that full-thickness biopsy of the large intestine should be avoided unless absolutely necessary and colonoscopy should be utilised preferentially in order to harvest colonic biopsy samples.

As a general rule, the use of enemas should be avoided in surgical patients because they can further deteriorate debilitated and/or anorexic patients, may cause colonic perforation, and liquefy intestinal contents which aids in the dissemination of contaminated material during surgery.

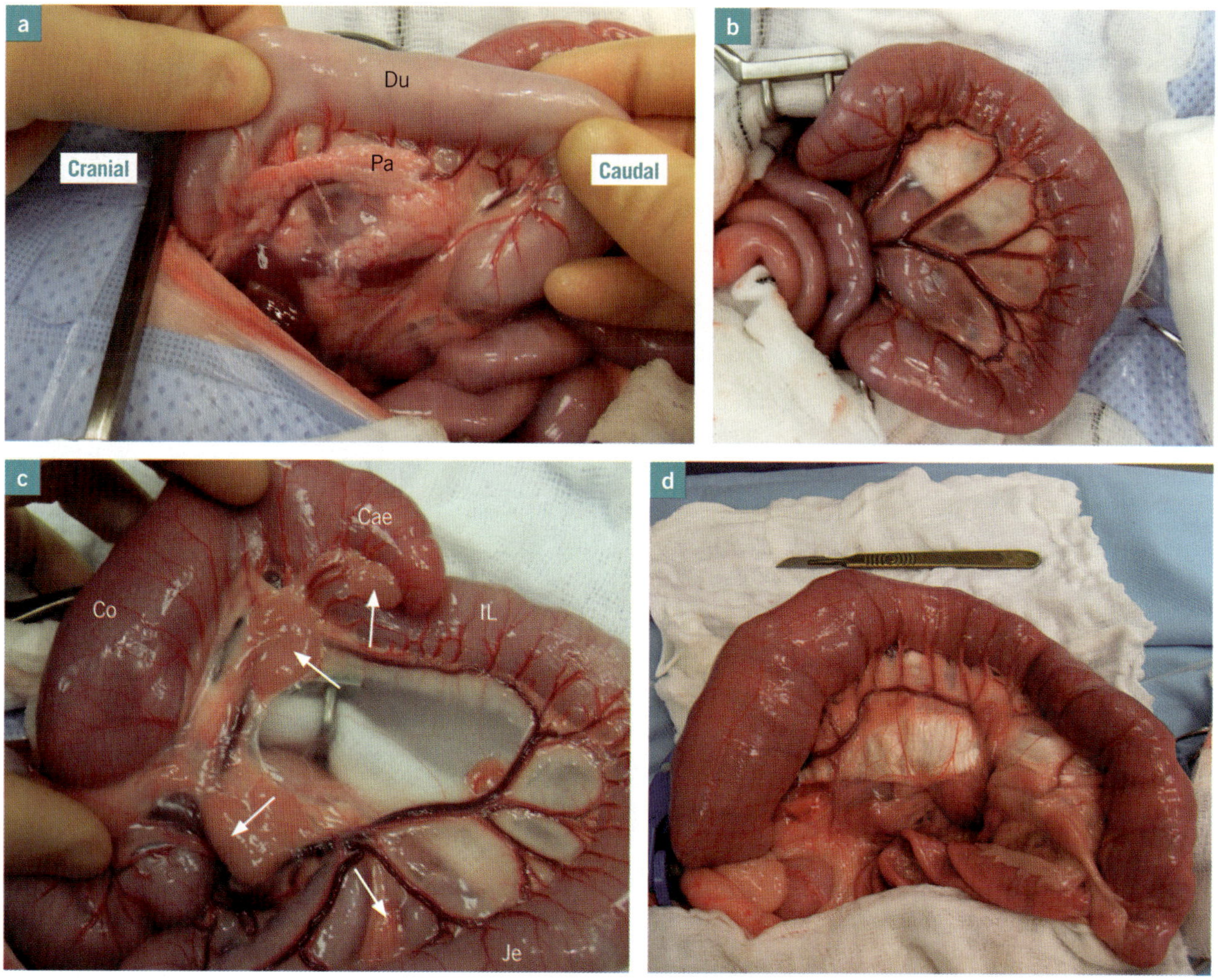

Figure 8.2. Intestinal anatomy. The duodenum (Du) extends from the pylorus to the jejunum and is relatively immobile, being intimately associated with the pancreas (Pa) (a). In the cat, the pancreatic duct enters the duodenum through the major duodenal papilla, which is the main (and often only) pancreatic duct opening into the duodenum. It enters the duodenum in partnership with the bile duct. Intraoperative image of the jejunum (b). Nearly all intestinal blood supply originates from the cranial mesenteric artery at the root of the mesentery and which divides into arcuate jejunal arteries along the mesenteric border of the gastrointestinal tract. Intraoperative image of the ileum (IL), caecum (Cae), and colon (Co) (c). In addition to the mesenteric blood supply, the ileum has an antimesenteric vessel, which is a branch of the caecal artery. The arrows indicate enlarged mesenteric lymph nodes. Intraoperative image of the descending colon in a patient with idiopathic megacolon (d). Note that the blood supply differs to the arcuate branches of the jejunum in image b. The large intestinal arterial blood supply arises from the cranial and caudal mesenteric arteries. With the exception of the colon immediately aboral to the caecum, where the blood supply remains arcuate, the majority of the colonic blood supply arises from the left colic artery, which runs in the mesenteric border parallel to the colon. Je, jejunum.

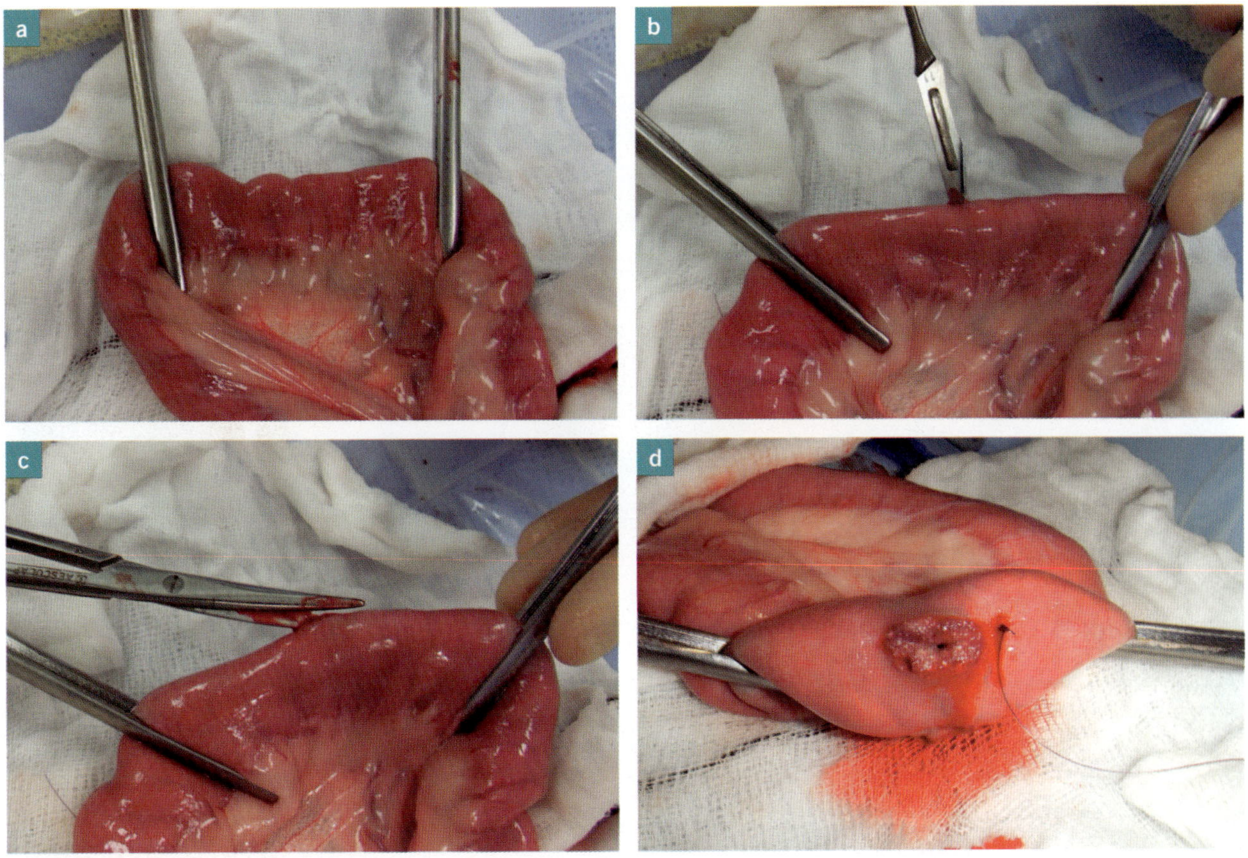

Figure 8.3. Full-thickness intestinal biopsy. Following exteriorisation and packing off the selected portion of intestine, the luminal contents are milked away from the proposed surgical site, and the lumen is closed using atraumatic Doyen bowel clamps or fingers placed 4–6 cm on either side of the proposed enterotomy site (a). There is no evidence for the superiority of Doyen vs. digital occlusion; both are equally atraumatic, and the choice depends on personal preference and the availability of spare hands. A full-thickness stab incision is made into the antimesenteric border of the isolated section of intestine (b). The incision is lengthened longitudinally using Metzenbaum scissors (c), and a full-thickness elliptical biopsy is removed and submitted for analysis. Handling of the tissue should ideally be performed with atraumatic DeBakey thumb forceps. Intestinal healing occurs in lag, proliferative, and maturation phases. The lag phase lasts 3–4 days: all the strength in the surgical wound at this stage comes from the suturing, which makes the technique crucial to avoiding leakage and dehiscence (which is most likely to occur in the first 72–96 hours postoperatively). It is imperative that optimal wound healing by primary intention is achieved, which requires accurate apposition of the wound edges. The author closes the intestinal wall using a full-thickness simple interrupted or simple continuous pattern, preferring the latter because it is more likely to achieve a watertight seal (d). These patterns reliably engage the collagen-rich, strength-holding submucosal layer, which is essential to achieve primary intention healing. Sutures should be placed sufficiently close together to achieve a watertight seal without crushing the tissue. The suture of choice is a monofilament absorbable suture material (e.g. poliglecaprone 25) on a swaged, taper-cut needle. Accurate apposition of the wound edges may necessitate trimming of the everted mucosa, as seen in image d. The author always starts the suture line just before the enterotomy site, as shown here, and completes the suture just after the enterotomy site, ensuring that a watertight seal is achieved along the entire suture length. ▶

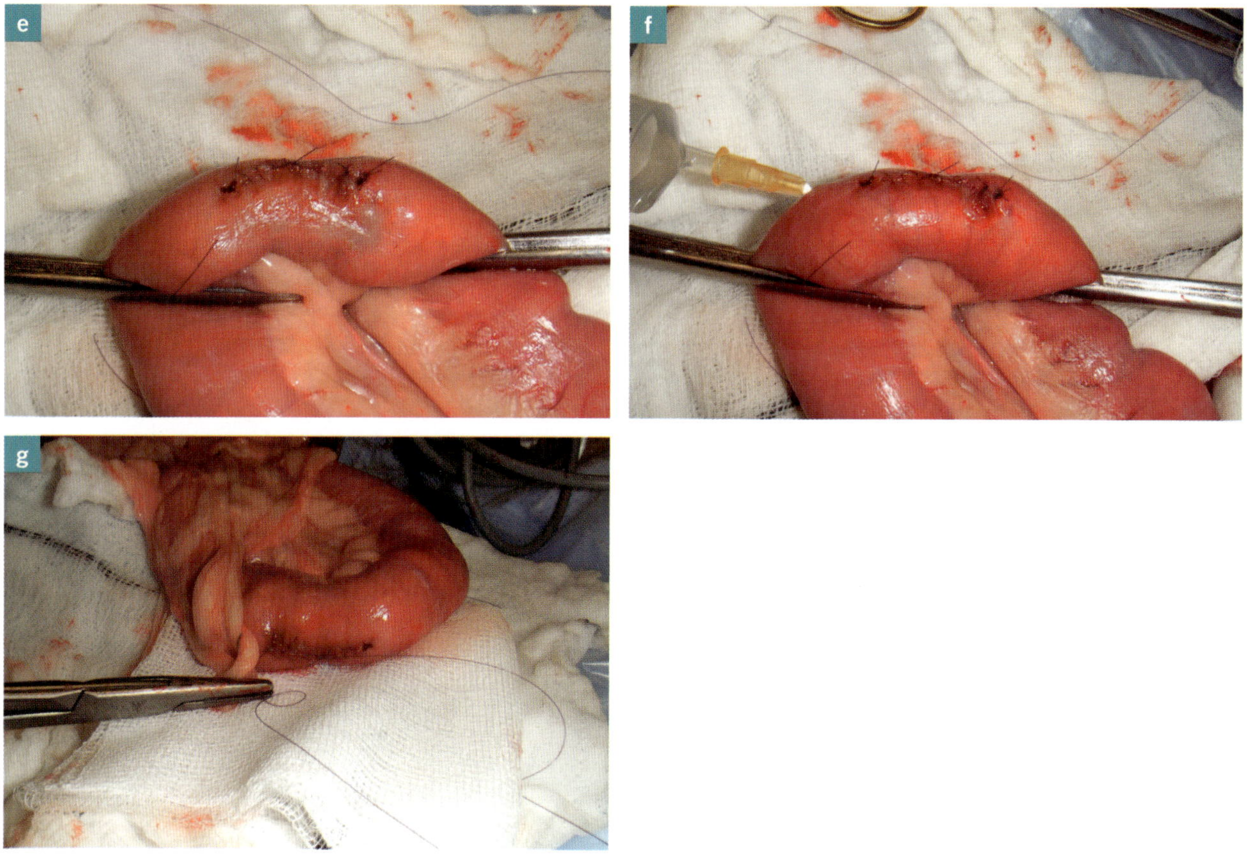

The enterotomy site after closure with a simple continuous suture pattern (e). Note the placement of a simple interrupted suture in the centre of the suture line, where the author was unhappy with the gross appearance of the closure at this site. Where there is concern over luminal narrowing, the surgeon may close the enterotomy in a transverse fashion, rather than longitudinally as shown here. The same principles for wound closure apply. The author always assesses the enterotomy seal by performing a leak test (f). The volume of saline which should be instilled into the lumen is unclear, but it is hypothesised that the volume should achieve the same targeted intraluminal pressure as generated during a peristaltic wave (15–25 mmHg [20–34 cm water] in the dog). In the canine jejunum, saline volumes of 16.3–19 ml (for digital occlusion) and 12.1–14.8 ml (Doyen occlusion) were required to achieve intraluminal pressures of 34 cm water during leak testing of a 10 cm segment containing a closed biopsy site.[18] Similar information is not available for the cat, so the author instils the intestinal lumen with sufficient saline to place the enterotomy site under "moderate" tension, as assessed subjectively. There is recent evidence that injection with a smaller syringe attached to a 22-gauge needle may lower the frequency of leakage from the injection site,[19] so the author now preferentially uses a 22-gauge needle. If any leakage of saline is identified from the suture line, the author places a simple interrupted suture at the offending site and repeats the leak test. Alternative reported methods for enterotomy closure include use of skin staplers[20] and adhesive,[21] although these have only been investigated in a small number of dogs and cannot be recommended at this stage. Once the enterotomy site is closed and confirmed to be watertight, omentalisation is recommended (g). The omentum's extensive vascular and lymphatic supply helps in restoring blood supply to the surgical site, as well as reducing infection, establishing lymphatic drainage and plugging small defects—although it should never be used as a replacement for good surgical principles. Some surgeons prefer to wrap the omentum around the suture line, others (including the author) like to suture the omentum to the surgical site (ensuring that the omental vascular supply is not occluded). There is no evidence that one approach is superior to the other. Following omentalisation, the laparotomy pads are removed, kit/gloves changed, and the abdominal cavity lavaged and closed in three layers.

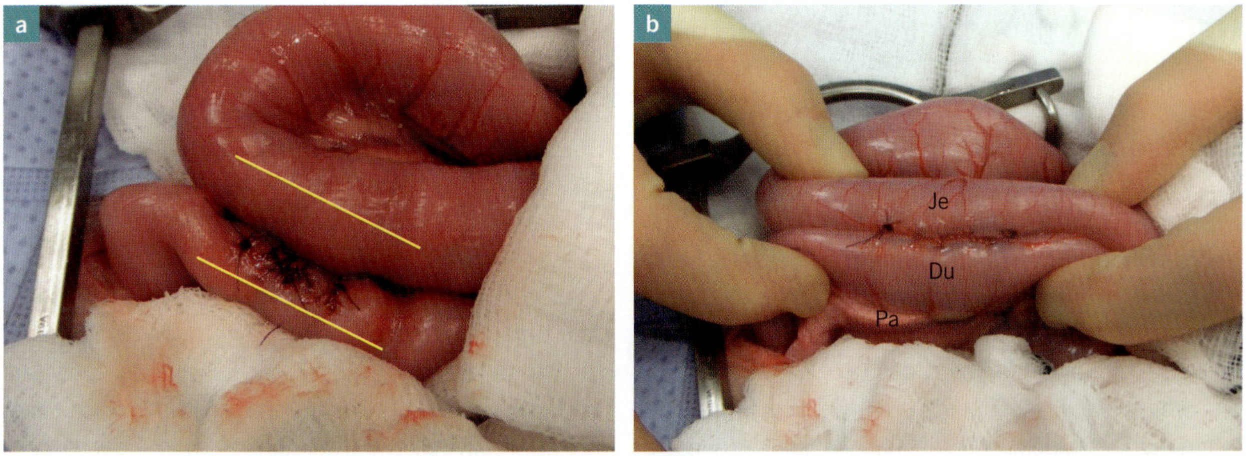

Figure 8.4. Placement of a serosal patch. The duodenum is a challenging area in which to perform a resection–anastomosis because of the intimate association with the pancreas (see Figure 8.2a). In this 11-year-old domestic shorthair cat, full-thickness duodenal biopsies were requested to investigate a prolonged history of vomiting and diarrhoea. Endoscopically obtained biopsy specimens were previously procured, but a diagnosis was not achieved. A full-thickness duodenal biopsy was performed, and the duodenal wall was noted to be very thickened and extremely friable. Poliglecaprone 25 sutures (1.5 and 2 metric) easily pulled through the intestinal wall, despite engagement of the submucosal layers. The enterotomy was closed and confirmed to be watertight (see Figure 8.3f). The author considered the repair to be suboptimal, but that it could not be improved with a resection–anastomosis of the site because of the location and because of the diffuse nature of the disease process. Therefore, placement of a serosal patch was considered necessary. In order to achieve this, a section of jejunum distant to the enterotomy site was selected and the antimesenteric borders of both sutured together medial to the enterotomy site, as seen in image a. The enterotomy site was covered with the serosa of the jejunal section by placing a second row of sutures between the mesenteric borders on the lateral side of the enterotomy (illustrated by the yellow lines). As with all intestinal surgery, the sutures should engage the submucosal layer of both sections of intestine. Completed serosal patch (b). The duodenum (Du) and the neighbouring pancreas (Pa) can be seen. The jejunum (Je) is visible laid on top of the duodenum, with the antimesenteric borders sutured together medially and laterally to the enterotomy site. In this patient, the repair was also omentalised.

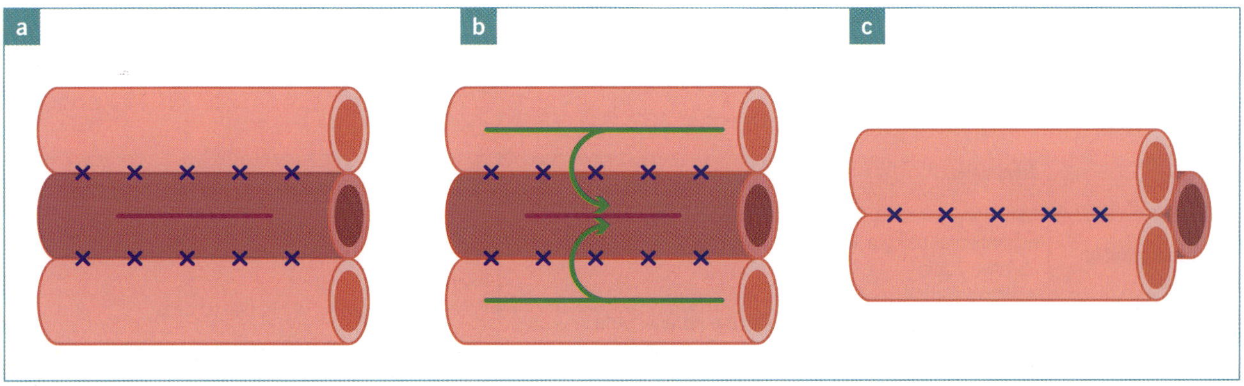

Figure 8.5. Diagram of the placement of a serosal patch. If there are concerns that the technique used in Figure 8.4 may create excessive luminal narrowing, two loops of intestine distant from the enterotomy site can be utilised to create the serosal patch. The section of intestine (dark pink) with the enterotomy site (purple line) is shown (a). The antimesenteric borders of two lengths of normal intestine (usually jejunum; light pink) have been sutured to the antimesenteric border of the enterotomy site (crosses), engaging the submucosa in both intestinal segments. It is important that the normal intestinal segments used are suitably distant to the enterotomy site, so that their use in the creation of a serosal patch does not generate kinks or obstruction in the gastrointestinal tract. The antimesenteric borders of the two portions of healthy intestine are sutured together (engaging the submucosa) along the green line, essentially encasing the enterotomy site in a cocoon of healthy serosa (b). The serosal patch is completed and now comprises two lengths of normal intestine completely surrounding the enterotomy site (c). Omentalisation can also be performed.

HEPATIC BIOPSY

Preoperative considerations

The liver is located in the cranial abdomen and is divided into the left lateral, left medial, quadrate, right medial, right lateral, and caudate lobes. Biopsy of the liver is commonly performed in cats and several methods have been reported (Table 8.3). Hepatic surgery carries a risk of haemorrhage which can potentially be life-threatening, therefore evaluation of coagulation profile, blood type, and crossmatching should be performed prior to surgery. In the author's experience, cats undergoing liver surgery may require particularly generous multimodal analgesia postoperatively compared with dogs, and the use of a feline-specific pain scoring system is strongly encouraged.

Cats should be closely monitored for haemorrhage following liver biopsy, regardless of the technique used. Major bleeding occurs in 56.7% of cats following percutaneous ultrasound-guided liver biopsy, and nonlethal bleeding complications occur in 16.7%.[22]

If liver biopsies are procured using a Tru-Cut, the devices should be semiautomatic. Automatic devices can result in severe shock which is unresponsive to resuscitation, theorised to be the result of a pressure wave causing intense vagotonia and shock.[23]

Open liver biopsy

Surgical biopsy allows the entire liver to be assessed, palpated, and sampled for histopathological analysis, culture, or copper analysis. When harvesting liver samples, it is imperative that multiple biopsies are taken from multiple liver lobes because disease processes can vary between lobes. At least six to eight samples are recommended. Peripheral samples may be procured using a guillotine technique (Fig. 8.6). Alternatively, a forceps technique can be utilised: a pair of haemostatic forceps is placed across the peripheral edge of a liver lobe, crushing the parenchyma, and the tissue distal to the forceps is transected with a scalpel. Usually haemorrhage is minimal with this technique, and no sutures are required. More centrally located samples can be harvested using a biopsy punch (Fig. 8.6).

Laparoscopic liver biopsy

Liver biopsies can be readily obtained laparoscopically from peripheral liver lobes. It is important that multiple samples are obtained from different lobes—a minimum of six to eight is recommended (Fig. 8.7).

PANCREATIC BIOPSY

The pancreas is situated caudal to the stomach and comprises right and left lobes and a central body (Fig. 8.2a). The splenic artery supplies the left limb of the pancreas,

Table 8.3. Methods for obtaining hepatic biopsy specimens.

	Advantages	Disadvantages
Ultrasonographic biopsy	Minimally invasive (can be undertaken by fine needle aspiration or using a Tru-Cut biopsy Relatively safe Ability to sample multiple liver lobes Easy to sample lesions deep within the parenchyma	Potentially poor diagnostic accuracy No direct visualisation of the liver to monitor/address haemorrhage Potential for seeding of neoplastic cells
Laparoscopic biopsy	Less invasive than an open approach Larger samples harvested compared with Tru-Cut Ability to sample multiple liver lobes Allows to visualise and address haemorrhage Can protect wound edges against potential seeding of neoplastic cells	Cannot safely sample central lesions Potential complications associated with abdominal insufflation May be more challenging if ascites, adhesions, or large volumes of intra-abdominal fat Specialised equipment and training required
Laparotomy	No specialised equipment required Ability to sample multiple liver lobes Allows to visualise and address haemorrhage Can procure very large samples Permits excisional biopsy of large mass lesions Can protect wound edges against potential seeding of neoplastic cells	Requires midline laparotomy (most invasive approach)

the cranial pancreaticoduodenal artery (from the hepatic artery) supplies the body and proximal right pancreatic limb, and the caudal pancreaticoduodenal artery supplies the distal right pancreatic limb. Unlike dogs, the majority of cats have a single pancreatic duct which joins with the bile duct and enters the duodenum at the major duodenal papilla.

Pancreatic biopsy should not be undertaken lightly, and the surgeon must be familiar with the local anatomy. It is essential that neither the duct nor the vascular systems are damaged during the procedure. Importantly, the gross appearance of the pancreas can be hugely variable and cannot be used to differentiate between disease processes (e.g. pancreatitis vs. neoplasia). Indeed, some cats with pancreatitis may not have grossly diseased pancreatic tissue. Biopsy of the pancreas can be performed via ultrasound guidance or via laparoscopy/laparotomy. In the presence of diffuse disease, the distal aspect of the right pancreatic limb is most accessible (using the duodenal manoeuvre, Fig. 8.2a) and should be preferentially biopsied. The most commonly utilised technique is a suture fracture technique as described in Figure 8.6. Importantly, the mesoduodenum should be closed and the wound covered with omentum

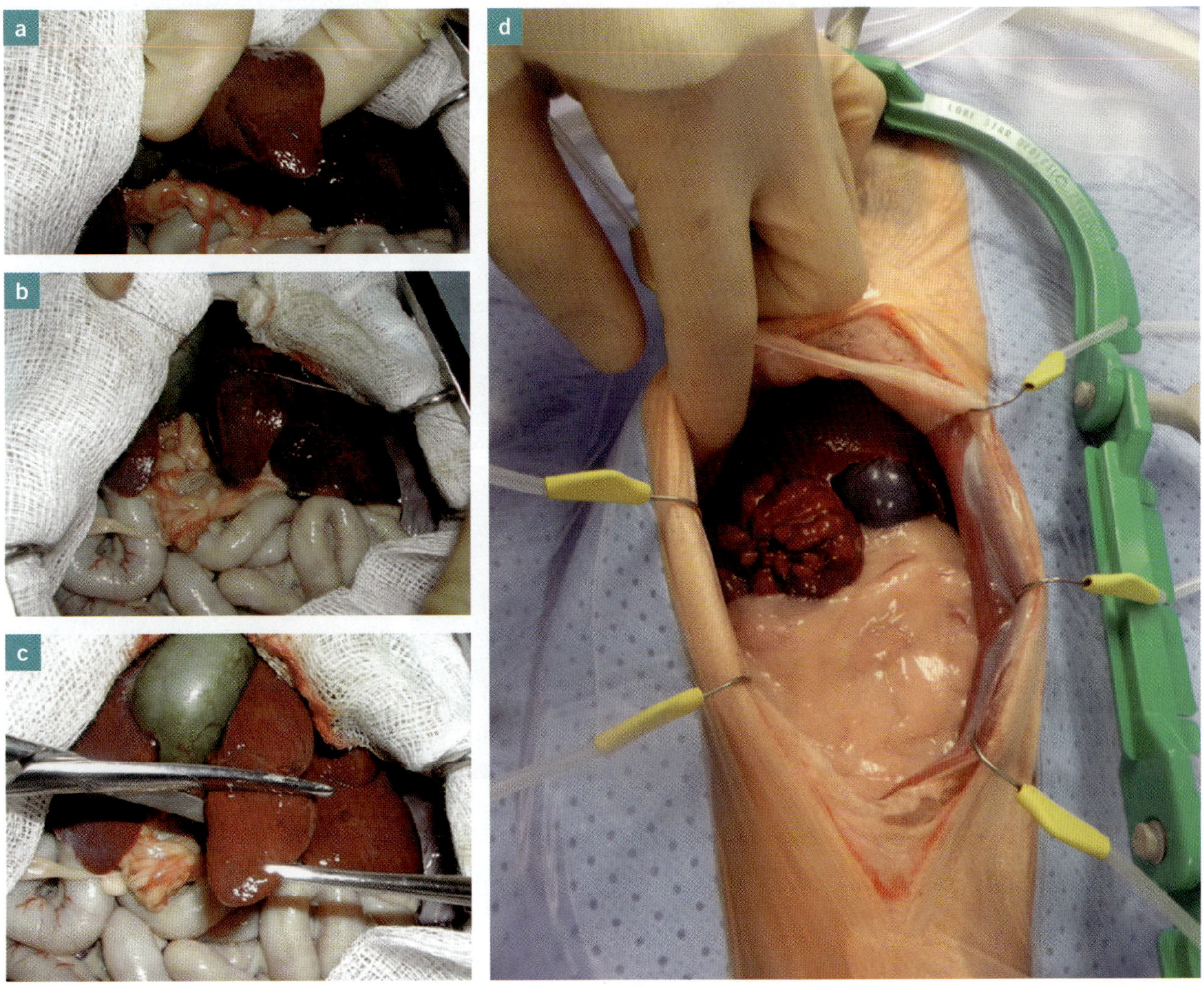

Figure 8.6. Open liver biopsy. The liver is approached via a midline laparotomy and packed off using sterile laparotomy pads. A peripheral lobe is isolated (a). In the author's experience, handling the liver using fingers is easier than using instruments when attempting to avoid damage to the parenchyma. A suture loop (monofilament absorbable) is placed around the periphery of the liver lobe and tied, crushing though the parenchyma and ligating the blood vessels and biliary ducts (b). The parenchyma distal to the suture is transected using Metzenbaum scissors or a scalpel blade (c). The guillotine method can also be utilised for larger peripheral liver masses, as seen in image d. In this case, an excisional biopsy would be appropriate. Note the use of a ring retractor, which is the author's preference during abdominal surgery in the cat. Images a–c courtesy of the University of Edinburgh, UK.

to minimise the risk of pancreatic leakage. Where the lesion is more focal, a small wedge biopsy or a Tru-Cut needle can be used.

Laparoscopic pancreatic biopsies can be performed with an approach similar to that illustrated in Figure 8.7; however, a punch biopsy forceps is preferentially utilised, taking care to avoid the vasculature along the dorsal surface (Fig. 8.2a).

If there is substantial pancreatitis, it is prudent to consider placement of an enteral feeding tube immediately postoperatively.

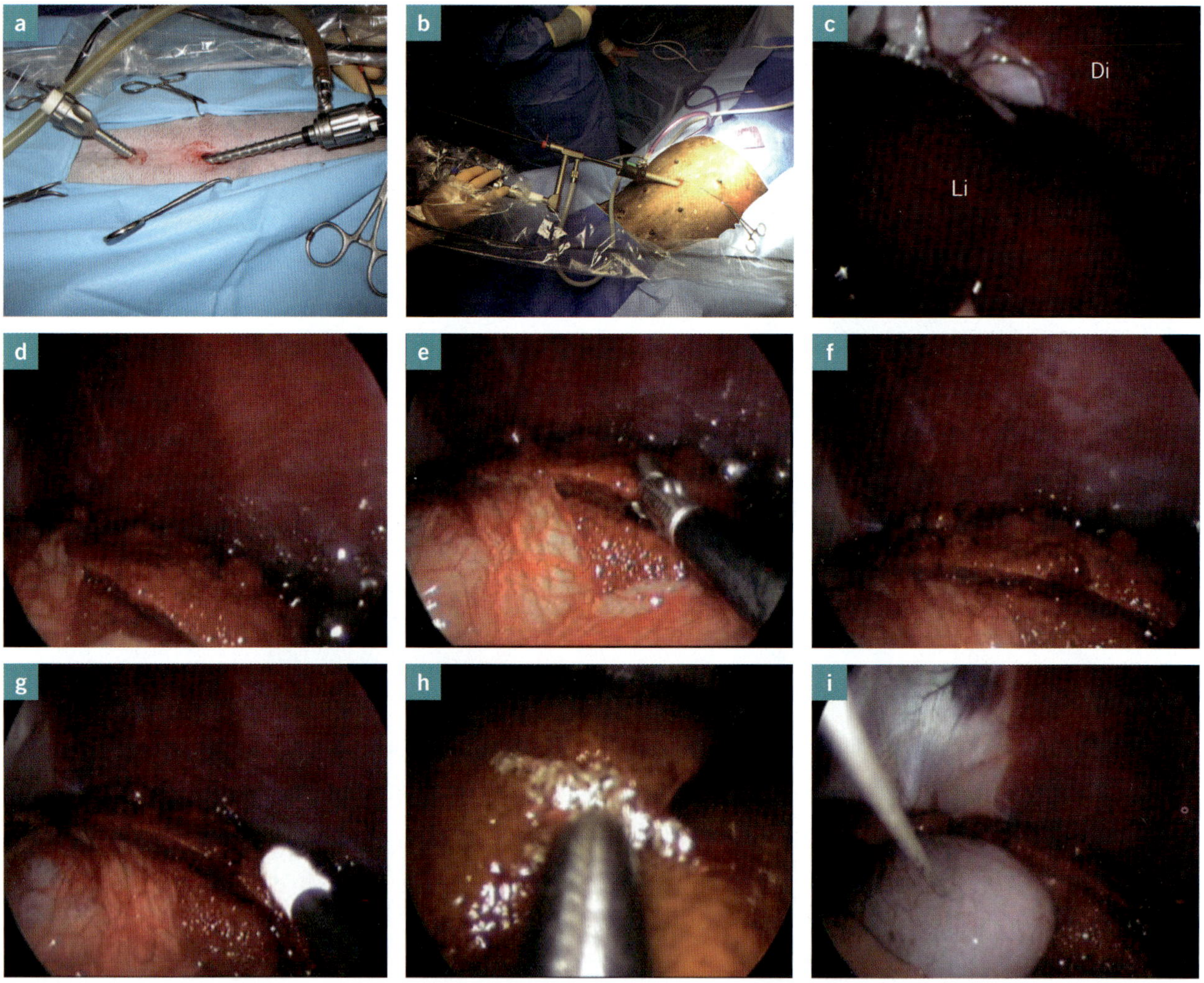

Figure 8.7. Laparoscopic liver biopsy. Laparoscopic liver biopsy is often performed via a two-port technique, using a camera (subumbilical) and an instrument (caudal midline or paramedian) port (a). To permit a less invasive approach, the author prefers to use a working laparoscope, which permits abdominal laparoscopic procedures to be completed through a single port (b). Visualisation of the cranial abdomen using a laparoscopic camera (c). The muscular and tendinous portions of the diaphragm (Di) can be seen. The liver (Li) appears grossly normal. Laparoscopic image of a diffusely nodular liver and ascites (d). To obtain a liver biopsy, laparoscopic cup biopsy forceps are passed through a port into the abdomen and used to grasp an edge of one liver lobe (e). The forceps are closed, twisted, and pulled, extracting a sample of liver parenchyma within the cup. The liver biopsy site after withdrawal of the cup biopsy forceps (f). The liver parenchymal defect can be seen near the centre of the image. Haemorrhage is minimal. If there is concern for haemorrhage, pressure can be applied using an endoscopic sponge (g). Alternatively, the site can be packed with collagen or cellulose sponges to aid haemostasis (h). Bile can also be sampled by inserting a needle into the gallbladder under laparoscopic guidance (i).

Take-home messages

- Surgical checklists and pain scores should be used as standard.
- Excisional biopsy of neoplastic masses should be avoided in most cases.
- Where neoplasia is suspected, biopsy tracts must not complicate future curative-intent surgery.

Gastrointestinal biopsy

- A potential complication of full-thickness gastrointestinal biopsy is septic peritonitis, which can be fatal. Alternative options (e.g. endoscopic biopsy) should be explored wherever possible.
- Colonic biopsy should be avoided unless absolutely required.
- Optimal healing requires observation of Halsted's principles, including a good blood supply, accurate mucosal apposition, and minimal surgical trauma.
- The submucosa is the strength-holding layer and should always be engaged by the sutures to provide a secure, watertight closure.
- The stomach can be closed in one or two layers; the intestine is usually closed in a single layer.
- Always omentalise the suture line of hollow organs, which will seal small sites of leakage and increase blood supply to the area, promoting healing.
- Consider covering surgical sites with a serosal patch if dehiscence is a concern.
- A synthetic, monofilament suture material is preferred for closure of full-thickness gastrointestinal biopsies. The author uses poliglecaprone 25, which is predictably absorbed by hydrolysis, produces minimal friction and drag, has minimal memory, and allows secure knots to be placed. Poliglecaprone 25 loses 20%–30% of its original tensile strength after 2 weeks and is completely absorbed by hydrolysis in 90 days.[24]
- Change kit and gloves following full-thickness gastrointestinal biopsy, particularly if neoplasia is suspected.

Hepatic biopsy

- Hepatic surgery carries a risk of haemorrhage which can potentially be life-threatening.
- Evaluation of coagulation profile, blood type, and crossmatching should be performed prior to surgery.
- When possible, laparoscopic liver biopsy is preferable over an open approach.
- It is imperative that multiple biopsy specimens are taken from multiple liver lobes because disease processes can vary between lobes.

Pancreatic biopsy

- Handle the pancreas gently to avoid causing pancreatitis.
- Because of the difficulty in diagnosing feline pancreatitis, biopsy may be indicated more often than is currently performed.
- Chronic pancreatitis is the most common finding on histopathological analysis of feline pancreatic biopsy samples.
- The right limb of the pancreas is preferentially biopsied in patients with diffuse disease, using a suture fracture technique.
- Reported complications following pancreatic biopsy in cats include pancreatitis, abdominal pain, nausea, pyrexia, inappetence, and recurrence of the primary disease process.[25]

REFERENCES

[1] National Cancer Institute. *NCI Dictionary of Cancer Terms.* "Biopsy", [accessed Jul 2020]. Available from: https://www.cancer.gov/publications/dictionaries/cancer-terms/def/biopsy/.

[2] Bowlt KL et al. Prospective study to investigate the use of fine needle aspiration techniques in UK veterinary practice. *J Small Anim Pract* 55:409, 2014.

[3] Bowlt Blacklock KL et al. A preliminary investigation of the effect of sample collection technique on the cell and RNA content of fine-needle aspirates of five canine tumours. *J Small Anim Pract* 59:211, 2018.

[4] Kilbane H, Oxtoby C, Tivers MS. Staff attitudes to and compliance with the use of a surgical safety checklist. *J Small Anim Pract* 61:332, 2020.

[5] Tivers M. Reducing surgical complications. *Vet Rec* 169:334, 2011.

[6] Tivers M. Reducing error and improving patient safety. *Vet Rec* 177:436, 2015.

[7] Gasson J. Reducing surgical complications using a safety checklist. *Vet Rec* 169:503, 2011.

[8] Gawande A. *The Checklist Manifesto: How to Get Things Right.* New York, Henry Holt and Company, 2009.

[9] Bergström A, Dimopoulou M, Eldh M. Reduction of surgical complications in dogs and cats by the use of a surgical safety checklist. *Vet Surg* 45:571, 2016.

[10] Evangelista MC et al. Facial expressions of pain in cats: the development and validation of a Feline Grimace Scale. *Sci Rep* 9:19128, 2019.

[11] Buisman M et al. The influence of demeanor on scores from two validated feline pain assessment scales during the perioperative period. *Vet Anaesth Analg* 44:646, 2017.

[12] Fossum TW. Surgery of the abdominal cavity. In: Fossum TW, editor. *Small Animal Surgery*, 5th ed. Philadelphia, Elsevier: 512, 2019.

[13] Blacklock KLB. Surgery of the abdominal cavity. In: Bergmann H, editor. *Improve International Manual of Small Animal Surgery Volume 1.* Sheffield, 5m Publishing, 2019.

[14] Lopez DJ et al. Effect of subcutaneous closure technique on incisional complications and postoperative pain in cats undergoing midline celiotomy: a randomized, blinded, controlled trial. *Vet Surg* 49:321, 2020.

[15] Swinbourne F et al. The incidence of surgical site dehiscence following full-thickness gastrointestinal biopsy in dogs and cats and associated risk factors. *J Small Anim Pract* 58:495, 2017.

[16] Greenfield CL, Walshaw R. Open peritoneal drainage for treatment of contaminated peritoneal cavity and septic peritonitis in dogs and cats: 24 cases (1980–1986). *J Am Vet Med Assoc* 191:100, 1987.

[17] Costello MF et al. Underlying cause, pathophysiologic abnormalities, and response to treatment in cats with septic peritonitis: 51 cases (1990–2001). *J Am Vet Med Assoc* 225:897, 2004.

[18] Saile K, Boothe HW, Boothe DM. Saline volume necessary to achieve predetermined intraluminal pressures during leak testing of small intestinal biopsy sites in the dog. *Vet Surg* 39:900, 2010.

[19] Brand KJ, Hess E, Risselada M. Effects of needle gauge and syringe size on small intestinal leakage at injection sites. *Vet Surg* 48:1237, 2019.

[20] Schwartz Z, Coolman BR. Disposable skin staplers for closure of linear gastrointestinal incisions in dogs. *Vet Surg* 47:285, 2018.

[21] Mutascio LM et al. Effects of a surgical sealant on leakage pressure and circumference of fresh canine cadaver small intestinal anastomoses. *Am J Vet Res* 79:1335, 2018.

[22] Pavlick M, Webster CR, Penninck DG. Bleeding risk and complications associated with percutaneous ultrasound-guided liver biopsy in cats. *J Feline Med Surg* 21:529, 2019.

[23] Proot SJ, Rothuizen J. High complication rate of an automatic Tru-Cut biopsy gun device for liver biopsy in cats. *J Vet Intern Med* 20:1327, 2006.

[24] Bezwada RS et al. Monocryl suture, a new ultra-pliable absorbable monofilament suture. *Biomaterials* 16:1141, 1995.

[25] Pratschke KM et al. Pancreatic surgical biopsy in 24 dogs and 19 cats: postoperative complications and clinical relevance of histological findings. *J Small Anim Pract* 56:60, 2015.

CHAPTER 9

Histopathology of gastrointestinal, pancreatic, and hepatobiliary tissues in cats

Mark R. Ackermann, Albert E. Jergens

The feline gastrointestinal (GI) tract, pancreas, and liver are essential for nutritional well-being, biometabolism, certain hormonal functions, and homoeostasis of a complex microbiome. Ducts lined by epithelium interconnect these organs and thus a lesion or disease condition can affect a single area or have generalised effects (e.g. triaditis). Many conditions can be physiological or even pathological and lack a gross and/or microscopic lesion. On the other hand, many diseases cause gross and/or microscopic lesions diagnostic of a specific disease, while other lesions may be insufficient for a definitive diagnosis. Thus, the histopathological features of the stomach, small and large intestines, caecum, pancreas and pancreatic duct, liver, gallbladder, and bile ducts are one piece of a larger diagnostic puzzle that has potential limitations when histopathological lesions alone are interpreted. Ancillary and supplemental tests along with recognition of salient clinical signs and other laboratory abnormalities are essential for the most complete and accurate diagnostic interpretation (Box 9.1, Table 9.1).

HISTOPATHOLOGY OF DISEASE CONDITIONS IN THE STOMACH AND INTESTINAL TRACT

Stomach

The feline stomach is monogastric and composed of cardiac, fundic, and antral regions leading to the pylorus. The epithelium lining the cardiac and fundic mucosa grossly forms folds or rugae that are composed of numerous glands lined by parietal and chief cells. Parietal cells (oxyntic cells) secrete acid necessary for pepsinogen activation. In cats, intrinsic factor, which is needed for vitamin B_{12} (cobalamin) absorption in the feline ileum, is produced by pancreas only unlike dogs and humans, in which parietal cells produce intrinsic factor. The fundic area also has enterochromaffin-like cells that contribute to acid production by release of histamine from parietal cells. Chief cells produce pepsinogen and chymosin. The antral mucosa lacks parietal and chief cells but does have antral D cells which produce somatostatin—the principal suppressor of gastric acid secretion—and gastric G cells that produce gastrin. Many conditions (e.g. hypergastrinaemia, obesity, drugs, gastric outlet obstruction) can alter gastric acid and intrinsic factor secretion.

The lamina propria of the stomach is limited in the cardiac and fundic areas compared to the antral/pyloric region, which has a more extensive and dense collagenous stroma. Occasional lymphocytes and rare plasma cells are present in the cardiac and fundic areas, and these immune cells are slightly increased in the antral/pyloric area. With antigenic stimulation in the gastric mucosa (e.g. *Helicobacter* sp. colonisation, *Ollulanus tricuspis* infestation), these cellular infiltrates can increase and sometimes form nodular aggregates. The distinction between this background/basal infiltration of lymphocytes vs. gastritis is not precise. Variable numbers of lymphocytes and plasma cells can be present depending on the extent of antigenic stimulation from luminal gastric contents, giving the appearance of inflammation, but they are actually due to a physiological response (Fig. 9.1).

Box 9.1. Sample collection concepts for histopathological assessment.

Gastrointestinal tract

Full-thickness sampling

Useful for:
- Lymphangiectasia (lymphatic vessels in tunica muscularis, subserosal area)
- Lymphoma/neoplasia
- Serosal/subserosal lesions (e.g. feline infectious peritonitis, myenteric ganglia assessment)

Downsides:
- Invasive
- Limited to a region and fewer samples
- Colon can be difficult to sample due to risk of dehiscence

Endoscopic sampling

Useful for:
- Multiple areas, colon
- Less invasive
- Assessment of many generalised disease conditions

Downsides:
- Mucosal area only is collected
- May miss patchy lesions or those deep within the mucosa
- Increased chance for distortion and procurement/processing artefacts

Sampling suggestions:
- Collect sample sufficient to include crypts and submucosa
- Take multiple samples per site (10 or more biopsies if possible)
- Orient properly; a cucumber slice provides a suitable surface to ensure orientation
- Do not crush
- Include other organs of significance (e.g. oesophagus, lymph node, pancreas, liver)
- Communicate to the pathologist:
  - Species, age, gender
  - Site of sample
  - Gross surgical or mucosal appearance
  - Condition/disease suspected
  - Major clinical findings
  - Major changes in clinical pathology
  - Major/pertinent ultrasonographic/radiological findings
  - Changes in behaviour, pertinent physical examination findings
  - Your differential diagnoses
  - Current or recent medications

Pancreas

Sampling suggestions:
- Avoid further damage to an injured pancreas
- Avoid affecting vascular flow to the pancreas
- Sample regions that can include islets
- Include peripancreatic adipose tissue near the pancreatic lesion

Liver

Sampling suggestions:
- Biopsy sample needs to include 15 or more portal triads
- Sample a minimum of three separate liver lobes and submit each separately
- Wedge biopsies or laparoscopic cup forceps biopsies are most useful
- Tru-Cut needle samples are more precise with ultrasonographic guidance but may contain inadequate number of triads
- Use a 16-gauge needle for percutaneous samples

Table 9.1. Selected special stains available for additional diagnostic information.

Stain	Elements being stained	Stain	Elements being stained
Warthin–Starry	*Helicobacter* sp.	**Masson's trichrome**	Fibrosis
Alcian blue	Goblet cells, mucin	**Perls' Prussian blue**	Iron
Gram	Bacteria (gram-negative, gram-positive)	**Rhodanine**	Copper
Periodic acid–Schiff (PAS)	Infectious agents, liver glycogen	**Giemsa and/or toluidine blue**	Mast cell tumours
Oil red O	Liver lipid in frozen sections but not formalin-fixed, paraffin-embedded samples	**Immunohistochemistry**	Lymphoma: • T cells: CD3 • B cells: CD79a, CD20, or PAX 5 Other neoplasms: • Plasma cells: MUM-1 • Epithelial cells: cytokeratin • Spindle cells (sarcoma): vimentin
Acid fast	*Mycobacteria* sp.		
Reticulin	Hepatic or pancreatic stroma/architecture		

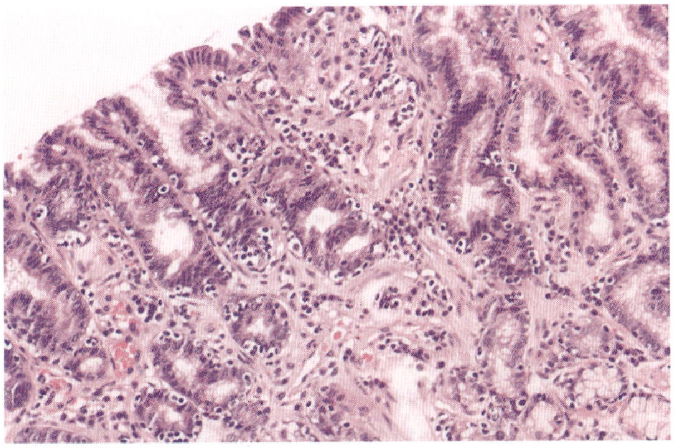

Figure 9.1. Stomach, lymphocytic gastritis. Modest diffuse infiltrates of lymphocytes and plasma cells in the lamina propria. Such infiltrates can be secondary to foreign bodies, infectious agents, or other causes. Haematoxylin–eosin stain. Image courtesy of Dr Pun Sriboonyapirat, Oregon State University, USA.

Congenital lesions

Siamese cats can develop pyloric stenosis which causes gastric outflow obstruction. Histologically, these lesions are often unremarkable other than mucosal thickening and a degree of smooth muscle hypertrophy. Kittens can also be born with umbilical or inguinal hernias.

Acquired lesions

A variety of risk factors are associated with gastric erosions and ulcers. These include stress, administration of nonsteroidal anti-inflammatory drugs, hairballs/foreign bodies, alterations in gastric motility and pH, and mucosal ischaemia. Ulcers are often covered by a small amounts of cell debris, fibrinopurulent inflammation, and fibrosis subjacent to the ulcer, along with variable infiltrates of lymphocytes, plasma cells, and occasional macrophages.

Helicobacter sp. can colonise the stomach of cats and localise in the gastric gland area due to its ability to survive in a low pH environment (Figs. 9.2 and 9.3). The role of gastric helicobacters causing gastritis and clinical disease is poorly understood. While initially considered a pathogen associated with gastric ulcers, these bacteria can colonise the stomach without causing significant lesions or GI signs. *Helicobacter* spp. has many virulence factors that can affect cell adhesion (BabA/B, sabA, OipA) and disrupt epithelial tight junctions (Ure A/B), and cytotoxin-associated gene A (CagA) which promotes p53 degradation causing inflammation and development of gastric cancer.[1]

Feline GI eosinophilic sclerosing fibroplasia can affect the stomach and/or intestines. Lesions are characterised by interconnecting trabeculae of fibrous connective tissue admixed with inflammatory infiltrates of eosinophils, lymphocytes, and plasma cells. These areas can be ulcerated with lesions extending into the submucosa.

Parasites of the cat stomach include *Ollulanus tricuspis*, *Physaloptera*, *Cylicospirura* spp., *Gnathostoma* spp., *Sarcina*-like bacteria, and *Cryptosporidium* sp. These parasites can evoke mild infiltrates of lymphocytes and plasma cells into the lamina propria along with eosinophils. This host response to parasitic infestation can damage the mucosal epithelium, contribute

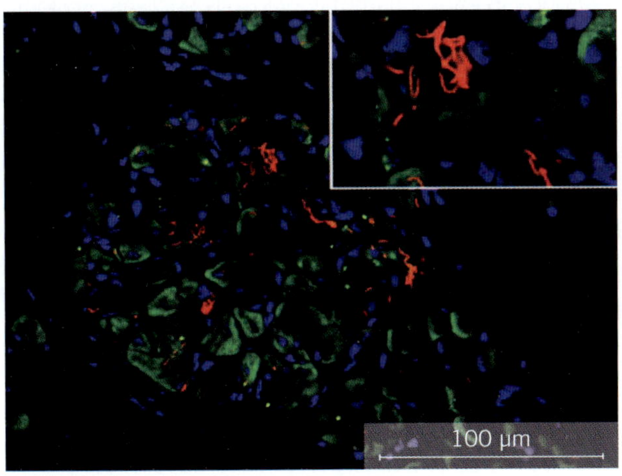

Figure 9.2. Stomach, fundic area, *Helicobacter* sp. Elongate spirochetes (stained red) between shadows of glandular epithelial cells. Fluorescent stain.

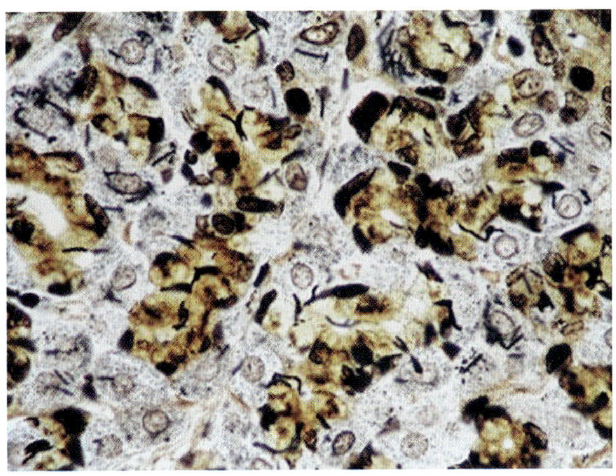

Figure 9.3. Stomach, fundic area, *Helicobacter* sp. Elongate spirochetes (stained black) between glandular epithelial cells. Warthin–Starry stain.

to variable degrees of mucosal hyperplasia, and create inflammation. *Cryptosporidium* sp. is a protozoon found in the subplasma membrane area of apical cytoplasm of enterocytes, but it can also be found in the cytoplasm of microfold (M) cells overlying Peyer's patches.

Gastric lymphoma

Feline lymphoma can occur in the stomach and/or involve the intestines and mesenteric lymph nodes. With gastric lymphoma, lesions are present in the mucosa but may extend into the submucosa and lamina propria. Lymphocytes are arranged in sheets of cells and there can be tingible body macrophages. While lymphoma can be difficult to differentiate from intense/severe lymphoplasmacytic inflammation in the small intestine, gastric lymphoma masses can be more distinct in the cardiac and fundic areas that typically have fewer lymphocytes and plasma cells as compared to the small and large intestines.

Gastric adenocarcinoma

A link between gastric carcinomas and *Helicobacter* sp. has been postulated but not clearly established.[2] In cats, gastric adenocarcinomas are uncommon. In one report of Persian cats, gastric adenocarcinoma was associated with chronic gastritis.[3] These masses have cuboid to polygonal cells arranged haphazardly or in variably sized and irregular small cysts and acini.

Gastric carcinoids

Carcinoid tumours may arise from neuroendocrine-like cells of the intestinal mucosa. Neoplastic cells have granules that contain serotonin and other endocrine substances that may evoke local and systemic effects. They are uncommon but aggressive tumours in cats and other species and generally carry a poor prognosis. Their biological behaviour is similar to that of adenocarcinomas, which metastasise via lymphatic vessels.[4] Carcinoid cells are often polygonal and form nests and small clusters microscopically.

Small intestine

The small intestine contains intestinal villi, but each segment has distinct functions. The duodenum receives pancreatic duct secretory products and bile from the liver that are vital to processing/degradation of nutrients along with carbohydrate enzymes such as lactase. The length of the jejunum allows abundant surface area for digestion to occur along with absorption of nutrients in the ileum. Some nutrients, such as vitamin B_{12}, are absorbed in the ileum; therefore, the loss of ileal absorptive function (e.g. severe distal intestinal disease, ileal resection) causes hypocobalaminaemia. Lacteals (main lymphatic vessels within villous tips) contribute to the uptake of lipids and fluids within the lamina propria. Cells lining the intestinal villi and crypts include enterocytes as well as Paneth cells, goblet cells, and other specialised epithelial subtypes such as enterochromaffin cells and M cells covering the dome epithelium in the ileum. Depending on the disease condition, villi may widen or shorten, crypts may elongate (hyperplasia) or dilate to form crypt abscesses, and lacteals can dilate and become distended (lymphangiectasia).

Like the stomach, the small intestine lamina propria has a basal/background level of lymphocytes and plasma cells that can increase or decrease physiologically depending on antigenic stimulation. Intraepithelial lymphocytes reside between enterocytes lining the villi and are often of gamma/delta T-cell origin, providing immune surveillance. In the ileum, submucosal areas can have nodular aggregates of lymphocytes that can become prominent with antigenic stimulation. These regions have a specialised dome epithelium containing M cells that can take up antigen/microbes and transport these products to proprial antigen presenting cells. During acute infections, neutrophilic infiltration responds to early inflammatory insults such as erosions, ulcerations, and the initial stages of microbial colonisation. As these injuries progress, additional infiltrates of lymphocytes and plasma cells and possibly macrophages and eosinophils accumulate at these sites. Further mucosal changes can include lacteal and lymphatic vessel dilation, oedema accumulation, and fibrosis.

Viral infections

Viral infections of the small intestine include those caused by the feline panleucopenia virus, feline coronavirus, feline infectious peritonitis (FIP) virus, and feline leukaemia virus (FeLV). Feline panleucopenia is caused by a parvovirus that damages the crypt and villous enterocytes, resulting in mucosal collapse, denuded villi, and infiltrates

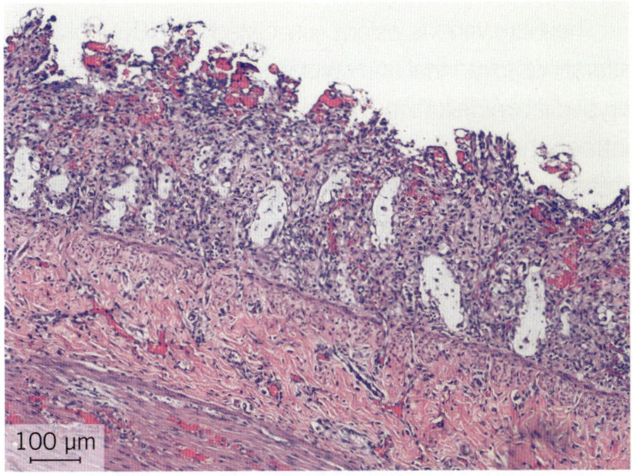

Figure 9.4. Jejunum, feline parvovirus (panleucopenia). The villi and some crypts are denuded of lining epithelial cells, resulting in diffuse partial collapse of the lamina propria. Many crypts are dilated and lined in areas by a few elongate enterocytes. The collapsed lamina propria contains occasional lymphocytes. Haematoxylin–eosin stain. Image courtesy of Dr Pun Sriboonyapirat, Oregon State University, USA.

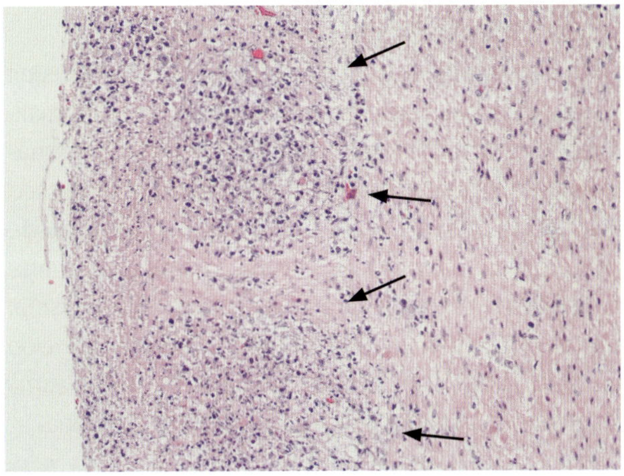

Figure 9.5. Jejunum, feline infectious peritonitis enteritis. Around a blood vessel, there are dense infiltrates of neutrophils admixed with macrophages and cell debris (arrows). The inflammatory cells extend to the adjacent serosa. The smooth muscle cells in nearby areas of tunica muscularis are mildly pale due to cytoplasmic vacuoles. Haematoxylin–eosin stain.

of lymphocytes and plasma cells over time (Fig. 9.4). The injured mucosa is also predisposed to colonisation by secondary bacteria such as *Escherichia coli.* FeLV infection occurs most commonly in middle-aged or older cats, causing lesions similar to those of feline panleucopenia. The feline coronavirus infects the villous epithelia and causes shortening and widening of villi, resulting in malabsorption. The wet form of FIP causes vasculitis with fluid accumulation in the abdominal cavity. Abdominal effusion along with fibrinous exudate can accumulate along the serosal lining. With the chronic, granulomatous form of FIP, perivascular areas can coalesce into dense infiltrates of macrophages admixed with neutrophils, lymphocytes, and plasma cells that obliterate/destroy the surrounding intestinal stroma/structure (Fig. 9.5). Some investigators hypothesise that the exudative (wet) and inflammatory (dry) forms of FIP are a continuum of the same disease condition/infection.[5]

Bacterial infections

Bacterial infections of the small intestine are often self-limiting but can include those caused by *E. coli, Clostridioides difficile* (former *Clostridium difficile*), *Clostridioides* (*Clostridium*) *perfringens, Clostridioides* (*Clostridium*) *jejuni, Salmonella*, and *Neorickettsia helminthoeca.* Various types of *E. coli* can colonise the intestine, causing acute inflammation with infiltrates of neutrophils. Enterotoxigenic *E. coli* attaches to epithelial cells by fimbriae and produces enterotoxins that cause diarrhoea in newborn kittens. Enteropathogenic *E. coli* (EPEC) does not produce Shiga-like toxins or enterotoxins but directly damages the mucosa by other mechanisms. EPEC is not common in cats, but cats can serve as a reservoir for human infection.[6] Enterohaemorrhagic *E. coli* (EHEC) and attaching and effacing *E. coli* (AEEC) do not occur in cats as often as they do in dogs.

Clostridioides sp. can proliferate secondary to alterations in the resident intestinal microbiota following broad-spectrum antibiotic administration. Affected cats develop fibrinonecrotic enteritis with enterocyte necrosis, haemorrhage, and accumulation of intraluminal fibrin admixed with seroproteinaceous fluid and neutrophils in response to enterotoxin secretion. The villous tips and body become necrotic, and the lamina propria retracts. Grossly, the entire intestinal wall can have congested blood vessels with areas of haemorrhage. *Clostridioides* (*Clostridium*) *difficile* releases Rho-glucosylating toxins TcdA and TcdB that depolymerise the actin cytoskeleton.[7] *Clostridioides* (*Clostridium*) *perfringens* can also colonise cats and cause enteritis.[8] Nontyphoidal *Salmonella* sp. infections are uncommon in cats and often subclinical. Consumption of raw meat diets rather than commercial diets increases the risk of *Salmonella* sp. infection in cats.

Parasitic infections

Similar to other species, cats can harbour and transmit various parasites. These include the family Ancylostomatidae (*Ancylostoma* spp. and *Uncinaria* spp.), nematodes of the genus *Strongyloides* (immunosuppressed and young cats),[9,10] *Dipylidium caninum*, trematode *Nanophyetus salmincola*, *Giardia*, *Cystoisospora*, and occasionally of the genera *Hammondia*, *Toxoplasma*, *Sarcocystis*, *Besnoitia*, and *Neospora*. Cats can develop granulomatous enteritis with infection by *Histoplasma capsulatum*, *Pythium insidiosum*, and mycobacteria.

Inflammatory bowel disease

Inflammatory bowel disease (IBD) is a group of chronic enteropathies that generally respond to sequential treatments such as dietary change, antibiotics, pro- and prebiotics, and/or immunosuppressive drugs.[11] While the cause of IBD is unknown, this disorder may result from interplay between mucosal immunity and the environment (e.g. diet, gut microbiota) in genetically susceptible hosts. Intestinal lymphoma (predominantly well-differentiated small-cell phenotype) is a common differential diagnosis in cats with chronic GI signs.

There are various lesions associated with IBD including alterations to luminal and cryptal epithelia, villous stunting, crypt dilation/distortion, lacteal dilation, fibrosis, increased intraepithelial lymphocytes, infiltration of lymphocytes, plasma cells, eosinophils, neutrophils, and macrophages into the lamina propria, and hyperplasia of the lymphoid follicles (Figs. 9.6 and 9.7). The lesions are graded by the World Small Animal Veterinary Association (WSAVA) histopathological scoring system to provide a measure of histopathological severity. Amongst these lesions, lacteal dilation in cats does not occur as commonly as in dogs but is found in severe cases of IBD and with lymphoma (Fig. 9.8). Crypt dilation is less common in cats with small intestinal disease. Distinguishing IBD from lymphoma can be challenging for both pathologists and clinicians. Especially difficult is differentiating intense infiltrates of lymphocytes, which can occur with severe IBD and/or various types of antigenic stimulation of immune cells in the intestinal mucosa. In general, IBD and inflammatory conditions have a mixture of lymphocytes and plasma cells that do not form large aggregates and lack significant cellular atypia and increased mitotic figures. Cats with IBD may also have reduced levels of interleukin (IL)-12p35

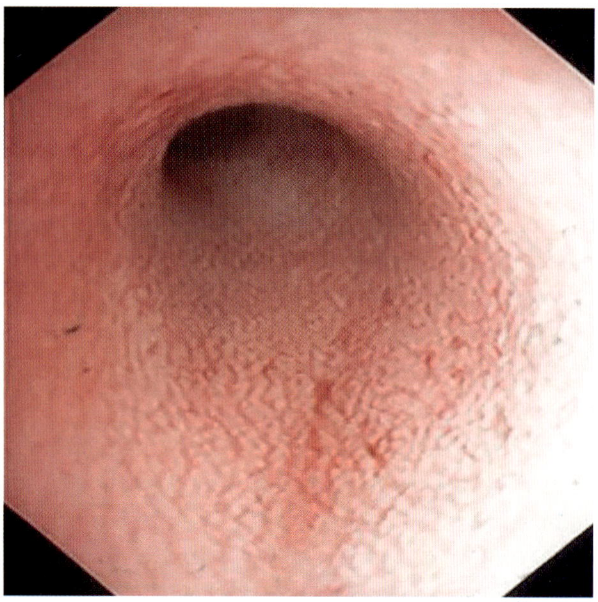

Figure 9.6. Duodenum, lymphoplasmacytic enteritis. Endoscopic image of the proximal duodenum in a 7-year-old domestic shorthair cat with severe lymphoplasmacytic enteritis. Numerous linear erosions are present on the duodenal mucosa and exhibit active haemorrhage.

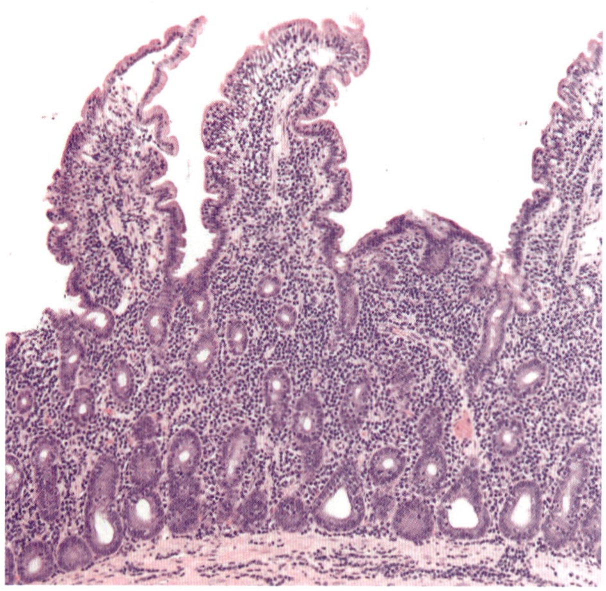

Figure 9.7. Duodenum, lymphoplasmacytic enteritis. The lamina propria has diffuse infiltrates of lymphocytes and plasma cells. There is moderate diffuse hyperplasia of crypts. Haematoxylin–eosin stain. Reprinted from Lidbury JA, Mooyottu S, Jergens AE. Triaditis: truth and consequences. *Vet Clin North Am Small Anim Pract* 50:1135, 2020, with permission from Elsevier.

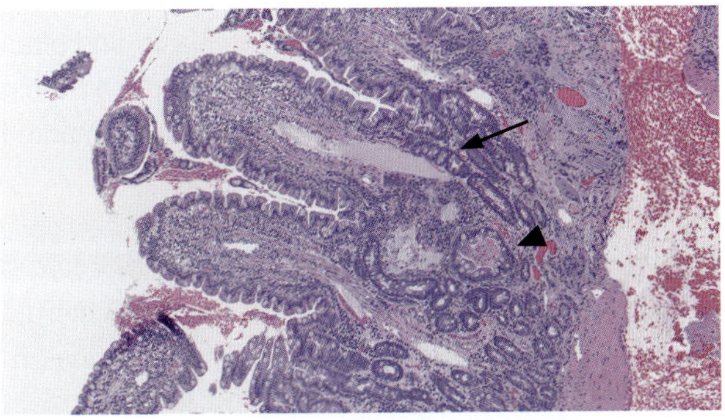

Figure 9.8. Duodenum, enteritis with dilated lacteals and crypts. Villi contain mild infiltrates of lymphocytes and plasma cells. There is mild dilation of lacteals (arrow), and multifocal crypts are moderately dilated (arrowhead). Haematoxylin–eosin stain.

and increased levels of IL-23, although a distinct helper T-cell profile has not been identified in feline IBD.[12]

Intestinal biopsy samples from clinically healthy client-owned cats may exhibit abnormalities on histopathology, immunohistochemistry, clonality testing, or some combination of these techniques, without apparent clinical relevance. Lesions can include small-cell lymphoma, lymphocytic enteritis, and pseudoclonality. With time, some cats can develop clinical signs of chronic enteropathy, while other cats can lack clinical signs for 219–869 days.[13] Many feline chronic enteropathies are managed with dietary modification and sequential use of drug therapy.[14,15]

Microbial dysbiosis

A variety of pathological conditions can initiate and/or exacerbate microbial dysbiosis including IBD, chronic enteropathies, acute diarrhoea, intestinal stasis, motility disorders, decreased gastric acid, exocrine pancreatic insufficiency, and antimicrobial use.[16,17] In turn, when dysbiosis occurs, it can initiate and/or exacerbate inflammation in the GI tract. Cats with IBD have increased mucosal-associated *Enterobacteriaceae* which are correlated to GI signs, histopathological abnormalities, and pro-inflammatory cytokine mRNA.[18] The dysbiosis in cats with acute and chronic enteropathy is characterised by decreased levels of *Bacteroidetes*, *Faecalibacterium* spp., and *Turicibacter* spp. and increased levels of *Enterobacteriaceae*.[19] These alterations result in decreased short-chain fatty acids and altered faecal bile acids, which further augment mucosal inflammation.

Food reactions and allergies

Adverse food reactions are due to a hypersensitivity reaction to a dietary ingredient often mediated by triggering of IgE-directed responses or metabolic (e.g. lactose intolerance), pharmacological (e.g. histamine in spoiled fish—tuna/mackerel—or methylxanthines in chocolate), toxic (bacterial toxins), or idiosyncratic reactions. Food allergens that elicit an immune response in humans include water-soluble and heat-stable glycoproteins having a molecular weight greater than 10 kDa. In cats, the most frequently reported food allergens are beef, chicken, and fish.[20] Importantly, cats may develop sensitivity to more than one dietary ingredient, which may include cereal grains. Histopathological findings in adverse food reactions and allergies are often subtle or difficult to identify but can include vascular congestion and increases in mucosal eosinophils and/or mast cells.

Intussusception

In the small and large intestine, the intestines can undergo telescoping of part of the bowel into a contiguous segment of bowel. This can occur physiologically and resolve, but in some conditions, the telescoped segment may remain with reduced venous blood flow, causing ischaemic necrosis. Histologically, these areas undergo extensive coagulative necrosis with haemorrhage, oedema, and vascular congestion. The reasons for intussusceptions are poorly understood but have been associated with GI parasites, foreign bodies, tumours, or chronic diarrhoea, and this disorder often involves the small intestines of young animals.

Small intestinal neoplasia

Lymphoma

Lymphoma is the most common GI tumour in cats. Salient histopathological features include lymphocytes that are of similar/uniform morphology, aggregates/masses of lymphocytes that expand the intestinal villous stroma and compress on adjacent structures, aggregates of intraepithelial lymphocytes, accumulations of lymphocytes that are uniform in appearance in the submucosa and/or tunica muscularis or serosa, increased mitotic figures, and nuclear atypia (Figs. 9.9 and 9.10). Immunohistochemical stains—$CD3^+$ (T cell) and $CD20^+$ (B cell)—may be helpful in identifying cellular homogeneity (i.e. clonality) that is

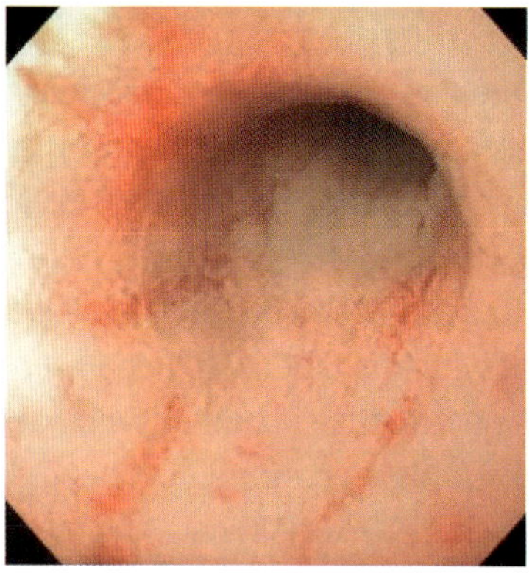

Figure 9.9. Duodenum, lymphoma. Endoscopic image of the distal duodenum in a 12-year-old domestic shorthair cat with well-differentiated gastrointestinal lymphoma. Note the numerous linear erosions present on the mucosal surface. Similar mucosal lesions were observed in the ileum and colon of this cat.

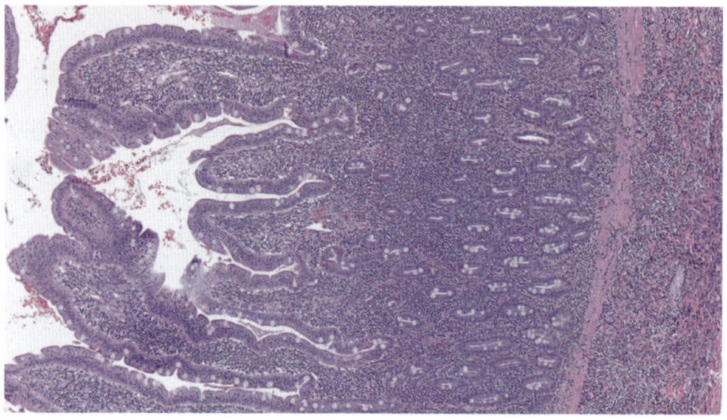

Figure 9.10. Duodenum, lymphoma, diffuse. Sheets of cells within the lamina propria of slightly widened villi. The cells of the mass extend into the submucosa. Haematoxylin–eosin stain.

useful in classifying types of lymphoma. Lymphoma in cats can occur spontaneously or may be associated with FeLV or other causes. Of these, most are of T-cell origin.[21,22] For enteric T-cell lymphoma, enteropathy-associated T-cell lymphoma (EATL) type II (small-cell) is the most common phenotype.[22] Mucosa-invading and intravascular bacteria can be present in feline small intestinal lymphoma but occur in a higher percentage of large-cell lymphomas.[23] Moreover, small-cell lymphoma occurs having a distinct mucosal dysbiosis (i.e. increased *Fusobacterium* sp.) associated with increased numbers of infiltrating CD11b^{+} cells and upregulated nuclear factor kappa B (NF-κB) expression as compared to cats with IBD.[24]

Adenocarcinomas

Intestinal adenocarcinomas are the second most common intestinal neoplasm of cats.[25] They generally carry a poor prognosis.[26] Histologically, tumour masses are composed of cells arranged in variably sized cysts and acini or haphazardly, and the cells are often polygonal to cuboidal with modest amounts of cytoplasm and often a single oval nucleus. Some cells can produce mucin and signet rings, while other tumours invoke a marked fibrous reaction.

Intestinal mast cell tumours

Mast cell tumours (MCTs) occur in the skin, internal organs such as spleen, and also the intestines unassociated with cutaneous masses.[27] Most MCTs occur in the small intestine at the ileocaecal junction and large intestine as well as the mesenteric lymph nodes. Their biological behaviour varies and is dependent on their degree of differentiation.[28] Feline MCTs infiltrate various areas of the intestine and appear as round cells with a central nucleus arranged in sheets. The cells of the mass can sometimes form granules. A subset of feline MCTs can form a fibrosing reaction in cats.

Leiomyomas/leiomyosarcomas

Leiomyomas and leiomyosarcomas arise from smooth muscle cells and often involve the tunica muscularis in the digestive tract.[29] They are uncommon tumours in cats, often locally invasive and slow-growing. Leiomyosarcomas should be differentiated from gastrointestinal stromal tumours (GISTs), which arise from the interstitial cells of Cajal, although GISTs in cats are also uncommon. With immunohistochemistry, GISTs can express CD117 antigen, while leiomyosarcomas do not express CD117 but can express smooth muscle actin. Histologically, leiomyosarcomas are composed of elongate cells with a cigar-shaped nucleus that can form interlacing bundles.

Carcinoids

Carcinoid tumours are uncommon in the intestine of cats but have been reported in the liver, bile duct, pancreas, stomach, and duodenum.[30] They arise from neuroendocrine cells and can be functional or nonfunctional in production of hormones such as gastrin, glucagon, and insulin-like substances. Histologically, cells are polygonal and form nests and packets subdivided by a fine fibrovascular stroma.

Mesotheliomas

Mesotheliomas arise from mesothelial cells lining the peritoneum and tunica vaginalis of the testis. These tumours are uncommon in cats. They often spread extensively before they are detected clinically. These masses can be difficult to differentiate from other types of tumours due to variability in cell arrangements and cellular phenotypes. Cells can be polygonal to elongate and irregular and arranged in papillary projections or irregular clusters or masses. Often immunohistochemistry or other diagnostic methods are needed for verification of mesothelioma diagnosis.[31]

Intestinal polyps

Rectal polyps are relatively common in dogs and humans but uncommon in cats. However, adenomatous polyps in the proximal duodenum can develop with a predisposition observed in cats of Asian ancestry.[32] Large polyps may cause pyloric outflow obstruction and lead to clinical signs (predominantly vomiting) that resolve with excision. Histologically, polyps are composed of mucosal papillary projections lined by epithelial cells that are often cuboidal. The epithelial cells often lack intervening goblet cells.

Amyloid deposition

Amyloid deposition in the intestinal tract is uncommon/rare in cats. If present, it can be secondary to a plasmacytoma (secondary or amyloid A [AA]) as reported in the duodenum of one cat.[33] Histologically, amyloid is an eosinophilic hypercellular substance that replaces nearby cells and stroma but evokes little host response.

Intestinal pseudoobstruction

Intestinal pseudoobstruction is an uncommon functional disturbance characterised by intestinal dysmotility without mechanical obstruction of the lumen. In cats, it has been associated with intestinal leiomyositis characterised by vacuolar degeneration, atrophy, and fibroblastic changes of the muscularis externa.[34] Intestinal pseudoobstruction has also been seen in a cat with myenteric ganglionitis, presumably causing intestinal dysmotility.[35]

Large intestine

The caecum, colon, and rectum of cats absorb water and electrolytes from food, form and store faeces, and have a complex microbiome that produces enzymes capable of degrading difficult-to-digest materials. The lining epithelium of the large intestine has increased number of goblet cells compared to the small intestine, with the lamina propria having variable numbers of lymphocytes and plasma cells in response to luminal stimuli. With disease conditions, such as IBD, infectious agents, or parasites, the numbers of lymphocytes and plasma cells are increased along with mucin production by goblet cells. As in the small intestine, severe inflammation, colonic masses, erosions, and ulceration can occur, resulting in frank blood present in the stool (haematochezia).

Infectious diseases

Granulomatous colitis and enteritis can be associated with GI and/or systemic mycobacterial infections in cats[36,37] and *E. coli*.[38] Other causes include *Pythium insidiosum*, *Histoplasma capsulatum*, FIP, mycotic enterocolitis, feline histiocytic colitis, and feline ulcerative colitis.[39]

Various types of inflammatory responses and mucosal injury may occur with *Trichuris* spp., *Strongyloides* spp., *Tritrichomonas blagburni* (*foetus*), *Entamoeba histolytica*, *Cystoisospora* spp., *E. coli*, and *Clostridium piliforme*.

T. blagburni is a protozoan parasite that causes refractory large bowel diarrhoea in cats.[40] *T. blagburni* organisms are tear-shaped to crescent and should be differentiated from *Giardia* sp. and a commensal trichomonad, *Pentatrichomonas hominis*. *T. blagburni* colonises the lumina of the inner and deeper portions of colonic glands, where it may be found intra- and extracellular and also within lymphatic vessels (Fig. 9.11). The colonic glands can dilate and undergo goblet cell hyperplasia with increased mucin production seen with infection. Varying infiltrates of lympho-

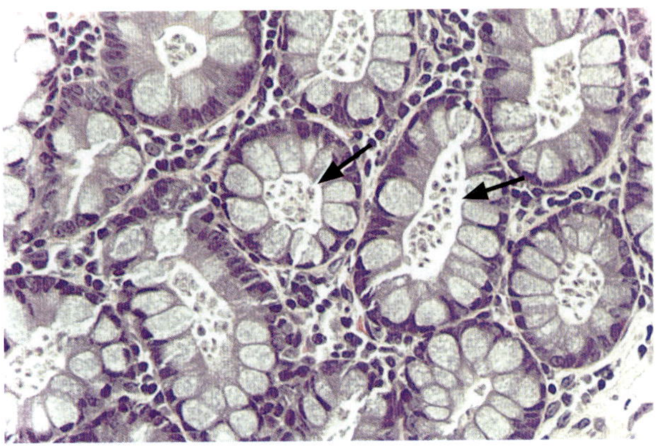

Figure 9.11. Colon, *Tritrichomas blagburni*. The colonic glands are dilated and contain numerous elongate to curviform pale structures within the gland lumen (arrows). Around these, the lamina propria contains lymphocytes and plasma cells. Haematoxylin–eosin stain.

cytes, plasma cells, and neutrophils may also be observed histologically depending on the stage of the infection.

Inflammatory bowel disease

Besides the small intestine, IBD can affect the large intestine of cats. Lesions typically include infiltrates of lymphocytes and plasma cells in the lamina propria along with mild to moderate dilation of glands and increased mucin production. There can also be increased deposition of collagenous stroma in the lamina propria. The mucosal surface may become thickened, with hyperplasia of the glands, and accompanied by epithelial erosions and ulceration with severe inflammatory disease.

Microbial dysbiosis

Like the small intestine, the large intestine has a complex microbiome composed of bacteria, bacteriophages, and other microbes. The microbiota is dynamic and responsive to diet, physiological changes, antibiotics, toxins, disease (infectious agents) conditions, and numerous other factors such as stress. Alterations in the microbiome can, in turn, impair the absorption of fluid and electrolytes, affecting intestinal function and causing large bowel diarrhoea.

Large intestinal neoplasia

Neoplastic conditions present in the stomach and small intestine can also occur in the large intestine, with the most common tumour being lymphoma. Neoplastic conditions in the GI tract are often multifocal and include the large intestine.

HISTOPATHOLOGY OF DISEASE CONDITIONS IN THE PANCREAS

The pancreas has both exocrine and endocrine functions that relate largely to nutrition and metabolism. The pancreatic acini perform exocrine functions via the release of trypsin, chymotrypsin, kallikrein, elastases, and carboxypeptidases which degrade proteins; lipase that breaks down fats; and amylase that facilitates starch digestion. These lytic enzymes pass from acini through intrapancreatic ducts to the pancreatic duct and enter the duodenal lumen. Other pancreatic secretory products are important for proper intestinal absorption of zinc and vitamin B_{12}. Pancreatic islets perform endocrine functions by releasing insulin, glucagon, gastrin, somatostatin, and other hormones that mediate glucose utilisation in peripheral tissues. These two major physiological functions can be altered by disease conditions affecting the acini and/or islets.

Pancreatitis

The cause(s) for pancreatitis in cats is poorly understood, although once initiated, pancreatic inflammation can result in refractory pain, altered digestion, and reduced quality of life.[41,42] It may also result in progressive exocrine and endocrine functional impairment. The specific causes of pancreatitis are diverse and include physical trauma, inadvertent surgical compression or vascular ligation (ischaemia), insecticides, toxins, toxoplasmosis, FIP, adverse drug reactions, component inflammation seen with triaditis, liver disease, and parasitic infections. Obstruction of the pancreatic duct can also occur by an intraluminal mass, pancreatolith, or cholelith blocking the common duct or by compression of the duct externally. While numerous differential diagnoses for pancreatitis exist, in many instances a definitive cause is not determined and a clinical diagnosis is made. Although pancreatic ducts have smooth muscle cells for constriction to prevent reflux, with inflammation in the duodenum caused by IBD, dysbiosis, or other conditions, it is possible that inflammation and/or microbial agents or products ascend the pancreatic duct. Alternatively, intestinal dysbiosis with enteric inflammation may allow bacteria to translocate across the inflamed intestines and travel haematogenously to the pancreas.[42] Cats have only a major pancreatic duct, which enters the duodenal papilla jointly with the hepatic bile duct. Thus, enteric inflammation ascending along the pancreatic duct may, concurrently, ascend into the biliary tree and cause hepatic inflammation. Histologically, the major pancreatic duct and intrahepatic ducts may harbour sparse lymphocytes in the lamina propria, while with chronic inflammation the number of these inflammatory cells increase and include plasma cells that can coalesce to form lymphocytic nodular aggregates.

Once pancreatic inflammation begins, pancreatic damage is exacerbated by further damage to acinar cells that release more digestive enzymes. In the initial/acute phase of pancreatitis, there are regions of necrosis with infiltrates of neutrophils and accumulations of seroproteinaceous fluid that contain cell debris. These inflammatory changes can extend to the peripancreatic adipose tissue, resulting in steatitis with infiltrates of neutrophils along with adipocyte saponification/mineralisation. In time, infiltrates of lymphocytes and plasma cells also occur. Acute pancreatitis can be missed clinically in affected cats since cats can have mild or nonspecific clinical signs, concomitant disorders, or inconclusive diagnostic test results.

Acute pancreatitis can be a continuum with chronic pancreatitis. With persistence of acute damage and inflammatory lesions, there are infiltrates of lymphocytes with lesser numbers of plasma cells and formation of trabeculae of fibrous connective tissue within lobules (Figs. 9.12 and 9.13). Pancreatic acini nearby these regions can become small and have reduced granules (atrophy); although with severe and long-term chronic pancreatitis, the remaining acinar cells can undergo some compensatory hyperplasia. Extensive fibrosis and inflammation can also efface/obliterate islets, promoting diabetes mellitus (DM).

Pancreatitis can occur with hepatic lipidosis, inflammatory liver disease, bile duct obstruction, DM, IBD, vitamin deficiency (B_{12}, folate), intestinal lymphoma, nephritis, pulmonary thromboembolism, and pleural and peritoneal effusions. Triaditis is a descriptive term defining an inflammatory triumvirate involving the pancreas, small intestine (e.g. IBD), and liver. Triaditis can occur in 50%–56% of cats diagnosed with pancreatitis and in 32%–50% of those with cholangitis/inflammatory liver disease.[43] In turn, metabolic alterations resulting from pancreatitis can trigger hepatic lipidosis.

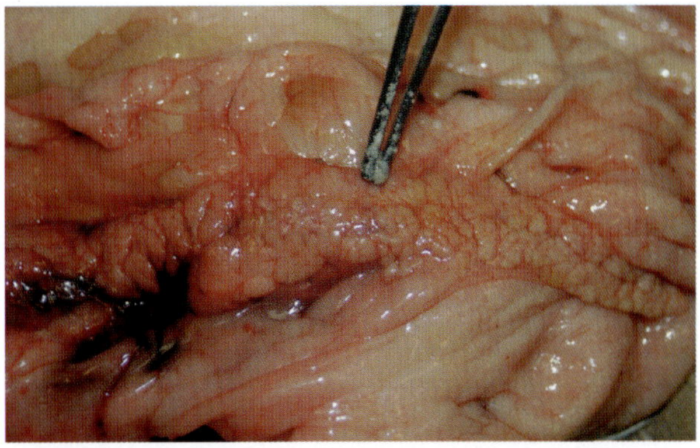

Figure 9.12. Pancreas. The pancreas (below forceps) has a nodular appearance grossly, and these undulations correspond to areas of fibrous trabeculae with inflammation microscopically. Image courtesy of Dr Pun Sriboonyapirat, Oregon State University, USA.

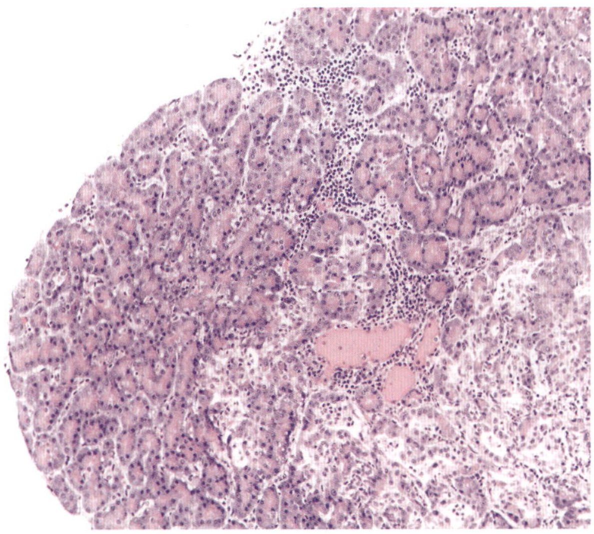

Figure 9.13. Pancreas, chronic lymphocytic pancreatitis. There are moderate multifocal infiltrates of lymphocytes and plasma cells and small trabeculae of fibrous connective tissues. Haematoxylin–eosin stain.

Pancreatic islet lesions and conditions

Cats can develop both type I and type II DM. Type I DM is associated with islet cell loss secondary to extensive inflammation or other causes of islet cell loss. Type II DM is associated with obesity and peripheral insulin resistance, with the accumulation of islet-associated polypeptide.

Type I DM in cats is rare. Lymphocytic infiltration of feline pancreatic islets with destruction/loss of β cells has been reported in only a few diabetic cats. There are no reports of naturally occurring autoantibodies to insulin or β cells causing diabetes in cats.[44]

Type II DM can occur secondary to endocrinopathies (e.g. hypersomatotropism, hypercortisolism), and it is associated with feline obesity as an apparent risk factor. With type II DM, there is both decreased effectiveness of insulin in peripheral tissues (insulin resistance) and failure of β cells to adequately produce insulin due loss of β-cell numbers and/or decreased function. In normal cats and cats with type II DM, there is production of islet amyloid polypeptide (IAPP), or amylin, which is a 37-amino–acid-long peptide secreted by the β-cell islets of Langerhans. IAPP acts locally in the islets to inhibit insulin and glucagon secretion and systemically at distant targets (satiety in brain and promoting gastric emptying).[45] IAPP can accumulate in the islets as amyloid, causing type II DM, with the accumulation causing continued loss of islet cells and decreased β-cell function. Histologically, affected islets are hypocellular due to deposition of eosinophilic hyaline amyloid material. Mature amyloid fibrils are relatively inert, but smaller oligomeric intermediates formed during fibrillogenesis may be cytotoxic (Fig. 9.14).

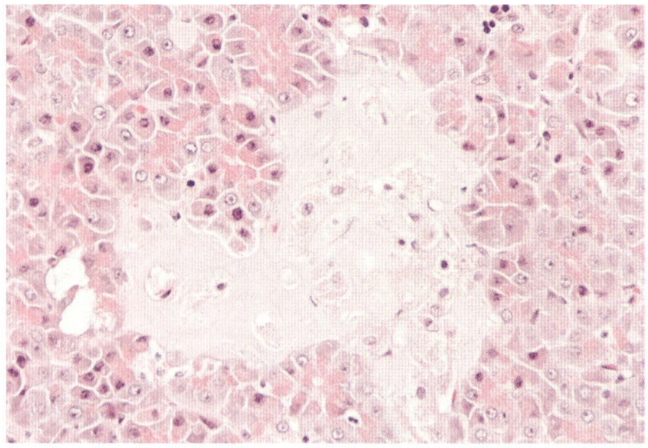

Figure 9.14. Pancreas, islet amyloid. The islet area is diffusely hypocellular due to deposition of a pale, homogeneous substance (amyloid; islet-associated polypeptide). Haematoxylin–eosin stain.

Pancreatic cysts and pseudocysts

Pancreatic cysts and pseudocysts are uncommon but can be associated with acute or chronic pancreatitis and DM, causing vomiting and anorexia in affected cats.[46]

Pancreatic neoplasia

Pancreatic nodular hyperplasia

Areas of pancreatic acini can undergo hyperplasia, in which there is proliferation of these cells into variably sized but often small lumen acini with increased cell density. They do not typically compress the surrounding acini/parenchyma to cause dysfunction. Pancreatic hyperplasia occurs with increasing age and is often an incidental finding in geriatric cats.

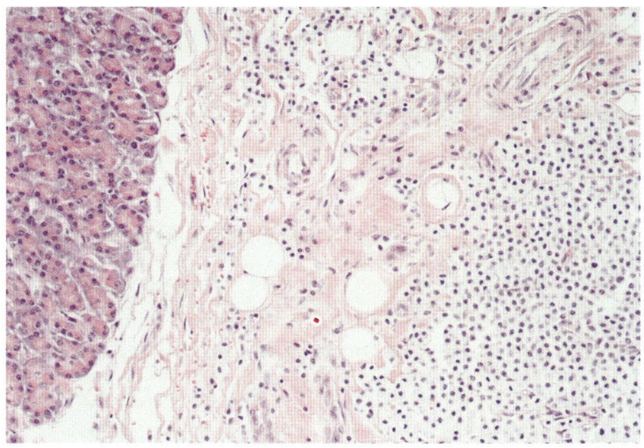

Figure 9.15. Pancreas, mast cell tumour. Nearby the pancreas (left of the image) are diffuse infiltrates of rounds cells phenotypically suggestive of mast cells. Haematoxylin–eosin stain

Ectopic spleen

Ectopic splenic tissue can be present in the mesentery near the pancreas. The reason for this occurrence is not fully understood but may occur secondary to abnormal embryological development or splenic fracturing by trauma.

Pancreatic exocrine adenomas

These masses are often solitary and compress the surrounding parenchyma. They are formed by pyramid-shaped acinar cells that often lack mitotic figures and are arranged in acini. Some of these structures can form cysts. Pancreatic adenomas often have a good prognosis and are treated by surgical excision.[47]

Pancreatic exocrine adenocarcinomas

Feline pancreatic exocrine carcinomas arise from ductal or acinar cells and have a high metastatic rate with poor outcome. In one study, the median survival rate was 97.5 days.[47] Histologically, the masses are composed of cuboidal to polygonal cells with increased mitotic figures (5–255/10 HPF) arranged haphazardly and variably sized and often irregular acini. They may also occur as sheets, nests, cysts, and cords with nearby fibrous tissue. Histopathological differentiation and mitotic rate may not be related to disease progression/survival.[47,48] Cyclooxygenase 2 (COX-2) enzymes can be upregulated in many human pancreatic exocrine carcinomas but are seen in only 25% of feline adenocarcinoma cases.

Endocrine tumours

Endocrine tumours, or islet cell tumours, are rare in cats. Those islet cell tumours identified have been of β-cell phenotype, producing insulin (insulinoma) and causing hypoglycaemia.[49]

Other neoplasms

Various other types of tumours can involve the pancreas, including lipomas, MCTs, and lymphoma (Fig. 9.15).

HISTOPATHOLOGY OF DISEASE CONDITIONS IN THE LIVER, GALLBLADDER, AND BILE DUCT

The liver has numerous functions related to metabolism, biometabolism, detoxification, protein synthesis (e.g. albumin, coagulation factors), and immunity. It receives blood from the digestive tract through the portal veins before passage to the rest of the body, participates in the synthesis and secretion of bile acids, and actively performs the biometabolism of chemicals, drugs, and toxins.

Hepatic parenchymal diseases

Diseases of the feline liver parenchyma include hepatocellular enlargement/swelling, amyloidosis, hepatocellular death (e.g. ischaemia, toxins), acute and chronic hepatitis, abscesses/granulomas, storage diseases, and others. Hepatocellular enlargement can be due to cell swelling (e.g. loss of ATPase pump activity) or accumulation of cytoplasmic glycogen and/or lipid as seen with vacuolar hepatopathy and feline hepatic lipidosis (FHL).

FHL occurs most commonly secondary to anorexia. Other causes include DM, pancreatitis, hepatobiliary inflammation, chronic enteropathies, as a component of triaditis, and neoplasia. FHL is defined by the accumulation of triglycerides in more than 80% of hepatocytes. Physiologically, protein and lipid metabolism in cats appears to be conditioned for a strict carnivorous diet, resulting in requirements for essential fatty acids and amino acids.[50] Cats are unable to synthesise linoleic acid and alpha-linoleic acid and have limited synthesis capacity for arachidonic acid (long-chain polyunsaturated fatty acid; LCPUFA), eicosapentanenoic acid, and docosahexaenoic acid due to decreased activities of the desaturase enzymes delta-5 and delta-6 in hepatocytes. LCPUFAs protect against lipid accumulation since they favour oxidation over triglyceride storage and facilitate glycogen synthesis. Coupled with these changes, hepatocytes in FHL have increased mitochondrial beta-oxidation of fatty acid and ketone formation with a potential reduction in L-carnitine transport of fatty acids into the mitochondria. With FHL, protein metabolism also decreases, and affected cats have over 50% reduction in alanine, arginine, citrulline, taurine, and methionine levels. Grossly, cats with FHL have enlarged livers (Fig. 9.16), and microscopically hepatocytes are enlarged due to clear cytoplasmic vacuoles that compress sinusoidal spaces (Fig. 9.17). Such cytoplasmic vacuoles can contain lipid and/or glycogen. Oil red O stain detects lipid but can be done only on frozen sections because xylene used in the processing of formalin-fixed, paraffin-embedded haematoxylin–eosin stained sections solubilises lipid. Glycogen can be detected with periodic acid–Schiff

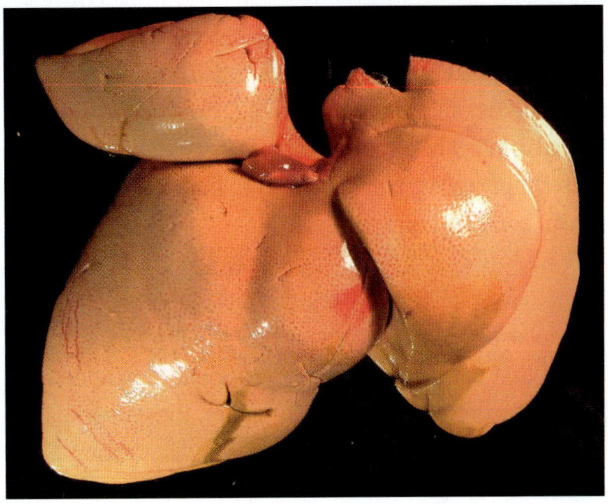

Figure 9.16. Liver, hepatic lipidosis. The liver is diffusely enlarged, pale, and yellow/tan due to diffuse lipidosis. Image courtesy of Dr Pun Sriboonyapirat, Oregon State University, USA.

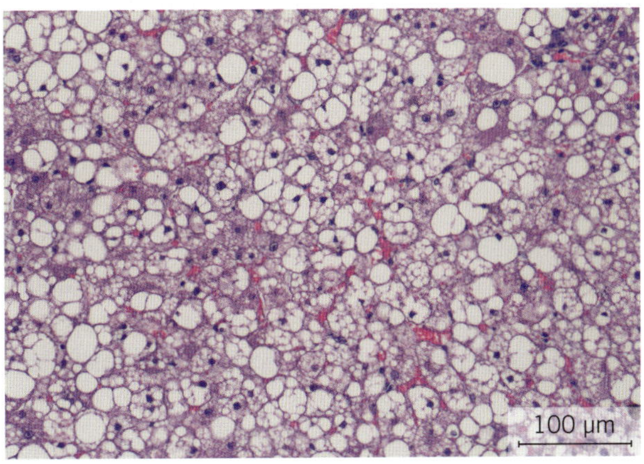

Figure 9.17. Liver, hepatic lipidosis. There is moderate diffuse enlargement of hepatocytes due to one to several variably sized vacuoles, resulting in compression of sinusoids. Haematoxylin–eosin stain. Image courtesy of Dr Pun Sriboonyapirat, Oregon State University, USA.

(PAS) stains (Table 9.1). Therapeutic approaches to FHL include aggressive enteral nutrition and supplementation with L-carnitine, vitamin B_{12}, taurine, N-acetylcysteine, and S-adenosylmethionine, with a recovery rate of 80%–85%.

Amyloid in the liver is largely secondary amyloid (serum amyloid A [SAA]) seen with chronic inflammation, with some breeds having a predisposition (Abyssinian, Siamese, and other breeds of Asian ancestry). Amyloid is a dense hypocellular hyaline/eosinophilic material found in the walls of vessels and the space of Disse in portal areas, resulting in hepatocellular atrophy. Hepatocellular death can occur secondary to hypoxia, toxins, infectious agents, and metabolic alterations. Infectious agents include feline herpesvirus, FIP virus, *E. coli*, *Salmonella* spp., *Clostridium piliforme* (Tyzzer's disease), and *Toxoplasma gondii*. Liver flukes of Opisthorchiidae or Dicrocoeliidae familes can also infect bile ducts and produce chronic cholangitis with lymphocytes, plasma cells, neutrophils, fibrosis, and portal bridging fibrosis if severe.

Vascular disorders

Vascular disorders in cats cause reduced flow of portal blood that decreases portal vein appearance, increases arteriolar profiles, dilates sinusoids, increases biliary hyperplasia, and results in hepatocellular atrophy. Such lesions can occur with congenital portosystemic shunts, portal vein hypoplasia, portal vein obstruction, and intrahepatic arteriovenous fistula.[51]

Biliary and gallbladder conditions

Feline bile contains nonsulphated primary bile acids and cholesterol conjugated to taurine. Taurine is an essential amino acid in cats due to their limited ability for taurine synthesis de novo. Bile secreted from hepatocytes into the canalicular area drains from the canals of Hering into interlobular and intrahepatic ducts and the common bile duct (CBD). Bile is stored in the gallbladder until it empties into the duodenum. The pancreatic duct joins the CBD before entering the duodenum; however, 20% of cats have an accessory pancreatic duct that enters the duodenum directly. Bile acids emulsify lipids and fat-soluble vitamins before 90% of total bile acids are reabsorbed in the ileum (i.e. enterohepatic circulation).

Cholestasis can be intrahepatic, with accumulation of bile in bile canaliculi or ducts secondary to fibrosis, cholangitis, drugs (e.g. methimazole, cyclosporin, rifampicin, cloxacillin), toxins, haemolysis, or endotoxins.[52] Microscopically, intrahepatic cholestasis has numerous biliary spicules in canaliculi or Kupffer cells. Extrahepatic cholestasis is due to impaired bile flow secondary to choleliths, inspissated bile (mucocele), or compression/obstruction secondary to neoplasia or inflammation of the gallbladder or CBD.

Inflammation of the biliary tree and gallbladder can occur secondary to pancreatitis, intestinal inflammation, and cholecystitis, resulting in acute/suppurative and lymphoplasmacytic inflammation. Neutrophilic cholangitis can be secondary to duodenal reflux of enteric contents into the biliary tree. Lymphocytic cholangitis in cats can result in marked portal/periportal infiltrates of lymphocytes and plasma cells that form numerous and sometime large nodular aggregates. The inflammatory intensity can be extensive enough that it can give the appearance of lymphoma (Fig. 9.18).

Cholecystitis

The causes for cholecystitis include microbial (bacterial) infection, endotoxaemia, cholelith formation, necrosis secondary to bile salts, impaired bile flow and sludge persistence, mucocele, and infarcts of the cystic artery. Neutrophilic cholecystitis can occur secondary to bacterial infections. Once initiated, gallbladder mucosa under-

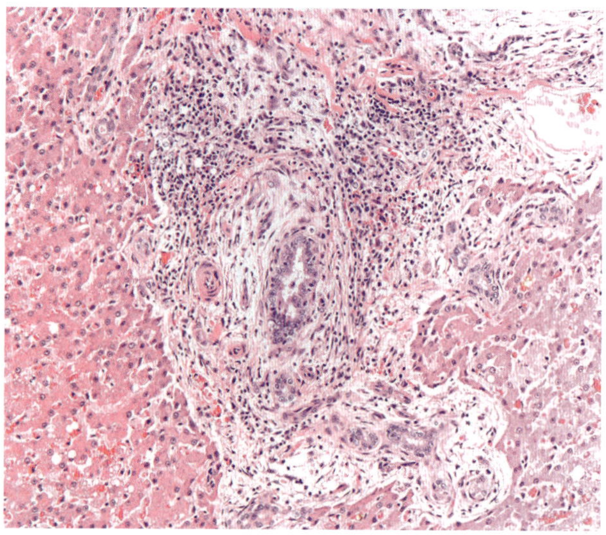

Figure 9.18. Liver, lymphocytic cholangiohepatitis. There are dense infiltrates of lymphocytes and plasma cells in and around the portal area. Haematoxylin–eosin stain.

goes hyperplasia, resulting in thickening and infiltration of lymphocytes and plasma cells. Ulcerated areas rapidly develop subjacent regions of fibrosis that also contain variable numbers of lymphocytes and plasma cells.

Proliferative lymphocytic cholecystitis

The mucosa of the gallbladder can also become thickened by hyperplasia and variable infiltrates of lymphocytes and plasma cells which may form nodular aggregates. This may occur secondary to persistent bacterial infection that triggers proliferation and inflammation.

Biliary cysts and biliary cystadenoma

Dilations of the primordial biliary ductular system arising from the ductal plate can form cysts and a fibrous response within the hepatic parenchyma. These lesions may also be associated with renal cysts in cats. Biliary cystadenomas containing irregularly sized benign cysts separated by a fibrous stroma are relatively common in cats. These occur at the edges of hepatic lobules in older cats and can be either focal or multifocal. They likely arise from small retention cysts associated with embryological maldevelopment of bile ducts.

Biliary neoplasia

Neoplastic conditions of the feline gallbladder and biliary tree include nodular hyperplasia, regenerative nodules, hepatocellular adenoma, hepatocellular carcinoma, cholangiocellular adenoma and adenocarcinoma, MCT, lymphoma, and metastatic neoplasms. Nodular hyperplasia is comprised of hepatocellular proliferation with normal trabecular/lobular architecture that compresses surrounding hepatocytes. Regenerative nodules result from proliferation of hepatocytes subsequent to chronic injury/inflammation and can be difficult to differentiate from adenoma. Adenomas are single, nonencapsulated masses that compress surrounding parenchyma. Hepatocellular carcinomas are uncommon and rarely metastasise. Cholangiocellular adenomas are uncommon, although cholangiocellular adenocarcinomas can occur and metastasise. They appear as white, firm masses that have a starburst appearance. The neoplastic cells form tubules and/or acini and vary from pleomorphic to biliary in appearance (Fig. 9.19).

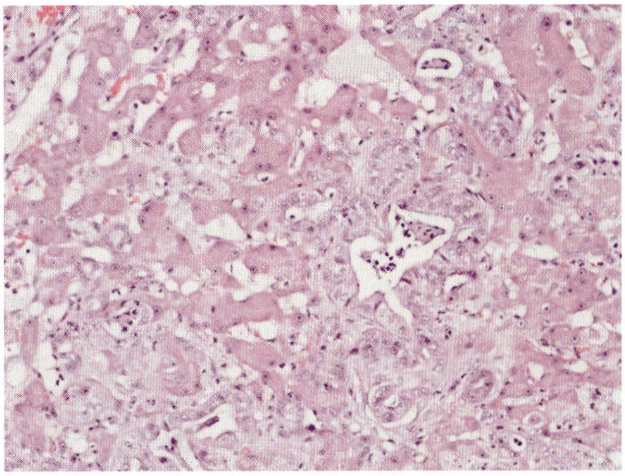

Figure 9.19. Liver, cholangiocellular carcinoma. Polygonal to cuboid cells of a mass arranged in variably sized acini surrounded by dense fibrous connective tissue and occasional regions of short trabeculae of hepatocytes. Haematoxylin–eosin stain.

Take-home messages

- Providing diagnostically adequate tissue samples with pertinent history and differential diagnoses will optimise histopathological interpretation.
- Numerous disorders affect the feline digestive tract, making it difficult to differentiate inflammation (inflammatory bowel disease) from alimentary tract lymphoma.
- Histopathological inflammation on intestinal biopsy specimens is required for diagnosis of feline inflammatory bowel disease. Multi-organ inflammation may involve the intestines, pancreas, and liver and is termed triaditis.
- Many different conditions affecting the digestive tract can alter metabolism and trigger hepatic lipidosis as a secondary event.
- Overlapping clinical signs and laboratory abnormalities obligates liver biopsy to differentiate suppurative from lymphocytic cholangitis.

REFERENCES

[1] Azer SA, Akhondi H. Gastritis. In: *StatPearls*. Treasure Island, StatPearls Publishing, 2020.

[2] von Babo V et al. Canine non-hematopoietic gastric neoplasia. Epidemiologic and diagnostic characteristics in 38 dogs with post-surgical outcome of five cases. *Tierarztl Prax Ausg K Kleintiere Heimtiere* 40:243, 2012.

[3] Dennis MM, Bennett N, Ehrhart EJ. Gastric adenocarcinoma and chronic gastritis in two related Persian cats. *Vet Pathol* 43:358, 2006.

[4] Rossmeisl JH Jr et al. Chronic vomiting associated with a gastric carcinoid in a cat. *J Am Anim Hosp Assoc* 38:61, 2002.

[5] Pedersen NC. An update on feline infectious peritonitis: virology and immunopathogenesis. *Vet J* 201:123, 2014.

[6] Morato EP et al. Domestic cats constitute a natural reservoir of human enteropathogenic *Escherichia coli* types. *Zoonoses Public Health* 56:229, 2009.

[7] Weese JS, Armstrong J. Outbreak of *Clostridium difficile*-associated disease in a small animal veterinary teaching hospital. *J Vet Intern Med* 17:813, 2003.

[8] Silva ROS et al. Isolation of *Clostridium perfringens* and *Clostridioides difficile* in diarrheic and nondiarrheic cats. *Anaerobe* 62:102164, 2020.

[9] Dillard KJ, Saari SA, Anttila M. *Strongyloides stercoralis* infection in a Finnish kennel. *Acta Vet Scand* 49:37, 2007.

[10] Wulcan JM et al. *Strongyloides* spp. in cats: a review of the literature and the first report of zoonotic *Strongyloides stercoralis* in colonic epithelial nodular hyperplasia in cats. *Parasit Vectors* 12:349, 2019.

[11] Jergens AE, Simpson KW. Inflammatory bowel disease in veterinary medicine. *Front Biosci (Elite Ed)* 4:1404, 2012.

[12] Heilmann RM, Suchodolski JS. Is inflammatory bowel disease in dogs and cats associated with a Th1 or Th2 polarization? *Vet Immunol Immunopathol* 168:131, 2015.

[13] Marsilio S et al. Results of histopathology, immunohistochemistry, and molecular clonality testing of small intestinal biopsy specimens from clinically healthy client-owned cats. *J Vet Intern Med* 33:551, 2019.

[14] Rudinsky AJ, Rowe JC, Parker VJ. Nutritional management of chronic enteropathies in dogs and cats. *J Am Vet Med Assoc* 253:570, 2018.

[15] Makielski K et al. Narrative review of therapies for chronic enteropathies in dogs and cats. *J Vet Intern Med* 33:11, 2019.

[16] Suchodolski JS. Diagnosis and interpretation of intestinal dysbiosis in dogs and cats. *Vet J* 215:30, 2016.

[17] Guard BC et al. Longitudinal assessment of microbial dysbiosis, fecal unconjugated bile acid concentrations, and disease activity in dogs with steroid-responsive chronic inflammatory enteropathy. *J Vet Intern Med* 33:1295, 2019.

[18] Janeczko S et al. The relationship of mucosal bacteria to duodenal histopathology, cytokine mRNA, and clinical disease activity in cats with inflammatory bowel disease. *Vet Microbiol* 128:178, 2008.

[19] Suchodolski JS et al. The fecal microbiome in cats with diarrhea. *PLoS One* 10:e0127378, 2015.

[20] Mueller RS, Unterer S. Adverse food reactions: pathogenesis, clinical signs, diagnosis and alternatives to elimination diets. *Vet J* 236:89, 2018.

[21] Moore PF, Rodriguez-Bertos A, Kass PH. Feline gastrointestinal lymphoma: mucosal architecture, immunophenotype, and molecular clonality. *Vet Pathol* 49:658, 2012.

[22] Carrasco V et al. Distinguishing intestinal lymphoma from inflammatory bowel disease in canine duodenal endoscopic biopsy samples. *Vet Pathol* 52:668, 2015.

[23] Hoehne SN et al. Identification of mucosa-invading and intravascular bacteria in feline small intestinal lymphoma. *Vet Pathol* 54:234, 2017.

[24] Garraway K et al. Relationship of the mucosal microbiota to gastrointestinal inflammation and small cell intestinal lymphoma in cats. *J Vet Intern Med* 32:1692, 2018.

[25] Munday JS, Löhr CV, Kiupel M. Tumors of the alimentary tract. In: Meuten DJ, editor. *Tumors in Domestic Animals*, 5th ed. Ames, John Wiley & Sons: 499, 2017.

[26] Smith AA, Frimberger AE, Moore AS. Retrospective study of survival time and prognostic factors for dogs with small intestinal adenocarcinoma treated by tumor excision with or without adjuvant chemotherapy. *J Am Vet Med Assoc* 254:243, 2019.

[27] Willard MD. Alimentary neoplasia in geriatric dogs and cats. *Vet Clin North Am Small Anim Pract* 42:693, 2012.

[28] Sabattini S et al. Feline intestinal mast cell tumours: clinicopathological characterisation and KIT mutation analysis. *J Feline Med Surg* 18:280, 2016.

[29] Hart K et al. A case of gastric leiomyosarcoma in a domestic shorthair cat. *JFMS Open Rep* 4:2055116918818912, 2018.

[30] Nabeta R et al. A case of feline primary duodenal carcinoid with intestinal hemorrhage. *J Vet Med Sci* 81:1086, 2019.

[31] Bacci B et al. Ten cases of feline mesothelioma: an immunohistochemical and ultrastructural study. *J Comp Pathol* 134:347, 2006.

[32] MacDonald JM, Mullen HS, Moroff SD. Adenomatous polyps of the duodenum in cats: 18 cases (1985–1990). *J Am Vet Med Assoc* 202:647, 1993.

[33] Tamura Y et al. Primary duodenal plasmacytoma with associated primary (amyloid light-chain) amyloidosis in a cat. *JFMS Open Rep* 6:2055116920957194, 2020.

[34] Harvey AM et al. Chronic intestinal pseudo-obstruction in a cat caused by visceral myopathy. *J Vet Intern Med* 19:111, 2005.

[35] Mortier J et al. Chronic intestinal pseudo-obstruction associated with enteric ganglionitis in a Persian cat. *JFMS Open Rep* 2:2055116916655173, 2016.

[36] Barandiaran S et al. Mycobacterioses in dogs and cats from Buenos Aires, Argentina. *J Vet Diagn Invest* 29:729, 2017.

[37] Gunn-Moore DA, Jenkins PA, Lucke VM. Feline tuberculosis: a literature review and discussion of 19 cases caused by an unusual mycobacterial variant. *Vet Rec* 138:53, 1996.

[38] Matsumoto I et al. *Escherichia coli*-induced granulomatous colitis in a cat. *JFMS Open Rep* 5:2055116919836537, 2019.

[39] Van Kruiningen HJ, Ryan MJ, Shindel NM. The classification of feline colitis. *J Comp Pathol* 93:275, 1983.

[40] Xenoulis PG et al. Intestinal *Tritrichomonas foetus* infection in cats: a retrospective study of 104 cases. *J Feline Med Surg* 15:1098, 2013.

[41] Bazelle J, Watson P. Pancreatitis in cats: is it acute, is it chronic, is it significant? *J Feline Med Surg* 16:395, 2014.

[42] Watson P. Pancreatitis in dogs and cats: definitions and pathophysiology. *J Small Anim Pract* 56:3, 2015.

[43] Simpson KW. Pancreatitis and triaditis in cats: causes and treatment. *J Small Anim Pract* 56:40, 2015.

[44] Gilor C et al. What's in a name? Classification of diabetes mellitus in veterinary medicine and why it matters. *J Vet Intern Med* 30:927, 2016.

[45] Westermark P, Andersson A, Westermark GT. Islet amyloid polypeptide, islet amyloid, and diabetes mellitus. *Physiol Rev* 91:795, 2011.

[46] Brückner M. Laparoscopic omentalization of a pancreatic cyst in a cat. *J Am Vet Med Assoc* 255:213, 2019.

[47] Törner K et al. Primary solid and cystic tumours of the exocrine pancreas in cats. *J Comp Pathol* 169:5, 2019.

[48] Linderman MJ et al. Feline exocrine pancreatic carcinoma: a retrospective study of 34 cases. *Vet Comp Oncol* 11:208, 2013.

[49] Jackson TC et al. Cellular and molecular characterization of a feline insulinoma. *J Vet Intern Med* 23:383, 2009.

[50] Valtolina C, Favier RP. Feline hepatic lipidosis. *Vet Clin North Am Small Anim Pract* 47:683, 2017.

[51] Cullen JM. Summary of the World Small Animal Veterinary Association standardization committee guide to classification of liver disease in dogs and cats. *Vet Clin North Am Small Anim Pract* 39:395, 2009.

[52] Otte CM, Penning LC, Rothuizen J. Feline biliary tree and gallbladder disease: aetiology, diagnosis and treatment. *J Feline Med Surg* 19:514, 2017.

CHAPTER 10

Feline oral inflammatory diseases

Karin Allenspach, Brenda Mulherin

FELINE CHRONIC GINGIVOSTOMATITIS

Feline chronic gingivostomatitis (FCGS) is a chronic, multifactorial condition that results in painful inflammation of the gingiva and nongingival mucosa, particularly in the palatoglossal folds of the oral cavity. The pathogenesis of FCGS is still unknown. It is thought to be caused by a hyperreactive immune response to either plaque bacteria in the oral cavity, plaque-retentive surfaces (the teeth themselves), or the periodontal ligament. Viral infections, most notably feline calicivirus (FCV), as well as bacterial overgrowth of gram-negative and anaerobic bacteria of the oral microbiome into the submucosa of the gingiva seem to be major drivers of the inflammation that may affect some cats more severely than others. These factors set off an inflammatory cascade that involves cytotoxic T-cell and B-cell infiltration into the oral mucosa, which leads to further inflammation, fostering a micromilieu that promotes further overgrowth of gram-negative anaerobes.

FCGS is a diagnosis of exclusion. On histological examination of biopsy samples, lymphoplasmacellular infiltration with few macrophages and neutrophils can be characteristic of the disease condition, but these findings are not conclusive for a diagnosis. Differential diagnoses to be considered in severe inflammation within the palatoglossal folds of the oral cavity include squamous cell carcinoma, eosinophilic granuloma complex (EGC), periodontitis (which often occurs concurrently with FCGS), and retained teeth with root resorption.

Frequently, treatment consists of partial- or full-mouth teeth extractions, which can result in partial or complete resolution in up to 60% of cases. However, many cats may need additional lifelong medical treatment with analgesic drugs, steroids, or cyclosporin. Recent publications also report some treatment success using recombinant feline interferon omega (rFeIFN-ω) or mesenchymal stem cell (MSC) treatment.

Epidemiology

FCGS is a relatively uncommon disease, with an estimated prevalence in the overall cat population of 0.2%–12%.[1] In a recent study evaluating about 300 cats with oral cavity lesions between 2010 and 2015, 63% of all lesions were identified as inflammatory vs. 37% that were neoplastic. FCGS commonly occurs concurrently with severe periodontitis, inflammatory root resorptions, and retained tooth roots identified on dental radiographs.[2] There is no age predilection for the condition.[1]

In several studies, an association with chronic FCV infection was observed in cats with FCGS,[3] as well as a higher rate of infection with feline immunodeficiency virus (FIV) than in the general population.[4–6] Concurrent infection with either of these viruses does not lend itself to a causative relationship between the disease conditions. With that being said, there is a correlation between cats infected with either of these viruses and the prognosis following surgical treatment. Furthermore, cats with more than one cat in the same living conditions (multicat household, shelters, etc.) were 70% more likely to develop FCGS than single-household cats.[7] The latter finding may point towards the possibility that repeated reinfections with FCV and other viruses play a role in the pathogenesis of FCGS.

Immunopathogenesis

Host immunopathology

Although most authors consider FCGS to be a multifactorial disease, the exact pathogenesis has not been elucidated. Evidence points in the direction of an overzealous immune response of the oral mucosa towards gram-negative anaerobic bacteria that produce plaque on the tooth surface. Chronic viral infections, such as FIV and FCV infections, have also been implicated.[5] This chronic inflammation results in a disease process that manifests in gingival inflammation and ulceration as well as a systemic inflammatory response syndrome. In the peripheral blood, hyperglobulinaemia and leucocytosis with neutrophilia can often be observed.[1] Furthermore, increased levels of alpha-1-acid glycoprotein point towards an increased acute phase reaction in many cats with FCGS.[8] With regard to local and peripheral immunoglobulin (Ig) levels, one study showed that IgG, IgM, and IgA levels were all increased in the blood of cats with FCGS. However, in saliva, IgA levels were decreased, while IgG and IgM levels were both increased.[9] The authors of the study hypothesised that the low IgA levels in the saliva of cats with FCGS may point towards reduced local immunity in the oral cavity. In addition, when flow cytometry was performed on peripheral blood, an increase in circulating cytotoxic $CD8^+$ T cells alongside a decrease in $CD21^+$ B cells was observed.[10]

Histopathological findings in the lesions of FCGS include primarily lymphoplasmacellular infiltrates, with some macrophages and pockets of neutrophils (microabscesses), the latter especially in areas of oral ulceration.[10] In particular, Mott cells, which are highly activated B cells, seem to be abundant in oral lesions of cats with FCGS. Immunohistochemistry was used to characterise the cellular infiltrate in several studies and found that $CD79^+$ and $CD20^+$ plasma cells and $CD8^+$ cytotoxic T cells were the main infiltrating cells.[10] The association with a cytotoxic T-cell response has been hypothesised to point towards an immune reaction directed against intracellular pathogens, such as viruses (e.g. FCV, FIV).

The cytokine profile of the oral lesions has also been evaluated in several studies. Overall, a predominance of T-helper (Th)1 cytokines, such as tumour necrosis factor (TNF), interferon gamma (IFN-γ), interleukin (IL)-1β, and IL-6, was found. In addition, in more recent studies, Th17 cytokines were also investigated and a strong expression of IL-17 and IL-17 receptor mRNA was found.[10] This is an interesting finding, as Th17 cytokines are also strongly implicated in the pathogenesis of Crohn's disease in people.[11] It is therefore possible that, similar to human inflammatory bowel disease, FCGS represents an overstimulation of the immune system to the resident oral microbiome. In one recent study, the mRNA expression profile of inflamed areas of cats with FCGS was analysed by PCR and was found to be enriched for genes associated with inflammatory nuclear factor kappa B (NF-κB) signalling, T-cell signalling, cell adhesion molecules, leucocyte trafficking, natural killer cell–associated cytotoxicity, and complement and coagulation cascades.[10] Moreover, the expression of mRNA for tight junction proteins was diminished, which altogether speaks for a strong Th1/Th17 cell response resulting in severe chronic inflammation and loosening of the oral mucosal barrier secondary to the inflammation.

Viral infections

Viral infections that have been consistently associated with the development of FCGS include FCV[3] and FIV infections.[6] Other virus infections, such as those caused by feline herpesvirus 1 and feline leukaemia virus (FeLV), have also been investigated but were not more frequently found in cats with FCGS than in healthy cats. The current thought is that FCV may play a causal role in the initiation of the disease,[5] which is then perpetuated by the overgrowth of resident oral bacteria and followed by an overzealous Th1/Th17 cell-mediated immune response. The additional presence of FIV infection intensifies the pathology, as FIV causes a decrease of $CD4^+$ helper cells in the periphery, therefore shifting the response even more towards a $CD8^+$ cytotoxic phenotype, and decreases the overall prognosis for resolution of clinical signs in the cat.

Bacteria

As mentioned before, the overall immunopathogenesis of FCGS is hypothesised to be an overreaction of the local oral immune system to resident bacteria and/or viruses. The oral microbiome in cats has been investigated in several studies. The normal oral microbiome in cats consists mainly of bacteria of the genera *Porphyromonas*, *Moraxella*, and *Fusobacterium*.[4] To the contrary, in FCGS, an overall increase in gram-negative and anaerobic bacteria and an associated decrease of species of the phylum *Proteobacteria* has been identified.[12,13,10] Specific families, such as *Peptostreptococcaceae*, and *Pasteurella* spp. are significantly overrepresented.[13,12] Furthermore, many commensal organisms of the normal feline oral microbiome, such as *Moraxella* spp., *Capnocytophaga* spp., *Actinobacillus* spp., amongst others, are decreased, leading to a dysbiosis of the oral microbiome. These findings are consistent with a shift of the microbiome in FCGS towards a more pro-inflammatory, gram-negative, and anaerobic bacterial biofilm encompassing plaque on the surface of the teeth and on the gingiva.[1,10] These bacteria produce pro-inflammatory cytokines, which results in inflammation of the gingiva. The pro-inflammatory milieu then favours the growth of even more gram-negative and proteolytic bacteria, which need amino acids and peptides for their growth. This then leads to a more anaerobic environment of the subgingiva. The pathogenesis of FCGS is reviewed in Figure 10.1.

Diagnosis

The history of cats with FCGS is consistent with severe oral pain and includes signs of ptyalism, anorexia, dysphagia/odynophagia, halitosis, and pawing at the mouth.[1] On physical examination, reddened, inflamed, ulcerative, and proliferative lesions are seen involving the buccal mucosa, gingiva, tongue, and lips, especially in the caudal areas of the oral cavity and the palatoglossal folds (Fig. 10.2).[14] Interestingly, in one study,

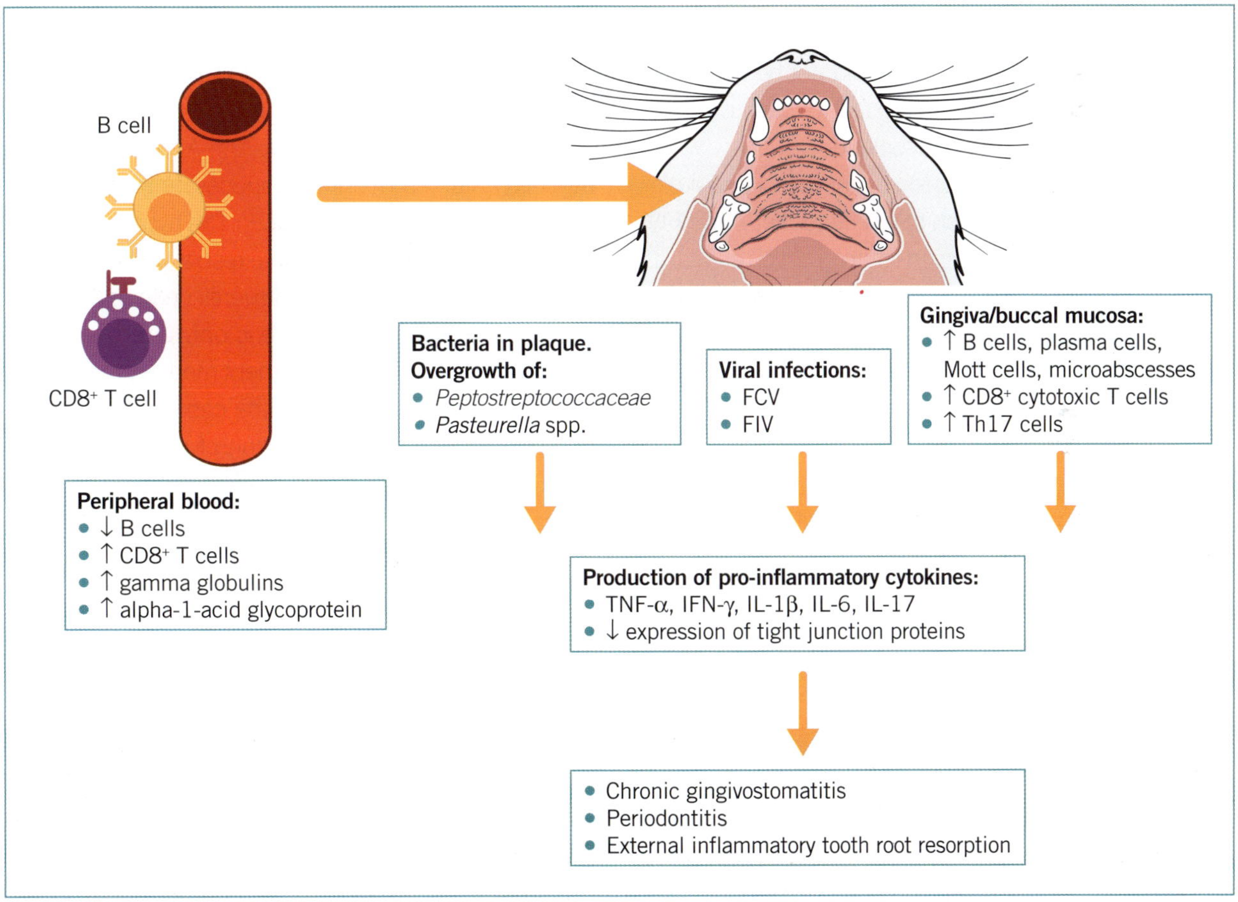

Figure 10.1. The pathogenesis of feline chronic gingivostomatitis (FCGS) is multifactorial. Chronic viral infections such as those caused by feline calicivirus (FCV) and feline immunodeficiency virus (FIV) have been identified as common underlying infections that predispose cats to the development of FCGS. The buildup of dental plaque subsequently leads to the overgrowth of some bacteria normally found in the oral cavity, such as *Peptostreptococcaceae* and *Pasteurella multocida*. These bacteria favour increased growth of gram-negative and anaerobic bacteria, which need amino acids and peptides for growth, therefore causing ulcerations in the oral mucosa. This pro-inflammatory milieu in the gingiva and oral mucosa leads to the recruitment of leucocytes, particularly neutrophils, B cells, cytotoxic CD8+ T cells, and T-helper cells type 17 (Th17 cells), to the oral mucosa, resulting in intense inflammation associated with increased cytokine release of tumour necrosis factor alpha (TNF-α), interferon gamma (IFN-γ), interleukin (IL)-1β, IL-6, and IL-17.

oesophagitis was found to be also present in almost all cats affected with FCGS that underwent upper gastrointestinal endoscopy.[15] The oesophagitis went into remission with treatment of the chronic gingivostomatitis and may therefore not need additional treatment unless there is excessive evidence of dysphagia and regurgitation. The differential diagnoses for FCGS include periodontitis, which can also occur concurrently with FCGS, tooth resorption, neoplasia, EGC, FCV infection, and caustic injury to the oral mucosa. An oral examination under anaesthesia is usually required, as the affected area is extremely painful. While anaesthetised, it is important to take dental radiographs to identify tooth resorption and retained teeth. Biopsy samples should then be obtained from the affected regions and will typically be reported as chronic lymphoplasmacytic and mixed inflammation with ulcerative lesions. Biopsy should not be used as a definitive diagnosis but rather as a tool to rule out a more insidious condition, such as neoplasia.

Performing a complete blood count (CBC) and a biochemistry profile, in addition to testing for FeLV and FIV, is important if there is suspicion for an infection as well as for confirming that the patient is a stable anaesthetic candidate. The CBC often shows leucocytosis with mature neutrophilia, although in FIV-positive cats, occasional leucopenia can also be identified.[10]

Treatment

Meticulous plaque control with frequent dental cleanings performed every 3–6 months combined with the institution of a dental home care regimen can help those patients that have a hyperimmune response to plaque within the oral cavity. Those patients that do not respond to a thorough dental cleaning and home care regimen progress to surgical management with either partial- (all premolar and molar teeth) or full-mouth teeth extractions. The treatment of FCGS frequently consists of surgical full-mouth teeth extractions.[14] This results in complete (1/3) and partial remission (1/3) in about 2/3 of affected cats.[6] The cats with FCGS that are unresponsive to surgical tooth extractions have been shown to be much more likely FIV positive and have a worse prognosis.

The cats in which tooth extractions do not result in remission need lifelong immunosuppressive or immunomodulatory medical treatment. Such medical treatment consists of the administration of systemic glucocorticoids at immunosuppressive doses. However, again, only about 50% of cats respond to this treatment after full-mouth teeth extraction. Cyclosporin has also been tried in a few cases and has shown to provide overall remission in 50%–80% of treated cases.[16,14] Another treatment modality that has been tried successfully is CO_2 laser ablation of proliferative mucosa.[17] The hypothesis is that the thermal ablation of the tissue results in the formation of avascular scar tissue which overall decreases inflammation. However, so far, there is only one single case report that describes this treatment modality in FCGS.[17] Recently, some reports describe cases that went into remission with the administration of rFeIFN-ω.[18,19] In a double-blind, randomised study evaluating a total of 39 cats treated with either prednisolone or daily oromucosal treatment with 0.1 MU of rFeIFN-ω, both groups had significantly improved oral lesions over 3 months of treatment; however, the difference between the two

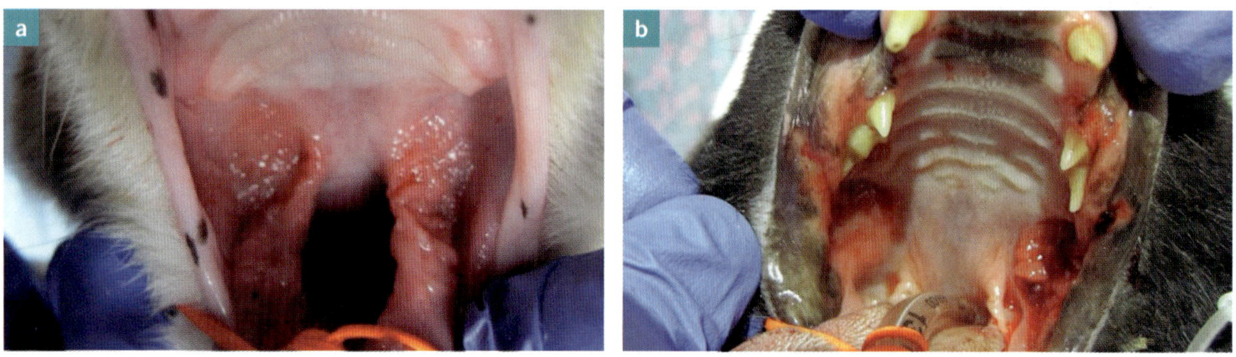

Figure 10.2. Typical lesions of feline chronic gingivostomatitis in the caudal oropharynx of cats. Inflammation and proliferation of the palatoglossal folds (a). Haemorrhagic ulceration of the mucosa of the gingiva, buccal mucosa, and palatoglossal folds (b).

groups was not significant.[19] Another novel treatment modality consists of the intravenous administration of adipose tissue–derived MSCs. MSCs have been shown to home to inflamed tissue and can have an anti-inflammatory effect locally, which can anecdotally lead to clinical remission in various chronic inflammatory conditions. In one recent study, 18 cats were enrolled in a multicentre, prospective, uncontrolled clinical trial, in which 6 cats also underwent a crossover treatment trial.[20] In this study, 10/13 cats that received autologous MSC transfusions experienced a partial or complete remission, and 3/5 cats had a clinical response after being transfused with allogeneic MSCs. Furthermore, the cats in the crossover trial had no clinical improvement during the time they were not receiving treatment. In addition, total serum globulin levels decreased along with the clinical signs in the cats that had a clinical response, and histopathological lesions resolved. Importantly, the time to clinical response was 3–6 months, meaning that cats needed to be followed up for a long time. Furthermore, 4 cats in this trial experienced extensive oedema formation in the forelimbs after the transfusion of MSCs, which occurred in the legs in which the catheter was placed. One cat even developed severe skin sloughing that needed surgical treatment. It is therefore recommended that if autologous stem cells are considered as a treatment for FCGS, since they appear to be associated with higher remission rates, central venous lines be utilised for the transfusion in order to avoid severe extravasation side effects.[20]

FELINE EOSINOPHILIC GRANULOMA COMPLEX

Pathogenesis

Feline EGC is a common condition in cats[21] that comprises inflammatory lesions occurring on the skin, mucocutaneous junctions, and, occasionally, in the oral cavity.[22] Clinical appearance of the lesions may vary from ulcerated lesions to linear, raised erythematous lesions frequently found on the face, caudal thighs, or in the oral cavity (Fig. 10.3).[23] The lesions are usually intensely pruritic but unpainful, and the cats are usually clinically

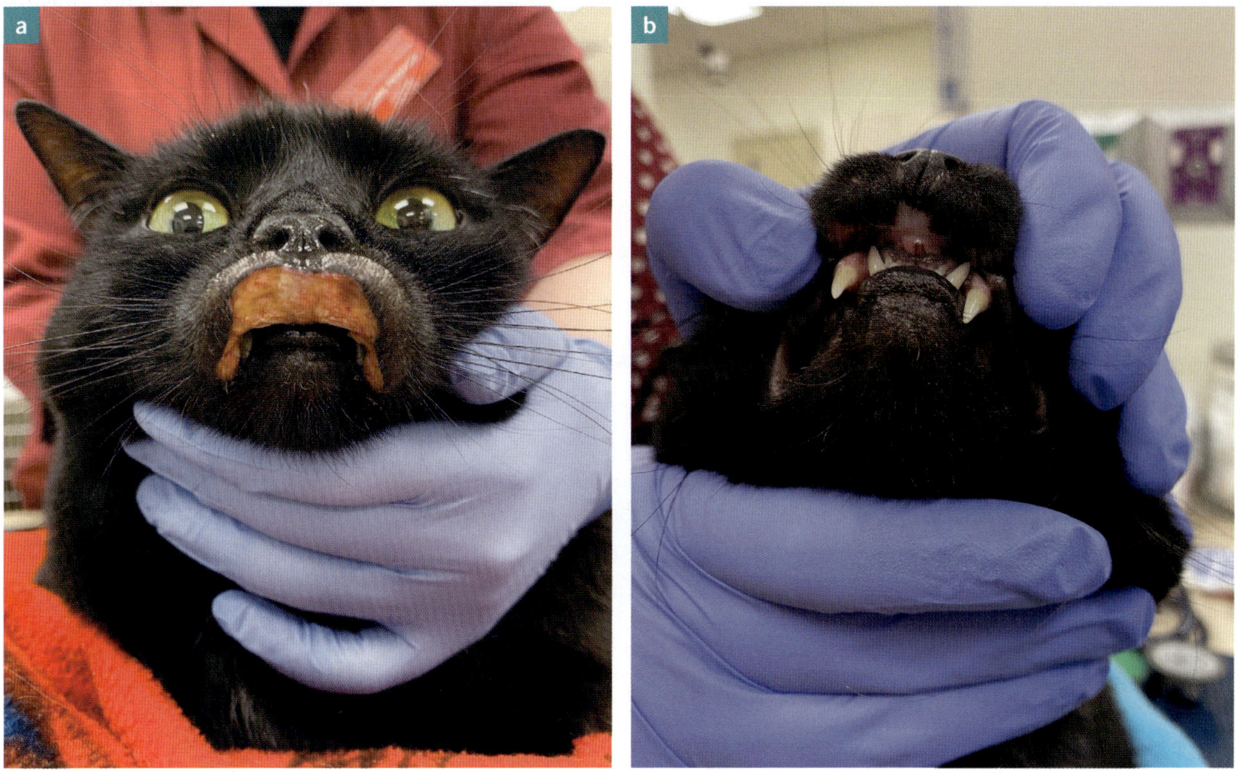

Figure 10.3. Typical aspect of an eosinophilic granuloma lesion at the mucocutaneous junction of the upper lip in a cat before (a) and after (b) treatment with immunosuppressive doses of steroids.

well and appear systemically unaffected. Histopathological examination of biopsied EGC lesions typically show infiltration with eosinophils, ulcerations, erosions, and flame figures, the latter consisting of foci of collagen surrounded by degranulated eosinophils.[24] EGC is, in most cases, thought to be triggered by an underlying allergic condition. Ectoparasites (fleas), food allergies, or atopic dermatitis are frequently diagnosed conditions in cats with EGC.[25,26] It is therefore important to try and identify such causes in the workup of the cases, as lesions often disappear through appropriate treatment of the underlying diseases.

Physical examination and diagnosis

Cats with EGC present with indolent ulcers or eosinophilic plaques that can be pathognomonic for the disease; however, occasionally, other diseases can produce similar lesions, such as neoplasia, FCGS (in the case of oral lesions), fungal infections, and immune-mediated diseases. A presumptive diagnosis can often be made by cytology of the lesions, which show large numbers of eosinophils. As mentioned, investigating potential underlying diseases is important; specifically, dermatologic investigations for ectoparasites and atopic dermatitis as well as elimination diets or hydrolysed diet trials for possible food allergy are indicated. In addition, especially if the cat shows systemic signs of being unwell, a CBC, serum biochemistry profile, urinalysis, and retroviral testing should be considered. A definitive diagnosis is made by histopathological examination of biopsy samples collected from the affected skin or oral lesions, which shows eosinophilic infiltration, epidermal hyperplasia, and erosions.[23]

Treatment

Treatment of EGC is directed at eliminating the underlying disease, if present.[22] If the lesions do not disappear despite managing the underlying disease, immunosuppressive doses of glucocorticoids are indicated and usually result in prompt remission. Care should be taken if cats are managed long-term with steroids, as complications such as development of diabetes mellitus are relatively common. Recent reports have also described some success with cyclosporin treatment,[27] as well as with chlorambucil or feline interferon omega.[28]

Take-home messages

- Feline chronic gingivostomatitis is a painful, multifactorial inflammatory condition that can be difficult to manage.
- Feline calicivirus, feline immunodeficiency virus, and bacterial overgrowth of plaque bacteria or an overzealous immune response to the teeth or periodontal ligament seem to play a role in the pathogenesis of the disease.
- The inflammation is driven by infiltration of B cells, $CD8^+$ T cells, and Th17 cells, which produce large amounts of pro-inflammatory cytokines.
- Treatment of feline chronic gingivostomatitis consists of meticulous plaque control or surgical removal of all teeth. However, in up to 30% of cases no improvement is achieved even with medical treatment after surgery.
- Novel treatments that may provide options for refractory cases include interferon omega and mesenchymal stem cells.
- Eosinophilic granuloma complex is a common disease in feline practice that can often be managed by treating underlying ectoparasites, food allergy, or atopic dermatitis. This disease also responds rapidly to immunosuppressive doses of steroids.

REFERENCES

[1] Lee DB, Verstraete FJM, Arzi B. An update on feline chronic gingivostomatitis. *Vet Clin North Am Small Anim Pract* 50:973, 2020.

[2] Farcas N et al. Dental radiographic findings in cats with chronic gingivostomatitis (2002–2012). *J Am Vet Med Assoc* 244:339, 2014.

[3] Nakanishi H et al. Prevalence of microorganisms associated with feline gingivostomatitis. *J Feline Med Surg* 21:103, 2019.

[4] Older CE et al. Influence of the FIV status and chronic gingivitis on feline oral microbiota. *Pathogens* 9:383, 2020.

[5] Belgard S et al. Relevance of feline calicivirus, feline immunodeficiency virus, feline leukemia virus, feline herpesvirus and *Bartonella henselae* in cats with chronic gingivostomatitis. *Berl Munch Tierarztl Wochenschr* 123:369, 2010.

[6] Druet I, Hennet P. Relationship between feline calicivirus load, oral lesions, and outcome in feline chronic gingivostomatitis (caudal stomatitis): retrospective study in 104 cats. *Front Vet Sci* 4:209, 2017.

[7] Afonso MM et al. A multi-national European cross-sectional study of feline calicivirus epidemiology, diversity and vaccine cross-reactivity. *Vaccine* 35:2753, 2017.

[8] Mestrinho LA et al. A pilot study to evaluate the serum Alpha-1 acid glycoprotein response in cats suffering from feline chronic gingivostomatitis. *BMC Vet Res* 16:390, 2020.

[9] Harley R, Gruffydd-Jones TJ, Day MJ. Salivary and serum immunoglobulin levels in cats with chronic gingivostomatitis. *Vet Rec* 152:125, 2003.

[10] Vapniarsky N et al. Histological, immunological, and genetic analysis of feline chronic gingivostomatitis. *Front Vet Sci* 7:310, 2020.

[11] Cho JH. Significant role of genetics in IBD: the *NOD2* gene. *Rev Gastroenterol Disord* 3 Suppl 1:S18, 2003.

[12] Rodrigues MX et al. The subgingival microbial community of feline periodontitis and gingivostomatitis: characterization and comparison between diseased and healthy cats. *Sci Rep* 9:12340, 2019.

[13] Dolieslager SM et al. Novel bacterial phylotypes associated with the healthy feline oral cavity and feline chronic gingivostomatitis. *Res Vet Sci* 94:428, 2013.

[14] Lyon KF. Gingivostomatitis. *Vet Clin North Am Small Anim Pract* 35:891, 2005.

[15] Kouki MI et al. Chronic gingivostomatitis with esophagitis in cats. *J Vet Intern Med* 31:1673, 2017.

[16] Lommer MJ. Efficacy of cyclosporine for chronic, refractory stomatitis in cats: a randomized, placebo-controlled, double-blinded clinical study. *J Vet Dent* 30:8, 2013.

[17] Lewis JR, Tsugawa AJ, Reiter AM. Use of CO_2 laser as an adjunctive treatment for caudal stomatitis in a cat. *J Vet Dent* 24:240, 2007.

[18] Southerden P, Gorrel C. Treatment of a case of refractory feline chronic gingivostomatitis with feline recombinant interferon omega. *J Small Anim Pract* 48:104, 2007.

[19] Yamaki S et al. Long-term follow-up study after administration of a canine interferon-α preparation for feline gingivitis. *J Vet Med Sci* 82:232, 2020.

[20] Arzi B et al. Therapeutic efficacy of fresh, allogeneic mesenchymal stem cells for severe refractory feline chronic gingivostomatitis. *Stem Cells Transl Med* 6:1710, 2017.

[21] Falcão F et al. Feline oral cavity lesions diagnosed by histopathology: a 6-year retrospective study in Portugal. *J Feline Med Surg* 22:977, 2020.

[22] Lommer MJ. Oral inflammation in small animals. *Vet Clin North Am Small Anim Pract* 43:555, 2013.

[23] Weissman A et al. Ultrasonographic and clinicopathological features of feline gastrointestinal eosinophilic sclerosing fibroplasia in four cats. *J Feline Med Surg* 15:148, 2013.

[24] Buckley L, Nuttall T. Feline eosinophilic granuloma complex(ities): some clinical clarification. *J Feline Med Surg* 14:471, 2012.

[25] Bryan J, Frank LA. Food allergy in the cat: a diagnosis by elimination. *J Feline Med Surg* 12:861, 2010.

[26] Ravens PA, Xu BJ, Vogelnest LJ. Feline atopic dermatitis: a retrospective study of 45 cases (2001–2012). *Vet Dermatol* 25:95, 2014.

[27] Hopke KP, Sargent SJ. Novel presentation of eosinophilic granuloma complex in a cat. *JFMS Open Rep* 5:2055116919891548, 2019.

[28] Foster AP. Immunomodulation and immunodeficiency. *Vet Dermatol* 15:115, 2004.

CHAPTER 11

Oesophageal diseases

Albert E. Jergens

The oesophagus transports food and liquids from the oral cavity to the stomach by means of muscular (peristaltic) contractions. While a relatively simple organ with regard to structure and function, it is surprisingly susceptible to a variety of pathophysiological processes including inflammation, motility disturbances, and mechanical obstruction (Box 11.1). The diagnosis of oesophageal disease relies heavily on the fundamentals of patient history, physical examination, and diagnostic imaging with or without contrast media. Oesophagoscopy is often indicated for diagnosis of cats with signs of oesophageal disease when radiography is inconclusive. Oesophagoscopy can also be used for therapeutic interventions including removal of foreign bodies, balloon catheter dilation of oesophageal strictures, and percutaneous endoscopic gastrostomy (PEG) tube placement. See Appendix for recommended dosages of drugs used for the treatment of oesophageal diseases.

Box 11.1. Oesophageal diseases in the cat.

Inflammatory disorders
- Oesophagitis*
- Oesophageal fistula

Motility disturbances
- Megaoesophagus
- Hiatal hernia
- Oesophageal diverticula
- Acquired dysmotility*

Mechanical obstruction
- Oesophageal foreign bodies*
- Oesophageal stricture*
- Vascular ring anomaly
- Oesophageal neoplasia

*Common in clinical practice.

STRUCTURE AND FUNCTION OF THE OESOPHAGUS

The oesophagus consists of the upper oesophageal sphincter (UOS), the tubular oesophageal body, and the lower oesophageal sphincter (LOS). It is composed of predominately striated muscle proximally, while the distal one-third of this organ contains transverse smooth muscle folds, resulting in the characteristic herringbone pattern in cats (Fig. 11.1). Motor function of the oesophagus is controlled by the extrinsic nervous system and branches of the vagus nerve. Neural coordination of swallowing is provided by somatic nerve connections from the nucleus ambiguus in the brainstem, autonomic nerves to the oesophageal smooth muscle, and general visceral afferent nerves responsive to oesophageal sensory receptors. The oesophageal phase of swallowing begins with relaxation of the UOS and passage of a bolus into the proximal oesophagus. Here, continuation of the primary peristaltic wave propels the bolus aborally towards the stomach. If the bolus fails to travel completely through the oesophagus, a secondary

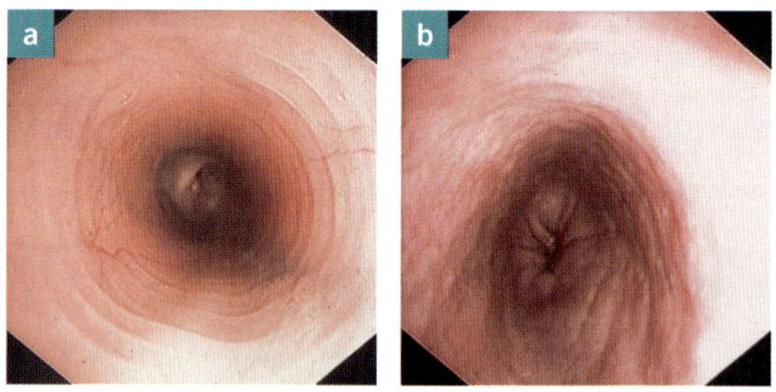

Figure 11.1. Endoscopic appearance of the normal oesophagus. Distal feline oesophagus (a). Note the transverse mucosal folds and prominent vascularity common to the cat. The lower oesophageal sphincter (LOS) is observed distally. Distal canine oesophagus (b). Dogs have longitudinal mucosal folds, lack marked mucosal vascularity, and have a more prominent LOS as compared to cats.

peristaltic wave, initiated by intraluminal distension, will complete bolus transport. The LOS relaxes in advance of bolus entry into the stomach and then immediately contracts and closes to prevent gastrooesophageal (GO) reflux.

DIAGNOSTIC EVALUATION (OVERVIEW)

History and clinical signs

A thorough history is important in identifying potential causes for oesophageal injury. The owner should be questioned about the possibility of ingested foreign bodies, oral medications (e.g. doxycycline, clindamycin), blunt abdominal trauma (hit by car), GO reflux (secondary to general anaesthesia or hiatal hernia), and possible ingestion of corrosive chemicals. Clinical signs indicative of oesophageal disease include regurgitation, dysphagia, odynophagia, salivation, repeated swallowing, gagging, vomiting, and retching. The regurgitated material is usually composed of undigested food, fluid, or frothy white foam (saliva). Acute onset of signs may be seen with oesophageal foreign bodies, oesophagitis, and developing strictures. Chronic regurgitation may be seen with motility disturbances, hiatal hernia, and neoplasia. With chronic disorders, systemic signs of anorexia, weight loss, and even a ravenous appetite can be observed. Tolerance of liquids vs. solid foods is suspicious for obstructive oesophageal diseases. Painful swallowing is seen with oesophagitis and oesophageal foreign bodies. Aspiration pneumonia secondary to regurgitation may cause fever, cough, dyspnoea, and tachypnoea.

Physical examination

The physical examination may be normal in cats with acute signs of oesophageal disease. Fever and pulmonary crackles heard on thoracic auscultation are suggestive of aspiration pneumonia. Cats with chronic disease may exhibit poor body condition associated with weight loss.

Cats with dysautonomia will commonly present with histories of progressive anorexia, weight loss, constipation, regurgitation, and/or vomiting. Abnormalities observed on the physical examination in these cats are unique and include dilated unresponsive pupils, prolapsed nictitating membranes, distended urinary bladder, dry mucous membranes, absent anal tone, bradycardia, and reduced lacrimation (see Chapter 22).[1]

Video 11.1. Oesophagoscopy in a lynx presenting with a history of anorexia. The endoscopic examination of the oesophagus is normal.

Diagnostic tests

The results of routine diagnostic tests are often normal in cats with oesophageal disease. The complete blood count (CBC) may detect neutrophilia and a left shift with aspiration pneumonia. Performance of a biochemical profile and urinalysis serves to rule out metabolic/systemic disorders and provide overall health assessment prior to general anaesthesia. Survey and contrast radiography are extremely useful for the diagnosis of many oesophageal diseases. Survey cervical and thoracic radiographs are initially obtained to identify the entire oesophagus and potential complications of oesophageal disease, such as aspiration pneumonia or pneumomediastinum (with oesophageal perforation). Disorders that may often be diagnosed on survey radiographs include radiopaque foreign bodies, megaoesophagus, oesophageal masses (outlined by air), diverticula (rare), and hiatal hernia. Contrast radiography of the oesophagus is indicated in animals with oesophageal disease when survey radiographs are normal or inconclusive. Static image barium radiographs (without fluoroscopy) are useful for documenting radiolucent foreign bodies, megaoesophagus, diverticula, and obstructive lesions (e.g. strictures, masses, vascular ring anomalies). Contrast videofluoroscopy, if available, provides dynamic assessment of the oropharyngeal, oesophageal (i.e. primary and secondary peristalsis), and GO phases of swallowing. Oesophagoscopy allows for direct visual assessment of diseases that disrupt the mucosa or obstruct the lumen (e.g. oesophagitis, foreign bodies, strictures, tumours) (Video 11.1). Oesophagoscopy is unreliable for the diagnosis of oesophageal motility disturbances. Oesophageal biopsy is uncommonly required except for oesophageal tumours. As biopsy of the oesophagus is difficult and often yields poor quality biopsies, endoscopic cytological specimens collected using a guarded (sheathed) cytology brush are most useful in diagnosing oesophageal neoplasia and eosinophilic oesophagitis.[2]

INFLAMMATORY DISORDERS

Oesophagitis

Oesophagitis denotes acute or chronic inflammation of the oesophageal mucosa that sometimes involves the underlying submucosa or muscularis. The oesophagus has a number of important barrier properties to prevent mucosal injury, such as stratified squamous epithelium with tight junctions, mucus gel, and bicarbonate ions. Disruption of this barrier function may result in mucosal inflammation, erosion, and/or ulceration involving these underlying structures.

Epidemiology and aetiology

The true prevalence of oesophagitis in cats is unknown, but it is a common diagnosis made in clinical practice. It results most commonly from GO reflux (secondary to general anaesthesia or hiatal hernia), injury from oesophageal foreign bodies, ingestion of corrosive substances or hot foods, oral medications (e.g. doxycycline, clindamycin), and inflammation associated with malignancy. The prolonged exposure of the oesophageal mucosa to gastric acid is an important cause of oesophagitis and potential stricture formation, particularly when the pH is below 4.0. Cats are also uniquely susceptible to doxycycline-associated oesophagitis and oesophageal stricture.[3] Therefore, routine administration of a water bolus (5 ml) after pill administration is recommended to promote oesophageal clearance.

History and physical examination

Cats with oesophagitis may have a history of recent general anaesthesia, ingestion of a foreign/corrosive substance, or doxycycline administration. Clinical signs often include hyporexia, food avoidance, painful swallowing, repeated swallowing, and drooling. The physical examination is usually normal except for excessive salivation.

Diagnostic investigation

Radiography is not useful for the detection of oesophagitis due to the subtle nature of the mucosal lesions. Oesophagitis is an endoscopic diagnosis made by visualising erythema, mucosal erosions, GO reflux, and/or increased friability with acute injury; while, granular surface texture, white areas of fibrosis, and strictures are most characteristic of chronic oesophagitis (Fig. 11.2). Endoscopic lesions of mucosal injury are generally found in the distal oesophagus near the LOS. However, oesophagitis associated with benign oesophageal stricture commonly occurs in the midthoracic oesophagus near the base of the heart. Eosinophilic oesophagitis is a rare form of oesophagitis that causes diffuse proliferative lesions of the mucosa diagnosed by endoscopic cytology and biopsy.

Management and treatment

Oesophagitis is often a presumptive diagnosis, with initial treatment aimed at removal of the underlying cause (i.e. GO reflux) if possible. There is clear evidence that treatment with proton pump inhibitors (PPIs; e.g. omeprazole) provides superior gastric acid suppression compared to H_2 receptor antagonists (e.g. ranitidine, famotidine) for acid-related oesophagitis. One strategy to reduce the severity of anaesthesia-associated GO reflux is to administer two oral doses of omeprazole (1 mg/kg) at 18–24 hours and 4 hours before anaesthetic induction.[4] Pretreatment with 5-HT_4 receptor agonists (e.g. cisapride, prucalopride), if available, may also reduce GO reflux by promoting gastric emptying and increasing LOS tone. Sucralfate is a mucosal protectant that binds to damaged mucosa and provides physical protection from acid peptic disease. While it would appear that sucralfate suspension would be of value in the treatment of oesophagitis, this practice is not supported by the available—weak—evidence.[5] There is no evidence that combining sucralfate with either a PPI or an H_2 receptor antagonist for treatment of oesophagitis is beneficial or indicated.

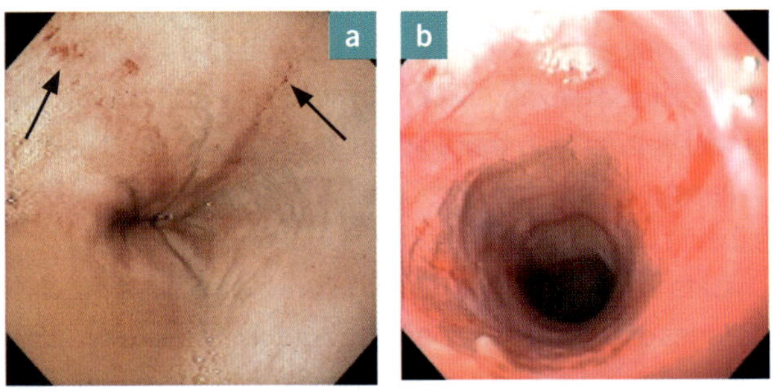

Figure 11.2. Oesophagitis in two different cats. Distal oesophagitis in a 4-year-old domestic shorthair cat (a). Multiple mucosal erosions are present (arrows) near the lower oesophageal sphincter along with moderate gastrooesophageal reflux. Moderate oesophagitis associated with benign oesophageal stricture and gastrooesophageal reflux in a 7-year-old domestic shorthair cat (b). Numerous erosions with active bleeding are present in the midoesophageal body.

Prognosis and outcome

The prognosis for mild acute oesophagitis is good, with most cats responding to PPI therapy. Cats with chronic oesophagitis may develop progressive stricture over time, with recurring regurgitation, weight loss, and malnutrition, which is best managed by balloon dilation of the stricture.

Oesophageal fistula

An oesophageal fistula is an abnormal communication between the oesophagus and adjacent structures, including the lungs or airways. Both congenital and acquired fistulae have been described in dogs but are rare in cats.

Epidemiology and aetiology

Most fistulae occur as acquired lesions resulting from foreign body ingestion, oesophageal perforation, and extension of inflammation into nearby tissues. Bones and grass awns are commonly incriminated. Sequelae of oesophagobronchial fistulae include localised pneumonias, pulmonary abscessation, and pleuritis.

History and physical examination

Signs reported in dogs with acquired fistulae include coughing that worsens after eating and drinking. Concurrent fever and dyspnoea may also be observed on physical examination. Regurgitation is not a salient feature of this disorder.

Diagnostic investigation

Survey thoracic radiographs reveal localised alveolar, bronchiolar, and/or interstitial lung patterns. Definitive diagnosis requires contrast radiography or oesophagoscopy to confirm the communicating tract. An oesophagram using dilute barium contrast will identify the fistula. Small fistulae may be missed by oesophagoscopy.

Management and treatment

Surgical excision and corrective repair are recommended for oesophagobronchial fistulae. Resection of the diseased lung is also recommended. Postoperative antibiotics are indicated when infection is obvious and are based on culture and sensitivity testing.

Prognosis and outcome

The prognosis is generally good with successful surgery.

MOTILITY DISORDERS

Megaoesophagus and dysmotility

Megaoesophagus describes generalised oesophageal dilation with hypomotility (i.e. lack of primary peristaltic waves) and is rare in cats. Disturbances in motility can be idiopathic or acquired and due to primary or secondary causes.

Epidemiology and aetiology

Congenital megaoesophagus is speculated to cause hypomotility due to delayed maturation of oesophageal function. Congenital idiopathic megaoesophagus has been reported in cats with pyloric dysfunction. Acquired myasthenia gravis (MG) may cause localised clinical signs of megaoesophagus and regurgitation with or without generalised weakness.[6] Oesophageal dysmotility can also occur in association with other disorders, including dysautonomia, GO reflux, hiatal hernia, oesophageal stricture, acquired MG, and mediastinal masses (e.g. thymoma, lymphoma).

History and physical examination

Regurgitation is the most reported clinical sign associated with megaoesophagus. The frequency of regurgitation varies from intermittent to several episodes observed in a day. The physical examination in cats with MG may reveal excessive salivation, regurgitation or dysphagia, weight loss, and generalised muscle weakness.

Diagnostic investigation

Routine CBC, biochemistry profile, and urinalysis should be performed to rule out secondary causes for megaoesophagus. Survey thoracic radiographs will be diagnostic for most cases of megaoesophagus and may confirm the presence of a cranial mediastinal mass. Contrast radiographs are uncommonly required but are useful in evaluating motility and the presence of an intraluminal mass or obstructive lesion. Oesophagoscopy is rarely indicated except to verify oesophagitis or an obstructive lesion. A positive acetylcholine receptor (AChR) antibody titre confirms a diagnosis of acquired MG.[7]

Management and treatment

Treatment of idiopathic megaoesophagus is largely supportive and focused on meeting the nutritional needs of the patient while managing secondary complications such as aspiration pneumonia (Table 11.1). Cats may be willing to eat, and their owners should choose the best dietary consistency (i.e. kibble vs. gruel vs. wet food) that minimises regurgitation episodes. In debilitated animals, placement of a PEG tube assures access for enteral nutrition.

Empirical antimicrobial therapy is indicated for aspiration pneumonia. Serotonin 5-HT_4 receptor agonists therapy may be beneficial in stimulating distal oesophageal motility. Cats with acquired MG confirmed by antibody titre can be treated with medical management, surgical management for mediastinal mass, or a combination of medical and surgical management.[6] Medical therapy alone involves the use of pyridostigmine and/or glucocorticoids depending on the clinical response and serial measures of AChR antibody titres.

Table 11.1. Treatment of feline megaoesophagus.

Problem	Therapy
Regurgitation of food/ water	Feed a semiliquid (slurry) diet Feed from an elevated position
Malnutrition	Feed a palatable, high-calorie diet Gastrostomy tube for enteral nutrition
Aspiration pneumonia	Use broad-spectrum antimicrobials to combat infection
Oesophageal motility disturbances	Cisapride for idiopathic megaoesophagus to stimulate distal oesophageal motility Pyridostigmine +/– prednisolone for acquired myasthenia gravis
Oesophagitis	Proton pump inhibitor (omeprazole*), sucralfate suspension, and cisapride

*Administer twice daily.

Prognosis and outcome

The prognosis for megaoesophagus depends on the underlying aetiology, presence of complications (e.g. aspiration pneumonia), and overall health status of the cat. In one retrospective study of 44 cats with diverse causes for oesophageal dysmotility, 78% of cats responded to medical therapy for oesophagitis.[8] A separate retrospective study evaluating risk factors and outcomes in cats with acquired MG showed that 58% of cats were euthanised for their disease.[6] There was a significant negative correlation between the value of the AChR antibody titre and the survival time in these cats. Spontaneous remission is not a characteristic feature of acquired MG in cats.

Hiatal hernia

Hiatal hernia is a protrusion of the abdominal viscera, most often the cardia and fundus of the stomach, through the oesophageal hiatus into the caudal mediastinum. While there are different forms of hiatal hernia, type I or sliding hiatal hernias are most common.

Epidemiology and aetiology

Sliding hiatal hernias may occur as a congenital or acquired lesion. Acquired hiatal hernias are most common, and their aetiology may relate to degeneration of the phrenooesophageal membrane over time, or they may be associated with airway obstruction.[9]

History and physical examination

Cats with hiatal hernia present with regurgitation, hypersalivation, vomiting, and odynophagia. Gastrointestinal signs are attributable to GO reflux and reflux oesophagitis. Airway obstruction (e.g. nasal polyp, rhinitis, stenotic nares, tachypnoea, dyspnoea) may occur concurrently with hiatal hernia in approximately one-third of cases.[9]

Diagnostic investigation

A diagnosis of hiatal hernia is based on findings from survey thoracic radiographs and contrast radiography, including fluoroscopy. Diagnostic imaging shows the presence of an air- or fluid-filled and often oval, soft tissue opacity within the caudodorsal thoracic cavity. Mild dilation of the oesophagus may or may not be present along with hiatal hernia. Oesophagoscopy confirms the presence of oesophagitis with cranial displacement of the LOS and an enlarged oesophageal hiatus.

Management and treatment

Both medical and surgical therapies are available for cats with hiatal hernia. Medical treatment is generally pursued first and includes a combination of acid suppressants (e.g. twice daily oral omeprazole), prokinetics (e.g. metoclopramide or 5-HT_4 receptor agonists to increase LOS tone and stimulate gastric emptying), and cytoprotective agents (e.g. sucralfate as a diffusion barrier agent). Surgical management includes phrenoplasty, oesophagopexy, and gastropexy, which may be performed in cats that do not respond to medical therapy.

Prognosis and outcome

While there is sparse evidence regarding the prognosis of cats with hiatal hernia, the prognosis for survival to discharge was excellent and overall survival was good for cats treated medically or surgically in one study.[9]

Oesophageal diverticula

Oesophageal diverticula are saclike outpouchings in the oesophageal wall that interfere with normal motility patterns. Both congenital and acquired diverticula have been reported. They are rare in dogs and cats.

Epidemiology and aetiology

Congenital diverticula occur in response to developmental abnormalities that permit herniation of the mucosa through the wall of the oesophagus. Acquired diverticula are subdivided into two types depending on the underlying pathogenesis. Traction diverticula often develop in the cranial and midoesophageal body in response to perioesophageal inflammation and fibrosis. Adhesions from the oesophageal wall to adjacent tissues (e.g. lung, bronchus, lymph node) contract and create sacculation. Traction diverticula have been associated with migrating foreign bodies in some instances. Pulsion diverticula are caused by disorders within the oesophagus that increase intraluminal pressure and disrupt normal motility, such as foreign bodies (e.g. trichobezoar) and stricture.[10] They may also develop in the cranial oesophagus as a consequence of vascular ring anomalies.

History and physical examination

The clinical signs of oesophageal diverticula are typical of other oesophageal disorders and include retching, regurgitation, and odynophagia. Signs are related to dysmotility and impaction of the diverticula with food and/or fluid.

Diagnostic investigation

Survey radiographs may show an air-filled or tissue density mass near to or involving the oesophagus. Contrast radiography will demonstrate a focal dilated segment of liquid barium pooling in the diverticulum. Diverticula are usually seen in the cranial mediastinal and epiphrenic portions of the oesophagus. Videofluoroscopy, if available, may detect a concurrent motility disturbance associated with the diverticulum. Oesophagoscopy confirms a saclike outpouching of the oesophageal lumen with erosions and adherent debris along the mucosa of the diverticulum. Small diverticula may only contain fluid. As diverticula are thin-walled structures, care should be taken during oesophagoscopy to avoid perforation.

Management and treatment

Small diverticula may be managed conservatively by feeding semiliquid diets (elevated feedings) to reduce further food entrapment in the pouch. Surgical excision with reconstruction of the oesophageal wall is required for treatment of large diverticula.

Prognosis and outcome

Cats with diverticula should be given a guarded prognosis since motility disturbances may persist following successful surgical correction. Stricture formation is a potential adverse event following corrective surgery.

OBSTRUCTIVE DISORDERS

Oesophageal foreign bodies

Lodged oesophageal foreign bodies in cats are a common reason for emergency visits in clinical practice. Linear foreign bodies (e.g. string, ribbon, shoe laces) and sewing needles are most commonly ingested by cats.[11]

Epidemiology and aetiology

The incidence of oesophageal foreign bodies in cats is considerably less than that observed in dogs. Oesophageal foreign bodies cause both mechanical obstruction and mucosal trauma that may result in serious consequences including oesophagitis, localised dysmotility, and perforation. The severity of oesophageal damage is dependent on the foreign body size, shape, angularity (with sharp points), and duration of obstruction.[12] Oesophageal foreign bodies should be considered medical emergencies, and prompt removal should be pursued.

History and physical examination

Owners may report a history of foreign body ingestion. In other instances, the ingestion may not have been witnessed, which delays definitive diagnosis. Clinical signs will depend on the severity and duration of the oesophageal obstruction. Large objects that result in complete obstruction will cause acute signs, while smaller objects that cause incomplete obstruction will have less intense signs over several days. Salient clinical signs include regurgitation, excessive salivation, odynophagia, anorexia, dysphagia, and retching.

Diagnostic investigation

A tentative diagnosis is made in cats presenting with oesophageal signs and a history of foreign body ingestion. Survey thoracic radiographs will detect radiopaque foreign bodies, but contrast radiography will be required to confirm radiolucent objects lodged in the oesophagus. Iodine contrast agents, instead of barium, should be used to avoid barium pleuritis if oesophageal perforation is suspected. Oesophagoscopy confirms a diagnosis and permits endoscopic removal of the foreign body in most instances.

Management and treatment

Oesophageal foreign bodies should be removed as soon as possible. Complications are directly linked to prolonged retention of the object and continued trauma to the oesophageal mucosa. Flexible (most common) or rigid endoscopic removal using retrieval forceps should be attempted first. While a variety of grasping forceps types are available, some combination of rat-tooth, tripod, snare, and basket forceps are most often used. Rat-tooth forceps permit removal of most small foreign bodies including linear foreign bodies, needles, and coins; tripod forceps are useful for soft, pliable objects like plastic and cloth; and basket forceps help to retrieve angular foreign objects such as bones (Fig. 11.3). Large foreign bodies that cannot be safely removed through the mouth may be pushed into the stomach for gastrostomy or left in place to be digested. Following endoscopic removal, the oesophagus should be visually evaluated for severity of the mucosal trauma and potential perforation. Survey thoracic radiographs will detect free air in the mediastinum or thorax if perforation is present. Animals with significant trauma will require enteral feeding through a gastrostomy tube placed at the time of endoscopy. Affected animals should be fasted for 24 hours after foreign body removal. Specific therapy for oesophagitis should include a PPI, with or without sucralfate suspension (clinician's preference), to reduce further mucosal injury. Antibiotics are indicated for ulceration or small perforations. If surgery is required after failed endoscopic retrieval of oesophageal foreign bodies, one recent study indicates that oesophagostomy is well tolerated and associated with a low incidence of complications.[13]

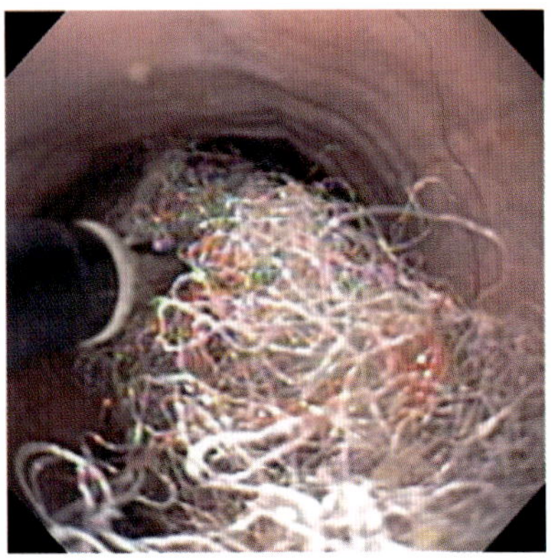

Figure 11.3. Oesophageal foreign body in a 2-year-old Persian cat. The oesophageal lumen contains abundant fine linear material (Easter grass) that is being removed using three-pronged (tripod) retrieval forceps.

Prognosis and outcome

The prognosis for most oesophageal foreign bodies is good with prompt and successful extraction. Animals with severe trauma are susceptible to post-extraction complications including fistulation, diverticula, or stricture.

Oesophageal stricture

Oesophageal stricture is a pathological narrowing of the oesophageal lumen. Strictures may be congenital (rare) or acquired secondary to severe mucosal injury.

Epidemiology and aetiology

Most strictures are acquired through chemical injury from swallowed substances, thermal injury from ingestion of hot foods, intraluminal trauma (e.g. oesophageal foreign bodies), GO reflux causing severe oesophagitis, complications of oesophageal surgery, and intraluminal (neoplasia) or extraluminal (abscess, granuloma) mass lesions.

History and physical examination

General anaesthesia and poor patient positioning during anaesthesia are significant risk factors for reflux oesophagitis and stricture. Cats are particularly susceptible to doxycycline-associated oesophagitis and stricture formation.[3] Clinical signs of progressive regurgitation and dysphagia are related to the rapidity and severity of the luminal narrowing. Cats often have a history of tolerating liquids better than solid meals. Some cats will have ravenous appetite related to inadequate caloric consumption. As stricture formation progresses, cats develop complete anorexia, weight loss, and malnutrition. The physical examination in the early disease course reveals mild weight loss, while salivation, regurgitation, and cachexia are observed in chronic untreated cases.

Diagnostic investigation

Survey thoracic radiographs fail to identify oesophageal strictures. Contrast radiography is required to delineate the number and location of strictures within the oesophagus. The typical lesion shows segmental or diffuse narrowing of the oesophageal lumen. There is often associated oesophageal dilation cranial to the stricture (Fig. 11.4). Oesophagoscopy confirms the site and severity of the stricture and allows for mucosal biopsy/cytological sampling of malignant stricture (Fig. 11.5). Differentiating a benign oesophageal stricture from other oesophageal disorders can sometimes be challenging and may require contrast radiography, endoscopy, and/or thoracic computed tomography.

Management and treatment

Mild benign strictures may be managed medically by feeding a semiliquid diet to provide adequate nutrition. In animals with a severe stricture, a gastrostomy tube may be placed at the time of oesophageal dilation to provide continuous enteral nutritional support. Oesophageal strictures are best managed by mechanical dilation using either bougienage tubes or balloon dilation catheters. Bougienage involves passing rigid tubes of increasing diameter longitudinally (aborally) through the stricture to mechanically dilate the site. Dilation occurs by progressive proximal-to-distal application of longitudinal and radial forces. Balloon dilation catheters are positioned within the stricture and then filled with fluid using an inflation gun with pressure gauge (Fig. 11.6). Here, balloon catheter dilation allows radial forces to be applied to mechanically dilate the area of oesophageal stenosis.

Oesophageal balloon dilation procedure

The procedure for balloon dilation is as follows. Confirm the number, length, and location of strictures using contrast radiography. Choose a balloon size that is 50%–

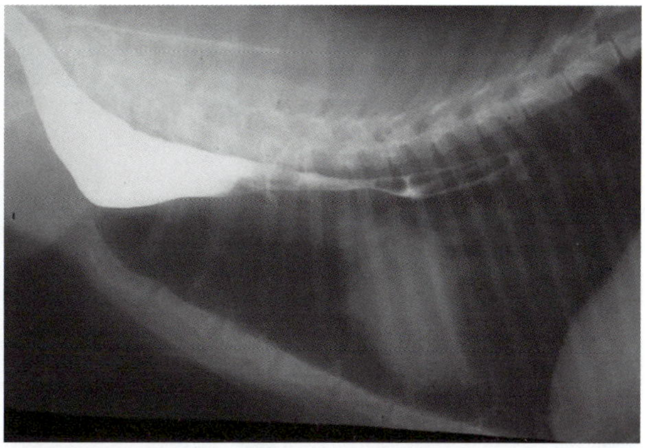

Figure 11.4. Barium contrast oesophagram (lateral projection) in a 1-year-old domestic longhair cat. The contrast bolus shows distinct narrowing over the base of the heart, with oesophageal dilation evident cranial to the heart at the thoracic inlet. Oesophagoscopy confirmed the presence of a benign oesophageal stricture.

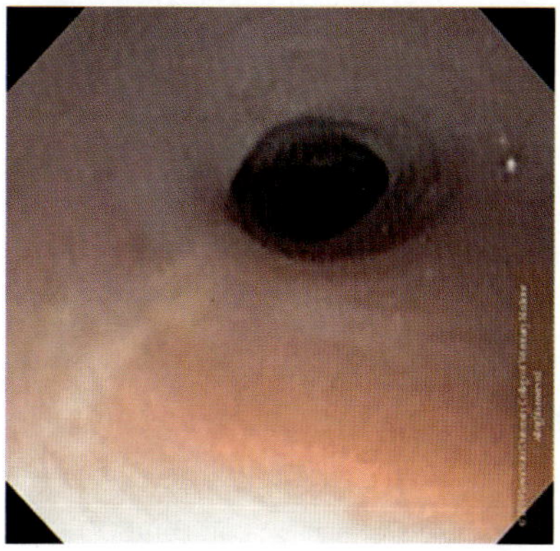

Figure 11.5. Endoscopic appearance of the benign oesophageal stricture observed by contrast radiography in Figure 11.4. The oesophageal lumen is narrowed by a single stricture having a luminal diameter of 4 mm.

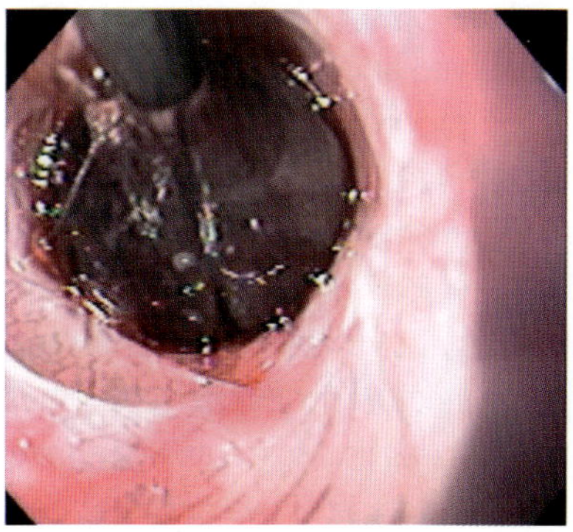

Figure 11.6. Oesophageal stricture dilation using an 18 mm fixed balloon catheter with an inflation gun and pressure gauge. The cat's stricture is being maximally dilated, with the fibrous rim of the stricture clearly evident along the ventral margin.

100% larger than the stricture as observed on contrast radiography. Using direct observation, pass the deflated balloon catheter alongside the endoscope insertion tube—rather than through the endoscope accessory channel—and measure the stricture diameter (predilation) using pinch biopsy forceps as reference. Correctly position the

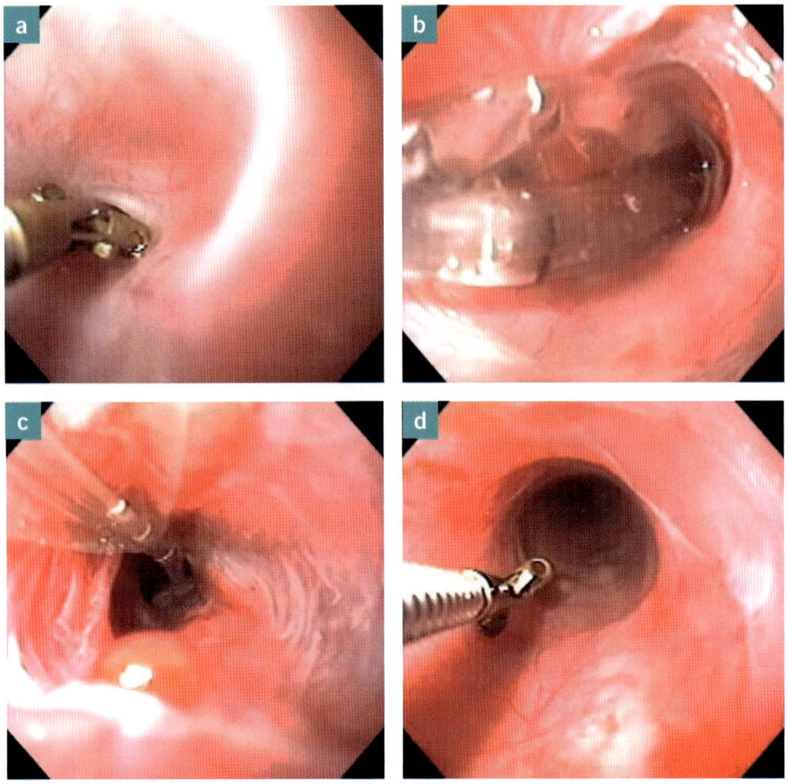

Figure 11.7. Technique for oesophageal stricture dilation in a 1-year-old Burmese cat using a balloon catheter. Predilation measurement of the stricture, which is less than 5 mm in diameter (a). Correctly positioned balloon catheter showing moderate dilation pressure exerted radially against the stricture (b). Balloon catheter deflation showing mucosal tearing (white fibrous tissue) and haemorrhage in response to sequential dilation episodes (c). Postdilation measurement of oesophageal lumen diameter (13 mm diameter) immediately distal to the stricture (d).

closed balloon catheter midway through the stricture and slowly distend the balloon with fluid, being careful to maintain optimal positioning within the stricture. Maintain dilation pressure for 2–3 minutes using an inflation gun pressure gauge to monitor consistent pressure. During active dilation, mucosal blanching, fibrous tearing, and haemorrhage will be observed and should be expected. Repeat the above dilation procedure two more times (a total of three dilations per anaesthetic event), increasing the balloon dilation catheter diameter each time if possible (Video 11.2). Measure the stricture diameter postdilation using the biopsy forceps (Fig. 11.7). Assess the remaining oesophagus aboral to the stricture for evidence of other lesions including active oesophagitis. Most cats will require repeat dilation procedures (average of two or three) performed at 24–48-hour intervals, as restricturing occurs rapidly (Fig. 11.8). The use of an indwelling oesophageal balloon dilation feeding tube (i.e. B-tube) for treatment of benign oesophageal stricture in cats has been recently described.[14] Placement of an oesophageal stent may be considered in cases of refractory stricture; however, this technique has been associated with a high complication rate and poor long-term outcome in dogs.[15]

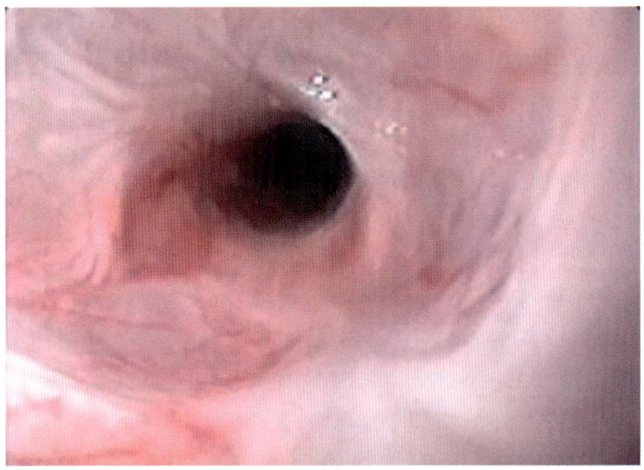

Figure 11.8. Oesophageal stricture 48 hours after a dilation procedure. Note the dramatic reduction of luminal diameter as observed in Figure 11.7. Strictures will require repeat dilation as early as 2 days after the initial dilation procedure. Four-quadrant triamcinolone injection locally into the mucosa surrounding the stricture performed before dilation will reduce the severity of restricture.

Video 11.2. Balloon dilation of a mid-oesophageal stricture. This stricture was associated with the ingestion of a foreign body which had been removed 3 weeks previously.

Postdilation treatment considerations

To minimise the extent of refibrosis, an intralesional steroid injection (triamcinolone, 1 mg) may be administered immediately prior to balloon dilation to reduce the risk of stricture recurrence.[16] Corticosteroids are used cautiously in patients having severe oesophagitis as a consequence of their disease or balloon dilation. Adjunctive medical therapy using PPIs as a gastrointestinal protectant, sucralfate (clinician's preference), and 5-HT_4 receptor agonists to increase LOS tone and promote gastric emptying will minimise GO reflux. Feeding with a semiliquid diet can be initiated 12–24 hours after balloon dilation. Placement of a PEG tube facilitates oesophageal rest and enteral feeding in animals with severe stricture.

Prognosis and outcome

The prognosis for benign oesophageal stricture is generally good with successful dilation. Multiple dilations will be necessary to achieve an adequate oesophageal lumen. Results indicate that oesophageal bougienage is safe and effective for stricture dilation, with outcomes similar to those reported for balloon dilation.[17] Perforation during balloon dilation is a potential possibility requiring emergency intervention. Owners should be counselled that a return to their pets' normal diet may not be possible and that feeding a semiliquid diet may be required. Malignant strictures carry a poor prognosis.

Vascular ring anomalies

Vascular ring anomalies are congenital malformations of the great vessels leaving the heart that entrap the oesophagus and trachea. Persistent right aortic arch (PRAA) is the most common vascular ring anomaly in the cat but is rare.

Epidemiology and aetiology

PRAA causes extraluminal compression of the oesophagus and/or trachea resulting in physical obstruction of the oesophageal lumen. While a heritable basis for this disorder in cats is suspected, it has not been proven.

History and physical examination

Clinical signs (e.g. repeated regurgitation, failure to thrive) usually manifest in kittens at the time of weaning. As kittens transition to solid food, regurgitation episodes increase in frequency and severity. Aspiration pneumonia with cough may occur as a result of frequent regurgitation. Physical examination reveals a thin animal, small in stature, and with a ravenous appetite.

Diagnostic investigation

A diagnosis of vascular ring anomaly is suspected based on supportive history and made on thoracic radiography. Survey radiography is inadequate for confirmation; however, barium contrast radiographs show oesophageal body dilation cranial to the base of the heart. In chronic cases, a small diverticulum may occur in the proximal oesophagus. The oesophagus caudal to the compression usually appears normal but may be mildly dilated. Oesophagoscopy may be performed to differentiate intraluminal stenosis (i.e. stricture) from extraluminal compression. With vascular ring anomalies, pulsations of blood through the major arteries are observed in the region of oesophageal narrowing, causing the narrowed lumen to "open and close". Another discriminating feature for vascular ring anomalies is their location over the base of the heart, while strictures may occur anywhere within the oesophageal body.

Management and treatment

Vascular ring anomaly (e.g. PRAA) is best treated by thoracotomy with ligation and dissection of the ligamentum arteriosum. Perioesophageal fibrosis should be reduced, and the luminal narrowing should be dilated with a balloon dilation catheter. Some animals may have persistent oesophageal hypomotility that remains following corrective surgery.

Prognosis and outcome

The prognosis for most animals is guarded with successful surgery, as motility disturbances and clinical signs may persist. Cat owners should be counselled on the need for elevated feedings using a blended or liquid diet.

Oesophageal neoplasia

Primary oesophageal tumours of the feline oesophagus are rare. Oesophageal tumours typically cause clinical signs as a result of mechanical obstruction.

Epidemiology and aetiology

Oesophageal tumours are predominantly seen in middle-aged and older cats. In the author's experience, the most common feline tumour types seen include squamous cell carcinoma and paraoesophageal lymphoma. Oesophageal tumours are typically locally invasive and may also be associated with concurrent motility disturbances.

History and physical examination

Primary clinical signs include intermittent or persistent regurgitation and progressive intolerance to solid foods vs. liquids. Other signs including dysphagia, halitosis, odynophagia, and weight loss are seen in chronic disease. The physical examination is mostly normal and may reveal weight loss.

Diagnostic investigation

Diagnosis begins with thoracic radiographs, which may show a soft tissue opacity (partially surrounded by air) within the oesophageal lumen. A barium contrast oesophagram will confirm a filling defect associated with the oesophageal mass (Fig. 11.9). Oesophagoscopy provides visualisation of the mass (sometimes associated with stricture) and permits acquisition of biopsy/brush cytological specimens, providing a definitive diagnosis (Fig. 11.10).

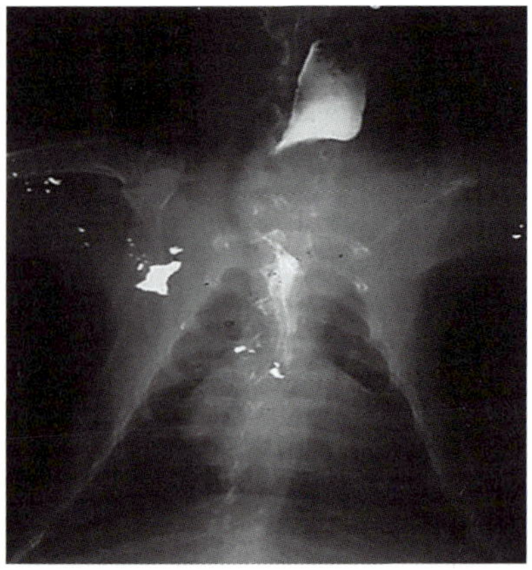

Figure 11.9. Barium contrast oesophagram (ventrodorsal projection) in a 9-year-old domestic shorthair cat. There is clear lateral deviation of the trachea and narrowing of the contrast bolus in the cranial oesophageal body. Miscellaneous metallic shrapnel is also present subcutaneously.

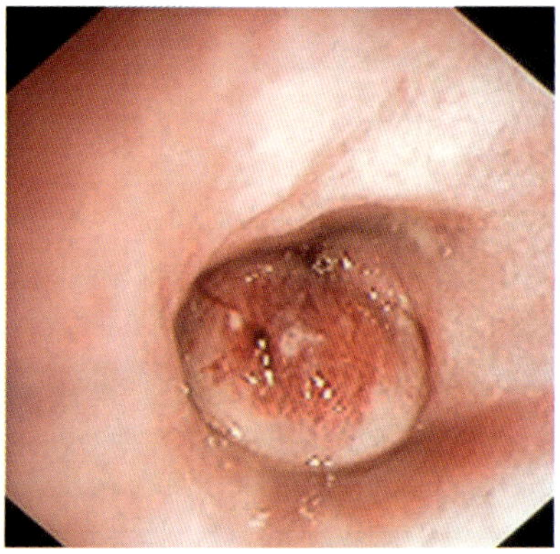

Figure 11.10. Endoscopic appearance of the large soft tissue mass seen in Figure 11.9, which occludes 90% of the oesophageal lumen. Brush cytology was consistent with a diagnosis of paraoesophageal lymphoma.

Management and treatment

Therapy for oesophageal tumours in cats is limited since the neoplasms have an insidious clinical course and disease burden is often advanced at diagnosis. Paraoesophageal lymphomas are often responsive to multidrug chemotherapy. Piroxicam may be used as palliative therapy in cats with primary oesophageal squamous cell carcinoma.[18]

Prognosis and outcome

The prognosis for cats with squamous cell carcinoma is poor. Cats with paraoesophageal lymphoma that respond to chemotherapy may survive for several months.

Take-home messages

- Oesophageal diseases are broadly classified as inflammatory, obstructive, or associated with dysmotility.
- Thoracic radiology (with or without contrast) and oesophagoscopy are important tools used to diagnose oesophageal disorders.
- The most common oesophageal diseases in the cat include oesophagitis, stricture, foreign body ingestion, and acquired dysmotility.
- Cats are uniquely susceptible to doxycycline-associated oesophagitis and oesophageal stricture.
- Oesophageal strictures are best managed by mechanical dilation using a balloon dilation catheter.
- Acquired myasthenia gravis may cause localised clinical signs of megaoesophagus and regurgitation with or without generalised weakness.

REFERENCES

[1] Sharp NJ. Feline dysautonomia. *Semin Vet Med Surg Small Anim* 5:67, 1990.

[2] Pera J, Palma D, Donovan TA. Eosinophilic esophagitis in a kitten. *J Am Anim Hosp Assoc* 53:214, 2017.

[3] German AJ et al. Oesophageal strictures in cats associated with doxycycline therapy. *J Feline Med Surg* 7:33, 2005.

[4] Garcia RS et al. Prevalence of gastroesophageal reflux in cats during anesthesia and effect of omeprazole on gastric pH. *J Vet Intern Med* 31:734, 2017.

[5] Marks SL et al. ACVIM consensus statement: support for rational administration of gastrointestinal protectants to dogs and cats. *J Vet Intern Med* 32:1823, 2018.

[6] Hague DW et al. Risk factors and outcomes in cats with acquired myasthenia gravis (2001–2012). *J Vet Intern Med* 29:1307, 2015.

[7] Shelton GD. Routine and specialized laboratory testing for the diagnosis of neuromuscular diseases in dogs and cats. *Vet Clin Pathol* 39:278, 2010.

[8] Moses L et al. Esophageal motility dysfunction in cats: a study of 44 cases. *J Am Anim Hosp Assoc* 36:309, 2000.

[9] Phillips H et al. Clinical findings, diagnostic test results, and treatment outcome in cats with hiatal hernia: 31 cases (1995–2018). *J Vet Intern Med* 33:1970, 2019.

[10] Durocher L, Johnson SE, Green E. Esophageal diverticulum associated with a trichobezoar in a cat. *J Am Anim Hosp Assoc* 45:142, 2009.

[11] Pratt CL, Reineke EL, Drobatz KJ. Sewing needle foreign body ingestion in dogs and cats: 65 cases (2000–2012). *J Am Vet Med Assoc* 245:302, 2014.

[12] Dollo V, Chambers G, Carothers M. Endoscopic retrieval of gastric and oesophageal foreign bodies in 52 cats. *J Small Anim Pract* 61:51, 2020.

[13] Deroy C et al. Removal of oesophageal foreign bodies: comparison between oesophagoscopy and oesophagotomy in 39 dogs. *J Small Anim Pract* 56:613, 2015.

[14] Tan DK et al. Prospective evaluation of an indwelling esophageal balloon dilatation feeding tube for treatment of benign esophageal strictures in dogs and cats. *J Vet Intern Med* 32:693, 2018.

[15] Lam N et al. Esophageal stenting for treatment of refractory benign esophageal strictures in dogs. *J Vet Intern Med* 27:1064, 2013.

[16] Leib MS et al. Endoscopic balloon dilation of benign esophageal strictures in dogs and cats. *J Vet Intern Med* 15:547, 2001.

[17] Bissett SA et al. Risk factors and outcome of bougienage for treatment of benign esophageal strictures in dogs and cats: 28 cases (1995–2004). *J Am Vet Med Assoc* 235:844, 2009.

[18] Berube D et al. Primary esophageal squamous cell carcinoma in a cat. *J Am Anim Hosp Assoc* 45:291, 2009.

CHAPTER 12

Pyloric diseases

Valérie Freiche, Fiona Da Riz

The pylorus acts as a valve in the distal part of the stomach and regulates the outflow of partially digested food from the stomach to the duodenum. It plays an essential role in mammalian digestion. In cats, the gastric wall is comprised of four layers, just like in all parts of the digestive tract: mucosal, submucosal, muscularis, and serosal layer. At the pylorus, the inner circular layer of the muscularis mucosae is ring-shaped and thickens to define the pyloric muscle (Fig. 12.1).[1,2]

Feline pyloric diseases are uncommon and remain poorly reported in the veterinary literature. Lesions affecting the pylorus may lead to marked gastric outflow obstruction and generate a clinical presentation primarily determined by acute and chronic vomiting according to different mechanisms: reduction or obstruction of the pyloric lumen potentially associated with mucosal lesions, or, less frequently, pyloric external compression by adjacent neoplasia or pancreatic

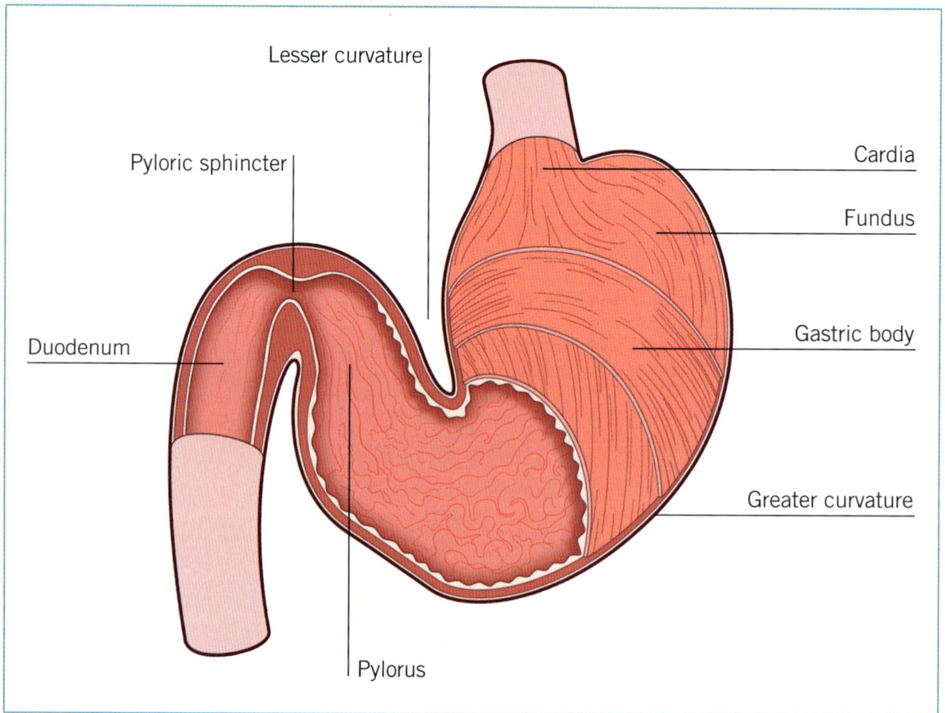

Figure 12.1. Anatomy of the feline stomach.

The authors express their grateful thanks to Dr Laurent Couturier, Centre de Vétérinaires Spécialistes AzurVet, Saint-Laurent du Var, France.

abscesses/pseudocysts. Pyloric diseases described in cats include:

- Congenital stenosis potentially associated with oesophageal dilation;[3–6]
- Acquired pyloric narrowing secondary to chronic inflammation;[1,7,8]
- Feline gastrointestinal eosinophilic sclerosing fibroplasia (FGESF);[10–13]
- Neoplasia: mainly intermediate- to high-grade lymphoma in this location (see Chapter 20), rarely smooth muscle tumours, and less likely carcinoma;[14]
- Benign adenomatous pyloroduodenal polyps[15,16] and hyperplastic gastritis;[17]
- Chronic hairball entrapment in the pylorus;
- Pyloric ulceration and perforation, mostly secondary to nonsteroidal anti-inflammatory drug (NSAID) administration.[18]

The aim of this chapter is to provide an overview of the different pyloric diseases in the cat and describe their diagnostic workup, highlighting the clinical and endoscopic findings, and approach to treatment.

EPIDEMIOLOGY AND AETIOLOGY

Epidemiology

Congenital pyloric stenosis—potentially associated with a megaoesophagus—has been described in young kittens. Siamese cats are overrepresented in the published studies.[3–6]

Acquired pyloric narrowing, pyloric perforation, and FGESF occur more frequently in adult cats. Considering the latter entity, a predominance of males was reported in a study conducted in 2014 describing 11 cases from Australia and 2 cases from the United Kingdom.[13] According to the authors of the study, FGESF can affect any breed (short-haired and long-haired), even if Ragdolls, Maine Coon, Maine Coon crossbreds, and Persians were regularly reported.[10,12,13,19] However, benign adenomatous pyloroduodenal polyps and pyloric neoplasia are reported in elderly cats. That said, some aggressive lymphoma cases can be diagnosed in young animals as well.

In addition, chronic hairballs can be detected in any adults, more frequently in medium- and long-haired cats.

Aetiopathogenesis

The aetiopathogenesis of many pyloric diseases is not yet totally elucidated. That said, any cause of pyloric narrowing may lead to acute to chronic hairball entrapment, even in short-haired cats.

Congenital pyloric stenosis

With regard to the association of pyloric and oesophageal dysfunction in cats, which was reported in a 1974 study,[3] the relationship between oesophageal and pyloric alterations is still unclear. An autonomic nervous dysfunction associated with a loss of the myenteric plexus of the gut has been suggested but was never definitively proven.

Acquired pyloric narrowing

The internal size of the pylorus can be challenging to assess. Despite being a sphincter with some degree of elasticity and contractility provided by the mucosal and muscularis layers, the pyloric lumen has limited dilation capacity. A recent retrospective study described 27 cats with chronic vomiting, in which the pylorus was abnormally narrow on visual inspection and could not be passed with an 8.6 mm endoscope, despite several attempts from an experienced endoscopist and in the absence of any other obstructive lesions.[8,9] In these cases, the pylorus appeared narrow and thickened and sometimes showed an extra mucosal fold (Fig. 12.2).

The reduction of pyloric diameter in these cases remains mild and therefore does not result in significant gastric distension or gastric retention, in contrast to cases of congenital pyloric stenosis, where pyloric obstruction and gastric retention syndrome are frequently seen.

Acquired mild pyloric narrowing may result from chronic changes in the mucosal and/or muscular layer characteristics, impairing the relaxing capacity of the pylorus. Histopathological analysis of pyloric biopsy samples in these cats suggests an underlying chronic inflammation. Further characterisation of the extent of fibrosis in such cases is currently under investigation at the authors' institution.

Feline gastrointestinal eosinophilic sclerosing fibroplasia

The aetiology of FGESF is still unknown. A strong antigenic stimulation has been hypothesised, suggesting a

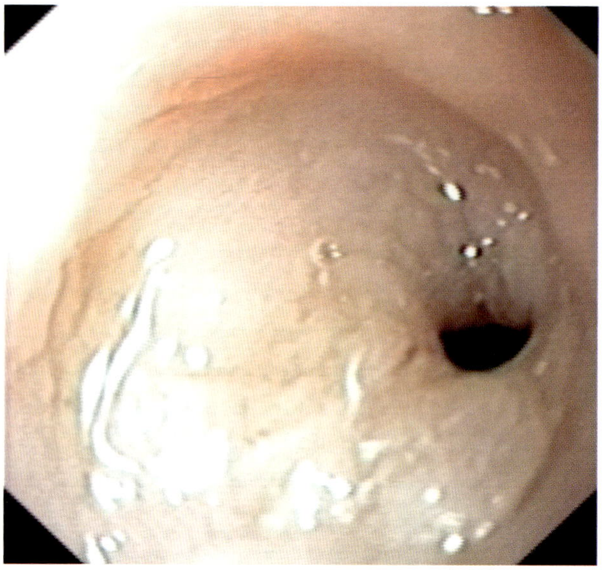

Figure 12.2. Endoscopic view of an acquired pyloric mucosal stenosis in a young female Oriental Shorthair cat presenting with chronic vomiting. The stomach was insufflated during the procedure. The mucosa is very abnormal, showing marked oedema and an irregular surface. The endoscopic view confirms the minimal diameter of both the pylorus and the pyloric canal.

genetic predisposition to develop eosinophilic inflammation in response to various antigens (e.g. bacteria, parasites).[13] Although bacteria were often identified in the mucosal lesions using a combination of cytology, histology, fluorescence in situ hybridisation (FISH), and tissue culture, it remains unclear if they are primarily invading the mucosa or if their role in the pathogenesis is secondary.[13] In fact, bacteria are only found in approximately half of the cases, and antibiotic treatment is not effective in all cases.[10,19]

More recently, other infectious agents have been identified, including nematodes (*Cylicospirura* spp.) in pumas and zygomycetes in a domestic cat.[10] Furthermore, the authors recently isolated *Rhizopus microsporus* from endoscopic biopsy specimens in a domestic shorthair cat diagnosed with FGESF.[12]

Neoplasia

Gastrointestinal (GI) lymphoma is overrepresented in cats (see Chapter 20). High-grade lymphoma and gastric adenocarcinoma have reportedly led to gastropyloric perforation in cats.[20,21]

Pyloric perforation

Local prostaglandin synthesis is inhibited by NSAIDs, leading to reduction of the prostaglandin-stimulated mucosal blood flow and mucous layer secretion.[21] According to some publications, the pyloroduodenal area is a particularly susceptible site for perforation in this context.[18]

HISTORY, PHYSICAL EXAMINATION, AND GASTROINTESTINAL LOCATION

History

The patient's history differs according to the cause of the pyloric disease. Main clinical signs reflect gastric outflow impairment. The most common clinical sign is therefore vomiting (frequently of food content), which can be acute to chronic. Other common clinical signs reported are anorexia or polyphagia, weight loss, or lack of weight gain. Excessive grooming has also been reported in cats diagnosed with FGESF.[13]

The history in these cases should therefore help to narrow the list of differential diagnoses: a congenital disorder should be suspected in a young kitten presenting with vomiting associated with lack of weight gain and polyphagia, while a neoplasia will be more likely in an elderly cat showing weight loss and anorexia.

Physical examination

Physical examination should be performed thoroughly. General activity, body condition score, mucous membrane colour, and capillary refill time should be noted. Assessment of the hydration status is always important in a vomiting cat. Careful abdominal palpation can help to detect any gastric dilation or intestinal/abdominal mass. In case of pyloric disease, abdominal palpation can be painful; however, the absence of pain should never lead to excluding this hypothesis.

Cardiopulmonary auscultation should also be performed in order to detect any cardiac murmurs which may prompt echocardiography if further investigations under general anaesthesia are planned. Furthermore, FGESF can sometimes also involve the thorax: pleural effusion and enlarged thoracic lymph nodes have recently been reported.[13]

DIAGNOSTIC INVESTIGATION

Differential diagnosis and diagnostic workup

As differential diagnoses of acute or chronic vomiting are numerous, these cases require a complete diagnostic workup. Metabolic diseases, hyperthyroidism, infectious processes, and inflammatory diseases may show the same clinical presentation and should be excluded first. Then, if a gastric and/or pyloric location are suspected, the most important investigations will include abdominal ultrasound and upper GI endoscopy. The diagnostic approach to pyloric diseases is detailed in the following paragraphs and illustrated in Figure 12.9.

Biochemistry and complete blood count

Haematology, biochemistry, and electrolyte panels represent an essential diagnostic step but may be nonspecific and nondiscriminatory.

Haematology

Haematologic changes can vary according to the disease context. In half of the FGESF cases reported, marked peripheral eosinophilia was noted.[10,11,19] Severe anaemia can sometimes be found in cats bleeding from benign adenomatous polyps.[16]

Biochemistry, electrolytes, and cobalamin

Modifications in biochemical parameters are highly variable depending on the underlying diagnosis. In cases of FGESF, hyperglobulinaemia is commonly detected. Both high serum total protein and hyperglobulinaemia were reported in a case series of FGESF, with the albumin:globulin ratio being less than 0.6 in 7/11 cases.[13]

Elevated serum urea concentration without elevation of creatinine serum concentration is consistent with GI bleeding, which can be found in various pyloric diseases, such as FGESF, ulcerated neoplasia, and benign adenomatous polyps, as well as in GI perforations.[13,16]

Cobalamin (vitamin B_{12}) serum concentration should also always be measured, as cobalamin is particularly important in cats, even if no distal intestinal lesion (e.g. in the ileum) is identified.

Radiography

Generally speaking, abdominal radiographs lack sensitivity in feline gastroenterology: their contribution to the diagnosis of pyloric diseases in cats is limited. In cases of congenital pyloric stenosis, radiographic findings reveal a gas- and fluid-distended stomach. Mineral opacities are suspicious for the persistence of ingesta in the stomach and could stem from gastric outflow obstruction.[6] Barium sulphate administration can reveal delayed gastric emptying.[5]

Thoracic radiographs may have a role in staging patients with neoplasia, although pulmonary metastasis of GI tumours is rare in veterinary patients. It can also be important in FGESF, as some of these cases have been found to also have thoracic lesions.[13]

Ultrasonography

Abdominal ultrasonography is an important step in the diagnostic workup. It allows the examination of the entire abdominal cavity and can help to detect any thickening of the intestinal or gastric wall as well as a loss of the normal layering of the intestine.

The dimensions and normal ultrasonographic features of the healthy feline pylorus have recently been reported.[2] The annular thickening of the muscularis layer is reported as a hypoechoic triangle in longitudinal section (Fig. 12.3).

Figure 12.3. Normal longitudinal ultrasonographic appearance of the feline pylorus. The muscularis layer is represented by a hypoechoic triangle (arrow). Image courtesy of Dr Laurent Couturier. Du, duodenum; PAn, pyloric antrum; PC, pyloric canal.

With regard to the stomach, chronic gastric outflow obstruction is characterised by severe fluid distension of the stomach and circumferential thickening of the pylorus.

Ultrasonographic differential diagnoses include:

- **Congenital pyloric stenosis.** Severe fluid distension of the stomach was reported in a 5-month-old kitten diagnosed with suspected congenital pyloric stenosis. Furthermore, a circumferentially thickened pyloric wall was noted.[6]
- **Acquired pyloric narrowing.** Thickening of the pyloric muscular layer may be documented in some cases, in addition to persistence of food in the stomach after prolonged fasting. However, in a small cohort of cats with suspected acquired pyloric narrowing, these ultrasonographic findings were not significantly different from those of cats with a normal pyloric diameter. In many cases of acquired pyloric narrowing, the ultrasonographic examination of the stomach is found to be normal.[9]
- **FGESF.** A focal thickening of the intestinal wall including a loss of wall stratification is generally identified on ultrasound. In addition, an isolated or multifocal abdominal lymphadenomegaly is generally seen in conjunction with the GI lesions. If there is no involvement of the pylorus, a gastric outflow obstruction may also result from the extent of the proximal duodenal lesions in cases of FGESF (Fig. 12.4).
- **Gastropyloric and duodenal neoplasia.** Although rare, high-grade lymphoma sometimes involves the pyloric sphincter. The ultrasonographic findings can be similar in cases of FGESF and high-grade lymphoma.

Fine needle aspiration (FNA) of the lesions can also be helpful, especially when neoplasia, FGESF, or polyps are suspected. If peritoneal effusion is present, FNA could also help to detect peritonitis secondary to perforation. Furthermore, chronic hairballs can be missed if food residues and gas within the gastric compartment impair the visualisation of the pyloric sphincter on ultrasound.

Gastrointestinal endoscopy

Endoscopic examination of the stomach is essential to assess all the stomach mucosa, including the antrum and pyloric area, as well as the proximal duodenal mucosa. Multiple intestinal samples for histopathological analysis should be obtained, as the macroscopic presentation may not reflect the histopathological diagnosis. Thus, a standardised procedure for upper GI endoscopy is recommended, such as the one described by the World Small Animal Veterinary Association (WSAVA) guidelines.[22] Premedication and anaesthesia should be chosen such that they do not interact with the lower oesophageal and pyloric sphincter tone.[23] Several premedication protocols (e.g. medetomidine and butorphanol) have been described and do not seem to affect the pyloric tone.[24]

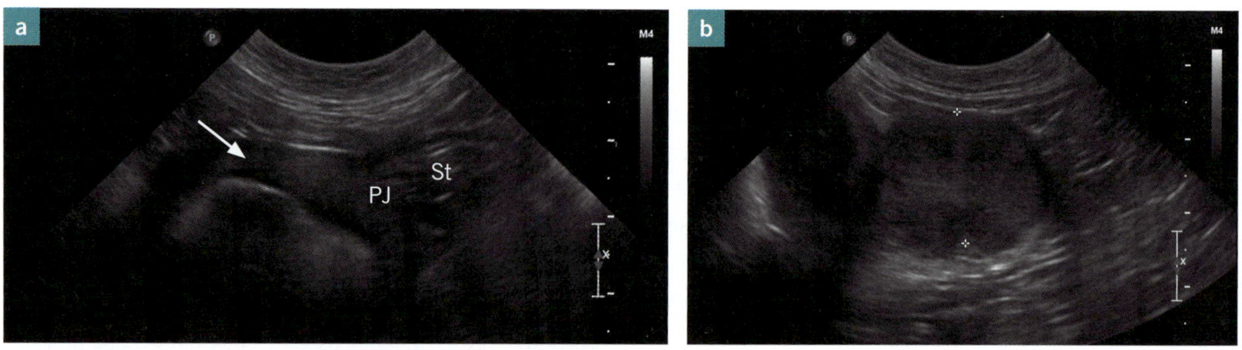

Figure 12.4. Ultrasonographic images of a 4.5-year-old neutered male Maine Coon cat presenting with marked anorexia and weight loss over the last 4 months. No vomiting was reported by the owners during the first 2 months. Upper gastrointestinal lesion of feline gastrointestinal eosinophilic sclerosing fibroplasia (a). The pyloroduodenal junction (PJ) is markedly abnormal and thickened. A loss of intestinal layering can also be noted, and the duodenal wall is thickened (arrow). Massively enlarged and hypoechoic pancreaticoduodenal lymph node (between callipers) (b). St, stomach.

Endoscopy can help detect lesions that may have been missed during ultrasonographic evaluation, such as trichobezoars, adenomatous polyps, erosions, or small ulcers, as well as diffuse mucosal infiltration (see Chapter 20).[16] After entering through the lower oesophageal sphincter (LOS), the first aim is to evaluate gastric contents, as any pyloric disease will likely impair gastric outflow. Any overinsufflation should be avoided in order to properly evaluate the mucosal surface. Next, the gastric mucosa is visualised. A retroflexion is needed to inspect the incisura angularis and the gastric part of the LOS. Then the endoscope is gently moved towards the antrum and the pyloric area. If the pylorus is normal, the pyloric sphincter is readily intubated with an 8.8 mm external diameter videoendoscope by an experienced endoscopist.[1,8] Until recently, the diagnosis of a suspected pyloric stenosis in cats was based on the association of clinical findings, radiographic and/or ultrasonographic findings, and endoscopic examination with exclusion of other causes by histological analysis of multiple biopsy specimens.[6] A recent study has now established an endoscopic method for semiquantitative measurement of the internal pyloric diameter in healthy cats. For this method, different biocompatible resin "olives" with diameters ranging from 4 to 12 mm were designed in order to measure the maximal internal pyloric diameter. The median internal pyloric diameter was 9 mm, with most cats being within ±1 mm of this measurement.[1]

An inability to intubate the pylorus should invoke the suspicion for pyloric stenosis with acquired lack of elasticity. Biopsy samples are required in the different areas of the stomach, pylorus, and duodenum. If the duodenum cannot be intubated, at least six duodenal biopsies should be obtained blindly by pyloric catheterisation using biopsy forceps.

Congenital pyloric stenosis

Upper endoscopy was performed on a 5-month-old kitten presenting with a congenital pyloric stenosis.[6] Endoscopic features included a dilated stomach and a shortened pyloric antrum. The diameter of the pylorus was estimated to measure 2 mm, which prompted the diagnosis of congenital pyloric stenosis.

Acquired pyloric stenosis

In the authors' experience, endoscopic examination of the pylorus in these cases usually reveals a loss of elasticity of the pyloric sphincter and reduced pyloric diameter, and sometimes hypertrophic mucosal folds. Usually the pyloric sphincter cannot be intubated. Acquired pyloric stenosis resulting from pyloric lack of elasticity may happen in cats with intestinal inflammatory diseases, such as chronic lymphoplasmacytic gastroduodenitis or small-cell lymphoma (Fig. 12.5). Any concurrent inflammatory process should be documented by both visual examination (ulcerations, oedema, erythema) and histopathological studies.

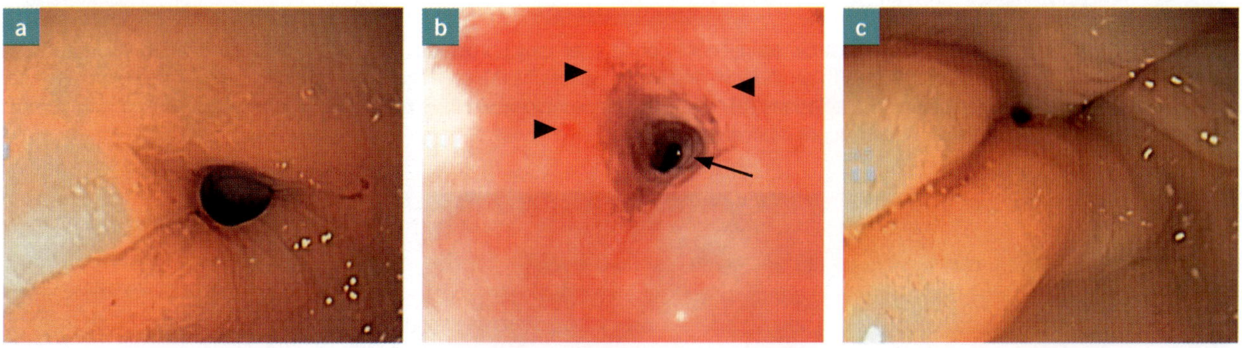

Figure 12.5. Upper intestinal endoscopy performed in a 7-year-old domestic shorthair cat presenting with chronic vomiting (a). The gastric cavity is properly inflated; however, the pyloric canal cannot be intubated by the 8.6 mm external diameter videogastroscope. Gastroduodenoscopy performed in a 6-year-old neutered male domestic shorthair cat suffering from acute vomiting in a context of chronic food-containing vomiting for 2 years (b). The macroscopic aspect of the antropyloric mucosa is considerably altered. Despite insufflation, the pyloric diameter is narrow (arrow), and erosions can be identified (arrowheads). Gastroscopy performed in a young cat referred for chronic delayed food vomiting (c). This pyloric close-up in normal conditions of insufflation shows persistent hypertrophic folds surrounding the pyloric sphincter. Multiple biopsy samples were performed and revealed a mixed inflammatory infiltrate associated with local fibrosis.

Feline gastrointestinal eosinophilic sclerosing fibroplasia

FGESF-related endoscopic lesions (Fig. 12.6) have recently been reported in five cases in which an ulcerated mass was observed in the stomach, which in most cases involved the pyloric wall and the proximal duodenum. FGESF has a characteristic appearance endoscopically with a dysplastic and proliferative macroscopic appearance: ulcerative lesions associated with FGESF usually display yellow-green discolouration.[12] Reexamination endoscopies were performed on two out of five cases and revealed a dramatic improvement of the lesions a few weeks after treatment initiation (antibiotics, corticosteroids 0.5–1 mg/kg/day, and cyclosporin 5 mg/kg/day).

Benign adenomatous polyps

Lesions can be located either in the antrum, in the pylorus itself, or in the proximal duodenum. If the pedicle is too extended, the polyp may enter the pyloric canal and completely obstruct gastric outflow (Fig. 12.7). Furthermore, compression of the major duodenal papilla by the polyp can also result in extrahepatic bile duct obstruction (EHBDO). As previously mentioned, despite being associated with a fairly good prognosis, polyps are also likely to lead to severe anaemia in elderly cats.

Foreign bodies: trichobezoars

Chronic hairballs are easily identified, entrapped through the pyloroduodenal junction; their extraction is possible with foreign body forceps (Fig. 12.8). The peripyloric mucosa should be evaluated for lesions after the foreign body removal, and biopsies are recommended.

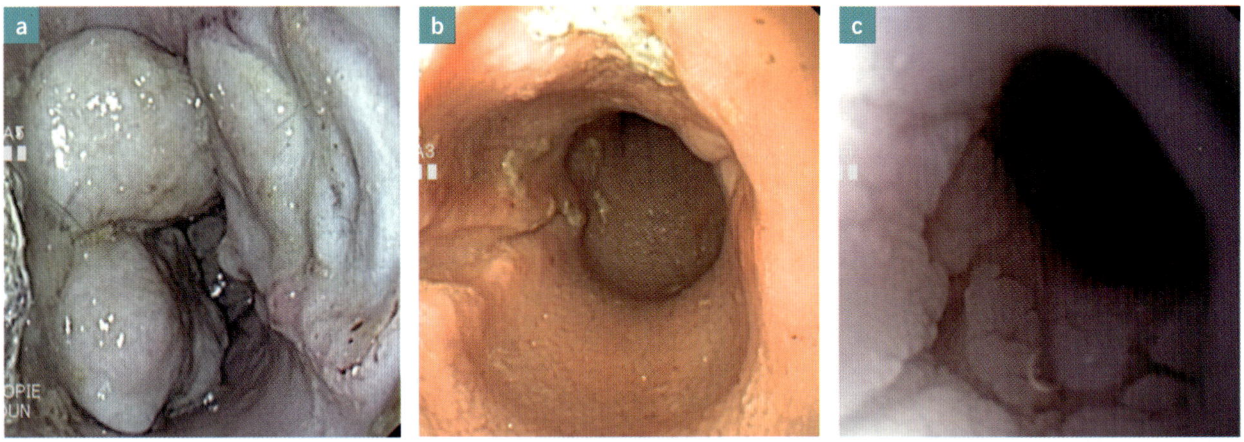

Figure 12.6. Endoscopic features of feline gastrointestinal eosinophilic sclerosing fibroplasia. In the cat previously reported in Figure 12.4, the pyloroduodenal area is abnormal, with both proliferative and ulcerative lesions (a); endoscopic reexamination performed 6 months after treatment shows a dramatic resolution of the lesions (b). Close-up endoscopic view of the pyloric canal in a cat presenting with chronic vomiting and weight loss (c). Note the significant mucosal irregularity.

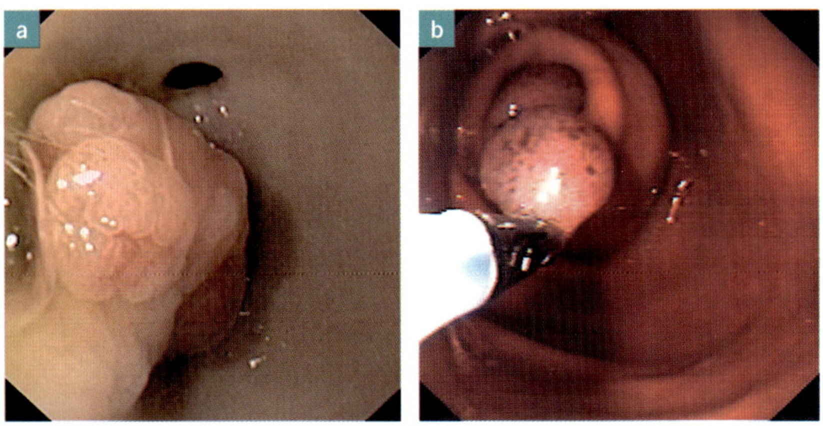

Figure 12.7. Endoscopic features of adenomatous antral polyps in elderly cats. A large polyp may be challenging to treat by endoscopic electrocoagulation due to the large size of its pedicle (a). Endoscopy performed in a cat presenting with prolonged postprandial vomiting, polyphagia, and weight loss (b). Gastric dilation was noted on previous abdominal radiographs. The endoscopic examination revealed a small polyp, which was completely inserted into the pyloric canal. A generalised gastric outflow obstruction was observed in this patient.

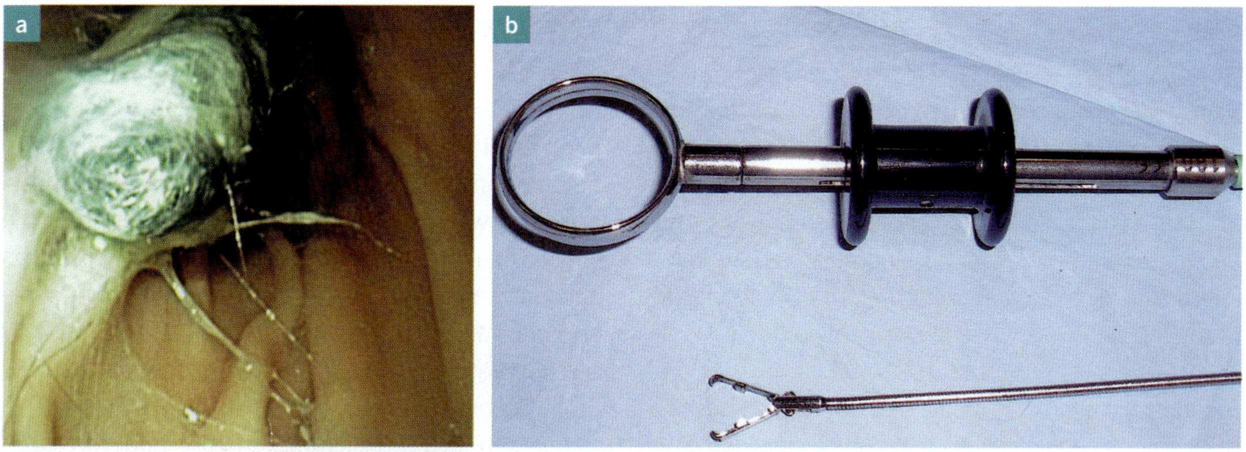

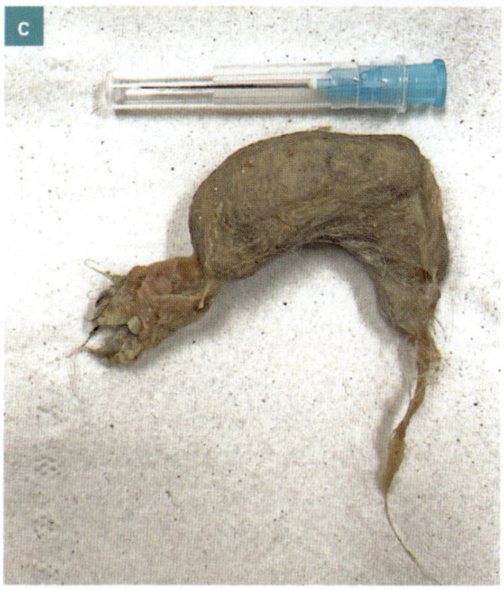

Figure 12.8. Hairball entrapment in a 5-year-old domestic shorthair cat presenting with chronic weight loss and chronic vomiting. Gastroscopy shows a huge hairball extending from the pyloric antrum to the proximal duodenum (a). Hairball extraction is performed during endoscopy using grasping forceps (b). Several attempts might be needed. Hairball aspect after removal (c).

Pyloric perforation resulting from nonsteroidal anti-inflammatory drug administration

Endoscopic examination is contraindicated when gastroduodenal perforation is suspected, since overinsufflation with air could generate a gastric tear and worsen the peritonitis.

Cytology and histology

Cytology

FNA for cytological evaluation is particularly indicated in cases of focal gastric or intestinal wall thickening with loss of layering, as well as in cases of significant (>5 mm) mesenteric lymphadenomegaly or in the presence of peritoneal effusion.

Cytology of GI masses aims at differentiating neoplastic conditions (particularly large-cell lymphoma) from inflammatory ones (particularly FGESF). Cytological characteristics of FGESF include large spindle cells, pink extracellular matrix, eosinophilic infiltrate, and neutrophilic components. Lymph node cytology may allow early detection of high-grade lymphoma. The probability of lymph node FNA leading to a diagnosis for high-grade lymphoma in the cat was reported to be 85.9% in one study.[25] However, 63% of false negatives were reported in cases of mesenteric lymph node T-cell neoplasms in cats,[26] which is likely due to the small-cell nature of these neoplasms. Cytology of peritoneal effusion is essential to rule out septic peritonitis (e.g. consequence of a perforated pyloroduodenal ulcer), neoplastic effusion, or feline infectious peritonitis.

Histology

Histology is an essential step of the diagnostic workup. Biopsy specimens should be placed in 10% neutral buffered formalin (pH 7.4) in preparation for histopathological analysis. Samples are processed by routine methods for histological examination, and sections need first to be stained with haematoxylin and eosin before being interpreted by a board-certified veterinary pathologist, according to the WSAVA recommendations.[22]

Amongst the previously mentioned pyloric diseases, the most challenging entities on histopathological diagnosis are the following:

- **Low-grade GI T-cell lymphoma** (see Chapter 20)**.** In this location, low-grade GI T-cell lymphoma is not frequent and is not likely to cause intestinal perforation. However, should it be present, it can be difficult to diagnose on histopathological examination because of the small-cell nature of this neoplasia and because of the common heterogeneous distribution of the neoplastic cells amongst the different areas of the biopsy samples.
- **FGESF.** The first descriptions of this disease confused it with extraskeletal osteosarcoma, sclerosing mast cell neoplasia, or fibrosarcoma.[13] In 2009, 25 cases were retrospectively analysed. Specific lesions included eosinophilic inflammation, trabeculae of dense collagen, and large reactive fibroblasts. The lesions were also characterised by marked infiltrates of eosinophils, masts cells, neutrophils, plasma cells, and lymphocytes.[19]

Fluorescence in situ hybridisation

FISH analysis is useful in order to identify mucosal-adherent or invading bacteria in some lesions, particularly when FGESF is suspected. A eubacterial probe is tested first; then, additional slides can be prepared for examination with specific probes to characterise bacteria such as *Escherichia coli* and clostridia species.

TREATMENT

Medical treatment

In cases of acquired pyloric stenosis, a combination of nutritional management, including feeding small meals preferably with wet and easily digestible food, and symptomatic treatments such as antiemetics, prokinetics, and anti-inflammatory doses of steroids can help to address an underlying chronic enteropathy and therefore may be effective to alleviate clinical signs and improve quality of life. Severe cases may require surgical correction.[8,9]

Cats with FGESF receiving immunomodulatory treatment have been shown to have a longer survival time than those receiving other treatments.[19] Antimicrobials may be necessary when microorganisms (bacteria or fungi) are found as well.

Conventional chemotherapy may be indicated in case of gastric lymphoma. Other types of pyloric tumours usually respond poorly to chemotherapeutic drugs.

Interventional endoscopic treatment

Interventional endoscopy is useful to treat benign adenomatous polyps when the pedicle is thin enough and if there is adequate visibility during endoscopy and to remove any foreign body entrapped though the pyloric sphincter. A coagulation profile should be performed prior to manipulation. Therapeutic endoscopy avoids surgery and allows for faster discharge from the hospital.

Surgical treatment

Surgical treatment indications are multiple in this context and depend on the aetiology of the disease. They include congenital pyloric stenosis, FGESF if the location of the lesion does not prevent surgical resection (e.g. unresectable ulcer, involvement of the major duodenal papilla), neoplasia if a subtotal gastric obstruction/compression is noted, benign adenomatous polyps, and pyloric perforation.

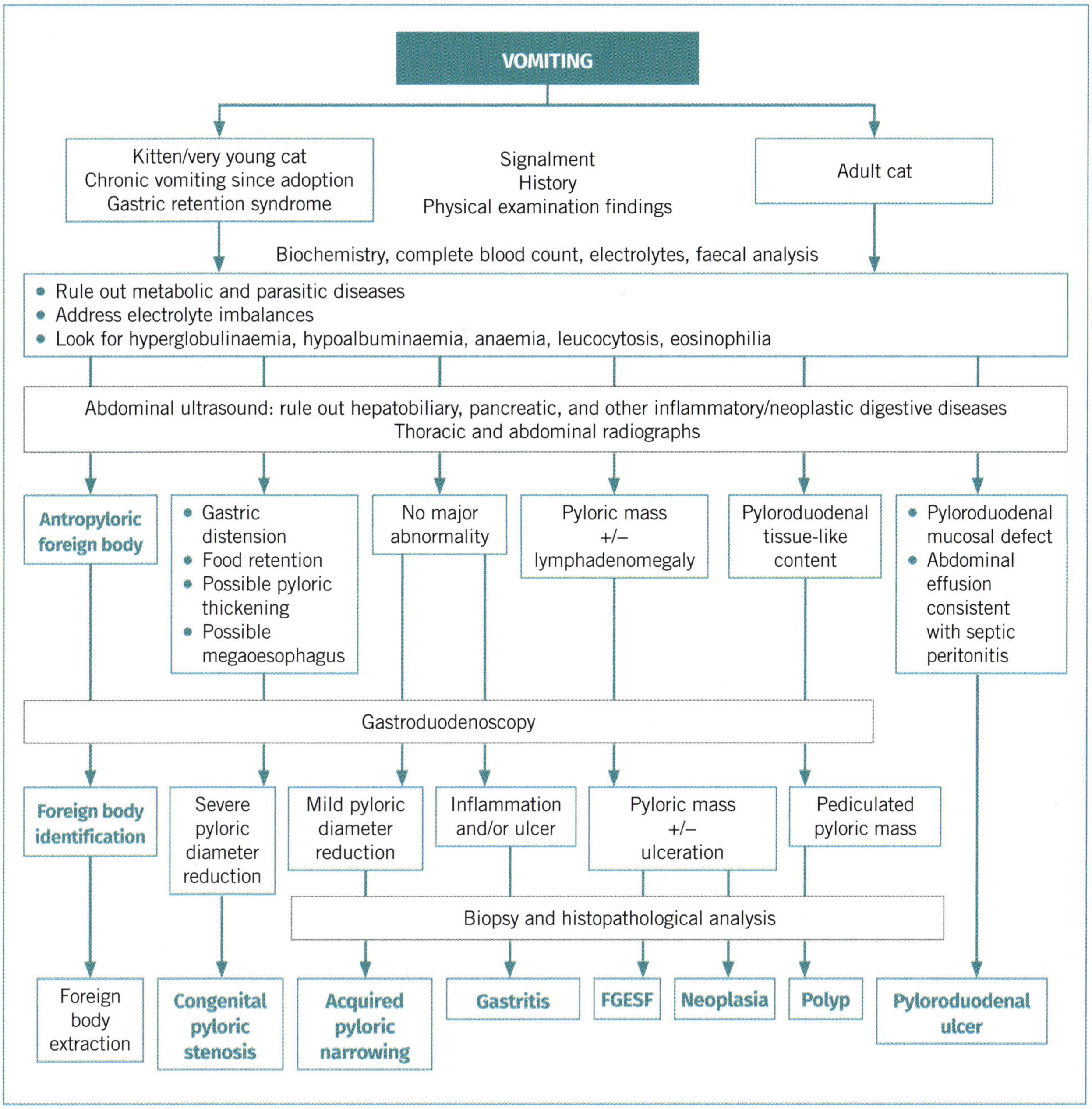

Figure 12.9. Diagnostic approach to pyloric diseases in cats with vomiting. FGESF, feline gastrointestinal eosinophilic sclerosing fibroplasia.

Adjuvant therapy

Nutritional management is an essential part of supportive care in feline pyloric diseases. As pyloric damage and/or dysfunction may impair food digestion, it is important to feed small amounts of easily digestible food frequently. GI or hypoallergenic diets are advised. Canned food is often associated with shorter transit time and may be better tolerated by some individuals.

PROGNOSIS

The prognosis is highly dependent on the underlying cause. Congenital pyloric stenosis carries a relatively good prognosis if surgical correction is performed, with good quality of life after surgical intervention. One exception is the occurrence of oesophageal dilation together with congenital pyloric stenosis, which was associated with a poor outcome in one study.[3]

The prognosis for cats with suspected acquired pyloric stenosis is fair to good with appropriate dietary and medical management. No published data are available on the median survival time of these cats; however, to the authors' knowledge, it is similar to that of cats with the underlying condition (often inflammatory bowel disease).[8,9]

FGESF is associated with a variable prognosis depending on the extent of lesions, the possibility of surgical resection, and the response to treatment. Cats responding to medical treatment or those being managed with a combination of surgery and medical treatment usually survive for several years after diagnosis.[13]

The prognosis for pyloric neoplasia is usually poor. Cats with intermediate- to high-grade lymphoma have a reported median survival time of 7–10 months if they respond to chemotherapy (35%–60%) (see Chapter 20). With other types of tumours, the prognosis varies depending on the possibility of complete surgical excision and metastatic spread.

Benign adenomatous pyloroduodenal polyps are usually associated with a good prognosis after either surgical or endoscopic excision of the polyps.

Pyloric ulceration can be a life-threatening condition if it results in septic peritonitis. One study reported a mortality rate of 71% after pyloric perforation in dogs and cats.[18] The prognosis is likely better for nonperforated ulcers with appropriate intensive medical care.

Take-home messages

- An important differential diagnosis for feline pyloric diseases is feline gastrointestinal eosinophilic sclerosing fibroplasia (FGESF).
- Other important differential diagnoses for feline pyloric diseases include acquired or congenital pyloric stenosis, neoplasia (mainly high-grade lymphoma concerning this localisation), benign pyloric and pyloroduodenal adenomatous polyps (rare), and foreign bodies.
- Clinical findings suggesting pyloric disease are compatible with a gastric retention syndrome and may include delayed vomiting of food, lethargy, diarrhoea, weight loss, anorexia, and excessive grooming.
- Ultrasonography is important to evaluate and measure the gastric and pyloric walls and their draining lymph nodes, even if some lesions may be missed (e.g. adenomatous polyps) or lead to misdiagnosis (e.g. FGESF may mimic neoplasia).
- Endoscopy is a key step in the investigation of pyloric diseases in cats to confirm diagnosis and allow sampling of the mucosa for histopathological analysis. Interventional endoscopy is needed to perform therapeutic measures (e.g. polyp extraction, foreign body removal).
- Treatment and prognosis depend on the aetiology and are therefore highly variable. When possible, surgery is the preferred treatment for some FGESF lesions, congenital pyloric stenosis, and adenomatous polyps. Diffuse lymphomatous intermediate- to high-grade lymphoma requires chemotherapy.

REFERENCES

[1] Lamoureux A et al. An endoscopic method for semi-quantitatively measuring internal pyloric diameter in healthy cats: a prospective study of 24 cases. *Res Vet Sci* 122:165, 2019.

[2] Couturier L et al. Ultrasonographic characterization of the feline cardia and pylorus in 34 healthy cats and three abnormal cats. *Vet Radiol Ultrasound* 53:342, 2012.

[3] Pearson H et al. Pyloric and oesophageal dysfunction in the cat. *J Small Anim Pract* 15:487, 1974.

[4] Twaddle AA. Congenital pyloric stenosis in two kittens corrected by pyloroplasty. *N Z Vet J* 19:26, 1971.

[5] Twaddle AA. Pyloric stenosis in three cats and its correction by pyloroplasty. *N Z Vet J* 18:15, 1970.

[6] Syrcle JA, Gambino JM, Kimberlin WW. Treatment of pyloric stenosis in a cat via pylorectomy and gastroduodenostomy (Billroth I procedure). *J Am Vet Med Assoc* 242:792, 2013.

[7] Leib MS et al. Endoscopic diagnosis of chronic hypertrophic pyloric gastropathy in dogs. *J Vet Intern Med* 7:335, 1993.

[8] Freiche V et al. Presumed acquired pyloric stenosis in cats: epidemiologic, clinical, histopathological and endoscopic data. A retrospective study of 34 cases. In: *Research Communications of the 26th ECVIM-CA Congress.* J Vet Intern Med 31:186, 2017.

[9] Freiche V et al. Endoscopic assessment of presumed acquired pyloric narrowing in cats: a retrospective study of 27 cases. *Res Vet Sci* 136:408, 2021.

[10] Grau-Roma L et al. A case of feline gastrointestinal eosinophilic sclerosing fibroplasia associated with phycomycetes. *J Comp Pathol* 151:318, 2014.

[11] Munday JS, Martinez AW, Soo M. A case of feline gastrointestinal eosinophilic sclerosing fibroplasia mimicking metastatic neoplasia. *N Z Vet J* 62:356, 2014.

[12] Tilmant CJMP et al. Endoscopic features of feline gastrointestinal eosinophilic sclerosing fibroplasia: a series of 4 cases. In: *Research Communications of the 30th ECVIM-CA Online Congress.* J Vet Intern Med 34:3058, 2020.

[13] Linton M et al. Feline gastrointestinal eosinophilic sclerosing fibroplasia: 13 cases and review of an emerging clinical entity. *J Feline Med Surg* 17:392, 2015.

[14] Hart K et al. A case of gastric leiomyosarcoma in a domestic shorthair cat. *JFMS Open Rep* 4:2055116918818912, 2018.

[15] Foy DS, Bach JF. Endoscopic polypectomy using endocautery in three dogs and one cat. *J Am Anim Hosp Assoc* 46:168, 2010.

[16] Daure E et al. Ultrasonographic and clinicopathological features of pyloroduodenal adenomatous polyps in cats. *J Feline Med Surg* 19:141, 2017.

[17] Barker EN et al. Hyperplastic and fibrosing gastropathy resembling Ménétrier disease in a cat. *JFMS Open Rep* 5:2055116919861248, 2019.

[18] Dayer T, Howard J, Spreng D. Septic peritonitis from pyloric and non-pyloric gastrointestinal perforation: prognostic factors in 44 dogs and 11 cats. *J Small Anim Pract* 54:625, 2013.

[19] Craig LE et al. Feline gastrointestinal eosinophilic sclerosing fibroplasia. *Vet Pathol* 46:63, 2009.

[20] Hinton LE et al. Spontaneous gastroduodenal perforation in 16 dogs and seven cats (1982–1999). *J Am Anim Hosp Assoc* 38:176, 2002.

[21] Bernardin F et al. Spontaneous gastrointestinal perforation in cats: a retrospective study of 13 cases. *J Feline Med Surg* 17:873, 2015.

[22] Washabau RJ et al. Endoscopic, biopsy, and histopathologic guidelines for the evaluation of gastrointestinal inflammation in companion animals. *J Vet Intern Med* 24:10, 2010.

[23] Smith AA et al. Evaluation of the effects of premedication on gastroduodenoscopy in cats. *J Am Vet Med Assoc* 225:540, 2004.

[24] Smith AL et al. Perioperative complications after full-thickness gastrointestinal surgery in cats with alimentary lymphoma. *Vet Surg* 40:849, 2011.

[25] Amores-Fuster I et al. The diagnostic utility of lymph node cytology samples in dogs and cats. *J Small Anim Pract* 56:125, 2015.

[26] Ku CK, Kass PH, Christopher MM. Cytologic–histologic concordance in the diagnosis of neoplasia in canine and feline lymph nodes: a retrospective study of 367 cases. *Vet Comp Oncol* 15:1206, 2017.

CHAPTER 13

Viral infections

Georgia Diakoudi, Vito Martella

Gastroenteritis is a common disease in domestic cats, particularly in young animals, cats with outdoor access, and cats living in shelters and other multianimal environments. Feline parvoviruses and feline coronaviruses are well-known viral agents of gastrointestinal (GI) disease in cats, but several other viruses have been detected in cats with enteritis including calicivirus, norovirus, rotavirus, astrovirus, and feline leukaemia virus. Over the last decade, next-generation sequencing and advances in metagenomic analysis have provided us with new insights into the faecal virome of cats, allowing the discovery of novel viruses for which the pathogenic potential remains to be elucidated (Table 13.1).

Table 13.1. List of viruses harboured in the intestinal tract of cats. Viruses for which vaccines are available are indicated.

Family	Genus	Species	Common name	Vaccination
Parvoviridae	*Protoparvovirus*	*Carnivore protoparvovirus 1*	Feline parvovirus	Core
		*Carnivore protoparvovirus 2**	Feline bufavirus	–
	Bocaparvovirus	*Carnivore bocaparvovirus 3* *Carnivore bocaparvovirus 4* *Carnivore bocaparvovirus 5*	Feline bocavirus	–
	Chaphamaparvovirus	*Feline chaphamaparvovirus*	Fechavirus	–
Coronaviridae	*Alphacoronavirus*	*Alphacoronavirus 1*	Feline coronavirus I	–
			Feline coronavirus II	Non-core
	Betacoronavirus	*SARS-related coronavirus*	SARS-CoV-2	–
Caliciviridae	*Norovirus*	–	Feline norovirus	–
	Vesivirus	*Feline calicivirus*	Feline calicivirus	Core
Astroviridae	*Mamastrovirus*	*Mamastrovirus 2* *Mamastrovirus* (unclassified)	Feline astrovirus	–
Reoviridae	*Rotavirus*	*Rotavirus A* *Rotavirus I*	Feline rotavirus	–
Picornaviridae	*Kobuvirus*	*Aichivirus A*	Feline kobuvirus	–
	Sakobuvirus	*Sakobuvirus A*	Feline sakobuvirus A	–
	Unclassified	Unclassified	Feline picornavirus	–
Circoviridae	Unclassified	Unclassified	Feline stool-associated circular virus	–
Polyomaviridae	Unclassified	Unclassified	Lyon-IARC polyomavirus	–

*Candidate novel species.

FELINE PARVOVIRUSES

Parvoviruses (family *Parvoviridae*) are small (23–28 nm), nonenveloped viruses with an icosahedral capsid. Their positive-sense, single-stranded DNA genome is of about 4–6 kb in length, with palindromic hairpin structures at the 5' and 3' ends that are essential for the replication of the virus. The *Parvoviridae* family is further divided into three subfamilies: *Densovirinae*, *Parvovirinae*, and *Hamaparvovirinae*. The subfamily *Parvovirinae* encloses the genera *Protoparvovirus* and *Bocaparvovirus*, which include well-described and novel parvoviruses detected in the feline intestinal tract (Table 13.1).

Feline parvovirus

Feline parvovirus (FPV)—genus *Protoparvovirus*—often referred to as feline panleucopenia virus, is currently classified within the species *Carnivore protoparvovirus 1*. The infection caused by FPV is the oldest known viral disease in cats.

The FPV genome (Fig. 13.1) contains two major open reading frames (ORFs) encoding the nonstructural proteins NS1 and NS2 and the structural proteins VP1 and VP2. Genetically, structurally, and antigenically, FPV is closely related to canine parvovirus type 2 (CPV-2), a virus that emerged suddenly in the late 1970s in dogs. CPV-2 likely evolved from FPV after cross-species transmission and adaptation in unknown wild carnivores that served as intermediate hosts. Shortly after its identification, CPV-2 started generating antigenic variants (i.e. CPV-2a, 2b, and 2c), which completely replaced the original CPV-2 type. Whilst the original antigenic type was not able to replicate in cats, the antigenic variants regained the ability to infect and replicate efficiently in cats, causing FPV-like disease. Panleucopenia in cats is caused in more than 90% of the cases by FPV, but in some studies nearly 80% of the cases of panleucopenia were due to CPV-2 variants. Mixed infections with FPV and CPV-2 variants have also been identified in cats.[1]

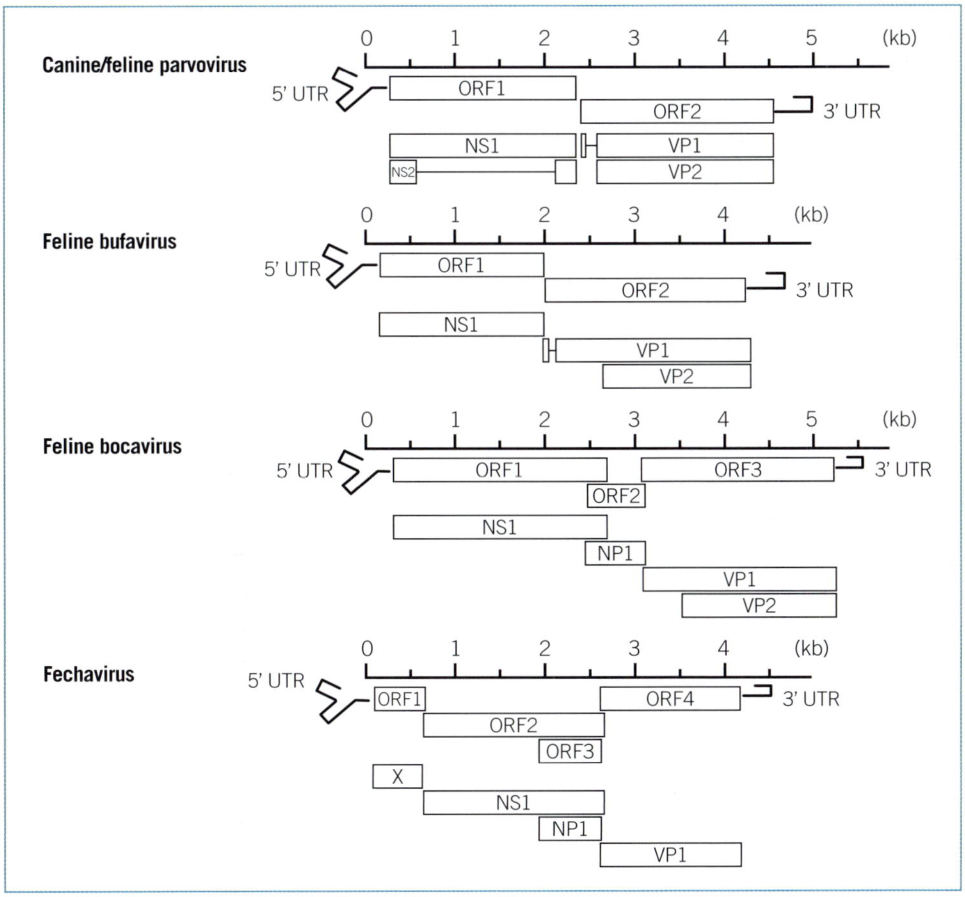

Figure 13.1. Genome organisation of different parvoviruses identified in cats. NP, nucleoprotein; NS, nonstructural protein; ORF, open reading frame; UTR, untranslated region; VP, viral protein.

FPV can infect and cause disease in all members of the family Felidae and some members of the families Mustelidae, Procyonidae, and Viverridae, including raccoons, minks, and ring-tailed cats. FPV is highly contagious and can be transmitted either directly, through the faecal–oral route by contact with faeces and body fluids of infected cats, or indirectly, through contaminated fomites or fleas. FPV is very stable in the environment and can survive for many months in organic material.

Shortly after (18–24 h) intranasal or oral infection, FPV replicates in the oropharyngeal lymphoid tissue and then spreads throughout the body by viraemia over the next 2–7 days. FPV has tropism for actively dividing cells, such as lymphoid tissue, bone marrow stem cells, and intestinal mucosa. As a result, FPV induces immunosuppression, severe leucopenia, and damages to the GI mucosa. The severity of the disease depends on several factors including age, immune status, and eventual coinfections with other pathogens.

In utero infection with FPV can lead to foetal death, abortion, and congenital abnormalities. In late prenatal and neonatal infection, the virus can replicate in various tissues and may cause cerebellar hypoplasia and ataxia in 2–3-week-old kittens. Other clinical signs of FPV infection in young and adult cats include high fever, lethargy, anorexia, vomiting, dehydration, and rapid weight loss. FPV is characterised by high morbidity and mortality rates. FPV-positive cats are usually prone to coinfection with other pathogens due to severe immunosuppression. Moreover, complications such as septicaemia, hypoglycaemia, haemorrhage, circulatory shock, and disseminated intravascular coagulation may be fatal.[1]

FPV infection is usually diagnosed based on signalment, history, clinical signs, complete blood count, serum biochemical testing, and a confirmatory test such as faecal antigen test, polymerase chain reaction (PCR), or virus isolation.

The most common abnormality in the blood smear or complete blood count is severe leucopenia with neutropenia and lymphopenia, observed in 65%–75% of FPV-infected cats. Thrombocytopenia and mild anaemia are described in 50%–55% of the cases.[2]

The most common abnormalities in serum biochemistry include hypoalbuminaemia, hypoglobulinaemia, hypocholesterolaemia, and electrolyte imbalance. In some cases, hyperglycaemia or hypoglycaemia as well as hyperbilirubinaemia or elevated aspartate aminotransferase (AST) or alanine aminotransferase (ALT) levels are present.[1,2]

Point-of-care immuno-based assays are commonly used in the diagnostics. DNA-based quantitative PCR (qPCR) assays are highly sensitive and specific.

Serology is used to assess maternally derived immunity and schedule vaccination. Haemagglutination inhibition is the standard method to detect antibodies against FPV.

Current vaccination guidelines worldwide include FPV in core vaccines. Both inactivated and attenuated live vaccines are available. Vaccine formulations with multiple antigens (i.e. FPV, feline calicivirus, and feline herpesvirus 1) are also available. Vaccines are usually administered starting at 6–8 weeks of age and then repeated every 3–4 weeks until 16 weeks of age. Vaccination against FPV generates a long-lasting humoral immunity, and it may also protect cats against CPV-2 infection. Despite the large adoption of vaccines worldwide, feline panleucopenia is still present in many countries.[2]

Since FPV is highly contagious, FPV-positive cats should be hospitalised and kept in quarantine for at least 2 weeks with strict hygienic measures. Symptomatic therapy along with appropriate nursing care can decrease mortality. Symptomatic therapy usually involves administration of broad-spectrum antibiotics for prevention of bacteraemia and sepsis, antiemetics combined with GI protectants and a highly digestible diet in cases of persisting vomiting, and intravenous fluid therapy to restore hydration and acid–base and electrolyte balance. Rarely, in cases of severe hypoproteinaemia and anaemia, fresh frozen plasma and whole blood transfusion might be required.[1]

Feline recombinant interferon omega and immune sera containing FPV antibodies are available. Both have been used in order to prevent infection in susceptible animals.

Feline bufavirus

In 2016, a novel protoparvovirus, similar to human bufaviruses and denominated canine bufavirus (CBuV), was identified in dogs with respiratory signs.[3] The virus was distantly related to FPV and CPV-2, sharing low nucleotide identities in the VP2 protein (less than 43%). CBuV was more common in juvenile dogs, and it was detected both in enteric and respiratory samples, but a possible association between respiratory signs and virus presence was observed.

By screening different collections of samples, bufavirus DNA was also detected in cats.[4] The virus was genetically similar (>99% at the nucleotide level) to CBuV. The feline bufavirus appeared as a common element of the feline virome, especially in juvenile cats, with an overall prevalence of 9.2%. The virus was more common in respiratory samples (9.5%–12.2%) than in enteric samples (2.2%).

Feline bocaviruses

Bocaviruses (genus *Bocaparvovirus*) possess an additional ORF between the nonstructural and the structural-coding regions of their genome that encodes the NP1 protein, a highly phosphorylated protein. Based on the current guidelines of the International Committee on Taxonomy of Viruses (ICTV), the genus *Bocaparvovirus* is classified into 21 species, with six species detected in carnivores: *Carnivore bocaparvovirus 1–6*. The feline bocaviruses (FBoVs) detected thus far have been classified in three species: *Carnivore bocaparvovirus 3–5*.[5–7]

Bocaviruses have been identified in several mammals including humans and nonhuman primates, dogs, pigs, bats, California sea lions, minks, rats, pine martens, and cats. Bocaviruses are transmitted through the faecal–oral route and have been associated with respiratory and intestinal diseases in humans, hepatitis in dogs, and encephalomyelitis in pigs.

FBoV (FBoV-1) was first identified in faecal, nasal, urine, kidney, and blood samples from cats during a large surveillance study in asymptomatic stray cats in Hong Kong.[5] The FBoV genomes shared the highest nucleotide identity (≤59.7%) to the minute virus of canines, forming a new species: *Carnivore bocaparvovirus 3*. Subsequently, other FBoVs have been identified using metagenomic analysis. A type 2 FBoV (FBoV-2), strain POR1, was identified in the faeces of a healthy cat in Portugal. The virus shared up to 70% amino acid identity in the *NS1* gene with the Hong Kong FBoV strain, and it has been classified as *Carnivore bocaparvovirus 4*.[6] A type 3 FBoV (FBoV-3), strain FBD1, was detected in faeces of sheltered cats in California. Strain FBD1 had up to 76% amino acid similarity to the other FBoVs in the NS1 and VP1 proteins, and it has been classified as *Carnivore bocaparvovirus 5*.[7]

The pathogenic role of FBoVs in cats remains unclear. FBoVs have been reported in both healthy animals and in cats with enteritis in different countries. Thus far, all three FBoV types have been detected in cats with gastroenteritis and in most cases in coinfections with other enteric viruses. FBoV-1 has also been detected in cats with acute haemorrhagic enteritis coinfected with FPV. The virus was identified in several organs such as the intestine, lymphoid nodes, lungs, and brain. These findings suggest the possibility of FBoV viraemia, as documented in humans and other animals.

For diagnostics, specific PCR assays targeting the *NS1* genomic region of the FBoV-1[5] and FBoV-2[6] and the *VP1* genomic region of the FBoV-3 have been designed.[7] Even though isolation in cell cultures is possible for many human and animal bocaviruses, efforts to cultivate FBoVs in different cell lines have been unsuccessful.[5]

Feline chaphamaparvovirus

Between November 2018 and January 2019, an outbreak of feline vomiting and diarrhoea occurred in a multifacility animal shelter in British Columbia, Canada. The samples tested negative for common enteric viral and bacterial pathogens. Upon viral metagenomics and PCR, the genome of a novel parvovirus, named fechavirus, was identified in 8/17 affected cats.[8] The closest relative (nucleotide identity of 74.2% at the genome level) was a parvovirus recently reported in canine faeces and named cachavirus, of the recently proposed genus *Chaphamaparvovirus*. NS1 and VP1 protein identities to the canine chaphamaparvovirus were 65.5% and 68.8%, respectively. Epidemiological investigation of disease signs, time of onset, and transfers of affected cats between three facilities supported a possible role for this new parvovirus in the observed highly contagious feline diarrhoea and vomiting disease.[8]

FELINE CORONAVIRUSES

Feline coronavirus (FCoV)—family *Coronaviridae*—is a common enteric pathogen of cats that in some cases leads to a fatal immune-mediated disease known as feline infectious peritonitis (FIP). The disease was first described in the early 1960s, although the viral aetiology was confirmed in 1968.

FCoV (subfamily *Coronavirinae*, genus *Alphacoronavirus*, species *Alphacoronavirus 1*) is a spherical, pleomorphic, enveloped virus with characteristic club-like spikes projecting from its surface. Their positive-sense, single-stranded RNA genome is of about 29 kb in length, one of the largest of all known viruses, and has 11 putative ORFs (Fig. 13.2a). Approximately two-thirds (≈20 kb) of the FCoV genome comprises two overlapping ORFs, 1a and 1b, encoding the main nonstructural protein. These proteins are involved in the synthesis of the viral RNA and, in some cases, in the interactions with the host cell. The remaining genome (≈10 kb) contains nine ORFs encoding four structural proteins: spike (S), envelope (E), membrane (M), and nucleocapsid (N); and five accessory proteins: 3 a–c and 7 a–b. The 3' UTR contains RNA structures that are essential for viral replication and synthesis.[9,10]

The S glycoprotein is composed by dome shaped peplomers that give the crown-like appearance of the virus and is considered the most important in terms of virus pathogenesis. It is essential for viral attachment and cell tropism as well as activation of the antibody response and cell-mediated immunity in the host. The M and E structural proteins are smaller surface glycoproteins important for virus maturation and assembly. The E protein seems to be essential in viral fitness, as studies have shown that coronaviruses with inactivation or deletion of the E protein are less virulent or lethal. The N structural protein is the only one present in the helical nucleocapsid. Its main role is to bind and protect the viral RNA, and it seems to be essential for viral transcription.

Thus far, the specific functions of the accessory proteins are not fully understood. However, the 3c protein seems to be important for viral replication and pathogenesis and is considered a key determinant in the switch from feline enteric coronavirus (FECV) to FIP virus (FIPV).[9] The 7a accessory protein is a type I interferon that seems to interfere with the antiviral immune response of the host, thereby protecting the coronavirus, whilst the 7b accessory protein is a glycoprotein that seems to induce antibody response in FCoV-infected cats.

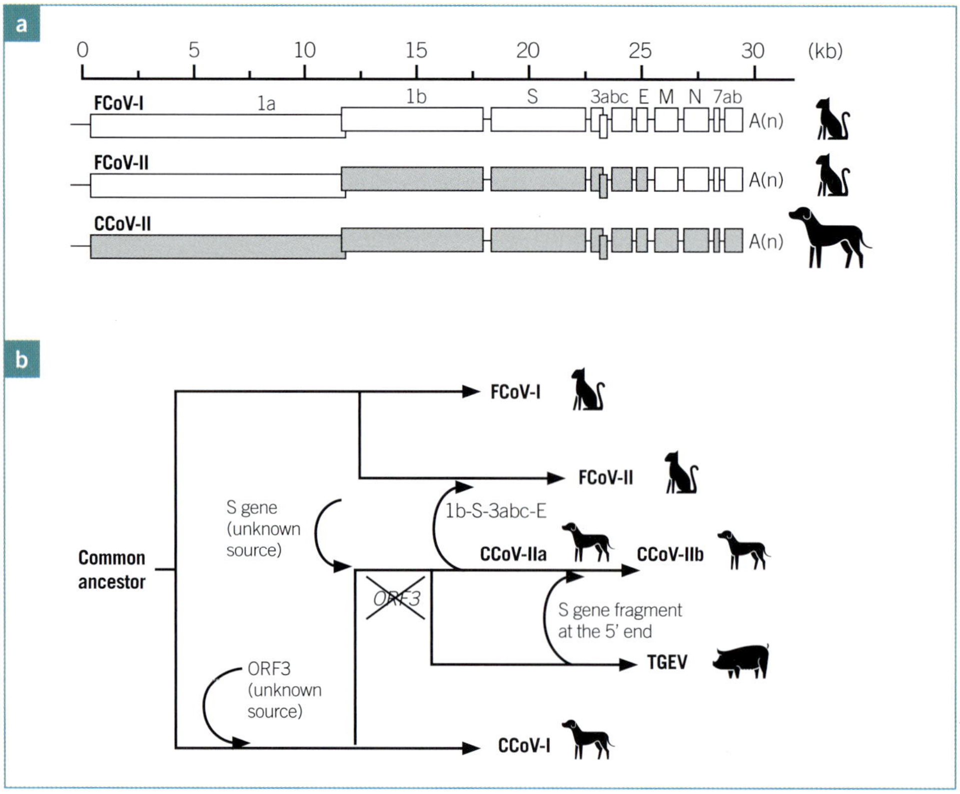

Figure 13.2. Evolution of alphacoronaviruses of cats and dogs. Feline coronavirus (FCoV) type II originated via recombination between FCoV-I and canine coronavirus (CCoV) type II (a). The evolution of alphacoronaviruses from domestic carnivores is the result of gain and loss of genes, recombination, and interspecies transmission (b). ORF, open reading frame; TGEV, transmissible gastroenteritis virus.

Two different FCoV genotypes have been identified: FCoV type I (FCoV-I) and FCoV type II (FCoV-II). The latter is the result of homologous recombination between FCoV-I and canine coronavirus (Fig. 13.2b). Most of the naturally occurring infections (80%–90%) in cats are caused by FCoV-I. Regardless of the genotype, FCoV exists as two different biotypes: the ubiquitous enteric biotype (FECV), which is usually asymptomatic, and the highly virulent biotype that causes FIP (FIPV). Cats can be infected by both FCoV-I and FCoV-II at the same time, and both genotypes are able to cause gastroenteric disease or fatal FIP.[9,10]

FCoVs and FIP-like disease have been reported in a variety of non-domestic felids, including cheetahs, wildcats, lynx, tigers, and lions, as well as in ferrets. FCoV is highly contagious, especially in multicat environments, and is usually transmitted indirectly through the faecal–oral route, mainly via litter trays. The virus can be successfully inactivated by most household detergents and disinfectants.[9,11]

FCoV-infected cats can either be asymptomatic or develop mild enteritis, but only a small percentage (5%) of cats with persistent FECV infection develop FIP. A major risk factor for developing FIP is age, as cats 3–16 months of age and older than 10 years are more prone to develop FIP. Breed and sex are also important risk factors, as Birman, Ragdoll, Bengal, Rex, Abyssinian, Himalayan, and British Shorthair breeds, as well as male cats, were found to be at higher risk of developing FIP. Other factors include genetics and host immune response, coinfection with feline leukaemia virus or feline immunodeficiency virus, and stress. After natural infection, cats start to shed the virus within the first week via faeces, and virus shedding may last from weeks to years (i.e. FECV carriers).[9,11]

The prevalence of the FECV biotype can reach 90%. FECV was thought to replicate only in the intestinal epithelium. Recently, FECV has been identified in blood monocytes and macrophages of cats with and without clinical signs. Instead, the FIPV biotype has a specific tropism for monocytes and macrophages, and it is believed to arise by mutations in the S protein or in the accessory genes, such as 3c.[9,10]

FIP can manifest as systemic serositis and vasculitis (effusive or wet form), as a multi-organ granulomatous disease (noneffusive or dry form), or as a combination of both.[11] These forms seem to be determined by the immune response of the cat. The wet form of FIP is often acute and characterised by thorax, pericardial, and abdominal effusions, which cause dyspnoea and/or abdominal distension.[9,11] In some cases, serositis can lead to scrotal enlargement. The dry form is more chronic and is usually associated with neurological, ocular, and/or dermatologic signs as well as nephromegaly. Occasionally, diffuse pyogranulomatous pneumonia as well as chronic diarrhoea and vomiting have been reported. Clinical signs of both effusive and noneffusive FIP involve fluctuating pyrexia, lethargy, anorexia, weight loss, generalised or regional lymphadenomegaly, and icterus.[11] Frequent clinical reexaminations of the affected cat are essential, as FIP clinical signs can change over time.[9]

Antemortem diagnosis of FIP is challenging since the most common clinical signs are not specific. Moreover, specific and sensitive assays are not available, and most tests cannot differentiate between FECV and FIPV. For this reason, diagnosis should be made based on a combination of signalment, history, clinical signs, and physical examination and laboratory findings.[11]

Haematologic abnormalities are frequent in cats with FIP. The most common alterations include anaemia, leucocytosis or leucopenia, microcytosis, lymphopenia, and thrombocytopenia. Serum biochemistry analysis might reveal hyperglobulinaemia, hypoalbuminaemia, electrolyte abnormalities, and elevated liver enzyme activities.[11] FIP-infected cats with neurological signs are more likely to have a cerebrospinal fluid with elevated protein content and pleocytosis. Part of the differential diagnosis is also the presence of idiopathic uveitis (i.e. ocular FIP).[10]

In the wet form of FIP, most of the cats show characteristic ascites and effusions. Ultrasonography and radiology might aid in the detection of effusions, and macroscopic and cytological examinations might contribute to the diagnosis of FIP. Several serological tests for identification of anti-FCoV antibodies with variable sensitivity and specificity are available, including indirect immunofluorescence antibody, virus neutralisation, ELISAs, and rapid immunochromatographic tests. The samples used for serological analysis are blood, effusions, and cerebrospinal fluid.

The gold standard for FIP diagnosis is immunohistochemical or immunofluorescence staining of intracellular FCoV antigens in samples of histopathological tissue lesions. Even though the differentiation between FECV and FIPV is not possible, positive antigen staining of macrophages in effusions confirms FIP infection.[10]

Moreover, highly sensitive reverse transcriptase (RT)-PCR and RT-qPCR assays can identify the presence of FCoV in biological samples including blood, effusions, faeces, saliva, cerebrospinal fluid, and tissues.

The development of vaccines against FIP has been complicated since vaccines might cause antibody-dependent disease enhancement, accelerating the virus uptake, and the development of FIP. An intranasal vaccine is available but not commonly used.[10] Supportive treatment with immunosuppressive drugs, like corticosteroids, and antivirals is used for reduction of inflammation and temporary remission of the disease.

No specific treatment is available, even though some novel drugs look promising. Thus far, the antiviral nucleoside analogue GS-441524 has been found to be safe and effective against FIP, even in cats with acute and neurological forms of the disease. Treatment with GS-441524 for at least 12 weeks lead to quick recovery and complete reversal of the FIP signs, even in cats with neurological signs when treated with higher doses. GS-441525 is similar to remdesevir (GS-5734), a molecule used for treatment of human patients with COVID-19, which is caused by a hypervirulent coronavirus. GS-5734 was also tested with good results in cats with FIP. Both GS-441524 and GS-5734 have not been licensed for animal use, as testing was interrupted out of fear that the cat research could impede the approval process for remdesivir in humans for treatment against Ebola virus. Illegal trading of GS-441524 has been reportedly increasing since the information on the existence of a lifesaving drug for cats with FIP started circulating the web.

Reduced transmission of disease can be achieved with proper hygiene (i.e. frequent cleaning of litter trays), by avoiding overcrowding in multicat environments, and with identification and removal of chronic shedders.

FELINE CALICIVIRUSES

Caliciviruses (family *Caliciviridae*) are currently classified into 11 genera. Caliciviruses can infect a wide variety of animals including mammals, birds, fish, and snakes.

Caliciviruses are small (30–35 nm), nonenveloped viruses with an icosahedral capsid. Their linear, positive-sense, single-stranded RNA genome is of about 7.4–8.3 kb in length, and it is covalently linked with a VPg protein at the 5' end, followed by two or three ORFs and a 3' UTR (Fig. 13.3). The virion RNA of caliciviruses is infectious, and its genome acts as an mRNA template. In cats, caliciviruses of two genera, *Vesivirus* and *Norovirus*, have been described.

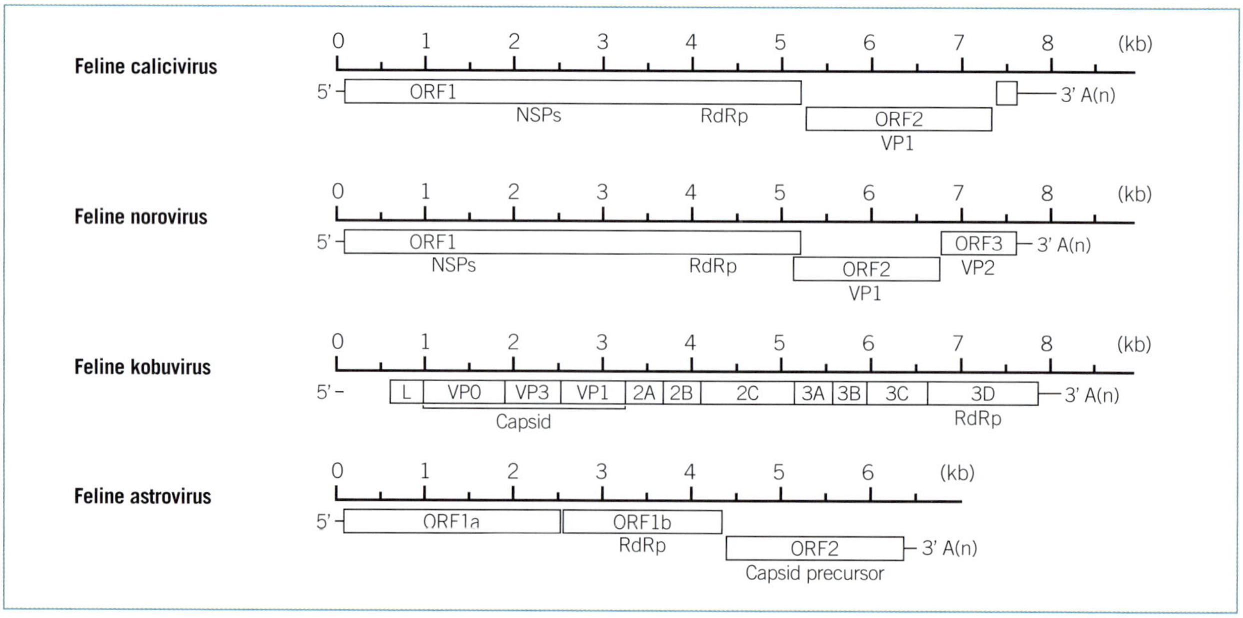

Figure 13.3. Genome organisation of calicivirus, norovirus, picornavirus (kobuvirus), and astrovirus identified in cats. NSP, nonstructural protein; ORF, open reading frame; RdRp, RNA-dependent RNA polymerase; VP, viral protein.

Feline norovirus

Noroviruses (NoVs)—genus *Norovirus*—are a major cause of acute gastroenteritis in children and adults worldwide. NoVs have been identified in a variety of mammals including cats, lions, dogs, cows, pigs, bats, sea lions, and harbour porpoises. Based on the ORF2, NoVs are currently classified into 10 genogroups (GI–GX) and 49 genotypes. NoVs belonging to genogroups GI, GII, GIV, GVIII, and GIX infect humans.

NoV (strain lion/Pistoia/387/06/ITA) was first identified in felids in 2006 in a 4-week-old lion cub that died of severe haemorrhagic enteritis at the zoo of Pistoia, Italy.[12] In 2007, a NoV (strain dog/Bari/170/07/ITA) was detected in a hospitalised 60-day-old mixed-breed puppy with diarrhoea and vomiting in Bari, Italy.[13] The canine virus shared 90.1% amino acid identity in the *VP1* genomic region with the strain lion/Pistoia/387/06/ITA (GIV.2 genotype). Subsequently, genetically similar and diverse canine NoV strains have been identified in dogs with and without gastroenteritis.

First evidence of NoV in cats was reported in a cat shelter in New York in 2012.[14] NoV RNA was identified in faecal samples from six 8-week-old cats with enteric symptoms. In the *VP1* genomic region, the feline NoV strain (CU081210E/2010/US) had 97.9% and 90.4% amino acid identity with the GIV.2 strain lion/Pistoia/387/06/ITA and the GIV.2 strain dog/Bari/170/07/ITA, respectively. Shortly after, feline NoVs were detected in a seemingly healthy cat in Japan (strain M49-1/2012/JPN)[15] and in a diarrhoeic cat in Italy (strain TE/77-13/ITA).[16] Sequence and phylogenetic analysis based on the ORF1 and ORF2 showed that both strains were more similar to canine GVI NoVs in the VP1 and highlighted a possible recombinant nature.

The pathogenesis of the feline NoVs remains to be determined. NoVs have been detected mainly in cats with signs of severe enteritis or vomiting,[16] but also in asymptomatic cats.[13,15] Moreover, in most cases feline NoVs were detected in cats coinfected with other enteric viruses.[16] Experimental infection with the GVI strain M49-1/2012/JPN in specific pathogen-free cats caused diarrhoea, and viral RNA was detected in the faeces and sera up to 56 days after infection.[15]

Diagnosis of feline NoVs can be achieved with RT-PCR assays using primers targeting highly conserved motifs of the RNA polymerase region. Since recombination is common within NoVs, virus characterisation should be based on both ORF1 and ORF2 regions. Seroepidemiologic studies have been performed using ELISA assays based on virus-like particles and have demonstrated that cats are largely exposed to NoV infection.

Feline calicivirus (*Vesivirus*)

The term "feline calicivirus" (FCV) usually refers to caliciviruses of the genus *Vesivirus*. FCV is a highly contagious pathogen and a common component of the feline virome.[17,18] FCV is considered strongly host-specific, as it infects only felids, even though FCV-like viruses have been reported in dogs with diarrhoea. The virus is shed in oral and nasal secretions of cats with acute infection, and shedding might last for months or years (long-term shedders). Cats are infected via the oral, nasal, and conjunctival routes, and the average prevalence of the virus in catteries and shelters reaches up to 40%, although there are reports of colonies with a FCV prevalence of up to 90%.[18]

After infection, the oropharynx is the first site of virus replication. After a few days transient viraemia occurs, and the virus can be detected in several tissues.[17] Many FCV-infected cats do not develop clinical signs. Clinical signs of acute FCV infection include fever, ulcers in the oral cavity, upper and lower respiratory tract disease—which might lead to pneumonia in some cases—chronic stomatitis, and limping syndrome.[18] The generalised and lethal forms of infection characterised by multi-organ involvement, subcutaneous oedema, and oral and cutaneous ulcers are referred to as virulent systemic disease (VSD). Overall, two distinct FCV phenotypes, respiratory and hypervirulent (i.e. VSD), are now commonly accepted by veterinary practitioners, animal care operators, and researchers/scientific literature.

Even though, FCV is mostly considered as an oral and respiratory disease, the virus was originally isolated from the GI tract of cats. FCV has also been hypothesised to have enteric tropism, as it has been identified and isolated from kittens with diarrhoea.

Using RT-PCR, the RNA of FCV was identified in 25.9% of stools of cats with enteritis and in no (0%) cats without diarrhoea or other clinical signs. Upon sequence analysis, the enteric viruses were found to be genetically heterogeneous and to differ amongst each other and from isolates of respiratory origin. The enteric isolates were found to be more resistant to low pH conditions, trypsin, and bile treatment than respiratory isolates. These findings are consistent with the hypothesis that some FCVs may acquire enteric tropism and eventually act as enteric pathogens.

Diagnosis of FCV is achieved by RT-PCR and RT-qPCR assays and virus isolation in feline cell lines. Detection of FCV antibodies can be achieved by ELISA and virus neutralisation assays. The FCV vaccine is considered a core vaccine for cats. Vaccination does not prevent infection or viral shedding and, in most cases, is challenged by virus antigenic variation. Treatment of FCV infection includes intensive nursing care and symptomatic therapy.[17,18]

OTHER FELINE ENTERIC VIRUSES

Feline astrovirus

Astroviruses (AstVs)—family *Astroviridae*—are small, nonenveloped, spherical viruses (28–30 nm in diameter) with a star-shaped structure. Their positive-sense, single-stranded RNA genome is of approximately 7 kb in length and comprises three ORFs: ORF1a (NS proteins), ORF1b (RdRp), and ORF2 (capsid protein) (Fig. 13.3). AstVs have been mostly associated with enteric infection in various mammalian and avian species. AstVs have been reported in cats, cheetahs, and tigers.

Feline astrovirus (FAstV) was first identified by electron microscopy in 1981 in a faecal sample from a domestic kitten with diarrhoea in the United States of America.[19] Since then, FAstVs have been detected in stool samples from cats all over the world, with a prevalence that ranges from 4.8% to 28.6%.[6,7] On molecular characterisation, FAstVs have been classified into the species *Mamastrovirus 2*. Sequence analysis based on the ORF2 of circulating FAstV strains has revealed distinct genetic clusters. Moreover, some FAstV strains were similar to AstVs of other animals like foxes, bats, and birds, indicating potential cross-species transmission of the virus.[6]

AstVs are transmitted through the faecal–oral route, and this could be a highly effective way of transmission in crowded cat environments (e.g. catteries, shelters).[7] The role of FAstVs as enteric pathogens in cats is not yet established. Experimental infection with FAstV in specific pathogen-free cats induced enteritis and viral shedding. FAstVs have also been reported in naturally infected cats with signs of diarrhoea or in cats coinfected with FPV.[19]

Feline rotaviruses

Rotaviruses (family *Reoviridae*, genus *Rotavirus*) are the leading viral cause of acute gastroenteritis in young children worldwide. Rotaviruses are currently classified into nine species (*Rotavirus A–J*) and have been recognised as important enteric pathogens in several mammals and birds. Their genome consists of 11 segments of double-stranded RNA that encodes six structural proteins (VP1–VP4, VP6, and VP7) and five or six NS proteins (NSP1–NSP5/NSP6). Rotaviruses of species A (RVAs) are common in humans and animals.

Antibodies for RVAs have been identified in cats.[20] Feline RVAs have been detected in faecal samples from both diarrhoeic and asymptomatic cats. Some of the studies have demonstrated an association between RVA infection and altered faecal quality (increased water content, altered stool conformation). Histological findings of RVA infection are swollen intestinal villi with mild infiltration by macrophages and neutrophils.[21]

Diagnosis was initially based on negative-stain electron microscopy and polyacrylamide gel electrophoresis. Currently, several RT-PCR and RT-qPCR methods have been developed. A *Rotavirus I* has been recently identified in the faeces of a diarrhoeic cat in North America.

Overall, feline RVAs rarely cause severe diarrhoea in cats and are not routinely screened in diarrhoeic cases. However, they have captured the attention since they are considered as causes of human disease. Human RVAs genetically homologous to feline RVAs have been detected worldwide, raising questions about the interspecies transmission and adaptation of rotaviruses as well as their zoonotic potential.

Feline picornaviruses

At least three different picornaviruses have been identified in cats. The first feline picornavirus (FePV) genome was described in 2012 from faecal and urine samples from stray cats in Hong Kong.[22] FePV is most closely related to members of the *Sapelovirus* genus and the unclassified bat picornavirus 3. Antibodies to FePV were detected in 33% of stray cats.

Subsequently, a feline kobuvirus (FeKoV)—genus *Kobuvirus*—was discovered in cats with diarrhoea in South Korea.[23] Kobuviruses (family *Picornaviridae*) are small, nonenveloped viruses with an icosahedral capsid. Their single-stranded, positive-sense RNA genome is 8.2–8.4 kb in length and encodes a VPg, which is attached to the 5' end of the genome, and a single polyprotein that is proteolytically processed to the mature polypeptides (Fig. 13.3). Kobuviruses have been identified in several mammals with or without diarrhoea. Based on their sequence similarities and genome organisation, the genus *Kobuvirus* is currently classified into six species: *Aichivirus A–F*.

Sequence analysis revealed that FeKoVs are mostly similar (82.1% nucleotide and 92.1% amino acid identities) to the canine kobuvirus strains.[23] FeKoV strains have been reported in faecal samples from both healthy and diarrhoeic cats in studies from Italy, China, and Korea. FeKoV strains are highly similar amongst each other and are currently classified into *Aichivirus A* species.

FeKoVs are shed in the faeces of infected animals and transmitted via the faecal–oral route. FeKoVs are more commonly detected in cats with diarrhoea rather than in asymptomatic cats. FeKoVs have been detected with a prevalence of 13.5%–28.8%, in most cases in cats coinfected with other enteric viruses. Kittens under 6 months old seem to be more susceptible to FeKoV infection.[23]

Detection of FeKoV can be achieved by RT-PCR using broadly reactive primers that target a highly conserved sequence within the *3D* genomic region, able to identify all members of the genus *Kobuvirus*. Even though isolation in cell cultures is possible for some kobuviruses, efforts to cultivate FeKoV in different cell lines have not been successful.

A third FePV was discovered in enteric samples (3.6%) from cats in Portugal.[6] The FePV was tentatively named feline sakobuvirus A (SakoV-A strain FFUP1). Over the entire polyprotein, the feline sakobuvirus A was slightly more related to members of the *Kobuvirus* genus (41%) than to members of the *Salivirus* genus (40%). The proposed name "Sakobuvirus" (Salivirus- and Kobuvirus-related virus) summarises the observed phylogenetic relationships.

EMERGING VIRUSES

Feline stool-associated circular virus

Circular replication-associated protein-encoding single-stranded (CRESS) DNA viruses are a type of single-stranded DNA viruses and are the smallest viruses that can infect animals. The major animal CRESS DNA viruses are circoviruses and cycloviruses, all of which belong to the family *Circoviridae*. Circoviruses and cycloviruses have been described in several insect, avian, and mammalian species, including carnivores. In dogs, circoviruses have been associated with clinical signs of severe haemorrhagic enteritis, vasculitis, and granulomatous lymphadenitis. Information about CRESS DNA viruses in cats is limited.[7,24] A cyclovirus was identified through metagenomic analysis in pooled faecal samples from healthy cats in a shelter in Davis, California.[7] More recently, a novel CRESS DNA virus, named feline stool-associated circular DNA virus (FeSCV), was detected in stool samples from diarrhoeic and healthy cats in a private cattery in Japan.[24] On phylogenetic analysis, the feline cyclovirus and FeSCV form distinct clusters within the *Circoviridae* family.

Lyon-IARC polyomavirus

Polyomaviruses (family *Polyomaviridae*) are nonenveloped, double-stranded DNA viruses of approximately 5 kb in length. Their natural hosts are primarily mammals and birds. Polyomaviruses are ubiquitous in the human population, and most of the infections occur early in life. Even though the majority of polyomavirus infections are asymptomatic, diseases are common amongst immunocompromised individuals (e.g. organ transplant recipients). Clinical signs of polyomavirus disease can vary based on the infected tissues, resulting in disorders such as brain disease, carcinoma, polyomavirus-associated nephropathy, and trichodysplasia spinulosa, a rare skin disease. Polyomaviruses have also been detected in faecal samples from both asymptomatic children and children with acute gastroenteritis, as well as in GI tissues of patients with malignant diseases.

In 2019, the genome of Lyon-IARC polyomavirus (LIPyV) was detected through metagenomics in 3/5 stool samples from cats with diarrhoea in Canada.[25] Coinfection with FPV was detected in only one of the samples. Sequence analysis indicated 97% nucleotide identity between the virus and reference human LIPyV genome. Originally, LIPyV was identified in human skin swabs, oral gargles, and one eyebrow hair sample from cancer-free patients. LIPyV shared the highest (≈65%) nucleotide identity with a polyomavirus identified in raccoons causing brain tumours.

Severe acute respiratory syndrome coronavirus 2

In December 2019, a novel severe acute respiratory syndrome coronavirus 2 (SARS-CoV-2) was identified in Wuhan, China, during an outbreak of pneumonia in humans. The disease was named COVID-19 (i.e. coronavirus disease 2019) and was declared a pandemic by the World Health Organization in March 2020. SARS-CoV-2 (family *Coronaviridae*) is classified into the subfamily *Orthocoronavirinae* and the *Betacoronavirus* genus and is genetically related to the original SARS-CoV-1. COVID-19 has been associated with mild to severe respiratory disease and death in humans, although nearly 90% of infections are asymptomatic.

Cats are susceptible to SARS-CoV-1, and SARS-CoV-2 has the same cell entry receptor as SARS-CoV-1: the angiotensin converting enzyme. Recently, cats have been found positive to SARS-CoV-2 on RT-PCR in Hong Kong, Belgium, France, Spain, Germany, United States of America, and Russia, mostly from households with infected human patients. Some animals were asymptomatic, some reportedly had dry coughs, and one cat showed severe clinical signs of diarrhoea, vomiting, and respiratory issues.[26] Serological investigation of cats in Wuhan demonstrated that the feline population had been exposed to SARS-CoV-2 during the outbreak.[27] SARS-CoV-2 has also been detected in tigers and lions in a New York zoo. The animals had dry cough and were likely infected by a presymptomatic caregiver.

Experimental infection of companion animals with SARS-CoV-2 revealed that cats are highly susceptible to COVID-19.[28] The experimentally infected cats had severe histological lesions in the nasal and tracheal mucosa epithelia and the lungs, while some of them died 3 days postinfection. Viral RNA was detected in several organs of the infected animals including tonsils, trachea, lungs, and small intestine as well as faecal samples, indicating that the virus can replicate efficiently in both the respiratory and digestive tracts.

Take-home messages

- Feline parvovirus is a major pathogen of cats that can induce immunosuppression, severe leucopenia, and damages to the gastrointestinal mucosa.
- Feline coronavirus exists as two different biotypes: the ubiquitous enteric biotype, which is asymptomatic or associated with mild enteritis, and the highly virulent biotype that causes a severe disease (feline infectious peritonitis).
- SARS-CoV-2, the coronavirus associated with COVID-19, has been detected repeatedly in cats with and without clinical signs and can infect cats experimentally.
- Other viruses have been associated with gastrointestinal disease in cats, including fechavirus, calicivirus (vesivirus, norovirus), astrovirus, and picornavirus (kobuvirus).

REFERENCES

[1] Barrs VR. Feline panleukopenia: a re-emergent disease. *Vet Clin North Am Small Anim Pract* 49:651, 2019.

[2] Kruse BD et al. Prognostic factors in cats with feline panleukopenia. *J Vet Intern Med* 24:1271, 2010.

[3] Martella V et al. Novel parvovirus related to primate bufaviruses in dogs. *Emerg Infect Dis* 24:1061, 2018.

[4] Diakoudi G et al. Identification of a novel parvovirus in domestic cats. *Vet Microbiol* 228:246, 2019.

[5] Lau SKP et al. Identification and characterization of bocaviruses in cats and dogs reveals a novel feline bocavirus and a novel genetic group of canine bocavirus. *J Gen Virol* 93:1573, 2012.

[6] Ng TF et al. Feline fecal virome reveals novel and prevalent enteric viruses. *Vet Microbiol* 171:102, 2014.

[7] Zhang W et al. Faecal virome of cats in an animal shelter. *J Gen Virol* 95:2553, 2014.

[8] Li Y et al. Virome of a feline outbreak of diarrhea and vomiting includes bocaviruses and a novel chapparvovirus. *Viruses* 12:506, 2020.

[9] Pedersen NC. A review of feline infectious peritonitis virus infection: 1963–2008. *J Feline Med Surg* 11:225, 2009.

[10] Kipar A, Meli ML. Feline infectious peritonitis: still an enigma? *Vet Pathol* 51:505, 2014.

[11] Addie D et al. Feline infectious peritonitis. ABCD guidelines on prevention and management. *J Feline Med Surg* 11:594, 2009.

[12] Martella V et al. Norovirus in captive lion cub (*Panthera leo*). *Emerg Infect Dis* 13:1071, 2007.

[13] Martella V et al. Detection and molecular characterization of a canine norovirus. *Emerg Infect Dis* 14:1306, 2008.

[14] Pinto P et al. Discovery and genomic characterization of noroviruses from a gastroenteritis outbreak in domestic cats in the US. *PLoS One* 7:e32739, 2012.

[15] Takano T et al. Molecular characterization and pathogenicity of a genogroup GVI feline norovirus. *Vet Microbiol* 178:201, 2015.

[16] Di Martino B et al. A novel feline norovirus in diarrheic cats. *Infect Genet Evol* 38:132, 2016.

[17] Radford AD et al. Feline calicivirus infection. ABCD guidelines on prevention and management. *J Feline Med Surg* 11:556, 2009.

[18] Pesavento PA, Chang KO, Parker JS. Molecular virology of feline calicivirus. *Vet Clin North Am Small Anim Pract* 38:775, 2008.

[19] Coyne KP et al. Lethal outbreak of disease associated with feline calicivirus infection in cats. *Vet Rec* 158:544, 2006.

[20] McNulty MS et al. Antibody to rotavirus in dogs and cats. *Vet Rec* 102:534, 1978.

[21] Greene CE. Feline enteric viral infections. In: Sykes JE, Greene CE, editors. *Infectious Diseases of the Dog and Cat*, 4th ed. St Louis, Elsevier Saunders: 80, 2012.

[22] Lau SK et al. Identification of a novel feline picornavirus from the domestic cat. *J Virol* 86:395, 2012.

[23] Chung JY et al. Detection and genetic characterization of feline kobuviruses. *Virus Genes* 47:559, 2013.

[24] Takano T et al. Novel single-stranded, circular DNA virus identified in cats in Japan. *Arch Virol* 163:3389, 2018.

[25] Fahsbender E et al. Lyon-IARC polyomavirus DNA in feces of diarrheic cats. *Microbiol Resour Announc* 8:e00550, 2019.

[26] Chini M. Coronavirus: Belgian cat infected by owner. *The Brussels Times*, Mar 2020 [accessed May 2020]. Available from: https://www.brusselstimes.com/news/belgium-all-news/103003/coronavirus-belgian-woman-infected-her-cat/

[27] Zhang Q et al. SARS-CoV-2 neutralizing serum antibodies in cats: a serological investigation. *bioRxiv*, 2020.

[28] Shi J et al. Susceptibility of ferrets, cats, dogs, and other domesticated animals to SARS-coronavirus 2. *Science* 368:1016, 2020.

CHAPTER 14

Bacterial infections

Conor O'Halloran, Danièlle Gunn-Moore

A number of bacterial species are potentially causative of, or contribute to, acute and chronic gastrointestinal (GI) disease in both kittens and adult cats. The UK Small Animal Veterinary Surveillance Network published data in 2019 suggesting that GI disease accounted for 2% of all instances that cats were presented to their general practitioners, representing thousands of animals across the period examined.[1] Although the prescription of systemic antimicrobials at initial examination declined from a recorded high of 40% in 2014, they were still prescribed to 25.7% of cats at the first consultation for GI signs in 2019.[1] This demonstrates that there is at least a perception that bacterial infection is a common cause of GI disease in domestic cats.

GENERAL PATHOGENESIS AND CLINICAL SIGNS

In most cases, for bacteria to cause diarrhoea, the following factors are required: the presence of the infectious agent (number of organisms, presence of virulence factors, etc.), host susceptibility (age, immune status, state of its GI tract, stress, etc.), and environmental pressure (housing conditions, stocking density, diet changes, antibiotics, recent surgery, etc.).

Subclinical carriage of a number of potentially pathogenic bacteria is common, especially in young animals. When disease is seen, it is most frequent in young animals (typically <6 months), especially if they are group housed, stressed (e.g. rescue or stray populations), or fed raw meat—which has become very popular in the United Kingdom, the United States of America, and Australia. The prevalence of infection may also vary depending on the geographical location, whether the cat is an indoor or outdoor animal, and whether or not it hunts and eats its prey. Episodes of disease may be seen in groups of kittens or cats and may be preceded by a stressful event such as environmental change, diet change, addition of new cats, or weaning.

Subclinical carriage means that potentially harmful organisms can be found in many apparently healthy animals. For example, depending on the population investigated and the method of testing, *Campylobacter* spp. (see below) can be found in up to 45% of cats, while *Salmonella* spp. (see below) are usually found in only 1%–2% of faecal samples from cats with diarrhoea. That said, one study found *Salmonella* spp. in 18% of samples from rescue kittens.

Some bacterial causes of diarrhoea are potentially zoonotic; therefore, when any animal presents with diarrhoea, owners should be given appropriate advice regarding hygiene and told to prevent contact between the affected animal and any immunocompromised individuals within the household.

CLOSTRIDIUM SPP.

Clostridium spp. are gram-positive anaerobic bacilli and include a number of pathogenic species including *Clostridium perfringens*, *Clostridioides* (*Clostridium*) *difficile* (*C. diff*), *Clostridium tetani*, and *Clostridium botulinum*.

C. perfringens and *C. diff* are considered common enteric pathogens of several animal species, including humans, although the pathogenesis and predisposing factors for disease differ between potential host species. Research investigating the significance of *C. perfringens* as a cause of significant enteric disease in veterinary medicine has expanded in recent years. *Clostridium* spp. can produce the highest number of toxins of any type of bacteria, and *C. perfringens* is both the largest toxin producer and the most widespread species, being found as part of the commensal microbiota of animals, including humans, as well as in soil. In their role as commensal organisms, these bacteria are involved in the deamination of amino acids, as well as in carbohydrate and amino acid fermentation.

Clostridial bacteria are classified according to the production of four major toxins: alpha (α), beta (β), epsilon (ε), and iota (ι). In addition to these toxins, they can also produce more than 15 other known toxin types, some of which act as additional virulence factors.

Epidemiology and aetiology

Clostridium spp. are geographically ubiquitous, as they are an abundant commensal organism of the feline GI tract and are also found in soil.[2]

The main cause of *C. perfringens*–associated disease is *C. perfringens* type A.[3] Prevalence studies offer differing estimates to the frequency of feline infections based on the geographical location, population studied, sample type examined, and laboratory techniques used; therefore, the prevalence of *C. perfringens* type A in the faeces of cats with diarrhoea varies between 20% and 80%. *C. perfringens* type F may also be a pathogen of cats; however, it has only very rarely been isolated from feline diarrhoeic faecal samples and has been identified at equal prevalence in the faeces of healthy cats.

Alpha toxin is the only toxin produced by all *C. perfringens* type A organisms. It can hydrolyse the phospholipids in the cell membranes of erythrocytes, leucocytes, epithelial cells, and endothelial cells, rendering it a haemolytic, cytotoxic, and endotoxic substance.[3] Overgrowth of this organism, particularly in the small intestine, leads to secretion of the alpha and other toxins, which have been shown to be fatal when purified and delivered intravenously to specific-pathogen-free laboratory mammals.

C. diff has not been established as a primary pathogen of cats. While human toxigenic *C. diff* strains have been frequently detected in rectal swabs of cats using the human ELISA for *C. diff* toxins, the performance of this assay has not been assessed for cats.

History and physical examination findings

Clinical history and physical examination findings for cats infected with *C. perfringens* or *C. diff* can be highly variable. Both organisms have been identified in the faeces of apparently healthy cats, making it unclear if this truly represents infection or if this is instead subclinical carriage, commensal colonisation, or transient shedding.

Clinical clostridial-associated diarrhoea is often described as large bowel in nature, having a watery faecal consistency, increased faecal mucus, increased defecation frequency, tenesmus, and haematochezia. Clinical signs are by no means pathognomonic, nor are they even suggestive of the genus over other pathogens, and a wide range of disease phenotypes have been attributed to the group, from mild self-limiting diarrhoea to rapidly fatal necrohaemorrhagic enteritis.

Diagnostic investigation

Faecal cytology

The microscopic detection of clostridial endospores in faecal smears has been used by some as a means of diagnosing *C. perfringens* infection. However, there is no evidence to indicate that this is an effective technique, as no studies have yet reported a correlation between the presence or number of spores and disease occurrence.

Faecal culture

Because of the high prevalence of *C. perfringens* in healthy cats, faecal culture is of limited utility. The most useful aspect of culture is often to rule out disease, because failure to isolate *C. perfringens* by a good diagnostic laboratory from a properly handled faecal sample indicates an extremely low likelihood of infection.

Endotoxin detection and molecular tests

The *C. perfringens* enterotoxin (CPE) can be identified using one of two immunoassays: a reverse passive latex agglutination assay (RPLAA) or an ELISA. However, neither test has been substantially investigated using feline samples. Both tests have reportedly low sensitivity and have been shown to yield positive results in samples from nondiarrhoeic cats. Whether or not this indicates poor test specificity or suggests that toxins can be present in the intestines (possibly at low levels) without inducing disease is unknown. This highlights the difficulties of interpreting such test results, which should therefore be considered suggestive of *Clostridium*-associated disease rather than definitive. Another important aspect to consider is that these tests only detect CPE and none of the many other *C. perfringens* toxins.

Faecal PCR tests (frequently available as multiplex panels) are offered by various diagnostic laboratories. However, as with culture, the high prevalence of *C. perfringens* and *C. diff* in healthy cats is a major limitation. Most commercial PCR assays target the alpha toxin gene. There are assays targeting less common toxin-encoding genes that are limited to more disease-causing strains, such as the CPE-encoding *cpe* gene, with potentially greater clinical relevance. However, there is inadequate evidence at this time to indicate that a single-species PCR test can be used diagnostically with confidence. These tests are often most useful as an adjunctive to other tests, with *cpe*-positive PCR results supporting a positive CPE ELISA or culture.

Coinfections of *C. perfringens* with other enteric pathogens, particularly feline coronavirus (FCoV), are common. One study analysing feline faecal samples using an eight-way multiplex PCR demonstrated that nearly two-thirds (62.5%) of test-positive faecal samples contained two or more species, and *C. perfringens* with FCoV was the most frequently documented two-way combination of coinfection.

In addition, particularly in cats, *Clostridiales* make up a large proportion of the healthy intestinal microbiome, especially in the large intestine. It is likely that in the coming years assessment of intestinal bacteria as an entire community or networks will become more of a diagnostic norm. This will likely be more informative regarding the significance of the presence of bacteria than traditional culture or PCR techniques (see Chapter 16).

Management and treatment

There is little evidence available to guide management or treatment decisions with respect to *C. perfringens*–related or *C. diff*–related disease. Specific therapy is only ever indicated in animals with chronic recalcitrant disease or acute cases with moderate to severe clinical signs. The usefulness of specific treatment (i.e. antibiotics) in mild diarrhoea due to *Clostridium* spp. is unknown, and it is difficult to assess given the difficulties in definitively diagnosing that diarrhoea is being caused by *C. perfringens* and the often self-limiting nature of the associated clinical signs. In accordance with good governance guidelines for the protection of antibiotic efficacy, antimicrobial agents are not required in these latter cases. Supportive treatment with probiotics, prebiotics, and/or an easily digested diet can be helpful.

Few studies have formally analysed the antimicrobial susceptibility profiles of cultured *C. perfringens* from cats (or dogs), but a recent study found isolates to be readily sensitive to amoxicillin–clavulanate, clindamycin, and erythromycin, with resistance to metronidazole and linezolid reported most frequently (4.6% and 5.5% of isolates, respectively).

Prognosis and outcome

The prognosis of infection is variable and related to the severity of clinical signs. In the majority of cases, disease is self-limiting and spontaneously resolves or else frequently responds well to supportive therapy (e.g. probiotics).

CAMPYLOBACTER SPP.

Campylobacter spp. are thin, gram-negative S-shaped or spiral rod-shaped bacilli.[4] *Campylobacter* spp. have the potential to be zoonotic causes of GI disease, albeit unlikely that they come from cats.[5] They can survive for weeks or even months in standing water and are an important cause of foodborne illness in humans, in particular when associated with poorly handled or underprepared poultry products.

Epidemiology and aetiology

More than a dozen *Campylobacter* species have been identified in the faeces of cats (and dogs), including animals with and without diarrhoea, being found in up to 58% of clinically healthy cats. *Campylobacter jejuni* is the most commonly cited as a causative agent of feline GI disease. The two *Campylobacter* species most frequently isolated from feline samples are *Campylobacter upsaliensis* and *Campylobacter helveticus*; however, there is not a clear association with disease, as they are often isolated at similar rates from healthy and diarrhoeic cats.[4] Young cats (<1 year old) have demonstrably higher carriage rates of *Campylobacter* spp. than older cats, although the clinical significance of this is unclear at the time of this writing.

History and physical examination findings

Campylobacter spp. colonise the jejunum, ileum, and colon but possess remarkably few virulence factors, meaning that the host immune response is the predominant deciding factor in the severity of clinical disease. Young kittens and immunocompromised cats are the most likely to be severely affected, with stress, overcrowding, and coinfection with other pathogens critical in contributing to clinical signs.

Diagnostic investigation

Routine haematology and serum biochemistry are frequently unremarkable or show only nonspecific changes. Animals with severe disease may show a neutrophilia or neutropenia with or without an increase in circulating band neutrophils (i.e. a left shift).

Microbiological assays include faecal microscopy, culture, and PCR testing.[5,6] Due to the high rates of carriage in healthy animals, the interpretation of positive test results is challenging. *Campylobacter* spp. can be grown on most routine bacteriological media, and selective media are available in most enteric panels that select for *Campylobacter* by using charcoal or blood-based agars that contain antimicrobials to eliminate contaminating bacteria. This gives culture excellent sensitivity and specificity. Similar accuracy can be achieved with PCR but more rapidly. Notably, a positive result from either technique does not necessarily imply that *Campylobacter* is the cause of any disease present.

Management and treatment

Uncomplicated cases are generally self-limiting and resolve with supportive therapy alone (e.g. probiotics, prebiotics, and/or an easily digested diet) or with extra fibre being added to the diet.[4,5] Even in the face of positive culture or PCR tests, targeted therapy may not be indicated and indeed may worsen the situation by causing further disruption to the gut microbiota. Antimicrobial treatment is only indicated for severely ill and/or immunocompromised cats or clinically unwell kittens. A macrolide such as erythromycin (10–20 mg/kg PO every 8 hours for 7 days) is usually effective. Enrofloxacin and metronidazole can induce drug resistance in *Campylobacter* spp. and should therefore be avoided.

Prognosis and outcome

The prognosis is generally considered good to excellent, depending on the severity of illness at presentation. Treatment failure may indicate resistance to the antibiotic used (see above) or infection with a nonpathogenic *Campylobacter* species in addition to an alternative cause. Recrudescence of infection following initial positive response has been documented occasionally in human patients.

SALMONELLA SPP.

Salmonella spp. are bacteria of significant importance to both animal and public health due to the zoonotic potential of the nontyphoidal serotypes, whose primary hosts are domestic and wild animals.[6] Humans usually become infected by eating poorly cooked contaminated food or via close direct or indirect contact with asymptomatic carriers or reservoirs.[6,7]

Epidemiology and aetiology

In pet cats (and dogs), the majority of reports of *Salmonella* infections are with serotypes of *Salmonella enterica* subsp. *enterica*, such as serovars *S. enterica* ser. Typhimurium, *S. enterica* ser. Dublin, and *S. enterica* ser. Enteritidis.[5] Major sources of infection are ingestion of faecally contaminated raw meat and offal, frequently by hunting wildlife reservoirs, particularly wild birds, leading to the condition known as "songbird fever" in cats.[6,7] The latter is particularly common when spring and winter birds arrive stressed at the end of their long migrations (i.e. March–April and September–November in the United Kingdom). In cats (and dogs), isolates belonging to *Salmonella enterica* group B serotypes are the most commonly isolated, being diagnosed in 69% of *Salmonella*-positive feline faecal samples. Since *Salmonella* spp. are not common commensals in cat faeces, when they are found, they are usually considered significant.

Diagnostic investigation

Diagnosis can be confirmed by isolation of the organism using selective culture protocols or detecting organism

DNA by PCR assays.[5] Genome sequencing is now routinely used in outbreak investigations to link cases of illness with similar bacteria and track them to the source.

Management and treatment

The treatment of clinical salmonellosis in cats (and dogs) depends on the severity of illness. Treatment is predominately supportive, including rehydration and replacement of lost electrolytes. In severe cases, plasma or blood transfusions may be necessary, as may parenteral feeding along with microenteral nutrition to support enterocyte healing in severe cases.[6]

The use of antibiotics for salmonellosis remains controversial. Although antibiotics often improve the clinical signs, their use can prolong the carrier state and, in some cases, may worsen the condition if the strain is resistant to the antibiotic used. There is also the risk of selecting for antibiotic resistance. Therefore, antibiotics should only be used if disease is considered severe (e.g. systemically unwell kittens, immunocompromised cats). In such cases, a faecal sample should be taken before treatment for diagnosis and antimicrobial susceptibility testing, even if treatment has to be started empirically before the result is available. Advocated empirical treatment currently includes combination therapy with amoxicillin (with or without clavulanic acid; 12.5 mg/kg PO every 12 hours) and a fluoroquinolone such as pradofloxacin (3–5 mg/kg PO every 24 hours) for 5–7 days. That said, the authors usually give amoxicillin–clavulanic acid pending the culture result, adding in pradofloxacin if salmonellosis is confirmed. The use of enrofloxacin should be avoided in all feline patients due to the risk of irreversible retinal toxicity, which has been reported in cats with apparently normal renal serum biochemistry even with short courses of treatment at low dose rates.

Because of the possibility of prolonged carriage, it is recommended that a further faecal sample is cultured after 2–3 weeks, and if positive, a third sample should be assessed. If there is very prolonged carriage, a long course of a suitable systemically active antibiotic to which the strain is sensitive could be considered on public health grounds in some circumstances, such as for hospice visiting cats or those owned by immunocompromised people. After such treatment, it is usual to test three further faecal samples 1–2 weeks apart to confirm successful clearance of infection.

Prognosis and outcome

The prognosis of infection is variable and related to the severity of clinical signs. In the majority of cases, the disease is self-limiting and spontaneously resolves; otherwise it frequently responds well to supportive therapy (e.g. probiotics, prebiotics, an easily digested diet). However, prognosis is guarded if the infection ascends the pancreatic duct and causes pancreatitis or if it ascends the common bile duct to the gallbladder and causes cholangitis and functional biliary stasis.

HELICOBACTER SPP.

Helicobacter spp. are gram-negative, spiral-shaped, mobile bacteria that colonise the GI tract of several mammalian and avian hosts. Although historically considered as pathogens of the stomach, there is a growing body of evidence that enteric forms of infection and disease also exist.

Epidemiology and aetiology

Various species of the genus *Helicobacter* have been isolated from the stomachs of cats, and mixed infections can be present, which sometimes complicate the diagnosis. These bacteria inhabit the mucosal lining of the stomach and can be found in the glandular cavities. The most common species found in cats are *H. felis* and *H. heilmannii*.[8] *H. pylori* has been isolated in the stomachs of cats and may potentially pose a zoonotic risk to humans, and vice versa; however, to date, this has only been assumed, not proven.[8]

A genetically novel helicobacter, *H. colefelis*, was isolated post-mortem from an 8-week-old domestic shorthair kitten that was euthanised due to severe diarrhoea. Histological examination of the intestine revealed a thick layer of bacteria that could not be cultured but that genetic analysis of the 16S ribosomal RNA gene sequence showed to be a distinct *Helicobacter* species, most closely related to *H. canis*. Just how pathogenic this new species is to cats is still debated. Attempts to induce diarrhoea by challenge with *H. colefelis* have so far failed, although cats do remain PCR positive.

Overall, subclinical infection with the aforementioned species of *Helicobacter* is suspected to be very common, whilst clinical signs can include vomiting, diarrhoea, anorexia, and lethargy, depending on which species and organ system are involved.

Diagnostic investigation

A number of diagnostic modalities exist including PCR of biopsy material (the preferred reference test), cytological examination of impression smears, histopathology of biopsy material, serological testing (which only indicates exposure and therefore is of limited clinical use), and culture of faecal samples or biopsy materials (although the sensitivity is very poor).[8]

For humans infected with *H. pylori*, the noninvasive test of choice is the urea breath test. *Helicobacter* spp. have high urease activity, and therefore when patients swallow urea labelled with an uncommon isotope, either radioactive carbon-14 or nonradioactive carbon-13, the subsequent detection of isotope-labelled carbon dioxide in exhaled breath indicates that urea was split; this indicates that urease, and hence *H. pylori*, is present. This technique has been used successfully in a research context examining 23 cats naturally infected with *H. heilmannii*.

Management and treatment

Various protocols exist for the attempted elimination of *Helicobacter*; however, bacteriological cure is difficult to achieve, and infection may last from months to years—in some cats, a lifetime. If treatment is deemed necessary, a 2–3-week course of omeprazole (1 mg/kg PO every 12 hours) with metronidazole (25 mg/kg PO every 12 hours) and clarithromycin (15 mg/kg PO every 12 hours), with or without amoxicillin (12.5 mg/kg PO every 12 hours), has been used most successfully.

Prognosis and outcome

The prognosis is generally considered to be favourable in all but the most severe cases.

ESCHERICHIA COLI

Escherichia coli is a pleomorphic, gram-negative, rod-shaped bacterium of the family *Enterobacteriaceae*. It is part of the normal gut microbiota; however, it can also be associated with enterocolitis when it has bacterial virulence factors or when the host has impaired local or systemic immunity.

Epidemiology and aetiology

There are more than 170 serovars of *E. coli* based on the identity of the bacterial O antigen (the external region of the bacterial wall lipopolysaccharide) and their flagellar (H) antigens (e.g. O157:H7). Disease-causing *E. coli* have been divided into characteristic pathovars, each of which is defined by a characteristic set of virulence factors that act in concert to result in the clinical, pathological, and epidemiological features of the disease. The seven pathovars described to date are: enteropathogenic (EPEC), enterotoxigenic (ETEC), enterohaemorrhagic (EHEC), necrotoxigenic (NTEC), enteroinvasive (EIEC), enteroaggregative (EAEC), and adherent–invasive (AIEC). The exact epidemiology of each of the pathovars in the context of companion animal species is not well understood. The bacterium normally resides in the intestines of most warm-blooded mammals, including cats, and is an opportunistic pathogen of the urogenital tract; only rarely does it cause significant GI disease. Normally, the presence of *E. coli* in the intestines is benign, and even beneficial, but in some kittens, it can cause severe disease.

Colibacillosis is most commonly seen in kittens in the first weeks of life and typically secondarily to the absence of adequate colostrum-derived antibodies. If a pregnant queen is infected with *E. coli*, the bacteria can invade the kittens' blood supply whilst in utero. Kittens can also acquire the infection during parturition or from feeding from their mother's inflamed mammary glands. Colibacillosis may lead to fatal septicaemia.

Diagnostic investigation

Care needs to be taken when submitting samples for microbiological culture, as false-positive results can occur when contaminated samples are submitted. When *E. coli* infection is suspected (e.g. if a queen has mastitis and a diarrhoeic kitten), selective MacConkey agar can be used. This may need to be specifically requested by clinicians (submission forms should be checked to see if this is standard or not), as it is not commonly included in the majority of faecal testing panels offered by most commercial laboratories due to the rarity of *E. coli* as a primary cause of diarrhoea in cats.

Management and treatment

Kittens with severe diarrhoea due to pathogenic *E. coli* require intravenous fluid therapy to counter fluid loss and electrolyte disturbances. It is important to monitor and treat for any resulting hypokalaemia. This bacterium usually has a broad sensitivity profile; therefore, amoxicillin is a good first-choice antibiotic (12.5 mg/kg PO every 12 hours). The use of antimicrobials to treat adult cats with diarrhoea and a positive *E. coli* culture is controversial due to the difficulties in convincingly discriminating pathogenic from commensal organisms on these tests.

Prognosis and outcome

The acute and severe nature of kitten colibacillosis, combined with the usual underlying immunodeficiency in these patients, can make this a very challenging condition to treat, and the prognosis is often guarded at best.

The possibility of zoonotic transmission and the emergence of multidrug-resistant strains of *E. coli* that may be shed by cats (and dogs) is a growing concern. A variety of drug resistance mechanisms have been identified, including efflux pumps and extended-spectrum beta-lactamase enzymes. There is emerging evidence that the strains shed by cats (and dogs), even when clinically healthy, can be shared amongst humans that reside in the same household, meaning that the transfer of plasmids carrying resistance genes between human and animal strains is possible even in the absence of zoonotic transmission per se. More studies are required to examine the frequency and clinical significance of this phenomenon for both human and animal health; in the meantime, this is further reason for the restricted use of antimicrobials in adult cats.

MYCOBACTERIUM SPP.

The genus *Mycobacterium* contains a number of species of nonmotile, acid-fast bacilli. They are most frequently classified into two categories: the *Mycobacterium tuberculosis* complex (MTBC) and the nontuberculous mycobacteria (NTM).[9] The MTBC are the group of mycobacteria which cause clinical tuberculosis; in cats, infection is usually due to either *M. bovis* (naturally found in cattle) or *M. microti* (naturally found in voles). These mycobacteria are considered to be obligate intracellular pathogens and represent a zoonotic risk to owners, although the risk is widely considered to be very low.[9]

NTM encompass all remaining mycobacteria. Not all of the NTM are inherently pathogenic and many are saprophytic species that may only represent opportunistic pathogens of cats. Groups of mycobacteria can be assigned to subsets of the NTM based on their laboratory growth characteristics. Rapidly growing mycobacteria (e.g. *M. smegmatis*) usually produce visible colonies on media growth plates in up to 7 days, whilst slow-growing mycobacteria (e.g. *M. avium*) typically require longer than 7 days to form visible colonies. The fastidious species are those that cannot—yet—be grown under laboratory conditions on synthetic growth media (e.g. *M. lepraemurium*).[10]

Epidemiology and aetiology

The incidence of mycobacterial infections in cats was estimated in the United Kingdom by a study published in 2013, which showed that 1% of all feline biopsy submissions demonstrated changes indicative of mycobacterial infection, and a third of those contained acid-fast organisms.[11]

An earlier study demonstrated a strong geographical distribution to the diagnoses of different mycobacterial infections within the United Kingdom. Infections with *M. microti* are the most frequently diagnosed in UK cats, comprising 19% of the submissions. These cases are predominately located throughout Scotland and the Scottish Borders as well as in urban areas such as London and South East England. The second most frequently diagnosed mycobacterial infection in UK cats is *M. bovis* (comprising 15% of submissions), and the incidence is highly associated with areas that have high rates of this infection in local cattle and wildlife populations; these areas include large parts of South West England and pockets across (South) Wales.[12]

Of the NTM, *M. avium* is cultured most frequently from cats in the United Kingdom. However, this may be skewed because it has similar growth characteristics to the MTBC mycobacteria and the culture system used in this study was that of the Animal and Plant Health Agency (APHA), Weybridge, which is optimised for the detection of *M. bovis* and therefore more likely to detect *M. avium* than other NTM. Feline infections with NTM species are most heavily associated with geographical locations in

North East England and the Midlands but have been sporadically reported all across the United Kingdom. Cats in Australia are much more frequently infected with other species of NTM such as *M. lepraemurium*.

Between 2018 and 2019, in the United Kingdom, there was an outbreak of GI tuberculosis in cats associated with the ingestion of a *M. bovis*–contaminated raw food product made from wild venison. This outbreak was important for a number of reasons; firstly, it led to cases appearing in geographical locations outside those outlined above, and secondly, since many of these cats were kept solely indoors, clinicians would not typically think of them being at risk for infection with *M. bovis*.[13]

History and physical examination findings

The most common clinical sign of mycobacterial infections in cats is a chronic nonhealing skin lesion or lesions which either do not or incompletely resolve with first-line antimicrobial agents such as amoxicillin or cefovecin (Fig. 14.1). A retrospective study found that 74% of feline mycobacterial infections present with dermatologic disease; many of these cases also had associated local lymphadenopathy.

GI tract pathology became an uncommon manifestation of mycobacterial disease in cats once pasteurisation of cow's milk became routine in many countries. Because the presumptive mechanism of infection in most cases of feline tuberculosis is via infected prey, many cats present with enlarged lymph nodes (e.g. retropharyngeal nodes). As granulomatous inflammation and/or granulomas then develop in the intestines, there is an impact on nutrient absorption, and therefore some cases will have intermittent or continuous diarrhoea.

GI mycobacteriosis is often a more clinically severe presentation than the cutaneous form, and cats are more likely to be generally unwell. The onset of clinical signs is gradual, and thus it is commonly more advanced by the time that cats are presented to the veterinary practice. Almost all cats are reported as being lethargic and hyporexic at presentation. On examination, weight loss is frequently notable and can be extremely severe; one case infected in the raw food–associated outbreak had lost 22.5% of its body weight over a 4-month period.[14]

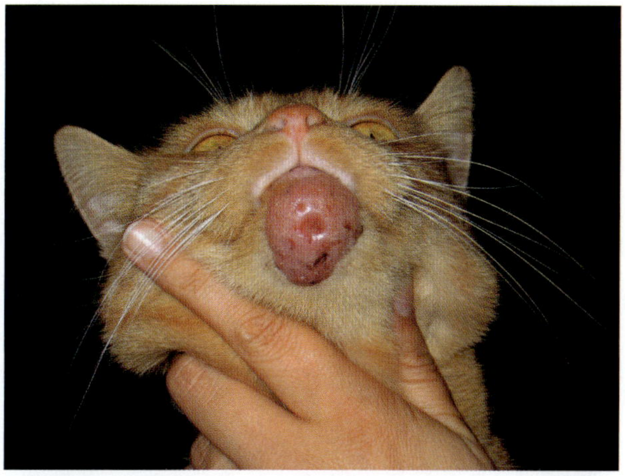

Figure 14.1. A cutaneous mass (granuloma) under the mandible of a 7-year-old neutered male domestic shorthair cat caused by infection with *Mycobacterium microti*. Image courtesy of Christoph Stork.

Diagnostic investigation

A diagnosis of mycobacteriosis can be challenging to achieve (Fig. 14.2). This is the case for a variety of reasons; however, several infectious agents can produce overlapping clinical signs, while different mycobacterial species carry different prognoses, optimal treatment choice, and zoonotic potential.

The exogenous retroviral status of cats should be established, as these viral infections are likely to be a poor prognostic indicator for any cat with mycobacteriosis. That said, positivity for feline immunodeficiency virus (FIV) and/or feline leukaemia virus (FeLV) has not been established as a predisposing factor for feline mycobacteriosis, as FIV and/or FeLV positivity is found in these cats at a similar prevalence to the national average for pet cats.

Radiography is useful for detecting systemic involvement, especially pulmonary dissemination, and for monitoring disease progression and treatment response (Fig. 14.3). While radiographic changes of mycobacterial infection are variable, pathology is most frequently seen in the thorax, typically consisting of a diffuse interstitial, alveolar, or bronchial pattern, with peribronchial and sternal lymph node involvement observed with increasing disease severity.[9] It is important to note that no pattern is pathognomonic for mycobacteriosis (e.g. it may also be consistent with a diagnosis of neoplasia or other infections, such as toxoplasmosis or infection with the lungworm *Aelurostrongylus abstrusus*) and that observed lung pathology can be mixed. Similar findings are seen with

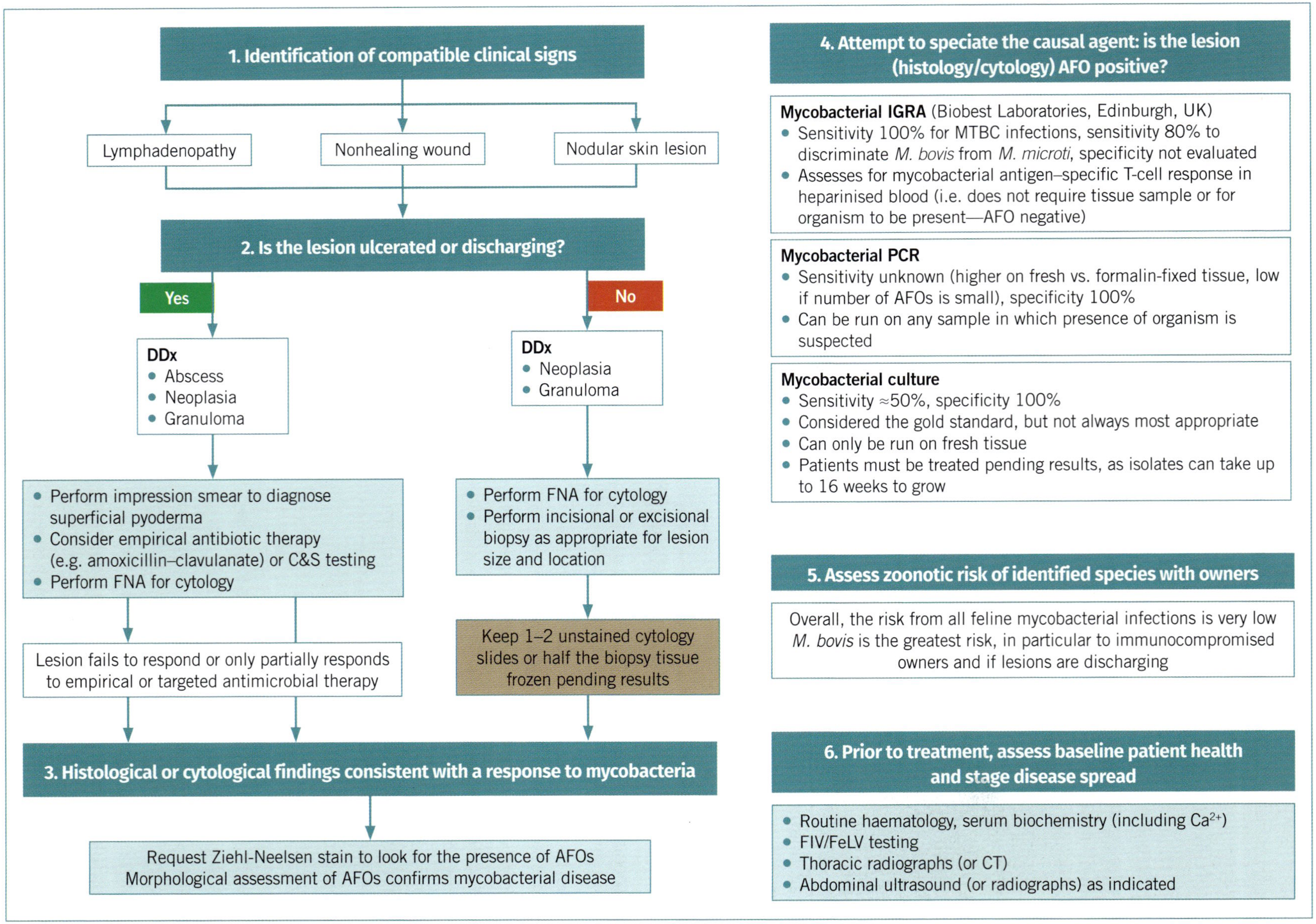

Figure 14.2. Diagnostic algorithm for suspected feline mycobacterial disease. AFO, acid-fast organism; C&S, culture and sensitivity; CT, computed tomography; DDx, differential diagnosis; FeLV, feline leukaemia virus; FIV, feline immunodeficiency virus; FNA, fine needle aspiration; IGRA, interferon gamma release assay; MTBC, *Mycobacterium tuberculosis* complex.

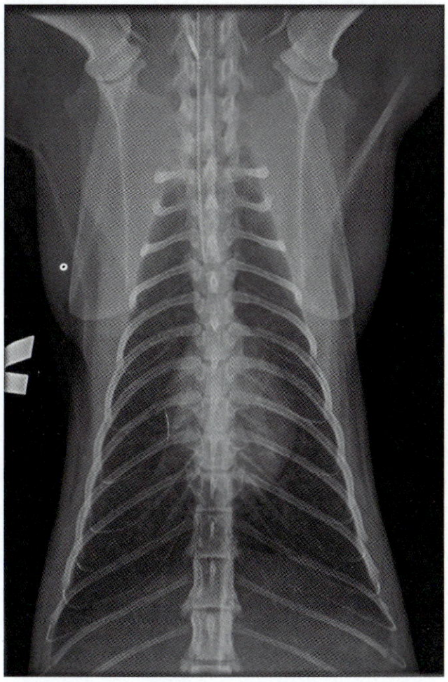

Figure 14.3. Dorsoventral thoracic radiograph of an adult neutered male cat infected with *Mycobacterium bovis*, showing typical diffuse changes throughout the lungs. Notably, the cat displayed no detectable respiratory abnormalities on clinical examination.

the use of computed tomography (CT) imaging, although the sensitivity of detection is increased with this modality. CT imaging can be done consciously in most patients using a Mousetrap as shown in Figure 14.4. If GI signs are present or if abdominal lymphadenomegaly is noted, abdominal ultrasonography can be extremely helpful to visualise and sample lesions.

Cytology can be very useful in the diagnosis of mycobacterial disease. Fine needle aspiration of the region of pathology, such as enlarged mesenteric lymph nodes, can be performed, and subsequent Romanowsky-type staining (e.g. Diff-Quik) may reveal the granulomatous to pyogranulomatous inflammation. In some samples, mycobacteria are detectable as negatively staining rods, or "ghost bacilli", within the cytoplasm of reactive macrophages (Fig. 14.5).[9]

Histopathology is frequently the mainstay of diagnostic investigation in these cases. Typical histopathological findings in most cats with mycobacteriosis include granulomatous inflammation with foamy, epithelioid, and/or palisading macrophages, occasionally with significant infiltration of lymphocytes distributed at the periphery of the granuloma. Ziehl-Neelsen staining may reveal highly variable numbers of mycobacteria.

The reference standard confirmatory test remains the isolation and speciation of mycobacteria following laboratory culture at a recognised reference laboratory. Although in the future molecular diagnostics will likely replace culture as the reference test, currently only a limited number of laboratories are able to offer PCR testing to provide a rapid, accurate diagnosis. The advantage of PCR is that it can be performed on fresh, frozen, or formalin-fixed paraffin-embedded tissue and Romanowsky-stained (but not Ziehl-Neelsen stained) cytology slides.

Matrix-assisted laser desorption/ionisation time-of-flight mass spectrometry (MALDI-TOF-MS) can identify bacterial organisms quickly and cheaply. Although primarily used for cultured samples, it is now being used directly on clinical samples in a limited number of laboratories around the world. The available spectral database for mycobacteria is steadily improving. Mycobacteria require prior inactivation and disruption of the mycolic acid–rich cell wall, both for biosafety reasons (in the case of the MTBC) and to liberate proteins within the cells. Success rates vary, but the differentiation between MTBC and NTM is usually very reliable.

The interferon gamma release assays (IGRAs) have been validated for use in cats. For the feline assay, peripheral blood mononuclear cells are isolated from heparinised peripheral blood samples obtained from cats with a high index of suspicion of mycobacterial disease (e.g. with clinical signs or histological findings indicative of mycobacterial infection). This test is currently commercially available only via Biobest Laboratories, Edinburgh, United Kingdom.

Management and treatment

Once the challenge of obtaining a diagnosis has been overcome (or while pending culture results, but based on clinical signs and histopathological findings), the next challenge for the clinician and owner is managing the mycobacterial infection. If treatment is to be attempted, it should be made clear from the outset that a prolonged course of multiantibiotic therapy is required to obtain a successful outcome, and success is dramatically influenced both by owner and patient compliance. Drug toxicity, particularly in feline cases, and the costs associated with medications and disease monitoring can make optimal regimes difficult to maintain.

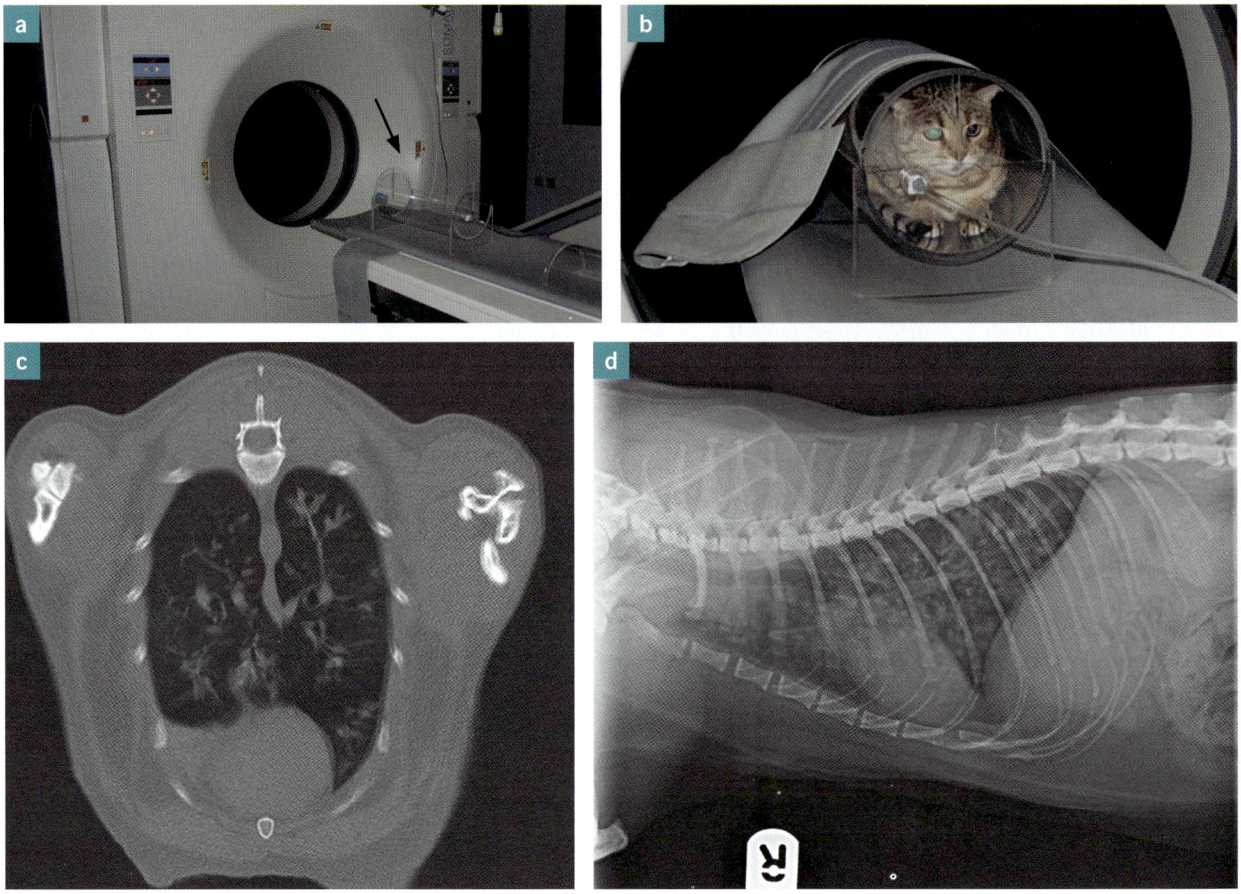

Figure 14.4. Feline patients can frequently be imaged consciously using a computed tomography (CT) Mousetrap to restrain them. This is a clear plastic cylinder (arrow) in which the cat can be placed and minimally restrained, with the lid secured with a strap and the tube supplemented with flow-by oxygen throughout the scan (a,b). In this example, the CT image (c) gives a much clearer image of the regions of pathology (caused by *Mycoplasma felis* infection), as compared to a laterolateral thoracic radiograph of the same cat (d). The radiograph shows a severe mixed bronchointerstitial nodular pattern with occasional areas of dystrophic mineralisation, while the CT image demonstrates a tree-in-bud pattern with occasional dystrophic mineralisation of the intraluminal contents, indicating chronic bronchiolar inflammation. Very similar changes can be seen caused by tuberculosis in cats; however, these images were used to demonstrate the advanced utility of CT when determining the exact nature of the pulmonary changes.

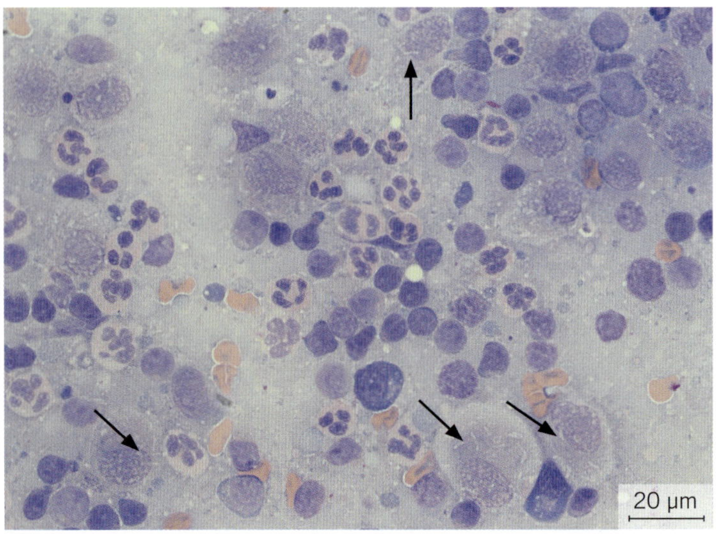

Figure 14.5. Cytological image of a Diff-Quick-stained fine needle aspiration sample obtained from the enlarged (pyogranulomatous) submandibular lymph node of a 4-year-old neutered female domestic shorthair cat infected with *Mycobacterium avium*. The arrows indicate mycobacteria which do not take up Romanowsky-type stains and thus appear as "ghost bacilli".

For single or small skin nodules, complete surgical resection may be curative. However, this cannot be guaranteed, and adjunctive medical therapy is usually indicated.

Standard first-line therapy (Table 14.1) comprises a fluoroquinolone, a macrolide/azalide, and rifampicin. The fluoroquinolone of choice is pradofloxacin (3–5 mg/kg PO every 24 hours) due to its excellent safety profile in the cat and its known in vitro activity against mycobacteria when compared to older quinolones.[14,15] Where this is not available, the use of moxifloxacin is advocated, as it has a very similar profile to pradofloxacin. Enrofloxacin should be avoided in cats due to its association with acute irreversible retinopathy. The macrolide/azalide of choice is azithromycin (7.5–15 mg/kg PO every 24 hours) due to once-daily dosing, which eases adherence to treatment in cats, plus its ability to concentrate within pulmonary macrophages, which can be useful in disseminated cases. An alternative choice is clarithromycin; however, this may require compounding for cats.

Rifampicin has long been a cornerstone of antituberculosis, and more general antimycobacterial, medical therapy. In cats, it is given at 5–15 mg/kg PO every 24 hours.[9] It has good efficacy against both extracellular mycobacteria and those slowly and persistently replicating within macrophages following phagocytosis. However, it should never be used as a monotherapy, as resistance develops rapidly. Rifampicin has the potential to be significantly hepatotoxic when used chronically. Before starting treatment, it is advisable to assess the patient's liver status including evaluation of serum biochemistry (and haematology). These tests should be repeated 2 weeks and then monthly after therapy is started or if any clinical signs appear which warrant investigation. Treatment with rifampicin should be stopped if circulating levels of liver enzymes significantly exceed the upper reference interval, hyperbilirubinaemia develops, or the patient develops clinical signs attributable to hepatic dysfunction (e.g. anorexia). If this occurs, rifampicin has to be discontinued, and liver support drugs should be given (e.g. S-adenosylmethionine [SAMe], N-acetylcysteine [NAC]). Once recovered, the rifampicin can be reintroduced at half of the previous dose, with close monitoring to ensure that the hepatopathy does not recur. Rifampicin is excreted in all bodily fluids and will cause urine, tears, and saliva to discolour to red orange. This is not clinically

Table 14.1. First-line antituberculosis medications for use in cats.

Drug	Dosage and route of administration	Contraindications	Side effects
Pradofloxacin	5–7.5 mg/kg PO every 24 h*	Cats <6 weeks of age due to potential adverse effects on cartilage Animals with epilepsy	Neutropenia with high doses or long courses.
Marbofloxacin	2 mg/kg PO every 24 h	As for pradofloxacin	Intermittent vomiting and transient diarrhoea on instigation of treatment.
Moxifloxacin	10 mg/kg PO every 24 h	As for pradofloxacin	Occasional vomiting. Ocular toxicity has not been thoroughly assessed.
Ciprofloxacin	5–15 mg/kg PO every 12 h	As for pradofloxacin	Occasional vomiting.
Azithromycin	5–15 mg/kg PO every 24 h*	Preexisting cardiopathy (especially arrhythmogenic diseases) Preexisting hepatopathy	Intermittent vomiting and diarrhoea possible but uncommon.
Clarithromycin	7.5 mg/kg PO every 12 h	Concurrent use of NSAIDs or antacids Preexisting hepatopathy	Pinnal erythema. Generalised erythema. Hepatotoxicity.
Rifampicin	5–15 mg/kg PO every 24 h	Preexisting hepatopathy Pregnant queens	Hepatotoxicity, induction of liver enzymes, anorexia, generalised erythema, and pruritus. CNS signs. Discolouration of body fluids.

CNS, central nervous system; NSAID, nonsteroidal anti-inflammatory drug.
*Recommended antituberculosis dosage outside the terms of the licence.

significant, but it can be distressing for clients who are unprepared, especially as the discolouration could be mistaken for haemorrhage. Deposition of the drug within the skin can cause irritation and, occasionally, hyperaesthesia. Chlorphenamine seems to have been helpful in reducing this skin irritation.

The duration of treatment depends on the clinical signs present at the time of diagnosis. Three months of triple therapy (at the doses outlined) should be considered a minimum in all cases.[9] Treatment should be extended for 2 months beyond the resolution of all clinical signs, including any pulmonary dissemination detectable on standard radiography. Treatment for cutaneous plus pulmonary disease is typically for 6 months. Monitoring for the resolution of pulmonary changes using CT studies is more difficult, as subtle changes such as minor scars remain detectable and may persist indefinitely beyond the need for treatment owing to the increased sensitivity of this imaging modality.

As ever, compliance with medication is frequently an issue in feline patients. Ease of dosing can be facilitated by selecting all liquid formulations of the drugs and drawing them into a single syringe immediately prior to administration. Mixing liquid drugs with a cat's usual diet is typically unrewarding, as these drugs are unpalatable to cats, especially rifampicin. In the United Kingdom, a combination of azithromycin and rifampicin is available as a single capsule suitable for cats in the weight range of 2.5–6 kg.

If oral dosing is not possible, drugs can be administered by placement of an oesophagostomy tube (Fig. 14.6). Clinical experience suggests that such tubes can be left in place for the entire duration of treatment without adverse effects and cut short (10 cm) to maximise patient comfort, supported by a specialised collar (KittyKollar). Such an approach appears to be very successful in maintaining patient compliance and the clients' relationship with their pets, and it also facilitates the administration of additional medications (e.g. SAMe, NAC) with ease (see also Chapter 40).

Prognosis and outcome

If dosing is maintained, the prognosis has been reported as being generally fair, with one review stating that 40% of cases reached and maintained complete clinical remission.[15] However, these data relate to a retrospective cohort, many of which were treated with what would now be considered to be suboptimal therapies, such as short courses of fluoroquinolone monotherapies. With the approach outlined above, clinical experience suggests a positive prognosis in close to 80% of feline tuberculosis cases, par-

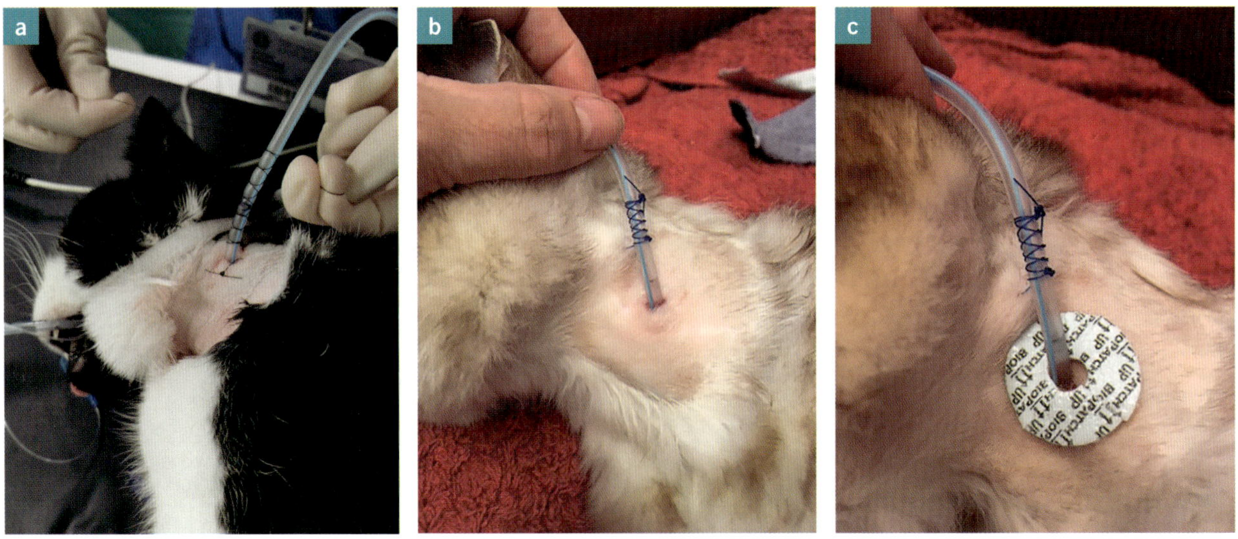

Figure 14.6. Oesophageal tube being secured with a Roman sandal suture (a). When placing an oesophageal tube, care should be taken to place the suture away from the wound (b). This makes it much easier to clean for the owner, reduces the risk of suture infection, and gives space for a protective disc (impregnated with chlorhexidine) to be placed around the tube (c), which reduces the risk of suture infection even further. The tube can then be covered by a KittyKollar—although expensive, these collars are washable and remove the need for other dressings.

ticularly those with cutaneous or pulmonary involvement. However, the authors' anecdotal evidence has not found such positive responses for GI mycobacterial infections, in which the prognosis has to be considered as guarded.

The treatment of NTM infections is generally more difficult and less rewarding than for tuberculous infections. This is because many of these organisms do not readily grow in laboratory conditions, and therefore it has not been possible to generate good sensitivity data across many clinical isolates. Additionally, the drug resistance patterns of these organisms vary widely, not just between species, but also between isolates of the same species. Furthermore, in vitro sensitivity results do not always correlate with in vitro drug activity, as some of the genes which confer resistance (e.g. to macrolides) are inducible and thus their presence does not necessarily correlate with observed sensitivity profiles. However, success has frequently been achieved with the same protocols as for tuberculous infections. Feline outcomes are not well documented, but human data show a strong correlation between the species of NTM organism and outcome, with the best outcomes achieved for *M. malmoense* and *M. kansasii* infections, probably due to their similarities to the MTBC. Worse outcomes are achieved in cases of *M. avium–intracellulare* complex (MAC) infections, and very poor outcomes result from *M. xenopi*, *M. simiae*, and particularly *M. abscessus*.

OTHER CAUSES OF GRANULOMATOUS ENTERITIS

Three bacterial genera, *Yersinia*, *Rhodococcus*, and *Nocardia*, can infrequently cause GI disease in cats.

Yersinia pestis is the causative agent of plague, to which cats in North America and Russia, where it is endemic, are highly susceptible. The most common presentation of plague in cats is bubonic plague, in which cats have fever, loss of appetite, lethargy, and enlarged lymph nodes that may be abscessed and draining. Ulcers in the mouth, skin abscesses, discharge from the eyes, diarrhoea, vomiting, and diffuse spreading inflammation of tissues beneath the skin have also been documented. High fever may be present. Cats with primary septicaemic plague have no obvious disease of the lymph nodes but have fever, lethargy, and poor appetite. Septic signs may also include diarrhoea, vomiting, tachycardia, weak pulse, and respiratory distress. Primary pneumonic plague has not been documented in cats, but secondary pneumonic plague can cause the signs of septicaemic plague along with a cough and other lung abnormalities.

Flea control is essential for prevention. Treatment cannot usually wait for confirmation of the diagnosis due to the rapid progression of the disease, especially for septicaemic patients. Appropriate protective equipment should be worn due to the significant zoonotic risk. Abscesses require drainage and flushing with a chlorhexidine solution. Parenteral administration of aminoglycoside antibiotics (e.g. gentamicin) is the treatment of choice for sick animals, whilst tetracyclines also have good efficacy against *Y. pestis*.

Rhodococcus equi is a common cause of diarrhoea in young foals. In cats, it can also cause a range of other clinical signs. One study of 40 feline cases found that 36 showed a pulmonary form of the disease, with 35 (87.5%) presenting with dyspnoea, while 4 cats presented with only cutaneous lesions. Leucocytosis with band neutrophilia, monocytosis, and thrombocytopenia were prominent findings on haematologic examination. Hyperproteinaemia with hypoalbuminaemia and hyperglobulinaemia were frequently revealed on routine serum biochemistry evaluation. Overall, the mortality rate was 67.5% in both forms. Cases have been too infrequently reported in cats to develop optimum treatment protocols. However, due to the similarities of *Rhodococcus* and *Mycobacterium*, with them previously being considered a single genus and the guidelines for the treatment of foals and humans, a similar treatment approach as to feline mycobacteriosis cases should be effective.

Nocardia spp. can, on very rare occasions, cause disease in cats including skin lesions resulting from inoculation via bite wounds, GI signs following ingestion of contaminated raw meat or prey, plus pneumonia or pyothorax. They are acid-fast organisms and thus can be visualised on cytological and/or histological samples, although molecular methods are generally required for a definitive diagnosis. Owing to the very small number of cases reported, treatment options have been poorly evaluated, but in one study of five cats, four were successfully treated: three with a trimethoprim–sulphonamide combination and one with clarithromycin.

TULARAEMIA

Tularaemia, also known as rabbit fever, is a bacterial disease caused by *Francisella tularensis* that can affect animals, including humans. It has been reported throughout North America but is more prevalent in the western United States of America. Cats can become infected by eating small animals such as rabbits or voles that carry the bacteria. Cats can also contract the disease if they are bitten by an infected tick or deer fly. When a cat becomes infected, they may display a variety of clinical signs that include fever, abscesses, oral ulcers, weight loss secondary to enteritis, pneumonia, and septicaemia.

The disease is only rarely encountered; it is not seen at all in the United Kingdom, Africa, South America, or Australia. In North America, tularaemia cases are scattered around the continent. It is most commonly seen in the late spring and summer.

Tularaemia generally causes an acute illness with high fever (40°C–41°C), enlarged and painful lymph nodes of the head and neck, abdominal pain, icterus, and in some cases diarrhoea and weight loss.

Routine blood work is usually not specific for this disease, and therefore diagnosis is based on the presence of antibodies against the bacteria in the blood. Any significant titre of antibody with compatible clinical signs is usually adequate for a presumptive diagnosis of the disease; however, a rising titre over a 2–4-week period is confirmatory. Most laboratories will not attempt blood cultures to isolate the organism because of the zoonotic risk of handling the blood; however, some laboratories do offer PCR testing on blood or tissues.

The prognosis is guarded for these cases, and early aggressive supportive therapy is essential if treatment is to be successful. Streptomycin is the antibiotic treatment of choice for severe cases and is normally given for 3 weeks to maximise the chances of successful elimination of the organism.

Take-home messages

- The role of most bacteria in causing gastrointestinal disease is often unclear (a positive culture for *Campylobacter* spp., *Clostridium* spp., or *Escherichia coli* does not mean that the bacterium is the cause of the diarrhoea). These bacteria are commensals, so it is important to look at the whole case to consider their potential relevance.
- Bacterial causes of diarrhoea are usually more common in young cats, immunocompromised individuals, those from multianimal households, and those fed raw food.
- Finding *Salmonella* spp. in a cat's faeces warrants further investigation because of its zoonotic potential; however, the use of antibiotics in its treatment is controversial.
- *Mycobacterium bovis* is the mycobacterium most likely to cause gastrointestinal disease, typically causing tuberculous granuloma within the mesenteric lymph nodes. When seen, it has usually been associated with feeding contaminated raw food.
- With the advent of more accurate culture systems and the use of advanced diagnostics (e.g. PCR, fluorescence in situ hybridisation), we are able to identify specific bacteria with ever more precision. This will hopefully allow us to gain a better understanding of exactly which bacteria cause disease and which do not.

REFERENCES

[1] Jones PH et al. Surveillance of diarrhoea in small animal practice through the Small Animal Veterinary Surveillance Network (SAVSNET). *Vet J* 201:412, 2014.

[2] Suchodolski JS. Companion animals symposium: microbes and gastrointestinal health of dogs and cats. *J Anim Sci* 89:1520, 2011.

[3] Popoff MR, Bouvet P. Genetic characteristics of toxigenic clostridia and toxin gene evolution. *Toxicon* 75:63, 2013.

[4] Thépault A et al. Dogs and cats: reservoirs for highly diverse *Campylobacter jejuni* and a potential source of human exposure. *Animals (Basel)* 10:838, 2020.

[5] Lappin MR et al. 2019 AAFP Feline Zoonoses Guidelines. *J Feline Med Surg* 21:1008, 2019.

[6] Weese JS. Bacterial enteritis in dogs and cats: diagnosis, therapy, and zoonotic potential. *Vet Clin North Am Small Anim Pract* 41:287, 2011.

[7] Oehler RL et al. "Down boy!" Infectious diseases spread by cats and dogs. *Infect Dis Clin Pract* 17:298, 2009.

[8] Thomson P et al. Detección de *Helicobacter* spp en la mucosa gástrica de felinos domésticos clínicamente sanos mediante la prueba rápida de ureasa e histopatología [Detection of *Helicobacter* spp in the gastric mucosa of clinically healthy domestic felines by the rapid urease test and histopathology]. *Rev Investig Vet Perú* 31:e19039, 2020.

[9] O'Halloran C, Gunn-Moore D. Mycobacteria in cats: an update. *In Pract* 39:399, 2017.

[10] O'Brien CR et al. Feline leprosy due to *Mycobacterium lepraemurium*: further clinical and molecular characterisation of 23 previously reported cases and an additional 42 cases. *J Feline Med Surg* 19:737, 2017.

[11] Gunn-Moore DA, Gaunt C, Shaw DJ. Incidence of mycobacterial infections in cats in Great Britain: estimate from feline tissue samples submitted to diagnostic laboratories. *Transbound Emerg Dis* 60:338, 2013.

[12] Gunn-Moore DA et al. Mycobacterial disease in cats in Great Britain: I. Culture results, geographical distribution and clinical presentation of 339 cases. *J Feline Med Surg* 13:934, 2011.

[13] O'Halloran C et al. Feline tuberculosis caused by *Mycobacterium bovis* infection of domestic UK cats associated with feeding a commercial raw food diet. *Transbound Emerg Dis*, 2020 [epub ahead of print].

[14] Gunn-Moore DA. Feline mycobacterial infections. *Vet J* 201:230, 2014.

[15] Gunn-Moore DA et al. Mycobacterial disease in a population of 339 cats in Great Britain: II. Histopathology of 225 cases, and treatment and outcome of 184 cases. *J Feline Med Surg* 13:945, 2011.

CHAPTER 15

Helminthic and protozoal diseases

Panagiotis G. Xenoulis

HELMINTHIC DISEASES OF THE STOMACH

Physaloptera spp.

Physaloptera spp. (e.g. *P. rara*, *P. praeputialis*) are nematode parasites that can occasionally affect cats.[1–5] Adult worms are about 2–6 cm long and are usually found in the stomach. These parasites have an indirect life cycle, with insects (e.g. crickets, beetles, and cockroaches that often feed on faeces) being the intermediate hosts. Paratenic hosts such as frogs, snakes, mice, and birds may play an important role in the infection of cats. Therefore, cats are infected during hunting. The clinical presentation of cats with *Physaloptera* spp. is not well characterised. Adult parasites attach to the mucosa of the stomach (often within the pylorus) and, in some cases, the proximal duodenum. The main clinical sign is vomiting, which can be severe and unresponsive to antiemetic treatment. Vomiting might also be chronic or intermittent. Infected cats are typically healthy otherwise.

Diagnosis can be challenging. The eggs of the parasite are transparent and, therefore, particularly difficult to see on faecal examination using flotation. In addition, the parasite burden is often low. Therefore, finding eggs (ova) of the parasite in the faeces is not consistent, and their absence cannot exclude infection. Diagnosis is often made during endoscopy for investigation of intractable vomiting, when direct visualisation of the parasites is possible. However, even one parasite can potentially cause severe vomiting, and it might not be easy to detect endoscopically. A treatment trial may be indicated in cases in which the diagnosis cannot be established. Treatment can be achieved with pyrantel pamoate, fenbendazole, or ivermectin (see Appendix for recommended dosages). Endoscopic removal is also therapeutic if the parasites can be identified during endoscopy.

Ollulanus tricuspis

Ollulanus tricuspis is a nematode parasite that lives in the mucosa of the stomach of the cat.[1–5] Adult worms are quite small (≈1 mm). Transmission from cat to cat is direct through consumption of vomitus. This parasite is more common in catteries, colony cats, and feral cats because the transmission is facilitated in those situations. Chronic vomiting is the main clinical sign, although some cats may be asymptomatic. In some cases, gastric inflammation might be severe and lead to haematemesis, significant weight loss, and dehydration.

Clinical diagnosis of infection is difficult. Direct faecal smears and faecal flotation methods are usually negative. Microscopic examination of vomited material (either by natural vomiting or by induced vomiting with xylazine) or stomach washings is considered the best diagnostic method, with a sensitivity of about 70%. The parasites may also be seen occasionally on histopathological examination of gastric biopsy samples. Treatment efficacy is questionable, but fenbendazole, pyrantel pamoate, and ivermectin have been shown to be effective (see Appendix for recommended dosages).

Gnathostoma spp.

Gnathostoma spp. (e.g. *G. spinigerum*, *G. procyonis*) are nematode parasites.[1–5] Adult worms (1–3 cm long) are attached to the mucosa of the stomach of the cat, where they usually form a large cyst of up to 2.5 cm in diameter that contains the worms. Their life cycle requires two intermediate hosts (copepods and fish, frogs, snakes, chickens, rodents, etc.), and cats are infected by eating one of the second intermediate hosts. Clinical signs are not well characterised, but vomiting and weight loss may be seen. In some cases, perforation of the gastric wall has been reported. Treatment might require surgical removal of the mass containing the adult parasites. The efficacy of medical treatment is unknown.

Aonchotheca putorii

Aonchotheca putorii is usually located in the mucus of the stomach of the cat, although it can also be seen in the small intestine.[1–5] Its size ranges between 3 and 8 mm. Hedgehogs appear to be the intermediate host, and cats are infected by ingestion of eggs of the parasite from soil contaminated with hedgehog faeces. Clinical signs are not well characterised but may include vomiting, haematemesis, anorexia, and weight loss. This parasite may cause ulcers and intestinal perforation. Histologically, severe hyperplastic gastritis can be seen. Faecal examination is usually negative. Histopathological examination of gastric biopsy samples may reveal adult parasites, while eggs might be observed in the mucus and in the lumen of pyloric glands. Therapeutically, surgery may be required to remove ulcers or perforated tissue, while ivermectin may be effective in eliminating the parasites.

HELMINTHIC AND PROTOZOAL DISEASES OF THE INTESTINE

Roundworms

Roundworms (ascarids) are amongst the most common parasites in cats around the world and include *Toxocara cati* and *Toxascaris leonina*.[1–6] The dog roundworm, *Toxocara canis*, can also rarely be found in the cat. Adult worms are 1–10 cm in length, or more, and are typically found in the small intestinal lumen. Cats can be infected either directly by ingestion of ova or indirectly by ingestion of paratenic hosts such as mice (larvae are found in the musculature), cockroaches, and earthworms. Ova can persist in the environment for long periods of time. In addition, transmammary transmission of *T. cati* through ingestion of milk from infected queens is common. Unlike *T. canis*, *T. cati* is unlikely to be transmitted transplacentally. After ingestion, the immature forms of *T. cati* (but not *T. leonina*) migrate through the liver and lungs (where they can cause hepatic fibrosis and significant pulmonary lesions) before settling in the small intestine.

Many infected cats and kittens are asymptomatic. In other cases, roundworms can cause or contribute to diarrhoea. Especially in young kittens, roundworms may cause diarrhoea (adult parasites are sometimes present in the faeces), vomiting (the vomitus often includes adult parasites), poor growth, weight loss, abdominal distension (potbellied appearance), abdominal pain, and even intestinal obstruction if adult parasites are numerous. Coughing might be seen in some cases as a result of pneumonitis due to *T. cati* larvae migration.

Diagnosis is usually straightforward because parasite ova are usually numerous in the faeces and can be easily identified by faecal flotation. In kittens, clinical signs may develop before eggs are detected in the faeces. Due to the high prevalence of roundworms in cats, many animals are treated regardless of whether parasitism has been confirmed.

Treatment of roundworms is relatively straightforward, and several anthelmintics have been shown to have almost 100% efficacy. These include pyrantel pamoate (which is safe for use in very young kittens), fenbendazole, ivermectin, milbemycin, and selamectin, amongst others (see Appendix for recommended dosages). In kittens, treatment should start at 6 weeks of age and repeated at 2-week intervals until the age of 3 months. Kittens should be treated even if faecal flotation is negative. Adult cats should be treated two or three times per year depending on exposure to the infectious forms of the parasite. The prognosis is generally excellent, except in very young kittens with severe infections that might lead to stunted growth or death.

Roundworms may infect humans and cause visceral and ocular larva migrans. Humans are infected by ingestion of ova. Therefore, treatment of kittens and adult cats should be aggressive, and parasite prevention should always be part of the feline preventive healthcare plan.

Tapeworms

Tapeworms are cestode parasites that are commonly found in the feline intestinal tract and have a worldwide distribution.[1–5] The most common tapeworm in cats is *Dipylidium caninum*, but several other species are also common. *D. caninum* has an indirect life cycle. Adult parasites are anchored to the small intestinal lumen and can reach a length of 70 cm. Segments of the adult parasites (proglottids) are passed in the faeces of infected cats (Fig. 15.1) and are then consumed by larval stages of the cat flea (*Ctenocephalides felis*). The cat becomes infected by ingesting infected fleas during the grooming process. *Joyeuxiella pasqualei* is another tapeworm found in the small intestinal lumen of the cat. It has two intermediate hosts: the first is currently unknown, and the second one is a reptile. *Taenia taeniaeformis* is acquired by ingestion of infected prey such as birds, rodent, and reptiles. *Echinococcus multilocularis* may also occasionally be found in the small intestine of cats. Unlike roundworms, tapeworms cannot be transmitted transplacentally nor transmammarily, and there is no extraintestinal migration.

The vast majority of cats infected with tapeworms are asymptomatic. Owners may often see proglottids crawling on the cat's perianal area or in the faeces (Fig. 15.2). Sometimes, owners will report dehydrated, shrivelled objects (i.e. dried proglottids) in the surrounding area of their cat's resting places. In some cases, there might be anal irritation associated with the presence of proglottids. In some cats, tapeworms may cause or contribute to diarrhoea or constipation. Very rarely, large numbers of tapeworms can cause intestinal obstruction.

D. caninum eggs are typically confined to the proglottids and, therefore, are not detected by routine faecal flotations. The eggs of *Echinococcus* spp. and those of some *Taenia* spp. may be found in the faeces. Tapeworms are usually diagnosed when the owner reports (e.g. "rice grains") or the veterinary practitioner sees proglottids in the faeces or in the perianal area. For species identification, it might be necessary to squash the proglottids so that the eggs are released and then identify the eggs using microscopy.

Praziquantel and epsiprantel are considered nearly 100% effective against all species of tapeworms (see Appendix for recommended dosages). However, a second treatment 1–2 weeks later may be acceptable in case not all the parasites were killed. Prevention of tapeworm infection and reinfection requires a vigorous flea control programme and access restriction to prey animals.

Hookworms

Hookworms are relatively commonly found in cats. Most common species include *Ancylostoma tubaeforme* (most common), *Ancylostoma braziliense*, and *Uncinaria stenocephala*.[1–5] They are 4–10 mm long. *U. stenocephala* is less common and less pathogenic in cats than *Ancylostoma* spp. Adult parasites are found in the small intestine, where they attach to the mucosa and ingest blood and/or plugs of mucosa depending on the species. The amount of blood loss can be significant, especially if the parasites are numerous and the patient is small in size. Cats are infected by ingestion of infected faeces or paratenic hosts (e.g. rodents), and the infective

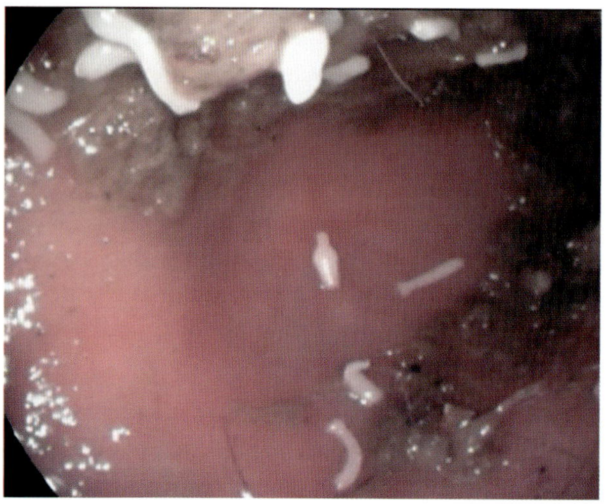

Figure 15.1. Endoscopic image showing several cestode proglottids in the large intestine of a cat.

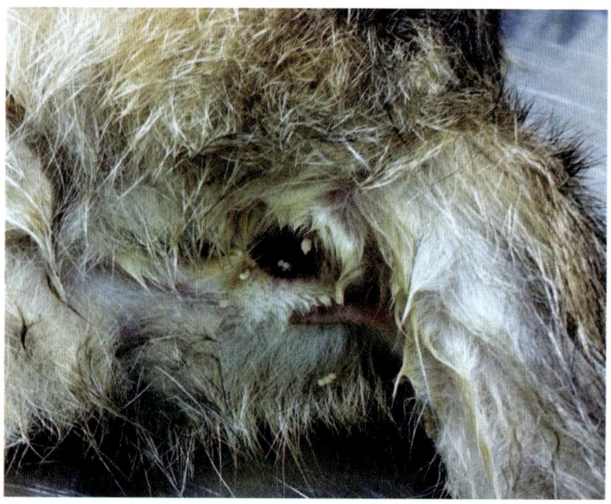

Figure 15.2. Several cestode proglottids are apparent in the perianal area of a cat.

larvae penetrate the gastric and intestinal walls, where they remain for 10–12 days before reentering the lumen. There is no extraintestinal migration, and transplacental or transmammary transmission does not occur. Infection can occasionally occur through skin penetration by the infective larvae, in which case they migrate through the lungs, up to the trachea, and down the oesophagus.

The infection may be asymptomatic. However, in cats with severe infections or in very young cats, clinical signs may be severe. Some cats present with combinations of diarrhoea (sometimes with melaena or frank blood), vomiting, weight loss, weakness, and various degrees of anaemia. Young cats with severe infections may present with life-threatening disease due to severe blood loss or iron-deficiency anaemia. In older animals, there might be iron-deficiency anaemia without any gastrointestinal signs. The presence of hookworms may potentiate the clinical signs of concurrent gastrointestinal disease or other infections.

Diagnosis is straightforward and is based on microscopic identification of parasite eggs by faecal flotation. Hookworms produce large numbers of eggs, and therefore the infection is easy to diagnose. Rarely, kittens may develop clinical signs before eggs are detected in the faeces. In these cases, ELISA identification of parasite antigens might be helpful.

Treatment is similar to that for roundworms, as the same anthelminthic drugs are effective for hookworms (see Appendix for recommended dosages). Treatment should be repeated after 3 weeks to kill the parasites that enter the intestinal lumen from the tissues. Some patients with severe anaemia may require a blood transfusion. The prognosis is generally good, with the exception of very young animals that are severely anaemic and debilitated.

Hookworms, particularly *A. braziliense*, may infect humans and cause cutaneous larva migrans.

Protozoa

Isospora spp. (coccidiosis)

Several *Isospora* species can infect cats, the most common being *I. felis* and *I. rivolta*.[1–5,7,8] Infected cats shed oocysts into the environment, which can survive for months. Oocysts are excreted unsporulated; sporulation occurs within 8–40 hours depending on the temperature. Cats are infected through oocyst-contaminated food or water or by grooming of contaminated body parts. They can also be infected by ingestion of paratenic hosts such as mice and rats. The prepatent period is 7–10 days.

The parasite affects mainly the villous cells of the ileum, but the duodenum and jejunum can also be affected. Most cats are resistant to infection and typically do not develop clinical signs, or they only show mild clinical signs. Exceptions are very young kittens, immunocompromised cats, stressed cats, and cats in multicat environments, with poor hygiene conditions and suboptimal nutrition. In these cases, coccidiosis might be associated with severe diarrhoea (often with mucus), haemorrhagic diarrhoea, and death especially in very young kittens. Also, concurrent viral or parasitic infections can lead to more severe clinical signs.

Diagnosis is based on identification of the parasite oocysts in direct faecal smears or by faecal flotation. Repeated faecal examinations may be necessary. Because many infected cats are asymptomatic, the presence of oocysts (especially in small numbers) does not ensure that the infection is the cause of the clinical signs. Adult cats with severe clinical signs from *Isospora* spp. should be investigated for risk factors and concurrent diseases. Differentiation of *Isospora* oocysts from those of other coccidia-like organisms might be difficult.

Drugs that can be used to effectively treat cats with clinical coccidiosis include sulphadimethoxine, trimethoprim–sulphonamide, ponazuril, and toltrazuril, amongst others (see Appendix for recommended dosages). Complete eradication of the parasite might not be necessary for improvement of the clinical signs, as host defence mechanisms might be able to restore intestinal health. The prognosis of infected cats is typically good to excellent. Removal of oocysts from the environment is important to avoid reinfections and infection of other cats.

Cryptosporidium spp.

Aetiology and pathophysiology

Cryptosporidium spp. may infect and cause disease in cats.[1–5,7] Currently, it is unclear whether disease in this species is caused by *C. felis* or *C. parvum*, or both. Cats are infected by ingestion of oocysts found in the faeces of infected cats or dogs, in the water, or in the soil. Faeces from infected animals contain the infectious form of the parasite when passed. The prepatent period in cats is about 10 days. The infection might be more common in multicat environments. *Cryptosporidium* spp. are mainly found in the mucosal epithelial cells at the tips of the small intestinal villi, while the crypts are typically not affected.

History and physical examination

Many cats, if not most, remain asymptomatic or only develop mild, self-limiting diarrhoea. In some cases, however, cryptosporidiosis can cause small intestinal diarrhoea, which can be severe. Most cats develop chronic or intermittent diarrhoea. Cats that are immunocompromised or have severe concurrent diseases (e.g. feline leukaemia virus [FeLV] infection, alimentary lymphoma, inflammatory bowel disease) or coinfections with other parasites (e.g. *Giardia*) may present with more severe clinical sings. However, severe disease can occur in cats with no identifiable concurrent immunosuppressive diseases. Severe cases usually develop haemorrhagic diarrhoea, anorexia, depression, weight loss, abdominal pain, and dehydration.

Diagnostic investigation

Diagnosis can be made by identification of oocysts via faecal flotation examination. However, oocysts are rather small (3.5–5 µm) and easy to miss. Therefore, experience in identifying *Cryptosporidium* spp. is important. Immunofluorescence assay (IFA), ELISA, or PCR using faecal material are useful for the diagnosis of cryptosporidiosis. PCR appears to be the most sensitive method, and PCR-based diarrhoea panels are used commonly and are convenient. Serological tests (ELISA) only indicate exposure and not current infection. Sometimes it is difficult to establish a cause–effect relationship with the clinical picture because many of the cats are asymptomatic. Cryptosporidiosis should be especially suspected if other infectious or parasitic causes have been excluded or if standard antiparasitic or symptomatic treatments have been ineffective. Diagnosis of cryptosporidiosis in cats should trigger diagnostic investigation for concurrent immunosuppressive diseases such as infection with FeLV or feline immunodeficiency virus (FIV).

Treatment

There is no treatment that is consistently effective and safe for cryptosporidiosis in cats.[1–5,7] Thankfully, most cases are asymptomatic and treatment is not needed. Paromomycin (125–165 mg/kg PO every 12 hours for 5 days) has been used with some success in cats, although efficacy is probably low and can potentially cause acute kidney injury and deafness. Azithromycin (7–15 mg/kg PO every 12 hours for 5–14 days) might be effective and is safe in this species. Tylosin (11 mg/kg PO every 12 hours for 4 weeks) may also be effective, but this is less certain. Nitazoxanide (25 mg/kg PO every 12 hours for 4 weeks) is effective in humans but might be toxic in cats (may cause vomiting and severe diarrhoea), and the efficacy is uncertain in the cat. For a summary of recommended dosages, see Appendix. In some cases, diarrhoea may persist despite treatment, and the prognosis is uncertain. Some cats may have to be euthanised due to persistent diarrhoea.

Zoonotic potential

Cryptosporidiosis is an important zoonosis, especially in immunocompromised individuals.[1–5,7] Although there have been reports linking feline cryptosporidiosis with human infection, this is highly questionable, and feline genotypes might not cause disease in humans or cause disease only in immunosuppressed individuals. Therefore, the role of cats in the transmission of *Cryptosporidium* to humans is currently undefined. Nevertheless, owners of cats diagnosed with cryptosporidiosis should be informed about the zoonotic potential of this parasite.

Giardia sp.

Aetiology and pathophysiology

Cats are commonly infected with the protozoan parasite *Giardia duodenalis* (also named *G. intestinalis* and *G. lamblia*).[1–5,7,9–11] There are seven genetic assemblances of *Giardia* (A–G) that are differentiated by genetic analysis using PCR. Cats are infected with assemblages A, B, and F, with the cat-specific assemblage F being found more frequently. People are mainly infected with assemblages A and B.

Cats are infected by ingestion of *Giardia* cysts found in the environment, where they can survive for months. After ingestion of the cysts, the trophozoites of the parasite develop in the small intestine and cause a clinical disease known as giardiasis. *Giardia* organisms cause damage to the epithelial cells of the distal small intestine, leading to villous blunting, inflammation, and malabsorption. Cysts are excreted in the faeces of infected animals (cats, amongst others), and sensitive hosts are infected either by ingesting faeces that contain cysts of the parasite or from contaminated food or water. The life cycle of *Giardia* is direct, and there is no extraintestinal migration nor transplacental or transmammary transmission.

Prevalence of infection

The prevalence of *Giardia* infection varies greatly depending on the population tested.[1–5,7,9–11] Depending on the study, the reported prevalence ranges between 1% and 31%, with the higher percentages seen in immunodeficient cats or cats that live in dense populations or that are presented at cats shows.

History and physical examination

Many cats with *Giardia* infections are asymptomatic.[1–5,7,9–11] Kittens and immunosuppressed cats are more likely to become infected and to develop clinical signs of giardiasis. Symptomatic patients may present with clinical signs that range from mild to severe. The most common clinical sign is diarrhoea, which can be acute or chronic. In many cases the diarrhoea is self-limiting, while in other cases it might be persistent or intermittent. Most commonly, the diarrhoea is small bowel in origin (typically "cow patty" without blood or mucus), but in some cases large bowel diarrhoea might be seen. Less commonly, cats with severe infection may develop weight loss, anorexia, dehydration, and/or vomiting. Clinical signs can develop before cysts are shed in the faeces (which usually takes 5–16 days).

Diagnostic investigation

Many cats infected with *Giardia* are asymptomatic. Therefore, identification of the microorganism in the faeces does not necessarily mean that *Giardia* is the cause of the clinical signs, or it might not be the only cause of the clinical signs. Testing of asymptomatic cats for *Giardia* is generally not recommended because many cats are asymptomatic; however, possible exceptions include catteries, multicat households, and households with immunocompromised people. Cats with severe clinical signs might be immunosuppressed and should be tested for FeLV and FIV.

Diagnosis of giardiasis in cats can be made using the methods listed below.[1–5,7,9–11] *Giardia* trophozoites can occasionally be seen on histopathological examination of small intestinal biopsy specimens. None of the diagnostic tests described below is 100% sensitive and specific for *Giardia*; therefore, it is highly recommended to use a combination of these methods to more confidently diagnose or rule out giardiasis.

- **Zinc sulphate faecal flotation.** Zinc sulphate solutions are the best choice for the identification of *Giardia* cysts in faeces and are commonly used in clinical practice. Centrifugal flotation is preferable compared to standing techniques. This method is cheap, provides fast results, and can be performed in-house. Since oocyst shedding occurs intermittently, random single faecal samples might be negative in infected patients. Therefore, at least three faecal samples should be examined over the course of 3–10 days in order to increase the sensitivity of the test (77% with one sample vs. 96% with three samples). Even when multiple samples are examined, false-negative results can occur, especially with inexperienced examiners. False-positive results can also occur due to particles in the faeces that might resemble *Giardia* cysts. Combining zinc sulphate faecal flotation with in-clinic *Giardia* ELISA tests is highly recommended, as this is believed to increase the sensitivity and specificity compared to any of these tests alone.
- **Faecal ELISA for *Giardia* antigens.** Faecal ELISA tests are available from several companies as in-clinic tests, as well as from diagnostic laboratories. These tests detect soluble *Giardia* antigens in faeces (fresh or refrigerated for a few days). Unlike *Giardia* cysts, *Giardia* antigens are constantly present in the faeces of infected animals and can be detected by ELISA assays. The in-clinic tests are used frequently and are quick and much easier to perform than faecal flotation techniques. An important advantage of in-clinic ELISA tests, compared to faecal flotation techniques, is that they do not require experienced technicians to be performed. Most faecal ELISA tests have high sensitivity

and specificity. However, there might be differences in their performance, and depending on the company some tests are more sensitive and specific than others. In a recent study, three in-clinic ELISA-based diagnostic tests for *Giardia* (VETCHEK ELISA, TECHLAB; SNAP *Giardia* Antigen Test, IDEXX Laboratories; and VetScan Giardia Antigen test, Abaxis) were compared using IFA as the gold standard and were all found to have a similar sensitivity (92.5%) and specificity (>95%). Combining in-clinic *Giardia* ELISA tests with zinc sulphate faecal flotation is highly recommended, as this is believed to increase the sensitivity and specificity compared to any of these tests alone.

- **Faecal IFA for *Giardia* antigens.** Faecal IFAs are also available for detecting *Giardia* cysts in faeces and are widely considered to be the most accurate diagnostic method for giardiasis because they are highly sensitive and specific. In several studies, IFA is used as the gold standard for the diagnosis of giardiasis. However, as with other tests, IFA is not 100% sensitive and specific. IFA testing requires sending faecal samples to specialised diagnostic laboratories.
- **PCR testing.** PCR testing is available for the detection of *Giardia* DNA in faecal samples. Some laboratories offer PCR testing that identifies the genotype of *Giardia* (A–G). PCR testing is highly specific for *Giardia* (≈100%), but its sensitivity is suboptimal (≈80%). Therefore, this test cannot be used to rule out giardiasis, and negative results do not exclude infection.
- **Direct faecal smear examination.** *Giardia* trophozoites and/or cysts may be detected by direct smear microscopic examination of faecal material or duodenal juice (collected during endoscopy or surgery). This method is simple, quick, and cheap but is associated with a low sensitivity (<50%), and therefore negative results do not exclude infection. *Giardia* trophozoites are highly motile, usually with a motion resembling a falling leaf. Trophozoite motility enhances the diagnosis; therefore, one should ensure that samples are fresh or refrigerated for a short period of time to assure trophozoite survival. *Giardia* trophozoites should be differentiated from those of *Tritrichomonas blagburni* (see section "*Tritrichomonas blagburni* (*foetus*)" in this chapter), although the two parasites might coexist in some animals.

Treatment

The drugs of choice for the treatment of giardiasis in cats are fenbendazole and metronidazole.[1–5,7,9–11] Fenbendazole is administered at 50 mg/kg PO every 24 hours for 5–7 days and is associated with minimal side effects. Metronidazole is administered at 20–25 mg/kg PO every 12 hours for 7 days. Side effects are rare at this dosage, but higher dosages have been associated with clinical signs of central nervous system toxicity such as weakness, ataxia, and seizures. For a summary of recommended dosages, see Appendix. The use of the two drugs in combination might be needed in resistant cases. Other medications might be effective but are generally not recommended or are not widely available.

None of the aforementioned medications are 100% effective in eliminating *Giardia*. It is also important to note that the clinical signs are self-limiting in many cases. The value of retesting patients whose clinical signs have resolved is of questionable value. Resistance of *Giardia* can occur in some cases. In immunosuppressed cats or cats with severe concurrent intestinal disease, elimination of the parasite might be very difficult, and repeated treatments might be required. Treatment of asymptomatic cats may be attempted in multicat households or households with immunosuppressed people.

Due to the difficulty in diagnosing giardiasis in some cases, therapeutic trials (e.g. fenbendazole for 5 days) are used commonly in clinical practice. However, the drugs used for giardiasis are not 100% effective, and therefore therapeutic failure does not rule out giardiasis.

Since *Giardia* cysts are resistant in the environment, reinfection of treated animals is common. Therefore, in addition to eliminating the parasite from the intestine, an effective treatment plan for giardiasis should also include decontamination of the environment. Animals should be bathed to remove cysts from their coat, and the environment should be disinfected using effective disinfectants such as quaternary ammonium compounds.

Prognosis

The prognosis is generally good for resolution of clinical signs. However, eliminating the parasite can be difficult. Elimination of the parasite and complete resolution of clinical signs in immunosuppressed cats or cats with concurrent severe intestinal disease might be particularly difficult.

Zoonotic potential

Giardia is a common and well-described pathogen in humans, especially in children.[1–5,7,9–11] Waterborne transmission is the main route of spread of giardiasis in humans. However, other routes of transmission are also important, including consumption of contaminated food and person-to-person transmission. There has been much debate regarding whether giardiasis is a zoonotic disease, and studies often show conflicting results. Recent studies have shown that cats have a significant prevalence of zoonotic *Giardia* genotype A (and, to a lesser degree, genotype B), suggesting that cats are be able to transmit the parasite to humans, with subsequent implications in public health. Because these genotypes are found primarily in humans, and no comprehensive studies to address zoonotic transmission of *G. duodenalis* are available yet, a potential role of cats in the transmission to humans cannot be conclusively excluded.

Tritrichomonas blagburni (foetus)

Over the past two decades, the protozoan parasite *Tritrichomonas blagburni* (formerly *T. foetus*) has emerged as a new and important cause of feline diarrhoea.[1–5,7,12–21] It is a relatively common infection that affects mainly the colon and distal ileum, causing chronic persistent or intermittent diarrhoea in susceptible cats.

Aetiology and pathophysiology

T. blagburni is a single-cell, highly motile, flagellated protozoan parasite that exists only as a trophozoite (there is no cyst stage).[1–5,7,12–21] *T. blagburni* isolates from cats are similar to, but genetically different from, isolates that cause infertility and abortions in cattle. The pathophysiological sequence is not fully understood, but organism, host, and environmental factors are likely involved. Infection occurs by direct faecal–oral transmission. *T. blagburni* trophozoites are present in the faeces of infected cats, where they can survive for several days if the faeces remain moist. Healthy cats are infected by ingestion of live *T. blagburni* trophozoites. Therefore, the source of infection is usually the litter tray, where the paws of healthy cats get in touch with the faeces of infected cats, and the trophozoites are ingested during grooming.

Prevalence of infection

Since the first reports of *T. blagburni* as a cause of diarrhoea in cats in the United States of America in 2003, the existence of *T. blagburni* has been reported in many countries around the world.[1–5,7,12–21] The prevalence of *T. blagburni* infection in cats depends mainly on the location (country), the cat population tested, and the diagnostic methods used. The reported prevalence of feline *T. blagburni* infection varies from 10% to 32%.

Signalment

Cats of any age, breed, or sex can be infected and develop clinical signs.[1–5,7,12–21] Infection associated with clinical sings is most commonly seen in young cats (<12 months of age), but older cats may also be infected and develop clinical signs. The reported age range for feline *T. blagburni* infection is 1 month–16 years. The infection is often asymptomatic in adult cats, and these cats may be an important source of infection for other cats. Purebred cats may be at increased risk for infection (dense housing conditions in catteries appear more likely factors than genetic predisposition). Densely populated environments (e.g. shelters, catteries, pet shops, multicat households) are an important risk factor for infection with *T. blagburni*.

History and physical examination

The clinical signs of *T. blagburni* infection in cats can vary greatly, ranging from asymptomatic infections to severe chronic refractory diarrhoea.[1–5,7,12–21] Adult cats may be less likely to develop clinical signs than younger cats. Clinical signs are often intermittent. The most common clinical sign is chronic persistent or recurrent diarrhoea, which is most commonly large bowel in origin and is characterised by increased frequency of defecation, and faeces might contain mucus or fresh blood (Fig. 15.3). Some cats may develop small bowel watery diarrhoea later in the disease course. The diarrhoea is often reported to be extremely malodorous. In cats with severe chronic diarrhoea, the anal region can become oedematous and painful, and involuntary dripping of faeces may occur. Tenesmus may also be seen. Most infected cats remain in good health and typically have a normal appetite, activity level, and body condition, unless concurrent diseases are present. Other clinical signs such as anorexia, depression, vomiting, weight loss, and fever may occur in some

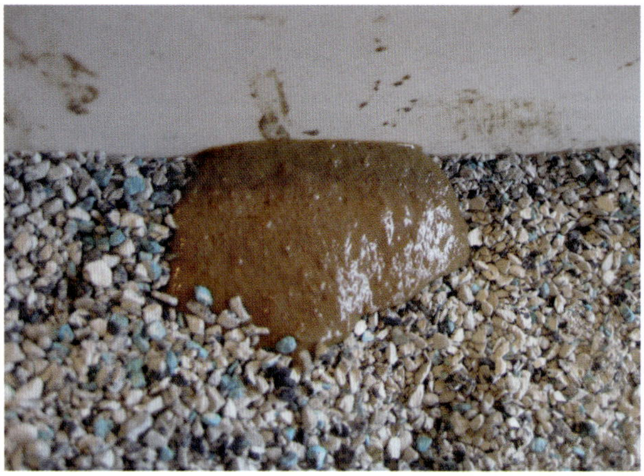

Figure 15.3. Typical appearance of the faeces of a cat with *Tritrichomonas blagburni* infection. The faeces are poorly formed and may or may not contain mucus or blood.

cats but are not very common. In fact, when such signs are present, they are more likely to be the result of concurrent diseases rather than the intestinal *T. blagburni* infection. Physical examination is usually normal unless other diseases are present.

If left untreated, *T. blagburni*–associated diarrhoea often persists intermittently for several months or years, or even for the rest of the animal's life. While in most cats diarrhoea usually resolves spontaneously at some point, this might take several months or years, and these cats will often experience recurrent bouts of diarrhoea after being exposed to stress (e.g. surgery, travel, adoption of a new animal, diet change). The majority of untreated cats remain infected even after clinical resolution of diarrhoea and can transmit the parasite to healthy cats.

Because many cats acquire the infection in catteries or pet shops, many owners report clinical signs since adoption or shortly thereafter (up to 60% of owners report diarrhoea since the time of adoption). The duration of diarrhoea ranges between 1 day and 8 years. The diarrhoea is typically refractory to standard antibiotic or antidiarrhoeal therapy or might improve initially but recur shortly after discontinuation of treatment.

Diagnostic investigation

Ideally, every cat with diarrhoea (especially with large bowel diarrhoea) should be tested for *T. blagburni* infection.[1–5,7,12–21] Young cats and cats from multicat environments seem to be at increased risk of infection, and testing is highly recommended in these cases. Similarly, cats with an incomplete response to standard antibiotic treatment or with a relapse after discontinuation of medication are highly suspicious for *T. blagburni* infection. Furthermore, cats that are unresponsive to treatment for suspected *Giardia* spp. infection should be tested for *T. blagburni* infection, as the two parasites often coexist and are often confused on routine faecal smear evaluation.

The differential diagnoses include giardiasis or enteritis due to other protozoan parasites, intestinal parasitism, infectious causes of colitis, infiltrative intestinal disease (inflammatory bowel disease, intestinal lymphoma), dietary intolerance or sensitivity, and intestinal dysbiosis (antibiotic-responsive diarrhoea).

Diagnosis of *T. blagburni* infection can be made with three methods: direct faecal smear examination, faecal culture, and PCR analysis of faecal material.[1–5,7,12–21] Diagnosis can also be made by histopathological examination of colonic biopsy specimens, but this method is not routinely used due to its invasiveness. Although none of the tests mentioned above is 100% sensitive and specific for diagnosing *T. blagburni* infection, PCR is the most sensitive and specific test and is currently recommended as the test of choice. Since *T. blagburni* does not have a cyst stage, faecal flotation and sedimentation techniques are rarely useful for the diagnosis of *T. blagburni* infection.

It has been shown that sampling methodology and sample quality play an important role in the correct diagnosis of *T. blagburni* infection. As a general rule, freshly voided diarrhoeic faecal samples (<6 hours old, ideally <2 hours old) that contain mucus or blood should be used because the microorganism is more likely to be present in these samples. Samples collected directly from the rectum either using the saline flush method or via faecal loop are likely to be more suitable for testing compared to freshly voided samples. In a recent study, faecal samples collected via faecal loop had increased probability of positive PCR test results compared to samples collected by colonic flush. When using diagnostic methods that require the microorganism to be alive (e.g. direct faecal smear, culture), the use of freshly voided samples or samples collected directly from the rectum are ideal. With PCR testing, fresh faecal samples might not be necessary because *T. blagburni* DNA is stable, and samples can be frozen before shipment. Dilution of the faecal material in saline has been recommended by some authors to reduce interference with PCR testing.

- **Direct faecal smear examination.** Direct examination of faecal smears should be performed in every cat with diarrhoea, not only to look for *T. blagburni* trophozoites but also for other infectious agents (e.g. *Giardia* spp.). This method is quick, cheap, and easy to perform. It is crucial that multiple faecal smears are examined to significantly increase the sensitivity of the method. It is also important to use multiple freshly voided diarrhoeic faecal samples or samples collected directly from the rectum in order to ensure survival of the microorganism. This is important because trophozoite motility facilitates its identification. If faecal samples are not freshly voided or are dried-out, refrigerated, or frozen, they will not contain live *T. blagburni* microorganisms, and this complicates diagnosis. Also, diarrhoeic faeces that contain mucus or blood are preferred because they are more likely to contain *T. blagburni* microorganisms. Some authors also recommend discontinuation of antibiotics a few days before sampling, although treatment was not associated with PCR testing results in a recent study.

  A small amount of fresh faeces is placed on a microscope slide, mixed with a drop of saline (0.9%), covered with a coverslip, and examined under a light microscope. Smears must be rather thin to ensure that the parasites are visible. After the slide has been checked for motile trophozoites, Lugol's solution, methylene blue, or Diff-Quick staining may be used to facilitate morphological identification of the microorganism (Fig. 15.4). *T. blagburni* trophozoites are characterised by rapid forward motion and can be seen at magnifications of at least ×100, although their structural characteristics are better seen at ×400. *T. blagburni* can be easily confused with *Giardia* spp. due to their similar size. The two microorganisms can be differentiated based on their structural features (unlike *Giardia* spp., *T. blagburni* has a single nucleus and an undulating membrane) and the characteristic rapid forward motion of *T. blagburni* (motility of *Giardia* resembles a falling leaf). However, experience and appropriate equipment are required for accurate differentiation. Faecal flotation and ELISA for *Giardia* help rule out other parasites and *Giardia*. *T. blagburni* can also be difficult to distinguish from the nonpathogenic *Pentatrichomonas hominis*, which is considered to be part of the normal microbiota in many animals. This means that if a microorganism that looks like *T. blagburni* is identified, one cannot be 100% confident that this is what it is based only on the microscopic appearance. The main limitation of direct faecal smear examination is its low sensitivity, which in one study was reported to be as low as 14%. Therefore, it is important to note that a negative faecal smear examination result (even if multiple smears are examined) does not exclude infection. Examination of multiple faecal smears is thought to increase the sensitivity of the method.
- **Culture.** *T. blagburni* can be cultured in-house (i.e. there is no need to send samples to a laboratory) using the commercially available culture system InPouch TF. Pouches should be inoculated with less than 0.1 g of freshly voided faeces (<2 hours old) and then incubated in the dark at 25°C for up to 12 days or at 37°C for 2 days. Incubation at 25°C is preferred by the author because overgrowth seems to be less common. Overgrowth will lead to death of the microorganisms and make their identification difficult or impossible. Pouches incubated at 25°C need to be evaluated under a light microscope every other day for the presence of *T. blagburni* trophozoites in order to avoid overgrowth. Positive results need to be confirmed by microscopic examination (Fig. 15.5). Results are usually obtained after 1–12 days of setting up a pouch. The growth of *Giardia* spp. and *P. hominis* is not supported by the culture media, and therefore a positive culture is highly suggestive of *T. blagburni* infection. Faecal culture is more sensitive than direct faecal smear examination (sensitivity of about 50% if performed correctly), but it can be negative if only small numbers of *T. blagburni* trophozoites are present in the faeces or if not performed correctly. Limitations of culture include its suboptimal sensitivity, difficulties in interpretation of results, the necessity of using freshly voided faeces, and the fact that results might not be available for up to 12 days.
- **PCR testing.** *T. blagburni* DNA can be amplified from feline faecal samples by PCR. PCR has been shown to be the most sensitive and specific method for detecting

T. blagburni in faecal samples and is currently considered the test of choice. Advantages of PCR testing compared to culture include a higher sensitivity and easier sample handling and storing because DNA is relatively stable under various temperature conditions. However, false-negative results may occur if the microorganism is not present in the faecal sample obtained. Therefore, the use of appropriate faecal samples to increase sensitivity (i.e. fresh diarrhoeic faeces or faeces collected directly from the colon by flushing sterile saline) is important. PCR for the detection of *T. blagburni* is widely available, and faecal samples can be stored and sent frozen to the laboratory for PCR testing.

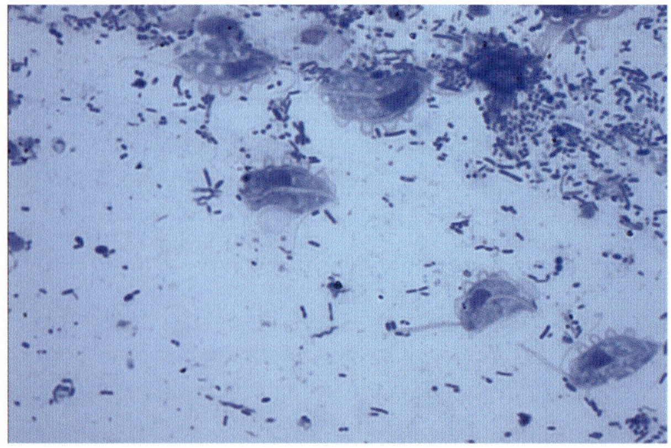

Figure 15.4. Microscopic image of *Tritrichomonas blagburni* microorganisms in a faecal smear from an infected cat. Note the single nucleus and the undulating membrane of each microorganism. The anterior flagella are also visible. Diff-Quick, ×400. Image courtesy of Dr Jody Gookin, North Carolina State University, USA.

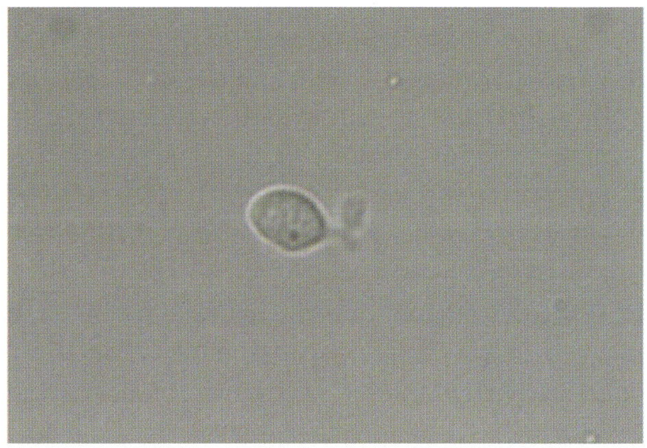

Figure 15.5. Microscopic image of a single *Tritrichomonas blagburni* microorganism from a culture.

Treatment

As mentioned previously, *T. blagburni*–associated diarrhoea often persists for several months or years if left untreated.[1–5,7,12–21] Although spontaneous resolution of clinical signs may occur, it can take several months, and these cats will often experience recurrent bouts of diarrhoea after being exposed to stress. In addition, most untreated cats remain infected and can transmit the parasite to healthy cats. Therefore, treatment of *T. blagburni*–associated diarrhoea is highly recommended.

T. blagburni–associated diarrhoea in cats does not respond to most antibiotics and antiparasitic agents currently available such as metronidazole, tylosin, erythromycin, enrofloxacin, amoxicillin, clindamycin, fenbendazole, and albendazole, amongst others. Temporary improvement may be seen initially with the use of these drugs, but the clinical signs almost always relapse after discontinuation of treatment. Currently, the only drug that has been shown to be effective against *T. blagburni* infection in cats both in vitro and in vivo is ronidazole. This drug is a 5-nitroimidazole (same group as metronidazole) and might be potentially carcinogenic. Therefore, human contact should be avoided (e.g. use of gloves when handling the drug or faeces from cats treated with this drug).

In most countries, ronidazole is not approved for use in companion animals and is rarely used in other animal species. Therefore, obtaining ronidazole for use in cats can represent a challenge for the small animal clinician. Powders containing ronidazole might be available in some countries and are typically intended to treat trichomoniasis in pigeons, but due to the extreme bitterness of ronidazole it is almost impossible to administer sufficient quantities of these formulations to cats. The safer, more accurate, and currently recommended method of administering ronidazole to cats is to use 100% pure, chemical grade ronidazole in capsule form obtained from specific pharmacies. Therefore, ronidazole should be purchased from reputable pharmacies after obtaining signed informed owner consent.

The most commonly used ronidazole treatment protocol for the treatment of *T. blagburni*–associated diarrhoea in cats is 30 mg/kg PO every 24 hours for 14 days (see Appendix). In some cases, clinical signs may relapse after discontinuation of treatment, and an additional treatment cycle is required. Neurological signs (e.g. depression, ataxia, weakness) can be seen in a small number of cats treated with ronidazole (especially if higher doses are used), but they usually resolve after discontinuation of the drug. Due to this potentially serious side effect, treatment with ronidazole should be reserved for cats with confirmed *T. blagburni* infection, and these cats should be closely monitored during treatment with ronidazole. For the same reason, therapeutic trials in cats with unconfirmed *T. blagburni* infections are not recommended.

Typically, *T. blagburni*–associated diarrhoea resolves or at least improves with ronidazole treatment. However, both in vivo and in vitro resistance of feline *T. blagburni* isolates to ronidazole has been shown, and therefore some cats may not respond to ronidazole treatment. Response to treatment should ideally be based on PCR testing 1–2 weeks after completion of the treatment. Since a negative PCR result does not definitively exclude the infection, other causes of diarrhoea should be considered in cats with a negative PCR result and persistence of clinical sings. Culture or direct faecal smear examination should not be used because these tests are even less sensitive, and negative results do not confirm parasitological cure. Because even asymptomatic cats may be infected, reinfection of treated cats is possible and sometimes difficult to prevent in multicat households if not all cats are receiving treatment. Finally, because coinfections with other parasites are relatively common (especially with *Giardia* sp.), identification and appropriate treatment of the coexisting parasitic infections is crucial.

It has been recommended that ronidazole should not be used in cats that are systemically severely ill, in very young kittens (<12 weeks of age), and in pregnant or nursing queens, as the safety of ronidazole in these cats is questionable. In a recent study of a group of pedigree cats with poor health conditions and *T. blagburni* and other parasitic infections in an animal shelter, rodinazole led to improvement of clinical signs. However, several cats developed neurological signs that disappeared when the treatment was discontinued. Other clinical signs such as anorexia, vomiting, and depression were also noted in some cats. The authors concluded that ronidazole can be used in cats with other systemic conditions if the benefit is high (e.g. if clinical resolution of signs will lead to adoption of the cat) and if there is close monitoring of the cats.

Zoonotic potential

Several trichomonad species, both pathogenic and nonpathogenic, have been found in humans. However, only a small number of isolated reports of *T. blagburni* infection in humans exist in the literature. These are almost exclusively described in people with severe concurrent diseases or immunosuppression. In addition, the contribution of *T. blagburni* infection in the clinical disease in those cases cannot always be confirmed.[1–5,7,12–21] The first report was a case of *T. blagburni*–associated meningoencephalitis in a recipient of allogeneic peripheral blood stem cell transplantation. In another case, *T. blagburni*–like microorganisms were identified in the bronchoalveolar lavage sample of a patient with AIDS. Infection of healthy humans by *T. blagburni* has not been reported, but it cannot be excluded. Therefore, people handling cats infected with *T. blagburni* should take measures to prevent possible transmission.

Take-home messages

- Helminthic and parasitic diseases are common in cats, and particularly common and clinically important in kittens and young cats.
- Diagnostic investigation for gastrointestinal disease should always include tests and therapeutic trials for intestinal parasites early in the diagnostic workup.
- Some of the gastrointestinal parasites mentioned in this chapter may be difficult to eliminate.
- Many of the gastrointestinal parasites of the cat are of zoonotic importance.

REFERENCES

[1] Bowman DD et al. *Feline Clinical Parasitology*. Ames, Iowa State University Press, 2002.

[2] Ettinger SJ, Feldman EC, Côté E, editors. *Textbook of Veterinary Internal Medicine*, 8th ed. St Louis, Elsevier, 2017.

[3] Norsworthy GD, editor. *The Feline Patient*, 5th ed. Hoboken, Wiley Blackwell, 2018.

[4] Washabau RJ, Day MJ, editors. *Canine and Feline Gastroenterology*. St Louis, Elsevier Saunders, 2013.

[5] Nagamori Y et al. Retrospective survey of parasitism identified in feces of client-owned cats in North America from 2007 through 2018. *Vet Parasitol* 277:109008, 2020.

[6] Rubinsky-Elefant G et al. Human toxocariasis: diagnosis, worldwide seroprevalences and clinical expression of the systemic and ocular forms. *Ann Trop Med Parasitol* 104:3, 2010.

[7] Scorza AV, Lappin MR. Gastrointestinal protozoal infections. In: August JR, editor. *Consultations in Feline Internal Medicine*, 6th ed. St Louis, Saunders Elsevier: 201, 2010.

[8] Dubey JP. A review of *Cystoisospora felis* and *C. rivolta*–induced coccidiosis in cats. *Vet Parasitol* 263:34, 2018.

[9] Ballweber LR et al. Giardiasis in dogs and cats: update on epidemiology and public health significance. *Trends Parasitol* 26:180, 2010.

[10] Gruffydd-Jones T et al. Giardiasis in cats: ABCD guidelines on prevention and management. *J Feline Med Surg* 15:650, 2013.

[11] Ramírez-Ocampo S et al. Prevalence of zoonotic and non-zoonotic genotypes of *Giardia intestinalis* in cats: a systematic review and meta-analysis. *Infez Med* 25:326, 2017.

[12] Gookin JL, Hanrahan K, Levy MG. The conundrum of feline trichomonosis: the more we learn the "trickier" it gets. *J Feline Med Surg* 19:261, 2017.

[13] Dąbrowska J et al. Whole genome sequencing of a feline strain of *Tritrichomonas foetus* reveals massive genetic differences to bovine and porcine isolates. *Int J Parasitol* 50:227, 2020.

[14] Hinney B et al. Efficacy and safety of ronidazole treatment against *Tritrichomonas foetus* in a cat colony with multiple disorders. *Vet Parasitol Reg Stud Reports* 18:100344, 2019.

[15] Zanzani SA et al. Coinfection with *Tritrichomonas foetus* and *Giardia duodenalis* in two cats with chronic diarrhea. *Case Rep Vet Med* 2016:5705168, 2016.

[16] Bissett SA et al. Feline diarrhoea associated with *Tritrichomonas* cf. *foetus* and *Giardia* co-infection in an Australian cattery. *Aust Vet J* 86:440, 2008.

[17] Foster DM et al. Outcome of cats with diarrhea and *Tritrichomonas foetus* infection. *J Am Vet Med Assoc* 225:888, 2004.

[18] Gookin JL et al. Prevalence of and risk factors for feline *Tritrichomonas foetus* and *Giardia* infection. *J Clin Microbiol* 42:2707, 2004.

[19] Gookin JL et al. Efficacy of ronidazole for treatment of feline *Tritrichomonas foetus* infection. *J Vet Intern Med* 20:536, 2006.

[20] Rosado TW, Specht A, Marks SL. Neurotoxicosis in 4 cats receiving ronidazole. *J Vet Intern Med* 21:328, 2007.

[21] Xenoulis PG et al. Intestinal *Tritrichomonas foetus* infection in cats: a retrospective study of 104 cases. *J Feline Med Surg* 15:1098, 2013.

CHAPTER 16

Microbiota and dysbiosis

Jan Suchodolski

The gastrointestinal (GI) tract harbours a highly diverse ecosystem consisting of various microorganisms (i.e. viruses, bacteria, fungi, and protozoa). This collection of microbes is termed intestinal microbiota when referring to the taxonomy (i.e. who is there?) and microbiome when referring to their gene content and function (i.e. what are they doing?). Of those microbes, bacteria are the largest component. A diverse and balanced intestinal microbiome plays an important role in maintaining host health, as it influences the immune system, defends against enteropathogens, and provides many metabolic and nutritional functions that directly benefit the host. These interactions between the intestinal microbiome and immune system are mediated through direct contact between bacterial components and immune cells (e.g. dendritic cells, toll-like receptors) and through microbiota-derived metabolites that activate immune function through various receptors. The commensal intestinal microbiome is of importance for the development and homoeostasis of gut structure and function, as shown by the fact that mice raised in a germ-free environment exhibit an altered epithelial architecture (e.g. decreased number of lymphoid follicles) and an underdeveloped immune system. The microbiota is important in early life for establishing oral tolerance in order to prevent onset of inappropriate immune responses against luminal bacteria and food antigens, which have been associated with chronic GI inflammation.

Recent research has shown that the intestinal microbiome also affects many other organ systems. Alterations in the intestinal microbiome are associated with intestinal disease, and also with various extraintestinal disorders such as diabetes mellitus, obesity, chronic kidney disease (CKD), and also neurological disorders.[1] At this point, many of the underlying mechanisms, and how they are applicable to clinical practice, remain unclear. Nevertheless, much progress has been made in understanding the intricate relationship between the host and the intestinal microbiome, and the important contributions of a balanced intestinal microbiome to health.

THE GUT MICROBIOME AS METABOLIC ORGAN

The intestinal microbiome is considered an important metabolic organ since bacteria produce metabolites that have direct beneficial effects on the host when in proper concentrations. For example, dietary carbohydrates are fermented by the intestinal microbiome into short-chain fatty acids (SCFAs), which are immunomodulatory and have various other functions (see below for more details). Other metabolites such as indole, from tryptophan degradation, and secondary bile acids (BAs) also have immunomodulatory properties and are important for strengthening the intestinal barrier function.[2]

Other external components such as drugs will be metabolised by the intestinal microbiome, and the byproducts are then absorbed by the host. These metabolites are mostly beneficial, but under certain circumstances, such as increased concentrations or when the normal microbiota is altered (intestinal dysbiosis), they can also have deleterious effects on the host, as some of these bacterial-derived metabolites may be toxic or irritating to the intestinal epithelial cells, causing inflammation or diarrhoea. Table 16.1 summarises some of the beneficial and deleterious effects of bacterial-derived metabolites, while below are some detailed examples for major metabolic pathways. Of particular interest is also that each animal has different abundances of bacterial taxa (Fig. 16.1). This individual composition may cause individual responses for each animal to diet, prebiotics, probiotics, and also how drugs are metabolised.

Short-chain fatty acids

Dietary fibres such as cellulose, pectin, and inulin are major nutrient sources for bacteria. Fermentation of these fibres by bacteria results in the production of SCFAs and other metabolites. SCFAs, primarily acetate, propionate,

Table 16.1. Examples of beneficial and deleterious metabolic pathways by the intestinal microbiome and effects on the feline host.

Source	Bacteria involved	Microbial metabolite	Effects on the host	
			Beneficial (in normal concentrations)	Potentially deleterious (in abnormal concentrations)
Carbohydrates from diet	Various (e.g. *Faecalibacterium* spp.)	Fermentation to SCFAs	Anti-inflammatory Barrier function Regulate intestinal motility Provide systemic and local energy	Abnormal SCFA ratio can activate virulence factors of enteropathogens
Primary BAs from liver	Mostly *Clostridium hiranonis* in cats	Transformation to secondary BAs	Anti-inflammatory Secondary BAs inhibit growth of *Clostridioides* (*Clostridium*) *difficile* Modulate glucose secretion	Increased primary BAs can lead to secretory diarrhoea Decreased secondary BAs leads to dysbiosis
Tryptophan from diet	Various	Indole metabolites	Anti-inflammatory. Maintain intestinal barrier function	In increased concentrations: cytotoxic, putrefactive Indoxyl sulphate acts as uraemic toxin
Tyrosine and phenylalanine from diet	Various	p-Cresol		Acts as uraemic toxin and leads to progression of chronic kidney disease

BA, bile acid; SCFA, short-chain fatty acid.

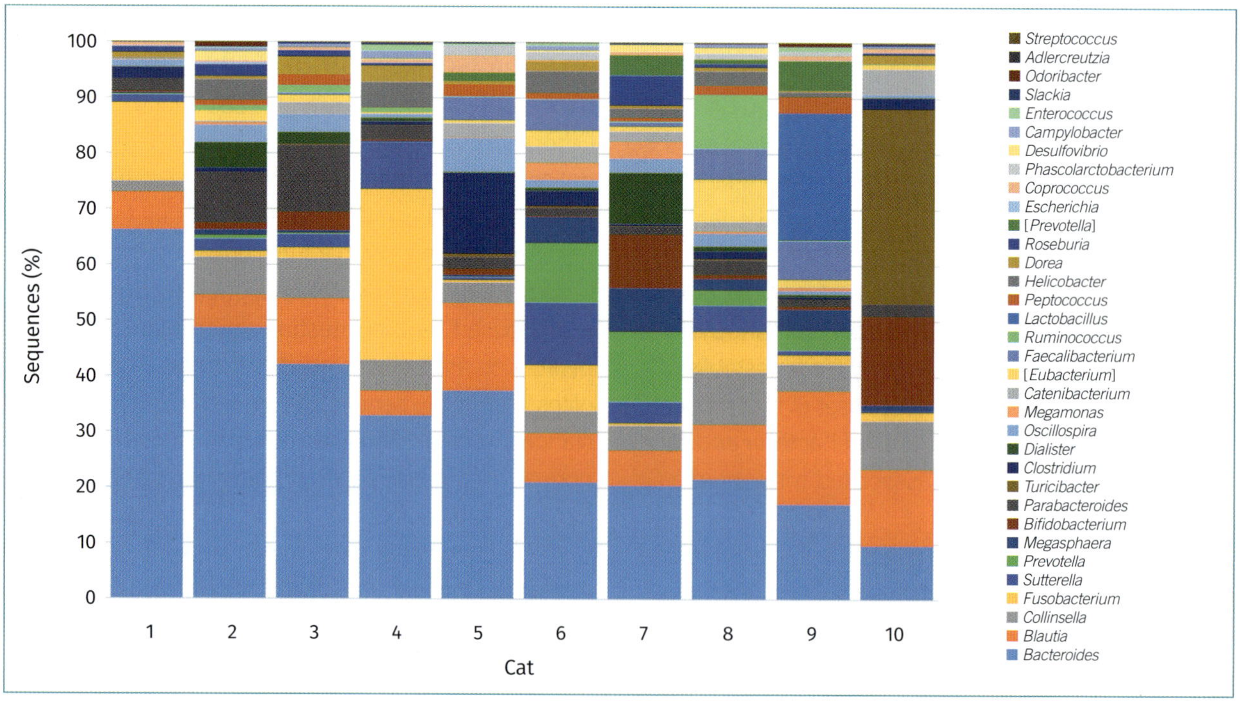

Figure 16.1. Predominant bacterial genera and individual differences in the faecal microbiota of healthy cats. Each healthy cat shows a unique distribution of bacteria in the colon. The individual microbiota composition will influence microbial function and therefore how each cat may respond to the same diet, fibres, and probiotics.

and butyrate, are produced through multiple pathways and through the combined efforts of various bacterial taxa. Approximately 90%–95% of the SCFAs produced in the intestinal lumen are then rapidly absorbed. The absorption of SCFAs leads to additional absorption of water, providing an antidiarrhoeal effect. Butyrate is an important energy source for epithelial cells in the intestine. There are additional health benefits, as SCFAs modulate intestinal motility, intestinal permeability, and decrease pro-inflammatory cytokines.

Bile acid metabolism

BA metabolism is an important pathway that involves microbiota transformation, with important implications on host health across various animal species, such as rodents, humans, dogs, and likely also cats.[3] Briefly, the primary BAs, cholic acid and chenodeoxycholic acid, are released into the intestinal lumen, aiding fat digestion. Reabsorption of BAs takes place in the ileum through the apical sodium-dependent bile acid transporter (ASBT), leading to enterohepatic circulation. A small proportion of BAs (5%–10%) enters the large intestine, where bacterial species (mostly *Clostridium hiranonis* in dogs and cats) convert the primary BAs to the secondary BAs deoxycholic acid and lithocholic acid. BAs are agonists for various receptors in the metabolism of cholesterol and carbohydrates. Furthermore, activation of the TGR5 receptor through secondary BAs, which is present on many cell types and various organs, results in downregulation of inflammation and secretion of glucagon-like peptide 1 (GLP-1), which helps in the regulation of insulin.

In humans and dogs with intestinal inflammation, an altered BA metabolism may contribute to diarrhoea. Approximately 50%–60% of dogs with chronic enteropathy (CE) have a decreased abundance of *C. hiranonis*, the main converter of primary to secondary BAs, and therefore decreased secondary BAs.[4] In preliminary studies, an altered BA metabolism has also been demonstrated in a subset of cats with CEs, although the prevalence appears to be lower compared to dogs, as a decreased abundance of *C. hiranonis* was observed in 13/60 (22%) cats (unpublished data).

In cats, use of broad-spectrum antibiotics such as clindamycin and amoxicillin–clavulanate has been shown to reduce the abundance of *C. hiranonis*, thereby preventing the conversion of primary to secondary BAs.[5]

ASSESSMENT OF THE INTESTINAL MICROBIOME

Obtaining a comprehensive assessment of the entire intestinal microbiome is challenging. It remains difficult to cultivate intestinal bacteria, as most species in the feline gut are strict or facultative anaerobes (e.g. *Bacteroidetes, Ruminococcus, Faecalibacterium, Fusobacterium, Clostridiales*).[6] Furthermore, there are differences in microbial composition along the upper and lower GI tract, and differences in luminal vs. mucosa-adherent bacterial populations. Moreover, there is much overlap in bacterial taxa present between healthy and diarrhoeic cats. Also, the same bacterial taxa may express, depending on the surrounding intestinal environment, different genes and therefore different virulence factors and metabolic functions. For example, a disrupted microbiota due to antibiotics or intestinal inflammation allows potential enteropathogens such as *Escherichia coli* to induce diarrhoea, as has been shown in kittens with experimentally induced *E. coli* infection.[7] In humans and dogs, the germination of *Clostridioides* (*Clostridium*) *difficile* (*C. diff*) spores is promoted by a disrupted microbiota and consequently a reduction in secondary and increase in primary BAs. When dysbiosis is present in dogs (e.g. due to intestinal inflammation or antibiotic use), it may lead to lack of *C. hiranonis*, lack of conversion from primary to secondary BAs, and therefore proliferation of *C. diff*. In an unpublished dataset from the author's laboratory, approximately 26% (315/1194) of dogs with chronic diarrhoea were positive for *C. diff*, and 80% of these lacked the BA-converting bacterium *C. hiranonis*. A similar relationship exists in cats, although cats with CE have a lower prevalence of *C. diff* (11%; 64/584) compared to dogs. Therefore, the overgrowth of *C. diff* may reflect the dysbiotic gut environment in CEs rather than being a primary cause of intestinal disease.

Bacterial culture

The majority of intestinal bacteria in the colon are strict anaerobes. In the small intestine, while dogs have a mix of aerobic and anaerobic bacteria, cats appear to have a more anaerobic flora.[8] Therefore, with the use of routine bacterial culture as performed in diagnostic laboratories, only a small percentage of bacteria can be grown. Hence, the actual number of bacterial taxa is vastly underestimated by bacterial culture, and consequently species that are cultured are often erroneously considered as being clinically more significant (e.g. *E. coli*). Therefore, bacterial culture has limited value when describing the intestinal microbiota and is not able to identify intestinal dysbiosis. However, bacterial culture remains an important test for antibiotic susceptibility of those few cultivable organisms that are known to be associated with intestinal infections (i.e. *Campylobacter jejuni* and *Salmonella* spp.).

Molecular methods

Culture-independent methods such as broad sequencing of the bacterial 16S rRNA gene allow for a more comprehensive characterisation of the intestinal microbiota, but these methods are mostly used for research studies only. While some companies offer such microbiome assessment tests on a commercial basis for individual animals, these have not been properly validated for diagnostic use in cats, and there are no standardised protocols for DNA extraction, selection of PCR primers, and sequencing platforms, making it difficult to properly compare results across the different commercial platforms. Furthermore, there are currently no published reference intervals for cats, making the interpretation of the results difficult.

Studies comparing the faecal microbiome of dogs and cats fed species-appropriate commercial diets found that cats had a larger number of bacterial species than dogs, hinting at a higher microbial diversity.[9] However, more studies are needed to confirm this finding. Based on 16S rRNA gene sequencing, the major bacterial groups found in the healthy feline intestine belong to the phyla *Bacteroidetes* (*Bacteroides*, *Prevotella*), *Firmicutes* (e.g. *Lactobacillales*, *Clostridiales*), and *Fusobacteria* (various *Fusobacterium* spp.) (Figs. 16.1 and 16.2). There is a difference in the proportion of these bacterial taxa along the length of the intestine, with *Lactobacillales* being more abundant in the jejunum and *Clostridiales* being more abundant in the colon.[10] The intestine of healthy cats also harbours various fungal organisms, with the majority of them belonging to the family Saccharomycetaceae.[9]

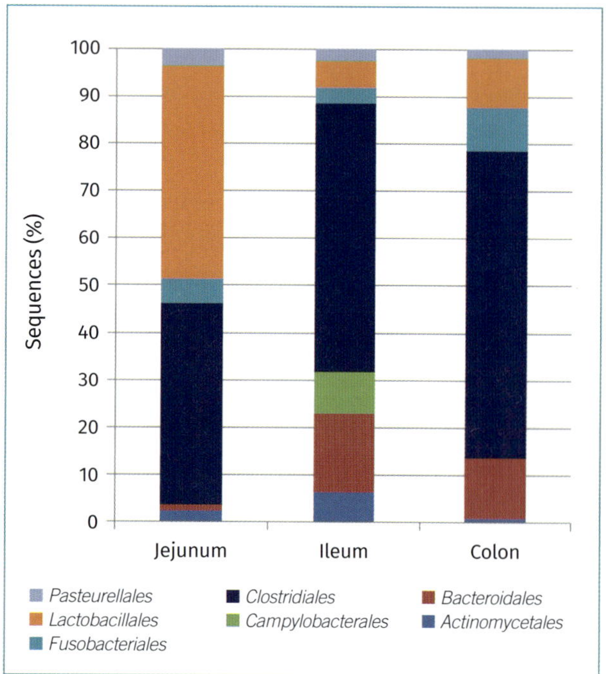

Figure 16.2. Variation in microbiota composition along the intestine of healthy cats.

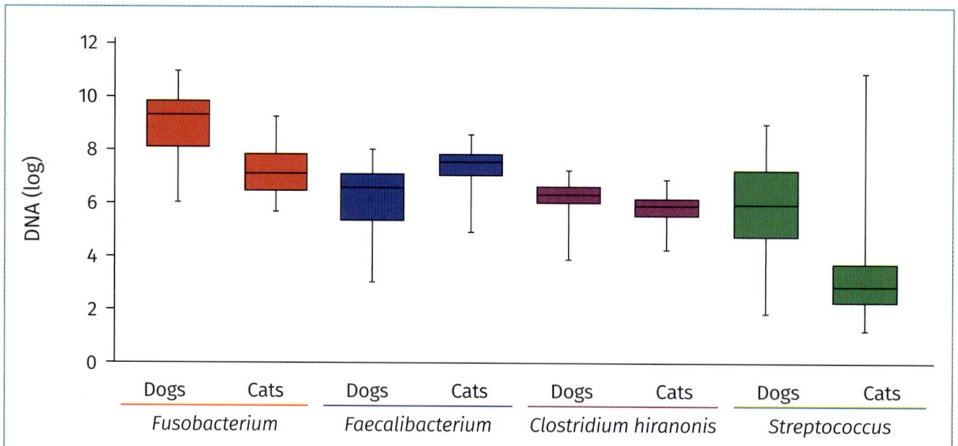

Figure 16.3. Differences in abundance of important bacterial taxa between dogs (n = 60) and cats (n = 60) evaluated by a validated quantitative polymerase chain reaction assay.

A rapid quantitative polymerase chain reaction (qPCR) assay that measures the abundance of key bacterial taxa within canine faecal samples and expresses the data as a dysbiosis index has been validated for use in dogs.[11] This assay allows for assessment of an abnormal microbiota. While this test has not yet been validated for clinical diagnostic use in cats, it allows to show the abundance of some important bacterial taxa in dogs and cats (Figs. 16.3 and 16.4), illustrating differences in microbial composition between both species. The clinical relevance of these differences is currently unknown.

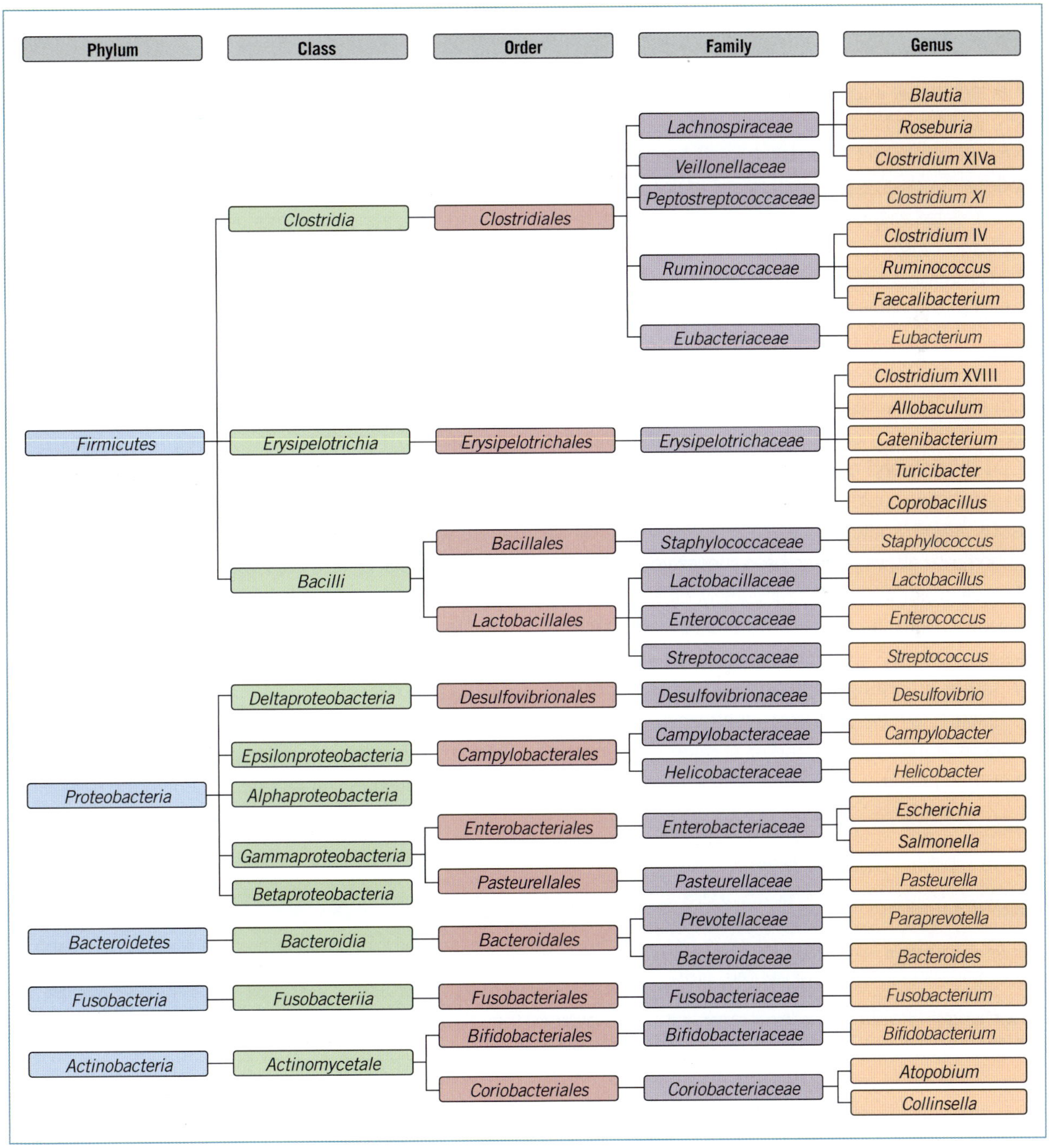

Figure 16.4. Cladogram showing the most important bacterial taxa present in the gastrointestinal tract of the cat.[12]

Emerging techniques for assessment of abnormal microbiota location or function

It becomes more apparent that some forms of intestinal disease are caused by mucosa-adherent or invasive bacterial populations. Intestinal biopsy, using fluorescence in situ hybridisation (FISH), allow to determine the localisation of bacteria within the intestinal tissue and whether they are mucosa adherent. Studies have shown that some cats with CEs have higher than normal attachment of bacteria to the intestinal mucosa. It has been shown that cats with inflammatory bowel disease (IBD) have increased numbers of *Enterobacteriaceae* adherent to the duodenal mucosa, and numbers of *Enterobacteriaceae* also correlated with changes in mucosal architecture.[13] *E. coli* and *Clostridium* spp. also correlated with intestinal inflammation, suggesting that alterations in intestinal bacteria contribute to the pathophysiology of IBD in cats. Cats with small-cell GI lymphoma had also increased numbers of mucosa-attached *Fusobacterium* sp. in the ileum and colon when compared to cats with IBD, and *Fusobacterium* sp. correlated with increased expression of CD11b$^+$ cells and nuclear factor kappa B (NF-κB).[14] This association could suggest a potential contribution of *Fusobacterium* sp. to the development of small-cell GI lymphoma in cats, as has also been suggested in humans, but requires further study. Unfortunately, FISH is currently not widely available, but may be a useful approach to assess mucosa-adherent bacteria in the future.

Another emerging approach to assess abnormal microbiota is to measure the concentration of microbial-derived metabolites as a marker of microbial function rather than changes in bacterial species. For example, an increase in serum trimethylamine N-oxide (TMAO), a bacterial product of microbial metabolism of dietary compounds (i.e. choline and L-carnitine), is associated with atherosclerosis and cardiovascular disease in humans and with chronic heart failure in dogs.[15] Bacterial metabolites such as p-cresol and indoxyl sulphate (Table 16.1) act as uraemic toxins, leading to further damage to the kidneys, and serum concentrations correlate with progression of CKD.[16]

MICROBIOTA DYSBIOSIS

Changes in the intestinal microbiota are defined as dysbiosis. This can include changes in the total bacterial abundance, increase in mucosa-adherent bacteria, and overall changes in total microbiota composition or in a few specific bacterial species. Furthermore, dysbiosis should also be understood as a potential change in microbiota function, with alterations in microbial-derived metabolites (Table 16.2). These metabolic changes can be associated with or without measurable shifts in microbiota composition. For example, decreases in bacterial groups that produce SCFAs correlated with a reduction in total amounts of SCFAs in dogs with CEs.[4] In contrast, while there was an increase in serum concentrations of the bacterial metabolites p-cresol and indoxyl sulphate in cats with CKD, this was not linked with measurable shifts in the faecal microbiota composition.[16]

Alterations of the intestinal microbiome

Alterations in the composition, diversity, and/or function is termed dysbiosis. It can be present in the small and/

Table 16.2. Different patterns of dysbiosis.

Major types of dysbiosis	Possible consequences
Abnormal substrate in intestinal lumen (e.g. undigested nutrients in maldigestion, inappropriate diets, drugs)	Increase in metabolites that lead to osmotic or secretory diarrhoea (e.g. conversion of dietary fatty acids to hydroxystearic acids) Microbial-derived metabolites of the drug mycophenolate mofetil cause diarrhoea
Loss of microbiota function due to loss of commensal bacteria (e.g. *Clostridium hiranonis*)	No conversion from primary to secondary bile acids leads to increase in *Clostridioides* (*Clostridium*) *difficile* abundance and dysbiosis
Increase in total bacterial abundance	More bacteria available for production of deleterious microbial metabolites Increased inflammatory immune response
Increase in mucosa-adherent bacteria	Increased attachment of bacteria to intestinal mucosa causes increased inflammatory immune response

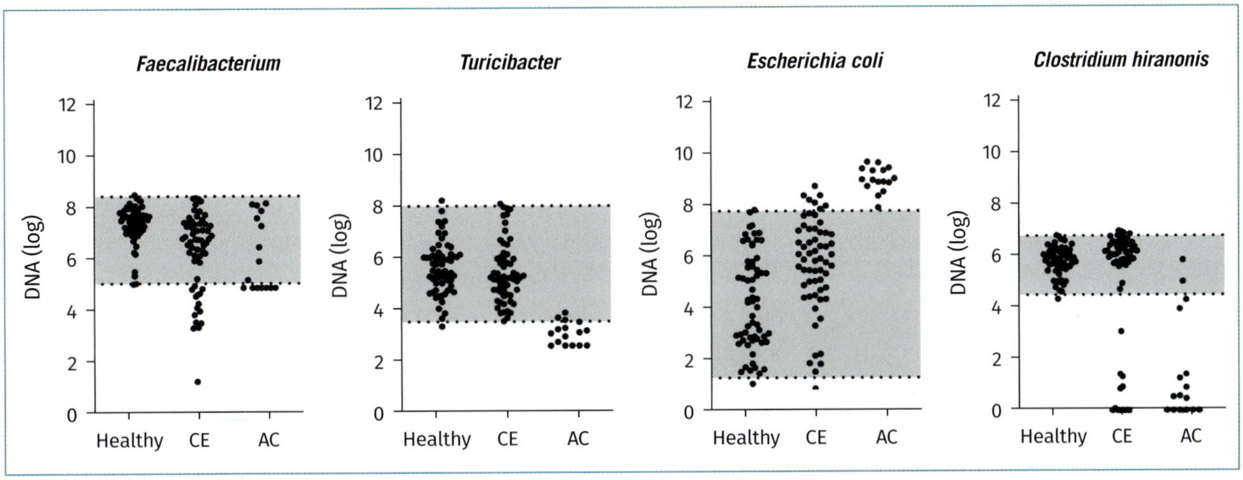

Figure 16.5. Differences in important bacterial taxa between healthy cats (n = 60), cats with chronic enteropathy (CE; n = 60), and healthy cats after 7 days of amoxicillin–clavulanate (AC; n = 16). The grey area in each graph corresponds to the reference interval. Only few cats with CE have an abundance of bacterial taxa outside the reference interval. In contrast, antibiotic administration has a major impact on many bacterial taxa.

or large intestine. To date, only few studies have been performed in cats, and therefore much remains to be determined regarding dysbiosis patterns in cats.

Administration of broad-spectrum antimicrobials such as metronidazole and tylosin have been shown to induce dysbiosis in healthy and diseased dogs.[17] While no studies with these two antimicrobials have been performed in cats, due to similarities in microbiota composition (i.e. presence of similar bacterial taxa), it is likely that the same antibiotics would also induce microbial alterations in cats. A few studies have specifically evaluated the impact of antimicrobials on the feline microbiota and metabolome in healthy cats. In one study, healthy cats received amoxicillin–clavulanate (62.5 mg/cat every 12 hours) for 7 days with either a probiotic (*Enterococcus faecium* SF68) or a placebo.[5] The antibiotic induced major changes in the intestinal microbiota in all cats, independent of whether they received the probiotic or the placebo. Figure 16.5 illustrates a decrease in the number of beneficial bacteria such as *Faecalibacterium*, *Turicibacter*, and *C. hiranonis*. In contrast, the abundance of *E. coli* increased during antibiotic administration. While most bacterial taxa returned to baseline levels 7 days after the end of administration, some taxa (e.g. *Peptococcus*, *Dialister*) remained altered at the end of the study. Antimicrobial administration was also associated with worsening faecal scores in up to 80% of cats. Cats receiving the probiotic had significantly better total diarrhoea scores but had the same microbial alterations as cats receiving the placebo. In another study, 16 healthy research cats received clindamycin (150 mg/day) for 21 days, with either a probiotic or a placebo.[18] Clindamycin induced major shifts in the microbiota and decreased microbial diversity in both treatment groups, with incomplete normalisation of some taxa even after 2 years. The numbers of *Bifidobacterium*, *Bacteroides*, *Blautia*, and *Faecalibacterium* were decreased, while *Clostridiaceae* and *Enterobacteriaceae* populations were increased. Furthermore, these microbial changes were associated with functional changes in the metabolome such as disruptions in the SCFA, BA, and indole pathways.

In dogs and humans, administration of the proton pump inhibitor omeprazole induces microbiota changes. In one study, omeprazole was administered to six healthy research cats.[19] While no changes in global microbiome structure or richness were observed, some bacterial taxa underwent transient changes: increases in *Streptococcus*, *Lactobacillus*, *Clostridium*, and *Faecalibacterium* and decreases in *Bifidobacterium*. No major changes were observed in the faecal metabolome during omeprazole administration.

Microbiome dysbiosis has been reported in cats with CEs. Earlier studies have enumerated bacterial taxa in faeces using FISH and reported decreased *Bifidobacte-*

rium and *Bacteroides* and increased *Desulfovibrio* abundances. Two studies evaluated the mucosa-adherent microbiota using FISH. One of these studies identified increased numbers of *E. coli* which correlated with intestinal inflammation in cats with IBD.[13] The other study observed increased numbers of mucosa-attached *Fusobacterium* sp. in the ileum and colon of cats with small-cell lymphoma when compared to cats with IBD.[14] Both studies suggested that the microbiota may play a role in IBD and small-cell lymphoma in cats, but further mechanistic studies are needed. Two studies evaluated the faecal microbiota of cats with CEs using 16S rRNA gene sequencing.[6,20] Both studies identified that the species richness was reduced in cats with CEs (Fig. 16.6). Only minor differences were observed in the overall microbiome structure, as there was strong overlap between samples from each group. Across both studies, common findings were decreased abundance of the SCFA-producing bacteria *Faecalibacterium*, *Bifidobacterium*, *Turicibacter*, and *Bacteroidaceae*, and increased abundance of *Enterobacteriaceae* and *Streptococcus*. Even though these findings have been confirmed in a validated qPCR assay for cats, overall, only few cats have altered abundances of these taxa outside the reference intervals for healthy cats, as seen in Figure 16.5. Decreased abundance of the BA-converting bacterium *C. hiranonis* is less common in cats than dogs with CEs (Fig. 16.5). This would suggest that cats with CEs have less frequently a faecal dysbiosis compared to dogs.

A few smaller studies have evaluated the faecal microbiome of obese cats. One study identified an increased *Firmicutes:Bacteroidetes* ratio in obese cats. After energy restriction, some members of the *Firmicutes* phylum were reduced. Another study evaluated the microbiota before and after caloric restriction with a moderate-protein, high-fibre diet and observed an increase in *Actinobacteria* and a decrease in *Bacteroidetes* abundances after weight loss. Clearly, more studies are needed to understand whether there is an association between intestinal microbiota and obesity in cats. In humans, the microbiota is thought to be a contributing factor to metabolic syndrome. In a study evaluating the faecal microbiota in diabetic cats,[21] cats with diabetes mellitus had lower bacterial diversity compared to lean cats, as

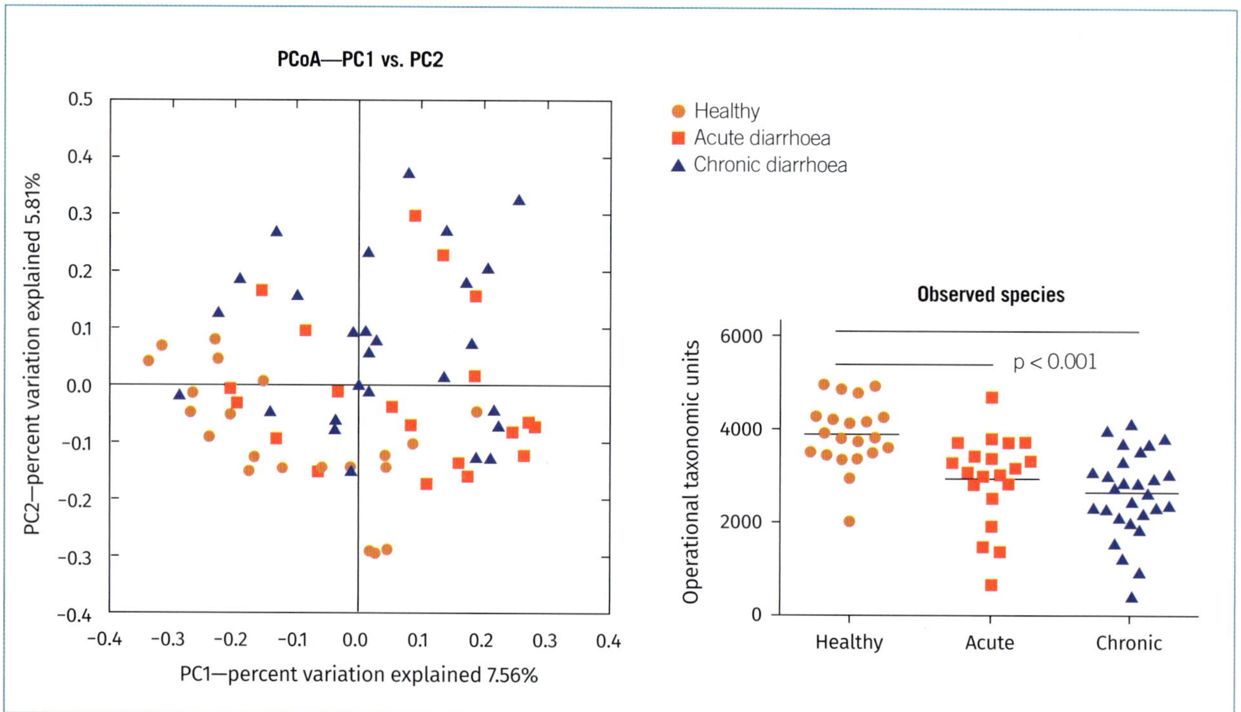

Figure 16.6. Comparison in microbiota structure (left) and microbial diversity (right) between healthy cats and cats with acute or chronic diarrhoea. Cats with intestinal disease have altered microbiota composition. Data based on Suchodolski et al. (2015).[20]

well as lower proportions of *Anaerotruncus*, *Dialister*, and SCFA-producing *Ruminococcaceae*. Serum fructosamine levels correlated negatively with the proportion of *Prevotellaceae* and positively with that of *Enterobacteriaceae*.

One study evaluating the faecal microbiota and selected bacterial-derived metabolites in cats with CKD found decreased microbial diversity in cats with CKD but no significant difference in the microbiota structure.[16] However, cats with CKD had increased serum concentration of the uraemic toxin indoxyl sulphate, which is derived from bacterial metabolism of the amino acid tryptophan, suggesting functional changes in the gut microbiome of cats with CKD.

THERAPEUTIC APPROACH TO DYSBIOSIS

The intestinal microbiome can be modulated by various complementary approaches, such as dietary modulation (see Chapter 39), antimicrobials (see Chapter 34), pre- and probiotics (see Chapter 36), and faecal microbiota transplantation (see Chapter 37). It is important to assess and, if possible, eliminate the underlying disease. Dietary modulation should always be part of the treatment. A highly digestible diet reduces undigested substrate within the intestinal lumen that would allow bacterial overgrowth. In addition, in CE, a novel or hydrolysed protein diet may reduce the host inflammatory response, a major driver of dysbiosis. In many cases of food-responsive enteropathy, this may be sufficient to achieve clinical response, with gradual improvement of mucosal inflammation and reduction of dysbiosis over several weeks or months (see Chapters 38 and 39 for more details).

Probiotics are live microorganisms that confer a health benefit to the host when administered in adequate amounts. Probiotics have only a minor impact on the total microbiota composition, but studies have shown that they may promote immune modulation, inhibit pathogens, and strengthen the intestinal barrier (see Chapter 36).

Prebiotics are indigestible carbohydrates that can be used selectively by microorganisms and therefore promote host health. In general, prebiotics can be classified as soluble vs. nonsoluble and fermentable vs. nonfermentable. Prebiotics are primarily fibre from the diet, such as fructooligosaccharides, pectins, inulin, resistant starches, beta-glucans, and various others. They may be of benefit to the host by selectively promoting growth and/or function of bacterial species already present in the colon. Dietary fibres have other functions in the GI tract. A commonly used fibre is psyllium, which has water- and BA-binding properties, thereby leading to improved faecal consistency and increased epithelial mucus production (see Chapter 36).

Antimicrobials are often used in chronic GI diseases and can lead to improvement of clinical signs, but some patients tend to relapse after antimicrobial cessation, often requiring long-term antimicrobial treatment. A possible explanation is that some animals with CE have increased bacterial load in the small intestine or increased numbers of mucosa-adherent bacteria,[13] causing a pro-inflammatory host response. Treatment with antibiotics leads to a reduction in the population of these bacteria and improvement of clinical signs. However, because the microbiome is an ecosystem, bacteria often regrow after antibiotic cessation, leading to relapse of clinical signs. Antibiotics also promote the development of antimicrobial resistance and often cause alterations in the intestinal microbiota that can last for weeks or months. Because of these negative effects, antibiotics should not be used as a first-line treatment in GI disease, but rather be considered in chronic patients that failed dietary and anti-inflammatory trials or in acute cases with signs of systemic inflammation (see Chapter 34).

Take-home messages

- The intestinal microbiome is an immune and metabolic organ with important influence on the gastrointestinal tract and other organ systems.
- Cats with chronic enteropathies appear to have less frequently a faecal dysbiosis, when compared to dogs.
- Increased abundance of mucosa-adherent bacteria in the intestine is associated with feline inflammatory bowel disease and small-cell lymphoma.
- Abnormal microbial function is associated with diabetes mellitus and chronic kidney disease.
- The therapeutic approach to intestinal dysbiosis needs to be evaluated in clinical studies.

REFERENCES

[1] Pilla R, Suchodolski JS. The role of the canine gut microbiome and metabolome in health and gastrointestinal disease. *Front Vet Sci* 6:498, 2020.

[2] Hang S et al. Bile acid metabolites control T_H17 and T_{reg} cell differentiation. *Nature* 576:143, 2019.

[3] Duboc H et al. Connecting dysbiosis, bile-acid dysmetabolism and gut inflammation in inflammatory bowel diseases. *Gut* 62:531, 2013.

[4] Minamoto Y et al. Fecal short-chain fatty acid concentrations and dysbiosis in dogs with chronic enteropathy. *J Vet Intern Med* 33:1608, 2019.

[5] Torres-Henderson C et al. Effect of *Enterococcus faecium* strain SF68 on gastrointestinal signs and fecal microbiome in cats administered amoxicillin-clavulanate. *Top Companion Anim Med* 32:104, 2017.

[6] Marsilio S et al. Characterization of the fecal microbiome in cats with inflammatory bowel disease or alimentary small cell lymphoma. *Sci Rep* 9:19208, 2019.

[7] Watson VE et al. Influence of the intestinal microbiota on disease susceptibility in kittens with experimentally-induced carriage of atypical enteropathogenic *Escherichia coli*. *Vet Microbiol* 231:197, 2019.

[8] Johnston K, Lamport A, Batt RM. An unexpected bacterial flora in the proximal small intestine of normal cats. *Vet Rec* 132:362, 1993.

[9] Handl S et al. Massive parallel 16S rRNA gene pyrosequencing reveals highly diverse fecal bacterial and fungal communities in healthy dogs and cats. *FEMS Microbiol Ecol* 76:301, 2011.

[10] Ritchie LE, Steiner JM, Suchodolski JS. Assessment of microbial diversity along the feline intestinal tract using 16S rRNA gene analysis. *FEMS Microbiol Ecol* 66:590, 2008.

[11] AlShawaqfeh MK et al. A dysbiosis index to assess microbial changes in fecal samples of dogs with chronic inflammatory enteropathy. *FEMS Microbiol Ecol* 93, 2017.

[12] Lyu Y et al. Past, present, and future of gastrointestinal microbiota research in cats. *Front Microbiol* 11:1661, 2020.

[13] Janeczko S et al. The relationship of mucosal bacteria to duodenal histopathology, cytokine mRNA, and clinical disease activity in cats with inflammatory bowel disease. *Vet Microbiol* 128:178, 2008.

[14] Garraway K et al. Relationship of the mucosal microbiota to gastrointestinal inflammation and small cell intestinal lymphoma in cats. *J Vet Intern Med* 32:1692, 2018.

[15] Karlin ET, Rush JE, Freeman LM. A pilot study investigating circulating trimethylamine N-oxide and its precursors in dogs with degenerative mitral valve disease with or without congestive heart failure. *J Vet Intern Med* 33:46, 2019.

[16] Summers SC et al. The fecal microbiome and serum concentrations of indoxyl sulfate and p-cresol sulfate in cats with chronic kidney disease. *J Vet Intern Med* 33:662, 2019.

[17] Pilla R et al. Effects of metronidazole on the fecal microbiome and metabolome in healthy dogs. *J Vet Intern Med* 34:1853, 2020.

[18] Whittemore JC et al. Short and long-term effects of a synbiotic on clinical signs, the fecal microbiome, and metabolomic profiles in healthy research cats receiving clindamycin: a randomized, controlled trial. *PeerJ* 6:e5130, 2018.

[19] Schmid SM et al. Omeprazole minimally alters the fecal microbial community in six cats: a pilot study. *Front Vet Sci* 5:79, 2018.

[20] Suchodolski JS et al. The fecal microbiome in cats with diarrhea. *PLoS One* 10:e0127378, 2015.

[21] Kieler IN et al. Diabetic cats have decreased gut microbial diversity and a lack of butyrate producing bacteria. *Sci Rep* 9:4822, 2019.

CHAPTER **17**

Pathogenesis of feline inflammatory bowel disease

Karin Allenspach, Chelsea Iennarella-Servantez

The pathogenesis of inflammatory bowel disease (IBD) in cats is unknown, although most evidence points to the involvement of a dysregulated immune response in the intestinal mucosa, a dysbiosis of the microbiome, and environmental factors (e.g. food antigens) playing a role in the development of the disease. In particular, a long-term dysbiosis of the microbiome is hypothesised to worsen the inflammation in the intestine, which can eventually lead to the development of low-grade intestinal T-cell lymphoma (LGITL). Furthermore, the possibility that ascending bacterial infections in cats with IBD can lead to the development of neutrophilic cholangiohepatitis and, possibly, pancreatitis (triaditis) needs to be considered in the workup of feline IBD cases.

Treatment for IBD in cats is directed at changing dietary food antigens by the use of elimination diets or hydrolysed diets. Immunosuppressive treatment with glucocorticosteroids is also warranted, which can be escalated to include low-dose chemotherapy treatment with chlorambucil to achieve clinical remission.

HOST IMMUNE FACTORS

Intestinal inflammation and expression of cytokines

In contrast to IBD and chronic enteropathies (CEs) in dogs, not many studies have investigated the involvement of specific cytokines in feline IBD. Most studies have attempted to discern a dominant expression profile of either T-helper (Th)1, Th2, or Th17 cytokines. These cytokines are pivotal host mucosal factors that can skew the immune response in order to adequately respond to a pathogen. In intestinal homoeostasis, or the normal case scenario, this usually means a dominant Th1 response resulting from intracellular infections (e.g. enteric viruses), a dominant Th2 response in the case of parasitic infections (e.g. helminths, protozoa), and a Th17 response in the case of bacterial infections. In the case of IBD, it is thought that these immune responses occur despite the fact that pathogens are absent and result in chronic idiopathic inflammation of the mucosa. In people with IBD, a predominant Th1 and Th17 cytokine profile has been identified in Crohn's disease, while a predominant Th2 cytokine profile is found in ulcerative colitis. In dogs with IBD, no particular mucosal cytokine profile has emerged, with the exception of interleukin (IL)-1β, an innate immunity cytokine that has consistently been found to be increased.[1] Similarly, studies on cytokine expression in the mucosa of cats with IBD have found conflicting results, and it is therefore still unclear whether there is a predominance of Th1 or Th2 cytokine expression in feline IBD.[2] For example, one study found increased transcription of genes encoding for both Th1 (IL-12p40, tumour necrosis factor alpha [TNF-α]) and Th2 cytokines (IL-6, IL-10, transforming growth factor beta [TGF-β]) and only concluded that an immune dysregulation is involved in feline IBD.[3] Another more recent study specifically evaluated Th1 and Th17 cytokines in the mucosa of cats with IBD and found an increase in IL-23p19 (Th17 cytokine) but a decrease in IL-12p35 (Th1 cytokine).[4] One pivotal paper by Janeczko et al. attempted a more comprehensive approach by evaluating histopathological severity, mucosa-adherent bacteria, and cytokine profiles in feline IBD.[5] An upregulation of IL-1, IL-8, and IL-12 mRNA was found and correlated with the number of mucosa-adherent *Enterobacteriaceae*, *Escherichia coli*, and *Clostridium* spp., but no distinct cytokine signature was seen. These findings would suggest that Th1 cytokines are more relevant in the pathogenesis of feline IBD, as is the innate cytokine IL-1, which has previously been found to be implicated in canine IBD as well. Interestingly, this study also found that mucosa-adherent bacteria, and particularly gram-negative bacteria, could play a role in the disease. These findings of increased bacteria attaching to the mucosa were later replicated in a study evaluating mucosa-adherent bacteria in cats diagnosed with either IBD or LGITL.[6] Furthermore, the study by Janeczko et al. also showed that mucosal architectural changes seem to be much more important in feline IBD than the inflammatory cell infiltrate itself. Another study that specifically evaluated mast cells in feline IBD found that these cells can be found in increased numbers in cats with IBD as compared to healthy cats.[7] This finding could be pointing towards a more pronounced Th2 cytokine pattern at least in some cases of feline IBD. Other factors that have been evaluated relate to the expression of P-glycoprotein, a drug efflux protein expressed in the intestine, and cyclooxygenase 2 (COX-2), an enzyme involved in the synthesis of pro-inflammatory prostaglandins,[8,9] both of which were found to be increased in feline IBD. This could point to the involvement of additional inflammatory pathways in feline IBD. The immunopathogenesis of feline IBD is explained in Figure 17.1.

Histopathology

Lymphoplasmacytic inflammatory bowel disease

The inflammation in feline IBD is most commonly lymphoplasmacytic, but various degrees of infiltration of eosinophils, neutrophils, and macrophages into the lamina propria can also be observed.[5,10] Interestingly, and similar to recent findings in canine IBD, the infiltration with various immune cells into the lamina propria may not be the most important histological finding. In fact, the World Small Animal Veterinary Association (WSAVA) Gastrointestinal Standardization Project has recognised that other factors, particularly mucosal architectural changes, are at least as important in the histological picture of feline IBD.[11] Such changes include villous stunting, crypt dilation and distortion, lacteal dilation, fibrosis, and increased intraepithelial lymphocyte counts. Lacteal dilation is seen much more rarely in cats with IBD as compared to canine IBD, but if it is present, it is usually associated with very severe IBD or LGITL.

Eosinophilic inflammatory bowel disease

Although eosinophilic IBD in cats is a condition that is seen much more rarely, there are a few case reports describing this form of intestinal inflammation. In general, clinical signs are similar to those reported in the lymphoplasmacytic form, with vomiting, diarrhoea, and weight loss being the most prominent clinical presentations. The definition of eosinophilic IBD is met when there is moderate to marked eosinophilic inflammation seen on histological examination (>10 eosinophils/HPF).[7] On physical examination, it is common to detect thickened intestinal loops on abdominal palpation. In addition, peripheral eosinophilia and/or eosinophilic infiltration in the mesenteric lymph nodes can also sometimes be found. On abdominal ultrasound, when compared to cases diagnosed with lymphoplasmacytic IBD, cases diagnosed with eosinophilic IBD had a greater mean jejunal wall thickness (3.34 mm ± 0.72 mm vs. 4.07 mm ± 0.58 mm, respectively) and an increased incidence of thickening of the muscularis layer of the mucosa (1/11 vs. 11/14, respectively).[12]

In some cases, when peripheral eosinophilia is present and various other organs are infiltrated with eosinophils, it has been proposed that eosinophilic IBD could be part of the feline hypereosinophilic syndrome.[13] Furthermore, feline gastrointestinal eosinophilic sclerosing fibroplasia should be a differential diagnosis, especially if isolated gastric ulcerative lesions are identified and consist of primarily eosinophilic infiltrates on histopathology.[14]

Inflammatory bowel disease and low-grade intestinal lymphoma

In recent years, LGITL in cats has been increasing in prevalence and is now one of the most common presentations of lymphoma in cats, representing 60%–70% of all alimentary lymphomas in this species.[15,16] For cross-reference, the clinical signs, diagnosis, treatment, and differential diagnosis of LGITL vs. IBD in cats are discussed in detail in Chapter 20.

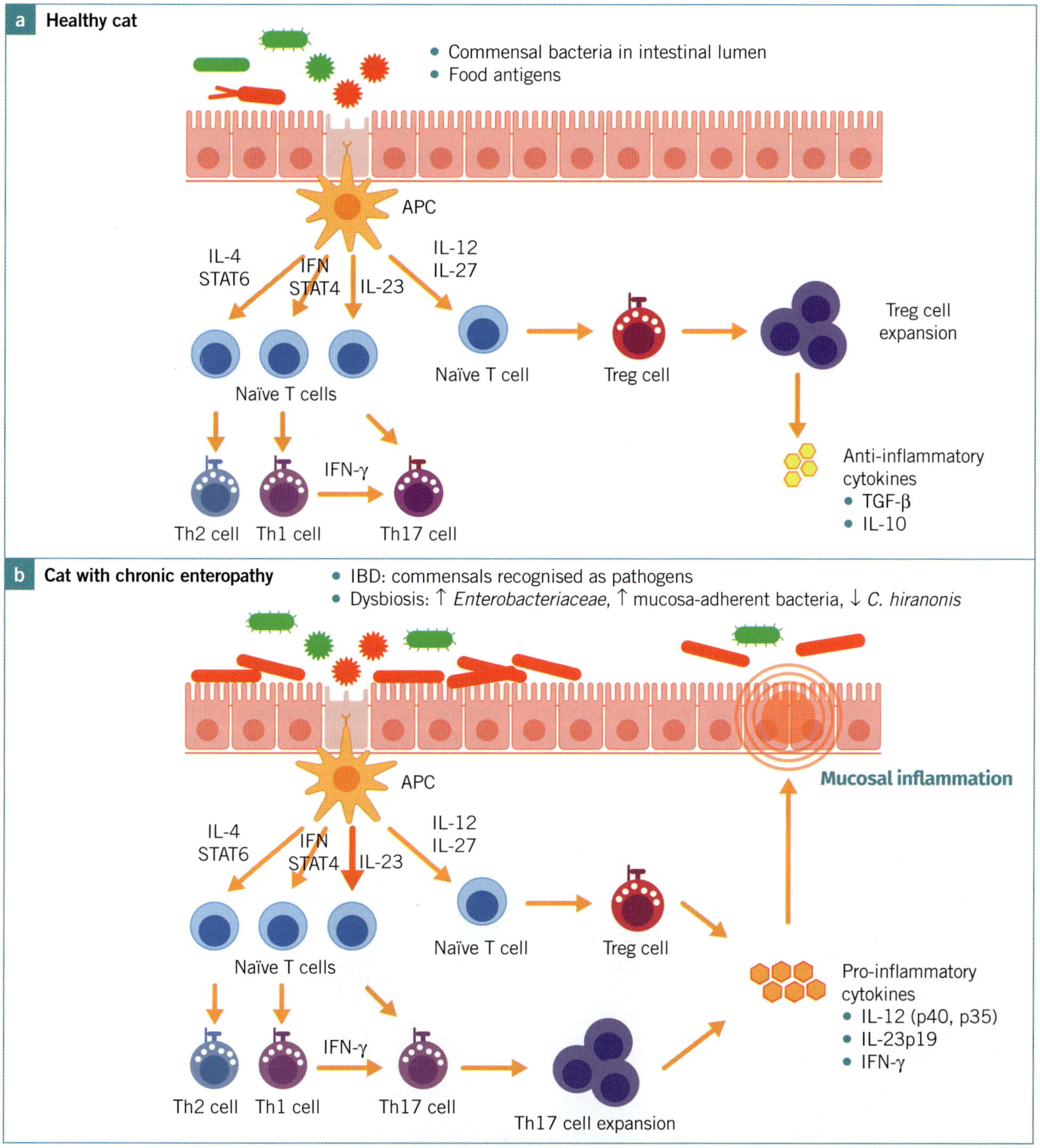

Figure 17.1. Current hypothesis of the immunopathogenesis of feline inflammatory bowel disease (IBD). In the normal intestinal mucosa (a), pattern recognition receptors on the surface of antigen presenting cells (APCs) sample signals from food antigens and commensal bacteria in the intestinal lumen, which trigger naïve T cells to differentiate primarily into regulatory T cells (Treg cells), producing anti-inflammatory cytokines such as transforming growth factor beta (TGF-β) and interleukin (IL)-10. Therefore, no or minimal mucosal inflammation is seen. In the case of feline chronic enteropathies (b), a severe microbiome dysbiosis drives the messaging towards a pro-inflammatory pathway of T-helper (Th) cell differentiation, resulting in the production of pro-inflammatory cytokines, mainly IL-12, IL-23p19, and interferon gamma (IFN-γ). The dysbiosis in feline IBD is characterised by an increase in *Enterobacteriaceae* as well as increased numbers of mucosa-adherent bacteria, mainly *Enterobacteriaceae* and *Fusobacteria*, which will further increase pro-inflammatory responses of the mucosa. In addition, bacteria with an anti-inflammatory action, such as *Clostridium hiranonis*, are decreased in feline IBD. The resulting inflammatory cytokines will lead to architectural changes in epithelial cells, such as increased leakage through tight junctions. This in turn will result in more bacteria attaching to and breaching the mucosal barrier, therefore leading to a vicious circle of inflammation. STAT, signal transducer and activator of transcription.

The exact aetiology of feline LGITL is unclear, although several possible underlying factors are being discussed. Retroviruses, including feline leukaemia virus (FeLV) and feline immunodeficiency virus (FIV), have historically been implicated in the development of lymphoma in cats. To the contrary, in LGITL, most reports show that cats are usually FeLV and FIV seronegative.[15] Some newer studies that have investigated latent FeLV and FIV infections using sensitive PCR methods did however find that provirus DNA sequences of these viruses can be detected in cats diagnosed with LGITL. Whether there is a direct association of retroviral infections and the development of LGITL is therefore unclear but seems less likely than for the large-cell lymphomas of cats. Herpesvirus infections, and specifically those caused by Felis catus gammaherpesvirus 1, have also been suggested as a possible aetiologic factor for cats developing LGITL, but no definitive conclusions can be made at this point. With regard to bacterial infections, there is more evidence available to link them to LGITL. One study found that the number of bacteria in the intestinal lumen of cats with LGITL was increased as compared to cats diagnosed with IBD.[17] In addition, the presence of mucosa-adherent and serosal bacteria, as well as bacteria in the peripheral blood, was only identified in cats with high-grade lymphoma and not in those with LGITL.[17] In a newer study that included a larger number of LGITL cases, mucosa-adherent *Fusobacterium* spp. were found to be increased in cats with LGITL when compared to cats with IBD (Fig. 17.2).[6] Taken together, these findings implicate that the microbiome dysbiosis that accompanies IBD in cats, and, in particular, mucosa-adherent bacteria and those that possibly invade the lamina propria and the vascular space, may play a role in the development of LGITL. Furthermore, it is also interesting to note that many cats diagnosed with LGITL also have concurrent IBD.[16] This is illustrated by the fact that in up to 60% of cats with LGITL, there can be focal pockets of clonal lymphocyte proliferations present within a polyclonal background.[15]

An interesting development in comparative medicine is the recent realisation that human indolent intestinal T-cell lymphoma seems to share many similarities with LGITL in cats.[15] Indolent intestinal T-cell lymphomas in humans are rare, and only a few case series have been described. The histological presentation of both diseases is typically comprised of a monomorphic population of small- to intermediate-sized T cells in the villi and lamina propria of the small intestine. In addition, T-cell infiltration into the epithelial layer of the mucosa is often seen, as is villous atrophy and crypt hyperplasia. Clinically, in the diseases in both species, patients seem to have prolonged survival; in fact, in people, indolent intestinal T-cell lymphoma is often not treated and can result in long-term persistent but

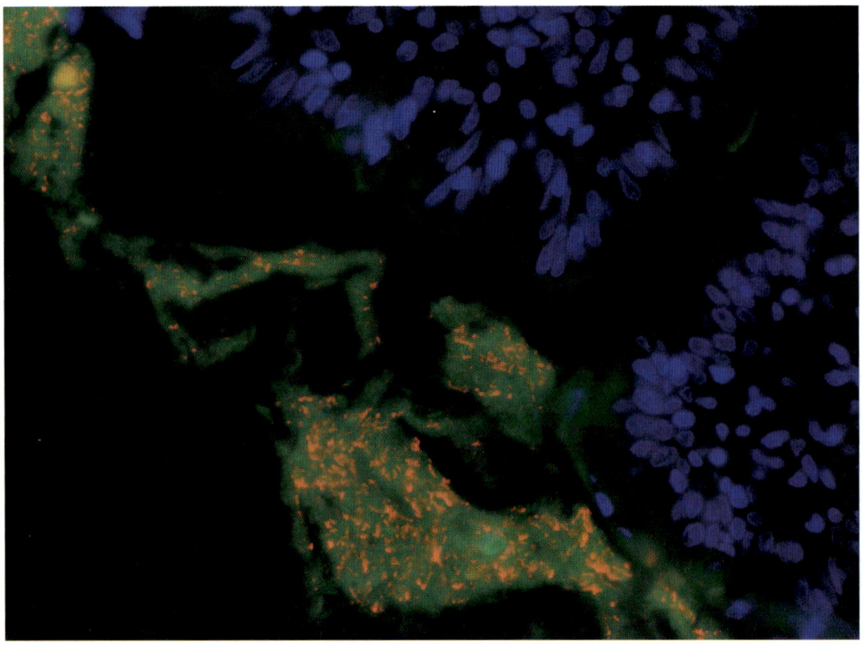

Figure 17.2. Cy3-labelled *Fusobacterium* spp. (labelled orange using fluorescence in situ hybridisation) localised within adherent mucus of an ileal biopsy specimen from a cat with low-grade intestinal T-cell lymphoma (LGITL). The mucus is occupied by other bacteria (total bacteria labelled green with FITC–Eub probe). The dark blue structures are epithelial cell nuclei stained with DAPI. The dysbiosis in feline inflammatory bowel disease is characterised by an increase of mucosa-adherent bacteria, such as *Fusobacterium* spp. The more fusobacteria can be found attached to the mucosa, the more likely it is that the cat displays a phenotype of LGITL. Image courtesy of Dr Kayode Garraway and Dr Albert E. Jergens, Iowa State University, USA.

minimal clinical signs.[15] It has therefore been suggested that the aetiology of both diseases could be overlapping. Interestingly, in human indolent intestinal T-cell lymphomas, an association has been found with some autoimmune diseases, specifically coeliac disease, which in some cases seem to have preceded the development of indolent intestinal T-cell lymphoma.[18] Specifically, the similarity of some histological findings, such as villous atrophy and crypt hyperplasia, is actually pathognomonic for coeliac disease in humans and occurs much more commonly in feline LGITL than in IBD.[19] This raises the suspicion that dietary antigens could be involved in the pathogenesis of both IBD and LGITL in cats. Immunohistochemical studies have also shown that both diseases are predominantly characterised by the presence of CD3 and CD4 positive infiltrates; however, Ki-67, a proliferation marker, is usually only minimally expressed. This latter finding fits well with the notion that both diseases are associated with slow clinical progression and long survival times. In addition, phosphorylated signal transducer and activator of transcription (phospho-STAT) 5 seems to be a marker that is commonly positive in both feline LGITL and in human indolent intestinal T-cell lymphoma, and it has recently been suggested as a potential novel marker to help differentiate LGITL from IBD in cats.

Genetics

Genetic defects in the recognition of commensal vs. pathogenic bacteria by the innate immune system play a pivotal role in disease pathogenesis in humans and dogs with IBD. Specific mutations in innate immunity receptors such as nucleotide-binding oligomerisation domain (NOD) 2, toll-like receptor (TLR) 4, and TLR5 have been identified as playing a role in human as well as canine IBD.[20] So far, there are no studies that have investigated genetic risk factors for IBD in cats, although some studies cite that Persian and Siamese cats could be predisposed. However, one recent study in Australia investigated associations between single nucleotide polymorphisms (SNPs) in the feline TLR4 receptors and an increased risk of developing infectious or inflammatory conditions in this species.[21] In this study, 22 SNPs were identified in the feline TLR4, with one SNP (c.869G>A) particularly associated with cats of the Burmese breed. Overall, however, the findings did not support a role of TLR4 dysfunction in breed predispositions to infectious or autoimmune diseases.[21]

Of interest, in some cases of indolent T-cell lymphoproliferative disorders of the gastrointestinal (GI) tract in people, which resemble the clinical disease of LGITL in cats, specific mutations, such as STAT3–Janus kinase (JAK) 2 fusion mutations, have been identified.[15] It is possible that such mutations also play a role in the pathogenesis of LGITL and/or IBD in cats, but, to date, no studies have been performed to investigate this.

MICROBIOME AND ENVIRONMENTAL FACTORS

Microbiome

The gut microbiome is defined as the diverse ecosystem found in the intestine of vertebrates and consists of various microorganisms (i.e. viruses, bacteria, fungi, and protozoa). The microbiome is an important aspect of GI health in mammals, and its composition is individually stable after transition from milk feeding to regular diet.[22] This therefore implicates, and it has been demonstrated in various studies, that the diet has a great effect on the composition of the microbiota. Importantly, the normal gut microbiome carries out numerous functions that result in the production of faecal metabolites, which are important for GI health. For example, in canines and felines, complex plant-based carbohydrates (i.e. fibres) are mostly digested by bacteria in the colon.[23] These bacteria belong predominantly to the genus *Faecalibacterium* and produce short-chain fatty acids (SCFAs) that serve important functions for the host. Specific SCFAs, in particular butyrate, have been shown to be anti-inflammatory, have positive effects on the intestinal barrier function, and provide an important source of energy for enterocytes and colonocytes. Other important functions of bacteria in the intestine relate to their ability to convert primary bile acids (BAs) into secondary BAs in the colon.[24] One of the most important bacteria for the conversion of primary into secondary BAs, particularly in cats, is *Clostridium hiranonis*.[25] Several studies have shown that the number of *C. hiranonis* in the microbiota of cats decreases after various insults, such as antibiotic usage or in CEs. Secondary BAs serve important functions in the GI immune system and in the metabolism of fat and glucose and have been shown to be anti-inflammatory. With a decrease in *C. hiranonis*, there is an imbalance of primary BAs vs. secondary BAs, with the amount of the latter in the intestinal lumen severely decreased. This then leads to metabolic derangements that can, at least in people, result in long-standing diarrhoea and even metabolic syndrome (Fig. 17.3).

Diet can also play an important part in the production of certain faecal metabolites, such as tryptophan.[26] Various bacteria have been found to be involved in metabolising tryptophan from the diet into indole. In dysbiosis, tryptophan is not converted to indole in an efficient manner, which results in cytotoxic effects on the enterocytes (Fig. 17.4).[27]

The advent of molecular methods has revolutionised the investigation of the microbiome. This is a significant advantage to culture of bacteria, since at least two-thirds of all bacteria in the intestine cannot be cultured and would be missed if only assessed by this method. To the contrary, 16S rRNA sequencing has become the most widely used method to enumerate which taxa are present in a sample. This method relies on the PCR amplification of a

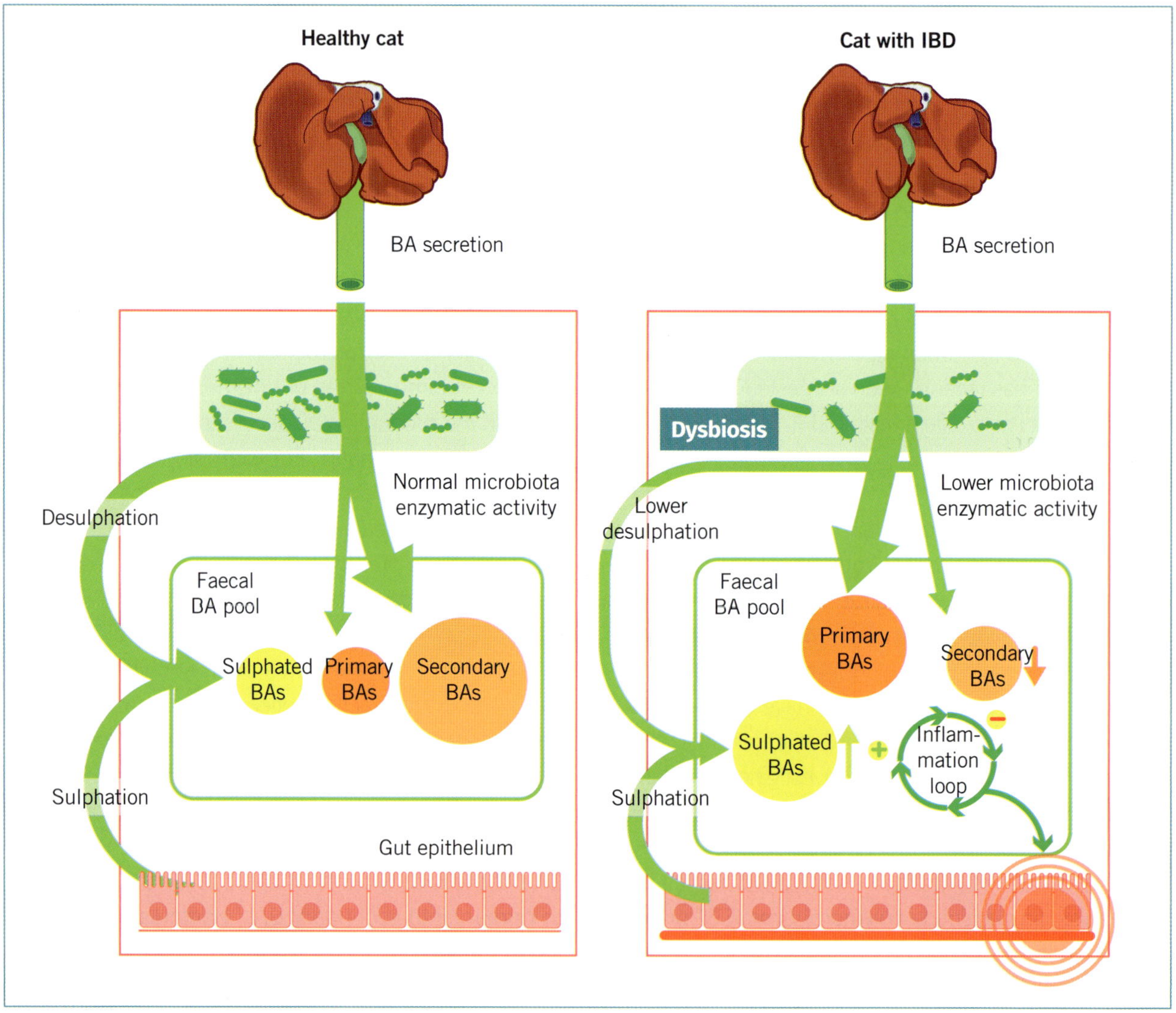

Figure 17.3. Bile acids (BAs) and their involvement in intestinal inflammation. BAs are produced in the liver from cholesterol and are secreted into the bile and delivered to the intestinal lumen in the duodenum, where they play an important role in the absorption of fat and fat-soluble vitamins. The normal intestinal microbiome converts primary BAs into secondary BAs. These secondary BAs act as important antimicrobial molecules in the intestine. However, if a dysbiosis present, as is the case in feline inflammatory bowel disease (IBD), there are not enough bacteria that convert primary to secondary BAs. This results in pro-inflammatory and permeability changes in the intestine, leading to chronic intestinal inflammation. Adapted from Duboc H et al. Connecting dysbiosis, bile-acid dysmetabolism and gut inflammation in inflammatory bowel diseases. *Gut* 62:531, 2013.

gene that is conserved across all bacteria (i.e. 16S rRNA), but not present in mammals, and whose hypervariable region allows for differentiation of the genetic material down to the species level. Importantly, while this method can identify a majority of taxa in a sample, it will not give any indication of the functions that these bacteria carry out. This is important to keep in mind, as bacterial species in the intestine are redundant and can take over specific functions of other bacteria that have diminished in number. Newer methods, such as shotgun metagenomic sequencing, allow a more granular assessment of the microbiome including their functional characteristics. Unfortunately, for cats, there is not much information available about these novel methods, and further research is warranted to elucidate specific changes in diseases such as CE. Another method to investigate the microbiota is fluorescence in situ hybridisation (FISH). This method stains bacterial DNA and can therefore be used to investigate spatial distribution of bacteria. Using this method, mucosa-adherent bacteria can be identified in intestinal biopsy samples.[6] Moreover, quantification of specific bacteria that indicate disease states has been recently suggested as an alternative to the above methods. Specifically, a dysbiosis index available at Texas A&M University, United States of America, has been proposed to be helpful in assessing dysbiotic changes in dogs, but this has not yet been validated for cats.[24] An alternative would be to quantify bacterial DNA for *C. hiranonis*, which, if decreased in numbers, has been associated with disease, specifically with CE in cats.[25]

The composition of the normal microbiome in healthy cats, measured using 16S rRNA methodology, consists mainly of the phyla *Bacteroidetes*, *Fusobacteria*, and *Firmicutes*. Several studies have investigated the changes of the microbiome in cats with CEs, in comparison to healthy cats and/or cats diagnosed with LGITL. These changes have collectively been termed dysbiosis and overlap with the dysbiosis found in people and dogs with CE.[25] The dominant changes are a decrease in microbial richness and diversity, with a concomitant decrease in the numbers of *Faecalibacterium* spp., *Bifidobacterium* spp., *Turicibacter* spp., and *Bacteroidaceae*, and increased abundances of *Enterobacteriaceae* (e.g. *E. coli*) and *Streptococcus* spp.

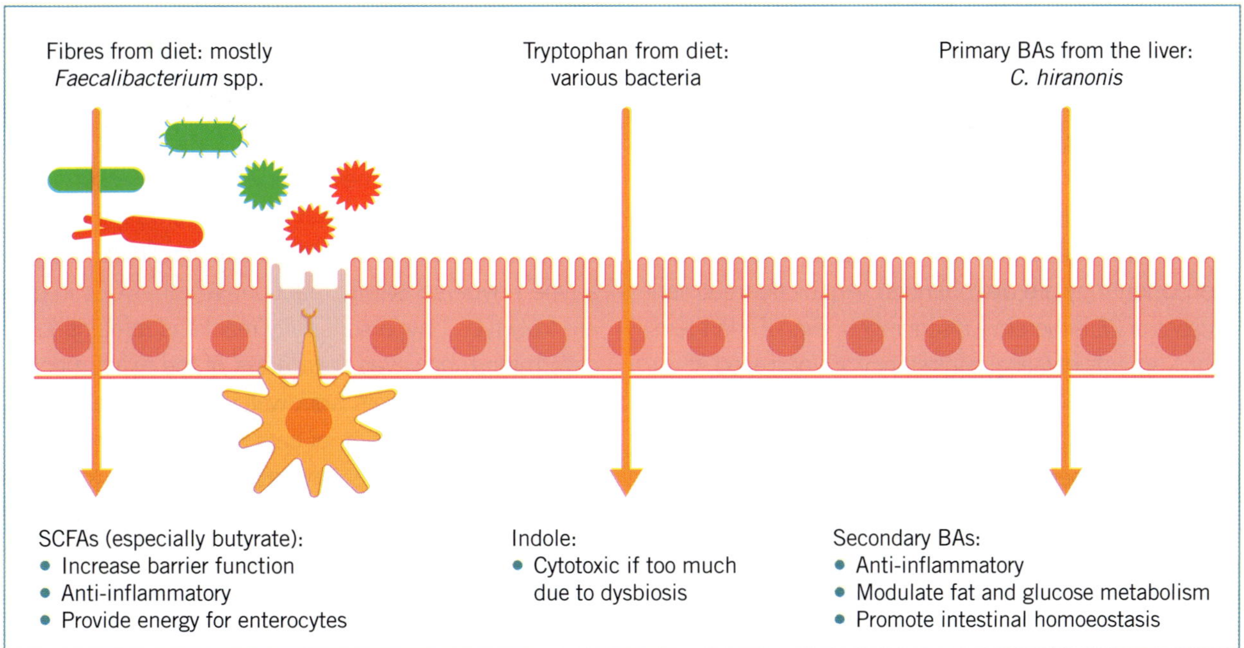

Figure 17.4. Dysbiosis in feline inflammatory bowel disease (IBD) is hypothesised to have numerous effects. Carbohydrates (fibres in prey animals) are primarily metabolised by *Faecalibacterium* spp. to anti-inflammatory short-chain fatty acids (SCFAs), such as butyrate, which are essential for normal colonocyte function. Tryptophan from the diet is metabolised to indole by various bacteria in the normal microbiome. If a dysbiosis is present, as in feline IBD, too much indole can be produced which is cytotoxic to the enterocytes. *Clostridium hiranonis* is a bacterium that is important in the conversion of primary bile acids (BAs) to secondary BAs, which have important anti-inflammatory effects in the intestine and modulate glucose and fat metabolism. The dysbiosis associated with feline IBD results in a severe decrease in *C. hiranonis* numbers, therefore decreasing the pool of secondary BAs and resulting in intestinal inflammation.

This indicates a reduction of diversity and numbers of beneficial anti-inflammatory species and an increase in potentially more pro-inflammatory species, such as *E. coli*. In another study that investigated the microbiome of cats with CE using FISH, mucosa-adherent *Enterobacteriaceae* populations were also found to be increased compared to those of healthy cats.[5] In another recent study, mucosa-adherent bacteria were investigated in cats with CE and in cats diagnosed with LGITL. In this study, an increase in ileal and colonic mucosa-adherent *Fusobacteria* could be found in cats with LGITL, as compared to cats with CE.[6] Taken together, these studies indicate that cats with CE likely have similar changes in their microbiome to those reported in dogs with CE, suggesting that gram-negative bacteria are abundantly present in these disease states, which leads to hyperreactivity to lipopolysaccharide in the mucosa and an overreaction of the immune system towards these bacteria. Hence, it is believed that the microbiome plays a pivotal role in the pathogenesis of CE in cats.

The notion that the dysbiosis in cats with CE (or dogs with CE, for that matter) can be treated by the administration of antibiotics is, however, fundamentally wrong. In fact, it has been shown that antibiotic treatment in healthy cats results in long-standing microbial dysbiosis, which is associated with a significant decrease in *C. hiranonis* numbers (which are important for the conversion of BAs) and increased numbers of *E. coli* (which cause increased inflammatory changes, as explained above). Furthermore, amelioration of diarrhoea is only seen during the administration of antibiotics, and recurrence is often seen when they are discontinued. Antibiotic treatment in cases of CE is therefore discouraged, even if short-term improvements of faecal consistency are achieved.[28]

Diet

Diet has long been known to have an effect on the microbiome composition. Since the microbiome has increasingly been recognised as a metabolically active organ, it makes sense that large shifts in the microbiome composition will affect the metabolome in the intestinal lumen and can therefore have significant effects on the health of the GI tract. Specifically, in cats with IBD, a dysbiosis can be detected that results in increased overall numbers of bacteria, *Enterobacteriaceae*, and *E. coli*.[5] This shift in the microbiome also leads to a functional defect in SCFAs, which is particularly obvious in cats with IBD.[29]

Macronutrient composition of the diet

With regard to macronutrient dietary composition, it has long been recognised that a restriction of fat content can be helpful in some cases of CE in dogs; however, in cats, fat restriction does not seem to have the same effect.[30] This may be the case because cats rely more on fat for energy and could possibly be more tolerant to higher dietary fat levels than dogs. Dietary fibres are plant-based carbohydrates that cannot be digested by mammalian enzymes. Fibre is important for the production of SCFAs, particularly butyrate, and therefore helps maintain normal colonocyte function. Consequently, some studies have found that dietary supplementation with fibre can be helpful in cats with CE.[27]

Elimination diets and hydrolysed diets

Another concept is the administration of elimination diets or hydrolysed diets to cats with CE. Encouragingly, it has been shown that up to 50% of cats with CE respond favourably to either elimination or hydrolysed diets within 2 weeks of starting the diet.[31–33] However, the mechanism of why hydrolysed diets work in cats with CE has not been sufficiently elucidated yet. One hypothesis stems from the idea that CEs share a common pathogenesis with type I food allergies. This theory states that the oligopeptides contained in hydrolysed diets are too small to effectively cross-link the IgE molecules on the surface of macrophages, and this will therefore stop the degranulation of mast cells and the resulting clinical signs in a type I hypersensitivity reaction. Whether CEs in cats are truly type I hypersensitivity reactions remains to be determined; however, regardless of the exact mechanism, hydrolysed diets work well in many cats with CE. Interestingly, up to 30% of cats that are switched back to their original diet after having responded to hydrolysed diets experience a relapse in clinical signs.[33] This fact highlights the possibility that food allergy may be more common in cats than in dogs with CE. It is also possible that hydrolysed diets are more easily digestible for cats, and this effect helps ameliorating the clinical signs seen in CEs. Some pet food manufacturers also claim that their hydrolysed diets are either vegetarian and/or soy-based, which has been shown to have immunomodulatory effects. The concept of type I hypersensitivity and hydrolysed diets is explained in Figure 17.5.

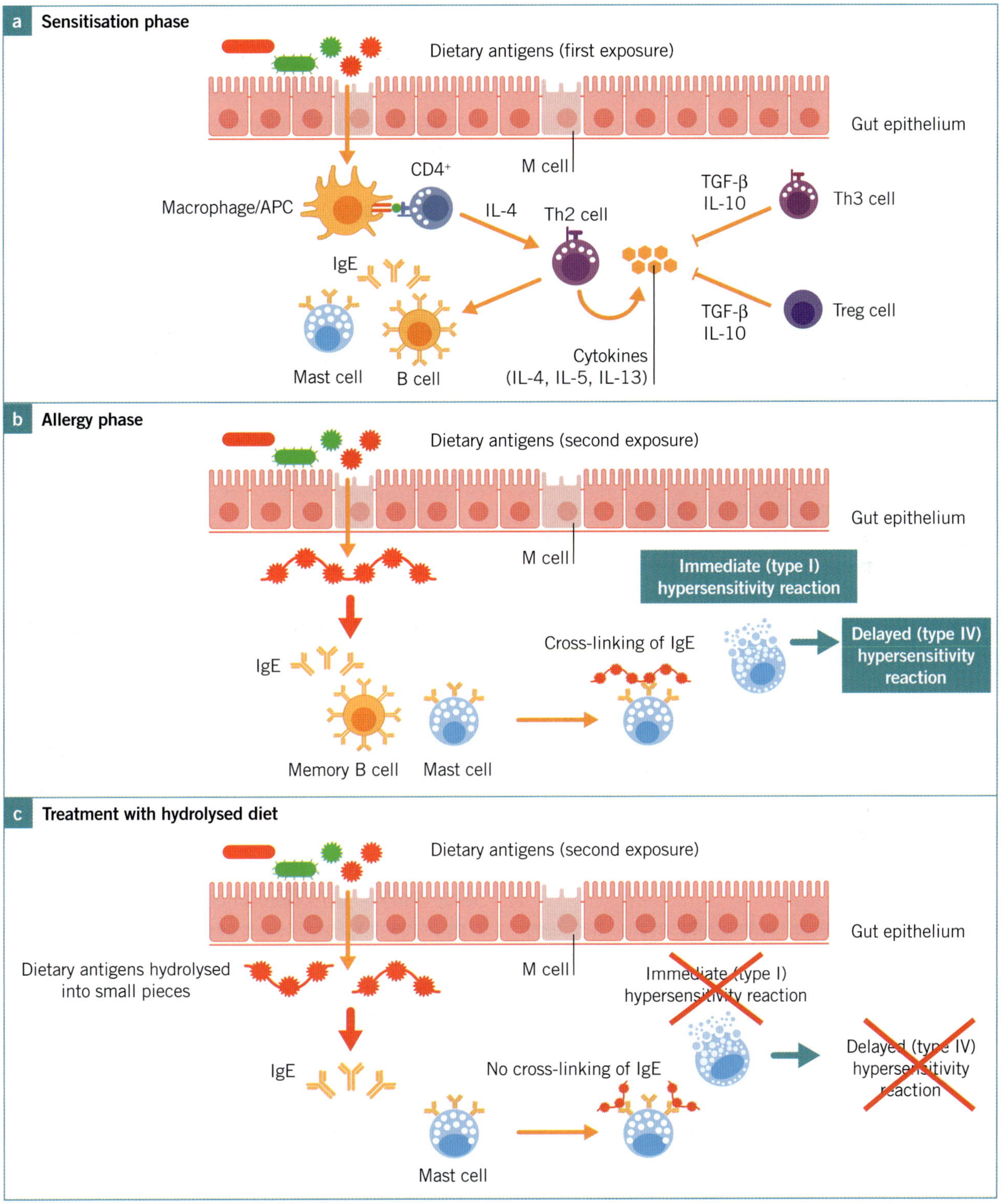

Figure 17.5. The concept of food allergy and hydrolysed diets in feline inflammatory bowel disease. Classically, type I hypersensitivity (i.e. food allergy mediated by immunoglobulin E [IgE]) develops starting from the first contact with the allergen when the naïve immune system is sensitised to produce an IgE response (a). The subsequent repetitive contact with that same allergen leads to an allergic reaction and clinical signs (b). The concept of breaking down proteins into smaller oligopeptides which will be too small to bridge two adjacent IgE molecules present on the surface of mast cells has been pivotal for the management of cow's milk allergy in infants, and this is exploited in hydrolysed diets (c). Hydrolysed diets have been found to be useful in the treatment of up to 50% of cats with chronic enteropathies. In addition, up to 30% of cats relapse when switched back to their previous diet, which implies a component of food allergy in about one-third of cats with chronic enteropathies.

Additional functional deficiencies

Several nutrients have been investigated in cats with CE and may influence GI health and the immune system in general.

Cobalamin

Serum cobalamin concentration has been recognised as an important factor in cats and is found to be decreased in CE or LGITL in up to 80% of cases.[34,35] Importantly, some studies have shown that if serum cobalamin concentrations are not corrected, the underlying disease may be refractory to treatment. It is therefore imperative that cats with chronic GI disease be supplemented with cobalamin. Some authors have gone as far as to suggest that all cats with GI disease should be supplemented with cobalamin because there is no risk of oversupplementation, as surplus levels are simply excreted through the urine and no adverse effects are expected. Several studies have also shown that cobalamin serum concentrations increase after subcutaneous or oral supplementation and correlate with clinical improvement in cats with CE.[34] For supplementation, it is recommended to administer 0.125–0.25 mg/cat/week SC for 4–6 weeks and then as needed to maintain normal serum concentrations. Alternatively, cobalamin can be given orally; if this route of administration is chosen, larger doses need to be given daily in order to maintain normal serum cobalamin concentrations.[36]

Vitamin D

Vitamin D is another essential nutrient that has been shown to be decreased in patients with GI disease, specifically in cats with CE.[37] Importantly, low serum vitamin D_3 concentrations have also been associated with a worse prognosis in cats with CE. It may therefore be prudent to measure vitamin D_3 serum concentrations in cats with CE and to supplement it in cats with subnormal levels. Vitamin D_3 is supplemented as calcitriol at 2.5–3.5 ng/kg/day orally for several weeks until serum concentrations normalise.

Amino acids

Plasma amino acid concentrations have been shown to be decreased in both humans with IBD and dogs with CE. A recent study in cats with CE has also shown decreases in several amino acid concentrations when compared to healthy cats, including arginine, histidine, lysine, methionine, phenylalanine, tryptophan, and taurine.[38] Tryptophan is particularly interesting, as its production in the intestine is influenced by the microbiome. In cats with CE and microbiome dysbiosis, tryptophan may not be efficiently converted to indole and can exert toxic effects on the enterocytes. On the other hand, low plasma concentrations of tryptophan are associated with a worse outcome in cats with CE. It has therefore been suggested that tryptophan supplementation may be indicated in some cats with deficiencies in this amino acid.

Other environmental factors

The notion that environmental factors play an important part in the development of chronic GI disease has been explored in several studies in humans with IBD and in dogs with CE. In people, it has been found that repeated exposure to antibiotic treatments in childhood significantly increases the risk of developing IBD later in life. In dogs with IBD, an association was found between an infection with parvovirus in early life and later development of CE. In cats, only few studies have been performed so far that evaluated factors in early life that could contribute to the development of chronic GI disease. One study explored early-life events, including diet, in 1212 cats presenting for GI signs later in life.[39] Interestingly, a significant association was found between cats being fed a diet that was not compliant with the WSAVA Global Nutrition Committee recommendations before 16 weeks of age and the frequency of visits to a veterinary practice for GI disease after that.[39] This implies that nutritional imbalances early in life could have consequences for the GI health in cats. Furthermore, several studies have shown an association between the administration of antimicrobials and a microbiome dysbiosis that can last for months after discontinuation of the antimicrobial treatment. It is therefore prudent to assume that frequent use of antibiotics may be detrimental to the GI health in cats and should be avoided unless specifically indicated.

Take-home messages

- Feline inflammatory bowel disease (IBD) is hypothesised to encompass a complex pathogenesis, with the intestinal microbiome, host factors, and dietary antigens playing important roles.
- The dysbiosis associated with feline IBD is characterised by increased overall numbers of bacteria and increased mucosa-adherent bacterial populations. In addition, *Clostridium hiranonis* numbers are decreased, which results in reduced conversion of primary to secondary bile acids, leading to perpetuated inflammation in the intestine.
- There is a strong indication that feline IBD and low-grade intestinal T-cell lymphoma (LGITL) are two sides of the spectrum of a single disease, with LGITL being on the severe side of the spectrum. It is hypothesised that increases in mucosa-adherent bacteria eventually lead to the development of pockets of clonal infiltrating lymphocytes which can result in diffuse LGITL.
- Diet is an important factor in the pathogenesis of IBD. Up to 50% of cats with IBD can be managed with a hydrolysed diet alone.

REFERENCES

[1] Hawes M et al. Interleukin-1β expression is increased in the duodenum of dogs with idiopathic inflammatory bowel disease. *Vet Rec* 183:536, 2018.

[2] Heilmann RM, Allenspach K. Pattern-recognition receptors: signaling pathways and dysregulation in canine chronic enteropathies—brief review. *J Vet Diagn Invest* 29:781, 2017.

[3] Nguyen Van N et al. Measurement of cytokine mRNA expression in intestinal biopsies of cats with inflammatory enteropathy using quantitative real-time RT-PCR. *Vet Immunol Immunopathol* 113:404, 2006.

[4] Waly NE et al. Measurement of IL-12 (p40, p35), IL-23p19, and IFN-γ mRNA in duodenal biopsies of cats with inflammatory enteropathy. *J Vet Intern Med* 28:42, 2014.

[5] Janeczko S et al. The relationship of mucosal bacteria to duodenal histopathology, cytokine mRNA, and clinical disease activity in cats with inflammatory bowel disease. *Vet Microbiol* 128:178, 2008.

[6] Garraway K et al. Relationship of the mucosal microbiota to gastrointestinal inflammation and small cell intestinal lymphoma in cats. *J Vet Intern Med* 32:1692, 2018.

[7] Kleinschmidt S et al. Characterization of mast cell numbers and subtypes in biopsies from the gastrointestinal tract of dogs with lymphocytic-plasmacytic or eosinophilic gastroenterocolitis. *Vet Immunol Immunopathol* 120:80, 2007.

[8] Castro-López J et al. Pilot study: duodenal *MDR1* and *COX2* gene expression in cats with inflammatory bowel disease and low-grade alimentary lymphoma. *J Feline Med Surg* 20:759, 2018.

[9] Castro-López J et al. Cyclooxygenase-2 immunoexpression in intestinal epithelium and lamina propria of cats with inflammatory bowel disease and low grade alimentary lymphoma. *BMC Vet Res* 14:158, 2018.

[10] Jergens AE. Feline idiopathic inflammatory bowel disease: what we know and what remains to be unraveled. *J Feline Med Surg* 14:445, 2012.

[11] Washabau RJ et al. Endoscopic, biopsy, and histopathologic guidelines for the evaluation of gastrointestinal inflammation in companion animals. *J Vet Intern Med* 24:10, 2010.

[12] Baez JL et al. Radiographic, ultrasonographic, and endoscopic findings in cats with inflammatory bowel disease of the stomach and small intestine: 33 cases (1990–1997). *J Am Vet Med Assoc* 215:349, 1999.

[13] Takeuchi Y et al. Hypereosinophilic syndrome in two cats. *J Vet Med Sci* 70:1085, 2008.

[14] Weissman A et al. Ultrasonographic and clinicopathological features of feline gastrointestinal eosinophilic sclerosing fibroplasia in four cats. *J Feline Med Surg* 15:148, 2013.

[15] Paulin MV et al. Feline low-grade alimentary lymphoma: an emerging entity and a potential animal model for human disease. *BMC Vet Res* 14:306, 2018.

[16] Marsilio S. Differentiating inflammatory bowel disease from alimentary lymphoma in cats: does it matter? *Vet Clin North Am Small Anim Pract* 51:93, 2021.

[17] Hoehne SN et al. Identification of mucosa-invading and intravascular bacteria in feline small intestinal lymphoma. *Vet Pathol* 54:234, 2017.

[18] Zanelli M et al. Indolent T-cell lymphoproliferative disorder of the gastrointestinal tract: a tricky diagnosis of a gastric case. *BMC Gastroenterol* 20:336, 2020.

[19] Fernández-Bañares F et al. Persistent villous atrophy in de novo adult patients with celiac disease and strict control of gluten-free diet adherence: a multicenter prospective study (CADER study). *Am J Gastroenterol*, 2021 [epub ahead of print].

[20] Kathrani A et al. TLR5 risk-associated haplotype for canine inflammatory bowel disease confers hyper-responsiveness to flagellin. *PLoS One* 7:e30117, 2012.

[21] Whitney J et al. Breed-specific variations in the coding region of toll-like receptor 4 in the domestic cat. *Vet Immunol Immunopathol* 209:61, 2019.

[22] Suchodolski JS. Intestinal microbiota of dogs and cats: a bigger world than we thought. *Vet Clin North Am Small Anim Pract* 41:261, 2011.

[23] Suchodolski JS. Companion animals symposium: microbes and gastrointestinal health of dogs and cats. *J Anim Sci* 89:1520, 2011.

[24] Guard BC et al. Longitudinal assessment of microbial dysbiosis, fecal unconjugated bile acid concentrations, and disease activity in dogs with steroid-responsive chronic inflammatory enteropathy. *J Vet Intern Med* 33:1295, 2019.

[25] Ziese AL, Suchodolski JS. Impact of changes in gastrointestinal microbiota in canine and feline digestive diseases. *Vet Clin North Am Small Anim Pract* 51:155, 2021.

[26] Sakai K et al. Decreased plasma amino acid concentrations in cats with chronic gastrointestinal diseases and their possible contribution in the inflammatory response. *Vet Immunol Immunopathol* 195:1, 2018.

[27] Kathrani A. Dietary and nutritional approaches to the management of chronic enteropathy in dogs and cats. *Vet Clin North Am Small Anim Pract* 51:123, 2021.

[28] Saettone V et al. State-of-the-art of the nutritional alternatives to the use of antibiotics in humans and monogastric animals. *Animals (Basel)* 10:2199, 2020.

[29] Minamoto Y et al. Feline gastrointestinal microbiota. *Anim Health Res Rev* 13:64, 2012.

[30] Laflamme DP, Xu H, Long GM. Effect of diets differing in fat content on chronic diarrhea in cats. *J Vet Intern Med* 25:230, 2011.

[31] Guilford WG et al. Food sensitivity in cats with chronic idiopathic gastrointestinal problems. *J Vet Intern Med* 15:7, 2001.

[32] Mandigers PJ, Biourge V, German AJ. Efficacy of a commercial hydrolysate diet in eight cats suffering from inflammatory bowel disease or adverse reaction to food. *Tijdschr Diergeneeskd* 135:668, 2010.

[33] Kathrani A et al. The use of hydrolysed diets for vomiting and/or diarrhoea in cats in primary veterinary practice. *J Small Anim Pract* 61:723, 2020.

[34] Simpson KW et al. Subnormal concentrations of serum cobalamin (vitamin B_{12}) in cats with gastrointestinal disease. *J Vet Intern Med* 15:26, 2001.

[35] Ruaux CG, Steiner JM, Williams DA. Early biochemical and clinical responses to cobalamin supplementation in cats with signs of gastrointestinal disease and severe hypocobalaminemia. *J Vet Intern Med* 19:155, 2005.

[36] Toresson L et al. Oral cobalamin supplementation in cats with hypocobalaminaemia: a retrospective study. *J Feline Med Surg* 19:1302, 2017.

[37] Lalor S et al. Cats with inflammatory bowel disease and intestinal small cell lymphoma have low serum concentrations of 25-hydroxyvitamin D. *J Vet Intern Med* 28:351, 2014.

[38] Kathrani A et al. Whole-blood taurine concentrations in cats with intestinal disease. *J Vet Intern Med* 31:1067, 2017.

[39] Kathrani A et al. Exploring early life events including diet in cats presenting for gastrointestinal signs in later life. *Vet Rec* 185:144, 2019.

CHAPTER 18

Classification, clinical staging, and treatment of feline chronic enteropathy

Fabio Procoli

Feline chronic enteropathy (FCE) is a term used to describe a spectrum of disorders characterised by gastrointestinal (GI) signs of more than 3 weeks duration for which extraintestinal and infectious/parasitic causes have been ruled out. Although its exact prevalence in primary and referral practice is unknown, FCE represents the most common cause of chronic GI signs in cats. The exact aetiopathogenesis of FCE is unknown. However, this syndrome is likely to be multifactorial, with the interplay of several key factors such as genetic susceptibility, dietary antigens, intestinal microbiota, intestinal barrier function, and innate and adaptive immune system. See Chapter 17 for more details on the aetiopathogenesis of FCE.

The diagnosis of FCE is one of exclusion and follows an extensive diagnostic workup aimed at ruling out other intestinal and extraintestinal causes of GI signs. Ultimately, it is based on intestinal mucosal histopathology and findings of mucosal inflammatory infiltrates and ultrastructural changes.[1]

No universal consensus exists with regard to the classification and treatment protocol of FCE. The majority of veterinary gastroenterologists subclassify FCE cases based on the response to sequential treatments into food-responsive enteropathy (FRE) and inflammatory bowel disease (IBD), also referred to as steroid-responsive enteropathy (SRE). Despite lacking evidence of an antibiotic-responsive phenotype of FCE (antibiotic-responsive enteropathy [ARE]), antibiotic use has been advocated historically by some either as a sole therapy (after a failed dietary trial) or in addition to diet and immunosuppressive drugs in cats with more severe clinical signs.[2] The proposed benefits of antibiotic therapy stemmed from their presumed immunomodulatory and anti-inflammatory properties. However, recent evidence shows that antibiotics cause detrimental and lasting effects on the intestinal microbiota of cats, which resemble those found in cats with FCE. If one adds the indisputable contributing role of indiscriminate antibiotic prescription to the global issue of antimicrobial resistance, it is easy to appreciate why safer alternatives to antibiotics need to be implemented when attempting to modulate intestinal microbiota in disease. Probiotics and faecal microbiota transplantation (FMT) are currently being evaluated for this purpose (for further details on these treatment modalities, see Chapters 36 and 37, respectively).

CLASSIFICATION

Despite the lack of a universally agreed classification of FCE, the majority of veterinary gastroenterologists, including the author, subclassify FCE in two phenotypes, namely FRE and IBD, based on the positive or negative response to a diet trial. It remains to be ascertained whether FRE and IBD represent phenotypic variations of the same complex multifactorial disease or whether they are different disease entities with different aetiologies. A prevailing hypothesis is that FCE is a multifactorial disease which involves a complex interaction of host genome, intestinal barrier, intestinal microbiota, dietary antigens, and the intestinal immune system; each of these factors might play a bigger or smaller role in each individual case (Fig. 18.1).

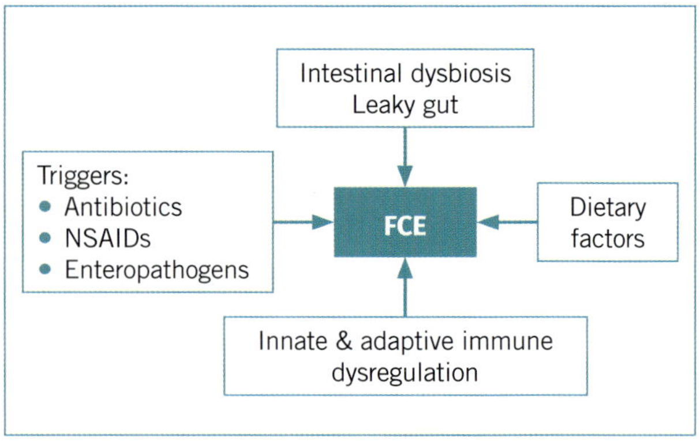

Figure 18.1. Pathogenesis of feline chronic enteropathy (FCE). FCE is a multifactorial disease thought to occur from the result of perturbations in the crosstalk between the immune system and the microbiome in a genetically susceptible host under the influence of intestinal luminal and environmental triggers, which are able to cause epithelial injury and/or increase intestinal permeability.

Food-responsive enteropathy

Strictly speaking, the term FRE should be reserved for cases of chronic GI signs of unknown cause with histopathological evidence of intestinal mucosal inflammation that, most importantly, have achieved swift clinical remission following a trial with a therapeutic (selected antigen, hydrolysed, or highly digestible) diet. The true prevalence of food-responsive FCE cases is not known. In a study involving 55 cats with idiopathic chronic GI signs,[3] food-responsive cases represented around 50% of total cases. However, of these cats, almost two-thirds were thought to suffer from food sensitivity rather than true enteropathy, as clinical signs relapsed following challenge with the original diet or selected food additives and resolved once again after reintroduction of the elimination diet. One-third of the food-responsive cases did not relapse following dietary challenge, therefore ruling out adverse food reaction (AFR) in these cases. Overall, it is not known whether all cases of feline FRE truly suffer from a complex multifactorial disease such FCE or whether they represent cases of AFRs, either immune-mediated (food allergy) or nonimmune-mediated (food intolerance). Irrespectively of the exact pathophysiology behind food responsiveness, FRE and AFRs are common disease entities, highlighting the role of dietary manipulation in the diagnosis and treatment of chronic GI signs in cats.

Inflammatory bowel disease

The term feline IBD was first introduced in the veterinary literature in the early 1990s to describe cases of cats with chronic recurrent GI signs and histopathological evidence of intestinal mucosal inflammation.[1] Subtypes of IBD were proposed based on the predominant cellular type of the inflammatory infiltrates, namely lymphocytic–plasmacytic enterocolitis (then most common), lymphocytic enteritis (to be distinguished from alimentary lymphoma), and eosinophilic enteritis. Up to 83% of these cases showed a complete or partial response to immunosuppressive doses of glucocorticoids.[4-6] Over time, the absolute significance of intestinal mucosal inflammation in the diagnosis of feline IBD has been questioned, with increasing attention being reserved to the histological evidence of mucosal ultrastructural abnormalities such as villous atrophy or fusion, lacteal and crypt dilation, and the presence of mucosal fibrosis,[2] which can be more indicative of chronic intestinal disease. Currently the term IBD is used interchangeably with SRE to indicate FCE cases that fail to respond to dietary intervention but achieve clinical remission (complete or partial) with immunosuppressive doses of glucocorticoids. The exact prevalence of feline IBD amongst all FCE cases is unknown, partly because in the majority of studies immunosuppressive therapy was almost invariably given in association with diets (selected antigen or hydrolysed), antibiotics, or other drugs (e.g. sulphasalazine).

Antibiotic-responsive enteropathy

Unlike in dogs, in which an antibiotic-responsive phenotype of chronic enteropathy (CE) has been described, ARE has not been clearly characterised in cats. Anecdotal reports of FCE cases that have responded favourably to antibiotic treatment alone do, however, exist. It is possible that these cats suffered from severe intestinal mucosal dysbiosis and the antibiotic successfully decreased the number of mucosa-associated bacteria, with subsequent amelioration of clinical signs. Alternatively, these cats suffered from an infection or overgrowth sustained by enteropathogenic bacteria. In a recent retrospective study of cats with a previous histological diagnosis of neutrophilic and lymphoplasmacytic IBD, archived intestinal biopsy samples were analysed using fluorescence in situ hybridisation (FISH) to detect bacterial DNA. The presence of mucosa-associated *Campylobacter coli* was demonstrated in 7/8 cases of neutrophilic inflammation, compared to 1/8 cases of lymphoplasmacytic IBD. A spatial association was found between the neutrophilic infiltrate and bacteria.[7] Lastly, rare cases of mucosa-adherent and invasive *Escherichia coli* (AIEC)–mediated granulomatous colitis have been described in cats[8] and have also been encountered by the author. However, the overall incidence of antibiotic-responsive cases in cats remains overwhelmingly low, supporting the current conviction amongst veterinary gastroenterologists that antibiotics should not be routinely used for diagnostic or therapeutic purposes without histological, immunohistochemical, or molecular evidence of granulomatous inflammation.

CLINICAL STAGING

Clinical staging of cats with FCE is fundamental to characterise disease localisation and severity, identify the presence of concurrent diseases (e.g. hepatobiliary and/or pancreatic), and detect complications arising secondarily to FCE. Clinical staging of FCE is based on the integration of signalment, clinical presentation, and findings from physical examination and clinical pathology with abdominal ultrasound, GI endoscopy, and eventually intestinal histopathology. Recently, a disease-specific clinical activity index has been validated for cats with FCE to allow reliable assessment of active disease burden and response to treatment.

Signalment and clinical presentation

FCE can affect cats of any breed, sex, and age. Although overlap exists in age at initial diagnosis between FRE and IBD, cats with FRE tend to be younger than cats with IBD, which are usually middle-aged. The clinical presentation of cats with FCE will depend on disease activity and severity, duration of clinical signs, previous treatment trials, and presence of concurrent diseases such as pancreatic and hepatic inflammatory diseases. Clinical signs can wax and wane, with periods of clinical remission alternating with disease flare-ups, or be progressive in nature. Often, reoccurrence of clinical signs can be triggered by dietary indiscretion or drugs such as nonsteroidal anti-inflammatory drugs or antibiotics. Clinical signs are attributed to mucosal architectural changes, inflammatory infiltrates, inflammatory mediators, and intestinal dysmotility. The most common presenting signs in cats with FCE are weight loss, followed by vomiting, reduced appetite or anorexia, and chronic diarrhoea. Unlike in dogs with CE, diarrhoea as the only presenting complaint is a rare occurrence in FCE. Vomiting can be of food or bile and may vary in severity and frequency. When reported, diarrhoea needs to be appropriately characterised and localised to either the small intestine, the large intestine, or both (mixed intestinal diarrhoea) (Table 18.1). In young cats, the occurrence of vomiting and large intestinal diarrhoea, especially if concurrent cutaneous signs are reported, is highly suspicious for FRE or AFRs (Fig. 18.2). Weight loss is commonly present in FCE cases (Fig. 18.3), and when associated with normal or increased food/caloric intake, it may indicate the presence of significant malabsorption. In addition to poor muscle and body condition scores, physical examination in cats with FCE may reveal segmental or diffusely thickened intestinal loops on abdominal palpation, as well as abdominal discomfort/pain that can often be localised to the cranial abdomen, indicating possible concurrent pancreatitis.

Table 18.1. Differences between small intestinal and large intestinal disease in cats.

Variable	Small intestinal disease	Large intestinal disease
Faecal volume	Increased	Reduced
Number of defecations	2–3	>3
Tenesmus	Rare	Common
Urgency	Rare	Common
Faecal mucus	Absent	Common
Faecal fat	Occasionally	Absent
Undigested food	Occasionally	Absent
Faecal fresh blood	Absent	Common
Melaena	Rare	Absent
Flatulence	Common	Absent
Vomiting	Common	Uncommon
Weight loss	Common	Rare

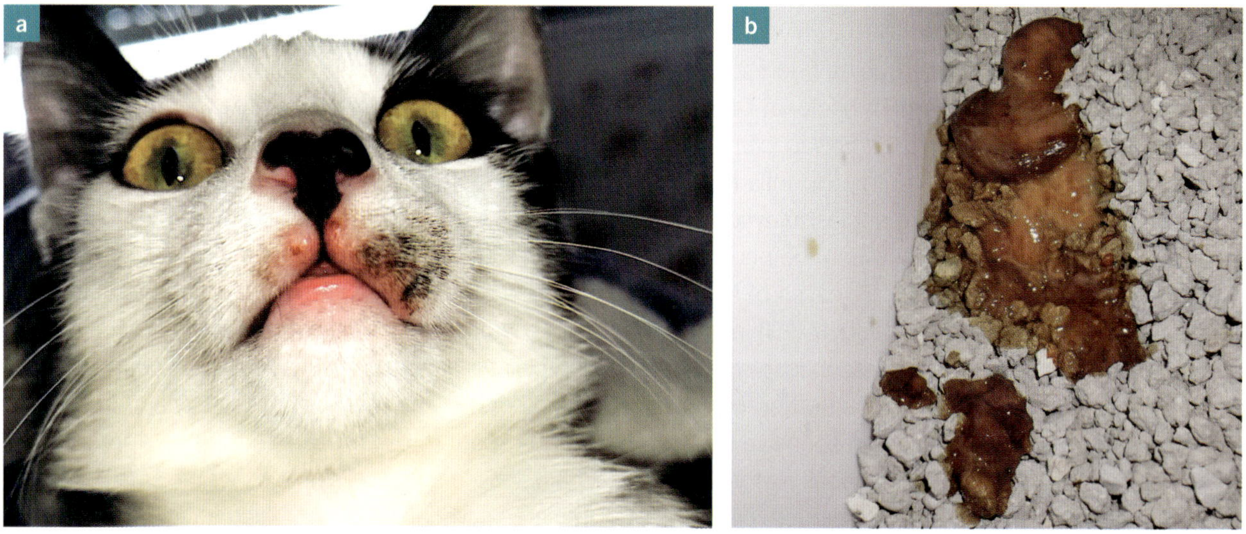

Figure 18.2. Young cat with adverse food reaction showing labial cutaneous lesions compatible with feline eosinophilic granuloma complex (a) and concurrent large intestinal diarrhoea with haematochezia and mucus (b). Cutaneous lesions and diarrhoea resolved swiftly after a trial with a hydrolysed diet.

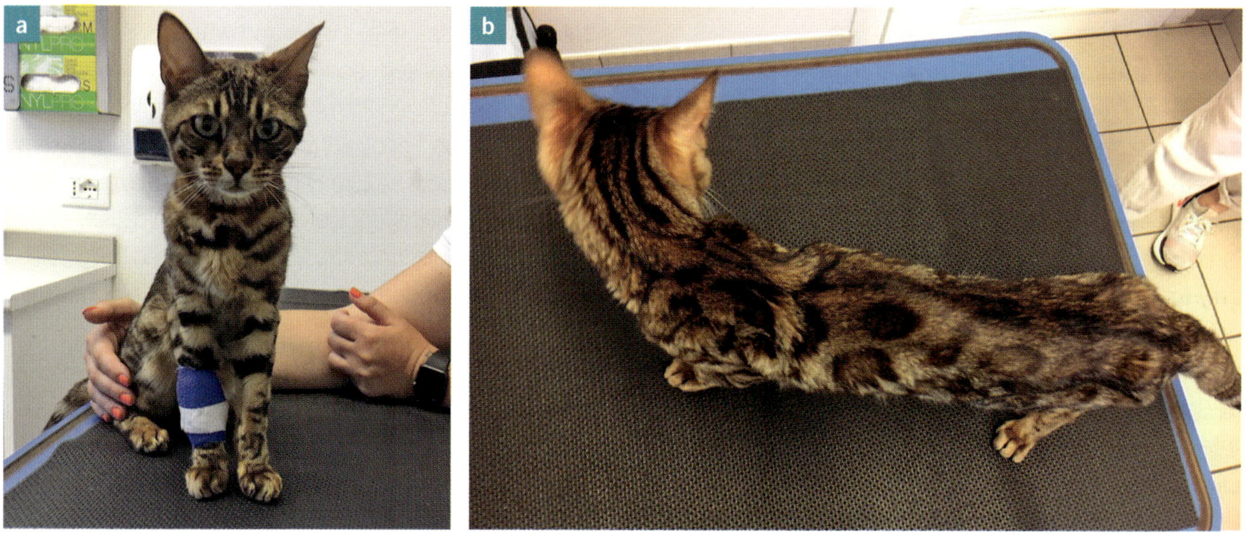

Figure 18.3. Young cat with feline chronic enteropathy showing severe weight loss and poor body condition despite an increased appetite.

Laboratory diagnostics

FCE is a diagnosis of exclusion, and as such, extensive clinicopathologic testing is required to rule out other intestinal and extraintestinal causes of chronic GI signs before considering GI biopsy (Table 18.2). Laboratory workup is helpful in clinical staging of FCE to evaluate the presence of markers of disease severity (e.g. hypoalbuminaemia, cobalamin deficiency, vitamin D deficiency) and guide supportive treatment. Lastly, blood work may allow identification of concurrent pancreatic or hepatic inflammatory disease (i.e. triaditis), which may influence the choice of intestinal biopsy collection modality, affect treatment choice, and ultimately have an impact on the outcome.

The most common haematologic abnormalities reported in cats with FCE include mild nonregenerative anaemia, mild to moderate mature neutrophilia, and mild eosinophilia. The latter was found to be more common in cats with food-responsive disease in a study including 55 cats with chronic GI signs.[3] Peripheral eosinophilia has also been reported in cats with eosinophilic enteritis,

Table 18.2. Main differential diagnoses for cats presenting with chronic recurrent gastrointestinal signs and diagnostic tests required for their diagnosis.

Disease	Diagnostic test
Exocrine pancreatic insufficiency	fTLI
Chronic endoparasite infestation (e.g. *Giardia* spp., *Cryptosporidium* spp., *Tritrichomonas blagburni* [*foetus*])	Faecal flotation, ELISA, IFA, PCR
Adverse food reaction (e.g. food allergy, food intolerance)	Elimination or hydrolysed diet trial and challenge
Gastrointestinal obstruction (e.g. luminal stenosis, CIPO)	Abdominal radiography, abdominal ultrasonography, endoscopy, histopathology
Gastrointestinal neoplasia (e.g. small- or large-cell lymphoma)	Abdominal ultrasonography, cytology, histopathology, IHC, PARR
Granulomatous colitis	PAS or GMS staining, FISH for AIEC or *Campylobacter* spp., culture and antimicrobial sensitivity, IHC or PCR for FCoV

AIEC, adherent–invasive *Escherichia coli*; CIPO, chronic intestinal pseudoobstruction; ELISA, enzyme-linked immunosorbent assay; FCoV, feline coronavirus; FISH, fluorescence in situ hybridisation; fTLI, feline trypsin-like immunoreactivity; GMS, Grocott–Gomori's methenamine silver; IFA, indirect immunofluorescence assay; IHC, immunohistochemistry; PARR, PCR for antigen receptor rearrangements; PAS, periodic acid–Schiff; PCR, polymerase chain reaction.

an histopathological variant of feline IBD.[9] Abnormalities found on serum biochemistry include: mild to moderate increase in liver enzymes activity (alanine aminotransferase [ALT] and alkaline phosphatase [ALP]), which likely reflects secondary reactive hepatopathy or concurrent inflammatory liver disease (provided that hyperthyroidism has been excluded); mild hypoalbuminaemia (more common in IBD than FRE), which could indicate downregulation of hepatic synthesis associated with acute phase syndrome or enteric loss of albumin; mild to moderate hyperglobulinaemia, which could indicate chronic antigenic stimulation or granulomatous inflammation; and mild hypophosphataemia secondary to malabsorption or loss through vomiting and diarrhoea. Although mild hypoalbuminaemia is reported in up to 39% of cats with IBD, the finding of significant (<2.0 g/dl) hypoalbuminaemia due to protein-losing enteropathy in a cat is strongly suggestive of alimentary lymphoma, as idiopathic protein-losing enteropathy has not been described in cats.

Other common abnormalities found during clinicopathologic testing in cats with chronic GI signs include hypocobalaminaemia, decreased or increased serum folate concentration, and increased serum feline pancreatic lipase immunoreactivity (fPLI) or 1,2-o-dilauryl-rac-glycero-3-glutaric acid-(6'-methylresorufin) ester (DGGR) lipase. Cobalamin (vitamin B_{12}) is a water-soluble vitamin derived from dietary proteins. Within the intestinal lumen, it is bound to intrinsic factor, which in the cat is of exclusive pancreatic origin. Then, cobalamin is absorbed in the ileum by binding to specific intrinsic factor–cobalamin receptors. In cats, hypocobalaminaemia can occur because of three main mechanisms: decreased intrinsic factor availability (e.g. exocrine pancreatic insufficiency, chronic pancreatitis), intestinal bacterial competition (e.g. intestinal dysbiosis), and reduced absorption due to ileal mucosal disease. At the cellular level, cobalamin is used for DNA synthesis; therefore, its deficiency can reduce enterocyte turnover and affect intestinal integrity, which contributes to the development of GI signs and weight loss. Irrespectively of the cause of hypocobalaminaemia, cobalamin supplementation is recommended, as it has been shown to improve appetite and faecal consistency in cobalamin-deficient cats.[10] The current recommendation is to supplement cobalamin as follows: 250 μg PO every 24 hours for 12 weeks or SC/IM every 7 days for 6 weeks, whenever serum concentrations are below 400 ng/l, which are believed to be associated with cellular deficiency. Unlike in dogs with CE, in which hypocobalaminaemia has been associated with clinical and histological severity and long-term outcome, hypocobalaminaemia in FCE is not associated with clinical or histological[11] severity nor outcome. This may be due to the fact that hypocobalaminaemia is highly prevalent amongst cats, with studies reporting it in up to 61% of cats with chronic GI signs.[12]

Folate is another water-soluble vitamin contained in several food sources and absorbed in the proximal small intestine, mostly the duodenum. Decreased serum folate concentrations can be caused by decreased dietary intake or decreased absorption due to proximal intestinal mucosal disease. The author does not routinely recommend supplementing folic acid to cats with GI signs and serum folate concentrations below the lower limit of the reference interval, mostly because a clear beneficial effect has not been demonstrated, and also because of the notorious difficulty for cat owners to administer oral medications to their cats. Increased serum folate concentrations can be seen with or without concurrent hypocobalaminaemia secondary to intestinal dysbiosis, which has been attributed to an increased ability of certain bacterial species to synthesise folate. However, hyperfolataemia is not synonymous of a positive response to antibiotic treatment.

The finding of increased fPLI or DGGR lipase in cats with FCE is common. It is not known whether such increases indicate concurrent clinically relevant pancreatitis or subclinical chronic antigenic stimulation of the pancreas secondary to small intestinal dysbiosis. A recent study found significantly increased fPLI in 16/23 cats with histologically diagnosed IBD and concurrent serum fPLI measurement.[13] Only 4 cats had ultrasonographic evidence of pancreatic disease, and pancreatic histopathology was not available for any of the cats. When dividing cats in groups based on the severity of serum fPLI increase (group with serum fPLI 6.9–11.9 µg/l; group with serum fPLI >12 µg/l), no differences were found between these two groups with regard to serum liver enzymes activities, clinical severity, pancreatic ultrasound findings, intestinal histopathology scores, treatment response rate, or clinical outcome. However, cats with serum fPLI above 12 µg/l were significantly more likely to be hypoalbuminaemic or hypocobalaminaemic. Although the clinical significance of increased serum fPLI or DGGR lipase in cats with FCE remains to be elucidated, the author recommends the institution of adequate pain control in cats with FCE if there is a suspicion of concurrent pancreatic disease. In addition, whenever full-thickness GI biopsy samples are being collected during the workup of chronic GI signs, whether by laparoscopy or laparotomy, the author recommends concurrent collection of pancreatic biopsy samples for histopathology if serum fPLI or DGGR lipase are increased.

Measurement of serum vitamin D concentrations in dogs and cats with CEs is not currently routinely performed, irrespective of ionised calcium concentrations. However, recent evidence in dogs with CE (with or without hypoalbuminaemia) suggests that hypovitaminosis D is relatively common and associated with histological severity and poor clinical outcome.[14,15] Similarly, a recent study found that cats with CE (IBD and small-cell lymphoma) had significantly lower serum vitamin D concentrations compared to healthy and hospitalised ill cats.[16] The mechanism by which hypovitaminosis D develops is not known, and its prognostic and therapeutic implications in cats with FCE need to be further investigated.

Clinical activity index

Clinical signs in cats with FCE are highly variable, and disease severity can differ greatly amongst cats, depending on the type of enteropathy, localisation, and extent of lesions in the GI tract. Defining disease activity in FCE is helpful in determining initial disease burden and, above all, in guiding assessment of treatment efficacy. Several clinical activity indices have been validated and applied in human and canine IBD and have been found to correlate with disease phenotype and with the likelihood of responding to different treatment strategies, as well as to predict clinical outcome. In 2010, a specific clinical activity index for cats with CE was developed and subsequently validated in a cohort of 23 cats with either FRE or IBD.[17] This index, called feline chronic enteropathy activity index (FCEAI), incorporated five clinical variables that were graded from 0 to 3 based on presence and severity, in addition to clinicopathologic and endoscopic abnormalities that were scored as 1 or 0 based on whether they were present or not (Table 18.3). The total FCEAI score ranged from 0 to 19. In the prospective validation study, the FCEAI was calculated at the time of diagnosis and 21 days following treatment in 17 cats with IBD and 6 cats with FRE and correlated well with a positive response to treatment in both groups. However, FCAEI at baseline did not distinguish between FCE disease phenotypes (mean FCEAI of the FRE group: 6.7, range 5–9; mean FCEAI of the IBD group: 8.2, range 4–13). The overall rate of clinical remission (defined as a reduction in FCEAI >75% from baseline) at 21 days in this cohort was 100%. However, as cats were only followed up in the short term, no information was given on the predictive ability of baseline FCEAI for treatment response and long-term clinical outcome. More studies with larger cohorts of patients are needed to further assess the prediction of treatment response and the prognostic value of FCEAI.

The role of abdominal ultrasonography in clinical staging

Abdominal ultrasonography is fundamental in the diagnostic workup and clinical staging of cats with chronic GI signs and suspected FCE and should be performed prior to considering collection of GI biopsy samples. Abdominal ultrasonography provides useful information regarding the GI tract (absolute and relative wall thickness and echogenicity), mesenteric lymph nodes (size, shape, and echogenicity), hepatobiliary system (volume, texture of the hepatic parenchyma, wall thickness and content of gallbladder, and diameter and content of intra- and extra-hepatic bile ducts), and pancreas (volume, echogenicity, and peripancreatic fat reactivity), in addition to the peritoneum and other abdominal organs.[18] Therefore, abdominal ultrasonography provides information about the presence of GI lesions, their location and distribution (segmental or diffuse), the presence of GI obstruction (partial or complete), and the presence of concurrent hepatobiliary and/or pancreatic inflammatory disease, which ultimately may prove useful in guiding the clinician in the choice of the best method of intestinal biopsy sample collection.

Historically, much attention has been given to finding a diffusely thickened muscularis propria (defined as a muscularis:submucosa ratio >1), which appeared to be more commonly associated with intestinal small-cell lymphoma (SCL) in elderly cats than FCE.[19] However, subsequent studies did not confirm such association and demonstrated a significant overlap in muscularis propria thickness across cats with FCE/IBD and SCL, as well as healthy cats.[20] A recent study sought to evaluate the ability of abdominal ultrasonography to predict the presence and location of histological lesions by small

Table 18.3. Feline chronic enteropathy activity index (FCEAI). Five subjective clinical variables are scored 0–3 according to their severity. Four clinicopathologic variables are scored 0 (normal) or 1 (increased/decreased). The presence of endoscopic mucosal lesions is recorded as 0 (absent) or 1 (present). The composite FCEAI score is obtained by adding each subtotal score and is proportional to the intestinal inflammatory activity.

Variable	0	1	2	3	Subtotal score
Attitude/activity	Normal	Slight decrease	Moderate decrease	Severe decrease	
Appetite	Normal	Slight decrease	Moderate decrease	Severe decrease	
Vomiting	None	Mild (1/week)	Moderate (2–3/week)	Severe (>3/week)	
Diarrhoea/frequency of defecation	Normal	Slightly soft faeces, blood, mucus, or slightly increased frequency (2–3/d)	Very soft faeces or moderately increased frequency (4–5/d)	Watery diarrhoea or severely increased frequency (>5/d)	
Weight loss	None	Mild (<5% loss)	Moderate (5%–10% loss)	Severe (>10% loss)	
Total protein	Normal	Increased			
ALT	Normal	Increased			
ALP	Normal	Increased			
Phosphorus	Normal	Decreased			
Endoscopic lesions (granularity, friability, ulcers/erosions)	Absent	Present			
Composite score					**Total (0–19)**

Adapted from Jergens AE et al. A clinical index for disease activity in cats with chronic enteropathy. *J Vet Intern Med* 24:1027, 2010.
ALP, alkaline phosphatase; ALT, alanine aminotransferase.

intestinal segment (duodenum, jejunum, ileum) and tissue layer (mucosa, muscularis propria, submucosa) in 166 cats that underwent concurrent abdominal ultrasonography and small intestinal full-thickness biopsy. Overall, the study showed a good positive predictive value for predicting histological lesions in all small intestinal segments but a poor negative predictive value, meaning that even if the ultrasound was normal, there could still be significant histological disease. While a good correlation was found with histopathology for mucosal ultrasonographic lesions (especially for the presence of a hyperechoic mucosal band indicating mucosal fibrosis), correlation was poor for muscularis and submucosal ultrasound lesions,[21] with the exception of muscularis thickening and histological evidence of eosinophilic lamina propria inflammation.

In light of the available evidence, clinicians should not use abdominal ultrasonography to distinguish FCE from SCL. Therefore, the decision to collect full-thickness biopsy samples based solely on ultrasound abnormalities affecting muscularis propria or submucosa is not advised. Nevertheless, abdominal ultrasonography still plays a very important role in the staging and diagnosis of FCE and as a guide for the best next diagnostic step. Cats with diffuse changes in the duodenum and proximal jejunum and/or the ileum may be good candidates for gastroduodenoscopy and ileocolonoscopy. By contrast, patients with segmental disease in the intestine that lies outside the range of the endoscope (i.e. jejunum), and/or in case of extramural abnormalities and changes in other organs, laparotomy or laparoscopy with collection of full-thickness biopsy samples should be considered. When choosing between full-thickness vs. endoscopic biopsy, one needs to consider the higher perioperative morbidity rate and the longer recovery time associated with full-thickness biopsy. The prevalence of major complications in cats undergoing full-thickness biopsy (i.e. biopsy site dehiscence and septic peritonitis) or GI endoscopy (i.e. iatrogenic intestinal perforation) is low according to recent studies. Finally, abdominal ultrasonography allows the collection of hepatosplenic, pancreatic, and nodal fine needle aspiration samples for the cytological evaluation of high-grade lymphoma (as cytology cannot differentiate between SCL and lymphoplasmacytic inflammation) and suppurative inflammation.

Intestinal histopathology to integrate clinical staging

Once all other common intestinal and extraintestinal causes of chronic GI signs have been excluded, histopathological examination of intestinal biopsy samples would be required to make a definitive diagnosis of FCE and to rule out SCL, a major differential diagnosis. However, in young cats with low clinical activity scores and normal appetite or those with large intestinal diarrhoea as their main clinical sign, a well conducted dietary trial with a hydrolysed or selected antigen diet should be carried out before collecting GI biopsy samples to rule out AFRs or FRE.

Historically, the histopathological diagnosis of FCE was based on finding mucosal lamina propria inflammation of varying severity.[1] Subtypes of FCE are identified based on the type of the main cellular infiltrate as lymphoplasmacytic (by far the most common), eosinophilic, and neutrophilic. Severe lymphoplasmacytic or predominantly lymphocytic FCE can be difficult to distinguish from SCL on histology alone, especially in cases with pronounced epitheliotropism, in which neoplastic lymphocytes mostly infiltrate the intestinal epithelium. Epitheliotropism in this context means that neoplastic lymphocytes are intersperse in the epithelial layer of the mucosa, more so than in the lamina propria. In such cases, evaluation of lymphocyte immunotype using antibodies against CD3 and CD79a via immunohistochemistry, with or without assessment of lymphocyte clonality using PCR for antigen receptor rearrangements (PARR), is recommended.[22] Further details can be found in Chapter 20. Intestinal mucosal infiltration with macrophages and/or neutrophils raises the suspicion for an infectious process, and special stains (e.g. periodic acid–Schiff, Grocott–Gomori's methenamine silver), culture, and/or FISH are indicated. While FISH is limited in its availability to a few academic/diagnostic laboratories, this molecular technique may be of clinical value by confirming the presence of increased mucosa-associated and invading bacteria (with or without accompanying neutrophilic infiltration), which may be best treated with antibiotics and/or probiotics. The presence of moderate to large numbers of eosinophils (with or without circulating eosinophilia) might suggest dietary sensitivity or intolerance or could indicate eosinophilic enteritis (a subtype of FCE) or hypereosinophilic syndrome, a syndrome characterised by multicentric eosinophilic organ infiltration with variable response to immunosuppressive therapy.[23] Although the nature and severity of the mucosal inflammatory infiltrate can be suggestive of the role played by dietary or microbial antigens, they do not correlate with clinical activity, nor do they have prognostic significance or predict response to different treatment strategies.

Recently, it has been recognised that changes in mucosal architecture, such as villous atrophy and fusion, epithelial injury, mucosal fibrosis, lacteal dilation, and crypt disease are clinically and diagnostically more relevant than mucosal inflammation, as they indicate significant GI disease and correlate with severity of GI signs and response to treatment. A recent study in cats with chronic GI signs showed that villus atrophy and fusion correlated with severity of clinical signs and degree of pro-inflammatory cytokine upregulation in the duodenal mucosa.[24]

Despite being universally considered as the diagnostic gold standard, intestinal histopathology has several pitfalls that need to be taken into account by the clinician. Firstly, interpretation of biopsies is notoriously subjective and is affected by significant interobserver variability.[25] Secondly, histopathological examination is greatly hampered by poor-quality biopsy samples (endoscopic and surgical) in addition to insufficient numbers, small size, inadequate depth, or other sampling artefacts of the specimens.[26] Lastly, inappropriate tissue handling and/or processing can lead to artefacts and poor sample orientation, which ultimately hampers meaningful histopathological interpretation.[27] Recently, written and pictorial guidelines have been published for histological interpretation and grading of GI lesions in dogs and cats in an attempt to reduce interobserver variability and improve the diagnostic accuracy and reliability of intestinal histopathology.[28,29] However, these guidelines have not been universally adopted by veterinary pathologists and commercial laboratories, and they are flawed by ongoing issues of diagnostic reliability.

Endoscopic vs. full-thickness gastrointestinal biopsy

Samples for histopathological diagnosis of IBD may be obtained endoscopically (mucosal biopsy) or by laparoscopy or exploratory laparotomy (full-thickness biopsy). Currently, controversy exists amongst veterinary gastroenterologists concerning the relative accuracy of endoscopic vs. full-thickness intestinal biopsies in differentiating FCE from SCL in cats. Each modality has intrinsic advantages and disadvantages that need to be critically evaluated by the clinician on a case-by-case basis (Table 18.4).

Endoscopy is a minimally invasive operator-dependent procedure that allows visual examination of duodenal and in some cases proximal jejunal and distal ileal mucosa, as well as the colonic mucosa. Endoscopy is the method preferred by the author, provided that extramural lesions and concurrent extraintestinal (hepatic and/or pancreatic) diseases have been excluded. The experience of the operator in recognising mucosal lesions is of great diagnostic value, as endoscopic lesions in cats with FCE have been shown to correlate well with clinical signs and histological severity.[17] A previous study concluded that endoscopic biopsy was less accurate than full-thickness biopsy in differentiating IBD from lymphoma in cats with chronic GI signs.[30] However, duodenal (endoscopic)

Table 18.4. Comparison of endoscopic vs. full-thickness gastrointestinal biopsies.

	Endoscopic	Full-thickness
Invasiveness	Minimal	Moderate/high
Recovery time	Hours	Days
Layers included in sample	Mucosa +/– submucosa	Mucosa, submucosa, muscularis, serosa
Gastrointestinal segments available for sampling	Stomach, duodenum (+/– proximal jejunum), ileum (if expert operator and suitable endoscope available), colon	Stomach, duodenum, jejunum, ileum, colon (not recommended)
Visual examination of mucosal lesions/ target biopsies	Yes	No
Number of collectable samples	Unlimited	1–2/gastrointestinal segment
Initiation of glucocorticoid therapy immediately after procedure	Yes	No, typically will need to wait 5–7 days
Evaluation of extraintestinal organs	No	Yes

assessment was limited to only 50% of the cats included in that study, and mucosal biopsy was performed blindly in one-third of cases. Because none of the cats in this study had endoscopic biopsy of the ileum performed, malignant infiltrates in the ileum could only be confirmed in full-thickness specimens obtained by laparotomy. In another study, the likelihood for diagnosis of alimentary lymphoma was greatest in cats undergoing multi-organ biopsy from all segments of the intestine and the mesenteric lymph nodes.[31] However, comparative data from endoscopic biopsies from the different intestinal segments was not available. A previous study showed that collecting ileal endoscopic biopsy samples significantly increased the probability of diagnosing SCL in cats.[32] However, in the latter study, the diagnosis was based solely on light microscopy evaluation of haematoxylin–eosin stained sections. A recent study that systematically incorporated use of immunohistochemistry and PARR in addition to light microscopy when evaluating biopsy samples found good agreement between duodenal and ileal diagnosis of FCE vs. SCL.[33]

Hepatic and pancreatic biopsy

Triaditis is the term used to describe concurrent inflammation of the pancreas, liver, and small intestine in cats.[34] However, the specific diseases of each organ that together constitute a diagnosis of triaditis remain to be defined. It is well established that cats are at increased risk of developing concurrent hepatobiliary, pancreatic, and small intestinal inflammation. This increased risk is thought to stem from the fact that the pancreatic duct and the common bile duct share a common tract before opening into the proximal duodenum in this species. This unique anatomic feature may allow for retrograde ascension of intestinal bacteria, whether associated with intestinal dysbiosis or not, into the pancreatic and biliary system, with subsequent antigenic stimulation or establishment of suppurative inflammation. Inflammation may also be a sequela of intestinal bacterial translocation and systemic bacteraemia.

The true prevalence of triaditis in cats with FCE is not known, as concurrent histopathology of all three sites would be required for diagnosis and is only rarely available. A recent prospective study involving 47 cats (27 symptomatic and 20 asymptomatic) that underwent concurrent small intestinal, hepatic, and pancreatic biopsies found that 8 (17%) cats had histological evidence of triaditis. Interestingly, triaditis was identified only in symptomatic cats (8/27, 29.6%), but not in clinically healthy cats. In the same study, 19 cats had inflammation involving at least two organs, more specifically 16 (34.0%) cats had concurrent IBD and cholangitis, but only 3 (6.4%) had concurrent IBD and pancreatitis.[35] A more recent study evaluated hepatic and pancreatic biopsy samples collected immediately prior to full-thickness small intestinal biopsy in 300 cats with chronic GI signs, of which 150 were diagnosed with FCE and 124 were diagnosed with SCL.[36] Hepatic lymphoma was diagnosed in 5/150 (3%) cats with FCE and in 10/124 (8%) cats with SCL. Cholangitis was diagnosed in 33/150 (22%) cats with FCE and in 28/124 (22%) cats with SCL. For the 164 cats that underwent pancreatic biopsy, 126 (77%) were normal or had nodular hyperplasia, 19 (11.5%) had amyloidosis, 9 (5.5%) had acinar atrophy, 5 (3%) had pancreatic lymphoma, and 5 (3%) had pancreatitis. Of the 10 cats with inflammatory or neoplastic pancreatic disease, 6 had presurgical Spec fPL concentrations within normal ranges (4/5 with lymphoma and 2/5 with pancreatitis). Of the 126 cats with normal pancreatic histology, 17 (13.5%) had presurgical Spec fPL concentrations over the cutoff diagnostic for pancreatitis of greater than or equal to 5.4 μg/l. Together, these studies show that inflammatory hepatic disease occurs very commonly in cats with FCE and that, rarely, cats with FCE will be diagnosed with low-grade hepatic lymphoma. On the contrary, histological evidence of pancreatitis appears rather uncommon in cats with a diagnosis of FCE.

The clinical significance of histological evidence of hepatic or pancreatic inflammation in cats diagnosed with FCE is currently equivocal. The author collects hepatic samples, in addition to bile by cholecystocentesis for cytology and culture, whenever full-thickness GI biopsy is performed, especially if significant hepatic enzyme elevation is present or ultrasonographic evidence of hepatobiliary disease is found. In the event of neutrophilic cholangitis, antimicrobial therapy (based on results of antibiotic susceptibility testing) is initiated in addition to a hydrolysed or elimination diet trial before considering immunosuppressive therapy (in the event that GI signs fail to respond to diet alone).

TREATMENT

Very few well-conducted randomised controlled trials have been published with regard to treatment of FCE. Historically, treatment strategies have been based on sequential trials with therapeutic diets, antibiotics, and immunosuppressive drugs, whereas combination therapy has been advocated in more severe clinical disease. However, scant to no evidence exists in support of the systematic use of antibiotics in cats with FCE. To the contrary, mounting evidence indicates that antibiotics induce a pattern of intestinal dysbiosis similar to that naturally found in enteropathic cats. If one considers the role of indiscriminate antibiotic use on the global emerging issue of antimicrobial resistance, it is easily understandable why alternative options to antibiotics are needed when attempting to modulate the intestinal microbiota in disease. The combination of prebiotics/probiotics and FMT are currently being evaluated for this purpose and are reviewed in-depth in Chapters 36 and 37, respectively. In this section, the author focuses on more established treatment strategies and proposes a new step-up therapeutic approach to cats with chronic predominantly small and large intestinal signs.

Therapeutic diets

A dietary trial is typically conducted after having excluded any other intestinal (e.g. infectious, neoplastic) and extraintestinal causes of GI signs and before proceeding to GI biopsy. Commercial diets available for this purpose include: single (and often novel) protein diets, hydrolysed protein diets, and low-residue diets (often referred to as "gastrointestinal diets").[37,38] The specifics of each diet type together with their advantages and disadvantages are shown in Table 18.5. No well-conducted and adequately powered randomised controlled trials have compared the relative efficacy or superiority of the different diet types in cats with FCE. Traditionally, single novel protein and hydrolysed diets have been preferred over gastrointestinal diets and have been considered an appropriate first choice. This conviction stemmed from the results of two prospective studies which evaluated the efficacy of single novel protein and/or hydrolysed diets in 55 and 23 cats with chronic GI signs, respectively.[3,17] These studies found a rate of diet-induced remission of 49% and 26%, respectively, and a no difference in efficacy was found between the two diets. In both studies, clinical remission was achieved swiftly within 7–10 days. A recent study compared two commercial dry gastrointestinal diets (traditionally considered best suited for the management of acute GI signs) in a group of 28 cats with chronic vomiting (without hypocobalaminaemia or hypoalbuminaemia).[39] Interestingly, the study showed that both diets significantly reduced vomiting in all cats within 2 weeks of starting the diet, indicating a possible role for the management and diagnostic workup of FCE also for gastrointestinal diets.

Table 18.5. Advantages and disadvantages of commercial therapeutic diets available for the management and diagnosis of feline chronic enteropathy.

Diet type	Advantages	Disadvantages
Low-residue (gastrointestinal)	Recently shown efficacy in cats with chronic gastrointestinal signs High digestibility High palatability Some formulas have higher total fibre	Mostly containing poultry proteins Anecdotally, lower efficacy compared to hydrolysed diets
Single novel protein	Proven efficacy in proportion of cats with chronic gastrointestinal signs High palatability Some formulas have higher total fibre content	Thorough dietary history required Contamination concerns with over-the-counter diets Lower efficacy in cats with chronic inflammatory enteropathy vs. adverse food reactions
Hydrolysed	Proven efficacy in proportion of cats with chronic gastrointestinal signs Thorough dietary history not always needed Anecdotally superior efficacy compared to single novel protein diet in cats with chronic inflammatory enteropathy	Possibly less palatable than gastrointestinal or single-protein diets Possibly more expensive than gastrointestinal or single-protein diets

The exact mechanisms by which therapeutic diets induce clinical remission in cats with FCE are unknown but are thought to include reduced immunogenicity of the dietary ingredients, improved digestibility, and modulation of the intestinal microbiota. Ideally, once clinical remission (defined as reduction in clinical activity score >75% from baseline) has been achieved, a challenge with the original diet would be required in order to rule out AFRs; however, most owners are reluctant to conduct such challenges, and cats are kept indefinitely on the therapeutic diet. In the event of a failed trial, providing that poor owner's compliance or access of the cat to other food can be excluded, it might be sensible to conduct a second trial with a different type of diet before considering collection of GI biopsy samples. This is especially important if a gastrointestinal or single-protein diet has been used first, the clinical severity is mild, or the cat is relatively young (Fig. 18.4).

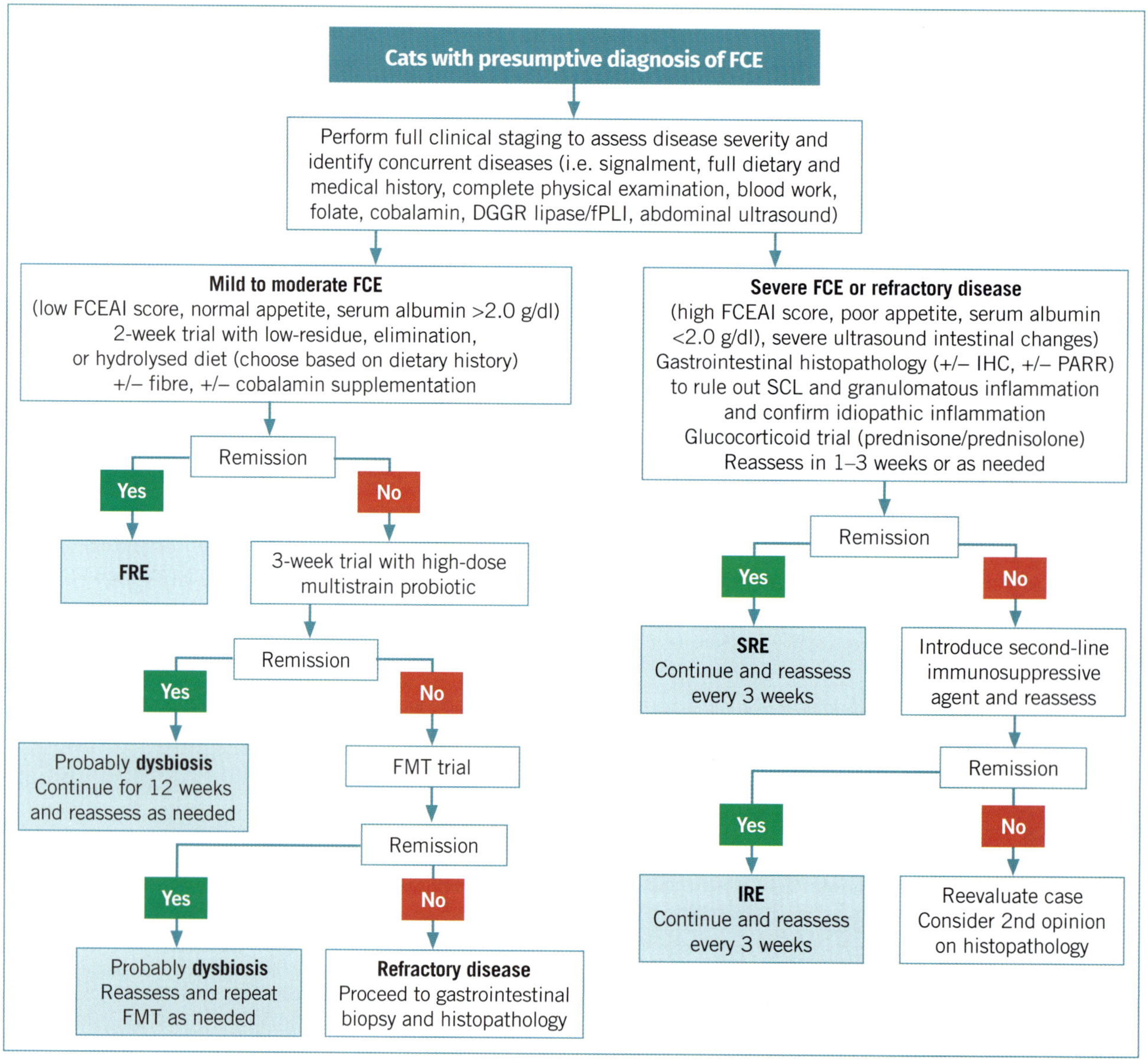

Figure 18.4. Diagnostic algorithm and staged therapeutic approach for cats presenting with chronic gastrointestinal signs with suspected feline chronic enteropathy (FCE). DGGR, 1,2-o-dilauryl-rac-glycero-3-glutaric acid-(6'-methylresorufin) ester; FCEAI, feline chronic enteropathy activity index; FMT, faecal microbiota transplantation; fPLI, feline pancreatic lipase immunoreactivity; FRE, food-responsive enteropathy; IHC, immunohistochemistry; IRE, immunosuppressant-responsive enteropathy; PARR, PCR for antigen receptor rearrangements; SCL, small-cell lymphoma; SRE, steroid-responsive enteropathy.

Immunosuppressive therapy

Immunosuppressive therapy is the mainstay treatment in FCE. It is usually based on the use of glucocorticoids (prednisone/prednisolone, dexamethasone, or budesonide) alone or, in cats with steroid-refractory disease, in association with chlorambucil (Fig. 18.4). Immunosuppressive therapy is usually initiated after one or two consecutive failed dietary trials or concurrently with diet in cats with severe clinical disease activity. Whilst cats (especially those with mild disease or of young age) should undergo dietary trials before considering GI biopsy, intestinal histopathology is recommended before commencing immunosuppressive treatment to ensure the presence of significant mucosal inflammation; to rule out granulomatous inflammation, which could indicate the presence of enteropathogens or bacterial translocation; and to rule out SCL, which would require combination therapy with glucocorticoids and chlorambucil.

Prednisolone (the active form of prednisone) is the most commonly used glucocorticoid for the management of FCE and is typically started at 2 mg/kg PO every 24 hours or divided in two doses every 12 hours. Even though cats are usually tolerant to steroid side effects, budesonide (3 mg/m^2 every 24 hours) has been anecdotally used as an alternative in patients intolerant to systemic steroids (e.g. cats with diabetes mellitus). Cats with severe malabsorption can benefit from initial treatment with subcutaneous injections of dexamethasone until the disease is better controlled. Only a few case-based studies have evaluated the efficacy of glucocorticoids in FCE. In the largest case-series with 60 cats with small and large intestinal FCE,[40] prednisone alone or in conjunction with other drugs induced complete or partial remission in 39/47 cats (83%) that had not responded to diet alone. However, extrapolation of reliable clinical data from this study is hampered by the fact that immunosuppressive therapy was invariably initiated together with diet and other drugs (e.g. salicylates, antimicrobials) and that evaluation of clinical remission was arbitrary. In another more recent prospective study, all of 17 cats with mild to moderate histological disease achieved complete remission (defined as a FCEAI score <75% from baseline) at 21 days of treatment with prednisolone as a sole agent.

In cases of FCE refractory to glucocorticoids, chlorambucil (an alkylating agent that cross-links DNA used to treat SCL) is usually added to the treatment regimen.[41] Chlorambucil is dosed at 2 mg/cat every 48 hours (every 72 hours in cats weighing <4 kg) and is usually very well tolerated by most cats, as it is only minimally myelosuppressive. An alternative dosing regimen of 20 mg/m^2 given every 14–21 days has also been used and might be considered for fractious cats that cannot be easily medicated by the owner. When using this 20 mg/m^2 protocol, regular (i.e. every 1–3 months) complete blood counts should be performed to rule out significant myelosuppression.

Antibiotics

The systematic use of antibiotics, alone or in combination with other treatment strategies, is not recommended in cats with chronic GI signs because of the low relative incidence of antibiotic-responsive cases, the impact that antibiotics have on the intestinal microbiota, and the recent rise of bacterial antibiotic resistance. Rarely, antibiotic therapy might be necessary to control cases of severe chronic mucosa-associated bacterial overgrowth or FISH positive cases of granulomatous colitis (see case-based example below).

Monitoring treatment efficacy

Unlike in human IBD, resolution or improvement of clinical signs is the main goal of treatment in cats with FCE. No studies in cats have evaluated the occurrence of mucosal (endoscopic) or histological remission after treatment. Therefore, it remains to be ascertained whether ongoing subclinical disease exists and whether this has implications on the long-term outcome or on the risk of developing SCL. As previously mentioned, a FCEAI specific for cats with chronic GI signs has been recently designed and prospectively validated in a small cohort of 23 cats. This index allows more reliable and repeatable assessment of clinical signs during treatment. Using this clinical activity index, complete remission is defined as a reduction in the FCEAI score of more than 75% from baseline (pretreatment), partial remission as a decline of 50%–75% from baseline, stable (refractory) disease as a reduction of 25%–49% from baseline, and treatment failure or progressive disease as a reduction of less than 25% from baseline. The response to treatment should be evaluated every 3–4 weeks. If complete remission is

Case-based example on rationale use of antibiotics for the treatment of feline chronic enteropathy

Signalment and anamnesis

Domestic shorthair cat, 14-month-old, male, neutered. Presented with chronic history of vomiting, weight loss, polyphagia, and severe large intestinal diarrhoea. Clinical signs refractory to sequential elimination and hydrolysed diet trials, anthelmintic treatment, multistrain probiotic therapy, and short course of prednisolone (2 mg/kg PO every 24 h).

Physical examination

Unremarkable, with the exception of severely reduced muscle and body condition scores and suboptimal body weight (2.2 kg).

Clinical staging

- Blood work: mild mature neutrophilia and mild hyperglobulinaemia
- Faecal flotation, *Giardia* spp. ELISA, and *Tritrichomonas blagburni* (*foetus*) PCR: negative
- Abdominal ultrasound: moderate diffuse thickening of the colonic wall, mild colic lymphadenopathy, and a minimal quantity of free peritoneal fluid
- Serum folate and cobalamin concentrations, feline trypsin-like immunoreactivity, and SNAP fPL: within normal limits

Upper and lower gastrointestinal endoscopy

Normal gastric fundic and pyloric mucosa, mildly increased multifocal duodenal friability, and severe diffuse colonic erosions. The ileum could not be intubated. Multiple visual mucosal samples were obtained from stomach, duodenum, and colon.

Histopathology

Normal fundic and pyloric mucosa, mild lymphoplasmacytic and neutrophilic duodenal inflammation with mild villous atrophy, and multifocally moderate pyogranulomatous and mild lymphoplasmacytic colitis with mild to moderate attenuation and degeneration of the surface epithelium (Figs. 18.5 and 18.6).

- Periodic acid–Schiff (PAS): mildly positive
- Grocott–Gomori's methenamine silver (GMS) stain, feline coronavirus immunohistochemistry, and *Prototheca* spp. and *Tritrichomonas blagburni* (*foetus*) PCR: negative

Fluorescence in situ hybridisation of colonic biopsies

In some areas, very large numbers of short rods in close apposition to the mucosa (Fig. 18.7). In other regions, rafts of superficially invasive rods in eroded ulcerated mucosa and in degenerating crypts (Fig. 18.8).

Bacterial culture of biopsy specimen

Negative for *Campylobacter* spp. and *Salmonella* spp. Scant growth of commensal *Escherichia coli*.

Final diagnosis

Idiopathic granulomatous inflammatory bowel disease associated with severe overgrowth of mucosa-adherent and invasive *Enterobacteriaceae* (microbial dysbiosis).

Treatment

Antibiotic therapy deemed necessary in this case to reduce mucosal bacterial load. Tylosin (5 mg/kg PO every 12 h) prescribed in association with a multistrain probiotic and a highly digestible fibre-enriched diet.

Follow-up and outcome

Clinical remission achieved 1 month after initiation of treatment, with resolution of vomiting and diarrhoea and significant weight gain. Antibiotic therapy discontinued. Probiotics and diet continued. Sustained clinical remission achieved despite discontinuation of antibiotics.

confirmed in cats with SRE, the dose of glucocorticoids is decreased by 25%–30% until the next follow-up. If partial remission is achieved, the current dose can be left unchanged, whilst in the event of refractory or progressive disease, chlorambucil is added to the treatment regimen.

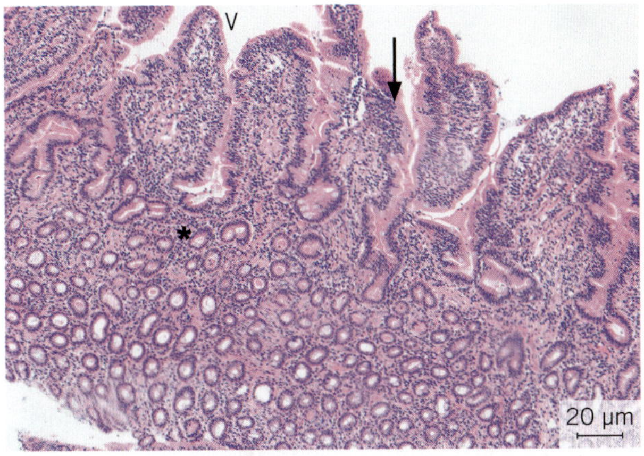

Figure 18.5. Duodenal biopsy specimen obtained endoscopically. Villi (V) appear to be mildly shortened. The epithelium is intact. Within the lamina propria, there are low numbers of lymphocytes, plasma cells, and occasionally neutrophils (asterisk). Mildly increased numbers of lymphocytes infiltrate the epithelium (arrow). Haematoxylin–eosin stain.

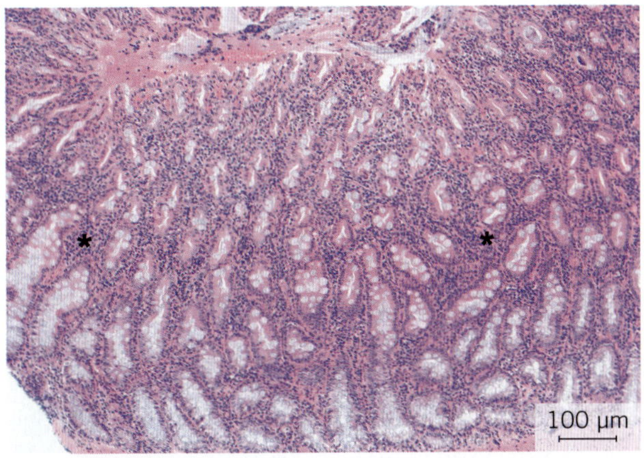

Figure 18.6. Colonic biopsy specimen obtained endoscopically. Within the lamina propria, there are low numbers of lymphocytes and plasma cells, and multifocally moderate numbers of neutrophils and macrophages (asterisks). Haematoxylin–eosin stain.

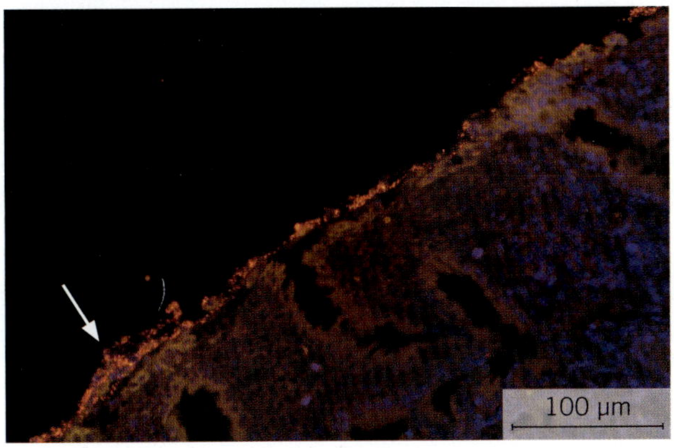

Figure 18.7. Colonic biopsy specimen showing mucosa-associated bacterial overgrowth. In close apposition to a markedly hypercellular mucosal epithelium, there are very large numbers of short rods (arrow). Fluorescence in situ hybridisation with eubacterial probe Cy3-EUB-338.

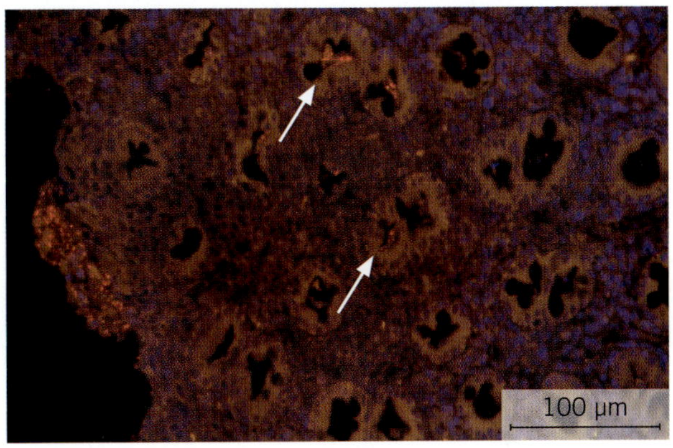

Figure 18.8. Colonic biopsy specimen showing mucosa-invading bacteria. Small rafts of invasive rods are seen within degenerating proprial crypts (arrows). Fluorescence in situ hybridisation with eubacterial probe Cy3-EUB-338.

PROGNOSIS

Little information is available regarding the long-term outcome of cats with FCE. In a recent study of cats with FCE and SCL with a median follow-up time of about 3 years, the proportion of cats with FCE alive at 1, 2, and 3 years was 84%, 75%, and 71%, respectively.[42] While many cats with FCE will respond favourably to dietary and immunosuppressive therapy, treatment failures may still occur. Some of the most common reasons for treatment failure include poor owner compliance in following dietary recommendations, presence of severe irreversible ultrastructural mucosal lesions, presence of concurrent disease (e.g. pancreatitis, cholangitis), and a missed diagnosis of SCL. If neutrophilic (bacterial) cholangitis is present in addition to FCE, antibiotic treatment (whenever possible chosen on the basis of culture and sensitivity results) of adequate duration (i.e. 4 weeks long) should be initiated prior to immunosuppressive treatment of FCE.

Take-home messages

- Feline chronic enteropathy (FCE) is a common cause of chronic gastrointestinal signs in cats. Unlike in dogs, only two main phenotypes of disease have been recognised: food-responsive enteropathy and inflammatory bowel disease. Small-cell lymphoma is the main differential diagnosis.
- Clinical staging in FCE is fundamental, as it allows identification of segmental disease, exclusion of concurrent diseases, and identification of complications from the disease.
- Intestinal histopathology remains the gold standard for the diagnosis of FCE, with equal relevance given to mucosal inflammatory infiltrates and ultrastructural abnormalities such as villous atrophy, epithelial injury, and mucosal fibrosis. In severe cases of inflammatory lymphocytic proprial or epithelial infiltrates, light microscopic evaluation of biopsy samples should be combined with immunohistochemistry and PCR for antigen receptor rearrangements (PARR) to exclude small-cell lymphoma.
- Treatment strategies for FCE are currently based on the sequential use of therapeutic diets and immunosuppressive drugs.
- Antibiotic-responsive enteropathy is not well characterised in cats; therefore, antibiotic trials for diagnostic purposes are no longer justified in cats with chronic gastrointestinal signs. Antibiotics should be reserved for cases with histological and molecular evidence of bacteria-associated granulomatous colitis or severe mucosal bacterial overgrowth.
- The role of probiotics and faecal microbiota transplantation in the management of FCE is currently under review but appears promising.

REFERENCES

[1] Willard MD. Feline inflammatory bowel disease: a review. *J Feline Med Surg* 1:155, 1999.

[2] Jergens AE. Feline idiopathic inflammatory bowel disease: what we know and what remains to be unraveled. *J Feline Med Surg* 14:445, 2012.

[3] Guilford WG et al. Food sensitivity in cats with chronic idiopathic gastrointestinal problems. *J Vet Intern Med* 15:7, 2001.

[4] Dennis JS, Kruger JM, Mullaney TP. Lymphocytic/plasmacytic gastroenteritis in cats: 14 cases (1985–1990). *J Am Vet Med Assoc* 200:1712, 1992.

[5] Dennis JS, Kruger JM, Mullaney TP. Lymphocytic/plasmacytic colitis in cats: 14 cases (1985–1990). *J Am Vet Med Assoc* 202:313, 1993.

[6] Jergens AE et al. Idiopathic inflammatory bowel disease in dogs and cats: 84 cases (1987–1990). *J Am Vet Med Assoc* 201:1603, 1992.

[7] Maunder CL et al. *Campylobacter* species and neutrophilic inflammatory bowel disease in cats. *J Vet Intern Med* 30:996, 2016.

[8] Leal RO et al. Granulomatous colitis: more than a canine disease? A case of *Escherichia coli*-associated granulomatous colitis in an adult cat. *JFMS Open Rep* 3:2055116917731168, 2017.

[9] Tucker S et al. Clinicopathological and ultrasonographic features of cats with eosinophilic enteritis. *J Feline Med Surg* 16:950, 2014.

[10] Ruaux CG, Steiner JM, Williams DA. Early biochemical and clinical responses to cobalamin supplementation in cats with signs of gastrointestinal disease and severe hypocobalaminemia. *J Vet Intern Med* 19:155, 2005.

[11] Maunder CL et al. Serum cobalamin concentrations in cats with gastrointestinal signs: correlation with histopathological findings and duration of clinical signs. *J Feline Med Surg* 14:686, 2012.

[12] Simpson KW et al. Subnormal concentrations of serum cobalamin (vitamin B_{12}) in cats with gastrointestinal disease. *J Vet Intern Med* 15:26, 2001.

[13] Bailey S et al. Comparisons between cats with normal and increased fPLI concentrations in cats diagnosed with inflammatory bowel disease. *J Small Anim Pract* 51:484, 2010.

[14] Allenspach K et al. Hypovitaminosis D is associated with negative outcome in dogs with protein losing enteropathy: a retrospective study of 43 cases. *BMC Vet Res* 13:96, 2017.

[15] Wennogle SA et al. Comparison of clinical, clinicopathologic, and histologic variables in dogs with chronic inflam-

matory enteropathy and low or normal serum 25-hydroxy-cholecalciferol concentrations. *J Vet Intern Med* 33:1995, 2019.

[16] LALOR S et al. Cats with inflammatory bowel disease and intestinal small cell lymphoma have low serum concentrations of 25-hydroxyvitamin D. *J Vet Intern Med* 28:351, 2014.

[17] JERGENS AE et al. A clinical index for disease activity in cats with chronic enteropathy. *J Vet Intern Med* 24:1027, 2010.

[18] GASCHEN L. Ultrasonography of small intestinal inflammatory and neoplastic diseases in dogs and cats. *Vet Clin North Am Small Anim Pract* 41:329, 2011.

[19] ZWINGENBERGER AL et al. Ultrasonographic evaluation of the muscularis propria in cats with diffuse small intestinal lymphoma or inflammatory bowel disease. *J Vet Intern Med* 24:289, 2010.

[20] DANIAUX LA et al. Ultrasonographic thickening of the muscularis propria in feline small intestinal small cell T-cell lymphoma and inflammatory bowel disease. *J Feline Med Surg* 16:89, 2014.

[21] GUTTIN T et al. Ability of ultrasonography to predict the presence and location of histologic lesions in the small intestine of cats. *J Vet Intern Med* 33:1278, 2019.

[22] MARSILIO S. Differentiating inflammatory bowel disease from alimentary lymphoma in cats: does it matter? *Vet Clin North Am Small Anim Pract* 51:93, 2021.

[23] MCEWEN SA, VALLI VE, HULLAND TJ. Hypereosinophilic syndrome in cats: a report of three cases. *Can J Comp Med* 49:248, 1985.

[24] JANECZKO S et al. The relationship of mucosal bacteria to duodenal histopathology, cytokine mRNA, and clinical disease activity in cats with inflammatory bowel disease. *Vet Microbiol* 128:178, 2008.

[25] WILLARD MD et al. Interobserver variation among histopathologic evaluations of intestinal tissues from dogs and cats. *J Am Vet Med Assoc* 220:1177, 2002.

[26] WILLARD MD et al. Effect of sample quality on the sensitivity of endoscopic biopsy for detecting gastric and duodenal lesions in dogs and cats. *J Vet Intern Med* 22:1084, 2008.

[27] WILLARD MD et al. Effect of tissue processing on assessment of endoscopic intestinal biopsies in dogs and cats. *J Vet Intern Med* 24:84, 2010.

[28] WASHABAU RJ et al. Endoscopic, biopsy, and histopathologic guidelines for the evaluation of gastrointestinal inflammation in companion animals. *J Vet Intern Med* 24:10, 2010.

[29] DAY MJ et al. Histopathological standards for the diagnosis of gastrointestinal inflammation in endoscopic biopsy samples from the dog and cat: a report from the World Small Animal Veterinary Association Gastrointestinal Standardization Group. *J Comp Pathol* 138 Suppl 1:S1, 2008.

[30] EVANS SE et al. Comparison of endoscopic and full-thickness biopsy specimens for diagnosis of inflammatory bowel disease and alimentary tract lymphoma in cats. *J Am Vet Med Assoc* 229:1447, 2006.

[31] KLEINSCHMIDT S et al. Chronic inflammatory and non-inflammatory diseases of the gastrointestinal tract in cats: diagnostic advantages of full-thickness intestinal and extraintestinal biopsies. *J Feline Med Surg* 12:97, 2010.

[32] SCOTT KD et al. Utility of endoscopic biopsies of the duodenum and ileum for diagnosis of inflammatory bowel disease and small cell lymphoma in cats. *J Vet Intern Med* 25:1253, 2011.

[33] CHOW B et al. Comprehensive comparison of upper and lower endoscopic small intestinal biopsy in cats with chronic enteropathy. *J Vet Intern Med* 35:190, 2021.

[34] SIMPSON KW. Pancreatitis and triaditis in cats: causes and treatment. *J Small Anim Pract* 56:40, 2015.

[35] FRAGKOU FC et al. Prevalence and clinicopathological features of triaditis in a prospective case series of symptomatic and asymptomatic cats. *J Vet Intern Med* 30:1031, 2016.

[36] NORSWORTHY GD et al. Prevalence and underlying causes of histologic abnormalities in cats suspected to have chronic small bowel disease: 300 cases (2008–2013). *J Am Vet Med Assoc* 247:629, 2015.

[37] KATHRANI A. Dietary and nutritional approaches to the management of chronic enteropathy in dogs and cats. *Vet Clin North Am Small Anim Pract* 51:123, 2021.

[38] MANDIGERS PJ, BIOURGE V, GERMAN AJ. Efficacy of a commercial hydrolysate diet in eight cats suffering from inflammatory bowel disease or adverse reaction to food. *Tijdschr Diergeneeskd* 135:668, 2010.

[39] PEREA SC et al. Evaluation of two dry commercial therapeutic diets for the management of feline chronic gastroenteropathy. *Front Vet Sci* 4:69, 2017.

[40] HART JR et al. Lymphocytic-plasmacytic enterocolitis in cats: 60 cases (1988–1990). *J Am Anim Hosp Assoc* 30:505, 1994.

[41] STEIN TJ et al. Treatment of feline gastrointestinal small-cell lymphoma with chlorambucil and glucocorticoids. *J Am Anim Hosp Assoc* 46:413, 2010.

[42] SABATTINI S et al. Differentiating feline inflammatory bowel disease from alimentary lymphoma in duodenal endoscopic biopsies. *J Small Anim Pract* 57:396, 2016.

CHAPTER 19

Feline gastrointestinal eosinophilic sclerosing fibroplasia

Michael Linton, Christine Griebsch

Feline gastrointestinal eosinophilic sclerosing fibroplasia (FGESF) refers to a clinical and pathological entity associated with eosinophilic mass(es) primarily confined to the gastrointestinal (GI) tract.[1,2] However, more recent case reports question the validity of the originally coined title given that lesions have been identified in extra-GI locations and possibly in other species.[3–6]

A large distribution of cases have been reported, with case reports/series originating in Oceania (Australia, New Zealand), North America (United States of America), Europe (Slovenia, Czech Republic, Spain, Finland, United Kingdom), and parts of Asia (Japan, South Korea).[1,2,4,6–11] Furthermore, there are unpublished case reports from Austria, Canada, and Sweden.

Based on reports the prognosis is guarded. However, this may be due to mismanagement because of an initial incorrect diagnosis and minimal available information in the literature on how to appropriately treat the condition.

On gross examination and prior to pathologists being made more aware of the entity, lesions were commonly confused as neoplasia or granuloma with misdiagnosis reported.[1,2] In a case series of 25 cats, 24% of cases were euthanised due to the gross appearance of the lesion at laparotomy.[1]

In 2009, one study coined the name and hypothesised that some cats have an uncharacterised genetic predisposition to develop eosinophilic inflammation in response to antigens, possibly from bacteria or parasites breaching the intestinal mucosa.[1] In the same year, cases were reported in Australia.[12] Bacteria have been identified in lesions using a range of diagnostic tools in some but not all cats.[1,2] Similar lesions found in the subcutis and abdomen of cats in Japan were proposed to be caused by methicillin-resistant *Staphylococcus* spp.[9] Other infectious agents have been associated with the condition, including zygomycetes in a domestic cat and nematodes in pumas (*Felis concolor*).[5,13]

Despite a number of interesting case reports and case series appearing in the literature, the aetiology of the disease is still unclear. Additionally, important questions remain unanswered, the most notable of which include:

- Is FGESF really a relatively new disease, or has it been around for longer than currently reported due to a history of misdiagnosis?
- If it is a new disease, then what has changed that led to its emergence?

Answers to these questions may provide the key to determining the aetiology of the disease which may aid diagnosis, therapy, and potentially prevention.

EPIDEMIOLOGY AND AETIOLOGY

The condition appears to primarily affect the domestic cat, although case reports suggest that it may not be limited to this species alone, with similar cases seen in pumas and a rat.[5,14] However, closer evaluation of histopathology from these species suggests variation and that lesions are not identical to those observed in domestic cats. Specifically, in the puma, the name "sclerosing fibroplasia" was proposed because of the relatively few eosinophils observed infiltrating the lesions, compared to cats. Additionally, all cases reported in pumas have had associated nematodes.[5] In the single case report of a rat, there were also relatively few eosinophils infiltrating the lesion and there was no formation of the trabecular sclerosing collagen fibroplasia as seen in cats, therefore the lesion was diagnosed as "fibroplasia".[14]

In a study by one of the authors, most cats were mature adults (median age 7 years), although cats of almost any age were affected (2–11 years).[2] In the literature, the youngest case reported is a 14-week-old neutered male Exotic Shorthair cross Persian that had a primary GI mass involving the duodenum.[1] A number of breeds have been reported, with domestic shorthair cats being the most prevalent. However, in the author's study, Ragdolls constituted 7/13 cases, and hence were considered predisposed, with males being more commonly reported than females.[2]

It has been hypothesised that affected cats suffer from immunological dysregulation triggered by one or more factors.[1,2] The factors which might be involved can only be speculated, but suggestions include dietary causes (food allergy or intolerance), dysbiosis of the gut microbiota, excessive ingestion of foreign material (e.g. hair), or the effect of other endo- or ectoparasites. In one domestic cat, FGESF was associated with fungi, showing numerous pleomorphic, nonparallel-walled, sparsely septate hyphae, characteristic of phycomycetes present within the collagen matrix.[8] In one cat, lymphoma developed at a site of FGESF.[15] It is unknown whether FGESF predisposed to the emergence of alimentary lymphoma in this cat or if they were unrelated.

The search to find a plausible causative microbial pathogen as an underlying cause of FGESF has been the focus of several studies.

Intralesional bacteria have been identified in a relatively high percentage of cases, with two case series reporting an incidence of 56% and 69%, respectively.[1,2] In one study, gram-positive cocci were identified in 23 of 27 cases.[9] It is noteworthy that many cases are not associated with infectious causes. This may reflect diagnostic limitations (not all tests were performed) or that infections are not solely involved in the pathogenesis of this syndrome. The location of most lesions to areas in close proximity to or in actual communication with areas containing normal bacterial flora makes conclusions regarding disease association complicated. Microscopically inflammation is focused around bacteria, suggesting that in some patients these bacteria may play a role in initiating or perpetuating the disease process.[1]

Alternatively, secondary infection with bacteria, protozoa, fungi, or other infectious agents may be facilitated by a breach in the mucosal integrity of the GI wall due to abnormal architecture from the FGESF lesion. These secondary infections presumably perpetuate the process, causing a vicious cycle of eosinophilic inflammation, fibroplasia, and eventually fibrosis.

In cats, eosinophilic inflammation is a defining feature of the condition. Eosinophils produce numerous mediators that can lead to tissue destruction (e.g. major basic protein [MBP], transforming growth factor beta [TGF-β], and interleukin [IL]-1β), while elaboration of IL-6 and MBP can result in fibroplasia and fibrosis. This leads to a self-perpetuating process presumably giving rise to various abdominal masses. These masses then cause structural alteration to the stomach, intestines, mesenteric lymph nodes, enteric nervous system, and lymphatic drainage, leading to vomiting, diarrhoea, and a poor appetite.[16] As mentioned, a notable difference between the intestinal nodules of the puma and domestic cat were the number of eosinophils within the lesions, suggesting that large numbers of eosinophils are not required for the development of this unique sclerotic response or that the current number of eosinophils is not representative of more acutely inflamed lesions.[5]

Interestingly, feline herpesvirus 1 is linked with an eosinophilic response in cats, especially eosinophilic dermatitis, conjunctivitis, and keratosis.[17,18] However, in one study, immunohistochemistry for feline herpesvirus 1 of FGESF lesions was negative in all cats tested (n = 12).[2]

Hyperglobulinaemia and a low albumin:globulin ratio are a common finding in cats with FGESF. A major differential diagnosis is feline infectious peritonitis (FIP). Additionally, pyogranulomatous lesions and mesenteric lymphadenomegaly are seen in both conditions. Immunohistochemistry is needed to differentiate between the two and was negative for coronavirus in all cats tested (n = 12) excluding FIP.[2]

As noted, Ragdolls seem to be overrepresented worldwide, with Ragdoll cases reported in the United States of America, the United Kingdom, Sweden, Japan, and Australia (published and unpublished).[2,12] This may be due to genetic predisposition to mount an unregulated immune response or may be due to their own unique behaviours (e.g. overgrooming predisposing to trichobezoar and GI trauma).

Subsequently, multifactorial events might play a role in the pathogenesis of FGESF. This might include genetic predisposition (e.g. immune dysregulation), ingestion of foreign material (e.g. plant matter, hair), penetration of foreign material into the GI mucosa especially at sites of increased peristaltic pressure such as the pylorus and ileocaecocolic junction, and subsequent secondary pathogen invasion perpetuating the process. Indeed, the pylorus and ileocaecocolic junction are the most common locations for FGESF.

HISTORY AND PHYSICAL EXAMINATION

Given that the majority of reported lesions are localised to the GI tract, it seems logical that the most common clinical signs reported are consistent with disease of these organs. However, because of occasional involvement in other organs or body cavities, the main presenting complaint can appear more obscure or misleading. Lastly, some cases reported have no prior clinical signs, and lesions were identified incidentally during physical examination being performed for another reason (e.g. vaccination).[2]

The most consistent historical features include chronic vomiting and/or diarrhoea. In one study, vomiting was the most common presenting sign (21/25, 84%).[1] There was wide variation in duration of signs, from days to years. Weight loss was the second most common presenting sign (15/22, 68%).[1] When chronic, these signs were typically ascribed to dietary hypersensitivity, food intolerance, or inflammatory bowel disease (IBD).[2] However, when histopathology was evaluated in the normal GI tract adjacent to a lesion, there was no evidence of eosinophilic enteritis or IBD.[2] In these cases, it would be informative to examine other portions of the GI tract to confirm or refute the presence of more widespread alimentary disease. Vomiting can occur relatively acutely (perhaps owing to complete or partial obstruction from the lesion).

Less common historical information includes excessive grooming (5/10, 50% in one study), anorexia (6/13, 46% in one study), coughing due to pleural effusion (seen in one case), and constipation due to mechanical obstruction of the colon by extra-GI lesions (seen in one case).[2,15,19]

One cat had an unusual presentation with incontinence, pollakiuria, vomiting, and weight loss. In this case, an abdominal mass was identified and localised to the jejunum. Fine needle aspiration of the bladder wall identified numerous eosinophils on cytology.[6] In addition, mycoplasma was cultured from the urine. The authors of that study speculated that the mycoplasma may be the cause of the cat's cystitis given that clinical signs of cystitis improved using fluroquinolones. The relationship between FGESF and mycoplasma cystitis in this case is uncertain because the mycoplasma was not identified at the intestinal sites.

If there is suspicion of FGESF (often after additional tests), then specific questions should be asked (if not already done). These include:

- GI anthelmintic history
- dietary history (e.g. access to bones) that may indicate if there has been a risk of intestinal trauma
- history of overgrooming or foreign body ingestion
- history of vomiting, diarrhoea, or comorbidities
- travel history (i.e. assess exposure to parasites)
- history of foreign body obstruction.

Physical examination findings will vary with lesion location. However, in two larger series, a palpable abdominal mass was identified in 100% and 85% of cats included in the study, respectively.[1,2] The mass has been further described as a firm, irregular, fixed abdominal mass, in some cases initially being mistaken for impacted faeces. Critically, when the mass lesions are subjected to palpation, aspiration, biopsy, or excision, they have a gritty hard feel likely due to abundant trabecula of mature organised collagen. Although not pathognomonic, this is a useful point of differentiation from other common intra-abdominal masses such as large-cell lymphoma, mast cell tumour (MCT) and nonscirrhous adenocarcinoma.

Abdominal discomfort may be appreciated. Ascites was seen in one case, and dyspnoea secondary to a pleural effusion was seen in another.[2,4]

Lesions are located at a number of sites both in the GI tract and at extra-GI tract locations (Table 19.1).

Table 19.1. Lesions in the gastrointestinal tract and at extragastrointestinal tract locations.

Lesion location	Number of cases	Studies
Ileocaecocolic and colic region	10/25 8/13	Craig et al.[1] Linton et al.[2]
Pylorus	12/25	Craig et al.[1]
Subcutaneous tissue or lymph nodes	9/27	Ozaki et al.[9]
Stomach (greater curvature)	1/13	Linton et al.[2]
Jejunum	3	Craig et al.[1] Brloznik et al.[6] Weissman et al.[15]
Mesentery	1	Kambe et al.[4]
Retroperitoneal space	1	Thieme et al.[19]
Pancreas	1	Craig et al.[1]
Liver	2	Weissman et al.[15]
Common bile duct with local spread to the proximal duodenum	2	Craig et al.[1] Weissman et al.[15]

DIAGNOSTIC INVESTIGATION

As noted before, history and physical examination findings may be relatively nonspecific. Therefore, diagnostic investigation for the "unwell cat", "vomiting cat", or "cat with a palpable abdominal mass" is often initially undertaken. Differential diagnoses for these signs are discussed in Chapters 1 and 2, and diagnostic workup can include a variety of laboratory tests (see Chapter 3) and diagnostic imaging procedures (see Chapter 5).

When there is a suspicion of FGESF, evaluation should involve the following:

- specific historical questions should be asked/physical examination (see above)
- serum haematology and biochemistry
- diagnostic imaging followed by cytology
- histopathology with special stains or immunohistochemistry as necessary
- microbial testing including special stains or fluorescence in situ hybridisation (FISH) as necessary and available.

Figure 19.5 provides a diagnostic algorythm for FGESF.

Haematology

On haematology, the most pertinent finding is an absolute eosinophilia seen in approximately 50% of cases. Differential diagnoses for eosinophilia include hypersensitivity reactions, infectious disease (most commonly parasitic, less commonly fungal, viral, bacterial, algal), neoplasia (i.e. MCT, lymphoma), and hypereosinophilic syndrome. In any cat with eosinophilia and an abdominal mass, FGESF should be considered.[20]

A nonspecific mild non- or preregenerative anaemia has been identified in some cases.[2]

Serum biochemistry

Hyperglobulinaemia is identified in approximately 50% of cases and is thought to be due to an inflammatory response. Serum protein electrophoresis (reported in two cases) revealed polyclonal gammopathy in both.[2,19]

Two cases had reported biliary obstruction due to infiltration from FGESF lesions of the common bile ducts, with hyperbilirubinaemia and elevated serum liver enzyme activities suggestive of hepatocellular damage in one case.[1,15]

In cats that were successfully treated, both eosinophilia and hyperglobulinaemia resolved.[2]

Diagnostic imaging

Diagnostic imaging is useful to determine the location of the lesion, which has implications for management and the exclusion of other intra-abdominal pathologies.

A number of imaging modalities is suitable, such as abdominal ultrasound, radiography, or a computed tomography (CT) scan. However, weighing up the benefit of cost, practicality, and availability, abdominal ultrasound would seem to be an appropriate first choice.

Ultrasonographic changes are nonspecific. Findings usually include a solitary mass with occasional (albeit rarer) involvement of other organs. For example, one case had a jejunal mass with hepatomegaly and liver nodules eventually characterised as FGESF lesions through histopathology.[15] Ultrasound can show mural thickening and loss of layering in the stomach, duodenum, jejunum, or colon (Fig. 19.1). In one case report, lesions were confined to the mesentery.[4] Regional lymph node enlargement is a common finding (7/25) (Fig. 19.2).[1] Histopathology from lymph nodes either suggests reactive changes or changes specific to FGESF.

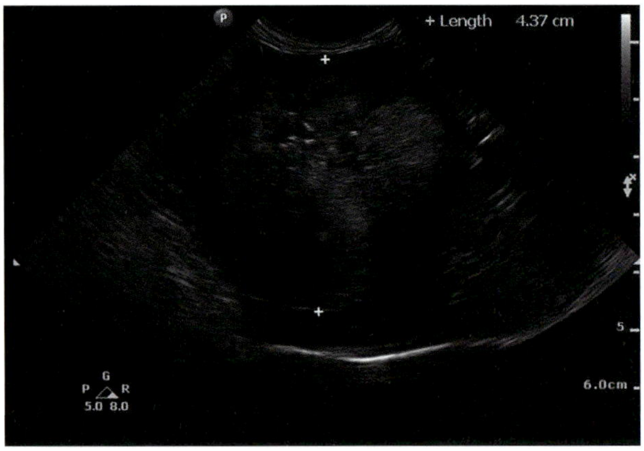

Figure 19.1. Ultrasound image from the pyloric lesion (between callipers). Note the loss of layering with the mixture of hypoechoic and hyperechoic regions within the tissue. It is thought that the hyperechoic regions correspond with the fibrotic zones described histologically.

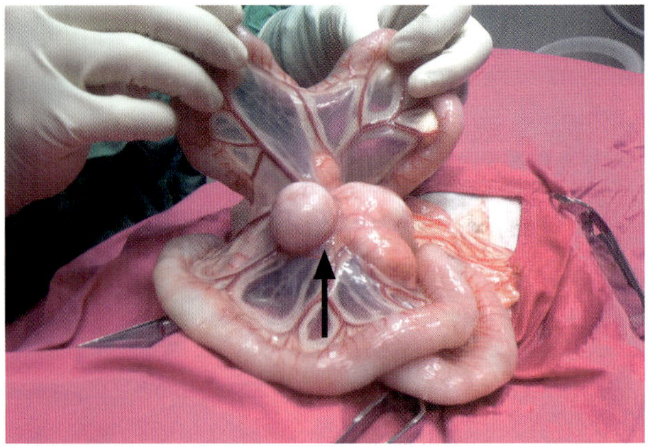

Figure 19.2. Note the marked enlargement of the lymph nodes (arrow) at the root of the mesentery. This is a common feature of feline gastrointestinal eosinophilic sclerosing fibroplasia and other disease entities such as lymphoblastic B-cell lymphoma. Image courtesy of Agnieszka Zoltowska, School of Veterinary Medicine and Science, University of Nottingham, UK (photograph taken whilst working at Your Vets, Coventry, UK).

CT scan may be useful for surgical planning and determining the origin of a lesion. One case report described CT scan findings for lesions localised in the mesentery.[4] Specifically, the FGESF was identified as a multilobulated, heterogeneous soft tissue mass. Multiple lobules of the mass were peripherally contrast enhancing with nonenhancing areas centrally. A few small mineral-attenuating foci were present within the centre of the mass. There was lymphadenomegaly with no contrast enhancement.

Cytology and histopathology

Cytology alone is generally nonspecific and cannot be used to a make a definitive diagnosis of FGESF. In some cases, it can be helpful to exclude differential diagnoses such as MCT and lymphoma.[10]

Histopathology is needed to confirm a diagnosis of FGESF. Given the extent of the disease process and heterogeneous nature of the condition, definitive staging and therapy require laparotomy with resection or biopsy of masses in most cases (Fig. 19.3). Other options include Tru-Cut biopsy or laparoscopy but carry their own inherent risks of complications.

When submitting a sample for histopathology it is critical to provide the pathologist with a succinct history, clinicopathologic findings, and the differential diagnoses considered to allow for adequate and thorough investigation.

Histopathology (including special stains/immunohistochemistry as detailed below) sections should be examined closely to exclude poorly differentiated cell neoplasia and atypical lymphoma and to search for foreign material (to exclude trichobezoars).

Histopathology has been well described.[1] In domestic cats, lesions were characterised by eosinophilic inflammation, large reactive fibroblasts, and trabeculae of dense collagen. Specifically, all lesions consisted of branching and anastomosing trabeculae of dense collagen separated by a densely cellular population of

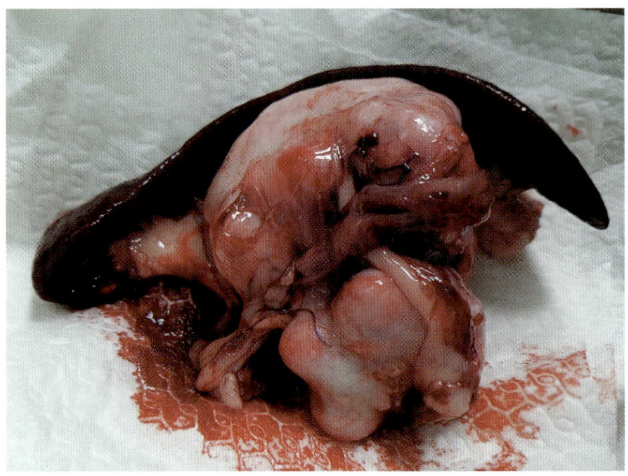

Figure 19.3. Image of a resected lymph node next to the splenic hilus. Histopathology was consistent with feline gastrointestinal eosinophilic sclerosing fibroplasia of the lymph node. Image courtesy of Ivo Stehlík, Pet Care Clinic, Prague, Czech Republic.

large spindle-shaped cells (Fig. 19.4). The trabecular collagen merged gradually into more typical granulation tissue at the periphery of the lesions. All lesions contained variably dense infiltrates of eosinophils, mast cells, and fewer neutrophils, lymphocytes, and plasma cells within the fibroplasia as well as within the surrounding tissues. Lesions were either transmural or affected the inner layers of the GI wall. Inflammation in the GI tissue is mixed but is predominantly eosinophilic. The presence of other inflammatory cells may be affected by other factors such as the presence or absence of bacteria. As noted, in more than 50% of cases bacterial colonies were present within microabscesses and necrotic foci within the lesion. In one study the bacteria included gram-negative rods, gram-positive rods, and gram-positive cocci.[1] In cats with intralesional bacteria, the dense collagen trabeculae formed irregular radiating and concentric bands around central microabscesses containing the bacteria.[1]

The authors suggest that, at a minimum, biopsies are collected from the GI tract (both at the site of a lesion and away from the lesion, even if the GI tract looks morphologically normal), any enlarged lymph nodes, liver, and from any other organ or area with gross evidence of disease.

Special histology stains and immunohistochemistry to differentiate from neoplasia

Based on histopathology, FGESF has been misdiagnosed as MCT, osteosarcoma, fibrosarcoma, and haematopoietic neoplasia.[1,2] This is not surprising given the similarity between some of these conditions.

Intestinal mast cell disease commonly involves the small intestines and is grossly characterised by marked transmural expansion by a firm, homogeneous tan mass with mucosal ulceration.[21] Like FGESF, mast cell disease has occasionally been associated with peripheral eosinophilia.[22] Histopathology of FGESF cases will often identify mast cells. Histopathology of MCTs can be relatively straightforward. However, in some cases, mast cells may be sparse with variable granule uptake, and differentiation between inflammation and neoplasia might be challenging.[21] In one case series, the diagnosis of FGESF or sclerosing MCTs was vigorously debated.[21,23–24] Clues may lie in the lesion location (the majority of FGESF are seen in the pylorus and ileocaecocolic junction), the presence of intralesional bacterial organisms, and lastly the response to therapy.[1,2,23–24]

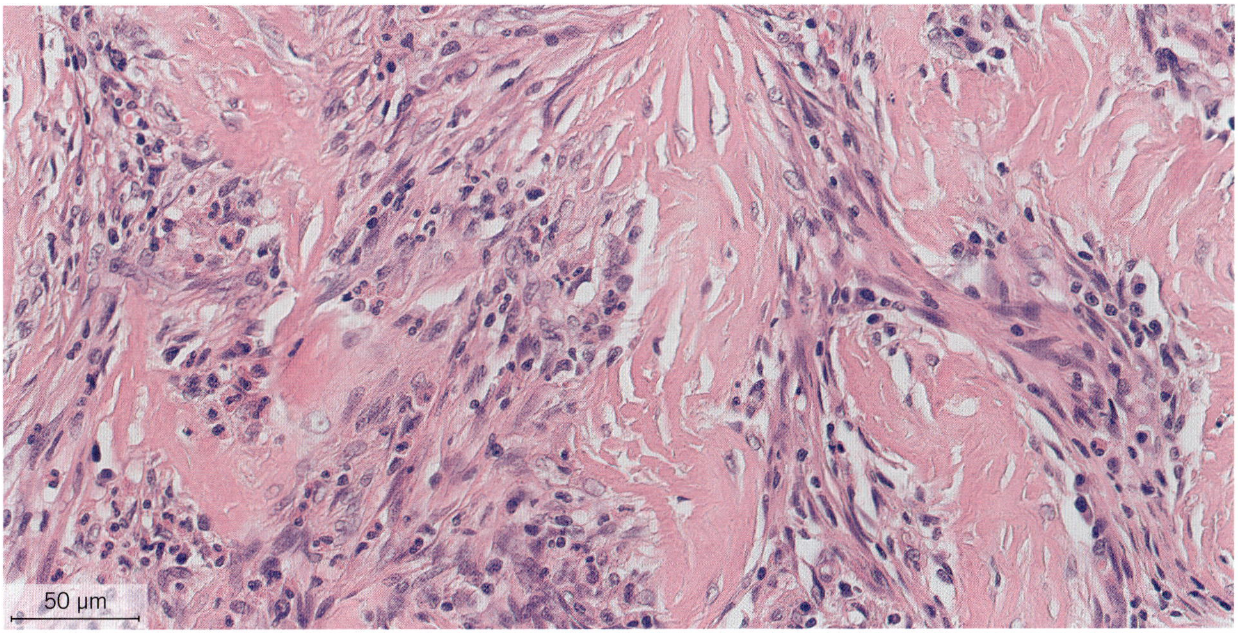

Figure 19.4. Histological image from a lymph node. The characteristic network of coarse collagen trabeculae (stained pink) throughout the lesion is an important distinguishing feature of feline gastrointestinal eosinophilic sclerosing fibroplasia. This abundance of collagen causes the hard, gritty texture of these lesions, which is most obvious during biopsy procedures (or during dissection at necropsy). Haematoxylin–eosin, ×40. Image courtesy of Dr Ladislav Novotný, Finn Pathologists, Harleston, UK.

Similar to mast cell neoplasia, lymphoma may also present as either nodular or diffuse disease, with transmural thickening associated with altered to absent GI wall layering. The most common solitary site is the ileocaecocolic junction. Special stains (CD3, CD79) can be utilised to determine the cell of origin and may help distinguish between FGESF and lymphoma if there is doubt based on histopathology.

In one case, macroscopic findings and ultrasound had characteristics of FGESF, lymphoma, and MCTs.[25] Immunohistochemistry was required to distinguish between these conditions. Antibodies used were CD3, CD79a, and CD117. These stains allowed a final diagnosis of T-cell lymphoma with reactive fibroplasia, effectively excluding FGESF. In this case, Giemsa staining and CD117 were negative and needed to exclude an interstitial MCT. The intense labelling with CD3 (associated with T-cell receptor) and the absence of positivity for CD79 (associated with B-cell antigen receptor) subsequently allowed the pathologist to make a diagnosis of T-cell lymphoma with extensive reactive fibroplasia.[25] In FGESF lesions, it would be expected that Giemsa and CD117 would be negative (excluding MCTs), as would strong staining with CD3 and CD79a (excluding lymphoma). Trichrome staining could be used and would be expected to stain positive, highlighting collagen in tissue sections.

Microbial testing including stains for pathogens

Multiple studies have identified bacteria in GI FGESF lesions. In one study, bacteria, including gram-negative rods, gram-positive cocci, and gram-positive rods, were found in the majority of cases.[1] In another study, similar eosinophilic sclerosing lesions were described in the subcutis and abdomen, with gram-positive cocci accompanying most lesions.[9] Additionally, bacteria were identified in a retroperitoneal FGESF mass in one case.[19]

Given the relatively common presence of pathogens identified intramurally, an investigative approach is recommended both for diagnostic and therapeutic purposes. Tests include:

- special stains for intralesional bacteria or other pathogens
- culture and sensitivity of FGESF tissue
- FISH.

Special stains to consider (but not limited to) include Giemsa (bacteria and protozoa), Gram stain (bacteria), methenamine silver (fungi), period acid–Schiff (fungi), and Ziehl–Neelsen stain (mycobacteria and nocardia).

On their own, each modality has limitations in detecting potential pathogens. For example, in one study, two cases negative for bacteria using FISH could be identified using histology and special stains.[2] This observation is supported by a human review where eubacterial FISH only identified 56% of bacteria on average (range 1%–100%).[26] Subsequently, a eubacterial probe is recommended initially to determine if bacteria are present within the walls of the biopsy specimen.[2] If there is fluorescence of bacteria, new slides can be prepared with specific probes to classify the species of bacteria, such as those specific for *Clostridium*, *Staphylococcus*, *Actinomyces*, *Escherichia coli*, and *Enterococcus*.[2] Despite a number of different bacteria have been cultured/identified and the current limited availability of specific probes, it may not always be possible to speciate the bacteria in every case with the current resources available.

Overall, to maximise diagnostic sensitivity, a combination of histopathology, special stains, immunohistochemistry, culture and sensitivity, and FISH is recommended.

However, it is noteworthy that up to 44% of cases are not associated with infection.[2] This might reflect diagnostic limitations (not all tests were performed) or that infections are not solely involved in the multifactorial pathogenesis of this syndrome.

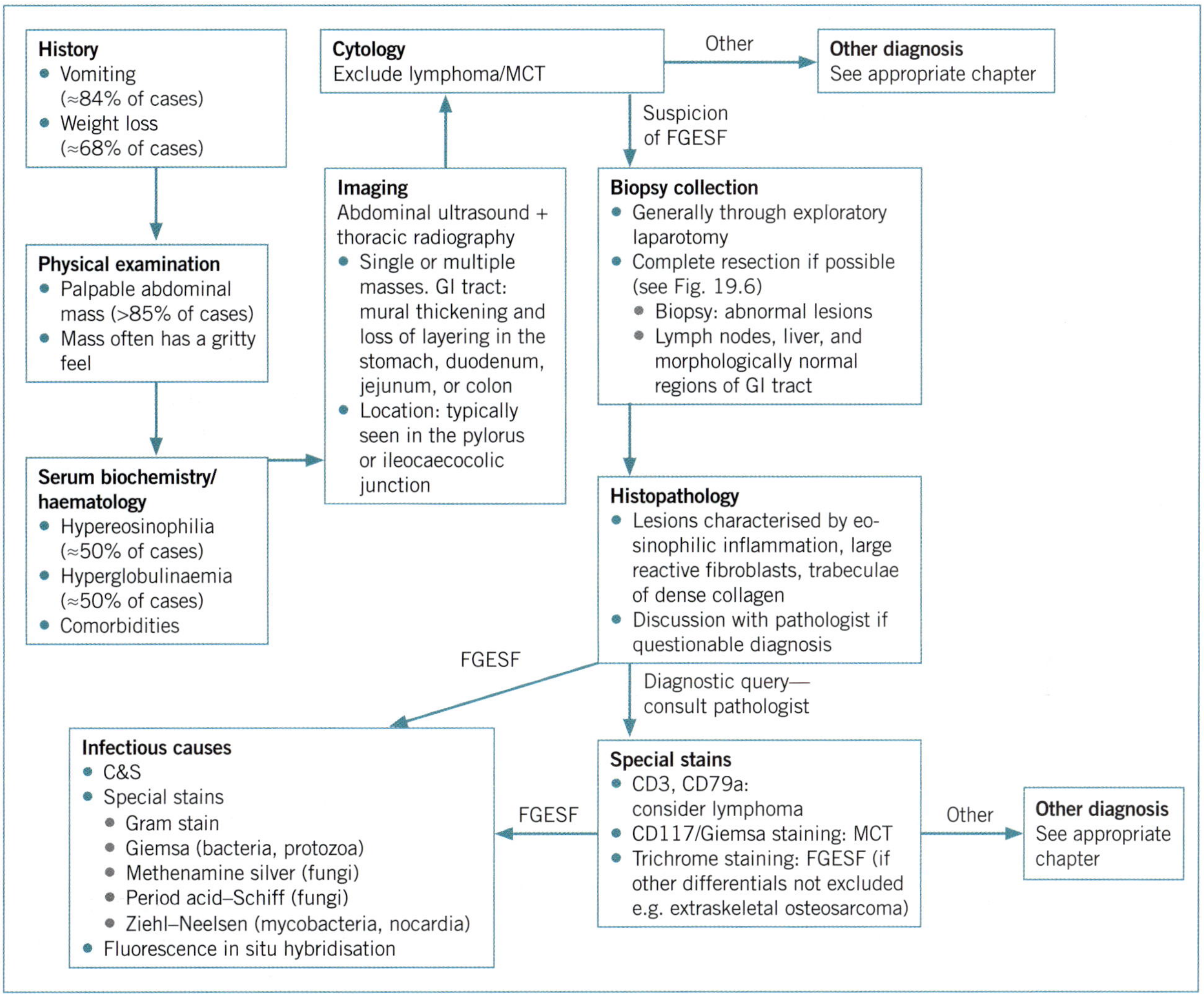

Figure 19.5. Diagnostic algorithm for feline gastrointestinal eosinophilic sclerosing fibroplasia (FGESF) cases. C&S, culture and sensitivity; GI, gastrointestinal. MCT, mast cell tumour.

TREATMENT

A number of therapeutic regimens have been trialled including surgery, various combinations of antimicrobial agents, corticosteroids, alkylating agents, GI tract protectants, analgesia, and dietary management. Notably, cases have responded very differently to both the same and different therapeutic regimens, although some trends are beginning to be appreciated.

Until more is known, a multimodal approach to therapy of FGESF would seem ideal (Fig. 19.6). That is, when possible, therapy should target the current extent of disease (surgical debulking), underlying cause, and any perpetuating factors (e.g. treating secondary infections, limiting the propensity towards immune dysregulation).

Immediate therapy

In some cases the disease process can be severe, leading to signs of full or partial intestinal obstruction which warrants immediate surgical intervention. The decision to perform surgery is also guided by the location of the lesion and the experience of the surgeon. Specifically, lesion location will influence whether surgical excision or debulking is possible. Masses in the pyloric region might not be amenable to surgical resection due to involvement of surrounding structures. For example, two cats showed apparent expansion of disease from the proximal duodenum to the bile duct.[1,15] Should surgical resection not be possible, treatment trials with antibiotics and immunosuppressive therapy can be considered in an attempt to decrease the size of the mass. Surgery might be considered at a later stage if still warranted.

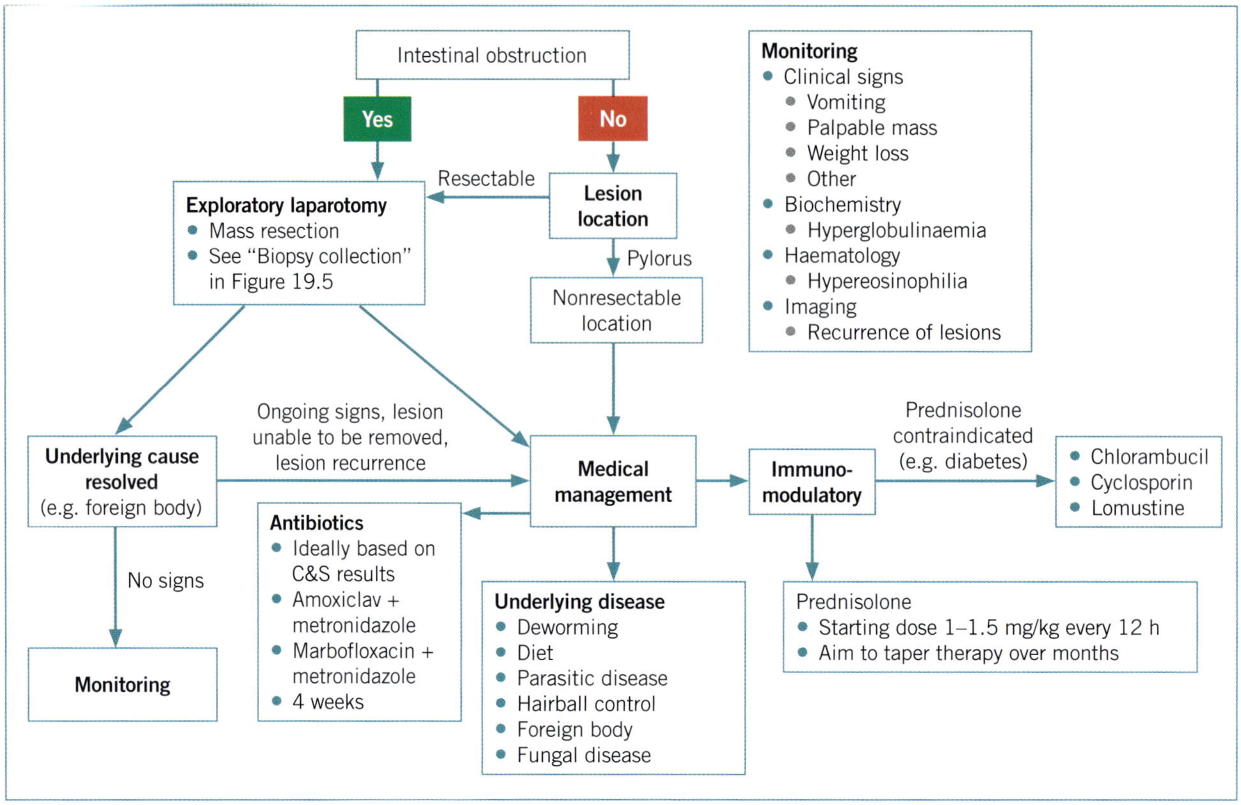

Figure 19.6. Treatment algorithm for feline gastrointestinal eosinophilic sclerosing fibroplasia cases. C&S, culture and sensitivity.

Long-term therapy

Glucocorticoids are currently the mainstay of treatment. These drugs can interfere with active cytokines, reducing survival times of eosinophils as well as dampening the release of eosinophilic granules. This aims to blunt the hyperactive immune response and therefore can reduce fibrosis. The use of cyclosporin, chlorambucil, hydroxyurea, or lomustine can be considered concurrently or alternatively to target the underlying immune dysregulation and in circumstances where prednisolone use is contraindicated. The duration of such therapy is unknown and appears to vary on a case by case basis; in some cats therapy can be discontinued after months, and others require indefinite therapy.

Parental antibiotics are recommended because of the high percentage of associated infection. One study recommended a combination of amoxicillin–clavulanate plus metronidazole or marbofloxacin plus metronidazole; however, these findings were not based on culture and sensitivity results.[2]

In one study, identified bacteria were gram-positive cocci in 23/27 cases.[9] Gram-positive cocci were identified as *Staphylococcus*, based on their morphological features and immunoreactivity.[9] In 15/17 lesions, the colonies expressed immunoreactivity to penicillin-binding protein 2, which is a drug-resistance gene product of methicillin-resistant *Staphylococcus* species, making susceptibility patterns ideal for appropriate antibiotic choice. However, given that in most cases lesions are associated with the GI tract, this may not be possible due to contamination.

Lastly, it would be logical to treat any apparent comorbidity that may be related to the underlying cause (e.g. fungal disease).

In summary, medical management is the mainstay of treatment in most cases, with the occasional exception. Surgery should be considered for all resectable masses. Nonresectable lesions may rely on medical treatment alone. Medical management involves a combination of prednisolone (starting dose 1 mg/kg PO every 12 hours) and antibiotics (empirical or based on culture and sensitivity results). Prednisolone can be tapered over months depending on response to therapy and monitoring. If prednisolone is contraindicated (e.g. diabetic patient), other agents can be considered possibly allowing for the exclusion of prednisolone in the treatment plan or allowing the dose to be minimised. Antibiotics are administered for at least 4 weeks. Any underlying disease should be treated.

OUTCOME AND PROGNOSIS

In a study of 25 cats, survival curves comparing treatment with surgical biopsy and prednisone (with or without antibiotics) (7/25 cats), treatment with surgical biopsy and antibiotics (8/25 cats), and treatment with only surgical biopsy (3/25 cats) were shown.[1] The longest survival times in this study were seen with cases treated with prednisone.[1] In another study, a trend towards improved survival times when prednisolone was included in the treatment regimen and when surgery was not the sole mode of therapy was seen.[2] However, the authors of this study note that this statement may be flawed because not all surgical cases survived sufficiently long enough (perhaps because of poor surgical case selection or surgeon experience) to receive systemic medications, which may have biased the outcomes.[2]

One case report described multiple firm masses in the sublumbar retroperitoneal space causing ventral displacement and compression of the descending colon, with extension of the masses into the pelvic canal. In this case, lesions were not amenable to surgery, and the cat was treated with a combination of prednisolone and antibiotics. Repeat evaluation and imaging at day 732 (postoperatively) revealed marked reduction in size of the abdominal mass, resolution of peripheral eosinophilia, and no clinical signs with continued prednisolone therapy (0.5 mg/kg PO every 24 hours).[19]

However, inconsistent response to prednisolone is seen. In one case report of treatment with prednisolone alone for a mass located at the proximal pylorus, the cat had a relatively poor outcome, with death reported at 56 days.[11]

Trends with other immunomodulatory drugs cannot be appreciated given the relative sparsity of reported use.

One case report of a lesion confined to the mesentery which was not surgically resectable was treated with a short course of prednisolone (22 days), antibiotics, and a prolonged course of cyclosporin (236 days). In this case, this regime resulted in a prolonged remission time.[4]

Administration of prednisolone and other immunosuppressive drugs requires monitoring for opportunistic infections. One cat treated with prednisolone and chlorambucil developed systemic toxoplasmosis.[2]

In contrast, in some cats immunomodulatory drugs were not used. In one case series, one animal had surgical resection (colonic mass) followed by a single dose of lomustine (due to an initial incorrect diagnosis of a MCT) followed by no further therapy. At the time of publication (43 months), the cat was still alive with no further clinical signs and no evidence of lesion recurrence.[15] In the same case series, another cat was reported alive 24 months after jejunal mass resection.[15]

However, surgical therapy alone appeared insufficient in one cat, with a new mass reported 1 year after initial resection.[6] Additionally, another animal was subject to multiple surgeries and antibiotics over a 10-year period and only appeared to be in remission through a combination of immunosupressive medication (prednisolone) and antibiotics (amoxicillin and clavulanic acid).[2]

Prognosis is hard to quantify due to marked inconsistencies in outcomes reported. Additionally, data may be severely skewed due to factors unrelated to the pathology itself. For instance, in one study, one case died postoperatively due to an unrelated comorbidity (cardiomyopathy), one case developed postoperative sepsis and was euthanised, one case treated in general practice was found dead 24 hours postoperatively, and one case was euthanised due to an incorrect diagnosis.[2] These are examples of why survival data should be evaluated cautiously.

Reasons for treatment failure may include failure to diagnose and treat an underlying disease, comorbidity or associated infection, inadequate medical management including tapering of immunosuppressive medication too fast, or inappropriate surgical case selection.

According to one study, lesion localisation was not associated with survival, with mean survival times not statistically different when cats with a lesion in the proximal GI tract (pylorus) were compared with those with lesions in the distal/aboral (ileocaecocolic junction or colon) portion.[1] However, the authors of this study comment that lesions in the pylorus tend to have a poorer prognosis.

This is possibly due to a decreased ability to remove the mass surgically and due to involvement of other local organs (e.g. biliary tract leading to biliary obstruction).

A prolonged survival is appreciated in cats surviving the first months after surgery. For example, survival times reported at the time of writing in one series was 1–10 years providing they survived the perioperative period.[2] Surviving cats have been managed with a number of different therapeutic regimens ranging from prolonged prednisolone use, dietary management only, to discontinuation of all therapy. Therapeutic decisions are based on ongoing monitoring.

Take-home messages

- There are no pathognomonic historical observations, physical examination findings, or routine laboratory results of feline gastrointestinal eosinophilic sclerosing fibroplasia (FGESF). However, a history of vomiting, weight loss, the finding of a firm gritty abdominal mass, and the presence of hypereosinophilia or hyperglobulinaemia are all footprints that may suggest FGESF.
- Abdominal lesions are usually palpable. Imaging usually localises lesions to the ileocaecocolic junction or stomach, although a number of less frequent locations (gastrointestinal and nongastrointestinal) have been identified.
- Clinicians should liaise with their pathologist to ensure that special stains are employed if there is any uncertainty with the definitive diagnosis based on histopathology alone.
- Bacteria have been isolated from lesions in a substantial proportion of cats, but not in all cases of FGESF. Their role in this disease is still uncertain.
- A multimodal approach to therapy would seem ideal, consisting of prednisolone, additional immunomodulatory agents, and antibiotics following surgical resection if feasible.

REFERENCES

[1] Craig LE et al. Feline gastrointestinal eosinophilic sclerosing fibroplasia. *Vet Pathol* 46:63, 2009.

[2] Linton M et al. Feline gastrointestinal eosinophilic sclerosing fibroplasia: 13 cases and review of an emerging clinical entity. *J Feline Med Surg* 17:392, 2015.

[3] Suzuki M, Onchi M, Ozaki M. A case of feline gastrointestinal eosinophilic sclerosing fibroplasia. *J Toxicol Pathol* 26:51, 2013.

[4] Kambe N et al. A case of feline gastrointestinal eosinophilic sclerosing fibroplasia limited to the mesentery. *J Small Anim Pract* 61:64, 2020.

[5] Eckstrand CD et al. Nematode-associated intramural alimentary nodules in pumas are histologically similar to gastrointestinal eosinophilic sclerosing fibroplasia of domestic cats. *J Comp Pathol* 148:405, 2013.

[6] Brloznik M et al. Recurrent feline gastrointestinal eosinophilic sclerosing fibroplasia and presumptive eosinophilic cystitis in a domestic short-haired cat: a case report. *Vet Med (Praha)* 62:295, 2017.

[7] Munday JS, Martinez AW, Soo M. A case of feline gastrointestinal eosinophilic sclerosing fibroplasia mimicking metastatic neoplasia. *N Z Vet J* 62:356, 2014.

[8] Grau-Roma L et al. A case of feline gastrointestinal eosinophilic sclerosing fibroplasia associated with phycomycetes. *J Comp Pathol* 151:318, 2014.

[9] Ozaki K et al. Abscess-forming inflammatory granulation tissue with Gram-positive cocci and prominent eosinophil infiltration in cats: possible infection of methicillin-resistant *Staphylococcus*. *Vet Pathol* 40:283, 2003.

[10] Sihvo HK et al. Pathology in practice. Severe chronic multifocal intramural fibrosing and eosinophilic enteritis, with occasional intralesional bacteria, consistent with feline gastrointestinal eosinophilic sclerosing fibroplasia. (FIESF). *J Am Vet Med Assoc* 238:585, 2011.

[11] Cho MJ, Kim MC, Seo KW. Feline gastrointestinal eosinophilic sclerosing fibroplasia in a Bengal cat. *J Vet Clin* 34:481, 2017.

[12] Nimmo JS, editor. *Three cases of feline gastrointestinal eosinophilic sclerosing fibroplasia (a newly recognised syndrome) in Ragdoll cats.* Fremantle, Western Australia, Aust Soc Vet Pathol, 2009.

[13] Catro-Lopez J, Fernandez M, de Sousa AR. A case of feline gastrointestinal eosinophilic sclerosing fibroplasia associated with zygomycetes fungi [abstract, ISFM Feline Congress. Budapest]. *J Feline Med Surg* 14:650, 2012.

[14] Kawasako K, Kanno T, Hamamura M. Jejunal fibroplasia in a rat. *J Vet Med Sci* 79:830, 2017.

[15] Weissman A et al. Ultrasonographic and clinicopathological features of feline gastrointestinal eosinophilic sclerosing fibroplasia in four cats. *J Feline Med Surg* 15:148. 2013.

[16] Batchelor DJ et al. Mechanisms, causes, investigation and management of vomiting disorders in cats: a literature review. *J Feline Med Surg* 15:237, 2013.

[17] Lee M, Bosward KL, Norris JM. Immunohistological evaluation of feline herpesvirus-1 infection in feline eosinophilic dermatoses or stomatitis. *J Feline Med Surg* 12:72, 2010.

[18] Dean E, Meunier V. Feline eosinophilic keratoconjunctivitis: a retrospective study of 45 cases (56 eyes). *J Feline Med Surg* 15:661, 2013.

[19] Thieme ME et al. Diagnosis and management of a case of retroperitoneal eosinophilic sclerosing fibroplasia in a cat. *JFMS Open Rep* 5:2055116919867178, 2019.

[20] Takeuchi Y et al. Intestinal T-cell lymphoma with severe hypereosinophilic syndrome in a cat. *J Vet Med Sci* 74:1057, 2012.

[21] Halsey CH, Powers BE, Kamstock DA. Feline intestinal sclerosing mast cell tumour: 50 cases (1997–2008). *Vet Comp Oncol* 8:72, 2010.

[22] O'Keefe DA et al. Systemic mastocytosis in 16 dogs. *J Vet Intern Med* 1:75, 1987.

[23] Gamble DA. Letters to the editor and rebuttal regarding the paper recently published in *Veterinary and Comparative Oncology*, "Feline intestinal sclerosing mast cell tumour: 50 cases (1997–2008) 2010; 8: 72–79" by C. H. C. Halsey, B. E. Powers and D. A. Kamstock. Letter to the editor #2. *Vet Comp Oncol* 8:235, 2010.

[24] Schulman FY, Lipscomb TP. Letters to the editor and rebuttal regarding the paper recently published in *Veterinary and Comparative Oncology*, "Feline intestinal sclerosing mast cell tumour: 50 cases (1997–2008) 2010; 8: 72–79" by C. H. C. Halsey, B. E. Powers and D. A. Kamstock. Letter to the editor #1. *Vet Comp Oncol* 8:234, 2010.

[25] Brosinski K et al. Diagnostic exercise: submucosal gastric masses in a cat. *Vet Pathol* 50:350, 2013.

[26] Bouvier T, Del Giorgio PA. Factors influencing the detection of bacterial cells using fluorescence in situ hybridization (FISH): a quantitative review of published reports. *FEMS Microbiol Ecol* 44:3, 2003.

CHAPTER 20

Gastrointestinal lymphoma

Valérie Freiche

Gastrointestinal lymphoma (GIL) is by far the most frequent digestive tract neoplasia in cats (Fig. 20.1). GIL is defined by the infiltration of neoplastic lymphocytes within the gastrointestinal (GI) tract with variable involvement of extraintestinal sites including draining lymph nodes, liver, spleen, and pancreas.[1,2] The gut-associated lymphoid tissue (GALT) is the primary site of neoplastic cell proliferation. The incidence of GIL has significantly increased over the two past decades.[2–4] Several subtypes have been defined according to the histological grade (low, intermediate, or high), or phenotype (T or B) of the neoplastic lymphocytes cell size (small or large).[3,5,6] GIL digestive distribution is variable, according to the lymphoma subtype (Table 20.1).

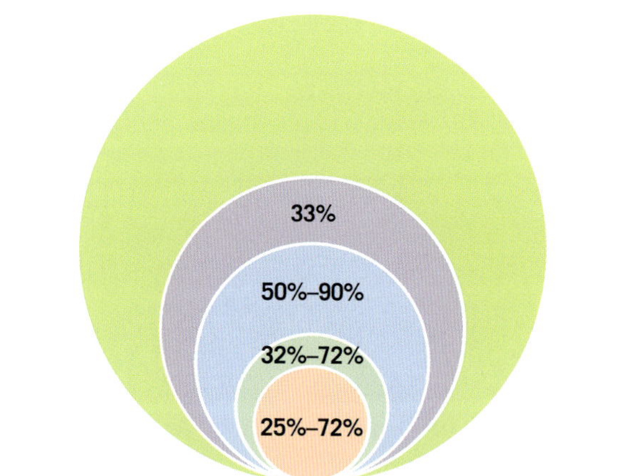

Figure 20.1. Feline gastrointestinal lymphomas amongst other neoplasia. Based on a diagram by Dr Mathieu Paulin, by kind permission of Les Éditions du Point Vétérinaire, France.

Clinical signs often lack specificity. Final diagnosis is based on cytology, histology, immunohistochemistry, and clonality testing. Due to the emergence of low-grade intestinal T-cell lymphoma (LGITL), a major challenge for the clinician is to distinguish chronic lymphoplasmacytic enteropathy (LPE) from LGITL, as many features of those entities may overlap.[1–4] Within this context, this chapter highlights this specific entity, which represents up to 75% of all GIL cases in cats.

Treatment and prognosis of GIL depend on the subtype of the disease. Oral chemotherapy can induce long-term survival in cats diagnosed with LGITL. In contrast, other subtypes of GIL require aggressive chemotherapy schemes. Prognosis can be poor in these cases, particularly in high-grade and large granular lymphocyte (LGL) lymphoma cases.

EPIDEMIOLOGY AND AETIOLOGY

Epidemiology

Lymphohaematopoietic tumours represent more than one-third of all feline malignant neoplasms, and 50%–90% of all lymphohaematopoietic tumours are lymphomas. Contrary to the canine species, GIL represents the most frequently diagnosed digestive tract neoplasia in cats, followed by adenocarcinomas, mastocytomas, and leiomyosarcomas.

No breed or sex predisposition has been reported, even though Siamese, Oriental, and males have been suggested to be overrepresented in some GIL studies.[4,7]

Aetiopathogenesis

The aetiopathogenesis of GIL remains poorly understood. The involvement of several factors is likely,

Table 20.1. Different subtypes of gastrointestinal lymphoma, main phenotype, and main digestive distribution.

Type		LGITL			IGIL			HGIL			LGLL		
GIL subtype		37%–75%			—			15%–54%			6%–7%		
Phenotype		T cell	B cell	NK cell	T cell	B cell	NK cell	T cell	B cell	NK cell	T cell	B cell	NK cell
		>90%	<10%	≈0%	—	—	≈0%	<50%	>50%	≈0%	>90%	≈0%	<10%
Most frequent localisations	Stomach	+/–			+			+++			+++		
	Small intestine	+++			+			+++			+++		
	Colon	+/–			+			+++			+++		
	Mesenteric lymph nodes	+++			+			+++			+++		
	Extraintestinal (lymph nodes, liver, spleen, bone marrow)	–			+			+			+++		
Prognosis		Favourable			Poor			Very poor			Very poor		

GIL, gastrointestinal lymphoma; HGIL, high-grade intestinal lymphoma; IGIL, intermediate-grade intestinal lymphoma; LGITL, low-grade intestinal T-cell lymphoma; LGLL, large granular lymphocyte lymphoma; NK, natural killer.

particularly when considering the relationship of GIL phenotype with histological grade. Factors that have been hypothesised to play a role are infectious agents, preexisting inflammatory bowel disease (IBD), genetic predisposition, geographical factors, diet composition, and other environmental factors.[1–4]

Infectious agents

Viruses

The risk of developing GIL is higher in cats infected with feline retroviruses (feline leukaemia virus [FeLV] or feline immunodeficiency virus [FIV]).[8] That said, this hypothesis has recently been challenged because most lymphocytic cancers in other species are nonretroviral, and the prevalence of feline leukaemia in Westernised countries has substantially decreased over the last 20 years.[4]

FeLV can infect the bone marrow, lymphoid tissue, and intestines. This retrovirus is suspected to be a major risk factor in the development of feline haematopoietic tumours, particularly mediastinal T-cell lymphoma.[4] The mechanisms by which FeLV causes neoplastic transformation result from virus genome insertion into the DNA of the host. In contrast to multicentric lymphoma, the exact role of FeLV in the development of GIL remains unclear since it is inconsistently identified in GIL cases. No circulating FeLV antigens are identified in most cases of GIL. One hypothesis is that FeLV may be present in a latent or replication-defective form in some of these cases.

Considering FIV infection, even if the topic has not been well documented, a partial loss of antitumoural immunity could induce indirect immune dysregulation and ultimately promote tumour development. FIV infection may increase the risk of developing different types of lymphomas, including GIL. Finally, it would be necessary to clearly establish the association between feline retroviruses and different subtypes of GIL, especially LGITL, given its increasing prevalence.

Felis catus gammaherpesvirus 1 (FcaGHV1) was more recently cited as a potential virus to promote the development of lymphoma.[4] Circulating FcaGHV1 DNA was associated with a significantly shorter survival time in cats diagnosed with lymphoma compared to FcaGHV1 qPCR negative cases. That said, low-grade intestinal lymphomas were not included in this study.

Bacteria

Chronic antigenic stimulation is a recognised potential oncogenic factor that promotes the development of gastric cancer in people. Logically, the impact of *Helicobacter* spp. has been studied in dogs and cats over the past decades, as these bacteria are often found in the stomach of companion animals. *Helicobacter pylori* infection is involved in mucosa-associated lymphoid tissue (MALT) lymphoma development in humans, but their pathogenic incidence remains poorly understood in companion animals. Gastric *Helicobacter heilmannii* was suspected to promote feline gastric lymphoma, but further studies are needed to define the precise role of *Helicobacter* spp. in the pathophysiology of gastric cancers in animals.

Microbial imbalances are implicated in the pathogenesis of approximately 20% of all human malignancies.[9] Mucosa-invasive bacteria have recently been identified in cats diagnosed with high-grade small intestinal lymphomas, while no bacteria were detected in LGITL cases.[10] That said, in a recent retrospective study,[9] bacterial groups were identified by fluorescence in situ hybridisation in GI biopsy specimens in 14 cats diagnosed with IBD vs. 14 cats identified with LGITL. Furthermore, bacterial expression was correlated to CD11b$^+$ and nuclear factor kappa B (NF-κB) expression. Compared with cats with IBD, cats with LGITL showed higher counts of *Fusobacterium* spp. and *Bacteroides* spp. Furthermore, the study established significant correlations between *Fusobacterium* spp. totals and CD11b$^+$ cell and NF-κB expression. Further studies are warranted to establish whether enteroinvasive or enteroadhesive bacteria opportunistically colonise the diseased, neoplastic intestinal mucosa and/or whether they potentially promote lymphomagenesis mechanisms.

Previous chronic enteropathies

Interestingly, some human low-grade GI T-cell lymphoma cases reported in the literature have had a history of Crohn's disease or autoimmune enteropathy. Chronic inflammation has been hypothesised to be a risk factor for the development of GIL, given the fact that concurrent IBD has been described in up to 60% of GIL cases.[4] Many authors highlight that IBD may precede, and thereupon promote, intestinal neoplasia in the feline species as well. In a recent study,[11,34] several arguments were pointed out to support a continuum between LPE and LGITL:

- duration of clinical signs statistically longer in cats diagnosed with LGITL compared with LPE cases;
- strong epitheliotropism may be seen in both LPE and LGITL;
- LGITL small lymphocytes appear in an apical-to-basal gradient, suggesting possible chronic antigenic stimulation;
- persistent cellular polymorphism infiltrates can be found in some LGITL cases;
- patchy lesions and nests can be seen in LGITL, even in a polymorphic background;
- monoclonality is seen in up to 40% of LPE cases;
- only minimal differences are seen between IBD and LGITL intestinal microbiome, and there is high similarity with the microbiome dysbiosis seen in human IBD.

A new model of lymphomagenesis has thus emerged from this comparative research and suggests a continuum of inflammatory enteropathy towards intestinal lymphoma (Fig. 20.2).[12]

Tobacco smoke and environmental factors

Chronic cigarette smoke exposure has been suggested to promote GIL.[4,8] More than 40 carcinogens and mutagens have been identified in environmental smoke. As companion animals share their owners' toxin exposures, it is legitimate to ask whether inhaled and hair tobacco smoke exposure could increase the risk of developing any type of lymphoma. Hair nicotine concentration has been measured as a biomarker in a recent prospective study.[13] Even though hair nicotine concentration was higher in the GIL group than in the control group, it failed to reach statistical significance; further research is needed in order to study environmental factors in cats suffering from GIL.

HISTORY, PHYSICAL EXAMINATION, AND GASTROINTESTINAL LOCATION

History

The history can vary, according to the lymphoma subtype:

- **LGITL.** As previously mentioned, GIL and particularly LGITL usually affect ageing cats (median age 13 years).[1–4,14] This entity is characterised by a slow onset and progression of clinical signs. In a recent prospective study involving 22 cases of LGITL and 22 cases of LPE,[11] the duration of clinical signs was statistically different in the two groups (median clinical signs duration of 365 days in LGITL vs. 106 days in LPE).

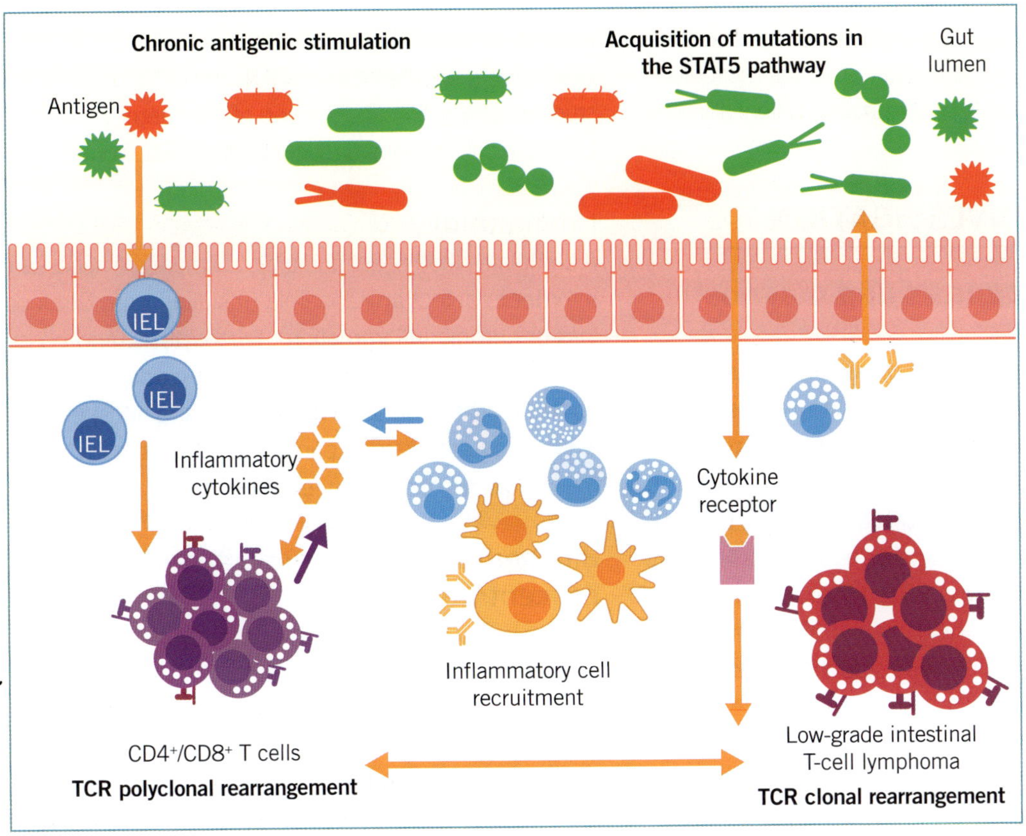

Figure 20.2. A novel model of lymphomagenesis illustrating a continuum of a chronic antigenic stimulation in an inflammatory background towards lymphomagenesis. IEL, intraepithelial lymphocyte; STAT5, signal transducer and activator of transcription 5; TCR, T-cell receptor.

- **Other subtypes of GIL.** Although GIL usually affects geriatric cats, high-grade lymphoma can also be identified in young animals, exhibiting more severe, recent, or acute clinical signs.

Physical examination

The clinical presentation of LGITL lacks specificity and is nonpathognomonic. The main clinical signs include weight loss, anorexia, and lethargy, while specific clinical signs comprise vomiting and diarrhoea. Hepatomegaly, splenomegaly, and polyuria/polydipsia are less frequently seen in this subtype. Abdominal palpation is an important part of the clinical examination, although an extensive clinical approach is required in this context. All the intestinal loops must be evaluated in terms of firmness and thickness. Small bowel infiltration is most frequently diffuse. Mesenteric lymph node evaluation is important as well: a mild enlargement is frequently seen, and firm lymph nodes may be palpated amongst intestinal loops. That said, the identification of markedly abnormal lymph nodes should evoke other differentials, such as intermediate- to high-grade lymphomas, mast cell tumours, or infectious diseases.

It is important to note that a normal clinical examination performed in an alert cat never rules out a low-grade intestinal lymphoma. Cats presenting with LPE can show exactly the same clinical features as cats presenting with LGITL.

Intermediate-grade, high-grade, or LGL lymphomas are more commonly associated with poor body condition: dehydration, weakness, anorexia, weight loss, icterus. Reported GI signs include vomiting and diarrhoea. Abdominal palpation may reveal mass lesions, marked lymphadenomegaly, ascites, and even peritonitis when the neoplasm leads to small bowel perforation. In contrast to LGITL, small bowel infiltration and thickness is often focal and localised.

Gastrointestinal location

LGITL can be found in all sections of the GI tract (Table 20.1). The disease can be multifocal or diffuse. The most common sites affected are the jejunum and the ileum, followed by the duodenum.[3] A gastric location is less frequent, and colonic infiltration is unlikely in this context. It is important to note that the GI distribution of LPE is quite similar to that of LGITL.

In contrast, other GIL subtypes are less frequent but can affect any intestinal segment as well as mesenteric lymph nodes, liver, spleen, pancreas, and potentially even the bone marrow.

DIAGNOSTIC INVESTIGATION

Differential diagnosis and diagnostic workup

In geriatric cats, diagnosing the disease requires a complete diagnostic workup, as endocrinopathies, metabolic diseases, infectious processes, and inflammatory diseases may present with similar clinical signs and may coexist with LGITL, thereby complicating the clinical presentation. The major diagnostic challenge is to differentiate LGITL from LPE. Moreover, it can be difficult to distinguish other forms of GIL from other more aggressive feline neoplasms such mastocytomas or carcinomas.

Classical diagnostic workup requires haematology and blood smear, serum biochemistry, total serum thyroxine concentration, vitamin levels (serum cobalamin, folate, and vitamin D), specific lipase and trypsinogen dosage, faecal and urine analyses, diagnostic imaging, and intestinal biopsy. Considering vitamin D, in a retrospective study,[15] the median serum 25(OH)D concentration was significantly lower in cats with LGITL or IBD compared to healthy cats, even if the mechanism leading to hypovitaminosis D was not elucidated.

Cats should also be tested for FeLV and FIV, given the associations previously reported with GIL. If diarrhoea is present, dietary trials are needed in order to rule out a food-responsive enteropathy. Hence, as previously mentioned, discriminating eosinophilic enteritis or lymphoplasmacytic enteritis from LGITL is challenging because all data may be confusing (clinical signs, diagnostic imaging results, pathological and histopathological findings). Even conventional immunohistochemistry and clonality testing may not be discriminatory tools, as will be discussed later in this chapter.

Laboratory data

Haematology and biochemistry results represent an important step in the diagnostic workup in order to exclude extraintestinal causes of chronic diarrhoea, but they are often nonspecific and nondiscriminatory, particularly if trying to differentiate LGITL from LPE. In a recent study involving 44 cats,[11] none of the haematologic nor biochemical data could discriminate LGITL from LPE.

Haematology

A complete blood count and a blood smear are necessary in order to detect any anaemia (resulting from GI blood loss or chronic inflammation), leucocytosis, and possible circulating lymphoblasts in a high-grade lymphoma context.[3] These data are usually mild and nonspecific,[8] while cats suffering from primary small intestinal lymphomas frequently exhibit anaemia.[16]

Biochemistry and serum vitamin concentration

Biochemistry is usually of low diagnostic yield for low-grade GIL as well as high-grade GIL. The most frequently reported abnormality in GIL is mild to moderate hypoalbuminaemia, which is more common in cats with high-grade and LGL lymphomas than in cats with intermediate-grade intestinal lymphoma and LGITL.[3] In another study,[14] hypoalbuminaemia was detected in 70% of cats with GIL, 49% of cats with LGITL, and 77% of cats with chronic enteropathies. In GIL, it is hypothesised that the loss of integrity of the small intestinal barrier may result in loss of albumin.[8] In dogs, it has been reported that cytokine interleukin (IL)-6 suppresses albumin synthesis and may be released by neoplastic cells. This has been speculated to contribute to the progressive hypoalbuminaemia observed in GIL.[4]

In severe cases, fluid and electrolytic imbalances can be identified as well; the most frequent abnormality in cats presenting with frequent vomiting and/or diarrhoea is hypokalaemia.

Hypocobalaminaemia is another concern in cats suffering from chronic enteropathies of any aetiology. Up to 80% of LGITL cases have been found to present with hypocobalaminaemia (reference >290 ng/l). This may be due to the distal location of the infiltrate (jejunum and ileum) in many cases of LGITL. Severe and more chronic hypocobalaminaemia can also lead to weakness in cats. In a prospective study involving 44 cases (22 LGITL cases and 22 LPE cases),[11] hypocobalaminaemia was significantly more severe in the low-grade lymphoma group.

Folate concentration may vary in cats diagnosed with GIL and is not pathognomonic of a distinct diagnosis. These cobalamin and folates perturbations have not been reported with other GIL subtypes.[3,4]

Faecal analysis

If small and/or large bowel diarrhoea is present, faecal tests that may be considered include faecal smears, flotation assays, and PCR assays or direct fluorescent antigen tests to rule out *Giardia, Tritrichomonas, Campylobacter*, and *Cryptosporidium* species. In cases of fever in cats presenting with haemorrhagic diarrhoea, although uncommon, infection with enteropathogenic bacteria should be considered as well (*Salmonella, Campylobacter, Clostridium* species).[3]

In a recent study,[17] the authors characterised the faecal microbiome of 38 healthy cats and 27 cats with chronic enteropathies (13 cats with IBD and 14 cats with LGITL). As depicted in humans, the host's microbiome may be disturbed in both LPE and LGITL cases. A dysbiosis is defined by a decreased diversity of the microbial community, a general decrease of species of the phyla *Bacteroidetes* and *Firmicutes*. Univariate analysis revealed a lower abundance of facultative anaerobic taxa of the phyla *Firmicutes, Actinobacteria*, and *Bacteroidetes* in cats with chronic enteropathy. No significant difference was found between the microbiome of cats with IBD and that of cats with LGITL. In addition, the dysbiosis seen in cats with both IBD and LGITL is very similar to that seen in people with IBD.[17]

Ultrasonography

Abdominal ultrasonography is a key step in the diagnostic workup. It allows both reliable examination of all abdominal organs and detection of diffuse or focal thickening as well as loss of the normal layering of the intestine. That said, minimal mucosal alterations may not be identified, particularly if they are located in the stomach or colon. The first goals of ultrasonography are to rule out an intestinal mass, organomegaly, and/or a peritoneal effusion.

Ultrasonographic images of the different lymphoma subtypes are presented Figure 20.3.

To date, ultrasonographic distinction between inflammatory disease and diffuse neoplastic infiltration is not possible: a diffuse thickening of the muscularis layer commonly defines both entities. For example, in a recent study involving 17 cats with IBD, 22 cats diagnosed with food-responsive enteropathy, and 17 cats with GIL, no significant differences in ultrasonographic findings were found between the three groups.[18] Although intestinal wall thickness reference values have been established in cats, clear diagnostic cutoffs for either LPE or LGITL have not been reported. The ratio of muscularis propria width to submucosal width can be helpful (≥0.5 is considered abnormal). However, abnormal ratios can be found in LPE, eosinophilic enteritis, and LGITL.[19] In one study,[20] older cats with muscularis layer thickening were more likely to be diagnosed with LGITL than IBD.

Moreover, mesenteric and ileocolic lymphadenomegaly are frequently noted on ultrasound: the regional lymph nodes may frequently appear hypoechoic, rounded, and thickened in inflammatory infiltrations (LPE and eosinophilic enteritis) as well as in LGITL. The diameter of mesenteric lymph nodes can vary; the average is 4–6 mm for jejunal lymph nodes and 5 mm for ileocaecal lymph nodes.[20] In GIL, alterations in the size of the mesenteric lymph nodes can be highly variable, ranging from minimal to considerably enlarged. Colic lymph nodes in LGITL cats were reported to be on average 1.6-fold larger in size than those from healthy cats, whereas an increased size of jejunal lymph nodes was not consistently associated with LGITL in a recent study.[19]

Fine needle aspiration (FNA) should be considered in case of any organomegaly, masses, and effusions in order to rule out aggressive forms of lymphomas and exclude other neoplasia (mast cell tumours, carcinomas).

In conclusion, LGITL should never be excluded based on a normal ultrasonographic examination, and histological analysis is always required in order to establish a definitive diagnosis.[4]

Endoscopy and laparotomy

Gastrointestinal endoscopy

Endoscopy of the GI tract is a minimally invasive technique that allows direct visualisation of the gastric, duodenal, and colonic mucosa. Multiple intestinal biopsy samples need to be collected, and at least 6–10 adequate samples should be obtained per intestinal site. Even if the jejunum is only partially reachable, or unreachable in case of pyloric narrowing in cats, blindly obtained biopsy

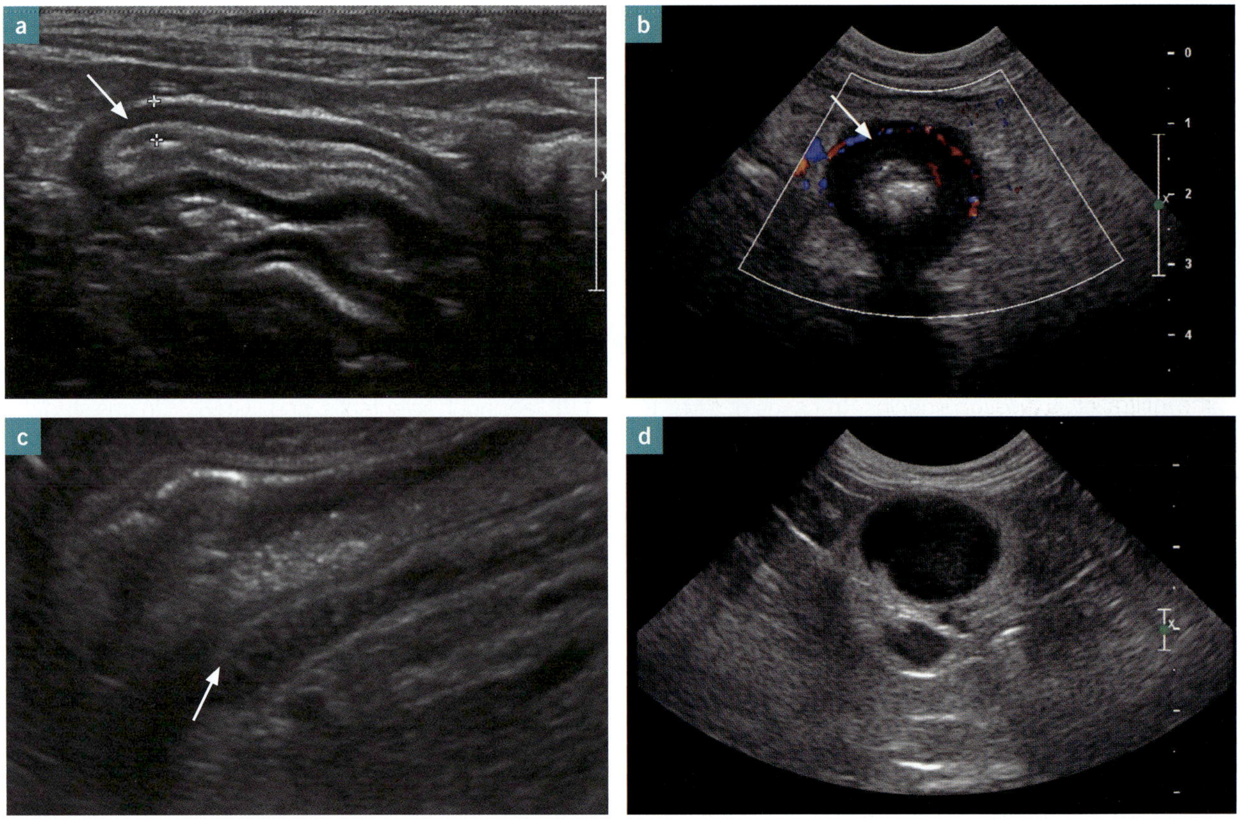

Figure 20.3. Ultrasonographic images of the different lymphoma subtypes. Diffuse thickened jejunal muscularis layer (arrow) in a cat diagnosed with low-grade intestinal T-cell lymphoma (a). High-grade lymphoma (b): intestinal mass, loss of digestive layering (arrow), and neoplastic vascularisation highlighted by Doppler ultrasonography. Intermediate-grade gastric lymphoma (c): a loss of layering (arrow) is identified, and the gastric wall is thickened. An enlarged gastric lymph node was also detected. In this case, examination of fine needle aspiration samples was inconclusive, and per-endoscopic gastric biopsy confirmed the diagnosis. Mesenteric lymph nodes in an 8-year-old spayed female cat presented with anorexia and vomiting for 3 weeks (d). This enlarged round-shaped lymph node is hypoechoic. Fine needle aspiration sample examination detected large granular neoplastic lymphocytes. Images courtesy of Dr Pascaline Pey, by kind permission of Les Éditions du Point Vétérinaire, France.

samples can be taken from the ileum.[4] In diffuse intestinal infiltrations, whatever their nature, mucosal lesions that were not identified by ultrasonographic examination are easily detected by endoscopy. In order to avoid misdiagnosis, the World Small Animal Veterinary Association (WSAVA) Gastrointestinal Standardization Group guidelines were established in order to promote a standardised interpretation of inflammatory changes in the GI mucosa of the dog and cat.[21] In cases of suspected LGITL, the indications for endoscopy must meet the following criteria:

- **LGITL.** As previously explained, the major challenge is to distinguish diffuse inflammatory infiltrations from LGITL. This indolent subtype of GIL tends to be mainly localised to the duodenum, ileum, and jejunum and is much less likely to be found in the gastric or colonic segments.[11] So far, no study has been able to establish the true percentage of the lymphomatous areas within the GI mucosa in cats. Moreover, it is the author's opinion that gastroduodenal inflammatory lesions are frequently associated with a diagnosis of jejunal LGITL. Unfortunately, a macroscopic distinction between inflammatory lesions (congestion, oedema, mucosal fibrosis) and LGITL lesions during endoscopy is impossible. Another concern is the quality of the samples and their interpretation. Numerous specimens need to be collected from each mucosal compartment with an adequate biopsy forceps, and samples need to be carefully mounted on a moisturised synthetic foam sponge and should never be floating free in formalin. Endoscopic biopsy specimens only include the mucosa and potentially, when deep samples are collected, parts of the submucosa. The epithelial origin of LGITL has recently been confirmed in a prospective study including 22 cases of LGITL and 22 cases of LPE.[11] An apical-to-basal gradient with more lymphoma cells in the apical regions of the villi was noted in 41% of the LGITL cases vs. 5% of the LPE cases, and no deep mucosal infiltration was noted in any of the LGITL cases. This means that, in most cases, LGITL can be diagnosed by endoscopy alone, since the infiltration is most obvious in the apical villus areas of the mucosa.

- **Other GILs.** Endoscopic diagnosis of other GILs is possible if the lesion of interest is reachable by endoscopy and include the following sites: gastric or duodenal mucosa, distal ileum mucosa, and colonic mucosa (the latter, however, is unlikely in GIL). The stomach is a frequent location for high-grade GIL. The macroscopic appearance of those neoplasms is quite specific: erosions and/or ulcerations are common features, as well as proliferative, thickened, discoloured, rigid folds. Figure 20.4 shows the endoscopic aspect of an aggressive B-cell lymphoma in the stomach of a young cat.

Exploratory laparotomy

Exploratory laparotomy allows direct inspection of all the intestinal segments but is more invasive than endoscopy (Fig. 20.5). Full-thickness samples are obtained from both the digestive tract and any other affected organs (lymph nodes, spleen, liver, pancreas). The procedure is generally safe, although a low incidence of postoperative leakage has been reported, particularly in more severely affected cases (e.g. those presenting with hypoalbuminaemia). Advantages and disadvantages of the surgical approach to taking biopsy samples are discussed below:

- **Suspected LGITL.** Because of the frequent lack of gross changes in cases with LGITL, it can be challenging to choose which part of the small intestine should be sampled. Thus, ultrasonographic findings can be helpful to identify the areas of the intestine that are thickened. In addition, "running the intestine" during the procedure can be helpful to identify local areas of thickening. If no specific areas of thickened intestine are identified, surgical biopsy samples should be collected from the jejunum and ileum.
- **Other subtypes of GIL.** The diagnosis of other subtypes can often be obtained cytologically via FNA of abnormal tissues. Main surgical indications for intermediate- to

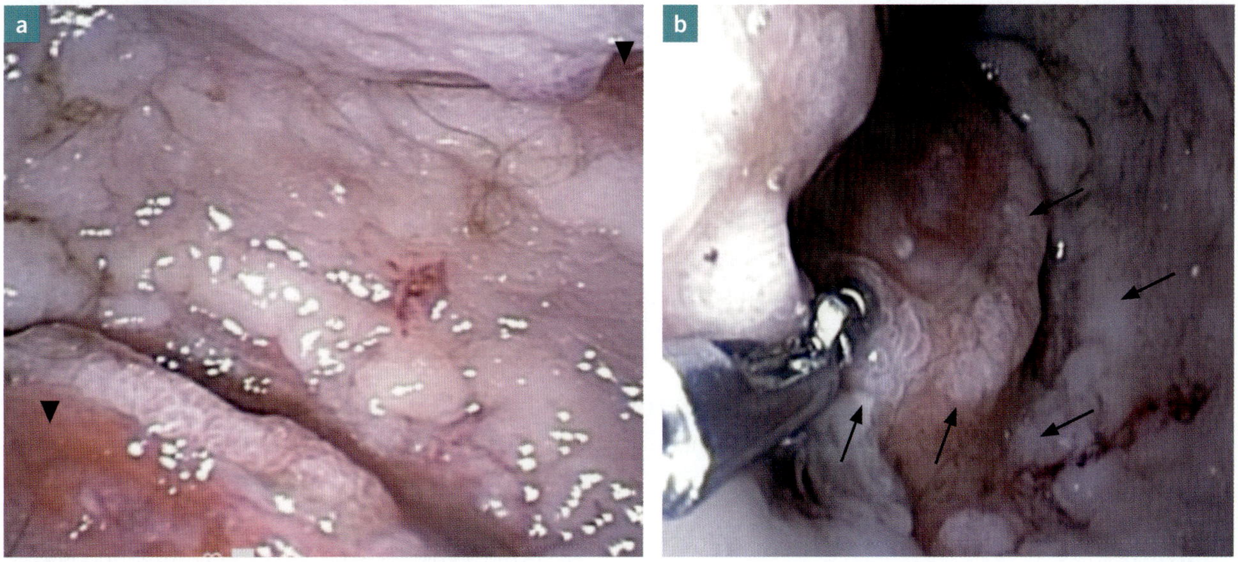

Figure 20.4. Endoscopic images of a highly aggressive B-cell gastric lymphoma in a 6-year-old spayed female cat presented with nonspecific clinical signs: slight weight loss in an overweight context, vomiting, and recent dysorexia. The gastric mucosal folds are extensively altered and do not flatten with air insufflation. The mucosa shows discolouration, huge thickening, and several ulcers (arrowheads) (a). A large ulcer is shown, surrounded by suspected neoplastic abnormal mucosa (b). Several biopsy samples were collected on its sides and all around (arrows).

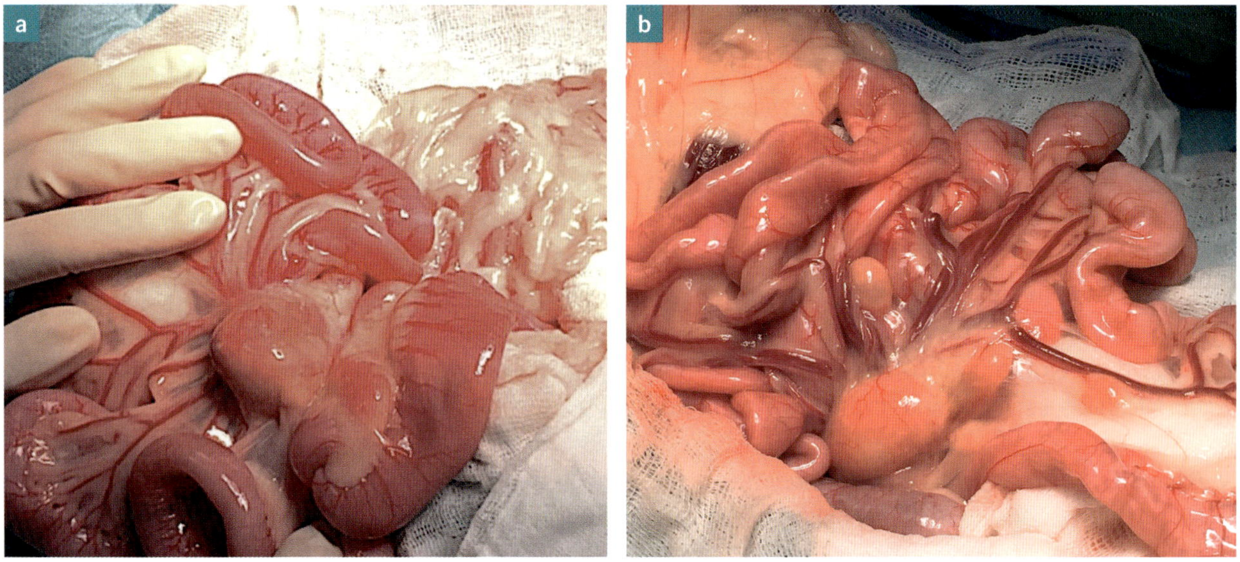

Figure 20.5. Macroscopic appearance of the intestine during exploratory laparotomy in two cats presented with the same history and expression and duration of clinical signs as well as similar paraclinical and ultrasonographic data. The enlarged mesenteric lymph node shown in the image had been previously detected by ultrasonographic examination (a). Biopsy samples collected from the jejunum and lymph nodes were analysed and revealed a severe lymphoplasmacytic enteritis. Although the intestine of the second cat has a similar macroscopic aspect (b), the final diagnosis was a low-grade intestinal T-cell lymphoma.

high-grade lymphomas include nonconclusive cytology obtained by FNA, obstructive lesions (mostly located in the small intestine), and peritonitis resulting from small bowel perforation.

Cytology and histology

Both cytological and histological assessment can be performed to diagnose GIL in cats.

Cytology

In regard to high-grade lymphomas and LGL lymphomas, an intestinal mass and enlarged mesenteric lymph nodes are frequently identified during ultrasonographic examination (Fig. 20.6). Thus, examination of samples obtained by FNA is an appropriate procedure to reach a diagnosis. In contrast, results of FNA examination on mesenteric lymph nodes are often unreliable for LGITL due to the presence of large numbers of small lymphocytes in the lymph nodes.

Histology

The gold standard to establish a diagnosis of GIL includes the combination of histology and immunohistochemistry, according to the guidelines of the WSAVA Gastrointestinal Standardization Group.

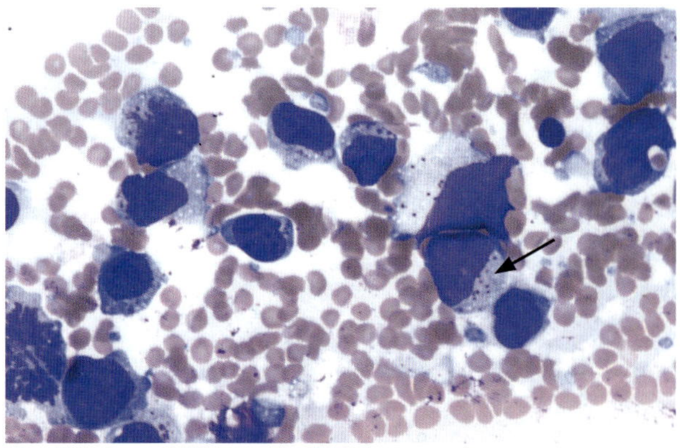

Figure 20.6. Fine needle aspiration cytology from a small intestinal mass in a 9-year-old castrated male cat diagnosed with a large granular lymphocyte lymphoma (May–Grünwald–Giemsa, ×1000). Large granular lymphocytes can be seen, with a purple basophilic cytoplasm containing large granules (arrow). Image courtesy of the Laboratoire d'anatomo-cytopathologie, Biopôle, École nationale vétérinaire d'Alfort, France.

LGITL histological lesions are defined by variable infiltration of the intestinal mucosa by a monomorphic population of small lymphocytes, mostly involving the epithelium but also the lamina propria and potentially the submucosa and muscularis.[6,22] Similarly, as described for clinical, ultrasonographic, endoscopic, and surgical findings, differentiating LGITL from LPE can represent a challenging task for pathologists. According to the 2016 revision of the World Health Organization (WHO) classification of lymphoid neoplasms,[23] several histological criteria are particularly relevant to distinguish those two entities:

- apical-to-basal gradient of infiltration: LGITL;
- epitheliotropism (homing of neoplastic T cells to the mucosal epithelium): LGITL;
- lamina propria cellularity: marked in LGITL;
- villous atrophy: stronger in LGITL;
- crypt characterisation (lymphocytic, neutrophilic cryptitis): lymphocytic cryptitis defines LGITL;
- lymphoid nests and plaques: LGITL;
- mixed lymphoid and plasmacytic inflammatory infiltrates, neutrophilic cryptitis, and/or abscesses: more pronounced in LPE, even if LGITL can exhibit polymorphism;
- depth of infiltration (submucosa–muscularis–serosa): LGITL spreads into the depth of the intestinal wall.

Mild cases of LGITL may be limited to infiltration of small T cells only into the epithelial layer. Plaques and nests were first defined by Kiupel et al. (Figs. 20.7 and 20.8).[24] An intraepithelial plaque is defined by five or more adjacent epithelial cells obscured by infiltrates of small T cells, while an intraepithelial nest shows five or more small T cells clustered within the villous epithelium. Nests and plaques may be identified in a polyclonal cellular background, and they should raise suspicion for the early emergence of a possible LGITL within a chronic inflammatory background. Whilst a predominant epitheliotropic T-cell infiltrate is not necessarily found in all intestinal lymphomas, it evokes a suspicion for LGITL rather than IBD. Furthermore, it has been suggested that performing a separate assessment of the epithelium and the lamina propria could improve the diagnostic accuracy of pathology and reduce interobserver discrepancy.[11]

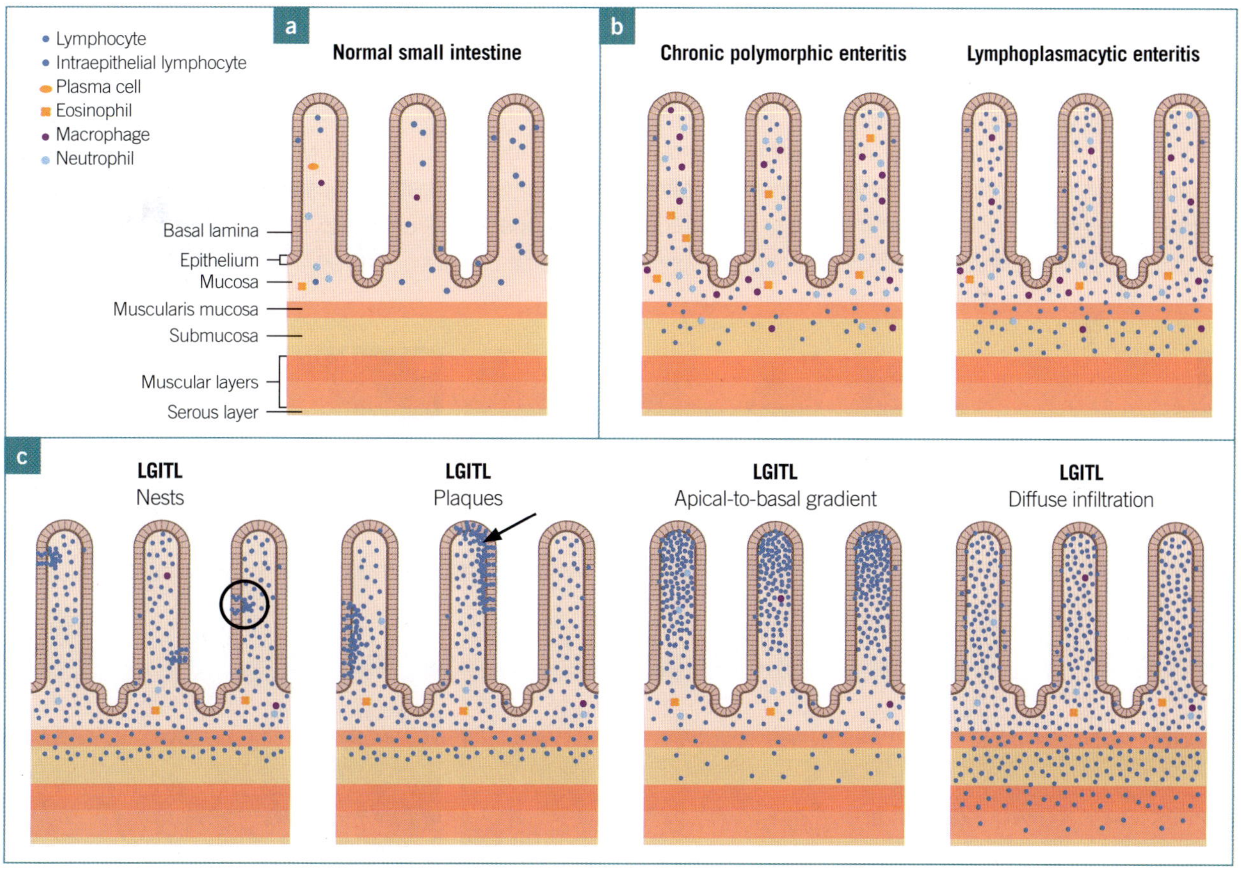

Figure 20.7. Schematic diagram of the intestine illustrating the histological criteria for the differential diagnosis of chronic enteritis and low-grade intestinal T-cell lymphoma (LGITL). Normal histological appearance of the small intestine (a). Histological differences between chronic polymorphic enteritis and lymphoplasmacytic enteritis (b). In LGITL, nests of lymphocytes (circle) are present within the epithelium (c); even in a mild polymorphism context, a LGITL may be suspected. Plaques (arrow), apical-to-basal gradient, and diffuse infiltration (small neoplastic lymphocytes invade the submucosa) are also characteristic of LGITL. Based on diagrams by Dr Mathieu Paulin.

A recent retrospective study investigated histology-guided mass spectrometry (HGMS) for the differentiation of 24 cats diagnosed with LPE from 30 cats diagnosed with LGITL.[25] Histopathology, immunohistochemistry, and clonality testing were available for all cats. A linear discriminate analysis (LDA) machine learning algorithm was developed to analyse the data. The respective sensitivity, specificity, and accuracy of the technique were over 87%. Further studies could document this new diagnostic tool.

In regard to other GIL subtypes, histology is required in intermediate- and high-grade lymphomas when cytology is undiagnostic and will, in most cases, allow to make a definitive diagnosis.

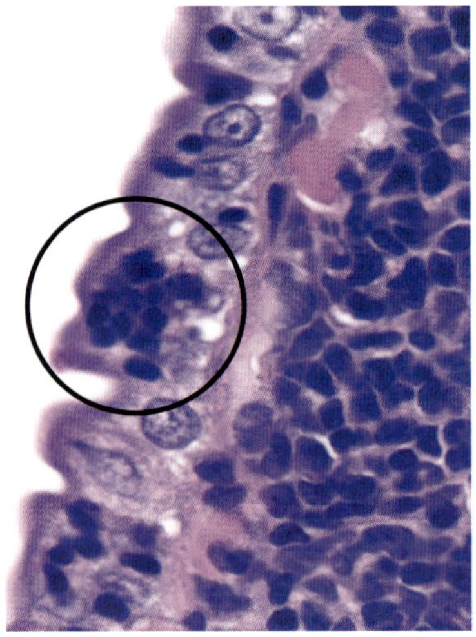

Figure 20.8. Intestinal villi infiltrated by small monomorphic lymphocytes. The circle indicates a nest. Image courtesy of the Laboratoire d'anatomo-cytopathologie, Biopôle, École nationale vétérinaire d'Alfort, France.

Immunohistochemistry

Immunohistochemistry enables the characterisation of the phenotype of the lymphoma (i.e. B or T cell). It is an essential complementary molecular technique in addition to standard histological examination which can help in differentiating LPE from LGITL (Fig. 20.9).[4,19,26] CD3 antibodies detect T cells, while CD20 and CD79 antibodies detect B cells, and CD57 antibodies detect natural killer (NK) cells.[6,26,27] Ki67 proliferation marker concentration increases during cell division and decreases after mitosis. This epitope could be of interest to determine the percentage of proliferating cells. In a recent prospective study,[12] Ki67 expression in lamina propria lymphocytes and intraepithelial lymphocytes was significantly increased in LGITL cases as compared with LPE cases. Hence, a 20% cutoff value was established to discriminate those two entities. To date, other feline-specific antibodies, such as CD4, CD8α, and CD8β, can only be used on fresh frozen biopsy samples, which limits their routine clinical application. They can be useful to define the exact immunosubphenotype of lymphomas. LGITL is of T-cell phenotype and stains positively with CD3 antibody in more than 90% of cases. The remaining 10% of cases exhibit a B-cell phenotype.[6,8,22]

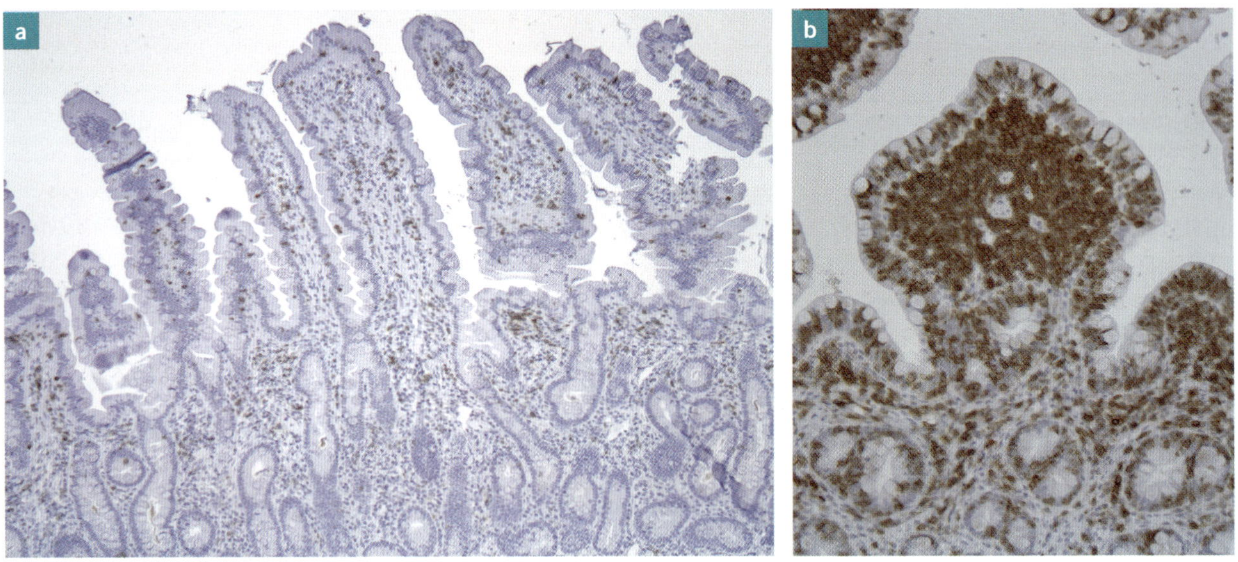

Figure 20.9. Immunohistochemical staining with CD3 antibody. In lymphoplasmacytic enteropathy, only a few cells express the epitope (a). In low-grade intestinal T-cell lymphoma, a strong expression of CD3 epitope can be seen (b). Furthermore, a major apical-to-basal gradient infiltrate of the lymphocyte is identified, exhibiting a strong epitheliotropism. Images courtesy of Dr Julie Bruneau, Service d'anatomopathologie, Hôpital Necker, Assistance Publique—Hôpitaux de Paris, France.

Clonality testing

Clonality testing is a diagnostic tool based on PCR targeting of the CDR3 region of the T-cell receptor gamma (TCR γ) gene for T cells and the immunoglobulin heavy chain (IGH) genes for B cells. In the feline species, this assay was first reported by Moore et al. in 2005.[20,22,28] The aim of the test, which is also called PCR for antigen receptor rearrangements (PARR), is to detect clonally expanded lymphocyte populations in the submitted samples. Clonality analysis has been presented as a gold standard test, with particular relevance in differentiating inflammatory infiltrations from LGITL in veterinary pathology.[6,29] Molecular detection of clonal TCR γ chain gene rearrangements can be performed either on DNA extracted from fresh frozen intestinal biopsy samples or from formalin-fixed paraffin-embedded tissue slides by multiplex PCR. Rearrangement is defined as monoclonal when only one peak is detected, oligoclonal when two to three peaks are detected, and polyclonal when no peaks or more than four peaks are detected. One to three peaks emerging from several minor peaks define monoclonality/oligoclonality in a polyclonal background. Regardless of phenotype (which is detected by immunohistochemistry, not by PARR), neoplastic lymphocytes may show clonal rearrangement of either or both the T- and B-cell antigen receptor genes. PARR cannot determine lymphocyte phenotype and, therefore, it never replaces immunohistochemical investigations. Some cases of mucosal T-cell lymphoma of the small-cell type have been found to also have clonal rearrangements of the IGH gene. This can result from malignant transformation and is called cross-lineage rearrangement. This phenomenon has previously been reported in both human and canine T-cell malignancies. The causes remain poorly elucidated.[24] Cross-lineage rearrangement was described in LGITL in a recent study and was reported in 8.6% of cases.[30]

In inflammatory lesions, PARR is expected to exhibit a polyclonal pattern, whereas in LGITL a clonal or oligoclonal TCR γ gene rearrangement is found in more than 90% of cases. The PCR-based clonality assay for routine diagnosis of feline TCR γ gene rearrangement has been shown in a previous study to have a diagnostic sensitivity and specificity close to 90%.[6] That said, the accuracy of this test can vary between laboratories, as different primers have been validated by different laboratories.

In a recent study,[29] Sabattini et al. recommended the assessment of clonality in duodenal endoscopic biopsy samples in order to improve the diagnostic ability to distinguish LGITL from LPE. In another recent prospective study,[11] molecular detection of TCR γ rearrangements revealed monoclonality in 19/22 cases (86%). Conversely, PARR was tested at the same time in 22 cats diagnosed with LPE. Monoclonality was found in 40% of the LPE cases, and 30% of cases displayed monoclonality in a polyclonal background. It has been speculated that in the case of monoclonality in LPE, this could result either from strong antigenic stimulation or from emerging clonal cells in a polyclonal background. A high percentage of clonality has been associated with severe inflammatory diseases in humans. Furthermore, the detection of a clonal lymphocyte population by PARR is not necessarily always indicative of neoplasia, since this can sometimes be found in response to unknown pathogens and concurrent malignancies. Hence, further studies are needed to clarify such cases. In summary, histological and immunophenotypic findings should remain the gold standard criteria to avoid the risks of a misdiagnosis. In this context, it is also important to state that reclassification of cases from LPE to LGITL solely based on PARR test results is not recommended. If a cat suspected with inflammatory lesions displays monoclonality, slides should be carefully reviewed by two different pathologists in order to check the different criteria listed above that help to diagnose LGITL histologically (epitheliotropism, villous atrophy, lymphocytic cryptitis, apical-to-basal gradient, etc.). In addition, CD3, CD20, and Ki67 markers can routinely be evaluated to aid in the differentiation of LPE and LGITL.

Low-grade intestinal T-cell lymphoma: a relevant model to study human indolent gastrointestinal lymphoproliferative disorders

Due to its diffuse infiltration of the epithelium and the lamina propria by monomorphic, medium-sized neoplastic T cells, LGITL was first compared to enteropathy-associated T-cell lymphoma in people (EATL; previously designated type I EATL) or monomorphic epitheliotropic intestinal T-cell lymphoma (MEITL; previously designated type II EATL).[6] Whilst EATL in humans is CD56 positive and shows an aggressive course, a recent study prospectively analysed CD56 in 22 cats diagnosed with LGITL and found that CD56 was negative in 100% of the feline cases.[11]

Therefore, and according to the latest WHO classification,[23] feline LGITL seems more likely to represent the feline equivalent of human indolent intestinal T-cell lymphoproliferative disorders (LPDs). Feline LGITL seems to share most clinical, paraclinical, histological, and phenotypic features with human LPDs.[34]

By contrast, phosphorylated signal transducer and activator of transcription (phospho-STAT) 3 was negative in 100% of the feline LGITL cases, while phospho-STAT5 was positive in 100% of the cases.[11] These results may suggest that the STAT5 intracellular pathway, rather than the STAT3 pathway, plays a key role in feline LGITL. The Janus kinase (JAK)–STAT pathway is known to regulate lymphocyte development, differentiation, and proliferation. Its deregulation has previously been identified as a major oncogenic mechanism in several T- and NK-leukaemia and lymphoma subtypes. Table 20.2 shows the comparative data between human LPDs and feline LGITL.

Additional workup and staging

The recommended additional workup and staging depends on the lymphoma subtype. Ultrasonography allows a reliable assessment of all abdominal organs. As previously discussed, in addition to mesenteric lymph node infiltration, liver, spleen, and pancreas infiltration may also be suspected. FNA is recommended in such cases, particularly in intermediate- to high-grade lymphomas, as organomegaly may not be consistent from case to case.

In regard to LGITL, neoplastic lymphocytes are mostly confined within the GI tract. Thoracic radiographs are

Table 20.2. Comparison between human indolent T-cell lymphoproliferative disorders of the gastrointestinal tract (GI-TLPDs) and feline low-grade gastrointestinal T-cell lymphoma (LGITL).

	Human indolent GI-TLPD	Feline LGITL
Epidemiology	Very rare	Increasing prevalence over the last two decades
Number of cases	57 cases over 25 years	22 cases over 24 months
Median age (years [range])	51.5 [15–77]	13 [8–16]
Median duration of clinical signs (days [range])	2562 [122–6222]	365 [62–1460]
Male	64%	73%
Clinical signs	Weight loss, diarrhoea, vomiting, abdominal pain	Weight loss, vomiting, diarrhoea, anorexia
Tumour location	Oral cavity, duodenum, jejunum, ileum, colon, liver	Stomach, duodenum, jejunum, ileum, liver
Histopathology	Normal or villous blunting Monomorphic infiltrate of small lymphocytes in the lamina propria	Villous atrophy (86%) Monomorphic infiltrate of small lymphocytes in the lamina propria
IEL	Variable degree of epitheliotropism	Strong epitheliotropism (86%)
Immunophenotype	$CD3^+$ (100%) $CD4^+/CD8^-$ (60%), $CD4^-/CD8^+$ (30%), $CD4^-/CD8^-$ (6%), $CD4^+/CD8^+$ (4%) $CD56^-$ Phospho-$STAT3^+$ (11%) Phospho-$STAT5^+$ (44%) Ki67 lamina propria <10%	$CD3^+$ (97%) $CD4^+/CD8^-$ (36%), $CD4^-/CD8^+$ (27%), $CD4^-/CD8^-$ (36%) $CD56^-$ (100%) Phospho-$STAT3^-$ (0%) Phospho-$STAT5^+$ (100%) Ki67 lamina propria 20%
Clonality (small intestine TCR)	Mainly clonal (94%)	Mainly clonal (86%)
Main differential diagnoses	Autoimmune enteropathy, inflammatory bowel disease, refractory coeliac sprue	Inflammatory bowel disease (e.g. lymphoplasmacytic chronic enteropathies)
Outcome	Indolent evolution (persistent disease at median follow-up of 5 years)	Indolent evolution (median survival time of 2 years)

IEL, intraepithelial lymphocyte; phospho-STAT, phosphorylated signal transducer and activator of transcription; TCR, T-cell receptor.

advisable when intermediate- to high-grade lymphomas are suspected, in order to detect enlarged thoracic lymph nodes or pleural effusion. Furthermore, a myelogram can detect potential bone marrow infiltration. A blood smear should always be performed and examined in order to identify circulating neoplastic cells. The classical staging criteria defined for other types of lymphoma cannot be reliably applied to classify GILs.

Flow chart for the diagnosis of gastrointestinal lymphoma in cats

As previously mentioned, the main challenge for clinicians is to differentiate LGITL from chronic inflammatory intestinal infiltrate (lymphoplasmacytic or eosinophilic). Figure 20.10 illustrates the different steps of investigations in a cat presenting with clinical signs consistent with a possible GIL.

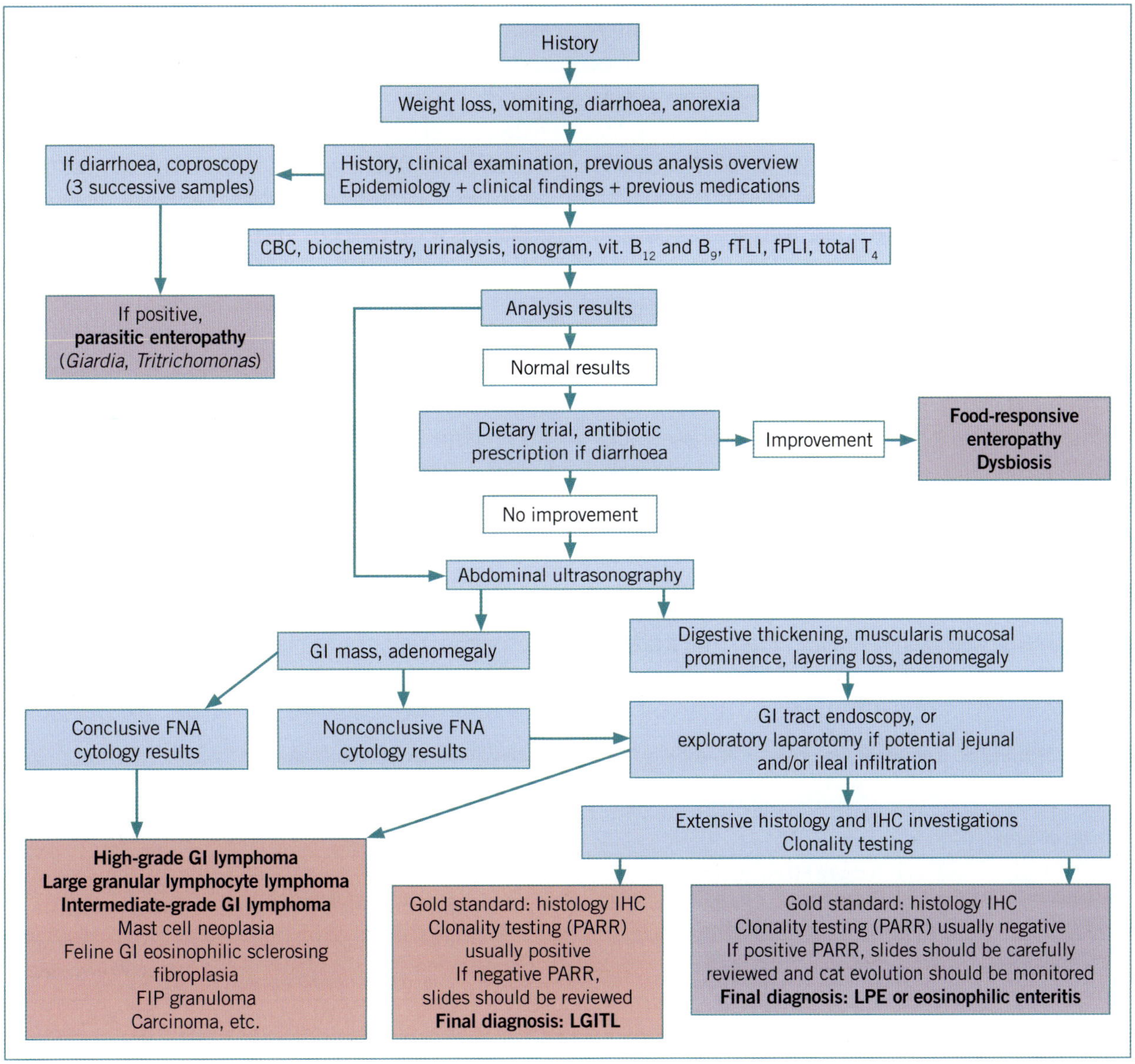

Figure 20.10. Diagnostic flow chart for feline gastrointestinal lymphoma. CBC, complete blood count; FIP, feline infectious peritonitis; FNA, fine needle aspiration; fPLI, feline pancreatic lipase immunoreactivity; fTLI, feline trypsin-like immunoreactivity; GI; gastrointestinal; IHC, immunohistochemistry; LGITL, low-grade intestinal T-cell lymphoma; LPE, lymphoplasmacytic enteropathy; PARR, PCR for antigen receptor rearrangements.

TREATMENT

Chemotherapy

The most effective treatment for GILs is systemic chemotherapy, as lymphoma is a systemic disease.

In cases of LGITL, according to different recommendations[1,8,27] and considering problems with treatment compliance in cats and their owners, the standard chemotherapeutic protocol combines two drugs: chlorambucil (pulsed administration or every other day, given orally every 24 hours) and prednisolone (3 mg/kg PO every 24 hours, tapering dose to 1 mg/kg PO once complete remission is achieved) or dexamethasone to initiate immunosuppression (up to 1–2 mg/kg every 12 hours). This therapeutic scheme is continued if no adverse effects occur, as no data have been reported concerning the optimal duration of chemotherapy. The different published protocols are summarised in Table 20.3. To the author's knowledge, even if side effects are uncommon, complete blood counts should be checked regularly. Transient anorexia or other GI signs may be noted in some individuals.

In regard to other GIL subtypes, a multiagent chemotherapy protocol is recommended in both intermediate- and high-grade lymphomas. A COP (cyclophosphamide, vincristine, prednisolone), L-COP (L-asparaginase, cyclophosphamide, vincristine, prednisolone), CHOP (cyclophosphamide, doxorubicin, vincristine, prednisolone) or L-CHOP (L-asparaginase, cyclophosphamide, doxorubicin, vincristine, prednisolone) protocol is most commonly implemented. If initiating a COP protocol, vincristine is administered weekly on weeks 1, 2, 3, and 4 at a dosage of 0.75 mg/m^2 IV, cyclophosphamide is given weekly on weeks 1 and 4 at a dosage of 300 mg/m^2 PO, and prednisolone is given daily at a dosage of 50 mg/m^2 PO. When doxorubicin is included in the chemotherapy protocol, the median survival time (MST) reaches 7–10 months.[2,31]

Main adverse effects include myelotoxicity (thrombocytopenia, leucopenia), weight loss, GI toxicity (anorexia, diarrhoea, vomiting), and renal and/or hepatic toxicity. A complete blood count should be performed prior to each chemotherapy. Treatment should be delayed for 1 week if the neutrophil count is under 1500 cells/µl.

Further studies including more homogeneous cases would be beneficial in the future, as to date many published studies describe different lymphoma localisations and/or mix different GIL subtypes.

Rescue protocol

If a relapse is diagnosed, other chemotherapy protocols are initiated: lomustine (CCNU) PO with or without corticosteroids, COP protocol, VELCAP-C (COP protocol) +/– L-asparaginase and doxorubicin, cyclophosphamide and prednisolone.[4] In one study,[32] 28 cats diagnosed with LGITL were treated with a combination of glucocorticoids and chlorambucil. A rescue protocol including prednisolone (5 mg every 48 hours) and cyclophosphamide (200–250 mg/m^2 PO every 2 weeks on days 1 and 3) was initiated. Based on resolution of clinical signs and normal abdominal palpation, the response rate was 100%. Three cats were lost to follow-up, while three cats died of unrelated diseases. The final cat relapsed 241 days after starting the rescue protocol. Further studies should prospectively investigate the outcome of cats by specific lymphoma subtype.

Table 20.3. Published therapeutic protocols for feline low-grade gastrointestinal T-cell lymphoma.

Study	Lingard et al. 2009[1]	Stein et al. 2010[32]	Fondacaro et al. 1999[14]	Kiselow et al. 2008[27]
Number of cases	12	28	29	41
Prednisolone	3 mg/kg PO every 24 h, tapering to 1–2 mg/kg once in remission	1–2 mg/kg PO every 24 h	10 mg/cat/day PO	5 mg/cat PO every 12–24 h
Chlorambucil	15 mg/m^2 PO every 24 h for 4 days every 3 weeks	20 mg/m^2 PO every 2 weeks	15 mg/m^2 PO every 24 h for 4 days every 3 weeks	2 mg/cat PO every 48 h
Number responding	—	27 (96%)	—	37 (95%)
Complete remission rate	—	—	20 (69%)	22 (56%)
Median remission time (days)	505	786	615	897
Median survival time (days)	513	—	510	704

Surgical resection

By definition, GILs are diffuse diseases, and surgical resection is not indicated to manage the lesions unless an obstructive mass or peritonitis is present. Furthermore, no benefit has been demonstrated in terms of survival when surgical resection of a nonobstructive mass was performed prior to chemotherapy.[8]

In regard to complications, in one study involving 20 cases of intermediate- and high-grade GIL, surgical resection had been performed prior to CHOP-based chemotherapy, and no postoperative surgical complications were reported.[7] Thus, cats diagnosed with GIL do not appear to present a higher risk of postoperative complications after full-thickness GI surgery.

Adjuvant therapy: dietary management, probiotics, and vitamins

Dietary management is an important concern in gastroenterology in general. A highly digestible diet is recommended in addition to medical treatment in all GIL cases. In neoplastic diseases, nutritional support is essential, and diet should be well accepted and tolerated. The impact of the disease is multifactorial: infiltration into the mucosa, malabsorption, malnutrition, vitamin deficiency, and side effects of treatments. In cats, lipids should ideally represent at least 50% of the energy source. Proteins of high biological value are recommended, while carbohydrates should be reduced. When anorexia is persistent, appetite stimulants are commonly prescribed (mirtazapine at 3.75 mg/cat PO every 3 days).[2,8] Capromorelin has recently been cited as a growth hormone secretagogue that increases food intake in anorexic cats.

Randomised studies should be conducted to highlight the potential benefits of prebiotic and probiotics in cats suffering from GIL. In a recent retrospective study, 0.25 mg cyanocobalamin tablets were given orally once daily in cats presenting with GI signs. Increases in serum cobalamin concentrations were documented after oral treatment in cats with hypocobalaminaemia.[33]

PROGNOSIS

The initial response to chemotherapy has been shown to be the most significant prognostic indicator.[8,14,31] Lethargy, anorexia, and vomiting at initial diagnosis are also considered to be negative prognostic factors, as well as FeLV and FIV status, anaemia, high concentration of lactate dehydrogenase (LDH), deeper infiltration of the gut wall, and a lack of or only partial clinical response.[1,8]

Most LGITL cases have a relatively good prognosis. It remains unclear as to whether, in the long-term, those case can progress to more aggressive forms of GIL. In the author's experience, and as noted in human LDPs, a few cats may develop more aggressive subtypes of GIL. However, no positive association has been found between different factors (including age, sex, weight, duration of clinical signs, presence of extraintestinal lesions, hypofolataemia, hypocobalaminaemia, and serum total protein concentration) and the response to treatment in cases with LGITL.[4,27] As previously discussed, the treatment is usually continued over several years.[4] Substantial remission and survival time periods (MST 19–29 months) have been reported in cats diagnosed with LGITL.[1,8,14] Commonly reported causes of death include comorbidities in senior cats, relapse of the disease, or the owner's request for euthanasia.[1,8]

Patients with high-grade GIL have a much shorter survival time (MST 7–10 months), while in cases of LGL lymphoma, MST is less than 70 days.

Take-home messages

- Gastrointestinal lymphoma is defined according to four different subtypes of increasing aggressiveness: low-grade gastrointestinal T-cell lymphoma (the most frequent and least aggressive form; an emerging disease), intermediate-grade gastrointestinal lymphoma, high-grade gastrointestinal lymphoma, and large granular lymphocyte lymphoma.
- A major challenge for clinicians is to distinguish low-grade intestinal T-cell lymphoma from lymphoplasmacytic enteritis given that their clinical, laboratory, diagnostic imaging, and histological presentations may overlap. Current data suggest a continuum between those two entities.
- A normal clinical examination performed in an alert cat never rules out a low-grade gastrointestinal lymphoma.
- A combination of conventional histopathology and immunohistochemistry remains the current gold standard to differentiate low-grade intestinal T-cell lymphoma from lymphoplasmacytic enteritis in cats. Clonality testing shows several limitations. Therefore, for now, clinicians should be cautious with regard to reclassifying cats previously diagnosed with inflammatory bowel disease to lymphoma based on PCR for antigen receptor rearrangements alone.
- Treatment and prognosis rely on the lymphoma subtype. Long survival time (>2 years) is reported for low-grade gastrointestinal lymphoma treated with oral chemotherapy. Other subtypes require conventional chemotherapy schemes. Prognosis can be very poor, notably for high-grade and large granular lymphocyte lymphoma cases.

REFERENCES

[1] Lingard AE et al. Low-grade alimentary lymphoma: clinicopathological findings and response to treatment in 17 cases. *J Feline Med Surg* 11:692, 2009.

[2] Ettinger SN. Principles of treatment for feline lymphoma. *Clin Tech Small Anim Pract* 18:98, 2003.

[3] Barrs VR, Beatty JA. Feline alimentary lymphoma: 1. Classification, risk factors, clinical signs and non-invasive diagnostics. *J Feline Med Surg* 14:182, 2012.

[4] Paulin MV et al. Feline low-grade alimentary lymphoma: an emerging entity and a potential animal model for human disease. *BMC Vet Res* 14:306, 2018.

[5] Wolfesberger B et al. Does categorisation of lymphoma subtypes according to the World Health Organization classification predict clinical outcome in cats? *J Feline Med Surg* 19:897, 2017.

[6] Moore PF, Rodriguez-Bertos A, Kass PH. Feline gastrointestinal lymphoma: mucosal architecture, immunophenotype, and molecular clonality. *Vet Pathol* 49:658, 2012.

[7] Gouldin ED et al. Feline discrete high-grade gastrointestinal lymphoma treated with surgical resection and adjuvant CHOP-based chemotherapy: retrospective study of 20 cases. *Vet Comp Oncol* 15:328, 2017.

[8] Barrs VR, Beatty JA. Feline alimentary lymphoma: 2. Further diagnostics, therapy and prognosis. *J Feline Med Surg* 14:191, 2012.

[9] Garraway K et al. Relationship of the mucosal microbiota to gastrointestinal inflammation and small cell intestinal lymphoma in cats. *J Vet Intern Med* 32:1692, 2018.

[10] Hoehne SN et al. Identification of mucosa-invading and intravascular bacteria in feline small intestinal lymphoma. *Vet Pathol* 54:234, 2017.

[11] Freiche V. *Novel extensive characterisation of feline low grade intestinal lymphoma*. 29th ECVIM-CA Congress, Milan, Italy, 2019.

[12] Freiche V et al. Feline T-cell low-grade intestinal lymphoma: a novel model of lymphomagenesis according to the One-Health concept. In: *2020 ACVIM Forum On Demand Research Abstract Program*. J Vet Intern Med 34:2830, 2020.

[13] Smith V et al. Hair nicotine concentration of cats with gastrointestinal lymphoma and unaffected control cases. *Vet Rec* 186:414, 2020.

[14] Fondacaro JV et al. Feline gastrointestinal lymphoma: 67 cases (1988–1996). *Eur J Comp Gastroenterol* 4:5, 1999.

[15] Lalor S et al. Cats with inflammatory bowel disease and intestinal small cell lymphoma have low serum concentrations of 25-hydroxyvitamin D. *J Vet Intern Med* 28:351, 2014.

[16] Sogame N, Risbon R, Burgess KE. Intestinal lymphoma in dogs: 84 cases (1997–2012). *J Am Vet Med Assoc* 252:440, 2018.

[17] Marsilio S et al. Characterization of the fecal microbiome in cats with inflammatory bowel disease or alimentary small cell lymphoma. *Sci Rep* 9:19208, 2019.

[18] Gianella P et al. Evaluation of clinicopathological features in cats with chronic gastrointestinal signs. *Pol J Vet Sci* 20:403, 2017.

[19] Daniaux LA et al. Ultrasonographic thickening of the muscularis propria in feline small intestinal small cell T-cell lymphoma and inflammatory bowel disease. *J Feline Med Surg* 16:89, 2014.

[20] Zwingenberger AL et al. Ultrasonographic evaluation of the muscularis propria in cats with diffuse small intestinal lymphoma or inflammatory bowel disease. *J Vet Intern Med* 24:289, 2010.

[21] Washabau RJ et al. Endoscopic, biopsy, and histopathologic guidelines for the evaluation of gastrointestinal inflammation in companion animals. *J Vet Intern Med* 24:10, 2010.

[22] Briscoe KA et al. Histopathological and immunohistochemical evaluation of 53 cases of feline lymphoplasmacytic enteritis and low-grade alimentary lymphoma. *J Comp Pathol* 145:187, 2011.

[23] Swerdlow SH et al. The 2016 revision of the World Health Organization classification of lymphoid neoplasms. *Blood* 127:2375, 2016.

[24] Kiupel M et al. Diagnostic algorithm to differentiate lymphoma from inflammation in feline small intestinal biopsy samples. *Vet Pathol* 48:212, 2011.

[25] Marsilio S et al. Differentiation of lymphocytic-plasmacytic enteropathy and small cell lymphoma in cats using histology-guided mass spectrometry. *J Vet Intern Med* 34:669, 2020.

[26] Waly NE et al. Immunohistochemical diagnosis of alimentary lymphomas and severe intestinal inflammation in cats. *J Comp Pathol* 133:253, 2005.

[27] Kiselow MA et al. Outcome of cats with low-grade lymphocytic lymphoma: 41 cases (1995–2005). *J Am Vet Med Assoc* 232:405, 2008.

[28] Moore PF et al. Characterization of feline T cell receptor gamma (TCRG) variable region genes for the molecular diagnosis of feline intestinal T cell lymphoma. *Vet Immunol Immunopathol* 106:167, 2005.

[29] Sabattini S et al. Differentiating feline inflammatory bowel disease from alimentary lymphoma in duodenal endoscopic biopsies. *J Small Anim Pract* 57:396, 2016.

[30] Andrews C et al. Cross lineage rearrangement in feline enteropathy-associated T-cell lymphoma. *Vet Pathol* 53:559, 2016.

[31] Vail DM et al. Feline lymphoma (145 cases): proliferation indices, cluster of differentiation 3 immunoreactivity, and their association with prognosis in 90 cats. *J Vet Intern Med* 12:349, 1998.

[32] Stein TJ et al. Treatment of feline gastrointestinal small-cell lymphoma with chlorambucil and glucocorticoids. *J Am Anim Hosp Assoc* 46:413, 2010.

[33] Toresson L et al. Oral cobalamin supplementation in cats with hypocobalaminaemia: a retrospective study. *J Feline Med Surg* 19:1302, 2017.

[34] Freiche V et al. Feline low-grade intestinal T cell lymphoma: a unique natural model of human indolent T cell lymphoproliferative disorder of the gastrointestinal tract. *Lab Invest* 101:794, 2021.

CHAPTER 21

Nonlymphomatous gastrointestinal tumours

David J. Argyle

Apart from oral tumours, tumours of the gastrointestinal (GI) tract in cats are uncommon, specific incidences being indicated below under specific disease syndromes. In addition, malignant disease of the GI tract in cats has been classically dominated by lymphoma, which is covered in Chapter 20. The aetiopathogenesis of GI malignancies in cats remains underresearched, but environmental pollutants, diets, and chemical agents have all been implicated as tumour initiators. However, the common denominators underpinning the malignant phenotype, as with most cancers in most species, are chronic inflammation and genomic instability.

CANCER BIOLOGY

The causes of cancer and cancer susceptibility in cats

Within the body, the maintenance of health relies on physiological homoeostasis, and the development of any disease is essentially the breakdown of physiological homoeostasis in the body. Cancer is a breakdown of cellular homoeostasis, in which there is a failure of cell birth, growth, propagation, and death to be adequately controlled by normal cellular mechanisms.[1] The classical stochastic model of carcinogenesis suggests that there is an initial insult to cellular DNA which causes a change (mutation) and survival advantage to that cell. The accumulation of such changes over time, each with a survival advantage, eventually leads to the cell escaping the normal cellular homoeostatic mechanisms, causing uncontrolled growth and proliferation. Ultimately, cells within the growing primary tumour can lose contact inhibition and invade the local tissues and eventually develop metastatic potential and spread to other sites. More recently, this stochastic model has been superseded by the stem cell model of cancer development.[1] In this model, cancer arises in true adult stem cells, and the tumour is driven by a small population of stem cells within the tumour that give rise to daughter cancer cells that make up the bulk population of the cancer. This is analogous to the maintenance of bodily organs by adult stem cells, such as the liver, brain, and heart. However, this carries huge therapeutic significance, as stem cells are characteristically resistant to conventional cancer treatments, and may explain the resistance of some cancers to treatment and eradication.[1] Cancer stem cells have been identified in feline cancers and may contribute to the poor prognosis in certain cancer types.

The true causes of cancer are incredibly difficult to define and are largely thought to be multifactorial (Fig. 21.1). However, fundamentally, the causes of cancer can be broadly divided into three areas:

- Infectious agents
- Physical agents
- Chemical agents

Many chemical (e.g. food additives, toxins) and physical agents (e.g. radiation, trauma) have been identified as potential initiators of the cancer phenotype by causing mutational changes in cellular DNA. A good example of this is the implication of injection trauma in cats in the development of injection-site sarcoma.[2] Infectious agents have also gained prominence in initiating cancer, either directly (by causing direct damage to DNA) or indirectly (by causing severe inflammation). The classical example in cats is feline leukaemia virus (FeLV) and its role in the development of haematologic malignancies. This is a directly oncogenic tumour virus and involves the integration of retroviral DNA into the host genome.[1] In terms of GI malignancies in cats, there is very little known about infectious causes of cancer beyond FeLV, but there has been some intense research around papillomavirus infection, which has focused in squamous cell tumours affecting the skin and upper GI tract, such as those found in the oral cavity (see below).[3]

The hallmarks of cancer, genomic instability, and inflammation

Despite the complexity of cancer as a disease, it has been convenient for researchers and clinicians to consider cancer as a disease (i.e. breakdown of cellular homoeostasis) that is brought about by the acquisition of eight fundamental characteristics that dictate malignant growth.[4] These can be acquired in any order during the progression to malignancy and are fundamental to the ability of cancer to persist in the body (Fig. 21.1):

- A self-sufficiency in growth (requiring no growth signalling)
- An insensitivity to anti-growth signals
- An ability to evade programmed cell death (apoptosis)
- Limitless replicative potential (mainly through reactivation of telomerase)
- An ability to sustain angiogenesis and maintain its own blood supply
- An ability to invade and metastasise to distant sites
- An ability to evade host immunity (cancer is "altered self" but often overcomes immune destruction)
- Changes in metabolism that allows the tumour to respire anaerobically, which is a massive drain on body energy and contributes to the catabolic state often experienced in cancer patients (cachexia)

Underlying the acquisition of these characteristics are two "enabling" characteristics which may be considered the common denominators seen in all cancer types: genomic instability and chronic inflammation (Fig. 21.1). Despite the commonality of cancer as a disease, considering the number of cells in the animal body, the development of a malignant cell is actually a very rare event. This is a result of the fastidious mechanisms that the cell has to repair DNA or to shut cells down if they develop major genetic lesions. For mutations, chromosomal translocations, or gene amplifications to be maintained in a cell, the genome must attain increased instability or mutability to overcome the redundant homoeostatic mechanisms that occur in the cell to prevent cancer from developing.

The link between cancer and inflammation is well known and is associated with unfavourable clinical prognoses in cancer patients.[3] Although inflammation normally functions to maintain tissue homoeostasis in response to tissue stressors (e.g. infection, tissue damage), clinical studies suggest a close association between chronic inflammation and tumorigenesis. Acute inflammation frequently precedes the development of protective adaptive immune responses to pathogens and cancer. Chronic inflammation, by contrast, has been shown to contribute to cancer initiation by generating genotoxic stress, to cancer promotion by inducing cellular proliferation, and to cancer progression by enhancing angiogenesis and tissue invasion. Chronic inflammation is now appreciated to orchestrate the tumour-promoting microenvironment that is intimately linked with tumorigenesis. Based on these observations, it has been proposed that inflammation and tumour immunity are mutually exclusive processes. The role of chronic inflammation is important, as it demonstrates the susceptibility of organ systems that are subject to chronic inflammation and also underscores a role for nonsteroidal anti-inflammatory drugs (NSAIDs) in the management of cancer beyond pain relief. This also provides a further link between host–pathogen interactions in infectious disease and a role for this in promoting the development of cancer, including the importance of the tissue environment. The gut is also unique in that it hosts a number of colonising organisms that make up the microbiome (see Chapter 16). This is a really important ecosystem that supports health of the host and normal immune function. The role of microbiome in cancer and in response to treatment is an intense area of research in human medicine and has the potential to offer new insights into cancer initiation and treatment in cats.[5] Many bacterial organisms have been identified as tumour promoting in mouse models of cancer, and dysbiosis of the oral microbiome has been associated with numerous human oral cancers, offering the potential as biomarkers of disease or opportunities for therapeutic intervention.[5–7]

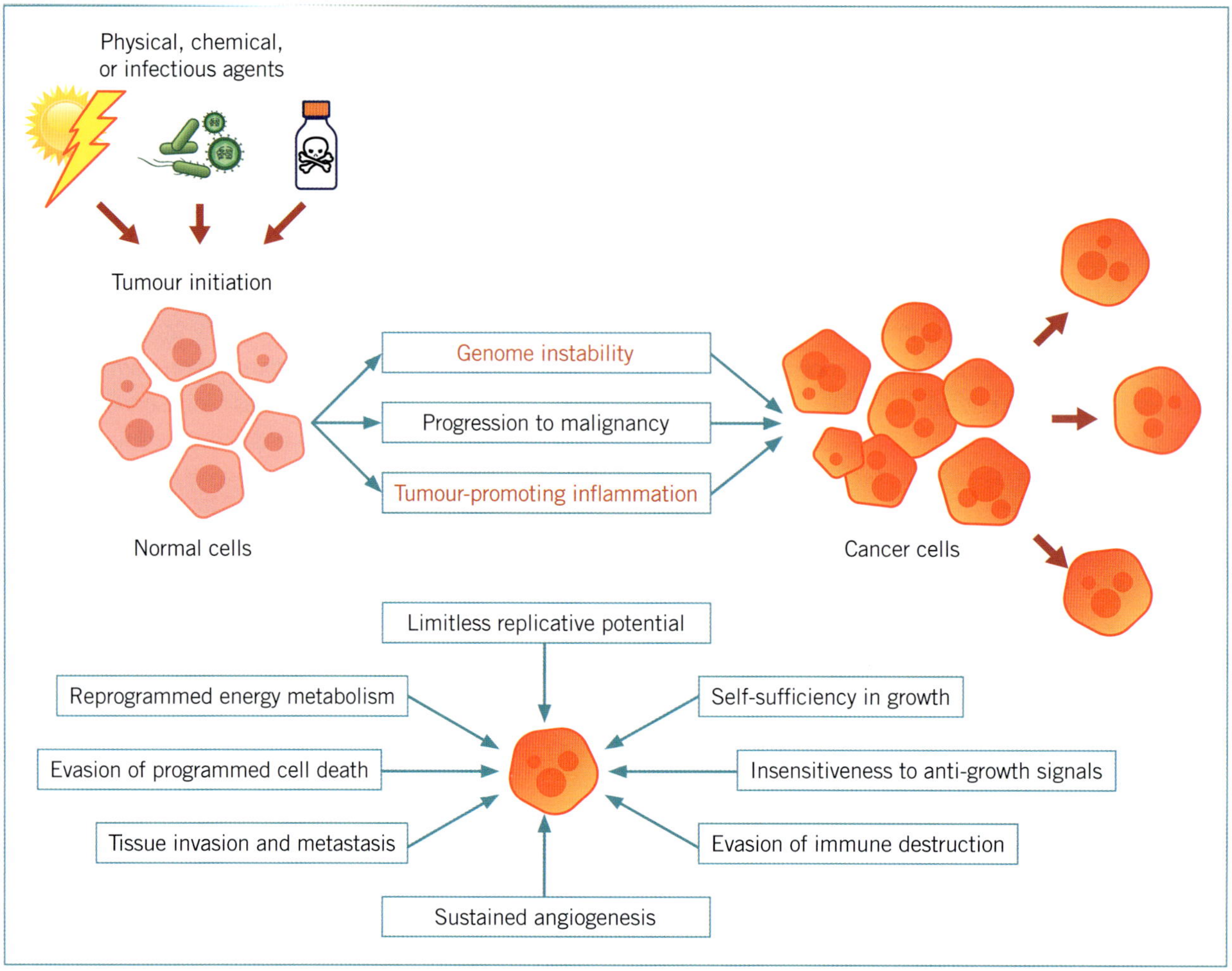

Figure 21.1. Schematic of cancer generation in cats. The effect of causal agents leads to tumour-promoting inflammation and an environment that propagates genomic instability. The acquisition of the core cancer traits leads to the generation of a cancer that is capable of invasion and metastasis.

GENERAL CLINICAL FEATURES AND CLINICAL APPROACH

The specific clinical features associated with each region of the GI tract are given below. However, in general, the clinical features reflect the relative position of the tumour in the GI tract. For example, tumours of the oesophagus classically present with regurgitation, whereas vomiting and/or diarrhoea are often associated with malignancies in more distal locations. In many instances, clinical signs can actually be incredibly vague, with weight loss, lethargy, and inappetence being common features. The sedentary lifestyle of cats and how they respond to disease also means that GI malignancies are often clinically detected at a very advanced stage of disease. As with all oncology cases, a logical approach to diagnosis and staging is followed. The aim of the diagnosis is to define the nature of the disease and its extent (i.e. local invasion and whether there is any metastatic disease to lymph nodes or distant organs). This is referred to as staging, which gives the clinician a baseline record of the disease and helps to define treatment options and prognosis. The standard approach is highlighted in Box 21.1 and Figure 21.2.

Box 21.1. Diagnostic workup and staging of gastrointestinal malignancies in cats.

Thorough clinical history (including diet, weight changes, and general health)

Clinical examination

Laboratory assessment

Changes in haematology parameters may include indicators of blood loss from the GI tract (e.g. microcytic, hypochromic anaemia), Heinz body anaemia can be an indicator of chronic intestinal obstruction in cats, and increases in blood urea levels can be an indicator of GI bleeding. Comprehensive laboratory screening will also provide a general health screen for organ systems in middle-aged to older cats. The author would also include FeLV and FIV screening.

Diagnostic imaging

Plain radiography is rarely of value in the principle diagnosis of GI malignancies and would normally require additional contrast studies (e.g. barium sulphate contrast passage assessments). These have largely been superseded by ultrasonographic assessment of potential primary lesions and lymph nodes or by three-dimensional imaging (e.g. CT scanning), where available. In addition, endoscopy is an invaluable tool in both visualisation of lesions of the mucosa and for biopsy retrieval.

Biopsy

This is the mainstay of tumour diagnosis. In the author's experience, percutaneous FNA samples of GI lesions suspected of being tumours are challenging to interpret and are rarely of value. Endoscopically retrieved specimens or full-thickness biopsy material retrieved surgically give far more reliable results. Significant care needs to be afforded for full-thickness biopsies due to the risk of perforation and release of gut material into body cavities.

Assessment of lymph nodes and metastatic disease

In evaluation of any distant spread, lymph node evaluation is best performed using either ultrasound or CT scanning. Cytological assessment of suspect nodes can be achieved with FNA. Evaluation of distant spread of any tumour can be achieved using three-view thoracic plain radiography (right and left lateral and dorsoventral views), abdominal ultrasound, and/or CT scanning.

Summary

Biopsy, coupled with evaluation of any local or distant spread, allows evaluation of the primary tumour (T), the local lymph nodes (L), and distant metastases (M). Staging can then be concluded, and specific values can be assigned to these three tumour compartments (TNM system), allowing the clinician to select the most appropriate therapeutic route and to be able to give a prognosis.

CT, computed tomography; FeLV, feline leukaemia virus; FIV, feline immunodeficiency virus; FNA, fine needle aspiration; GI, gastrointestinal.

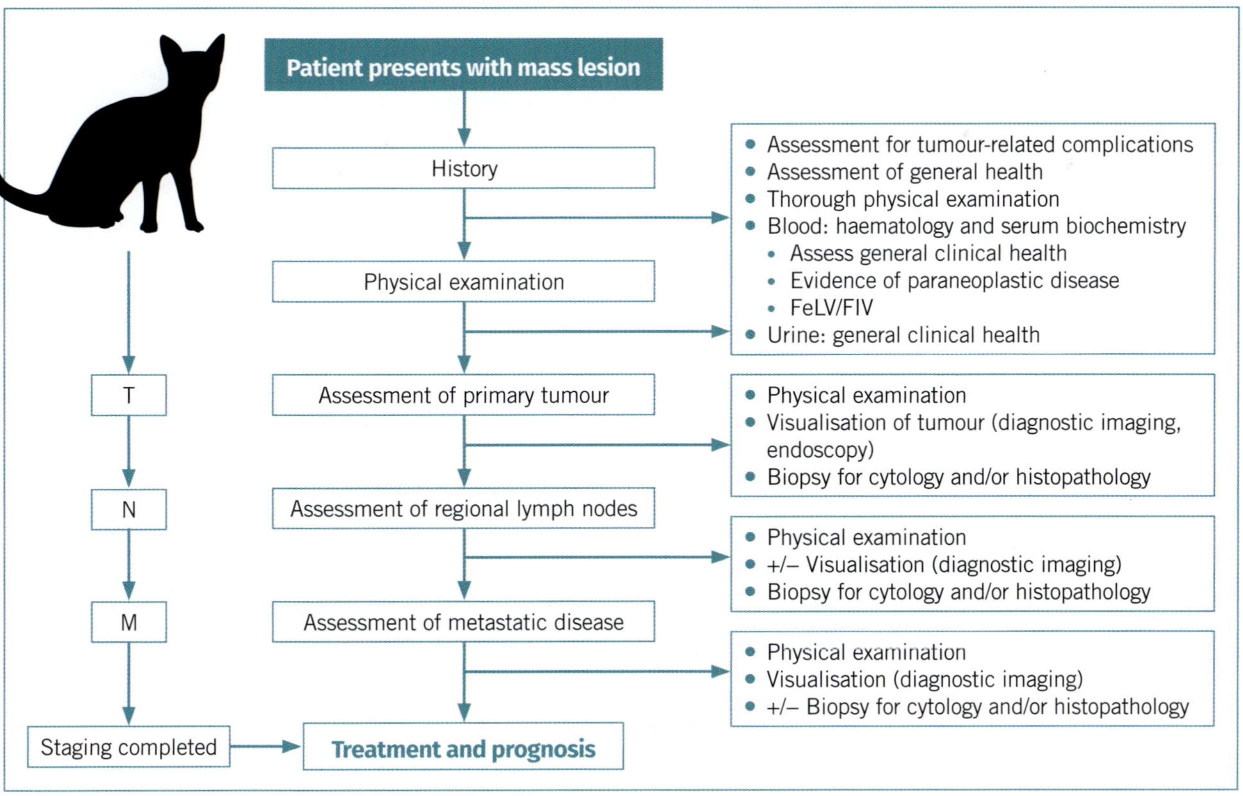

Figure 21.2. Flow chart showing the stages in cancer staging that allows veterinary clinicians to determine the prognosis and most appropriate treatment options. FeLV, feline leukaemia virus; FIV, feline immunodeficiency virus.

Treatment options

Surgery is the mainstay of managing nonlymphomatous GI malignancies in cats. Beyond surgery, there is a paucity of other appropriate treatment modalities for the treatment of nonlymphomatous GI tumours in cats. The feline species is underresearched, and there is a lack of large-scale data sets that would allow for evaluation of classical or experimental therapies. Sadly, most reports in the literature are either anecdotal or represent only very small numbers of studies with limited patient numbers.

Broadly speaking, cancer treatment modalities include:
- surgery (usually used for managing primary tumours)
- radiotherapy (usually confined to the management of primary tumours)
- chemotherapy (usually confined to managing disseminated disease).

Radiotherapy for GI malignancies is not well researched in veterinary medicine and has many limitations due to the potential side effects on highly sensitive normal GI structures. Equally, the value of chemotherapy is poorly explored in veterinary GI oncology (beyond lymphoma), with only anecdotal reports in the literature. The exception to this is the adjunctive radiation and/or chemotherapeutic regimes sometimes used for oral tumours in cats described specifically below. More recently, small-molecule inhibitors, such as the tyrosine kinase (TK) inhibitors, have gained some prominence in the veterinary oncology literature. The obvious target in GI oncology would be GI stromal tumours, which are rare tumours thought to arise from the cells of Cajal and are CD117 positive (which is a target for some TK inhibitors). Their use in these tumours has been anecdotal and without large-scale success. Facts that have to be taken into account when considering treatment options for cats with nonlymphomatous GI tract neoplasms are summarised in Box 21.2.

Box 21.2. Considerations when defining treatment options for cancer in cats.

- Is the clinical challenge one of managing primary disease or secondary disease, or both?
- Surgery and radiotherapy are the main modalities for treating primary disease, but chemotherapy is largely used for managing secondary disease.
- Surgery is the most important treatment modality for gastrointestinal malignancies of nonlymphomatous origin in cats.
- Chemotherapy for cats with such tumours is poorly described and with little evidence that there are positive therapeutic benefits.
- Small-molecule inhibitors may have a role in limited tumour types, such as those which are $CD177^{+}$. However, clinical evidence is limited.
- Radiotherapy is poorly described in such tumours but may have a palliative role in the management of oral tumours.

SPECIFIC TUMOUR TYPES

Oral tumours

Oral cancer in cats is not uncommon (around 3% of all tumours) and is dominated by two major cancer types, squamous cell carcinoma (SCC) and fibrosarcoma, the former being the most common diagnosis (70% of all oral tumours vs. 20% for fibrosarcoma).[16] Other tumour types are recognised (e.g. melanoma, osteosarcoma) but are much rarer. SCC and fibrosarcoma represent a significant therapeutic dilemma in cats, as both carry a poor prognosis and are far more challenging to manage than equivalent diseases identified in dogs.

Feline oral squamous cell carcinoma

Aetiopathogenesis

Feline oral squamous cell carcinoma (FOSCC) is a disease that is locally aggressive and invasive but slow to metastasise.[8] In dogs, the degree of malignancy is dependent on the site of occurrence of the tumour, with rostral tumours having a more favourable prognosis than more caudal tumours (e.g. tonsillar carcinoma). In cats, this is not the case, and FOSCC tends to carry a poor prognosis irrespective of the site of occurrence (Fig. 21.3). Tonsillar SCC is rare in cats compared to dogs, with the major sites being mandible, maxilla, and sublingual.

Epidemiologically, risk factors for FOSCC in cats have been identified and include flea collars and the feeding of wet diets, specifically canned tuna.[8] The pathological link between these factors and FOSCC is, as yet, to be determined.

Over the past 30 years, there has been increasing interest in the role of viruses in the development of epithelial cancers in cats. However, there appears to be minimal association of papillomavirus with FOSCC, in

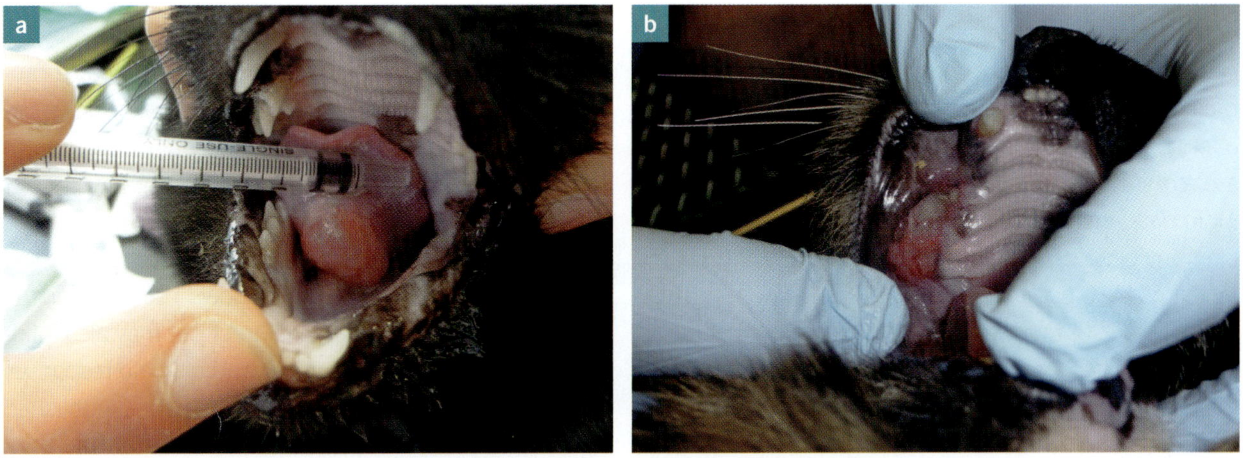

Figure 21.3. Examples of sublingual (a) and maxillary (b) feline oral squamous cell carcinoma.

which there has been no real identification of either virus or the hallmarks of viral-induced malignancy associated with classical papillomavirus infections. In a more recent study, a broader approach to virus discover was taken to try and identify viral association with FOSCC.[9] Even with this more sophisticated approach, no real association with virus infection could be identified, and it was concluded that environmental and genetic causes were more likely. In human oncology, a parallel disease (head and neck squamous cell carcinoma [HNSCC]) can be divided into two basic types which are either virus positive (human papillomavirus) or virus negative. Virus-positive patients have a much better outcome that virus-negative ones, which may be due to immune activation by viral antigens. FOSCC would seem to be more akin to the virus-negative HNSCC.

Despite the poor prognosis of this disease in cats, there are very few research studies addressing the biology and treatment. More focused molecular studies have suggested that an oncogene called epidermal growth factor receptor (EGFR) may have a central role in maintaining the cancer phenotype and may represent a target for therapy.[10] This may be through the direct targeting of this receptor or by potentiating the activity of conventional therapies such as radiotherapy.[10–12]

Diagnosis

Ptyalism, anorexia, oral bleeding, halitosis, and facial asymmetry in an older cat (mean age >12 years) may alert owner and veterinary clinician to the possibility of an oral tumour. The general approach to diagnosis is followed, as in Box 21.1. Biopsy is critical, as there is a need to be able to distinguish this tumour from inflammatory dental lesions, which are common in cats. Although intraoral radiology is possible, the most appropriate imaging technique for oral tumours is computed tomography (CT), as this will give a more accurate analysis of invasion into bone and extent of disease, which in turn will allow a more accurate assessment of prognosis and feasibility of surgical resection. FOSCC rarely spreads beyond the primary site, but assessment of the local mandibular lymph nodes (palpation and fine needle aspiration) and assessment of the thorax (radiography in three views or as part of the CT scanning) completes the diagnostic workup for the purpose of staging.

Treatment and prognosis

FOSCC is locally invasive but slow to metastasise, and the clinical challenge is one of controlling primary disease rather than metastatic disease. The key treatment modalities are therefore considered surgery and/or radiotherapy, which rely on the accurate imaging provided by CT scanning.

The overall prognosis for FOSCC is poor, however, and cats that are untreated or treated by one modality alone (e.g. surgery) have an average survival time of around 3 months, with 1-year survival times being less than 10%.[13] The most promising survival times have been achieved using surgery (when the lesion is in the mandible and more amenable to wide resection) and followed by radiotherapy. This requires referral to a specialist and still, based on limited cases series, offers only survival times of around 1 year to 14 months. Recent case studies have suggested that accelerated radiation protocols combined with carboplatin chemotherapy may offer some survival advantage, but larger-scale studies are required.[14]

To date, there are no chemotherapy drugs that really offer any benefits in FOSCC. Cyclooxygenase 2 (COX-2) inhibitors have been suggested as a palliative approach to treat FOSCC, but less than 10% of tumours actually express COX-2. Despite this, some studies have shown that the use of NSAIDs, with or without toceranib (a TK inhibitor), had a measurable biological response and resulted in prolonged mean survival times. Although complete and partial responses were rare, around 50% of cats in this study achieved stable disease. However, these studies were not prospective and involved small numbers of cases, hence results should be treated with caution until large-scale prospective studies are available.[15] As stated above, the identification of EGFR as a major oncogenic driver may offer a new therapeutic avenue using targeted drugs or antibodies, but the ultimate development of resistance is still a clinical barrier to cure. The use of oncogenic targeting as a sensitising treatment for radiation is an exciting possibility that should be explored in the future. In all cases, pain medication and nutritional support are essential and should be a major part of therapeutic planning.

Oral fibrosarcoma

Fibrosarcoma represents about 20% of feline oral tumours. Like SCC, it is a disease that is locally invasive but rarely metastasises (lung metastasis is recognised in a small proportion of cases), making the goal of treatment the control of primary disease. It is a disease that predominantly affects the gingiva and causes invasion into the underlying bone. The approach and staging assessments are identical to those of SCC and allow the clinician to determine the extent of primary disease and the feasibility of surgical resection. Resection of oral fibrosarcomas with adequate margins is a major challenge in cats but carries a better (although still only fair) prognosis compared to FOSCC. Prognosis will depend on the accessibility of the tumour to a good surgical resection with adequate margins. Combination with postoperative radiotherapy may improve this for easily accessible tumours.

The oral microbiome and cancer

The normal microbial flora in the oral cavity has a profound effect on the host in terms of promoting a healthy oral cavity and normal immune function. Little is known about the oral microbiome in cats with cancer and its effect on tumour initiation or tumour outcomes. There is now a clear link between periodontal disease in people and the development of oral cancer. The microbiome influences the health of the GI tract but may also influence the progression of cancer and ultimate responses to treatment on several levels (Fig. 21.4). A published meta-analysis indicates that periodontal bacterial infections (e.g. caused by *Porphyromonas gingivalis*) increased the incidence of oral cancer and also reduced overall survival. Understanding this bacterial ecosystem may help to develop new approaches to treatment or even prevention.[5–7]

Oesophageal tumours

Tumours of the oesophagus are incredibly rare in cats, with limited reports in the literature. As expected, the ones that have been described are SCCs arising from the oesophageal squamous epithelia. Other primary mesenchymal tumours are similarly rare, but metastasis of non-GI malignancies has been described. Primary oesophageal cancer has been described as occurring in middle-aged to older cats and mainly affecting the distal oesophagus. Clinical features include regurgitation, weight loss, lethargy, and dullness. Surgery would be the treatment of choice, although this represents major challenges and risks. Usually, by the time this disease is diagnosed (using a combination of radiography and endoscopy/endoscopic biopsy), the window of surgical opportunity has closed. Downstaging (i.e. shrinking the tumour to a size more amenable to surgery) using chemotherapy, prior to surgery, is a technique used in human medicine but has not been used in the feline species. It is likely that side effects of chemotherapy, in this instance, would far outweigh the clinical benefit of performing this. In humans, Barrett's oesophagus is a premalignant lesion that is identified as a precursor to oesophageal cancer but has not been identified in cats.

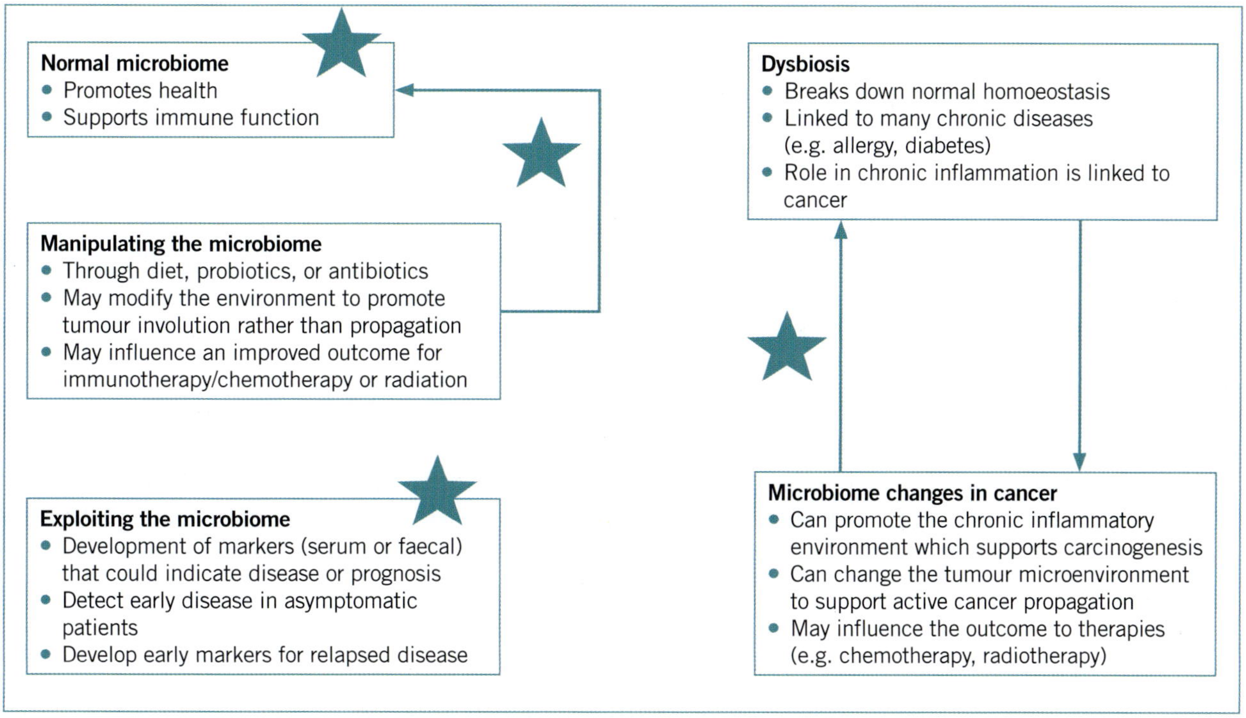

Figure 21.4. Aspects around the connection between cancer development and the microbiome. The stars indicate where the microbiome can be harnessed for diagnostic and therapeutic purposes.

Gastric tumours

Gastric cancer is rare in cats, and the most commonly diagnosed form is lymphoma (see Chapter 20). Beyond lymphoma, the most common gastric malignancy is gastric adenocarcinoma. Benign smooth muscle tumours (leiomyoma) have been reported in the literature but are rare. Although it is often quoted that vomiting is a prominent clinical feature of gastric cancer, it is the author's experience that this disease often follows an insidious course of general lethargy and malaise with inappetence and weight loss. Bleeding into the gastric mucosa can lead to blood loss and iron-deficiency anaemia (hypochromic and microcytic), coupled with anaemia of chronic disease, and can lead the patient to be quite debilitated.

Diagnosis of gastric cancer is usually by endoscopy and mucosal pinch biopsy (or surgical exploration and biopsy). In the majority of cases, lesions have become extensive by the time the diagnosis is achieved. In addition, extension into the mesentery and lymph nodes may have occurred. If any treatment is to be attempted, accurate and extensive staging needs to be performed as described above.

Gastric adenocarcinoma in human patients carries a grave prognosis, with only a 5% survival at 5 years irrespective of treatment.[16] Although adjuvant chemotherapy protocols have been described in human oncology, the therapeutic long-term benefit has not been realised. Studies in cats are limited to anecdotal reports, but in the vast majority of cases, the stage of disease precludes any definitive treatment beyond palliation. In rare cases, if lesions are small, surgical excision could be attempted, but this should be performed by a specialist surgeon and the potential side effects and complications of extensive gastric surgery should be fully explained to the owners. The value of any adjuvant chemotherapy has not been explored, aside from anecdotes in feline oncology. Small benign tumours or polyps may be cured with surgery, but the prognosis of patients with even small adenocarcinomas would have to be considered poor.

Rare cases of GI stromal tumours have been described in cats, and theoretically these may have sensitivity to TK inhibitors based upon their expression of CD117.[17] However, research on TK inhibitors is very limited, and there is little experience with these drugs in feline GI oncology.

A role of *Helicobacter*

Species of *Helicobacter* have been intensely studied in human gastric and intestinal oncology for nearly three decades since the revolutionary work that was carried out directly linking this infection to the development of malignancy.[16] *H. pylori* can alter the levels of reactive nitrogen and oxygen species, promoting conditions which are tumorigenic in people. In human medicine, this has led to the use of antibiotics to prevent or manage GI *H. pylori* colonisation. *Helicobacter*-like organisms have also gained attention in canine and feline GI oncology, and some work has identified colonisation in some cancer-associated lesions.[18] At present, these studies are still quite limited and there is no causal link between their colonisation and the development of GI cancer in cats. A recent study did suggest that *Helicobacter* spp. may be involved in large intestinal carcinoma development in cats. However, this study was limited to 55 cases, and the presence of these bacteria may still only reflect normal commensal colonisation.[18]

Intestinal tumours

Intestinal tumours in cats are also predominantly lymphoma. Beyond lymphoma, adenocarcinomas followed by mast cell tumours (MCTs) dominate, but all of these should also be considered uncommon in the grand scheme of feline oncology. Occurring mainly in older cats, with no sex predilection, epidemiology suggests that Siamese breeds may have an increased susceptibility to developing intestinal tumours, although these studies are limited by numbers.

Intestinal adenocarcinoma

Clinical features

The clinical features of intestinal tumours are reflective of the site of occurrence. Adenocarcinoma is more likely to occur in the small intestine rather than the large intestine in cats, and proximal lesions are more likely to be associated with vomiting. Anorexia and weight loss are common clinical features, and any clinical presentation in cats suggesting small bowel disease should be investigated.

Diagnosis

The basic diagnostic workup described above is relevant to intestinal tumours as well. In terms of imaging, it is the author's experience that abdominal ultrasound offers a good opportunity to assess the nature and extent of disease and the status of the regional lymph nodes. Percutaneous and ultrasound-guided fine needle aspiration samples can yield a positive diagnosis, but sometimes this may require exploratory laparotomy. Intestinal adenocarcinoma can invade locally, affect local mesenteric lymph nodes, and metastasise to the liver and spleen. Equally, there is a possibility of developing transcoelomic spread and widespread carcinomatosis. In these cases, ascites may be present.

Treatment and prognosis

For cats with small intestinal adenocarcinoma with no evidence of metastasis, surgical resection is the treatment of choice. There appears to be significant perioperative risk of dying (sepsis, wound breakdown, and peritonitis) in comparison to dogs. However, if cats live beyond 2 weeks after surgery, there are reports of mean survival times of up to around 15 months.[19] For cats with large intestinal tumours, the best opportunity for longer-term control is a subtotal colectomy followed by adjuvant doxorubicin chemotherapy (around 9 months mean survival time). With surgery alone, survival is around 4–5 months.[20]

Intestinal mast cell disease

As the third most common intestinal tumour in cats, MCT is largely a disease of older cats, with no sex predilection. Most cats will present with a history of vomiting, diarrhoea, anorexia, and a palpable abdominal mass. Diagnosis is achieved as above and can usually be confirmed by percutaneous fine needle aspiration of the intestine. If the cat has a peritoneal effusion, there may be mast cells present, but peripheral mastocytosis is not a feature (unlike splenic MCT in cats).[21,22] This disease has high metastatic potential, and the prognosis is often dictated by histological appearance and the mitotic index.[21] The treatment of choice is surgery with wide surgical margins (>5 cm). Cats with poorly differentiated tumours and a mitotic index greater than 2 have a poor prognosis (mean survival time <6 months), but there have been reports of cases which have a lower mitotic index and treated with surgery and/or TK inhibitors (+/– corticosteroids) having survival times out to 18 months.[21] Sclerosing MCT is a recently described variant which is highly metastatic and carries a grave prognosis.[22]

CONCLUSIONS AND FUTURE DEVELOPMENTS

The field of feline oncology has not changed dramatically in the past 30 years. However, it was previously dominated by lymphoma and leukaemia because of FeLV infections. The fall in lymphoma cases has made more prominent other cancer types in cats, especially SCC. Veterinary oncologists have been limited previously by the lack of effective chemotherapy drugs and a limited evidence base specific to cats. However, there is a cause for optimism as we move forward into twenty-first-century feline oncology:

- Our ability for large-scale genetic studies in cats and in cancers offers greater insight to understand the disease, susceptibility, and the development of new therapies.
- The ability to increase large cohort studies and to integrate and interrogate large data sets means that drug discovery and opportunities for prevention may become much easier. Equally, as the cost of these technologies falls, it may become possible to take a precision medicine approach to feline oncology to improve outcomes for individual patients.
- Hopefully, this research also allows the development and identification of early biomarkers of disease so that treatments can be initiated at an early stage or recurrence of disease can be recognised earlier.
- The cost of producing drugs and antibodies is falling, and this will contribute to better outcomes in cats.
- Veterinary clinicians have to stop thinking that cats are small dogs, and treat them as a separate species when considering new and evolving therapies.

Despite the fact that the field is hampered by a lack of research funding and by an unwillingness of drug companies to invest in feline-specific therapeutics, with the advent of large data sets and more economical ways of developing and producing drugs, there should be optimism that this could also change.

Take-home messages

- Cancer is a genetic disease: there are major changes to the normal DNA in cells. This is passed to daughter cells during cell division and leads to a breakdown of cellular homoeostasis.
- There is strong evidence that cancer is a stem cell disease in which cancer stem cells maintain the cancer phenotype and contribute to the resistance to therapy.
- It is likely that some cats may have inherited genetic susceptibility to some cancer types, but this needs further research.
- Genetic instability and inflammation are the common denominators underpinning the cancer phenotype.
- Infectious, physical, and chemical agents can contribute to cancer initiation and promotion. Equally, the microbiome may play a major role in the gastrointestinal tract in cats in terms of initiation and promotion of cancer and response to treatments. However, research in this area is still lacking in this species.
- Nonlymphomatous gastrointestinal tract tumours are dominated by oral tumours, squamous cell carcinoma, and fibrosarcoma. See Chapter 20 for lymphoma.
- Nonlymphomatous gastric and intestinal tumours are rare in cats.
- Intestinal mast cell tumours occur in cats and carry a poor prognosis.

REFERENCES

[1] Argyle DJ, Blacking T. From viruses to cancer stem cells: dissecting the pathways to malignancy. *Vet J* 177:311, 2008.

[2] Raposo TP et al. Inflammation and cancer: till death tears them apart. *Vet J* 205:161, 2015.

[3] Munday JS, Sharp CR, Beatty JA. Novel viruses: update on the significance of papillomavirus infections in cats. *J Feline Med Surg* 21:409, 2019.

[4] Hanahan D, Weinberg RA. Hallmarks of cancer: the next generation. *Cell* 144:646, 2011.

[5] Lyu Y et al. Past, present, and future of gastrointestinal microbiota research in cats. *Front Microbiol* 11:1661, 2020.

[6] Irfan M, Delgado RZR, Frias-Lopez J. The oral microbiome and cancer. *Front Immunol* 11:591088, 2020.

[7] Corbella S et al. Is periodontitis a risk indicator for cancer? A meta-analysis. *PLoS One* 13:e0195683, 2018.

[8] Bilgic O et al. Feline oral squamous cell carcinoma: clinical manifestations and literature review. *J Vet Dent* 32:30, 2015.

[9] Chu S et al. A virome sequencing approach to feline oral squamous cell carcinoma to evaluate viral causative factors. *Vet Microbiol* 240:108491, 2020.

[10] Bergkvist GT et al. Expression of epidermal growth factor receptor (EGFR) and Ki67 in feline oral squamous cell carcinomas (FOSCC). *Vet Comp Oncol* 9:106, 2011.

[11] Bergkvist GT et al. Studies on the inhibition of feline EGFR in squamous cell carcinoma: enhancement of radiosensitivity and rescue of resistance to small molecule inhibitors. *Cancer Biol Ther* 11:927, 2011.

[12] Gray ME et al. Dual targeting of EGFR and ERBB2 pathways produces a synergistic effect on cancer cell proliferation and migration in vitro. *Vet Comp Oncol* 15:890, 2017.

[13] Northrup NC et al. Outcomes of cats with oral tumors treated with mandibulectomy: 42 cases. *J Am Anim Hosp Assoc* 42:350, 2006.

[14] Fidel JL et al. A nine-day accelerated radiation protocol for feline squamous cell carcinoma. *Vet Radiol Ultrasound* 48:482, 2007.

[15] Olmsted GA et al. Tolerability of toceranib phosphate (Palladia) when used in conjunction with other therapies in 35 cats with feline oral squamous cell carcinoma: 2009–2013. *J Feline Med Surg* 19:568, 2017.

[16] Kim J, Wang TC. *Helicobacter pylori* and gastric cancer. *Gastrointest Endosc Clin N Am* 31:451, 2021.

[17] McGregor O, Moore AS, Yeomans S. Management of a feline gastric stromal cell tumour with toceranib phosphate: a case study. *Aust Vet J* 98:181, 2020.

[18] Swennes AG et al. Enterohepatic *Helicobacter* spp. in cats with non-haematopoietic intestinal carcinoma: a survey of 55 cases. *J Med Microbiol* 65:814, 2016.

[19] Cribb AE. Feline gastrointestinal adenocarcinoma: a review and retrospective study. *Can Vet J* 29:709, 1988.

[20] Slawienski MJ et al. Malignant colonic neoplasia in cats: 46 cases (1990–1996). *J Am Vet Med Assoc* 211:878, 1997.

[21] Barrett LE et al. Outcome following treatment of feline gastrointestinal mast cell tumours. *Vet Comp Oncol* 16:188, 2018.

[22] Halsey CH, Powers BE, Kamstock DA. Feline intestinal sclerosing mast cell tumour: 50 cases (1997–2008). *Vet Comp Oncol* 8:72, 2010.

CHAPTER **22**

Dysmotility of the upper gastrointestinal tract

Conor O'Halloran, Danièlle Gunn-Moore

Disorders of upper gastrointestinal (GI) motility include those affecting the oesophagus, stomach, and small intestine. These areas can be affected individually or as part of a generalised motility disorder. The overall prevalence of these disorders is largely unknown, as there is a lack of data to accurately estimate their rate of occurrence.

The focus of this chapter is on nonobstructive upper GI motility disorders, as these are generally harder to diagnose than obstructive disorders and the clinical signs may be subtle unless pathology is severe (Table 22.1). Obstructive disorders of the upper GI tract include foreign bodies, strictures (see Chapter 11), stenoses (e.g. pyloric; see Chapter 12), and luminal neoplasia (see Chapters 20 and 21). These are thought to be quite common conditions and relatively straightforward to diagnose with imaging (see Chapters 5–8).

OESOPHAGEAL HYPOMOTILITY

After the upper oesophageal sphincter, the feline oesophagus is comprised of two spirally arranged muscularis layers that wind in opposite directions. The muscles consist of striated muscle fibres in the proximal third (cervical segment) and then transition into smooth muscle distal to this (the thoracic segment). A thickening of the muscle occurs at the gastrooesophageal junction that functions as the lower oesophageal sphincter. Motility is regulated by neurons originating in the nucleus ambiguous of the brainstem, and sensory innervation of the oesophagus arises via neurons from the solitary tract nucleus in the medulla oblongata; both nuclei are linked together by a web of interneurons. The vagus nerve and its branches connect the muscular layers of the oesophagus to the higher brain centres. Pathology along any part of these pathways can result in dysmotility of the oesophagus, which is seen clinically almost exclusively as hypomotility, and gives rise to the clinical signs of oesophageal disease.

Oesophageal motility in the cat is far weaker than in the dog, with 100% of tablets and 83% of capsules given by dry swallow failing to reach the stomach within a minute. With time, tablets will pass slowly to the stomach; however, capsules become stuck, dissolving in situ.[1]

Administering tablets in a "pill delivery treat" fails to reduce the average transit time from ≈60 seconds, while the use of a flavoured liquid flush reduces the average transit times of a tablet and a capsule to 36 and 16 seconds, respectively. This slow oesophageal motility predisposes to iatrogenic tablet- and capsule-associated oesophagitis and secondary stricture formation; it also predisposes to the retention of oesophageal foreign bodies and possibly to general anaesthesia–associated gastric reflux.

Epidemiology and aetiology

In general, nonobstructive oesophageal motility diseases are thought to be rare in cats. Studies produced by referral hospitals and specialist veterinary centres report prevalence rates of 0.05%–1% within their admitted hospital

Table 22.1. Differential diagnoses for nonobstructive causes of upper gastrointestinal tract dysmotility.

Section of the upper gastrointestinal tract	Differential diagnoses
Oesophagus (see also Chapter 11): hypomotility and/or megaoesophagus	Idiopathic functional hypomotility and/or megaoesophagus* Primary functional dysmotility (e.g. in Siamese and Bengal cats)* Oesophagitis (e.g. iatrogenic caused by acidic medication; associated with chronic vomiting, oesophageal foreign body, or rare congenital defects such as gastric heterotopia) Toxicity causing megaoesophagus (e.g. lead poisoning, botulism) Congenital defect (e.g. vascular ring anomaly) Type 1 (sliding) hiatal hernia Feline dysautonomia Myasthenia gravis +/– thymoma Toxoplasmosis Systemic inflammation
Stomach: delayed gastric emptying	Primary functional disorder (e.g. primary functional dysmotility is often associated with functional pyloric outflow tract obstruction typically in Siamese and Bengal cats)* Exaggerated interdigestive hypomotility (leading to hairball formation) Foreign body Subsequent to gastrotomy or other abdominal surgical procedures Acute or chronic infectious gastritis (e.g. due to *Helicobacter* infection) Secondary to abdominal effusion (e.g. cardiogenic ascites, effusive or wet FIP). Secondary to IBD (see Chapters 17 and 18) Secondary to alimentary lymphoma, usually of the small intestine (see Chapter 20) Feline dysautonomia Extragastric/systemic inflammation (e.g. pancreatitis, chronic kidney disease, hyperthyroidism, diabetes mellitus)
Small intestine: hypomotility, atony or ileus of the small intestine, hypermotility (mostly due to infectious causes), or a combination (oral and aboral movement of a foreign body)	Chronic enteritis of any cause including inflammatory (e.g. IBD) or infectious (e.g. salmonellosis) Parasitosis (e.g. nematodes such as *Ollanulus tricuspis*; see Chapter 15) Reactive ileus following abdominal surgery Foreign body Granuloma (e.g. infections such as mycobacteriosis) Neoplasia (e.g. lymphoma, adenocarcinoma, mast cell neoplasia of the small intestine; see Chapters 20 and 21) Sclerosis (e.g. FGESF; see Chapter 19) Radiation-induced enteropathy Feline dysautonomia Secondary to peritoneal disease (e.g. septic peritonitis, FIP, neoplasia such as carcinomatosis) Local or systemic inflammation (e.g. pancreatitis; see Chapter 24)

FGESF, feline gastrointestinal eosinophilic sclerosing fibroplasia; FIP, feline infectious peritonitis; IBD, inflammatory bowel disease.
*It is unclear whether primary functional dysmotility, for example in Oriental and Bengal cats, is a separate condition or a subgroup of idiopathic functional hypomotility and/or megaoesophagus.

populations;[2] however, it is unknown how this translates back into the feline population at large, as only the most severe cases are likely to be referred.

History and physical examination findings

The major clinical signs of oesophageal dysmotility include regurgitation, dysphagia, odynophagia (pain when swallowing), hypersalivation, hyporexia, and weight loss. Vomiting may be seen following regurgitation if the presence of regurgitated material in the pharynx triggers the vomiting reflex. Respiratory signs may occur secondary to gastrooesophageal reflux, which in severe cases can result in aspiration pneumonia.

Diagnostic investigation

The underlying cause of oesophageal hypomotility can be hard to establish, and many cases are classed as idiopathic. Primary diagnoses may include focal dysmotility of the oesophagus, such as megaoesophagus and type 1 (sliding) hiatal hernias, or generalised motility disorders such as feline dysautonomia. Oesophageal dysmotility can also occur secondary to oesophagitis (e.g. associated with an oesophageal foreign body—or following its removal), be associated with chronic vomiting or rare congenital defects (e.g. gastric heterotopia), or, perhaps most commonly, occur following the administration of acidic medications like doxycycline hyclate, clindamycin, nonsteroidal anti-inflammatory drugs, alendronate, or methotrexate. Oesophageal dysmotility and/or megaoesophagus can also be associated with toxicity, such as lead poisoning or botulism, or with severe systemic inflammatory responses (e.g. anaphylaxis).

Diagnostic tests that are useful in the identification of oesophageal dysmotility include survey radiographs of the length of the oesophagus and contrast studies. These should, ideally, be dynamic fluoroscopic feeding studies, which remain the gold standard for the assessment of oesophageal motility (see Chapters 5 and 11).

Before undertaking these studies, it is imperative to consider the risks vs. benefits of the procedure. Importantly, many underlying motility issues that these studies would aim to diagnose place the patients at risk of regurgitation and iatrogenic aspiration pneumonia. Aspiration of barium can be particularly damaging to the lungs, as macrophages are unable to remove it, even after extended periods.

Endoscopy can be used to visualise obstructive disease or oesophagitis. Abdominal ultrasonography can be useful for confirming sliding hiatal hernias, especially when forward pressure is applied to the abdominal contents while holding the ultrasound probe to image the lower oesophageal area.

Management and treatment

Some causes of oesophageal dysmotility can be avoided entirely by using nonirritant formulations of medications (e.g. doxycycline monohydrate rather than doxycycline hyclate—a grilled chicken–flavoured paste that also appears significantly more palatable has recently been marketed in the United Kingdom) or by using increasingly available liquid or paste formulations of medicines instead of tablets or capsules (e.g. liquid meloxicam).[2,3]

The best treatment for oesophagitis is prevention, avoiding known risky medications whenever possible and mitigating when not (e.g. by crushing tablets). Once established, oesophagitis is treated by giving sucralfate liquid; however, this is difficult to administer to cats.

Since oesophagitis is painful, appropriate analgesia needs to be considered. Oral nonsteroidal anti-inflammatory medications should be discontinued, especially if they were part of the inciting cause, and alternative analgesia should be introduced (e.g. sublingual buprenorphine).

Although it may initially seem that feeding cats with oesophagitis a soft or liquid diet might be more comfortable, these cats need to be fed solid food to prevent oesophageal stricture formation.

Once oesophageal hypomotility has been demonstrated, obstruction has been excluded, and oesophagitis either treated or excluded on oesophagoscopy, there is no single straightforward treatment option.[2,3] Owners will have to trial different food consistencies which enable adequate nutritional intake (which can be variable amongst patients) and use gravity to help prevent gastric reflux by ensuring that the cat remains upright for a few minutes after eating. While most cats cope best being fed small balls of wet food, occasional cats cope best being fed a slurry. Positional feeding is less easily achieved in cats, compared to dogs, as few cats are willing to sit in a "begging chair". That said, some cats will learn to be fed on steps (Fig. 22.1), or while being held up against one owner so its front feet are on the owner's shoulder while another owner offers the food.

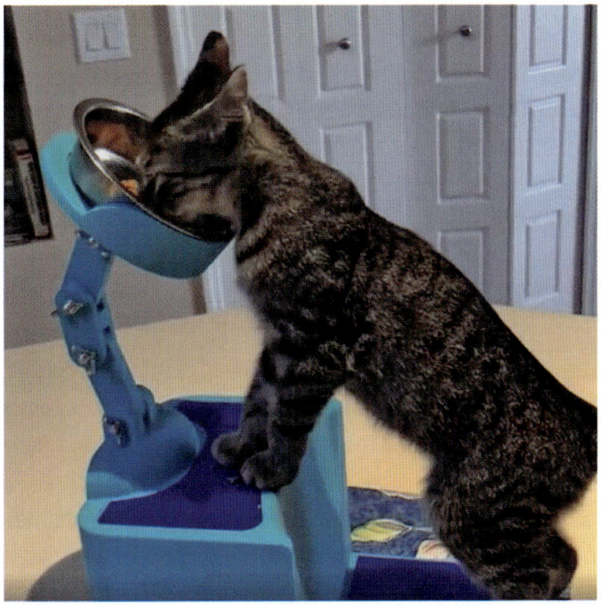

Figure 22.1. Kitten with oesophageal hypomotility being fed from a raised bowl to reduce the risk of regurgitation.

Prokinetic drugs may help in some cases of idiopathic or primary oesophageal dysmotility. Cisapride solution, transdermal cisapride gel, or liquid metoclopramide are available in different countries. They may stimulate oesophageal peristalsis in the distal two-thirds, where smooth muscle is present (i.e. within the thoracic segment). Cisapride is more potent than metoclopramide in cats and is usually the preferred drug.

Since inadequate nutritional intake is common, many of these cats will also need a gastrostomy tube or a percutaneous endoscopic gastrostomy (PEG) tube (see Chapter 40).

Prognosis and outcome

The prognosis is variable depending on the underlying pathology. Many cases are irreversible and require lifelong adapted feeding practices and/or medication.

MEGAOESOPHAGUS

In people, megaoesophagus is most commonly secondary to chronic body-wide inflammation; for example, in Chagas disease, megaoesophagus occurs following the chronic (up to 20 years) inflammatory response to the parasite *Trypanosoma cruzi*. In contrast, megaoesophagus in domestic mammals is far more frequently idiopathic, and no infectious causes have been identified to date in cats.

Epidemiology and aetiology

Megaoesophagus occurs when the oesophagus becomes weak, flaccid, and therefore is not able to propel ingesta adequately from the oropharynx into the stomach. It is a rare condition of cats and most instances are idiopathic cases, many of them occurring congenitally. Siamese and Bengal cats may be more frequently affected than other breeds; alternatively, the condition in these breeds may be a separate subgroup of congenital idiopathic megaoesophagus. The most frequent cause of acquired megaoesophagus in the cat is feline dysautonomia (see below), and other causes, such as myasthenia gravis, occur very infrequently in this species. When myasthenia gravis is present, it is more common in Abyssinian or Somali cats, sometimes associated with concurrent thymoma (the incidence of thymoma in cats with myasthenia gravis is 26%). Rare cases may occur due to toxoplasmosis or chronic lead or organophosphate poisoning.

History and physical examination findings

The main presenting sign of megaoesophagus is regurgitation; however, this may be reported as vomiting by some owners. Occasional cases may present with bilateral nasal discharge or aspiration pneumonia. Cats are frequently cachectic and can have either a ravenous appetite or hyporexia/anorexia. Ptyalism and halitosis may be reported by owners or be present on examination. Affected kittens generally display a markedly reduced growth rate.

Diagnostic investigation

Diagnosis of megaoesophagus is made by survey radiographs of the oesophagus, with static or dynamic contrast studies adding sensitivity (if needed) in cases where they can be performed safely. Care must be taken with contrast studies. It would be usual to perform barium studies assessing the passage of liquid barium and then of barium mixed in food. However, liquid barium carries a significant risk of aspiration pneumonia in these cases and therefore should only be used with great care, if at all. Indeed, if the megaoesophagus is clear on the survey radiograph, contrast studies should not be performed.

Management and treatment

Treatment of acquired cases of megaoesophagus relies on the diagnosis and management of the underlying cause, while congenital cases usually require lifelong management techniques such as feeding from a raised bowl. Since inadequate nutritional intake is common, many of these cases need to have a gastrostomy tube or PEG tube placed.

As with oesophageal hypomotility, prokinetic drugs (cisapride is usually the preferred drug) may help in some cases.

Prognosis and outcome

The long-term prognosis for cats with congenital megaoesophagus is generally considered to be reasonable, providing that successful management techniques can be implemented. GI motility of Siamese and Bengal cats with congenital megaoesophagus and functional pyloric outflow tract obstruction typically improves following Y–V pyloroplasty. For acquired cases of megaoesophagus, the long-term prognosis depends on the severity of the causative disease and on whether or not it can be reversed (e.g. successful management of dysautonomia is challenging and depends on the severity of the case). Megaoesophagus associated with myasthenia gravis will sometimes resolve following initial medical management of the myasthenia gravis (using anticholinesterase medication, such as pyridostigmine, and corticosteroids or other immunosuppressive drugs—immunosuppressive drugs should only be given if really necessary, as they can exacerbate weakness) or, if present, following successful removal of a thymoma.

DELAYED GASTRIC EMPTYING

The control of gastric emptying is regulated by the myenteric plexus and the interstitial cells of Cajal that have a pacemaker function. In healthy animals, the rate of gastric emptying is heavily influenced by the nutrient composition of the meal (protein being the quickest to exit, followed by carbohydrate and then fats), its moisture content (liquid meals progress fastest, followed by wet foods and then dry biscuits), the size of the meal (small meals pass faster than large ones), and even the shape of the biscuits (triangular kibble has been shown to be emptied more slowly than round kibble).[4]

Epidemiology and aetiology

Primary functional gastric motility disorders appear to be rare in cats, apart from the usually low-grade functional delayed gastric emptying that is involved in the formation of hairballs.[5] Cats are unique in completely lacking coordinated interdigestive gastric motility which, in other species, is responsible for the expulsion of indigestible material from the stomach into the small intestine. This deficit is present in all cats and may promote the accumulation of hair within the stomach and prevent its passage into the small intestine, ultimately leading to the retention of fur and the formation of a gastric hairball. Hairballs are most likely to be formed when there is low-grade GI dysfunction that exacerbates the natural functional deficit and/or when overgrooming occurs for a dermatologic or psychological reason, particularly in long-haired cats.

In cats, delayed gastric emptying frequently occurs as a sequela to inflammatory disorders such as intestinal parasitosis (e.g. *Toxascaris leonina, Toxocara cati*), inflammatory bowel disease (IBD), and alimentary lymphoma, as well as in cases of inflammation in other abdominal organs leading to paralytic ileus, most commonly seen with pancreatitis, septic peritonitis, or following intestinal surgery.

History and physical examination findings

No clinical signs are pathognomonic for delayed gastric emptying, nor does it induce any clinical signs of itself but rather may result in clinical signs associated with nausea such as excessive salivation, lip licking, or lip smacking. Affected cats may vomit at excessively long intervals after a meal and may show projectile vomiting if functional gastric obstruction develops. Gas accumulation in the stomach causes some cats to have increased eructation, which is hard for most owners to notice, whereas vomiting, anorexia, hyporexia, and chronic weight loss may be more obvious.

On physical examination, if any findings are present, they may be subtle. Occasionally, distension of the abdomen or discomfort on palpation can be noted.

Diagnostic investigation

In a general practice setting, survey radiographs may show a markedly distended stomach, but they are most often normal even if functional gastric hypomotility is present. Liquid-contrast gastrograms can provide information relating to gastric emptying times. A dose of 12 ml/kg barium suspension (or alternative contrast medium) can be given orally when the stomach is empty, and radiographs are taken at set times after ingestion. In a healthy cat, barium should start to reach the duodenum after 30 minutes and have completely emptied from the stomach 3 hours after ingestion. The main limitation of this technique is that because the contrast is given in liquid form, this may artificially shorten the transit time compared with a cat's normal solid food diet. Since these patients could have oesophageal dysmotility, giving liquid barium carries a significant risk of aspiration. Altered protocols to mix contrast media with food to overcome these problems have been tried, but the technique remains insensitive.

A further improvement has been sought with the use of barium-impregnated polyethylene spheres (BIPS) of graduated diameter sizes; however, studies have shown poor correlation with other techniques, and therefore the clinical utility of BIPS has been questioned.

Similarly, ultrasonography can be used to measure the cross-sectional diameter of the antrum of the stomach and estimate the antral volume.[6] As the stomach empties postprandially, the antrum reduces in size and returns to fasted values.

Research studies use radioactive scintigraphy as the reference standard test for measuring the gastric emptying time of cats. The cat is fed a solid meal containing radiolabelled technetium-99m (^{99m}Tc), and postprandial scans are performed at set intervals to measure the quantity of radioactive material remaining in the stomach. The half-life (the time at which the radiation in the stomach is reduced by 50%) is plotted to give an accurate evaluation of the rate of gastric emptying. Feline evaluation of breath tests indicated that the ^{13}C-sodium acetate breath test can be a valid alternative to ^{99m}Tc radioscintigraphy in healthy cats.[7]

Management and treatment

Primary gastric dysmotility associated with GI dysmotility of Siamese and Bengal cats is usually seen with congenital megaoesophagus and a functional pyloric outflow tract obstruction, and gastric retention and projectile vomiting may improve following Y–V pyloroplasty. Medical interventions are discussed below.

The management of secondary gastric dysmotility and reduced emptying times relies on the identification and successful treatment or stabilisation of the inciting cause. As with primary motility issues, management can take the form of dietary alterations such as feeding liquidised meals or reducing the fat content and calorific density of solid foods (although, notably, these alterations can reduce the palatability for cats). Medical interventions centre on the use of prokinetics including cisapride, metoclopramide, and, occasionally, erythromycin.

Prognosis and outcome

The long-term prognosis for cats affected congenitally with delayed gastric emptying is generally considered to be reasonable, providing that successful medical or surgical management techniques can be implemented. For acquired cases, the long-term prognosis depends on the severity of the causative disease and the response to causative as well as symptomatic treatment.

MOTILITY DISORDERS OF THE SMALL INTESTINE

A small number of intestinal transit disorders have been documented in domestic cats. Vomiting, diarrhoea, hyporexia, and weight loss are the most important clinical signs associated with these conditions.

Enteritis and mechanical and reactive ileus are the most common small intestinal motility problems seen in feline patients. Enteritis (e.g. acute with infections [see Chapter 14], or chronic with IBD) causes a disruption to the phasic peristaltic contractions of the intestine, which usually resolves with the successful treatment or control of the inflammation.

IBD is a common cause of chronic GI tract inflammation. Infiltration of the intestinal wall with inflammatory cells can be used to identify IBD and/or its progression to (small-cell) lymphoma by histopathology. Management of IBD frequently includes the exclusion of parasitosis, monitoring of vitamin B_{12} levels, dietary modification (e.g. hydrolysed diet such as Purina Pro Plan Veterinary Diets HA), and long-term medication, usually corticosteroids such as prednisolone tapered to the lowest effective dose that controls the clinical signs (see Chapter 18).

Many disorders arising from outside the GI tract, often inflammatory and most commonly pancreatitis (see Chapter 24), can also cause paralytic ileus. Current treatment options focus on effective management of the condition rather than cure and include intravenous fluid therapy to ensure adequate hydration, analgesia, antiemetics for cats that are vomiting, and nutritional support including appetite stimulants (e.g. mirtazapine) and in some cases the placement of feeding tubes.

Less common diagnoses include pseudoobstruction (which can occur after surgical manipulation of the intestines), nematode infections such as those caused by *Toxascaris leonina* or *Toxocara cati* (which can be treated with anthelmintic medications such as moxidectin; see Chapter 15), intestinal sclerosis or scaring after surgery or after the passage of a foreign body, feline GI eosinophilic sclerosing fibroplasia (see Chapter 19), and radiation-induced enteritis. The latter is a common side effect of radiation therapy for oncological treatment that occurs in up to 50% of therapy patients. External beam radiation therapy using a linear accelerator to produce ionising radiation in form of photons or charged particles can damage both normal and malignant cells. During G_2 and M phases of mitosis, cells are more vulnerable to radiation, especially rapid-proliferating cells (e.g. cells in the intestinal mucosa). When tissue stem cells are injured, the replacement of normal functional cells is reduced, as in the case of damage to the stem cells of the intestinal crypts, which leads to the reduction of intestinal epithelial cells and, consequently, to loss of integrity of the mucosal barrier. Medical treatment should be the first approach to treat radiation-induced GI clinical signs.

FELINE DYSAUTONOMIA

Feline dysautonomia, previously referred to as Key–Gaskell syndrome, is the term used to describe a syndrome of disease caused by a generalised dysfunction of the autonomic nervous system (ANS) and characterised by neuronal degeneration. Many cases of feline dysautonomia were described during the 1980s and 1990s, mainly in the United Kingdom, after the first description of the condition by Key and Gaskell in 1982 in Scotland.[8,9,10] The incidence rate decreased after large numbers of cases were reported during that initial "outbreak", with far fewer cases reported since then. Although no age or breed predispositions have been identified, review studies show highest case numbers amongst domestic shorthair cats (presumably because of their high overall frequency within the general cat population). The majority of affected animals are young adults, almost exclusively younger than 7 years old at the onset of clinical signs.[8]

Epidemiology and aetiology

Dysautonomia has been reported globally and in a variety of species, including cats. The aetiology remains uncertain, although a possible association with *Clostridium botulinum* (type C/D) neurotoxin has been described in cats. Dysautonomic cats have been reported to be deficient in sulphur-containing amino acids (methionine and cysteine/cystine) despite an adequate dietary intake. It has been hypothesised that this deficiency was due to the consumption of an unidentified and/or completely novel dietary neurotoxic mycotoxin or xenobiotic that resulted in the clinical signs of dysautonomia.

Several "outbreaks" of dysautonomia have been reported, indicating possible contagion, interaction with, and/or ingestion of contaminated food or of an as yet unidentified environmental toxin. To date, most reported feline cases have occurred in the United Kingdom (particularly Scotland), Scandinavia, and midwestern United States of America. However, the significance that this geographical range, and in particular the fairly consistent latitude, may have with respect to aetiology is unknown. Similar regional hotspots in prevalence exist across the United Kingdom in numbers of equine grass sickness cases, which may indicate that these two conditions share a common aetiology.

History and physical examination findings

Because the pathogenesis of this disease lies within the ANS, the clinical signs in cats are associated with its acute loss or chronic decline in function. Commonly reported clinical signs include depression, anorexia or hyporexia, dysphagia, dysuria, regurgitation or vomiting, constipation or occasionally diarrhoea, dilated and unresponsive pupils, third eyelid protrusion, reduced lacrimation, orthostatic hypotension, and sustained bradycardia without sinus arrhythmia (referred to by some authors as a "metronomic heart rate"). Dry nares and mucosae are particularly common. Reduced anal tone has also been described, although less often, likely caused by denervation of the internal anal sphincter, which is autonomically innervated. Non-ANS signs such as ataxia and proprioceptive deficits have also been described. If systemic blood pressure is assessed, it tends to be low-normal for being in a veterinary clinic and, like the heart rate, is described as "metronomic" (i.e. not increasing when the cat is stressed).

A large-scale retrospective review of presenting clinical signs published in 2020 found that nearly all dysautonomic cats and dogs (92%) of the 53 examined displayed hyporexia, while vomiting or regurgitation were the second most frequently noted clinical signs, documented in 85% of the cases.[8]

Diagnostic investigation

Currently, dysautonomia is almost exclusively definitively diagnosed by the postmortem identification of pathognomonic lesions in the ventral horns of the spinal cord, the autonomic ganglia, and/or the brainstem nuclei. A histopathological antemortem diagnosis can sometimes be made on full-thickness intestinal biopsies, although the sensitivity is unknown and it is limited in its practicality, as many of these cats are too ill to be anaesthetised. Histopathological findings in acute cases include neuronal chromatolytic degeneration and nuclear pyknosis, while neuronal loss and proliferation of satellite cells are seen in more chronic cases.

Diagnostic tests that can support an antemortem diagnosis are those that assess ANS functionality (Fig. 22.2). Most commonly used is the Schirmer tear test (STT). In one review, the STT results were found to be abnormal (<15 mm in 60 seconds) in at least one eye in 90% of the cats examined.[8] However, this test is not specific for autonomic dysfunction, and several authors have questioned the accuracy of a 15 mm cutoff for normal tear production in the cat, suggesting that completely healthy cats can have STT values of as low as 9 mm in 60 seconds, or even less.

Since pupil diameter is tightly controlled by the ANS, testing the pupil response to pharmacological agents can give a more specific indication about ANS dysfunction. Pilocarpine is a cholinergic agonist (parasympathomimetic), and a pilocarpine response test has frequently been reported as useful in aiding in this diagnosis. However, it is important to note that there is no standardised test protocol available, and therefore interpretation is based on the subjective decision by the attending clinician. For the pilocarpine response test, a baseline pupil diameter measurement is taken to see if pupil reactivity is possible; this is ideally performed under both light

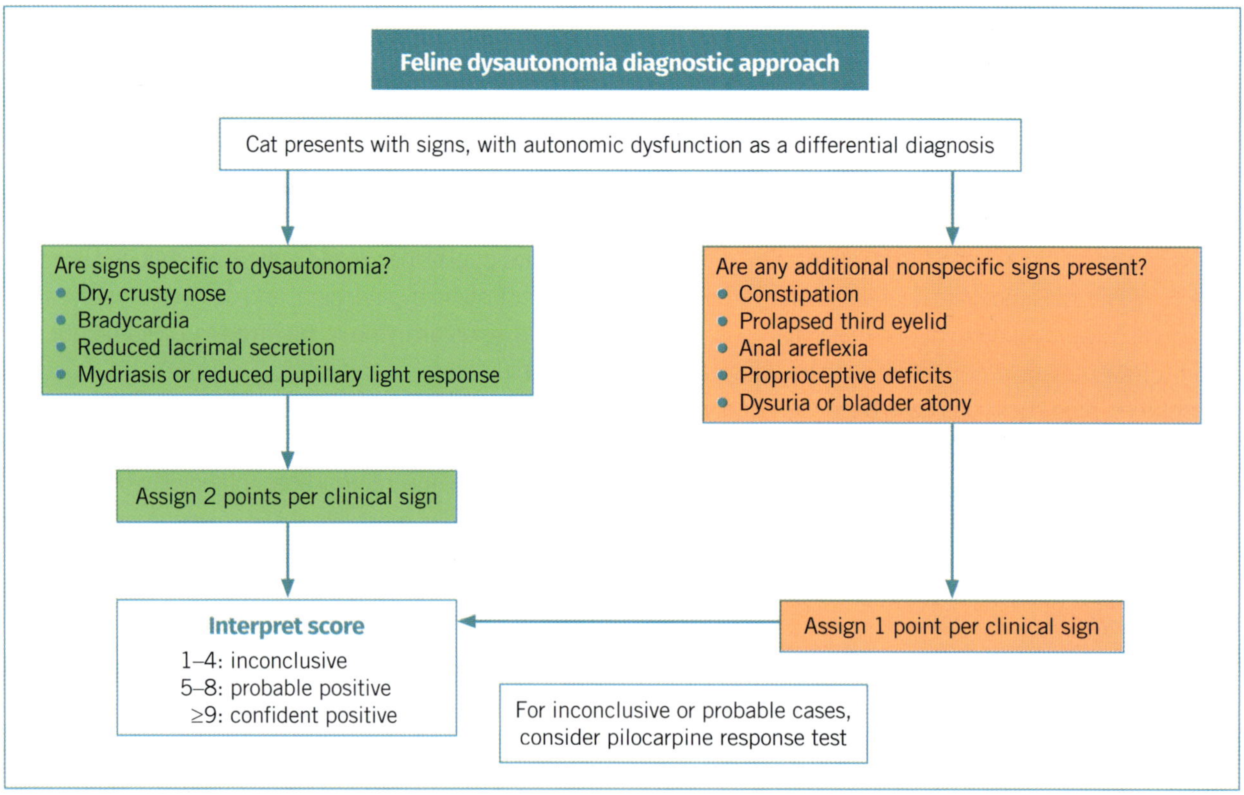

Figure 22.2. Scoring system for the clinical signs that are commonly associated with feline dysautonomia. The clinical features are divided into two groups: the first (in green) consists of features that are frequently encountered in feline dysautonomia but are otherwise uncommon in the cat; features in the second group (in orange) are less frequently encountered in the condition and may be more likely to be associated with other disorders. In combination, however, the features in the second group occurring together are suggestive of feline dysautonomia. Adapted from Wheeler SJ, editor. *Manual of Small Animal Neurology*. Cheltenham, British Small Animal Veterinary Association, 1982.

and dark conditions, approximately 200 and 0.25 lux, respectively. A weak solution of 0.05%–0.1% pilocarpine is then instilled onto the cornea of the eyes and the pupil diameter measurement repeated 15–30 minutes later. The pupil of a healthy cat (i.e. with a normal ANS) will dilate under low light conditions and will not constrict following the administration of the low-concentration pilocarpine. If the pupil constricts, this is consistent with denervation hypersensitivity and suggestive of dysautonomia (Fig. 22.3). The ocular pilocarpine response test was used as a diagnostic aid in 22 cats and was reported to be consistent with dysautonomia by the attending clinician in 19 cases (86%), suggesting it may have a high sensitivity and probably the highest of the currently available antemortem tests.[8]

Atropine, a direct-acting parasympatholytic agent, blocks the action of acetylcholine at the muscarinic receptors in the parasympathetic nervous system. Under normal circumstances, when given by intravenous or intramuscular injection, it causes an increase in heart rate as the sympathetic nervous system becomes dominant. Dysautonomia can cause a loss of sympathetic innervation to the heart leading to the observed bradycardia, either absolute bradycardia or inappropriately low rates for a given situation (e.g. when cats are stressed by being in a veterinary clinic). No change in heart rate is seen in response to the administration of atropine in cats with feline dysautonomia.

An occasionally reported but seemingly rarely used test is the cutaneous histamine test. As ANS functionality is disrupted, the capillaries in the skin are unable to respond to histamine, and therefore there is no visible reaction to histamine injection in the skin of dysautonomic cats.

Diagnostic imaging typically shows findings expected based on the progression of the disease. Moderate to severe megaoesophagus is frequently noted (Fig. 22.4), less commonly with concurrent aspiration pneumonia (which is less frequently seen than in affected dogs). The stomach experiences delayed emptying, leading to dilation with gas or ingesta (Fig. 22.5). Abdominal ultrasonography can demonstrate hypomotile intestines, again sometimes associated with dilation. The reduced innervation to the urinary bladder can lead to urine retention, which can be seen on either radiographic or ultrasound

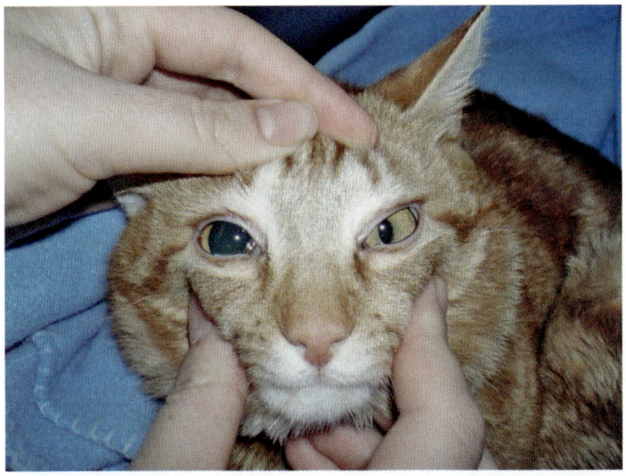

Figure 22.3. Positive pilocarpine response (abnormal constriction) in the left eye of a 3-year-old neutered male domestic shorthair cat with feline dysautonomia.

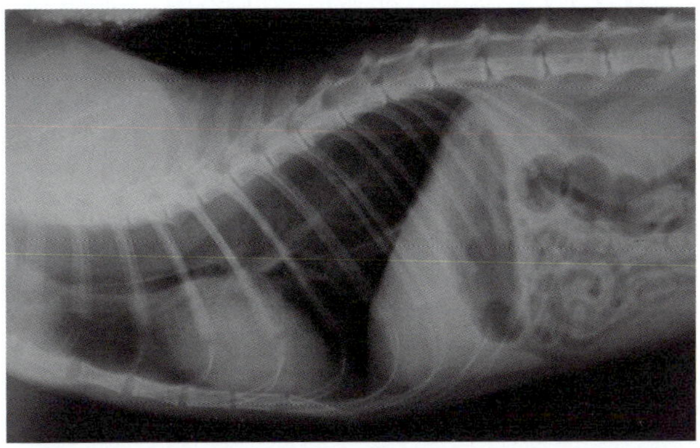

Figure 22.4. Laterolateral thoracic radiograph of a 3-year-old neutered male domestic shorthair cat with feline dysautonomia showing megaoesophagus and gastrointestinal gas retention.

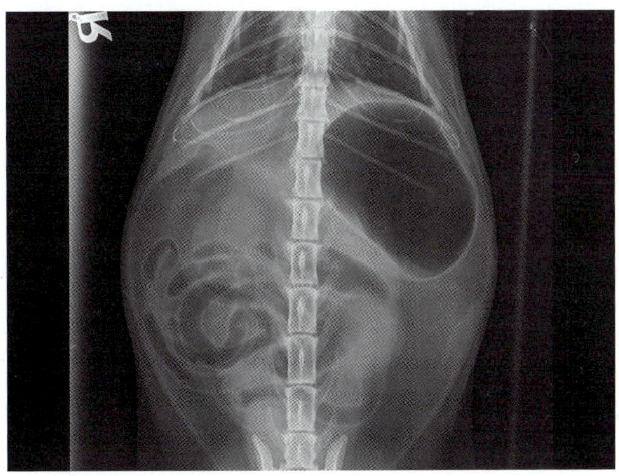

Figure 22.5. Ventrodorsal radiograph of a 7-year-old neutered male domestic longhair cat showing marked gaseous dilation of the stomach and mild gaseous dilation of the intestines due to feline dysautonomia.

imaging (Fig. 22.6). Functional evaluation by fluoroscopy consistently demonstrates oesophageal dysmotility including hypomotility, contrast retention, retrograde peristalsis, gastrooesophageal reflux, contrast pooling at the thoracic inlet, contrast pooling caudal to the base of the heart, and overall delayed transit times.

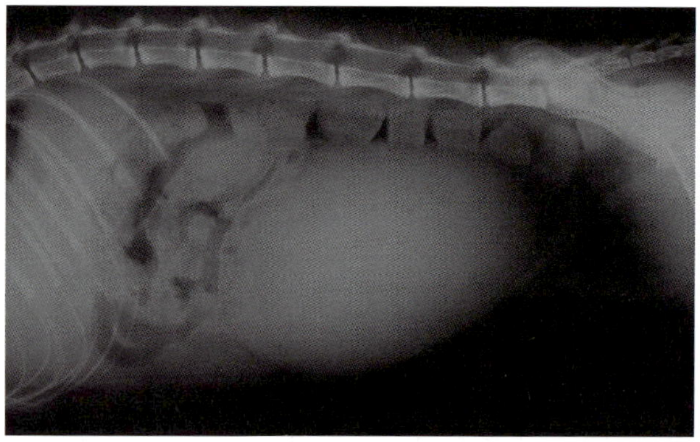

Figure 22.6. Laterolateral abdominal radiograph of the same 3-year-old neutered male domestic shorthair cat with feline dysautonomia as seen in Figure 22.4, showing urinary bladder distension and accumulation of faecal matter in the colon (constipation).

Management and treatment

As the aetiology of dysautonomia is yet to be established, current treatment is exclusively supportive and symptomatic. To date, no studies have included sufficient numbers of cats to determine with confidence which interventions are the most effective, and therefore treatment choice is empirical based on the presenting clinical signs of individual patients and their severity.

For ocular signs and cats with reduced STT values, eye lubrication and tear replacement applied every 4–6 hours can help prevent the formation of corneal ulcers and reduce patient discomfort.

Prokinetic medications are commonly needed for animals with signs associated with GI dysmotility. Cisapride or metoclopramide can be used to increase the rate of gastric emptying, whilst polyethylene glycol is frequently given to manage constipation, if present. Cisapride, as a serotonin agonist, is more potent than metoclopramide, which is a dopamine antagonist, in treating delayed gastric emptying in dysautonomic feline patients.

Maropitant can be prescribed to reduce nausea/vomiting and provide visceral analgesia for the pain that may accompany ileus and bloat. Mirtazapine can be given as an additional appetite stimulant and can help increase food intake in hyporexic patients. For anorexic patients, it may be necessary to use feeding tubes to ensure adequate nutritional intake and avoid hepatic lipidosis. However, PEG tubes are usually needed, as oesophageal dysmotility may preclude nasogastric or oesophageal tubes.

Dysautonomic patients are at significant anaesthetic risk during PEG tube placement, from gastric reflux to poorly controllable blood pressure, heart rate, and/or body temperature.

Gastroprotection may help some cats. Cytoprotective agents such as liquid sucralfate increase the resistance of the gastric and oesophageal mucosae to acid injury; however, most cats resist taking them. Famotidine and/or short courses of omeprazole can be employed as gastroprotectants as needed.

Urinary retention can present a significant problem in cats with dysautonomia. Bethanechol is a parasympathomimetic choline carbamate that selectively stimulates muscarinic receptors without any effect on nicotinic receptors. Unlike acetylcholine, bethanechol is not hydrolysed by cholinesterase and therefore has a significantly longer duration of action. Bethanechol acts on the detrusor muscle to initiate micturition and also has some effect on the GI tract that can benefit dysautonomic patients. Prazosin and phenoxybenzamine are α_1-adrenergic receptor blockers that cause smooth muscle relaxation, prevent spasm, and facilitate micturition. However, since phenoxybenzamine typically takes 5 days to gain efficacy, and these cats are usually critically unwell, prazosin is the drug of choice. The recommendation that prazosin should always be started before bethanechol to prevent iatrogenic urinary obstruction (as the latter constricts the urethra as well as the bladder) should still be followed in dysautonomic patients, but it may be an unfounded concern due to pathological changes in the ANS.

A major limiting factor when trying to treat cases of dysautonomia is that each cat is affected differently, with different patterns of nerve damage. Hence, case by case decisions and empirical treatment attempts have to be undertaken and the response observed in each individual patient.

Prognosis and outcome

The prognosis for feline dysautonomia is generally poor. In one study, 7/9 cats were euthanised 2–5 days after presentation to a referral centre. In another study, 70% of the cats had died or had been euthanised by 18 months after the diagnosis. Of the 34 cats included in the review study mentioned above, only 10 (29%) survived to discharge and 3 of those were euthanised within 8 days of discharge due to progressive signs consistent with dysautonomia.[8] However, 7/34 cats (21%) achieved complete and long-term (>2 years) resolution of dysautonomia. Other reports support this finding. Cats showing mild clinical signs or signs limited to a particular organ system have the best chance for long-term survival, but exact prognostic variables are unknown.

Importantly, most of the cases included in the literature are those which are treated at referral centres. It is therefore likely that milder cases are treated successfully in general practice, and the long-term prognosis may not be as poor as reported. Furthermore, given the challenges associated with reaching a definitive diagnosis and the fact that spontaneous regression has been reported in some animals, it is likely that mildly affected individuals are treated symptomatically, often without dysautonomia ever being considered as the underlying cause due to the lack of clinical severity or progression. It is important for clinicians to be aware of dysautonomia as a differential diagnosis in cats with GI signs in order to prevent unnecessary diagnostic tests being performed, some of which may have an associated morbidity.

Take-home messages

- Dysmotility disorders affecting individual sections of the feline gastrointestinal tract are generally rare. Generalised dysmotility is most commonly caused by feline dysautonomia, which has had a variable incidence historically from very rare to relatively common.
- Feline dysautonomic patients frequently display a range of clinical signs, none of which are pathognomonic, making an antemortem diagnosis challenging.
- The presence of ocular signs (inappropriate mydriasis, third eyelid prolapse) and dry nares and mucosae in combination with bradycardia, lower urinary tract signs, or megaoesophagus/regurgitation are highly supportive of dysautonomia.
- Feline dysautonomia currently remains a relatively rarely diagnosed condition, with a reportedly high mortality rate.
- The cause of feline dysautonomia remains unknown, but the occurrence of disease "outbreaks" may indicate a novel infectious agent or the exposure to a common toxin or environmental contaminant.
- Prospective long-term studies are required to gain more information about the best way to treat feline dysautonomia, but the rarity of this disease will make this challenging.

REFERENCES

[1] Westfall DS et al. Evaluation of esophageal transit of tablets and capsules in 30 cats. *J Vet Intern Med* 15:467, 2001.

[2] Frowde PE et al. Oesophageal disease in 33 cats. *J Feline Med Surg* 13:564, 2011.

[3] Xiang H et al. Feline oesophagus. *J Med Imaging Radiat Oncol* 62 Suppl 1:73, 2018.

[4] Armbrust LJ et al. Gastric emptying in cats using foods varying in fiber content and kibble shapes. *Vet Radiol Ultrasound* 44:339, 2003.

[5] Weber M et al. Influence of the dietary fibre levels on faecal hair excretion after 14 days in short and long-haired domestic cats. *Vet Med Sci* 1:30, 2015.

[6] Husnik R et al. Validation of ultrasonography for assessment of gastric emptying time in healthy cats by radionuclide scintigraphy. *J Vet Intern Med* 31:394, 2017.

[7] Schmitz S et al. Direct comparison of solid-phase gastric emptying times assessed by means of a carbon isotope-labeled sodium acetate breath test and technetium Tc 99m albumin colloid radioscintigraphy in healthy cats. *Am J Vet Res* 75:648, 2014.

[8] Clarke KE et al. Dysautonomia in 53 cats and dogs: retrospective review of clinical data and outcome. *Vet Rec* 187:e118, 2020.

[9] Edney ATB, Gaskell CJ, Sharp NJH. Waltham symposium no. 6 feline dysautonomia—an emerging disease. *J Small Anim Pract* 28:333, 1987.

[10] Key TJ, Gaskell CJ. Puzzling syndrome in cats associated with pupillary dilatation. *Vet Rec* 110:160, 1982.

CHAPTER 23

Constipation and megacolon

Frédéric P. Gaschen

INTRODUCTION

Anatomy of the large intestine

The length of the feline large intestine was found to vary between individual cats (31.6 ± 5.1 cm); however, it was remarkably consistent when expressed as a percentage of the total intestinal length (20.9% ± 2.0%) in a study of 28 healthy cats.[1] Unlike in dogs, the caecum in cats is a short, cone-like structure with no compartmentalisation, and the ascending colon is often proportionally shorter. It is followed aborally by the right flexure, the transverse colon, the left flexure, the descending colon, which represents the longest large intestinal segment, and the rectum.

Colonic smooth muscle is organised in an inner circular muscular layer that forms a tight circumferential spiral along the course of the colon and an incomplete outer longitudinal muscle layer. It is innervated by the enteric nervous system, which consists of thousands of small ganglia located within the colonic wall that are organised in the myenteric and submucosal plexuses, and by extrinsic nerves that connect the gut to the extraintestinal ganglia and the central nervous system. Muscular activity is regulated by neurons located in the myenteric plexus and in the external layer of the submucosal plexus. Extrinsic nerves modulate colonic motility. While sympathetic fibres have a suppressive effect on colonic muscular activity, parasympathetic fibres may exert both excitatory effects during colonic propulsive activity and inhibitory effects that allow an increase in colonic compliance.

Colonic motility

Colonic motility has been studied in cats decades ago, first as a model for human physiology, then in an attempt to elucidate the mechanisms leading to feline megacolon. In addition to these observations, it is thought that more recent knowledge gained from other species (dogs, humans) can be applied to cats as well.[2] Overall, colonic motility facilitates the main functions of each segment of the colon: absorption of water and electrolytes in the ascending and transverse colon and faecal storage and evacuation in the descending colon (Fig. 23.1).

Electrical activity in the feline colon consists of two main patterns: slow waves, occurring in all segments at a frequency of 5–6/minute, and spikes.[3] Slow waves are generated by the vast network of interstitial cells of Cajal located in the myenteric plexus and circular muscle layers. They stimulate Ca^{2+} entry by activating voltage-dependent Ca^{2+} channels in smooth muscle cells. This induces electromechanical coupling by causing phosphorylation of the myosin light chains, cross-bridge cycling, and contraction.

In the ascending and transverse segments, contractile activity consists of slow rhythmic contractions directly associated with slow waves. Spikes may greatly increase Ca^{2+} entry when superimposed onto slow waves. Spikes are associated with slow waves in the ascending and transverse colon and generally occur independently in the descending colon. Profound circular contractions in the descending colon appear to be triggered by bursts of spikes.

Colonic motility includes propagating and nonpropagating contractions. Nonpropagating contractions (also called stationary or segmenting contractions) occur mostly in the ascending and transverse colon, where they mix the intraluminal contents and indirectly promote water and electrolyte absorption. Their frequency parallels that of slow wave electrical activity. Nonpropa-

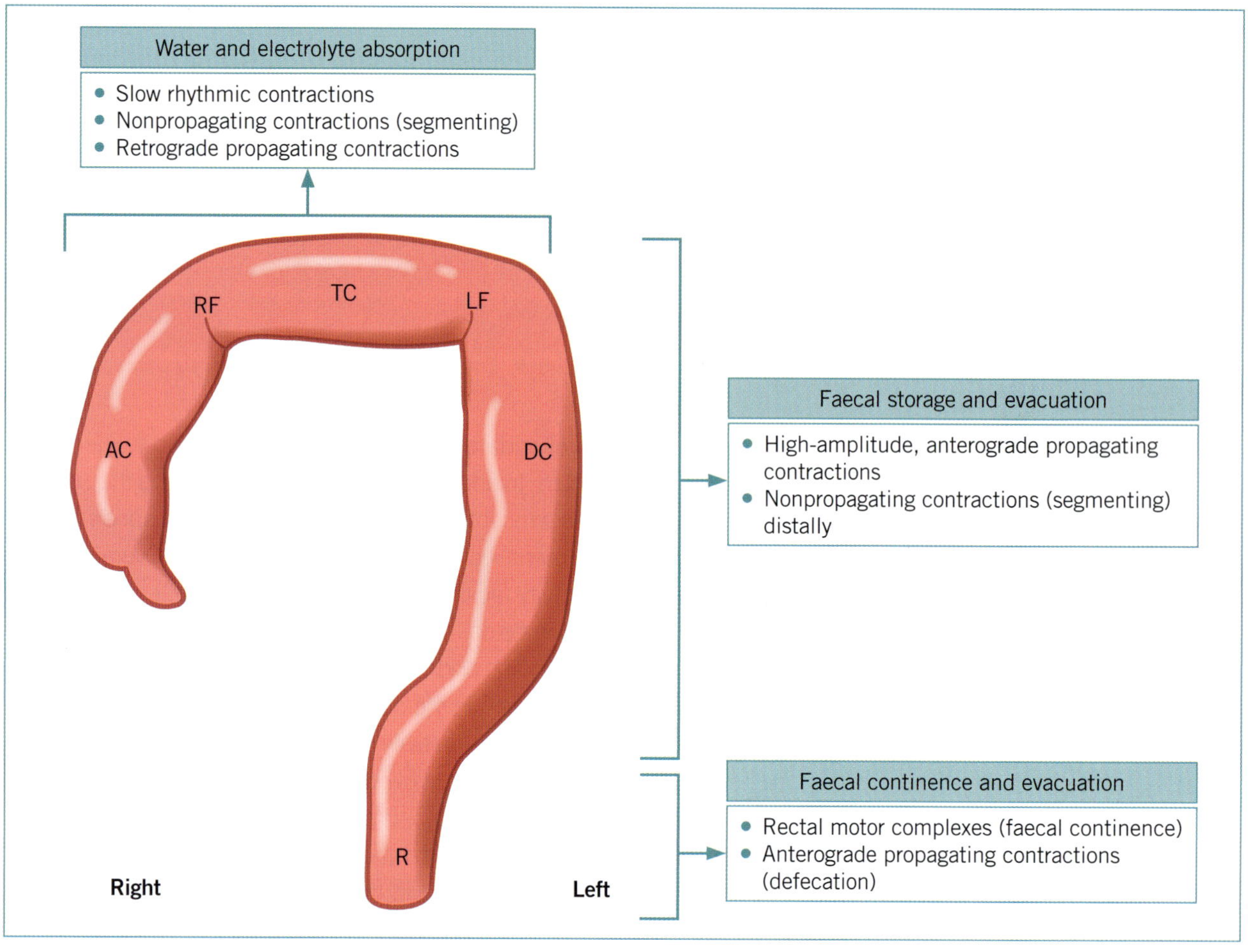

Figure 23.1. Schematic drawing of the colon of a cat in dorsal recumbency showing the motility patterns and function of the feline large intestine. The blue boxes summarise the function of each large intestinal segment, and the white boxes list the motility patterns known to occur in each segment. AC, ascending colon; DC, descending colon; LF, left flexure; R, rectum; RF, right flexure; TC, transverse colon.

gating contractions also occur in the distal colon, where, in conjunction with rectal motor complexes, they promote faecal continence. Propagating contractions are lumen-occlusive events that move in anterograde or sometimes in retrograde direction. Retrograde (orad) propagating contractions are limited to the ascending colon and only expand over short distances. High-amplitude propagating contractions (also called giant or mass movement contractions) occur in the descending colon several times per day and propagate over longer distances, ultimately leading to defecation. This type of contraction can be induced by luminal distension and by mucosal stimuli such as the irritant laxative bisacodyl.

Distension of the rectum initiates the defecation reflex. At that time, increased propulsive colonic and rectal motility move the faeces towards the anus, and the internal anal sphincter relaxes. Voluntary relaxation of the external anal sphincter is required so that defecation can occur. The pelvic nerve plays an essential role in the voluntary control of defecation.

Anterograde propagating colonic motility is increased postprandially. This gastrocolonic response is at first mediated by extrinsic enteric nerves in response to gastric dilation and then by release of enteropeptides in the vasculature following arrival of chyme in the distal small intestine. The gastrocolonic response commonly leads to postprandial defecation.

In healthy cats, large bowel transit time (LBTT) was shown to be 40 hours when measured using radiopaque spheres.[4]

AETIOLOGY AND EPIDEMIOLOGY

Definitions

Several terms are used to describe cats with less frequent or absent defecation. Constipation refers to cats experiencing one or two episodes during which they display clinical signs and can be easily treated with appropriate measures. Obstipation refers to cats experiencing chronic recurring constipation that has become refractory to treatment due to permanent loss of colonic function. A presumptive diagnosis of obstipation is made when a chronically constipated cat has failed to respond to several treatment attempts using different approaches. Finally, cats affected with dilated megacolon have permanently lost colonic function and show colonic dilation and hypomotility, and megacolon may in fact be the end stage of constipation and obstipation with a total loss of motility (Fig. 23.2). Even though it may create confusion, the term megacolon is also used to describe a severely dilated colon on abdominal radiographs.

Aetiology

Constipation is a frequent problem in human medicine, and the American Gastroenterology Association (AGA) has published a technical review that explains the concept of normal-transit constipation (NTC) and slow-transit constipation (STC).[5] Patients are diagnosed with STC following intraluminal assessment of colonic motility with manometry and a barostat, although the technique appears to have limitations for definitive differentiation between normal and abnormal colonic motility. Besides motility disorders, sensory disturbances, such as reduced rectal sensation, may cause constipation as well. Defecatory disorders are an additional cause of constipation due to abnormalities in the defecation response.[5]

In feline medicine, diagnostic tools used in people such as colonic manometry and barostat testing are not practical nor available. Nevertheless, it is important to differentiate obstructive and nonobstructive causes of constipation, as management of these two categories differ greatly.

Obstructive constipation should be ruled out first. It is usually associated with tenesmus and dyschezia, at least in the initial stages, and the passage of smaller size faeces (e.g. ribbon-like). Optimally, its management should focus on elimination of the obstruction, even though this is not applicable to all cases. Causes include obstruction of the colonic or rectal lumen by foreign bodies and space-occupying lesions originating from the gut wall (e.g. polyp, adenocarcinoma, lymphoma, mast cell tumour) or impinging on the large intestine from adjacent structures. Pelvic fractures with displacement may cause narrowing of the pelvic canal, and most cats with severe narrowing (around 50% or more) developed chronic constipation in one study.[6] However, a recent study following 43 cats with pelvic fractures long-term reported mild to moderate chronic constipation in only 19% of cases with no clear relationship to severity of pelvic canal narrowing, and all cases could be successfully managed medically.[7] Furthermore, perianal bite wounds or abscesses are

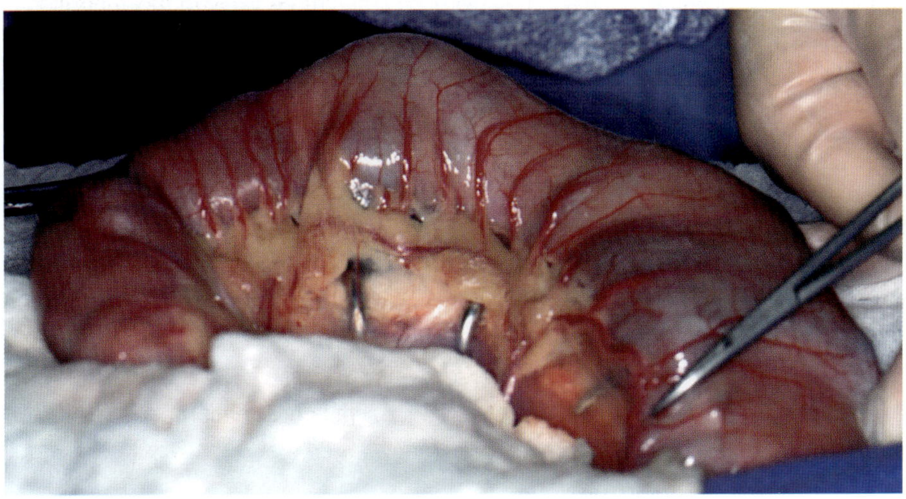

Figure 23.2. Feline megacolon. Dilated colon filled with faeces in a cat with chronic recurring obstipation that had become refractory to medical treatment. The colon was exteriorised from the abdominal cavity prior to subtotal colectomy. Image courtesy of Dr Howard B. Seim III, Colorado State University, USA.

painful and may cause dyschezia and possibly acute constipation.

Diseases associated with nonobstructive feline constipation are listed in Box 23.1. The list is remarkably succinct in comparison to similar documents summarising diseases and drugs known to be associated with constipation in people.[5] Dehydration may lead to enhanced faecal water absorption in the proximal colon, a mechanism thought to play an important role in cats with chronic kidney disease (CKD). Some veterinary practitioners believe that other diseases associated with polyuria and polydipsia may predispose to constipation as well; however, there is no evidence in the literature to substantiate this, and the author has not recognised this to be true in his practice. Also, electrolyte imbalances such as hypokalaemia (which may also occur with CKD) and hypercalcaemia may decrease the contractile properties of the colonic smooth muscle and should be ruled out in constipated cats.

Finally, the reported aetiologies for 120 cats diagnosed with chronic obstipation collected in a review of the literature performed more than 20 years ago included idiopathic megacolon (63%), pelvic canal stenosis (23%), nerve injury (6%), and Manx cats sacral cord deformity (5%). Therefore, the majority of cases were idiopathic, orthopaedic, or neurological in origin.[8]

Box 23.1. Causes of nonobstructive constipation in cats.

Neuromuscular disorders

Congenital
- Agenesis/hypogenesis of coccygeal vertebrae in Manx cats[19]
- Large intestinal hypoganglionosis (Hirschsprung's disease)

Acquired
- Lumbosacral disc disease
- Dysautonomia
- Prolonged colonic distension (e.g. secondary to chronic obstructive disease)
- Idiopathic megacolon

Nonneurological comorbidities
- Overweight[10]
- Age[9,10]
- Chronic kidney disease[20]
- Electrolyte imbalances: hypokalaemia, hypercalcaemia
- Dehydration
- Hypoadrenocorticism
- Congenital or juvenile-onset hypothyroidism

Drugs (tentative)
- Sucralfate in cats with chronic kidney disease
- Drugs known to cause chronic constipation in people that are used in cats: chronic use of opioid agonists, anticholinergics, diuretics, barium sulphate; however, there is no documented evidence of constipation with these drugs in cats

Behaviour and environment
- Soiled litter tray
- Inactivity
- Hospitalisation
- Change in environment

Epidemiology

In people, the overall prevalence of constipation in adults is 16%, while it reaches 33.5% after 60 years of age with an overall female:male ratio of 1.5. Risk factors include lower socioeconomic status, less self-reported physical activity, medications, depression, and stressful life events.

Unfortunately, there is no similar epidemiologically sound and detailed data for feline constipation. Based on visual faecal scores obtained from nearly 1700 faecal samples from cats housed in UK shelters, a study reported hard faeces suggestive of constipation in 5.6% of samples, and prevalence seemed to increase with age.[9] The study relied solely on faecal appearance and may have significantly overestimated the prevalence of constipation, as hard faeces can also be passed by cats that are not truly constipated as per the prevailing definition. Recently, a retrospective study reviewed 189 cats presented to a large urban emergency facility for constipation or obstipation and identified several risk factors in their cohort when comparing it to control cats presented to the emergency facility for causes unrelated to constipation. When compared to controls, constipated cats were older and had a higher body condition score (overweight). Also, they were 20 times more likely to have a previous history of constipation and 3.8 times more likely to have CKD than controls.[10]

Finally, an older study reported a prevalence of 0.23% for the diagnosis of megacolon amongst all cat diagnoses in US and Canadian veterinary colleges in 1989. However, megacolon is likely only the tip of the iceberg, and nowadays most cases of feline constipation are probably well managed in primary care practice and not in referral institutions. In the author's opinion, constipation can be considered a feline disease of relatively low but not negligible incidence, while obstipation and megacolon seem to occur rarely.

HISTORY AND PHYSICAL EXAMINATION

Signalment

The median age of 189 cats presented to an emergency facility for constipation was 10 years, ranging from 3 weeks to 21 years, and there was no sex predisposition.[10] In an older review of 120 cats with the more severe conditions of obstipation and megacolon described in the literature prior to 1997, the mean age was 5.8 years, suggesting that idiopathic megacolon is a disease of middle-aged rather than old cats, and male cats seemed to be more frequently affected (70% males vs. 30% females).[8] In these two cohorts, domestic shorthair and longhair cats represented the vast majority of cases, and no breed predisposition could be identified.

History

Owners of cats presented for constipation usually observed reduced, absent, or painful defecation for days to months. Constipated cats may assume a defecation posture in the litter tray for prolonged periods of time or make multiple unproductive attempts to defecate (dyschezia). Depending on the cause of the problem, particularly if an obstruction is present or if the faeces are very hard, defecation may be painful. In severe cases of nonobstructive constipation or in cats with obstipation and megacolon, the urge to defecate may have disappeared. Rectal prolapse may be observed in some cats. If cats are able to pass faeces, these are usually hard and dry, and may be found either in or outside the litter tray. In the presence of an obstruction in the caudal part of the distal colon or in the rectum, ribbon-like faeces may be passed. Occasionally, constipated cats may intermittently pass diarrhoeic faeces, sometimes with haematochezia, and owners may be confused as to what is happening. These signs are attributed to mucosal damage caused by the stationary, hard, dry faeces and the pressure they may exert on the colonic and rectal wall. Cats with severe and prolonged constipation or obstipation may ultimately develop signs of systemic illness, such as lethargy, hyporexia, weight loss, and vomiting. These are thought to result from the effects of the long-standing colonic obstruction and possibly from a disrupted mucosal barrier in the colon. Finally, clinical signs of any associated comorbidity can also be present, such as polyuria and polydipsia in cats with CKD. It is noteworthy that dysuria and stranguria, occurring for instance in cats with urolithiasis or acute/chronic lower urinary tract signs, may be misinterpreted as constipation by some owners.

Physical examination

Physical examination is often mostly unremarkable in a cat experiencing a first episode of mild constipation. However, cats with chronic moderate to severe constipation, obstipation, or megacolon most commonly have a palpably enlarged descending colon filled with hard to very hard faeces and may display pain on abdominal palpation. Mild to moderate mesenteric lymphadenopathy may be present as well. On occasion, the abnormal colon may be misinterpreted as a large abdominal neoplasm. Findings resulting from the systemic impact of prolonged constipation and colonic impaction, such as lethargy, malaise, dehydration, and weight loss, may also be observed. Finally, changes associated with comorbidities, such as pelvic pain and asymmetry due to pelvic fractures, may be noticed as well.

Concurrent presence of bradycardia, urinary and faecal incontinence, regurgitation, prolapsed nictitating membrane, mydriasis, and/or decreased tear production suggest generalised autonomic dysfunction and a diagnosis of feline dysautonomia, a rare disease of cats.

DIAGNOSTIC INVESTIGATION

The veterinary practitioner needs to evaluate the full history and determine if the cat is constipated or obstipated and assess the severity of the colonic impaction. These criteria will determine the extent of the recommended diagnostic investigation and management (Fig. 23.3).

All constipated cats should undergo a detailed visual inspection of the perineal and anal regions and a rectal palpation under sedation or general anaesthesia to carefully examine the anus, the rectum, and possibly the caudal end of the distal colon with a well lubricated gloved finger matching the size of the cat's anus and rectum. Particular attention should be paid to anal sacs (inflammation or abscess); presence of perineal hernia (possibly with rectal diverticulum—rare in cats), colorectal stricture, foreign body, polyp, or neoplasia; and narrowing of the pelvic canal due to displaced pelvic bones.

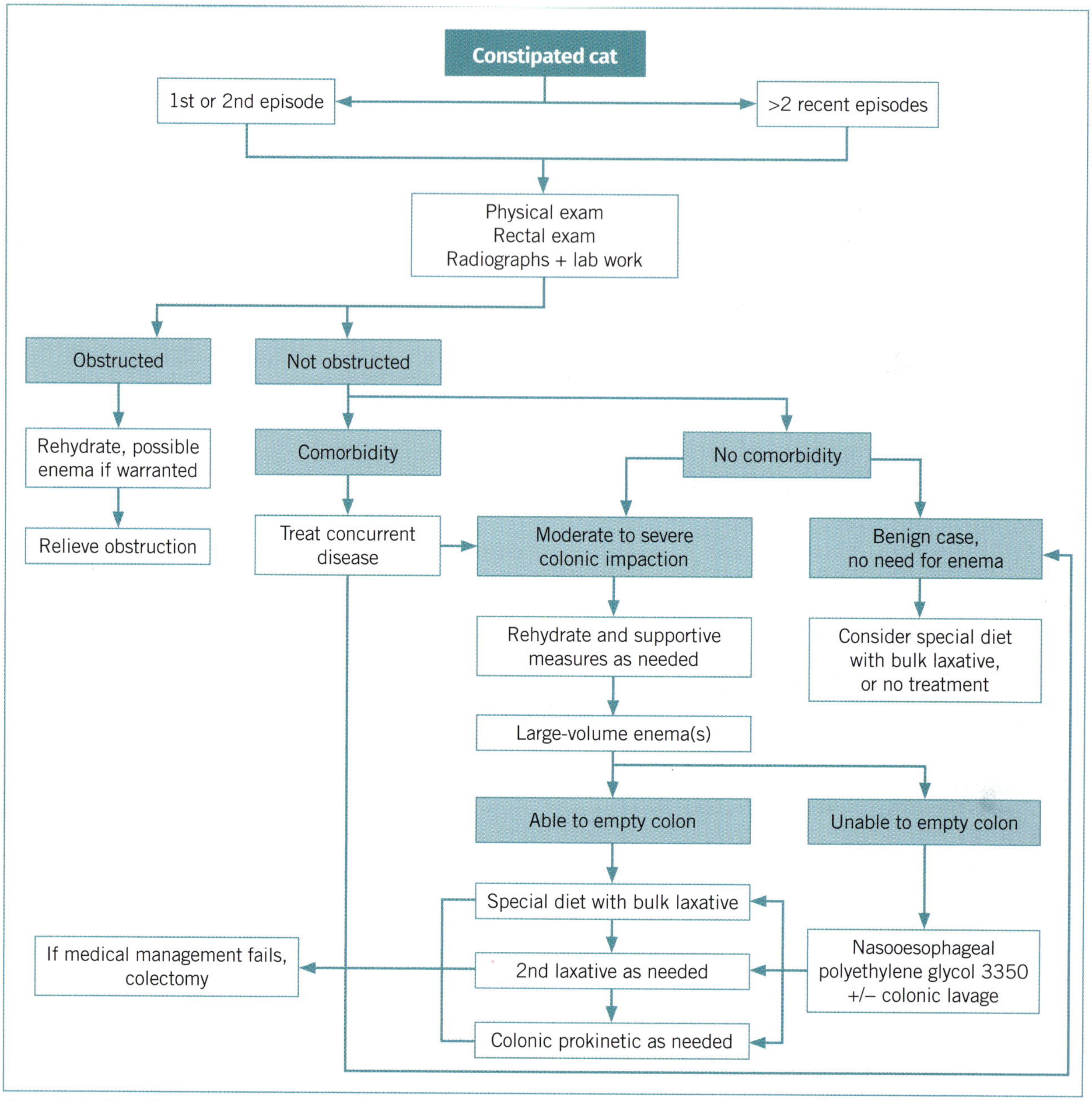

Figure 23.3. Simplified approach to the constipated cat.

Constipated cats also benefit from abdominal radiographs to assess the extent of colonic dilation, the presence of other abdominal masses, and the integrity of the bony structures of the pelvis and lumbosacral and coccygeal spine (Figs. 23.4–23.6). In a study of 39 cats with constipation or megacolon, a ratio was calculated between maximal colon diameter and length of the fifth lumbar vertebra (L5) on lateral radiographs. A value greater than 1.48 was a good indicator of megacolon, while all cats with a ratio greater than 1.62 had megacolon (Fig. 23.6).[11]

In addition, since many constipated cats are old, a minimal database including complete blood count, biochemistry panel, and urinalysis should be obtained in search for comorbidities that may be associated with constipation, such as CKD, hypokalaemia, or hypercalcaemia, or without such known association.

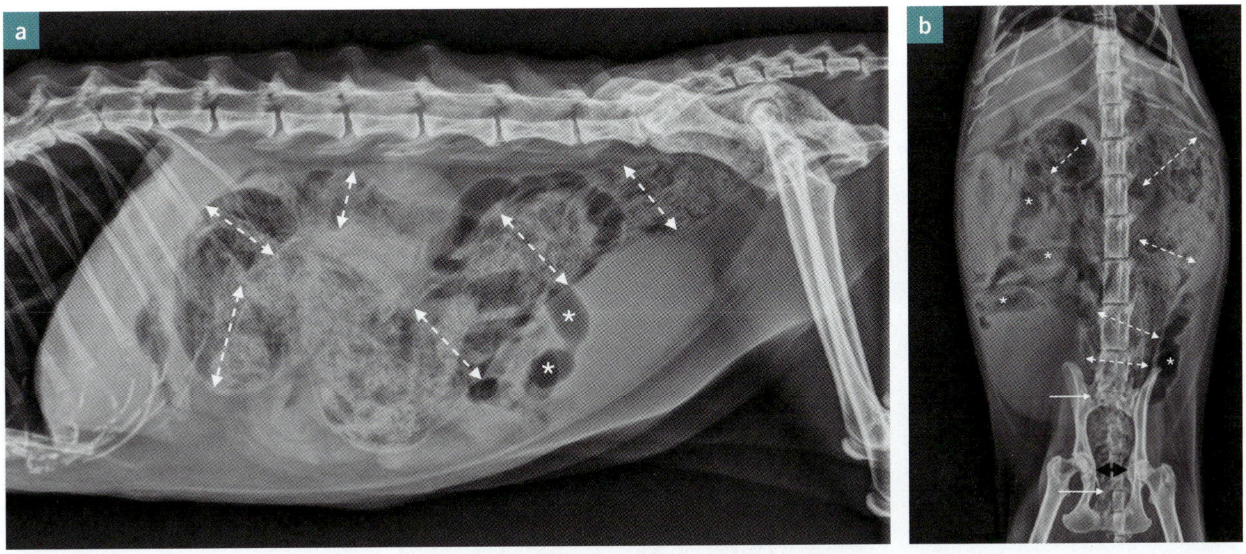

Figure 23.4. Right lateral (a) and ventrodorsal (b) radiographic views of an adult cat with a severely dilated colon (dashed double-headed arrows) due to narrowing of the pelvic canal resulting from old, right-sided pelvic fractures of the ilium and pubis with sacroiliac luxation (solid white arrows). The pelvic canal is narrowed by approximately 50% (double-headed black arrows). A few jejunal segments in the caudal abdomen are mildly dilated and contain gas (asterisks), which is a common finding when the colon is obstructed with faeces. Images courtesy of Dr Lorrie Gaschen, Louisiana State University, USA.

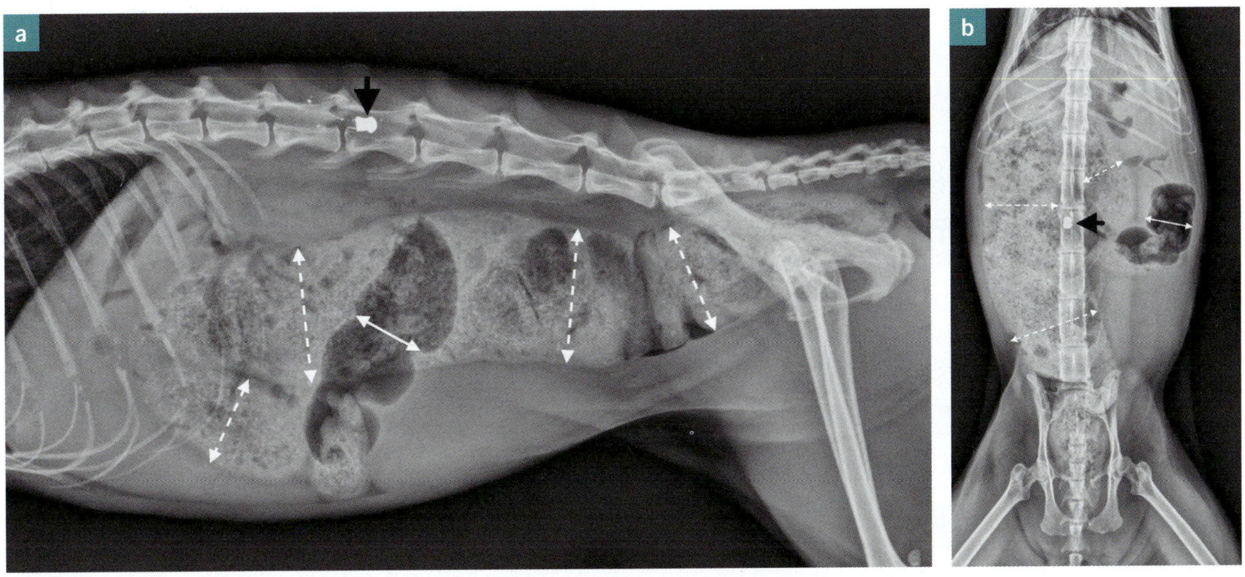

Figure 23.5. Right lateral (a) and ventrodorsal (b) radiographic views of a 4-year-old spayed female domestic shorthair cat that had been paraplegic after being shot in the spine at 1 year of age. The cat had lower motor neuron deficits in the hindlimbs and had developed chronic recurrent constipation that was successfully managed with diet and oral laxatives until 1 week prior to presentation. Ballistic foreign material is visible at the level of L3 (black arrow). The colon is severely dilated with faecal material (dashed double-headed arrows) and is displaced to the right of the spine. The colon can shift from its normal position on the left side due to the weight of the faeces. The ascending colon is shifted to the right for the same reason (solid double-headed arrow). There is poor serosal detail in the rest of the abdomen, which is likely due to a combination of thin body condition and mass effect created by the large colon. Images courtesy of Dr Lorrie Gaschen, Louisiana State University, USA.

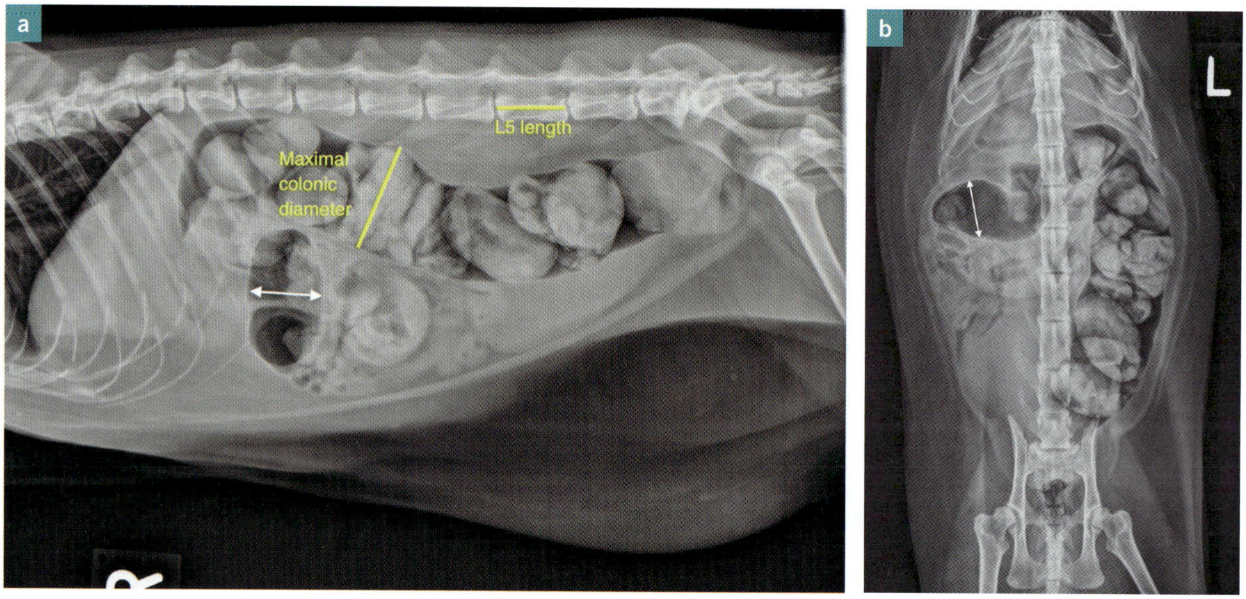

Figure 23.6. Right lateral (a) and ventrodorsal (b) radiographic views of a 10-year-old overweight neutered male cat with chronic constipation. The colon is severely dilated and filled with large faecal balls that are of mixed soft tissue and mineral opacity due to desiccation. The ratio between maximal colonic diameter and length of the L5 vertebra is approximately 1.5 and suggestive but not diagnostic of megacolon. The ascending colon is gas dilated (solid double-headed arrow). The opacity and shape of the faecal balls in combination with the large size of the colon lead to a diagnosis of nonobstructive constipation with possible megacolon. Following a saline–lactulose enema, the cat was successfully managed for several years with a combination of psyllium-enriched diet, oral laxatives, and cisapride. Images courtesy of Dr Lorrie Gaschen, Louisiana State University, USA.

If extracolonic abdominal lesions are identified on the radiographs or if the minimal database is indicative of abdominal disease in addition to colonic impaction, further exams, such as abdominal ultrasound with possible cytological evaluation of fine needle aspirates, should be considered. Abdominal ultrasonography may additionally reveal enlarged regional lymph nodes attributable to the presence of chronic inflammation associated with constipation/obstipation.

MANAGEMENT AND TREATMENT

The management of a constipated cat can be divided in immediate measures to relieve the colonic impaction and further treatment to prevent its recurrence.

Immediate measures

Cats experiencing rare episodes of mild constipation and impaction may not require any immediate treatment and be managed well in the home environment with diet and oral laxatives (see below). However, constipated cats with significant colonic impaction should receive basic supportive treatment as needed, including intravenous fluid therapy to address dehydration and electrolyte abnormalities. Rectal palpation and abdominal radiographs (see above) under sedation are best done after the cat has been stabilised.

Once it has been determined that an enema could be safely administered, a large-volume enema with isotonic fluids warmed to body temperature should be prepared. It is always safer to sedate cats before the administration of a large-volume enema, even though some may tolerate the enema without sedation. In obstipated cats, larger enema volumes may be needed, and the procedure may take more time. Therefore, the risk of vomiting in response to acute rectal and colonic distension is higher, and it is of paramount importance to place an endotracheal tube to prevent aspiration pneumonia. Cats showing abdominal pain were less likely to defecate after receiving an enema when compared to nonpainful cats.[10]

The reader is referred to the video in Chapter 37 for a description of the actual procedure, since the techniques for colonic administration of faecal microbiota transplantation and enema are similar. However, it should be noted that the recommended initial catheter diameter for enemas is 12 Fr, even though larger catheters can also be used if they can be safely introduced into the descending colon. The cat should be placed on a wet table for the procedure. A mixture of isotonic electrolyte solution (5–10 ml/kg) with lactulose (5 ml total) and water-soluble lubricant or mineral oil (5 ml total) has anecdotally been found to work well under these circumstances. Larger volumes can be used for colonic lavage in obstipated cats. Tap water could be used as well; however, cats with severe impaction are likely to have some degree of colonic mucosal damage, which makes the use of isotonic fluids preferable.

For mild to moderate constipation, some veterinary practitioners prefer using small-volume enemas. Several types of small-volume enemas are available specifically for cats and dogs, or some products marketed for people can be safely used. Their names and composition vary in each country. Safe small-volume enemas usually contain one or several laxatives such as dioctyl sodium succinate (DSS, also called docusate sodium), glycerine, sodium citrate, sorbitol, mineral oil, or other mild laxatives. Mineral oil and DSS should not be used together, as the combination could increase absorption of mineral oil. Very importantly, small-volume enemas containing sodium phosphate (e.g. Fleet Saline Enema, Practo Clyss) should never be used in cats, as they may cause severe hypernatraemia, hyperphosphataemia, and hypocalcaemia.[21]

In the past, manual fractioning and evacuation was recommended in severely impacted cats, using various instruments to remove hardened faeces (faecoliths), with the risk of damaging or even perforating the colonic wall. However, there is now a better option that can be used even when the faeces present in the colon are very hard. Administration of the osmotic laxative polyethylene glycol 3350 via nasooesophageal or nasogastric tube results in spontaneous defecation in many obstipated cats without need for invasive colonic procedures. In the most severely impacted cats, it allows to soften faeces enough so that they can be massaged out of the colon during a final large-volume enema/colonic lavage procedure (Fig. 23.7). In a small study of nine constipated/obstipated cats, the polyethylene glycol 3350 solution that is typically used for colonic cleansing prior to colonoscopy was administered as a constant-rate infusion at a dose of 6–10 ml/kg/h to a total dose of 40–150 ml/kg (median total dose 80 ml/kg) and resulted in significant spontaneous defecation within 5–24 hours (median 8 hours).[12] If a long and potentially traumatic faecal evacuation is required, some authors recommend administering a short course of antibiotics (e.g. metronidazole 7.5–15 mg/kg PO every 12 hours) to reduce the risk of bacterial translocation during or after the procedure.

In some cases, for instance in overweight or obese cats in which abdominal palpation is difficult, it may be

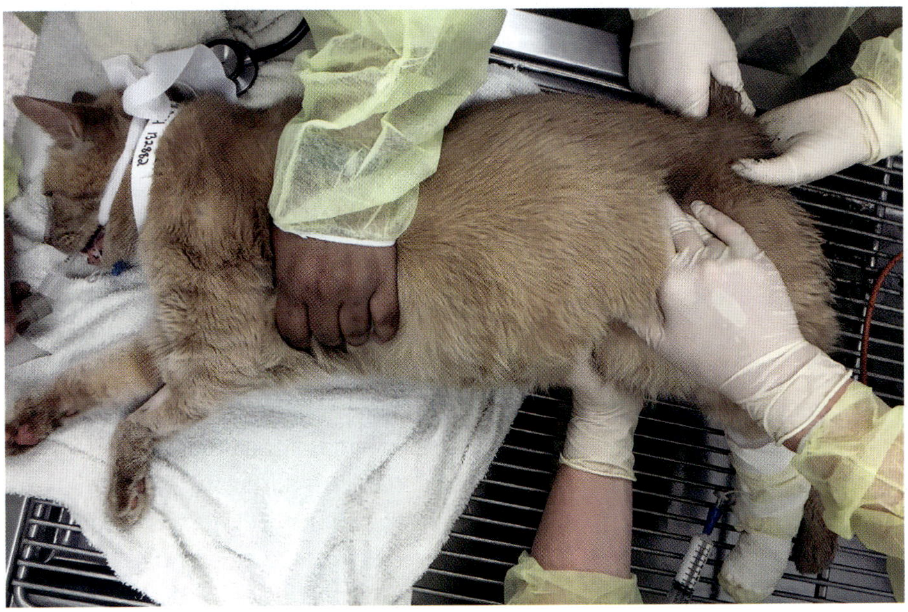

Figure 23.7. Colonic lavage and faecal evacuation in a 6-year-old neutered male domestic shorthair cat with chronic obstipation and severe colonic impaction. The cat was administered intravenous fluids and polyethylene glycol 3350 as a constant-rate infusion via naso-oesophageal catheter for 12 hours and then anaesthetised for faecal evacuation. The faeces had become softer and easier to massage out. While one person massaged the descending colon, another person administered several large-volume enemas and facilitated the exit of faecal material through the rectum, and a third person monitored anaesthesia. Note that an endotracheal tube was in place.

very useful to repeat radiographs after enemas or colonic lavage and faecal evacuation to better evaluate the success of the procedure.

Long-term management

For cats with underlying disorders, adequate management of constipation depends on proper treatment or management of the primary disease. Potential environmental issues resulting in the cat avoiding the litter tray should be addressed. In cats with obstructive constipation due to pelvic fractures and narrowing of the pelvic canal, pelvic osteotomy may be required to reestablish passage of faeces.[13] Similarly, in cats with nonobstructive constipation associated with dehydration secondary to CKD, proper management of fluid and electrolyte balance is essential for limiting recurrences and may necessitate regular administration of subcutaneous fluids by the owners.

Once existing underlying issues have been addressed and the impacted large intestine has been emptied, a stepwise approach is recommended (Fig. 23.3). It consists in first prescribing bulk laxatives such as psyllium or other sources of fibre. In an uncontrolled study of 66 chronically constipated cats fed a commercial moderate-fibre, psyllium-enriched diet, the cats did not experience any recurrence of constipation over 2 months of treatment, and in many cats other medications (other laxatives, prokinetics) could be decreased or even discontinued during that period.[14] If psyllium does not seem to work, commonly administered oral laxatives for long-term management include osmotic laxatives such as lactulose (liquid) and polyethylene glycol 3350 (powder). See Appendix for recommended dosages of laxatives that can be used in chronically constipated cats.

Some owners are able to regularly administer rectal suppositories or small-volume enemas (see above) to their chronically constipated cats, and this may be a useful component of long-term treatment in cats that do not respond to bulk or osmotic laxatives. Paediatric laxative rectal suppositories available in drug stores usually contain DSS, glycerine, or bisacodyl and are applied to effect (start with one paediatric suppository to effect). However, most cats do not tolerate rectal insertion of suppositories or enemas in their home environment, and this option should not be further pursued if this is the case because of the risks of owners being harmed, and the potential for rectal or colonic perforation.

There is an undisputed connection between mucosal and luminal microbiota and colonic motility. A recent pilot study of 10 chronically constipated or obstipated cats showed that a highly concentrated multistrain probiotic administered orally daily for 90 days resulted in softer faeces being produced in 7 cats after a median treatment duration of 38 days. Furthermore, treated cats appeared to show improvement in neuronal lesions of the colonic enteric nervous system.[15] While it delivered promising results, this study remains very preliminary, and further investigations are required to confirm the value of probiotics in the treatment of feline constipation.

In cats that are refractory to the abovementioned treatments, the next step is to use drugs that promote colonic motility. All commonly used colonic prokinetics are agonists of the 5-HT_4 (serotonin type 4) receptors located in neurons of the submucosal and myenteric plexuses. These presynaptic receptors are proexcitatory and, when activated, ultimately cause the release of acetylcholine and other neurotransmitters at neuromuscular junctions. The most commonly used feline colonic prokinetic in the United States of America and Canada is cisapride, which was withdrawn from the human pharmaceutical market more than two decades ago because of increased risk of fatal reentry cardiac arrhythmias in people, but this does not seem to be a cause of concern in cats. Cisapride was shown to stimulate contractions in smooth muscle strips from healthy cats and from cats with idiopathic megacolon in vitro.[16] Even though there are no studies documenting its effect in vivo, there is a large body of anecdotal evidence supporting its use in the stepwise approach of chronically constipated cats. The drug can be obtained from compounding pharmacies in the United States of America, Canada, and in some other countries but is not universally available. Mosapride is another 5-HT_4 agonist that is available in some Asian countries. It was shown to prevent recurrence of constipation in a pilot study of 15 chronically constipated cats that were refractory to diet and laxatives.[17] Tegaserod, another 5-HT_4 agonist with good effect on colonic motility in people and in dogs, was also withdrawn from the human pharmaceutical market in 2007 for causing cardiac arrhythmias. There are no reports on its effects on feline colonic motility, and the use of this drug in cats cannot be recommended at this time. Prucalopride is the only 5-HT_4 agonist that is currently licensed as a gastrointestinal prokinetic for people in North America, Europe, Australia, and New Zealand. It has prokinetic properties on all segments of the canine gastrointestinal tract and has been shown to elicit defecation within 1 hour of oral administration in 5 of 12 healthy cats. Unfortunately, there is no in vitro or clinical data about its efficacy in constipated cats. Consequently, although the drug holds promise, no further recommendations can be made at this time for its use in constipated cats.

Colectomy

In cats with intractable chronic recurring obstipation or megacolon, surgical resection of the colon needs to be considered. Many cats may be well controlled medically for months to years, and ultimately become refractory to conservative treatment and develop megacolon. Different techniques for colectomy have been used successfully in these cats.[18] A description of the procedures can be found in the surgical literature (Fig. 23.2). Diarrhoea is a common immediate postoperative complication that usually resolves within 1–6 weeks. Other more life-threatening complications include septic peritonitis and dehiscence of the intestinal anastomosis, which require immediate attention and an aggressive approach.[18]

PROGNOSIS AND OUTCOME

Many cats experience one or two episodes of constipation without further recurrence. However, some cats will progress to a state of chronic constipation that over the course of months to years may lead to recurring obstipation and megacolon. In cats with obstructive constipation due to pelvic narrowing, resolution of the obstruction within the first 6 months is associated with sufficient regain of colonic motility, whereas the issue generally becomes irreversible after that window of time.[13] While there are no published data to support this, it is generally believed that in cats with nonobstructive constipation early use of prokinetics in addition to diet and one or more laxatives may delay or prevent the occurrence of megacolon and the necessity for colectomy.

Take-home messages

- Constipation is a relatively infrequent disease in cats, and many affected cats experience one or two episodes of constipation followed by full recovery.
- In some cats with nonobstructive constipation, the initial episodes may be followed by chronic recurring constipation that, over a period of months to years, may lead to obstipation and decreased or absent ability of the colon to contract (megacolon).
- The initial diagnostic workup aims at differentiating obstructive from nonobstructive causes of constipation, as their respective managements are very different, and at identifying any underlying disease predisposing to nonobstructive constipation.
- For obstructive constipation, removal of the source of obstruction (e.g. foreign body, colorectal stricture, pelvic fractures narrowing down the pelvic canal) is the best course of action.
- Chronic recurring nonobstructive constipation is usually managed with a combination of enemas at the veterinary practice, diet, laxatives, and prokinetic drugs used in a stepwise manner. Cases refractory to medical management should undergo colectomy.

REFERENCES

[1] Sturgess CP et al. A gross and microscopical morphometric evaluation of feline large intestinal anatomy. *J Comp Pathol* 124:255, 2001.

[2] Bharucha AE, Hasler WL. Motility of the small intestine and colon. In: Podolsky DK et al., editors. *Yamada's Textbook of Gastroenterology*. Oxford, John Wiley & Sons: 367, 2016.

[3] Wienbeck M. The electrical activity of the cat colon in vivo. I. The normal electrical activity and its relationship to contractile activity. *Res Exp Med (Berl)* 158:268, 1972.

[4] Fucci V et al. Large bowel transit times using radiopaque markers in normal cats. *J Am Anim Hosp Assoc* 31:473, 1995.

[5] Bharucha AE, Pemberton JH, Locke GR 3rd. American Gastroenterological Association technical review on constipation. *Gastroenterology* 144:218, 2013.

[6] Hamilton MH, Evans DA, Langley-Hobbs SJ. Feline ilial fractures: assessment of screw loosening and pelvic canal narrowing after lateral plating. *Vet Surg* 38:326, 2009.

[7] Meeson RL, Geddes AT. Management and long-term outcome of pelvic fractures: a retrospective study of 43 cats. *J Feline Med Surg* 19:36, 2017.

[8] Washabau RJ, Hasler AH. Constipation, obstipation, and megacolon. In: August JR, editor. *Consultations in Feline Internal Medicine*. Philadelphia, WB Saunders: 104, 1997.

[9] German AC, Cunliffe NA, Morgan KL. Faecal consistency and risk factors for diarrhoea and constipation in cats in UK rehoming shelters. *J Feline Med Surg* 19:57, 2017.

[10] Benjamin SE, Drobatz KJ. Retrospective evaluation of risk factors and treatment outcome predictors in cats presenting to the emergency room for constipation. *J Feline Med Surg* 22:153, 2020.

[11] Trevail T et al. Radiographic diameter of the colon in normal and constipated cats and in cats with megacolon. *Vet Radiol Ultrasound* 52:516, 2011.

[12] Carr AP, Gaunt MC. Constipation resolution with administration of polyethylene glycol solution in cats. *J Vet Intern Med* 24:753, 2010.

[13] Schrader SC. Pelvic osteotomy as a treatment for obstipation in cats with acquired stenosis of the pelvic canal: six cases (1978–1989). *J Am Vet Med Assoc* 200:208, 1992.

[14] Freiche V et al. Uncontrolled study assessing the impact of a psyllium-enriched extruded dry diet on faecal consistency in cats with constipation. *J Feline Med Surg* 13:903, 2011.

[15] Rossi G et al. Effects of a probiotic (SLAB51™) on clinical and histologic variables and microbiota of cats with chronic constipation/megacolon: a pilot study. *Benef Microbes* 9:101, 2018.

[16] Hasler AH, Washabau RJ. Cisapride stimulates contraction of idiopathic megacolonic smooth muscle in cats. *J Vet Intern Med* 11:313, 1997.

[17] Kang JH et al. Use of mosapride citrate in cats with chronic constipation. WSAVA/FECAVA/BSAVA World Congress 2012.

[18] White RN. Surgical management of constipation. *J Feline Med Surg* 4:129, 2002.

[19] Deforest ME, Basrur PK. Malformations and the Manx syndrome in cats. *Can Vet J* 20:304, 1979.

[20] Quimby JM. Update on medical management of clinical manifestations of chronic kidney disease. *Vet Clin North Am Small Anim Pract* 46:1163, 2016.

[21] Atkins CE, Tyler R, Greenlee P. Clinical, biochemical, acid-base, and electrolyte abnormalities in cats after hypertonic sodium phosphate enema administration. *Am J Vet Res* 46:980, 1985.

CHAPTER 24

Pancreatic necrosis and inflammation

Panagiotis G. Xenoulis, Joerg M. Steiner

Pancreatitis is the most common disorder of the exocrine pancreas in cats.[1] Although many cases can be mild and self-limiting, some cats can develop severe disease that is associated with significant mortality. Despite that, little progress has been made with regard to elucidating the aetiology and pathophysiology of this disorder in cats, its diagnosis remains challenging, and its management is almost exclusively based on supportive and symptomatic care. It has been suggested that, similarly to humans, the majority of cases of feline pancreatitis remain undiagnosed. However, with the widespread use of more sensitive and specific diagnostic modalities and with increased awareness by clinicians, it is now being diagnosed with increasing frequency.

CLASSIFICATION AND DEFINITIONS

Classification of feline pancreatitis has not been universally standardised, and therefore there is often confusion with regard to the terminology used. Feline pancreatitis is most commonly classified based exclusively on histopathological criteria, and several studies have described and categorised the histopathological features of the pancreas in cats with pancreatitis.[1–4] There are two main distinct forms of pancreatitis in cats: acute and chronic. The main histopathological feature that differentiates the two forms is the presence of permanent histopathological lesions, which occurs in chronic pancreatitis but not in acute pancreatitis. The predominant histopathological features of acute pancreatitis are neutrophilic inflammation, peripancreatic fat necrosis, and, in cases of severe disease, pancreatic necrosis (Fig. 24.1). Some authors have further differentiated interstitial and necrotising pancreatitis, but this differentiation is often only possible post-mortem.

In contrast to acute pancreatitis, chronic pancreatitis is characterised by permanent histopathological lesions as well as lymphocytic–plasmacytic infiltration.[1–5] Fibrosis and acinar atrophy represent the main permanent histopathological changes that define chronic pancreatitis (Fig. 24.2). It should be noted that some cats show histopathological evidence of both acute and chronic pancreatitis (e.g. necrosis and concurrent fibrosis or a mixed inflammatory infiltrate). Although some authors classify these cases according to their predominant histopathological features as having either acute or chronic pancreatitis, others classify them as having both acute and chronic pancreatitis concurrently (e.g. acute on chronic pancreatitis). The term chronic active pancreatitis has been used to describe the combination of acute and chronic histopathological changes in cats with pancreatitis.

EPIDEMIOLOGY

Although pancreatitis has been established as a clinically significant disease in cats, its exact prevalence is unknown. Early necropsy studies reported a prevalence of feline pancreatitis ranging from 0.6% to 2.4% of all cats examined. However, more recent findings suggest that the prevalence of feline pancreatitis is much higher. In one study, thorough histopathological examination of pancreases from 115 healthy and diseased cats presented for postmortem examination revealed that pan-

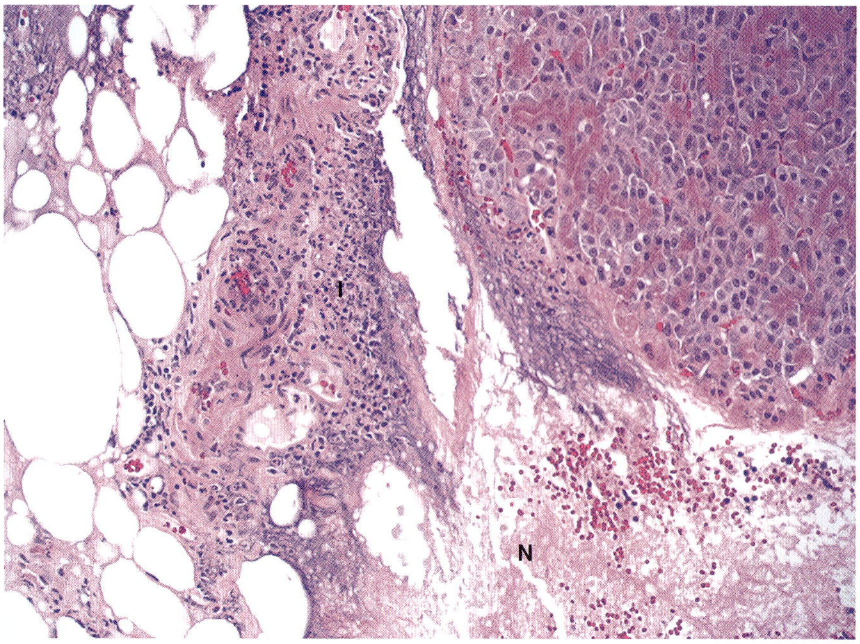

Figure 24.1. Microscopic appearance of the pancreas in a cat with acute pancreatitis. There are areas of extensive pancreatic necrosis (N) and neutrophilic infiltration (I). No fibrosis or atrophy is present. Haematoxylin–eosin stain, ×20. Image courtesy of Dr B. Porter, Texas A&M University, USA.

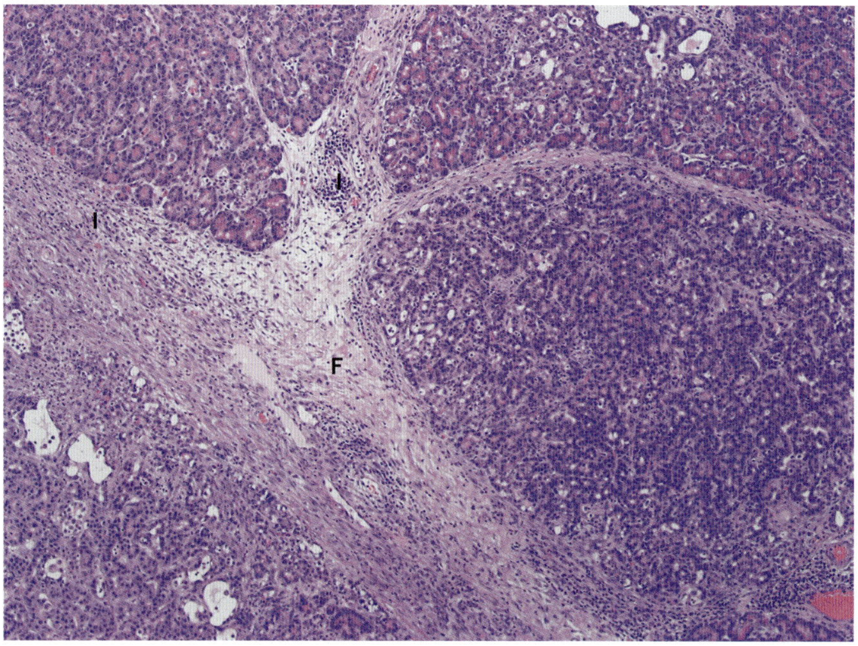

Figure 24.2. Microscopic appearance of the pancreas in a cat with chronic pancreatitis. There is extensive fibrosis (F) replacing large areas of the normal pancreatic parenchyma. There is also marked lymphocytic infiltration (I) of the pancreas. Haematoxylin–eosin stain, ×20. Image courtesy of Dr S. J. Newman, University of Tennessee, USA.

creatitis was present in 67% of cases, thus establishing pancreatitis as a common pathological condition in cats.[4] However, the fact that in the same study histopathological evidence of pancreatitis was found in 45% of apparently healthy cats raises concerns regarding the clinical significance of histopathological findings of pancreatic inflammation in cats, especially when these findings are mild.[4] This underlines the necessity for establishment of universally accepted histopathological criteria for diagnosing pancreatitis in cats.

In cats, chronic pancreatitis is considered to be more common than acute pancreatitis and has been reported in 65%–89% of all pancreatitis cases.[1,6] A necropsy study is in agreement with these findings, as chronic pancreatitis was found in 50.4% and acute pancreatitis in 6.1% of 115 cats presented for necropsy, including clinically healthy cats.[4] Concurrent evidence of both acute and chronic pancreatitis in the same animal (chronic active pancreatitis) has been reported in 9.6%–44% of cases.

AETIOLOGY AND RISK FACTORS

In the vast majority of cats with pancreatitis, an underlying initiating factor cannot be identified, and pancreatitis is considered to be idiopathic.[1,7] In a recent retrospective study, pancreatitis was considered to be idiopathic in 87% of cats hospitalised for this condition.[7] It is currently unclear whether acute and chronic pancreatitis are distinct disease entities or whether chronic pancreatitis results from recurrent attacks of acute pancreatitis, although it seems likely that both can occur. Risk factors that have been associated with the development of pancreatitis in cats are summarised in Box 24.1.

Many cats with pancreatitis have concurrent diseases. Several studies have shown an association of pancreatitis, inflammatory bowel disease (IBD), and cholangitis in cats.[6,8,9] Different combinations of these disorders may occur, and the term triaditis has been used to describe the coexistence of the three of them. In general, 50%–67% of cats with pancreatitis have triaditis.[6,8,9] Also, 50%–80% of cats with cholangitis have pancreatitis with or without IBD.[6,8,9] In a recent prospective study that included both sick and healthy cats, histopathological evidence of pancreatitis was found much more commonly in combination with IBD (25%) or with IBD and cholangitis (i.e. triaditis; 67%), rather than pancreatitis by itself (8%) or pancreatitis with cholangitis (0%).[6] In the same study, out of 40 cats with IBD, 8% also had pancreatitis, 20% had triaditis, and 40% had cholangitis, while the remaining 32% had IBD alone. In contrast, in another recent study, histopathological evidence of pancreatitis was found in only 3% of cats with intestinal infiltrative disease (e.g. IBD, lymphoma, etc.).[10] However, it should be pointed out that a direct comparison amongst studies and the determination of the exact prevalence of coexistence of pancreatitis, cholangitis, and/or IBD is problematic owing mainly to differences in study design (e.g. postmortem vs. antemortem studies) and histopathological classification used.

At the time of this writing, it is uncertain which disease occurs first and what role pancreatitis plays in the pathogenesis of the other disorders. One could speculate that chronic vomiting, which is the most common clinical sign of IBD in cats, could permit reflux of duodenal fluid into the pancreaticobiliary ductal system (the major pancreatic duct and the common bile duct fuse together and constitute a common anatomical and physiological structure in cats), and this could potentially lead to pancreatitis and cholangitis. Due to the common coexistence of the three pathological conditions, cats with known IBD and/or biliary disease should be considered at risk for developing pancreatitis.

An association between diabetes mellitus (DM) and pancreatitis has also been identified in several studies. The exact nature of this association has not yet been determined, but it is likely that DM may be predisposing to pancreatitis, as the inflammation does not spare the islets of Langerhans (see section "Complications of pancreatitis" in this chapter). In addition, experimental hyperglycaemia has been shown to induce pancreatic inflammation in cats.[11]

Some more important risk factors for pancreatitis in cats include trauma (e.g. traffic accidents, high-rise syndrome), ischaemia (e.g. due to hypotension during general anaesthesia), or hypercalcaemia. Other less commonly suspected risk factors include pancreatic tumours,

Box 24.1. Factors that have been implicated in the aetiology of pancreatitis in cats.

Common factors
- Inflammatory bowel disease
- Biliary tract disease (cholangitis, obstruction)
- Ischaemia (e.g. hypotension, anaesthesia)
- Trauma (e.g. car accident, high-rise syndrome)

Uncommon factors
- Pancreatic duct obstruction (e.g. neoplasia)
- Organophosphates
- Hypercalcaemia
- Drugs
- Infectious agents (rare)
  - *Toxoplasma gondii*
  - *Eurytrema procyonis* (pancreatic fluke)
  - *Amphimerus pseudofelineus* (liver fluke)
  - Feline calicivirus (virulent strain)
  - Feline parvovirus
  - Feline herpesvirus

pancreatic ductal obstructions (e.g. as a result of intra- or extrapancreatic neoplasia), and organophosphate poisoning (e.g. fenthion).[1] Several systemic infectious diseases have been reported or suspected to be occasionally associated with pancreatitis, but none has been reported as an important cause of pancreatitis in cats. Hepatic (e.g. *Amphimerus pseudofelineus*) or pancreatic flukes (e.g. *Eurytrema procyonis*) can also cause pancreatitis in cats, but these cases are exceedingly rare. Recently, an association between feline pancreatitis and immune-mediated haemolytic anaemia has been reported, although it is currently unknown exactly how these two conditions are connected pathophysiologically and which disease occurs first. Other risk factors reported to have an association with pancreatitis in dogs such as obesity, high-fat diets, dietary indiscretion, and drug administration (other than fenthion) have not been reported in cats, although there is anecdotal evidence that high-fat diets may also play a role in the development of pancreatitis in cats.

PATHOPHYSIOLOGY

The initiating events that lead to acute pancreatitis take place in the acinar cell. Retention and intracellular activation of zymogens (i.e. pancreatic enzyme precursors stored in zymogen granules) as well as disruption of the paracellular barrier in the pancreatic duct that allows its contents to leak into the paracellular space are the main intracellular events that lead to the development of acute pancreatitis. Once intracellular activation of pancreatic enzymes has taken place, autodigestion of the acinar cell follows, and activated enzymes escape into the pancreatic tissue (leading to local effects), the peritoneal cavity, and the systemic circulation (potentially contributing to systemic effects). Local effects vary and can range from mild interstitial oedema to severe acinar cell necrosis, haemorrhage, and peripancreatic fat necrosis. Acinar cell injury leads to recruitment and activation of inflammatory cells (mostly neutrophils and macrophages), which release pro-inflammatory cytokines and other inflammatory mediators (e.g. interleukin [IL]-1, IL-2, IL-6, IL-18, tumour necrosis factor alpha, substance P, platelet-activating factor) that play a crucial role in modulating systemic manifestations. Such manifestations include cardiovascular shock, disseminated intravascular coagulation, systemic inflammatory response syndrome, and multi-organ failure, and they are seen in cases of severe acute pancreatitis.

DIAGNOSIS

Over the past two decades, the development of new diagnostic modalities and the publication of several studies that evaluated the performance of various diagnostic tests for the diagnosis of pancreatitis in cats have provided clinicians with useful information, and pancreatitis has been diagnosed much more frequently than in the past. Despite this, accurate premortem diagnosis or rule out of pancreatitis in cats is often challenging. Feline pancreatitis should be suspected on the basis of suggestive historical and physical examination findings and routine clinical pathology. The diagnosis should be confirmed by more specific diagnostic tests. A diagnostic algorithm for feline pancreatitis is shown in Figure 24.3. Detailed and up-to-date reviews on the diagnosis of pancreatitis in cats have recently been published.[12,13]

Signalment

Cats of any age, breed, or sex can develop pancreatitis. Older cats appear to be more likely to develop pancreatitis, especially the chronic form, although the age range reported is very wide (5 weeks–20 years). Domestic shorthair and Siamese cats have been reported to be at increased risk in some studies, but this has not been confirmed in other studies.

Clinical features

Acute and chronic pancreatitis in cats cannot be differentiated based on clinical signs or the duration of illness.[3] Although both acute and chronic pancreatitis can range in severity from mild to severe, chronic pancreatitis is more commonly mild, while acute pancreatitis is more commonly severe. Severe pancreatitis is associated with systemic signs and local and systemic complications. Mild cases of pancreatitis are believed to often remain subclinical or be associated with mild clinical signs that are often not detected by the owners (e.g. mild or occasional hyporexia and low-grade weight loss in cats with chronic pancreatitis).[4] When clinical signs are present, they are usually nonspecific. By far, the most common clinical

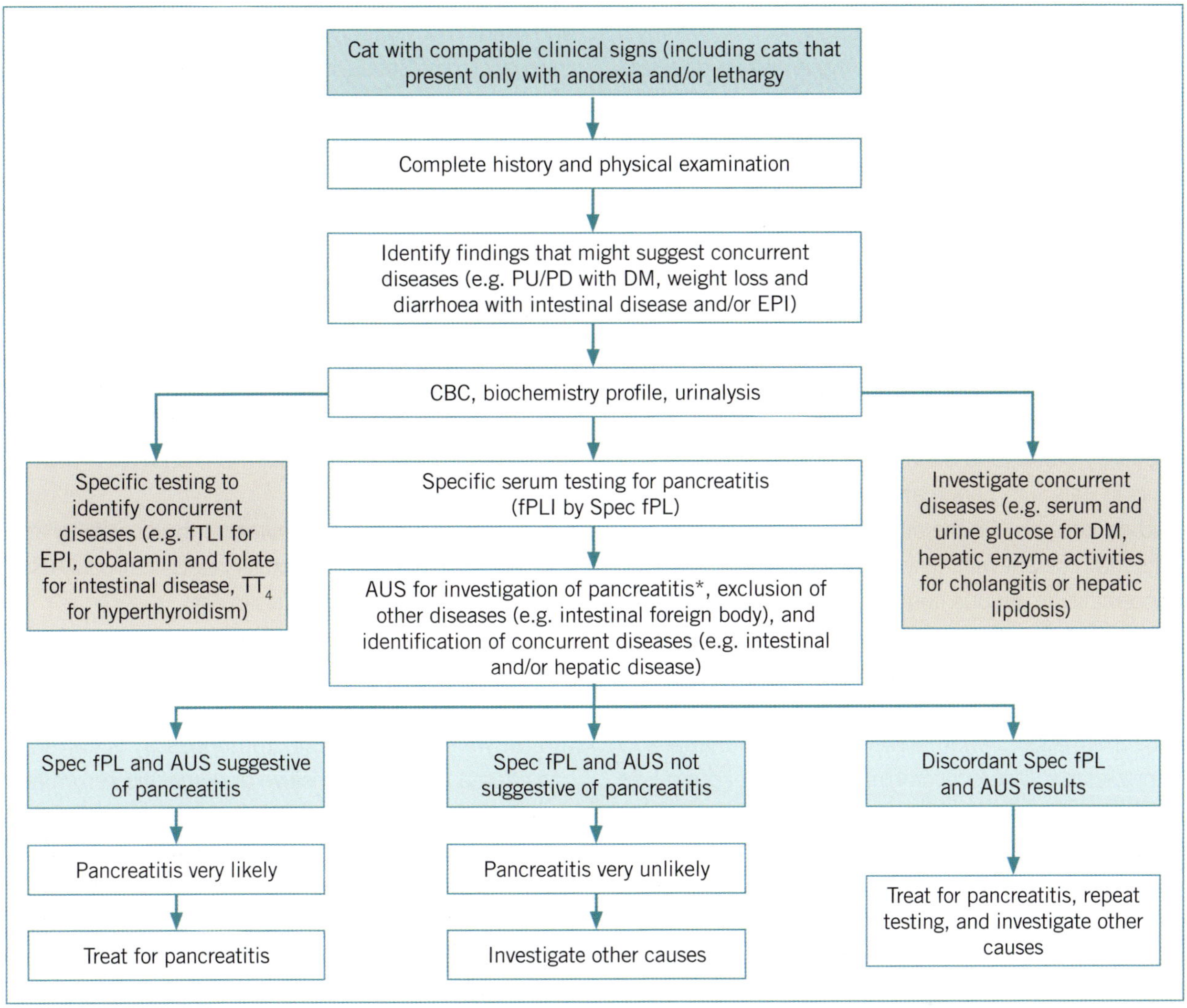

Figure 24.3. Algorithm for the diagnosis of pancreatitis in the cat. AUS, abdominal ultrasound; CBC, complete blood count; DM, diabetes mellitus; EPI, exocrine pancreatic insufficiency; fPL, feline pancreatic lipase; fPLI, feline pancreatic lipase immunoreactivity; fTLI, feline trypsin-like immunoreactivity; PU/PD, polyuria and polydipsia; TT_4, total thyroxine.
*Abdominal ultrasonography has low sensitivity in cats with chronic pancreatitis.

signs in cats with acute or chronic pancreatitis are hyporexia or anorexia (62%–97%) and lethargy (28%–100%), which can be seen in a wide range of other diseases.[3,4,7,8] Less frequently seen clinical signs include vomiting (35%–61%), weight loss (21%–61%), and diarrhoea (11%–33%). It is important to note that vomiting and abdominal pain, which are common and considered suggestive of pancreatitis in dogs, are considerably less common in cats with pancreatitis. For example, in one study, abdominal pain was reported in only 22% of 157 cats hospitalised for pancreatitis.[7] The most common physical examination findings in cats with pancreatitis include dehydration, pallor, and icterus. Tachypnoea and/or dyspnoea, hypothermia/fever, tachycardia, signs of abdominal pain, and/or a palpable abdominal mass may also be noted. Severe systemic complications may occasionally be seen in cats with severe pancreatitis and may include disseminated intravascular coagulation, pulmonary thromboembolism, cardiovascular shock, and multi-organ failure. In two studies, 26% of 46 cats with disseminated intravascular coagulation and 11.8% of 17 cats with pulmonary thromboembolism had pancreatitis as the underlying condition. Finally, other clinical signs may be seen as a consequence of concurrent diseases (e.g. polyuria/polydipsia in cats with DM, weight loss and unformed faeces in cats with exocrine pancreatic insufficiency).

Routine clinical pathology

A complete blood count, serum biochemistry profile, and urinalysis should always be performed in cats suspected of having pancreatitis. Although the findings of these tests are nonspecific and cannot confirm or rule out pancreatitis, they are useful for the diagnosis and exclusion of other differential diagnoses and give important information about the general condition of the animal. These tests also help recognise specific abnormalities (e.g. electrolyte disturbances), the correction of which is crucial for the management of the cat.

The results of the complete blood count, serum biochemistry profile, and urinalysis are often within normal limits in cats with pancreatitis, especially in those with mild pancreatitis. On the other hand, cats with pancreatitis may present with almost any kind of haematologic abnormality in various combinations, including leucocytosis or, less commonly, leucopenia, regenerative or nonregenerative anaemia or haemoconcentration, and thrombocytopenia or thrombocytosis.[2,3,7,8] Biochemical abnormalities, when present, are also variable and unpredictable. Different combinations of increases in liver enzyme activities and hyperbilirubinaemia are common and, when present, should raise the suspicion for pancreatitis. In some cases, these findings might be associated with extrahepatic bile duct obstruction (EHBDO), while in others it might suggest concurrent cholangitis or hepatic lipidosis. Increases in serum creatinine, blood urea nitrogen (BUN), or symmetric dimethylarginine concentrations are variably present and most often associated with dehydration due to vomiting, diarrhoea, and/or decreased water intake. In severe cases, azotaemia might be the result of concurrent renal disease. Other possible findings include hypercholesterolaemia, hypoalbuminaemia, and hyperglycaemia. The latter can be transient or permanent, in which case, it reflects concurrent DM.[2,3,7,8]

A variety of electrolyte abnormalities may be present in cats with pancreatitis, with hypocalcaemia and hypokalaemia being the most common.[3,7,14] Up to 60% of cats with pancreatitis have hypocalcaemia, and therefore this finding should always raise the suspicion for pancreatitis in cats with compatible clinical signs. Subnormal ionised plasma calcium concentrations (≤1 mmol/l) in cats with pancreatitis have been shown to be associated with a poor prognosis.[14] Cats with chronic pancreatitis and triaditis or concurrent IBD may also have cobalamin deficiency. Because hypocobalaminaemic cats with gastrointestinal (GI) disease can benefit from cobalamin supplementation, serum cobalamin should be measured in cats suspected of having pancreatitis.

It should be noted that laboratory findings similar to those described above have been found in cats with a histologically normal pancreas, indicating that these findings are not specific for pancreatitis and, in some cases, may be the result of concurrent diseases rather than pancreatitis per se.

Serum tests for pancreatic function and pathology

Table 24.1 provides an overview of the sensitivity and specificity of the different laboratory tests commonly used for the diagnosis of pancreatitis in cats.

Pancreatic lipase immunoreactivity

Measuring feline pancreatic lipase immunoreactivity (fPLI) by a species-specific immunoassay is currently considered the most sensitive and specific serum test for the diagnosis of pancreatitis in cats. Pancreatic lipase is a pancreatic enzyme synthesised in the acinar cells and normally secreted into the pancreatic ductal system through which it reaches the duodenum, with only minimal amounts entering the circulation. However, during pancreatitis, larger amounts enter the circulation and can be quantified by a fPLI immunoassay. The advantages of this assay over the traditional lipase activity assays rely on two facts: pancreatic lipase is exclusively of pancreatic origin, and, in contrast to the traditional activity assays for lipase, which indiscriminately measure the activities of lipases of multiple cellular origins, immunoassays exclusively measure the concentration of pancreatic lipase in serum based on its unique three-dimensional structure.[12] Therefore, fPLI immunoassays have inherent advantages over the traditional serum lipase activity assays that make them more suitable for specific evaluation of the exocrine pancreas in cats.

The originally developed immunoassay for the measurement of fPLI has been replaced by a more widely available immunoassay (Spec fPL).[12] The reference interval of this assay is 0–3.5 µg/l, with a grey zone in the interpretation of the results (3.6–5.3 µg/l); values in the grey zone are nondiagnostic, and further testing or retesting is recommended. Concentrations greater than or equal to 5.4 µg/l (measured by Spec fPL) are considered highly suggestive of pancreatitis.[12] A recent study suggested that serum fPLI concentrations (measured by Spec fPL) have high individuality and that population-based reference intervals may fail to detect clinically significant differences in pancreatic physiology in cats. Use of subject-based reference intervals might be more useful for this test, but this requires further research.

Studies in cats with both experimental and spontaneous pancreatitis have repeatedly shown that serum fPLI is one of the most sensitive and specific serum markers currently available for the diagnosis of feline pancreatitis.[8,15–17] In a recent retrospective study of 274 cats, Spec fPL was reported to have a sensitivity of about 76% in cats with definite or probable pancreatitis.[16] In another clinical study of 182 cats, the sensitivity of measuring serum fPLI concentrations by Spec fPL was reported to be 79%.[18] In a study that included primarily cats with chronic pancreatitis that also had an acute histopathological component, serum fPLI measurement was found to be 100% sensitive for histopathologically moderate to severe pancreatitis.[8] In the same study, the sensitivity of the test was 54% for histopathologically mild pancreatitis, with an overall sensitivity of 67%. For comparison, the overall sensitivity of the feline trypsin-like immunoreactivity (fTLI) assay in the same study was only 28%. Similar results were reported in a histopathological study from Germany, in which fPLI assay sensitivity ranged from 57% to 82%, depending on the histopathological severity of pancreatitis and the cutoff for fPLI.[17] It must be noted that patients with end-stage chronic pancreatitis, where pancreatic fibrosis and atrophy are the predominant histopathological features, may not show leakage of pancreatic enzymes, and therefore the sensitivity of the fPLI assay is believed to be lower for chronic pancreatitis (without concurrent acute pancreatitis) than for acute pancreatitis.[13] Therefore, false-negative results exist, especially in cats with end-stage or mild chronic pancreatitis.[17]

Similar to its sensitivity, the specificity of serum fPLI measurement for the diagnosis of feline pancreatitis is very high, with reported values of 67%–100%.[8,16,18] In a recent clinical study of 274 cats, Spec fPL had a specificity of about 90%.[16] In another clinical study of 182 cats, the specificity of fPLI measurement was 82%.[18] In another study, azotaemia as a result of experimentally induced chronic renal failure did not have any clinically significant effect on serum fPLI concentrations.[19] Finally, other pancreatic conditions, such as pancreatic neoplasia, that are often associated with concurrent pancreatitis can lead to increased serum fPLI concentrations.[17]

A rapid, in-clinic, semiquantitative test (SNAP fPL) for the estimation of feline pancreatic lipase in serum has recently been developed.[12,20] It incorporates a reference spot that corresponds to the upper limit of the reference interval and a sample spot that is visually compared to the reference spot. Therefore, the results of this test are considered either normal (less intense than the reference spot) or abnormal (equally to or more intense than the reference spot). In the latter case, the actual fPLI concentration may be in the grey zone or consistent with the diagnosis of pancreatitis. This cannot be determined with certainty, however, using the in-clinic assay, and further testing using the quantitative reference method is recommended. The manufacturer indicates that this test has an 82%–92% agreement with the Spec fPL assay. In a recent clinical study, the agreement between SNAP fPL and Spec fPL was 97.5% for negative results and 90% for positive results, suggesting that overall there is a high agreement between the two methods.[15] This study concluded that the SNAP fPL was a valuable tool to exclude or include pancreatitis as a differential diagnosis in an emergency setting.[15] However, abnormal results could be in the grey zone or consistent with the diagnosis of pancreatitis, and further testing using the quantitative Spec fPL assay would be necessary. Another patient-side assay, the VCheck fPL, is available in parts of Asia. This species-specific assay has not been assessed in the primary literature; however, the VCheck cPL for use in dogs failed analytic validation.[21]

Trypsin-like immunoreactivity

Trypsin-like immunoreactivity (TLI) is a species-specific immunoassay that measures trypsinogen (and trypsin) in serum. Serum fTLI measurement has been evaluated for the diagnosis of spontaneous feline pancreatitis, and several cutoff values for pancreatitis have been suggested. The main limitation of fTLI is that when cutoff values allowing adequate specificity of the assay are used (e.g. 100 µg/l), the sensitivity of the fTLI assay for the diagnosis of pancreatitis in cats is low (28%–33%).[8,13] Although serum fTLI is considered to be specific for pancreatitis (i.e. trypsin is theoretically produced exclusively by the pancreatic acinar cells), its specificity has been questioned because high fTLI concentrations have been reported in cats with no demonstrable pancreatic disease (although localised lesions might have been missed on histopathology) that had other GI disorders (e.g. IBD, GI lymphoma) or azotaemia. In the face of availability of tests with better performance, the fTLI assay is currently considered to be of limited usefulness for diagnosing pancreatitis in cats.[13]

Amylase and lipase

Serum amylase and lipase activities have been evaluated in both experimental and spontaneous feline pancreatitis. Results of clinical studies suggest that traditional catalytic assays for the measurement of serum amylase and lipase activities are of no clinical value in cats and should not be used for the diagnosis of feline pancreatitis due to unacceptably low specificity and sensitivity.[13]

DGGR assay

More recently developed colourimetric lipase activity assays, such as the 1,2-o-dilauryl-rac-glycero-3-glutaric acid-(6'-methylresorufin) ester (DGGR) assay, have shown better performance than traditional catalytic assays. Supposedly, this substrate is more specific for pancreatic lipase that traditional catalytic assays, and some studies that compared DGGR assays with Spec fPL have suggested similar performance between the two.[22–24] However, it should be noted that there are various DGGR-based assays for serum lipase activity, and they differ dramatically due to changes in added compounds (e.g. colipase, bile acids) and assay conditions (e.g. pH). The analyser used can also have an impact on test results. Moreover, none of the currently available DGGR-based assays have been shown to be more specific for the measurement of pancreatic lipase than more traditional serum lipase activity assays. For example, a recent experimental study in cats showed that DGGR is not only hydrolysed by pancreatic lipase but also by lipoprotein lipase or hepatic lipase, or both. These extrapancreatic lipases may contribute to a lack of analytic specificity of this assay.[35] In the same study, there was no significant effect of heparin on serum fPLI concentrations (measured by Spec fPL). Therefore, further studies are needed before DGGR lipase assays can be recommended for the routine use of diagnosing pancreatitis in cats.

Diagnostic imaging

Table 24.1 provides an overview of the sensitivity and specificity of the imaging techniques commonly used for the diagnosis of pancreatitis in cats.

Radiography

Conclusive diagnosis or exclusion of pancreatitis is not possible based on abdominal radiography alone, but radiography may be used as an initial approach for cats suspected of having pancreatitis because it is relatively inexpensive and useful for the diagnosis and/or exclusion of other diseases that may cause similar clinical signs. Abdominal radiography lacks both specificity and sensitivity in identifying pancreatitis in cats.[3,13] In the majority of cases of feline pancreatitis, abdominal radiographs are normal or display nonspecific findings. Also, differentiation of acute and chronic pancreatitis is not possible on the basis of abdominal radiography.[3] The most common radiographic finding in cats with pancreatitis is decreased detail and contrast in the cranial abdomen possibly due to abdominal effusion, which is reported in 30%–50% of cases.[3] Other radiological findings that might be identified less frequently in cats with pancreatitis include dilation of the small intestine (due to fluid or gas), hepatomegaly, and presence of a cranial abdominal mass.[3,13] The more typical findings (i.e. increased opacity of the right cranial abdomen, displacement of abdominal organs) reported in dogs with pancreatitis have rarely been reported in cats with pancreatitis. In any case, in cats suspected of having pancreatitis, radiography should always be followed by more sensitive and specific tests.

Ultrasonography

Abdominal ultrasound is currently considered the imaging modality of choice for the diagnosis of pancreatitis in dogs and cats.[13] Furthermore, abdominal ultrasound is useful for the diagnosis or to rule out other diseases that cause similar clinical signs. It is of utmost importance to recognise the fact that the performance of abdominal ultrasonography for the diagnosis of pancreatitis is highly dependent on the expertise of the ultrasonographer and the quality of the equipment used. In most reported studies, abdominal ultrasonography has been performed at teaching hospitals by board-certified radiologists with a special interest in pancreatic ultrasonography, and therefore the performance of abdominal ultrasound for diagnosing pancreatitis is expected to be considerably lower when performed by clinicians with less experience. Also, the severity of the disease affects the sensitivity and specificity of ultrasonography. The sensitivity of ultrasonography for diagnosing necrotising pancreatitis in cats is far higher than for mild chronic pancreatitis.

The reported sensitivity of abdominal ultrasonography for the diagnosis of feline pancreatitis is generally low (11%–35%), with only one study reporting a sensitivity of 67%.[13] In one study, when only cases with moderate to severe pancreatitis were included in the analysis, the sensitivity was 80%. Differentiation of acute and chronic pancreatitis is not possible based on ultrasound examination.[3] All the aforementioned studies used histopathology as the gold standard for diagnosing pancreatitis. This wide range of reported sensitivity likely reflects differences in the level of suspicion or skill of the ultrasonographer, the equipment used, and the severity of lesions and highlights the lack of standardised diagnostic criteria.[13] However, it should be noted that these studies were published more than a decade ago. Since then, there have been significant advances in both the quality of the equipment and the knowledge concerning the frequency of pancreatitis, and the level of suspicion for pancreatitis in small animal medicine has increased. Therefore, the performance of ultrasonography is expected to have improved since those reports were published.

Other more recent studies have evaluated the agreement between serum fPLI concentration and ultrasonography, and the results often show conflicting results. In one study, the sensitivity and specificity of pancreatic ultrasonography in cats with increased serum fPLI and clinical signs indicative of pancreatitis was 84% and 75%, respectively.[25] In another study, a significant agreement was found between serum fPLI concentration and abdominal ultrasonography for the diagnosis of traumatic pancreatitis in a group of cats with high-rise syndrome. However, in another study, a poor to fair agreement was reported between serum fPLI concentration and ultrasonography in cats with a suspicion of pancreatitis.[23] Finally, in another study, only 25% of cats with increased fPLI concentrations had ultrasonographic evidence of pancreatitis.[26] Based on these studies, it is impossible to determine which diagnostic test is more accurate (i.e. fPLI assay or ultrasonography), and therefore the results should be interpreted with caution.

The sensitivity of abdominal ultrasound reported in the aforementioned studies clearly indicates that a normal pancreas on ultrasound examination cannot rule out pancreatitis. This can happen in cases of acute pancreatitis but is particularly true in cases of chronic or mild pancreatitis, where pancreatic changes are minimal. In cases where ultrasonographic examination of the pancreas is unremarkable but clinical suspicion of pancreatitis is high, it is recommended to repeat the ultrasound examination 1–4 days later, as this time period might be sufficient for ultrasonographic changes to appear.

The specificity of abdominal ultrasound for diagnosing feline pancreatitis is considered relatively high when stringent criteria are used. However, other diseases of the pancreas (e.g. neoplasia, hyperplastic nodules, oedema due to portal hypertension or hypoalbuminaemia) may display similar ultrasonographic findings and cannot be differentiated from pancreatitis in many cases.[13,27]

The most common and relatively specific ultrasonographic findings in cats with pancreatitis are hypoechogenicity of the pancreas (suggesting pancreatic necrosis or oedema) and increased peripancreatic echogenicity (indicating peripancreatic fat necrosis) (Fig. 24.4).[2,3,7,22–24] Changes in echogenicity of the pancreas are probably the most useful for the diagnosis of feline pancreatitis, but they are not always present. Abdominal effusion or peripancreatic free fluid is also commonly seen but is even less specific for pancreatitis. Other possible ultrasonographic findings in cats with pancreatitis include an enlarged pancreas, irregular pancreatic margins, cavitary lesions of the pancreas (e.g. pseudocysts), and calcification of the pancreas.[2,3,7,22–24] It has been suggested that dilation of the pancreatic duct is suggestive of pancreatitis in cats, but recent studies have not confirmed this hypothesis. Instead, it was shown that the diameter of the pancreatic duct in healthy cats increases with age. On occasion, hyperechoic areas of the pancreas can be identified, possibly indicating the presence of pancreatic fibrosis.[13,24]

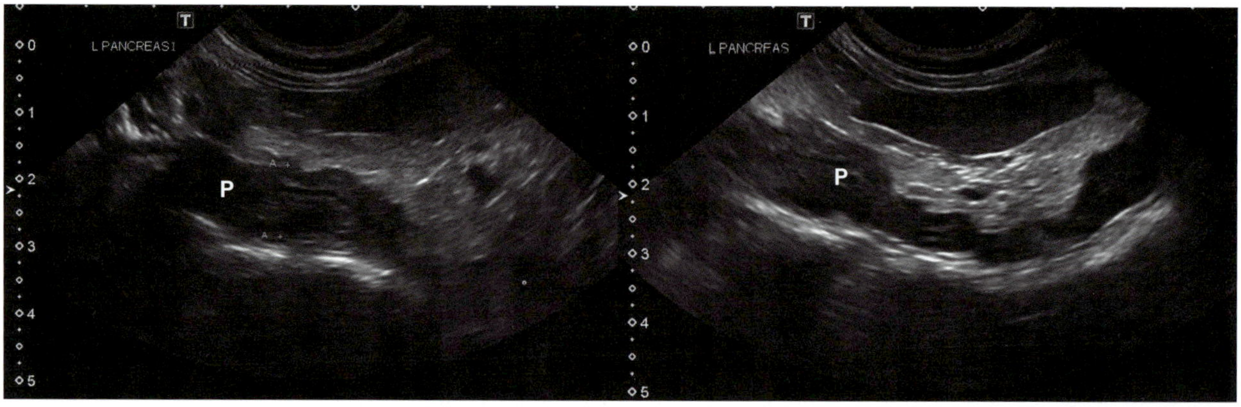

Figure 24.4. Sagittal ultrasound images from a 14-year-old spayed female domestic shorthair cat diagnosed with triaditis: cholangitis, cholecystitis, inflammatory bowel disease, and pancreatitis. The left limb of the pancreas (P) shows enlargement in thickness and length. The pancreas is diffusely hypoechoic, surrounded by hyperechoic peripancreatic mesentery. The pancreas is also irregularly marginated. These findings represent acute pancreatitis. Image courtesy of Dr L. Gaschen, Louisiana State University, USA.

Other imaging modalities

In one older study, computed tomography performed in cats with histologically confirmed pancreatitis showed a very low sensitivity (20%).[8] However, with additional studies and improvement of equipment and knowledge, this diagnostic modality may prove more useful in the future. Other imaging modalities (e.g. endoscopic retrograde cholangiopancreatography [ERCP], endoscopic ultrasonography) have been used in healthy cats as well as in cats with pancreatitis with varying results. Also, a recent study evaluated the usefulness of magnetic resonance imaging and magnetic resonance cholangiopancreatography (MRCP) for the diagnosis of pancreatitis in cats and reported promising results. However, due to the lack of standardised criteria for the diagnosis of pancreatitis, the complexity of these imaging modalities, the necessity for general anaesthesia, the limited availability, and the cost of the equipment, none of the above methods can currently be recommended for the routine diagnosis of feline pancreatitis.

Cytology

Fine needle aspiration (FNA) of the pancreas and cytological examination of the aspirated material is a minimally invasive technique that can be used for the diagnosis and differentiation of pancreatitis and other exocrine pancreatic diseases in cats (Table 24.1). It is usually performed either under ultrasonographic guidance or during laparotomy. In a recent study, in which ultrasound-guided pancreatic aspiration was performed in 73 cats, the procedure was found to be safe, and the aspirated material was diagnostic in 67% of the samples obtained.[28] However, ultrasound-guided pancreatic aspiration may be somewhat technically demanding, especially for the general practitioner. In the same study, there was an 86% agreement with histopathology in the small number of cats for which histopathology was also available.[28] This is encouraging, but to date there are no other studies that have evaluated the sensitivity and specificity of this diagnostic modality for the diagnosis of feline pancreatitis.

It is logical to assume that the finding of inflammatory cells within the aspirated material from the pancreas should be specific for pancreatitis. Pancreatic acinar cells constitute the majority of the cells found in FNA smears from a normal pancreas. In animals with acute pancreatitis, the cytological picture is mainly characterised by the presence of intact and degenerated neutrophils and degenerated pancreatic acinar cells (Fig. 24.5). In animals with chronic pancreatitis, small numbers of lymphocytes are usually present, and the specimen is often characterised by low cellularity, possibly due to replacement of the normal pancreatic tissue by fibrotic tissue. It should be highlighted that, as for histopathology, localised lesions might be missed. Thus, negative FNA cytology results are not sufficient to rule out pancreatitis.

Gross pathology and histopathology

Direct visualisation of the pancreas is possible during exploratory laparotomy or laparoscopy or during necropsy. When certain gross pancreatic lesions are present,

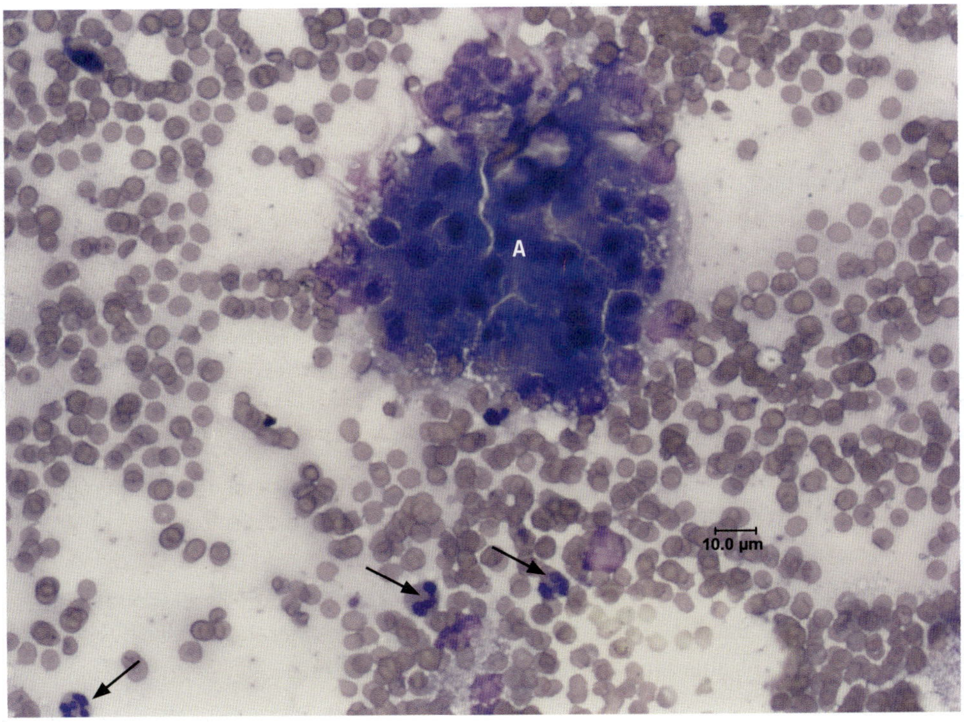

Figure 24.5. Microscopic image of a fine needle aspiration sample obtained from a feline pancreas with pancreatitis. There is mild to moderate neutrophilic inflammation, as indicated by the presence of neutrophils (arrows). A cluster of normal acinar cells (A) can be seen. Diff-Quick, ×500. Image courtesy of Dr P. J. Armstrong, University of Minnesota, USA.

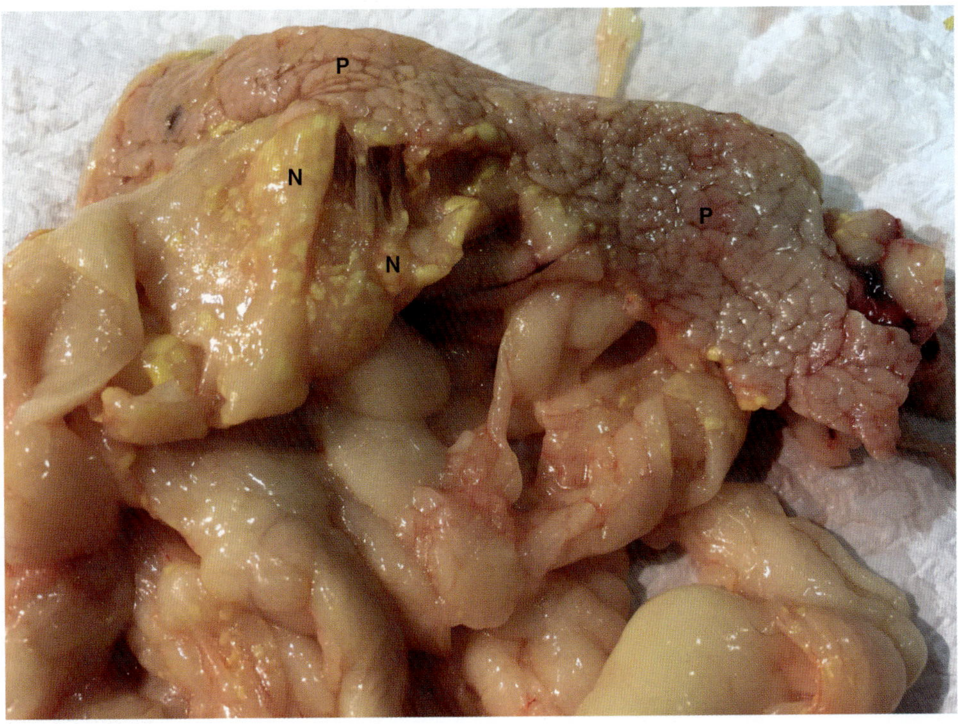

Figure 24.6. Gross appearance of the pancreas of a cat with pancreatitis. The pancreas (P) appears oedematous, granular, and haemorrhagic, and there is extensive peripancreatic fat necrosis (N). These macroscopic changes are highly suggestive of pancreatitis.

they are highly suggestive of pancreatitis and are usually the preferred sites for biopsy collection. Such lesions have been reported in up to 85% of cats with pancreatitis and may include pancreatic oedema, pancreatic haemorrhage and congestion, pancreatic nodules or plaques, pancreatic necrosis, peripancreatic fat necrosis (saponified fat), and a dull granular capsular surface (Fig. 24.6).[2,6]

At present, a definitive diagnosis of pancreatitis can only be made by histopathological examination of the pancreas (Table 24.1).[13] Histopathology is also the only diagnostic modality by which definitive differentiation of acute and chronic pancreatitis is possible, and a histopathological scoring system, which reflects on the severity of the lesions of acute and chronic pancreatitis, has recently been proposed in cats.[4] However, several limitations are associated with pancreatic histopathology as a definitive tool for pancreatitis. Firstly, determining the clinical significance of the histopathological findings may be quite challenging. In a recent study, histopathological lesions of pancreatitis (mostly chronic) were found in 67% of all cats examined, including 45% of healthy cats.[4] These findings suggest that pancreatitis, especially the chronic form, is often subclinical. Thus, extreme caution should be taken not to overinterpret histopathological lesions, especially if these are mild, as they might constitute an incidental finding and may not reflect on the cause of the clinical signs at the time of presentation. Secondly, definitive exclusion of pancreatitis based on histopathology is not possible because inflammatory lesions of the pancreas are often localised and can easily be missed.[4] Thus, multiple sections from every portion of the pancreas must be evaluated in order to increase the likelihood of identifying microscopic lesions. Negative results of histopathology must therefore be interpreted with caution, especially when only one section of the pancreas has been examined. A higher likelihood to detect lesions in the left pancreatic limb has been reported in cats.[4] Lastly, pancreatic histopathology requires invasive procedures (typically surgery), which are expensive and potentially detrimental in cats that are severely debilitated. However, in one study of 300 cats, 164 of which underwent pancreatic biopsy (along with intestinal and hepatic biopsies), no clinically important consequences were noted.[10]

Table 24.1. Reported sensitivities and specificities of commonly used tests for the diagnosis of feline pancreatitis.[13]

Diagnostic test	Sensitivity (%)	Specificity (%)	Comments
Pancreatic enzymes			
Serum feline pancreatic lipase immunoreactivity (Spec fPL)	54–100	91–100	Highly sensitive and specific. Most accurate serum test for pancreatitis currently available.
Serum feline trypsin-like immunoreactivity	28–64	82	Low sensitivity. Normal concentrations do not exclude pancreatitis. Renal failure and intestinal disease might give false-positive results. High concentrations in the absence of renal or intestinal disease are suggestive of pancreatitis.
Serum amylase	Low	Low	Not useful for the diagnosis of pancreatitis.
Serum lipase	Low	Low	Not useful for the diagnosis of pancreatitis.
Serum DGGR	67	79–100	Likely highly sensitive and specific. Performs similar to the Spec fPL assay.
Imaging			
Abdominal radiography	Low	Low	Not useful for the diagnosis or exclusion of pancreatitis. Useful for the evaluation of other diseases.
Abdominal ultrasonography	11–67	Relatively high	Useful for the diagnosis of pancreatitis. It is very operator- and equipment-dependent. Relatively high specificity if stringent criteria are met. Negative results do not rule out pancreatitis.
Pancreatic biopsy			
Cytology	Unknown	Unknown (can be high)	Minimally invasive. Specificity is believed to be high, but pancreatic lesions might be missed if they are localised, thereby decreasing sensitivity.
Histopathology	Can be high	High	The gold standard for confirmation of pancreatitis. However, it is invasive, expensive, and cannot be performed in severely compromised patients. Since lesions are often highly localised, multiple biopsy samples must be evaluated before pancreatitis can be ruled out (potentially low sensitivity if only one biopsy sample is evaluated).

DGGR, 1,2-o-dilauryl-rac-glycero-3-glutaric acid-(6'-methylresorufin) ester; fPL, feline pancreatic lipase.

Because more than 50% of cats with pancreatitis also have concurrent inflammation of the liver and/or intestines (i.e. triaditis), hepatic and intestinal biopsies should also be considered in cats undergoing pancreatic biopsy. Likewise, cats with IBD and/or cholangitis undergoing surgery for intestinal and/or hepatic biopsies should ideally also have their pancreas biopsied.[6,10]

MANAGEMENT OF SEVERE (ACUTE) PANCREATITIS

As mentioned previously, acute and chronic pancreatitis in cats cannot be differentiated based on clinical signs or the duration of illness.[3] Despite this, treatment of feline pancreatitis is based almost exclusively on supportive care. See Appendix for a summary of recommended dosages of the medications mentioned below. Although in most cases of pancreatitis the aetiology remains unknown, any potential risk factors (e.g. hypercalcaemia, IBD, parasites), should be investigated and, if possible, properly managed.

Fluid and electrolyte therapy

Cats with severe pancreatitis are often presented with variable degrees of dehydration or hypovolaemia, or both, due to ongoing anorexia, vomiting, and/or diarrhoea. Aggressive intravenous fluid therapy is very important in severely dehydrated or hypovolaemic animals and should be initiated as soon as possible, as maintenance of tissue and pancreatic perfusion is crucial in these cases. However, close monitoring is required in order not to overhydrate the patient. Crystalloid fluids (e.g. lactated Ringer's solution and 0.9% NaCl) are usually the preferred choice, but administration of colloid fluids (e.g. hetastarch) might be indicated in cases of severe hypoalbuminaemia or hypotension. Fresh frozen plasma might also be used in cases of hypoalbuminaemia (it also contains protease inhibitors and coagulation factors), although no studies have evaluated the usefulness of this approach in cats with pancreatitis. Whole blood transfusion might be indicated in cases with severe anaemia.

Hypokalaemia is often present as a result of potassium loss due to combinations of diarrhoea, vomiting, fluid therapy, and anorexia or food being withheld (a practice that is outdated, see below). Therefore, serum potassium should be monitored throughout hospitalisation, and potassium must be added to the intravenous fluids if necessary (starting at 20–30 mEq/l KCl). Hypocalcaemia is also common in cats with pancreatitis and is associated with a poor prognosis.[14] When moderate to severe hypocalcaemia is present, 10% calcium gluconate (60–90 mg/kg IV over 12–24 hours) may be given, and serum total and/or ionised calcium should be monitored during therapy. Other electrolyte and acid–base balance disturbances should also be identified and corrected.

Nutritional therapy

Traditionally, nutritional strategies in patients with acute pancreatitis were aimed at reducing pancreatic stimulation, enzyme release, and, consequently, pancreatic autodigestion by withholding food (a practice commonly referred to as "resting the pancreas"). However, experimental animal studies and studies in humans suggest that pancreatitis itself is in fact associated with reduced enzyme secretion and that enteral feeding has no stimulatory effects on pancreatic secretion. Furthermore, there is mounting evidence that humans and dogs with acute pancreatitis actually benefit from early enteral nutritional support. Studies have also shown that enteral nutrition is superior to total parenteral nutrition in the treatment of acute pancreatitis in humans and other animals, and enteral nutrition has now become the gold standard of nutritional management in humans with acute pancreatitis. Lack of enteral nutrition adversely affects intestinal motility and GI barrier function, disrupts the normal intestinal microbiota, and can cause villous atrophy. Therefore, it is hypothesised that early enteral nutrition promotes gut health and immunity and reduces ileus, vomiting, and bacterial translocation.

In dogs with naturally occurring or experimentally induced acute pancreatitis, early enteral nutrition (by means of oesophagostomy or jejunostomy tubes) did not exacerbate the clinical signs of pancreatitis and, in some cases, had beneficial effects. In a recent study, early enteral nutrition in 10 dogs with naturally occurring severe acute pancreatitis delivered proximal to the pylorus was well tolerated and resulted in fewer complications than parenteral nutrition.[29]

Unfortunately, there are currently no clinical trials evaluating different nutritional approaches in cats with pancreatitis, and therefore evidence-based recommendations based on cats cannot be made. However, given the evidence available from studies in humans, dogs, and experimental animals, it appears safe to assume that cats with pancreatitis likely also benefit from early enteral nutrition. This is particularly important because cats have considerably higher dietary protein requirements than dogs or humans and, therefore, are more prone to protein malnutrition during anorexia or prolonged fasting. In addition, because the vast majority of cats with acute pancreatitis are presented with a history of anorexia of several days' duration, additional food restriction could induce or worsen hepatic lipidosis. In the only study to date that evaluated the use of feeding tubes in cats with pancreatitis, nasogastric tube feeding was tolerated well, with no worsening of clinical signs.[30]

In general, cats with pancreatitis that do not vomit should be fed orally. In cats that do not vomit but are anorexic, some form of feeding tube should be used (see below). Appetite stimulants might be used in anorexic cats but might not lead to adequate caloric intake, especially in severe cases. Mirtazapine is a good option and also has antiemetic properties. In cases of severe vomiting, there is risk for aspiration pneumonia, and oral intake of food or feeding tube placement should probably be delayed until vomiting is controlled with antiemetics. This period should be as short as possible; therefore, antiemetic treatment should be aggressive. After vomiting is controlled, small amounts of water or food can be introduced, and if vomiting does not recur, a feeding tube can be placed if needed.

With regard to the choice of feeding tube, studies in cats are lacking, and recommendations are based on clinical experience and evidence from humans and other animal species. It is important to note that there is no evidence to support the use of postpyloric feeding in patients with acute pancreatitis, and therefore achieving postpyloric feeding should not be an absolute goal in cats with acute pancreatitis. Nasogastric or nasooesophageal tubes are easily placed and do not require general anaesthesia. Thus, they can be used for short-term nutritional support in severely ill cats in which general anaesthesia is contraindicated. They have been reported to be well tolerated and associated with only few clinically significant complications. The main disadvantage of these tubes is their small diameter, which results in frequent obstructions. Placement of oesophagostomy tubes requires short general anaesthesia and represents an excellent option for cats with pancreatitis. Complications are uncommon and usually mild provided that tube placement is confirmed both visually and radiographically or endoscopically prior to anaesthetic recovery. In a recent study, complications were reported in 35% of 248 cases and included stoma site infection (12%), removal of the tube (17%), and tube blockage (3%).[31] Gastrostomy tube placement requires more invasive procedures (surgery or endoscopy) and might be associated with more complications. Therefore, less invasive methods are preferred by the authors, and gastrostomy tubes are typically reserved for animals that undergo surgery for other reasons (e.g. exploratory laparotomy, biopsy, biliary tract obstruction). However, because of their larger diameter, they can be used for longer periods of time when this is necessary. Finally, jejunostomy tubes offer the theoretical advantage that they are placed distal to the site of pancreatic stimulation and might also be better tolerated in cats with intractable vomiting. As with gastrostomy tubes, jejunostomy tubes typically require laparotomy for placement, and therefore they are typically reserved for animals that might require laparotomy for other reasons.

With regard to the appropriate diet that should be used in cats with pancreatitis, evidence-based information is lacking. Hyperlipidaemia, high-fat diets, obesity, and dietary indiscretion are considered risk factors for pancreatitis in dogs, and lifelong fat restriction is usually recommended in dogs with pancreatitis. A relationship between pancreatitis and hyperlipidaemia, high-fat diets, or obesity has not been reported in cats. Cats have higher protein requirements and appear to digest and use high levels of dietary fat better than dogs. In a retrospective study of 55 cats with acute pancreatitis, a liquid high-lipid diet (45% of caloric density as lipids) fed through a nasogastric tube was well tolerated. Having said this, anecdotally, there is a group of cats that will develop pancreatitis a few weeks after having been switched to a high-fat diet and will improve when switched to a diet with a lower fat content. Therefore, it would appear prudent to avoid diets that are particularly high in fat, but more studies on the subject are needed to more clearly delineate the impact of dietary fat in cats with acute or chronic pancreatitis.

Analgesic therapy

Although uncommonly confirmed clinically, abdominal pain is believed to be present in the majority of cats with pancreatitis. The low incidence of abdominal pain reported in cats with pancreatitis likely reflects our inability to detect abdominal pain in this species. Pain induces several physiological changes, including decreased appetite, decreased GI motility, decreased regional blood flow to several abdominal organs (including the pancreas), and possibly a catabolic state. Thus, analgesic therapy should be an important component of the management of cats with pancreatitis, even when pain is not clinically suspected.

Pain management in cats with pancreatitis is typically achieved with opioids. Administration of an injectable opioid such as buprenorphine (0.01–0.03 mg/kg IV, IM, or SC every 4–8 hours), fentanyl (0.005–0.01 mg/kg IV, IM, or SC every 2 hours; or constant-rate infusion at 0.002–0.006 mg/kg/h), or meperidine (2–5 mg/kg IM or SC every 2–4 hours) is effective and provides fast results. Butorphanol (0.2–0.4 mg/kg IV or SC every 2–6 hours) can also be used, but its effectiveness in reducing pain in cats has been questioned, and this drug should probably be reserved for cases with mild to moderate pain. Fentanyl patches (25 µg/h, patch with half exposed, every 3–4 days) are safe and practical for providing a longer duration of analgesia, but they should be used only after analgesia has been achieved by use of injectable opioids, as it takes longer for transdermal preparations to achieve analgesia. Multimodal analgesic therapy may be indicated in some cases with severe pain and may include intravenous infusion of ketamine (0.6 mg/kg/h) and/or lidocaine (0.1 mg/kg/h; use with caution for possible lidocaine toxicity) with morphine. The effectiveness of nonsteroidal anti-inflammatory drugs is questionable in cats with acute pancreatitis, and they should ideally be avoided, as these animals are often dehydrated or hypovolaemic and therefore at risk for GI ulceration and renal injury.

Antiemetic therapy

Antiemetic therapy is indicated in the majority of cats with acute pancreatitis. The need for antiemetic therapy is obvious when vomiting is present, but antiemetic therapy may also be indicated when vomiting is absent. Many cats with pancreatitis do not vomit, but the vast majority of them are believed to experience nausea, which is extremely difficult to diagnose clinically. Nausea is believed to contribute to anorexia and weight loss and may lead to prolonged hospitalisation and a worse prognosis.

Maropitant (1 mg/kg PO or SC every 24 hours), a neurokinin-1 (NK_1) receptor antagonist, is a very potent and safe antiemetic that is often used as a first-line antiemetic in cats with pancreatitis. There is also evidence that maropitant has analgesic properties, making this drug very attractive for use in patients with pancreatitis. Furthermore, recent evidence in experimental models of pancreatitis have suggested that maropitant may also have anti-inflammatory properties, thereby potentially reducing pancreatic inflammation. Other good antiemetic choices include 5-HT_3 antagonists such as ondansetron (0.1–0.2 mg/kg, slow IV, every 6–12 hours). Dopaminergic antagonists, such as metoclopramide (0.2–0.5 mg/kg IV, IM, SC, or PO every 6–8 hours), are considered less effective in treating nausea and vomiting in cats but might be useful in enhancing upper GI motility. Constant-rate infusion of metoclopramide (1–2 mg/kg/day IV) may be more effective in treating vomiting and nausea in cats. Experimental studies have indicated that dopamine may ameliorate pancreatitis in cats, and therefore dopaminergic antagonists might be contraindicated in cats with pancreatitis, although this has not been confirmed in clinical studies. In cats with intractable vomiting, combinations of different antiemetics can be used. Finally, mirtazapine is a tetracyclic antidepressant that is commonly used as an appetite stimulant in cats and also has some antiemetic properties, mainly by antagonising 5-HT_3 receptors, and can be useful in the treatment of cats with pancreatitis.

Gastric acid suppression therapy

No studies have evaluated the benefit of gastric acid suppression in cats with pancreatitis, and the 2018 ACVIM consensus statement on the use of gastric acid suppressants in dogs and cats states that "there is no evidence that acid suppression treatment is beneficial or indicated in the management of dogs or cats with pancreatitis, unless the animal has concurrent evidence of gastroduodenal ulceration and erosion".[32]

Antibiotic therapy

There is currently very limited information regarding the role of bacteria in feline pancreatitis. In a preliminary study using fluorescence in situ hybridisation, 35% of cats with moderate to severe pancreatitis had evidence of pancreatic infection, possibly as a result of intestinal bacterial translocation. However, the clinical significance of these findings remains unknown. Thus, the routine use of antibiotics in cats with pancreatitis is currently unsubstantiated. In some cases, however, clinically important infectious complications of the pancreas may occur and can be associated with a poor prognosis. Therefore, antibiotics are recommended if infectious complications have been identified (e.g. infected pancreatic abscess) or are suspected (e.g. left shift, persistent fever, and shock). Cefotaxime (20–80 mg/kg IV or IM every 6 hours), enrofloxacin (5 mg/kg IM or PO every 12 hours), marbofloxacin (2.5–5 mg/kg PO, SC, or IV, off-label use), and ampicillin sodium (10–20 mg/kg IV, IM, or SC every 6–8 hours) are considered good antibiotic choices because they seem to penetrate well into the pancreatic tissue. It should be noted, however, that antibiotics are rarely indicated in cats with pancreatitis, even when severe. Antibiotics should also be used in cats in which concurrent diseases (e.g. neutrophilic cholangitis) necessitate their use.

Surgical treatment

Experience with surgical treatment of pancreatitis in cats is limited. In general, surgical treatment is indicated in cases in which pancreatitis is complicated by an infectious fluid accumulation, such as a pancreatic abscess. However, it should be noted that most feline pancreatic abscesses reported in the literature have been sterile and thus would not usually be treated by surgical intervention. In addition, surgical treatment may be indicated in cases with a suspicion for complete EHBDO due to pancreatitis, but again this is exceedingly rare. In one retrospective study at an emergency and referral practice, surgical intervention was deemed necessary in 8 (≈4%) of 203 cats with acute pancreatitis, and surgery was performed for EHBDO (6 cats), pancreatic abscess (3 cats), and pancreatic necrosis (1 cat), but it is unclear whether the clinical course of disease in these cats would have been different without surgical intervention.

Other management strategies

A plethora of other therapeutic agents, including but not limited to dopamine, histamine type 1 receptor antagonists, somatostatin, anticholinergics, and antioxidants, have been recommended by some authors and are occasionally used for the management of feline pancreatitis. However, there is currently no clinical evidence that any of these agents are beneficial in spontaneous cases of feline pancreatitis. Thus, the authors do not currently recommend the use of any of these agents until more evidence on their efficacy and safety is available. It should be noted that a new drug for the treatment of acute pancreatitis, fuzapladib, has been recently approved in Japan for the treatment of acute pancreatitis in dogs. However, at the time of this writing, no data are available for use of this drug in cats.

MANAGEMENT OF MILD (CHRONIC) PANCREATITIS

Chronic pancreatitis is usually considered to be mild and can be managed on an outpatient basis in most cases. As mentioned for severe pancreatitis, the presence of possible risk factors, such as hypercalcaemia or a drug history, should be evaluated and managed accordingly if identified. Also, it should be kept in mind that a large percentage of cats with pancreatitis (especially chronic) have concurrent intestinal and/or hepatic inflammation or DM, and these concurrent conditions should be investigated and, if diagnosed, managed accordingly. However, it is often impossible to determine which disease is responsible for the clinical signs in each cat. As mentioned above, if a cat is currently on a high-fat diet, especially if switched recently, it may be prudent to switch the cat to a diet that is lower in fat content.

Many cats with chronic pancreatitis have hyporexia or even anorexia. These patients may benefit from antiemetic medication, such as an NK_1 antagonist (e.g. maropitant) or a $5\text{-}HT_3$ antagonist (e.g. ondansetron), and an appetite stimulant (e.g. mirtazapine in cats, capromorelin in dogs) may also be useful. Finally, an analgesic maybe indicated in patients that appear to have abdominal pain.

At least some cases of feline chronic pancreatitis are believed to have an autoimmune basis. In these cases, corticosteroid or cyclosporin treatment may be used if symptomatic treatment is not sufficient. However, the benefits of such an approach remain unproven. Corticosteroids or cyclosporin are also often used to manage concurrent intestinal and/or hepatic disease. Diet modification, like that implemented for the management of intestinal disease in cats, may also be tried in cats with chronic pancreatitis.

Regardless of the management, progress of the disease should always be monitored. Just as in human patients with chronic pancreatitis, cats with chronic pancreatitis are at risk for developing episodes of severe pancreatitis at any time or exocrine pancreatic insufficiency and DM later in life.

COMPLICATIONS OF PANCREATITIS

Diabetes mellitus

Extension of inflammation from the exocrine to the endocrine pancreas can lead to progressive destruction of the islets of Langerhans, impaired beta cell function, and subsequently DM. Both clinical and histopathological studies have investigated the association between pancreatitis and DM in cats, and it is fairly well established that DM and pancreatitis often coexist. In clinical studies, 31%–83% of cats with DM were found to have clinical evidence of pancreatitis (based on fPLI/Spec fPL measurements and/or abdominal ultrasonography).[33,34] Pancreatitis was asymptomatic in the vast majority of cases in those studies. Results from necropsy studies are conflicting; histological evidence of pancreatitis was found in 51%–57% of cats with DM, but in a recent study, histological evidence of pancreatitis was not more common in diabetic cats compared to control cats, although this study had several limitations. In many cases where DM and pancreatitis coexist, it is impossible to determine which disease came first. It is likely that a bidirectional association exists and although pancreatitis can lead to DM in some cases, pancreatitis might be the result of DM in other cases. Insulin therapy is necessary in cases in which pancreatitis is complicated by DM, and good glycaemic control may be particularly difficult to achieve in these animals as long as pancreatic inflammation is present.

Pancreatic complications

Pancreatic complications are uncommon in cats with pancreatitis and mainly include pancreatic fluid collections (i.e. pancreatic pseudocysts, pancreatic abscesses, and pancreatic pseudobladders). It needs to be pointed out that the terminology used to describe these fluid collections in cats is outdated, often confusing, and not in line with the current human medicine literature. Pancreatic pseudocysts have been reported relatively more frequently than other complications and are defined as collections of fluid containing mainly pancreatic juice and debris, which are enclosed by a wall of fibrous or granulation tissue (lacking the epithelial lining characteristic of true cysts), and they are usually sterile. Pancreatic abscesses, defined as collections of purulent material containing little or no pancreatic necrosis that may or may not be infected, have been reported in a very small number of cats. Pancreatolithiasis (pancreatic stones) and pancreatic pseudobladder (cystic dilation of the pancreatic duct) have been reported in one cat with chronic pancreatitis. Due to the very small number of reported cases, the aetiology, clinical presentation, diagnosis, and treatment are poorly defined. Clinical signs of pancreatic complications of pancreatitis are practically indistinguishable from those of pancreatitis itself and typically persist despite treatment for pancreatitis. Thus, the presence of pancreatic complications must be ruled out in cases in which clinical signs persist despite proper management of pancreatitis.

Pancreatic fluid collections are usually identified during ultrasonographic examination of the pancreas. Evaluation of the fluid is very useful for diagnosing, differentiating, and managing pancreatic fluid collections. The diagnosis is usually based on cytological and bacteriologic analysis of material obtained through ultrasound-guided FNA (usually initial approach) or surgery. Histopathology may be required for definitive diagnosis and differentiation of pseudocysts and abscesses. In some cases, small pseudocysts might spontaneously resolve. Ultrasound-guided FNA of the cystic fluid may be used for the management of small pseudocysts. Repeated ultrasound-guided aspiration might be required. In some cases, however, clinical signs may persist or worsen despite treatment, and enlargement of the pseudocyst may occur over time. In these cases, surgical intervention can be considered.

Surgical intervention is almost always indicated when an infected fluid collection is identified.

Extrahepatic bile duct obstruction

Pancreatic enlargement during acute pancreatitis can result in compression and temporary obstruction of the common bile duct (i.e. EHBDO) that typically causes severe icterus and distension of the biliary tree. EHBDO is considered a relatively frequent sequela of acute pancreatitis in cats and appears to be the most common reason for surgical intervention in cats with pancreatitis. However, most cases of EHBDO as a result of pancreatitis resolve spontaneously with appropriate treatment for pancreatitis, and surgery is not indicated. Nevertheless, if the obstruction persists for more than 2 weeks, the biliary system may need to be decompressed. The gallbladder can be drained intermittently through needle aspiration under ultrasonographic guidance or continuously via surgical stent placement. Surgical techniques have also been described.

Hepatic lipidosis

Hepatic lipidosis has been reported to develop as a result of prolonged anorexia associated with pancreatitis in cats. This is of particular importance because the development of hepatic lipidosis in cats with pancreatitis is considered a factor of poor prognosis, once again highlighting the need for aggressive nutritional support in these patients.

Exocrine pancreatic insufficiency

Chronic pancreatitis is associated with pancreatic atrophy, which ultimately leads to insufficient acinar function for digestion of macronutrients, leading to exocrine pancreatic insufficiency. See Chapter 25 for further information on exocrine pancreatic insufficiency.

PROGNOSIS

The prognosis for cats with pancreatitis varies widely and cannot always be predicted. In patients with a single episode of mild and uncomplicated pancreatitis, the prognosis is usually good. In cats that have severe disease, frequent acute episodes, or complicating diseases, the prognosis should always be guarded. In cats with acute pancreatitis, a decreased serum ionised calcium concentration (<1 mmol/l) or concurrent hepatic lipidosis have been reported to be associated with a poor prognosis. Other factors such as hypoglycaemia, azotaemia, and withholding antibiotic treatment have shown weak negative associations with prognosis, but additional research is required.[7]

PANCREATIC CYSTS

Pancreatic cysts are rare in cats; only three cases have been reported to date. In contrast to pancreatic pseudocysts, pancreatic cysts are lined by a single layer of cuboidal epithelial cells and usually do not develop as a complication of pancreatic inflammation. A congenital pancreatic cyst was reported as an incidental finding in an adult cat, while multiple pancreatic cysts were reported in a cat with polycystic kidney disease and multiple renal and hepatic cysts. In the third report, multiple recurrent pancreatic cysts with associated pancreatic inflammation, atrophy, and subsequent DM were described. Based on this report, pancreatic cysts may be of clinical significance in some cases.

PANCREATIC NODULAR HYPERPLASIA

Pancreatic nodular hyperplasia is considered a common finding in older cats. It is characterised by the presence of multiple nodules throughout the pancreatic parenchyma, and it is typically an incidental finding during imaging (e.g. ultrasound, computed tomography), surgery, or necropsy. Nodular hyperplasia is not expected to lead to any changes in the measurement of serum pancreatic enzymes and does not cause any functional changes or clinical signs. Ultrasonographic findings in cats with pancreatic nodular hyperplasia (i.e. hypoechoic nodules and pancreatic enlargement) can be very similar to those seen in cats with pancreatitis or malignant neoplasia of the pancreas, and therefore cytology and/or histopathology are required for definitive differentiation. Although there is a tendency for multiple pancreatic nodules to be considered compatible with benign lesions, this feature has also been described in cats with a pancreatic adenocarcinoma.

Take-home messages

- Pancreatitis should be considered in any cat with inappetence, lethargy, weight loss, vomiting, or apparent abdominal pain of unknown cause. However, many cats with pancreatitis do not show overt clinical signs.
- Ultrasonography remains the recommended primary imaging modality for feline pancreatic disease. Ultrasound-guided fine needle aspiration of the feline pancreas is considered a safe procedure, with complication rates similar to those following aspiration of other organs.
- To date, measurement of serum lipase activity, regardless of the substrate being used, lacks specificity for pancreatic lipase, while measurement of feline pancreatic lipase immunoreactivity is specific for pancreatic lipase, with the sensitivity for the diagnosis of pancreatitis being dependent on disease severity.
- The management of acute pancreatitis is mainly supportive and symptomatic and includes fluid therapy, analgesics, antiemetics, enteral nutrition, and other management strategies as needed. Antibiotics and antacids should not be used routinely but only when an infection or gastrointestinal ulcer is diagnosed or heavily suspected.
- The management of chronic pancreatitis involves evaluating the patient for risk factors and for common concurrent conditions, instituting symptomatic therapy, monitoring, and potentially using immunosuppressive therapy.

REFERENCES

[1] Xenoulis PG, Steiner JM. Current concepts in feline pancreatitis. *Top Companion Anim Med* 23:185, 2008.

[2] Saunders HM et al. Ultrasonographic findings in cats with clinical, gross pathologic, and histologic evidence of acute pancreatic necrosis: 20 cases (1994–2001). *J Am Vet Med Assoc* 221:1724, 2002.

[3] Ferreri JA et al. Clinical differentiation of acute necrotizing from chronic nonsuppurative pancreatitis in cats: 63 cases (1996–2001). *J Am Vet Med Assoc* 223:469, 2003.

[4] De Cock HE et al. Prevalence and histopathologic characteristics of pancreatitis in cats. *Vet Pathol* 44:39, 2007.

[5] Swift NC et al. Evaluation of serum feline trypsin-like immunoreactivity for the diagnosis of pancreatitis in cats. *J Am Vet Med Assoc* 217:37, 2000.

[6] Fragkou FC et al. Prevalence and clinicopathological features of triaditis in a prospective case series of symptomatic and asymptomatic cats. *J Vet Intern Med* 30:1031, 2016.

[7] Nivy R et al. A retrospective study of 157 hospitalized cats with pancreatitis in a tertiary care center: clinical, imaging and laboratory findings, potential prognostic markers and outcome. *J Vet Intern Med* 32:1874, 2018.

[8] Forman MA et al. Evaluation of serum feline pancreatic lipase immunoreactivity and helical computed tomography versus conventional testing for the diagnosis of feline pancreatitis. *J Vet Intern Med* 18:807, 2004.

[9] Twedt DC et al. Evaluation of fluorescence in situ hybridization for the detection of bacteria in feline inflammatory liver disease. *J Feline Med Surg* 16:109, 2014.

[10] Norsworthy GD et al. Prevalence and underlying causes of histologic abnormalities in cats suspected to have chronic small bowel disease: 300 cases (2008–2013). *J Am Vet Med Assoc* 247:629, 2015.

[11] Zini E et al. Role of hyperglycemia in the pathogenesis of pancreatitis in cats. *J Vet Intern Med* 23:696, 2009.

[12] Xenoulis PG, Steiner JM. Canine and feline pancreatic lipase immunoreactivity. *Vet Clin Pathol* 41:312, 2012.

[13] Xenoulis PG. Diagnosis of pancreatitis in dogs and cats. *J Small Anim Pract* 56:13, 2015.

[14] Kimmel SE, Washabau RJ, Drobatz KJ. Incidence and prognostic value of low plasma ionized calcium concentration in cats with acute pancreatitis: 46 cases (1996–1998). *J Am Vet Med Assoc* 219:1105, 2001.

[15] Schnauss F, Hanisch F, Burgener IA. Diagnosis of feline pancreatitis with SNAP fPL and Spec fPL. *J Feline Med Surg* 21:700, 2019.

[16] Lee C, Kathrani A, Maddison J. Retrospective study of the diagnostic utility of Spec fPL in the assessment of 274 sick cats. *J Vet Intern Med* 34:1406, 2020.

[17] Törner K et al. Histopathology and feline pancreatic lipase immunoreactivity in inflammatory, hyperplastic and neoplastic pancreatic diseases in cats. *J Comp Pathol* 174:63, 2020.

[18] Forman MA et al. Evaluation of feline pancreas-specific lipase (Spec fPL™) for the diagnosis of feline pancreatitis. *J Vet Intern Med* 23:733, 2009.

[19] Xenoulis PG et al. Serum fPLI and Spec fPL concentrations in cats with experimentally induced chronic renal failure. *J Vet Intern Med* 23:758, 2009.

[20] Xenoulis PG, Steiner JM. SNAP tests for pancreatitis in dogs and cats: SNAP canine pancreatic lipase and SNAP feline pancreatic lipase. *Top Companion Anim Med* 31:134, 2016.

[21] Cridge H et al. Comparative repeatability of pancreatic lipase assays in the commercial and in-house laboratory environments. *J Vet Intern Med* 34:1150, 2020.

[22] Oppliger S et al. Agreement of the serum Spec fPL™ and 1,2-o-dilauryl-rac-glycero-3-glutaric acid-(6'-methylresorufin) ester lipase assay for the determination of serum lipase in cats with suspicion of pancreatitis. *J Vet Intern Med* 27:1077, 2013.

[23] Oppliger S et al. Agreement of serum feline pancreas-specific lipase and colorimetric lipase assays with pancreatic ultrasonographic findings in cats with suspicion of pancreatitis: 161 cases (2008–2012). *J Am Vet Med Assoc* 244:1060, 2014.

[24] Oppliger S et al. Comparison of serum Spec fPL(™) and 1,2-o-dilauryl-rac-glycero-3-glutaric acid-(6'-methylresorufin) ester assay in 60 cats using standardized assessment of pancreatic histology. *J Vet Intern Med* 30:764, 2016.

[25] Williams JM et al. Ultrasonographic findings of the pancreas in cats with elevated serum pancreatic lipase immunoreactivity. *J Vet Intern Med* 27:913, 2013.

[26] Bailey S et al. Comparisons between cats with normal and increased fPLI concentrations in cats diagnosed with inflammatory bowel disease. *J Small Anim Pract* 51:484, 2010.

[27] Hecht S, Penninck DG, Keating JH. Imaging findings in pancreatic neoplasia and nodular hyperplasia in 19 cats. *Vet Radiol Ultrasound* 48:45, 2007.

[28] Crain SK et al. Safety of ultrasound-guided fine-needle aspiration of the feline pancreas: a case-control study. *J Feline Med Surg* 17:858, 2015.

[29] Mansfield CS et al. A pilot study to assess tolerability of early enteral nutrition via esophagostomy tube feeding in dogs with severe acute pancreatitis. *J Vet Intern Med* 25:419, 2011.

[30] Klaus JA, Rudloff E, Kirby R. Nasogastric tube feeding in cats with suspected acute pancreatitis: 55 cases (2001–2006). *J Vet Emerg Crit Care (San Antonio)* 19:337, 2009.

[31] Breheny CR et al. Esophageal feeding tube placement and the associated complications in 248 cats. *J Vet Intern Med* 33:1306, 2019.

[32] Marks SL et al. ACVIM consensus statement: support for rational administration of gastrointestinal protectants to dogs and cats. *J Vet Intern Med* 32:1823, 2018.

[33] Forcada Y et al. Determination of serum fPLI concentrations in cats with diabetes mellitus. *J Feline Med Surg* 10:480, 2008.

[34] Zini E et al. Longitudinal evaluation of serum pancreatic enzymes and ultrasonographic findings in diabetic cats without clinically relevant pancreatitis at diagnosis. *J Vet Intern Med* 29:589, 2015.

[35] Lim SY et al. The 1,2-o-dilauryl-rac-glycero-3-glutaric acid-(6'-methylresorufin) ester (DGGR) lipase assay in cats and dogs is not specific for pancreatic lipase. *Vet Clin Pathol* 49:607, 2020.

CHAPTER 25

Exocrine pancreatic insufficiency

Panagiotis G. Xenoulis

Exocrine pancreatic insufficiency (EPI) is caused by inadequate production of pancreatic enzymes from pancreatic acinar cells, leading to maldigestion and subsequent clinical signs such as weight loss and diarrhoea. EPI has previously been considered rare in the cat, but it is now recognised that most cases of feline EPI escaped diagnosis in the past due to the lack of sensitive and specific diagnostic tests, low awareness for the disease, and its coexistence with other gastrointestinal (GI) conditions that cause similar clinical signs. The literature on feline EPI is sparse, consisting of 10 cases of confirmed or suspected EPI published between 1975 and 2009[1,2] as well as two small case series that included a total of 36 cases.[3,4] Recently, a retrospective, survey-based study that evaluated 150 cats with EPI diagnosed based on low trypsin-like immunoreactivity (TLI) concentrations was published.[2]

EPIDEMIOLOGY

The true prevalence of feline EPI is unknown. Feline EPI has traditionally been believed to be rare in the cat. Of 180648 cats that entered the Veterinary Medical Data Base from the early 1980s to the early 1990s, only 11 (0.006%) were diagnosed with EPI.[1] However, since the introduction of feline trypsin-like immunoreactivity (fTLI) in 1995,[5] considerably more cats have been diagnosed with EPI. In a recent study, the Gastrointestinal Laboratory's database at Texas A&M University, United States of America, was searched over an approximately 2-year period between 2008 and 2010, and 1094 of 46529 serum samples from cats submitted for fTLI measurement had fTLI concentrations diagnostic of EPI (2.4%).[2] Although the above two percentages are not comparable due to being from different populations, and despite the fact that the population used in the second study is skewed because it reflects cats with GI signs and a possible suspicion of EPI, it appears that EPI is a condition that is not uncommon in cats with GI signs. Whether this reflects a true increase in prevalence or merely a reflection of greater index of suspicion and better means for arriving at a diagnosis is unknown. Therefore, although its true prevalence remains unknown, EPI does occur in cats and should be suspected in cases with a compatible clinical picture (see below).

AETIOLOGY AND PATHOPHYSIOLOGY

No studies have specifically investigated the potential causes of EPI in the cat. Chronic pancreatitis leading to gradual and extensive destruction of the acinar cells has been traditionally cited as almost the sole cause of EPI in cats. However, this was based on a small number of case reports of cats diagnosed with EPI in the past.[1,6] Although chronic pancreatitis is still believed to be the most common cause of feline EPI, other aetiologies may also exist. In recent studies, several cats were diagnosed with EPI at a young age, making chronic pancreatitis a less likely cause and suggesting that different aetiologies may exists in those cases.[2] The reason for this is that it is believed that longer time is needed for chronic inflammation to lead to almost complete destruction of the exocrine portion of the pancreas, although this has not been proven. Alternatively, chronic pancreatitis may destroy enough pancreatic tissue to produce EPI in a shorter period of time than previously assumed. Other potential aetiologies for EPI could include pancreatic acinar atrophy, pancreatic hypoplasia or aplasia, pressure atrophy due to pancreatic duct obstruction, and *Eurytrema procyonis* infestation (reported in a small number of cases).[1] Pancreatic acinar atrophy, the most common cause of EPI in dogs, has been reported in a very small number of cats with EPI but may be underdiagnosed. Most other potential causes of EPI cited above have currently not been reported in cats. Isolated pancreatic lipase deficiency has recently been reported as a cause of EPI in dogs (while other pancreatic enzymes are normally produced),[7] but this has not been reported in cats. A flow chart with the different causes of feline EPI is shown in Figure 25.1. The exocrine pancreas has an exceptional functional reserve, and clinical signs of EPI are believed to develop only when more than 90% of the secretory capacity of the exocrine pancreas is lost.[1] Regardless of the cause, insufficient production and secretion of pancreatic enzymes in the small intestine leads to maldigestion of nutrients. The large amount of undigested nutrients in the intestine may lead to osmotic diarrhoea, while decreased absorption of nutrients causes weight loss.

Of major importance is the pathophysiological association between pancreatic function and cobalamin absorption. The intrinsic factor is a cobalamin-binding protein that facilitates cobalamin absorption in the ileum. In contrast to dogs, in which the intrinsic factor is also produced in the stomach, the intrinsic factor in cats is produced exclusively in the exocrine pancreas. Therefore, EPI leads to reduced production and secretion of intrinsic factor, resulting in decreased intestinal absorption of cobalamin. This results in hypocobalaminaemia and cobalamin deficiency.[8]

In cases in which EPI is a result of chronic pancreatitis, destruction of the endocrine portion of the pancreas may lead to concurrent diabetes mellitus. Additionally, many cats with EPI may have concurrent pancreatic inflammation, inflammatory intestinal disease, and/or hepatic disease.

SIGNALMENT

There is no significant breed or sex predisposition.[2] The median age of cats with EPI is about 8 years, but the age range is wide: from 3 months to 19 years.[2] This is important because EPI has been traditionally considered a disease of middle-aged to older cats. EPI should be considered in cats of any age.

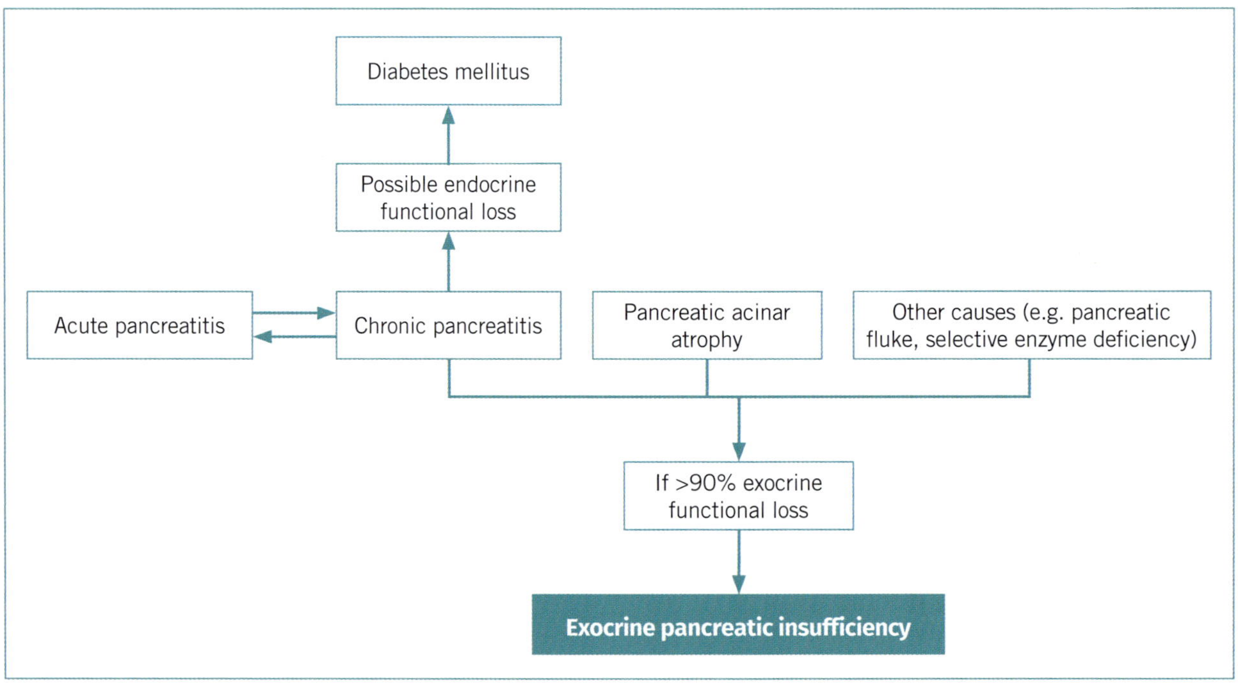

Figure 25.1. Aetiology of feline exocrine pancreatic insufficiency.

CLINICAL SIGNS

The clinical signs of cats with EPI are nonspecific and often seen in diseases diagnosed more commonly than EPI in clinical practice (e.g. hyperthyroidism, chronic enteropathies, pancreatitis, chronic kidney disease). Weight loss was by far the most common clinical sign and was present in more than 90% of 150 cats in one study (Fig. 25.2).[2] In the same study, weight loss was the only clinical sign in 5% of the cats. Loose stools occurred in only 62% of those cats, with two-thirds of them having occasional watery diarrhoea (Fig. 25.3). This is in contrast with the typical "EPI dog", in which loose stools are reported in the vast majority of cases (95% in one study).[9] Other clinical signs include poor haircoat (50%), polyphagia (42%), anorexia (42%), lethargy (40%), vomiting (19%), and greasy soiling of the haircoat.[2] Some of the reported clinical signs (e.g. anorexia, depression, vomiting) are not typical of EPI and are more likely to be associated with concurrent diseases (e.g. concurrent inflammation of the intestine, liver, and/or pancreas) than with EPI per se. There has been one report of a cat with EPI that developed D-lactic acidosis presumably due to increased bacterial fermentation in the intestine as a result of bacterial overgrowth, which presented with clinical signs of weakness, lethargy, and ataxia.[10] This is considered to be rare.

It is clear that the clinical presentation of many cats with EPI differs from the typical presentation seen in dogs. Clinical signs are more subtle and less specific in cats, and, therefore, EPI should be suspected in cases with unexplained weight loss or anorexia, even when diarrhoea or polyphagia are not present (see Chapters 1 and 2 for differential diagnoses).

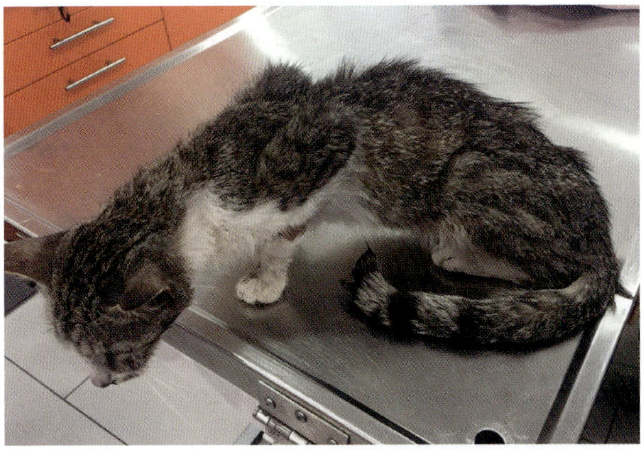

Figure 25.2. This cat was diagnosed with exocrine pancreatic insufficiency and inflammatory bowel disease. The cat is thin (body condition score 2/9) despite having a normal appetite.

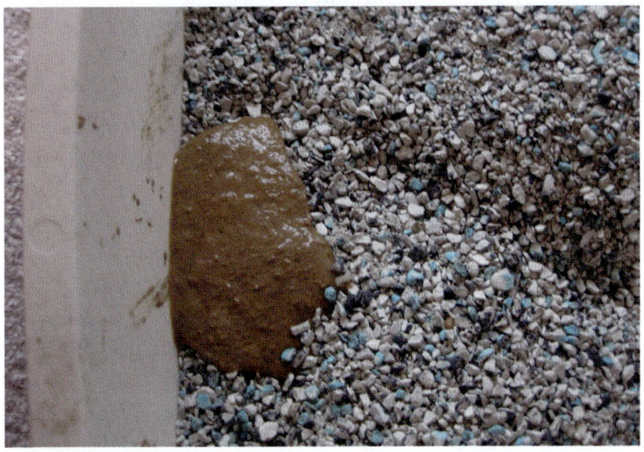

Figure 25.3. Faeces from the cat in Figure 25.2. Note the loose and greasy appearance.

DIAGNOSIS

EPI is initially suspected based on clinical presentation (see above). Cats with GI inflammatory diseases may also have EPI. Cats with chronic GI diseases (e.g. inflammatory bowel disease) that do not respond to appropriate treatment may have concurrent EPI that remains undiagnosed. Therefore, in a cat diagnosed with a chronic enteropathy or another GI disease that continues to lose weight or have loose stools despite appropriate treatment, EPI should be in the differential diagnoses list.

Results of a complete blood count and serum biochemical profile are usually normal or show nonspecific changes. However, due to concurrent diseases, several haematologic and biochemical changes may be present reflecting those diseases (e.g. anaemia, increased liver enzyme activities, hyperglycaemia, hypoalbuminaemia). None of these findings are specific for EPI (see Chapters 3 and 4).

Serum cobalamin concentrations are decreased in the majority of cats with EPI (80%–100%).[2] There is evidence that tissue cobalamin is depleted before hypocobalaminaemia develops, and, therefore, even normocobalaminaemic cats could have cellular cobalamin deficiency.[8] Although common in cats with EPI, hypocobalaminaemia is not specific for EPI, as it is commonly present in cats with other conditions (e.g. inflammatory bowel disease, GI lymphoma, hyperthyroidism).[8]

EPI is a functional disease and requires a functional diagnosis (see also Chapter 4).[1] The gold standard for the diagnosis is the measurement of serum fTLI concentration (85%–100% specificity; sensitivity unknown but considered to be high).[1–3] Ideally, fasting samples should be obtained for serum fTLI measurement. Since the TLI assays are species-specific, assays developed and validated for dogs or humans are not appropriate for use in cats. The TLI assays detect the trypsinogen produced by the exocrine pancreas that circulates in the blood. In case of EPI, due to significant reduction of the functional capacity of the exocrine pancreas, serum trypsinogen concentration is reduced, and this is reflected as a subnormal serum fTLI concentration. Currently, the only validated assay for fTLI is offered by the Gastrointestinal Laboratory at Texas A&M University. The reference range of this assay is 12–82 µg/l; values less than or equal to 8 µg/l are considered diagnostic for EPI. Some cats with GI clinical signs have serum fTLI concentrations in the questionable range (8–12 µg/l). These cats should be retested a few weeks or months later to check whether fTLI concentrations have normalised or are in the diagnostic range for EPI. Because trypsinogen is excreted by the kidney, serum fTLI concentrations may be falsely increased in cats with decreased kidney function.[11] Therefore, a diagnosis of EPI may be hampered in some cats with azotaemia due to chronic kidney disease. In cats in which EPI is suspected and are azotaemic, reevaluation of serum fTLI concentrations after improvement of azotaemia may be needed. Other functional biomarkers (e.g. faecal elastase) for diagnosing feline EPI might be available in some countries, but their diagnostic accuracy has not been evaluated and cannot be currently recommended.

Imaging modalities (radiographs, ultrasound, computed tomography) are not helpful for the diagnosis of EPI in cats because they do not reflect the functional capacity of the pancreas (see Chapter 6). However, imaging can be useful for the diagnosis or exclusion of concurrent diseases or diseases that can cause similar clinical signs. Gross appearance of a small pancreas and histopathology are also not useful for a diagnosis of EPI because they do not reflect the functional capacity of the pancreas.

TREATMENT

An overview of the pancreatic enzymes used in the treatment of feline EPI is provided in Table 25.1. For other medications that might be used in cats with EPI, see Appendix.

Enzyme replacement therapy

As in dogs, the mainstay of treatment in cats with EPI is pancreatic enzyme supplementation. There are several commercial products (dried extracts of porcine pancreas) available, but no studies have evaluated the efficacy of different products and preparations in cats. In a recent study, no difference was identified with regard to the specific product or type of pancreatic enzyme used for the treatment of feline EPI, and, therefore, all products might be equally effective.[2] Although older studies in dogs supported the use of powdered products, while enteric-coated products were considered less effective, a recent prospective, placebo-controlled study showed that enteric-coated products may be more efficacious.[12] Raw pancreas from beef, pork, or game may also be used.[1] The author's personal preference is powdered or enteric-coated products.

Regardless of the product used, pancreatic enzymes should be added to each meal and thoroughly mixed with food. The dose for each product has not been established, and it is titrated for each cat based on response to treatment. An initial dose of one teaspoon of pancreatic enzyme powder per meal seems appropriate.[1] Enteric-coated products could be used at an initial dose of 300 mg of pancreatin per day (divided in each meal). Response to treatment is expected to be quick, with resolution of loose stools usually within the first week. After resolution of clinical signs, gradual reduction to the lowest effective dose should be attempted. If raw pancreas is used, about 50 g per meal is appropriate as an initial dose, with dose adjustments as needed. Raw pancreas should be kept frozen in portions of 50 g until use (it can be kept frozen for several months without losing efficacy). However, it should be made clear to the owners that feeding raw pancreas may be associated with a small risk of infectious and parasitic disease transmission (e.g. bovine spongiform encephalitis, Aujeszky's disease, *Echinococcus* spp.).[1]

Table 25.1. Pancreatic enzymes used in the treatment of feline exocrine pancreatic insufficiency.

Product	Dosage regimen	Comments
Powder	0.5–1 teaspoon/meal	Mix with food just prior to feeding Rarely, may cause oral bleeding and irritation; in these cases, dose reduction is indicated
Enteric-coated formulations	300 mg of pancreatin per day (divided in each meal)	Give with food Titrate to the minimum effective dose after clinical signs resolve
Raw pancreas	30–90 g/meal	Can be kept frozen for several months without losing efficacy Small risk of infectious/parasitic disease transmission

Due to their ability to break down protein and fat, pancreatic enzymes can cause oral or oesophageal irritation and ulcers if they remain long enough in contact with the mucosa. Therefore, powdered pancreatic enzymes should be mixed thoroughly with food, while administration of tablets or capsules should be followed by food or water consumption to reduce the risk of stomatitis and oesophagitis.[1]

Cobalamin supplementation

Cobalamin supplementation is also of major importance and has been shown to favourably affect response to treatment both in cats with EPI and in cats with chronic enteropathies, two conditions that often coexist.[2,13] Cobalamin deficiency can lead to intestinal inflammation and villous atrophy, disturbance of various biochemical pathways, and malabsorption of nutrients such as folate.[8] In a study of cats with GI disease and severe hypocobalaminaemia, cobalamin supplementation led to significant increases in body weight and improvement of vomiting and diarrhoea.[13] In another study of 150 cats with EPI, cobalamin supplementation favourably affected the response to treatment, even in cats with normal serum cobalamin concentrations.[2] Finally, hypocobalaminaemia associated with certain GI diseases in dogs has been shown to be a negative prognostic factor, and hypocobalaminaemia in dogs with EPI was associated with shorter survival.[14,15]

The exact serum cobalamin concentration that indicates cellular cobalamin deficiency and designates the need for cobalamin supplementation is currently unknown and hampered by the fact that reference intervals of serum cobalamin concentrations vary greatly amongst laboratories. The use of markers of cobalamin deficiency such as serum methylmalonic acid concentrations is more useful, but testing for these markers is only routinely available in some countries.[16]

In addition to cats with hypocobalaminaemia, in which cobalamin supplementation is clearly indicated, some normocobalaminaemic cats with EPI (especially those with results at the lower limit of the reference interval) could benefit from cobalamin supplementation, possibly because these cats have cellular cobalamin deficiency.[2,8,16] Due to the fact that virtually all cats with EPI either have or are prone to develop cobalamin deficiency due to lack of intrinsic factor, it might be recommended that cats with EPI should be supplemented with cobalamin regardless of their serum cobalamin concentration.

Due to lack of intrinsic factor and the resulting impaired cobalamin absorption by the GI tract, parenteral cobalamin supplementation is typically recommended.[1,8] Studies on the pharmacokinetics of parenteral cobalamin supplementation in cats with and without GI disease indicate that the serum half-life of cobalamin is 5 and 13 days, respectively.[17] Protocols on cobalamin supplementation in cats with GI disease have been published, and efficacy may be variable depending upon the underlying disease, the frequency of administration, and the formulation used.[1,8] No studies have specifically evaluated cobalamin supplementation protocols in cats with EPI. The author currently recommends that cobalamin is administered in the form of hydroxocobalamin (preferably) or cyanocobalamin at a total dose of 250 µg (500 µg for cats weighing more than 5 kg) per cat, SC or IM, every 1–2 weeks for 6–8 weeks, making monthly rechecks of serum cobalamin concentrations. When these become normal, cobalamin is administered at monthly intervals, and serum cobalamin reevaluations are performed every 3 months. Many cats will require long-term cobalamin supplementation despite enzyme replacement treatment for EPI.

Recent evidence indicates that oral cobalamin supplementation may be as effective as parenteral cobalamin administration for correcting cobalamin deficiency in cats with GI disease.[18] However, no studies have specifically evaluated the efficacy of oral cobalamin supplementation in cats with EPI. Therefore, the author currently recommends parenteral administration of cobalamin in all cats with EPI. If this is not possible, 250 μg (per cat) of hydroxocobalamin or cyanocobalamin may be given orally daily for 2–3 months, and subsequent reevaluations of serum cobalamin concentrations should be performed.

Antibiotics and intestinal microbiota modification

Antibiotic use was not found to affect response to treatment in cats with EPI in one study.[2] Antibiotics are often used in the treatment of canine EPI to control concurrent intestinal dysbiosis, although no clear benefit has been shown in some studies.[19] However, disturbances of the microbiota in cats with EPI have not been fully described or confirmed, and, therefore, antibiotic use is of unknown benefit in these cases. Given the difficulty in identifying small intestinal dysbiosis in cats, and because many cats may have concurrent small intestinal disease, a trial with antibiotics may be considered in patients that do not respond to enzyme and cobalamin supplementation. Metronidazole (15 mg/kg PO every 12 hours) or tylosin (20 mg/kg PO every 12 hours) are good choices, but both are very bitter and, depending on the country, palatable formulations for cats might not be available. Due to the possibility of inducing intestinal dysbiosis (see Chapter 16), and because efficacy is questionable, antibiotics should not be used routinely in cats with EPI.

Probiotics may also be able to control intestinal dysbiosis (see Chapter 36), but no studies are available. Faecal microbiota transplantation is gaining ground as a means of intestinal microbiota modification, and, although studies in cats are lacking, it is used more and more commonly in clinical practice (see Chapter 37).

Dietary recommendations

No evidence-based dietary recommendations can be made for cats with EPI (see also Chapter 39). A good-quality, high-protein maintenance diet would seem appropriate in most cases, unless concurrent diseases are present that make necessary the use of specific clinical diets. In the past, low-fat diets have been recommended for the management of EPI, especially in dogs, but no studies exist in cats.

Other treatments

Some authors recommend using a proton pump inhibitor (e.g. omeprazole, pantoprazole) concurrently with pancreatic enzyme replacement therapy to reduce gastric acidity and decrease enzyme inhibition in the stomach.[19] However, the benefits of such treatment are unknown, and most cats seem to respond well without such intervention. Cats that do not respond well to pancreatic enzyme and cobalamin supplementation may be put on a proton pump inhibitor therapy to see if this will change the response to treatment (see also Chapter 33).

There have been occasional reports of cats with EPI that presented with coagulopathy that responded to vitamin K supplementation.[20] Although believed to be very rare, if a bleeding diathesis is noted in a cat with EPI, coagulation parameters should be measured and vitamin K supplementation should be initiated.

PROGNOSIS

Overall, response to treatment is considered good in 60% of cases, and cats with EPI that are treated appropriately typically have an excellent prognosis and a good quality of life.[2] Only 13% of cases have been reported to have a poor response to treatment.[2] The reason that some cats do not respond well to treatment for EPI is not clear. Lack of or partial response to treatment might be due to lack of cobalamin administration or the presence of inadequately managed concurrent diseases (e.g. chronic enteropathies, liver disease). All cats that do not respond to appropriate treatment should be reevaluated for important concurrent diseases, or the diagnosis of EPI should be questioned.

Take-home messages

- Exocrine pancreatic insufficiency (EPI) should be considered in any cat with weight loss and/or loose stools, although many cats may also have inappetence, lethargy, vomiting, and polyuria/polydipsia due to the presence of concurrent diseases.
- Serum feline trypsin-like immunoreactivity concentration is considered the gold standard for the diagnosis of feline EPI, as it has high sensitivity and specificity. Serum amylase or lipase activity, serum feline pancreatic lipase immunoreactivity, imaging, or histopathology are not useful for the diagnosis of EPI in cats.
- The management of EPI in cats is mainly based on pancreatic enzyme and cobalamin supplementation. Antibiotics or proton pump inhibitors may occasionally be tried if pancreatic enzyme and cobalamin supplementation are not effective.
- All cats that do not respond to appropriate treatment should be reevaluated for important concurrent diseases, or the diagnosis of EPI should be questioned.

REFERENCES

[1] Steiner JM. Exocrine pancreatic insufficiency in the cat. *Top Companion Anim Med* 27:113, 2012.

[2] Xenoulis PG et al. Feline exocrine pancreatic insufficiency: a retrospective study of 150 cases. *J Vet Intern Med* 30:1790, 2016.

[3] Steiner JM, Williams DA. Serum feline trypsin-like immunoreactivity in cats with exocrine pancreatic insufficiency. *J Vet Intern Med* 14:627, 2000.

[4] Thompson KA et al. Feline exocrine pancreatic insufficiency: 16 cases (1992–2007). *J Feline Med Surg* 11:935, 2009.

[5] Steiner JM, Medinger TL, Williams DA. Development and validation of a radioimmunoassay for feline trypsin-like immunoreactivity. *Am J Vet Res* 57:1417, 1996.

[6] Williams DA. The pancreas. In: Guilford WG et al., editors. *Strombeck's Small Animal Gastroenterology*, 3rd ed. Philadelphia, WB Saunders: 381, 1996.

[7] Xenoulis PG et al. Suspected isolated pancreatic lipase deficiency in a dog. *J Vet Intern Med* 21:1113, 2007.

[8] Ruaux CG. Cobalamin in companion animals: diagnostic marker, deficiency states and therapeutic implications. *Vet J* 196:145, 2013.

[9] Batchelor DJ et al. Breed associations for canine exocrine pancreatic insufficiency. *J Vet Intern Med* 21:207, 2007.

[10] Packer RA et al. D-lactic acidosis secondary to exocrine pancreatic insufficiency in a cat. *J Vet Intern Med* 19:106, 2005.

[11] Steiner JM, Finco DR, Williams DA. Serum feline trypsin-like immunoreactivity (fTLI) in cats with experimentally induced chronic renal failure. Abstract. *J Vet Intern Med* 16:385, 2002.

[12] Mas A et al. A blinded randomised controlled trial to determine the effect of enteric coating on enzyme treatment for canine exocrine pancreatic efficiency. *BMC Vet Res* 8:127, 2012.

[13] Ruaux CG et al. Early biochemical and clinical responses to cobalamin supplementation in cats with signs of gastrointestinal disease and severe hypocobalaminemia. *J Vet Intern Med* 19:155, 2005.

[14] Soetart N et al. Serum cobalamin and folate as prognostic factors in canine exocrine pancreatic insufficiency: an observational cohort study of 299 dogs. *Vet J* 243:15, 2019.

[15] Volkmann M et al. Chronic diarrhea in dogs—retrospective study in 136 cases. *J Vet Intern Med* 31:1043, 2017.

[16] Worhunsky P et al. The relationship of serum cobalamin to methylmalonic acid concentrations and clinical variables in cats. *J Vet Intern Med* 27:1056, 2013.

[17] Simpson KW et al. Subnormal concentrations of serum cobalamin (vitamin B_{12}) in cats with gastrointestinal disease. *J Vet Intern Med* 15:26, 2001.

[18] Toresson L et al. Oral cobalamin supplementation in cats with hypocobalaminaemia: a retrospective study. *J Feline Med Surg* 19:1302, 2017.

[19] Batchelor DJ et al. Prognostic factors in canine exocrine pancreatic insufficiency: prolonged survival is likely if clinical remission is achieved. *J Vet Intern Med* 21:54, 2007.

[20] Perry LA et al. Exocrine pancreatic insufficiency with associated coagulopathy in a cat. *J Am Anim Hosp Assoc* 27:109, 1991.

CHAPTER 26

Hepatic vascular disorders

Mickey S. Tivers, Vicky J. Lipscomb

The liver has a unique vascular arrangement, with blood supplied by both the hepatic artery and hepatic portal vein and drained by the hepatic vein. The hepatic portal vein drains blood from the cranial and caudal mesenteric veins, the splenic vein (left gastric vein), and the gastroduodenal vein. It supplies the liver with approximately 75% of the afferent blood flow and 50% of the oxygen supply.

Hepatic vascular disorders are characterised by an abnormal liver blood supply, with reduced portal blood flow, typically resulting in hepatic insufficiency. These disorders can be congenital or acquired. The most common abnormality in cats is a congenital portosystemic shunt (CPSS). Other congenital conditions include hepatic arteriovenous malformation (HAVM), primary portal vein hypoplasia (PPVH), and peliosis hepatis. Multiple acquired shunts (MAS) occur as a result of portal hypertension (PH) secondary to congenital or acquired liver disease.

CONGENITAL PORTOSYSTEMIC SHUNTS

Epidemiology and aetiology

CPSSs are seen less commonly in cats compared with dogs, although they are rarer still in humans. In 1995, the incidence was reported to be 2.5 per 10000 cats seen in referral practice.[1] A more recent study found that 48 out of 1217 (3.8%) liver biopsy samples from cats submitted for histopathology were consistent with a CPSS.[2] The incidence of CPSS in the general cat population is unclear, but it remains an uncommon yet fascinating condition.

The liver performs many important functions including the metabolism of toxins, such as ammonia, absorbed from the gastrointestinal (GI) tract and delivered by the portal vein. A CPSS is an aberrant vessel that forms a communication between the portal and systemic blood systems. The abnormal vessel allows blood from the portal vasculature (draining the stomach, small intestine, spleen, and pancreas) to bypass the liver and flow directly into the systemic circulation. Thus, waste products and toxins accumulate in the systemic circulation, causing hepatic encephalopathy (HE) and associated clinical signs. Importantly, the liver requires normal portal blood flow and factors derived from the gut and pancreas for normal growth and development. Due to the shunt, the liver in affected cats is not stimulated to develop in a normal fashion, resulting in liver hypoplasia and effective hepatic insufficiency. Histopathology of the liver in cats with CPSS is similar to that of dogs and shows changes characteristic of reduced portal perfusion, including portal vein hypoplasia, arteriole hyperplasia, biliary hyperplasia, hepatocellular degeneration, and periportal fibrosis (Fig. 26.1).[3]

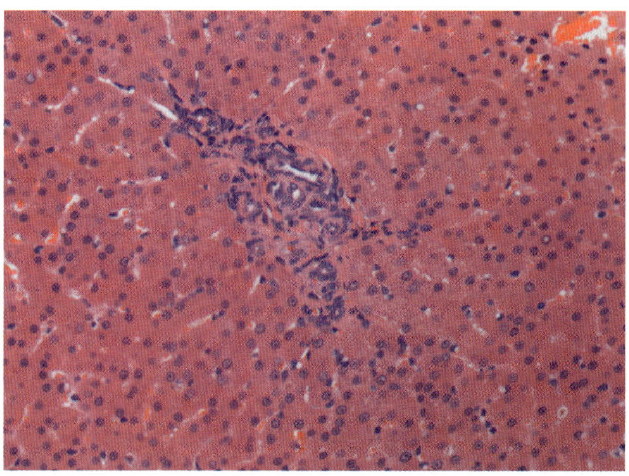

Figure 26.1. Photomicrograph of a hepatic biopsy from a cat with an extrahepatic congenital portosystemic shunt (×200 magnification). The characteristic changes of portal vein hypoperfusion can be seen, including absence of portal venules and the proliferation of arterioles and biliary tracts.

CPSSs have two general types: extrahepatic and intrahepatic. Extrahepatic are more common. In one study of 50 cats with CPSS, 40 were extrahepatic and 10 were intrahepatic.[4] Extrahepatic shunts take the form of an abnormal vessel branching from a tributary of the portal vein, outside of the liver parenchyma. The shunt vessel inserts on the vena cava (in a pre- or posthepatic location), the azygous vein, or the phrenic vein. The most common morphologies are splenocaval, left gastrophrenic, and left gastrocaval, responsible for 92% of extrahepatic CPSSs in cats (Fig. 26.2).[5] Other morphologies in cats include gastroazygous and left colic.[5]

In intrahepatic CPSSs, the abnormal vessel connects an intrahepatic branch of the portal vein to the vena cava and lies either partially or completely within the liver parenchyma. Intrahepatic CPSSs can be divided into three forms depending on the liver lobe involved: right divisional (right lateral and caudate liver lobes), central divisional (right medial and quadrate liver lobes), and left divisional (left medial and lateral liver lobes). The majority of intrahepatic CPSSs in cats are left divisional and are typically a patent ductus venosus, caused by failure of this normal embryonic vessel to close after birth (Fig. 26.3).[6] Right and central divisional shunts have also been reported in cats, but the origin of these morphologies remains unclear.

History and physical examination

Most cats diagnosed with CPSS are domestic shorthair cats, although this may represent the fact that this is the most common cat in the general population. Several clinical studies have suggested that Persian, Himalayan, and Siamese breeds are predisposed to CPSS.[6] A recent study of liver biopsy samples identified that domestic shorthair cats were at significantly reduced risk of having a CPSS, with the British Shorthair breed having a significantly increased risk.[2] A hereditary basis for CPSSs has been reported in various breeds of dog, however there are no such reports in cats. It has been suggested that male cats are more commonly affected than females, although this has not been a consistent finding.[6]

Clinical signs in cats with CPSSs are variable and nonspecific, affecting the nervous, digestive, and urinary systems. Most cats (93%–100%) demonstrate neurological abnormalities due to HE (see Chapter 28), including reduced mentation, altered behaviour, ataxia, head pressing, circling, tremors, blindness, seizures, and coma.[6] Signs of HE can range from very mild to

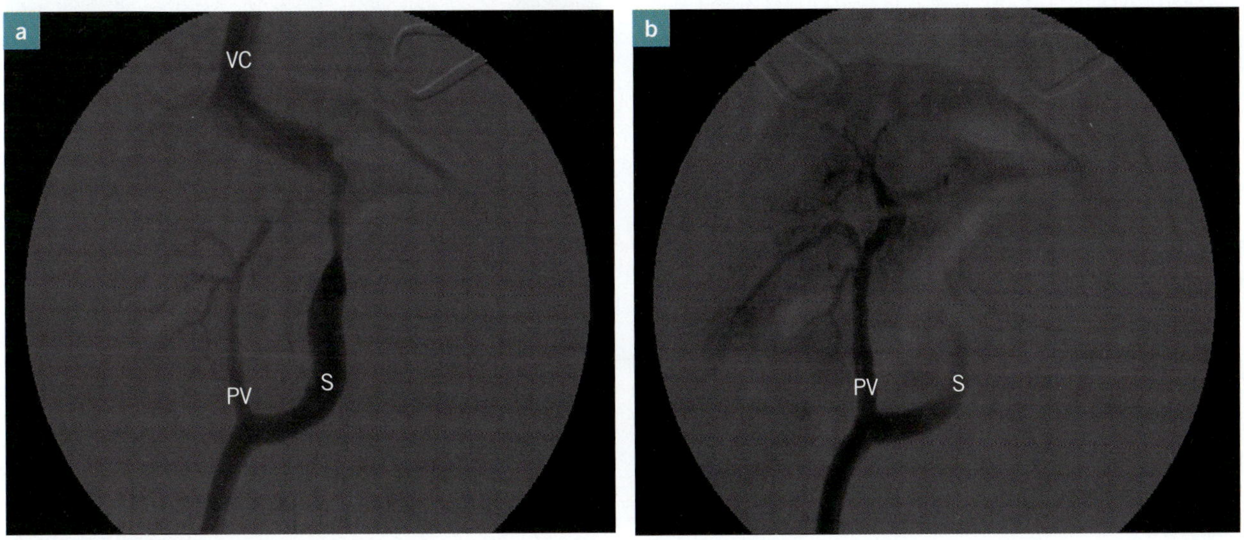

Figure 26.2. Intraoperative mesenteric portovenograms from a cat with an extrahepatic congenital portosystemic shunt. The cat is in dorsal recumbency, with cranial to the top of the images. Contrast has been injected through a catheter in a jejunal vein under fluoroscopic guidance with digital subtraction. Pre-attenuation portovenogram (a) showing a left gastric vein extrahepatic congenital portosystemic shunt (S) inserting on the posthepatic vena cava (VC). The majority of blood flow is through the large shunt, with faint opacification of the portal vein (PV) and intrahepatic vasculature. Repeat portovenogram following temporary complete occlusion of the shunt (b). There is increased opacification of the intrahepatic vasculature and no contrast flow through the shunt.

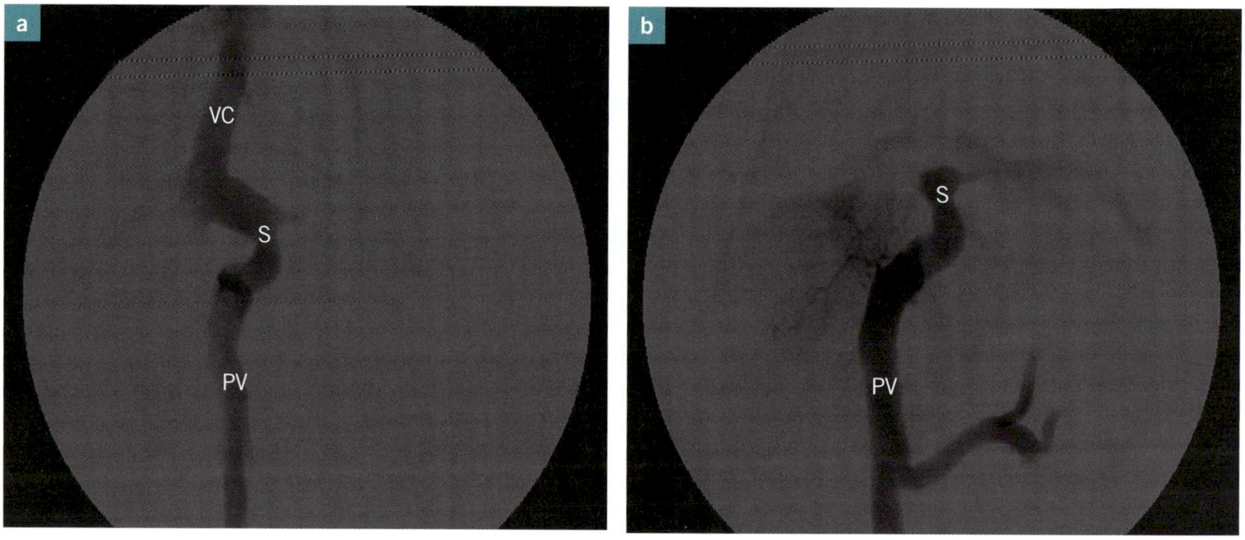

Figure 26.3. Intraoperative mesenteric portovenograms from a cat with an intrahepatic congenital portosystemic shunt. The cat is in dorsal recumbency, with cranial to the top of the images. Contrast has been injected through a catheter in a jejunal vein under fluoroscopic guidance with digital subtraction. Pre-attenuation portovenogram (a) showing a left divisional intrahepatic congenital portosystemic shunt (S). There is no opacification of the intrahepatic vasculature. Repeat portovenogram following temporary complete occlusion of the shunt (b). There is increased opacification of the intrahepatic vasculature and no contrast flow through the shunt. PV, portal vein; VC, vena cava.

extremely severe, may be intermittent, and can also wax and wane. They can be induced or deteriorate as a result of feeding, GI bleeding, anaesthesia, or azotaemia. Cats can be presented as emergencies due to an acute encephalopathic crisis.

Cats with CPSSs commonly demonstrate marked ptyalism/hypersalivation, which is seen in 67%–84%.[6] The cause of the ptyalism is unclear but may be related to HE or GI derangement. Copper-coloured irises have also been associated with CPSSs in 13%–64% of cats, although the reason for this is unclear (Fig. 26.4).[6]

Most cats demonstrate clinical signs when immature, and a CPSS is typically diagnosed before 6 months of age. Cats are often small or stunted, with poor weight gain and a low body condition score. However, a CPSS can be diagnosed in a mature cat, either due to late onset of clinical signs or as an apparently incidental finding, with abnormalities identified on routine blood testing.

Other clinical signs include polyuria and polydipsia (PU/PD) and those associated with the GI and urinary tracts. However, these are less common in cats compared to dogs. GI signs can include vomiting, diarrhoea, inappetence, and weight loss and are seen in 24%–71% of cats.[6] Urinary tract signs can include dysuria and haematuria related to ammonium urate urolithiasis and are reported in 8%–39% of cats.[6]

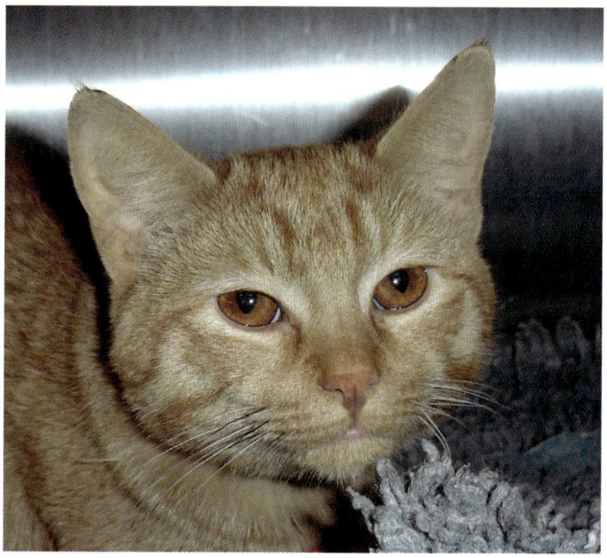

Figure 26.4. Image of a cat with copper-coloured irises associated with an extrahepatic congenital portosystemic shunt. This is a common clinical finding in cats with congenital portosystemic shunts.

Diagnostic investigation

Laboratory investigation

The first step in the investigation of a cat with a suspected CPSS is routine haematology and biochemistry and liver function testing, typically dynamic serum bile acids (BAs) and/or plasma ammonia.

Biochemical changes relate to decreased liver function as a result of the shunt. Reduced urea is the most common abnormality, reported in 61%–100% of cats.[6] Urea is low due to reduced synthesis in the liver as the product of ammonia metabolism (Krebs–Henseleit urea cycle). It may also be low due to recent fluid therapy, PU/PD, or a restricted protein diet. Creatinine may also be reduced due to low muscle mass in small or stunted cats. Decreases in albumin, total protein, and glucose can be seen in cats with CPSS, but these changes are less common than in dogs. These decreases reflect hepatic insufficiency due to the shunt. Although hypoglycaemia is uncommon in cats, glucose should be checked, as severe hypoglycaemia can cause neurological signs. Alkaline phosphatase (ALP) and alanine aminotransferase (ALT) may be normal or moderately increased, possibly as a result of hypoxic hepatocellular damage due to reduced liver perfusion.

The most common abnormality on haematology is microcytosis (mean corpuscular volume below reference interval), reported in approximately 25%–54% of cats.[6] Unlike in dogs, anaemia is very uncommon in cats (0%–15%).[6] These abnormalities are thought to be related to impaired iron metabolism. A recent study explored the complete blood count parameters in 42 cats prior to CPSS surgery.[7] Microcytosis was present in 76.2% of cats, although only one cat (2.4%) was anaemic. Changes in white blood cell parameters were very uncommon: lymphocytosis in 2.4% and lymphopenia in 19.1% of cats. Microcytosis was significantly improved after surgery (although not resolved), suggesting that these changes are partly reversible with improved hepatic portal blood flow and presumably improved liver function. This study also investigated clotting times in cats with CPSSs prior to surgery and found that prothrombin time (PT) and activated partial thromboplastin time (aPTT) were increased in 87.5% and 68.8%, respectively. Despite this, none of the cats demonstrated a clinical coagulopathy, and there were no surgical complications associated with bleeding.

Cats may have a low specific gravity on urinalysis, particularly if they have PU/PD. Cats with shunts have impairment of normal uric acid metabolism in the liver. This results in an increase in serum uric acid, which is excreted in the urine and forms ammonium biurate crystals. These crystals can be seen on urine sediment examination in 20%–43% of cats.[6] They are golden in colour and have a thorn apple shape when seen under the microscope.

Routine haematology, biochemistry, and urinalysis are useful in the investigation of cats with suspected CPSSs, particularly to rule out other differential diagnoses and to increase the index of suspicion. However, changes are typically mild and nonspecific and, in some cats, significant abnormalities are absent. Liver functions tests are therefore indicated to further investigate cats.

A BA stimulation test is an easily performed method for assessing liver function and is very reliable for diagnosing portosystemic shunting. BAs are synthesised in the liver and stored in the gallbladder. They are released into the duodenum in response to the ingestion of food and are subsequently reabsorbed from the ileum. The liver takes up bile from the blood very rapidly following absorption from the intestines. Therefore, only minor and transient increases in serum BAs are seen in a normal animal. However, in a cat with CPSS or MAS, BAs that are reabsorbed from the intestine are diverted into the systemic circulation, bypassing the liver and causing prolonged and high serum BA concentrations. The sensitivity of preprandial and postprandial BAs in cats has been reported as 58%–100% and 100%, respectively, with a specificity of 84% for fasting BAs.[6] Cats with CPSSs may have normal preprandial BAs but increased postprandial BAs, highlighting the importance of the postprandial sample.[8]

Fasting ammonia is increased in the majority of cats with CPSSs but can occasionally be within the reference interval, and thus a normal result should not rule out a CPSS.[6] As ammonia is normally metabolised by the liver, resting ammonia levels represent a crude estimate of liver function. As ammonia is very labile, samples must be frozen and analysed very quickly or measured on a point-of-care analyser. The sensitivity and specificity of ammonia levels for the diagnosis of CPSS in cats has been reported as 83% and 86%, respectively.[9]

Imaging

Once portosystemic shunting is suspected, imaging is necessary to confirm the diagnosis of a CPSS, determine its precise anatomy, and rule out other diagnoses such as HAVM, PPVH, or liver disease with MAS (see the corresponding sections in this chapter for more details).

Abdominal ultrasonography is very useful to screen for the presence of a CPSS and provides broad information regarding its morphology. It is relatively inexpensive, noninvasive, and can be performed on conscious or sedated cats. It has been reported to be 100% accurate for the diagnosis of CPSSs in cats, but it is very operator dependent, and lower accuracy (45%–50%) has also been described.[6] Ultrasonography can identify details regarding shunt morphology, including whether it is extrahepatic or intrahepatic. If ultrasonography fails to confirm a suspected CPSS or does not provide sufficient morphological information to allow adequate surgical planning, then computed tomography angiography (CTA) is recommended as the gold standard for CPSS assessment. However, in the authors' experience, ultrasonography, performed by an experienced operator, is sufficient to diagnose and plan surgery for nearly all CPSSs in cats.

Rectal portal scintigraphy with technetium pertechnetate ($^{99}Tc^{m}O_4^-$) can be used to investigate suspected CPSSs in cats and has been associated with good sensitivity and specificity.[6] However, scintigraphy is not widely available and has been superseded by ultrasonography and CTA in most instances.

CTA is the gold standard for the investigation of CPSSs, providing a definitive diagnosis as well as very detailed information regarding shunt morphology and intrahepatic vasculature development. Importantly, it is minimally invasive and can be performed prior to surgical management. However, it is relatively expensive and requires heavy sedation or general anaesthesia.

A variety of different contrast radiographic techniques have been used in cats with shunts both to confirm the diagnosis and to facilitate surgery.[6] Preoperative techniques have been replaced by ultrasonography or CTA. However, intraoperative mesenteric portovenography (IOMP) using fluoroscopy is still utilised by some veterinary surgeons as an adjunct to surgical management (Figs. 26.2 and 26.3). IOMP allows confirmation of the shunt during surgery, provides information on the morphology of the shunt, and rules out a second CPSS or MAS. Its use may be particularly important for cats that have not had preoperative CTA. In addition, IOMP during temporary complete shunt occlusion allows assessment of the degree of intrahepatic portal blood flow, which can help determine whether a CPSS will tolerate complete acute ligation, and confirms correct identification of the shunt and its branches during surgery and thus optimal placement of any attenuation.[10]

Management and treatment

Medical management

Medical management is designed to control the signs of HE with a combination of an appropriate diet, lactulose, and antibiotics (see Chapter 28). This works primarily by modifying the gut environment to reduce the production and absorption of ammonia and other toxins. Sometimes cats suffer from severe signs of HE, and this can result in collapse, coma, or seizures/status epilepticus. Deterioration in clinical signs can be precipitated by an anaesthetic episode or other trigger in a cat being medically managed or with occult disease. See Chapter 28 for emergency investigation and management of severe HE.

It is important to remember that although medical management may control the signs of HE, the underlying condition (shunting) remains untreated. Cats therefore have ongoing hepatic insufficiency, and lifelong medical treatment is needed, with concerns over residual clinical signs and the risk of relapse. Although some individuals can have a good long-term outcome with medical management alone, there is very limited information on long-term medical management in cats. Studies have shown an incomplete response to medical management in 52%–68% of cats prior to surgery, suggesting that it may not be a good long-term solution for some.[4,10] In dogs, surgical management is associated with a significantly better survival rate and a reduced frequency of ongoing clinical signs compared with medical treatment.[11]

Surgical management is recommended for most cats with CPSSs in order to close the shunt and improve or restore liver function.[6] However, surgery is not without risk, and this must be considered when determining the optimum treatment for an individual. Medical management is typically used when surgery is not feasible for technical or financial reasons or is declined by the cat's owner. It is recommended that animals should have 2–4 weeks stabilisation with medical management prior to surgery.

Surgical treatment

Surgery aims to attenuate the shunting vessel to redirect blood flow to the liver via the portal vein and therefore improve or restore normal liver function. Several different surgical procedures are recommended for the treatment of CPSSs in cats including suture ligation, ameroid constrictors (ACs), thin film bands (TFBs), and endovascular coils.[12] There is limited information in the literature to recommend one method over another, and all have potential advantages and disadvantages.

Suture ligation

Historically, surgical treatment involved partial or complete suture ligation of the shunting vessel. In many cats with CPSSs, the hepatic portal vasculature is poorly developed/ hypoplastic. This means that they are not able to tolerate complete acute attenuation of their shunt, as the liver is unable to accommodate the increased portal blood flow. The increased flow causes PH, which is fatal if the attenuation is maintained. Careful intraoperative assessment using objective and subjective measurement of portal pressures and IOMP to determine portal blood flow before and after temporary complete attenuation of the shunt can be used to determine whether the cat can tolerate complete ligation or not (Fig. 26.5).[12] Complete acute ligation of the CPSS is possible in approximately 29%–43% of cats, although it may be less likely in intrahepatic CPSSs compared with extrahepatic.[12] Cats that can tolerate complete CPSS attenuation have a better long-term outcome, as those treated with partial ligation are at greater risk of persistence of clinical signs or relapse due to persistent shunting.[12] For those that cannot tolerate a complete ligation, one method is to perform partial ligation and then repeat surgery approximately 3 months later.[10,13] This allows the liver to develop in the intervening period, and most cats are able to tolerate complete ligation at the second surgery. The disadvantage of this approach is the increased cost and morbidity of a second surgery, although typically it is well tolerated. For this reason, most veterinary surgeons prefer the use of a gradual attenuation device.

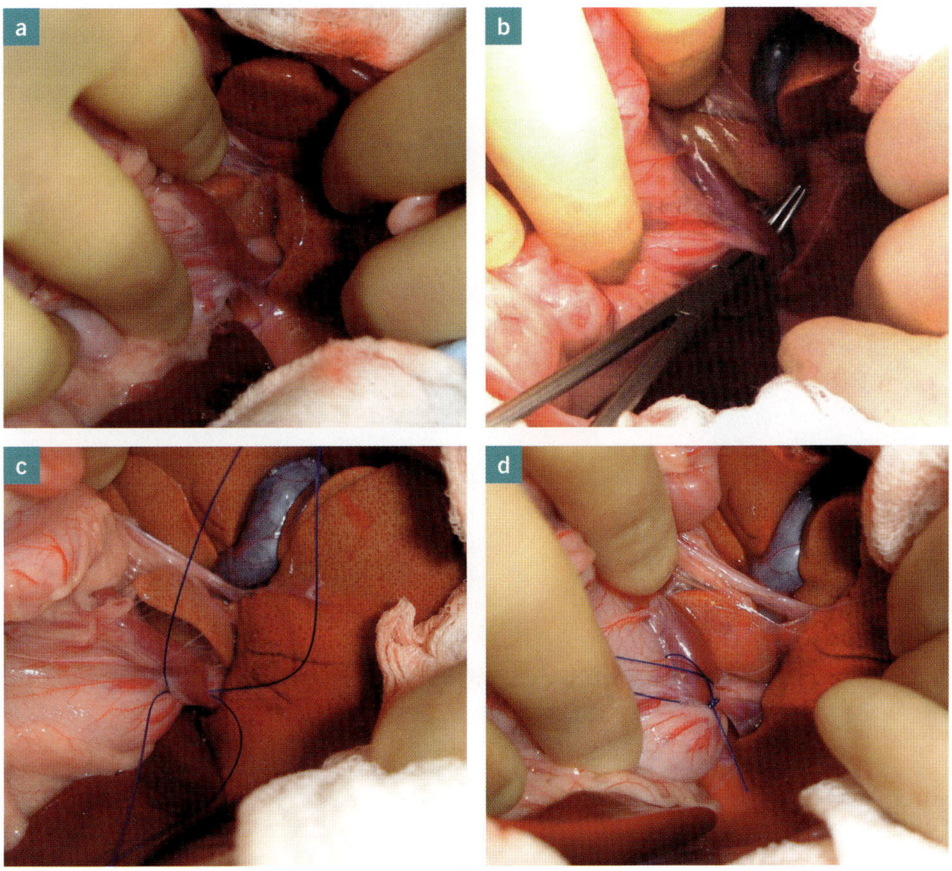

Figure 26.5. Intraoperative images of a cat with a left gastric vein extrahepatic congenital portosystemic shunt. The stomach is retracted caudoventrally to reveal the shunting vessel in the region of the gastric cardia (a). Mixter forceps are used to carefully dissect around the shunt (b). Two lengths of polypropylene suture are passed around the shunting vessel to allow temporary occlusion and subsequent ligation (c). Intraoperative assessment determined that this cat could tolerate complete occlusion of the shunt, and the suture is tied tightly (d).

Gradual attenuation

Gradual attenuation techniques have been developed in response to the risk of PH with suture ligation and the inability to completely close all shunts acutely. The most common treatments for cats with CPSSs are placement of an AC or TFB, both of which are considered simple to use (Figs. 26.6 and 26.7). The aim of these methods is to completely close the shunt over a period of weeks, whilst avoiding the risk of PH or the need for a second surgery. However, there is no control over the rate of attenuation, and in some cats too rapid attenuation may lead to the development of MAS. There is also the possibility that attenuation may be incomplete, with persistent shunting through the original vessel. The exact rate of complete attenuation with these techniques is unknown in cats, but studies have shown that persistent shunting can occur with both.

Surgical treatment of intrahepatic congenital portosystemic shunts

Intrahepatic CPSSs are more challenging to treat surgically than extrahepatic shunts due to their location within the liver parenchyma. Despite this, surgery can be performed safely and successfully. In the authors' experience, most shunts (particularly left divisional ones) can be attenuated posthepatically, either directly or via ligation of the draining hepatic vein. There is limited data on intrahepatic CPSSs in cats in the literature and most have been treated with suture ligation, although AC and TFB placement are described. ACs and TFBs may be harder to place where access is limited. Intraoperative haemorrhage is a potential concern for intrahepatic shunts, and it is prudent for cats to be blood typed prior to surgery and for blood to be available.

In dogs, endovascular coil embolisation of intrahepatic CPSSs has been developed as a minimally invasive technique to reduce morbidity and mortality associated with open surgery. Coils are inserted into the shunt via a catheter placed through the jugular vein. A wire stent is placed in the vena cava to maintain the coils within the shunt vessel and prevent migration. The coils typically provide acute partial closure of the vessel via thrombosis, although further closure may occur over time. Nevertheless, some animals require repeat procedures to add more coils to achieve complete shunt closure. Successful coil embolisation of a left divisional intrahepatic CPSS

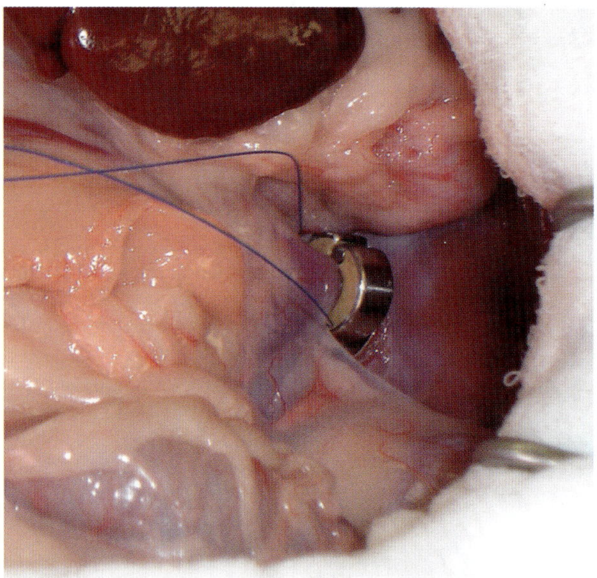

Figure 26.6. Intraoperative image of a cat with a portoazygous extrahepatic congenital portosystemic shunt. An ameroid constrictor is placed around the shunt at the point that it passes through the diaphragm. Note the length of loose polypropylene suture around the shunt; this will be left in situ and can be used to facilitate further attenuation at revision surgery if necessary.

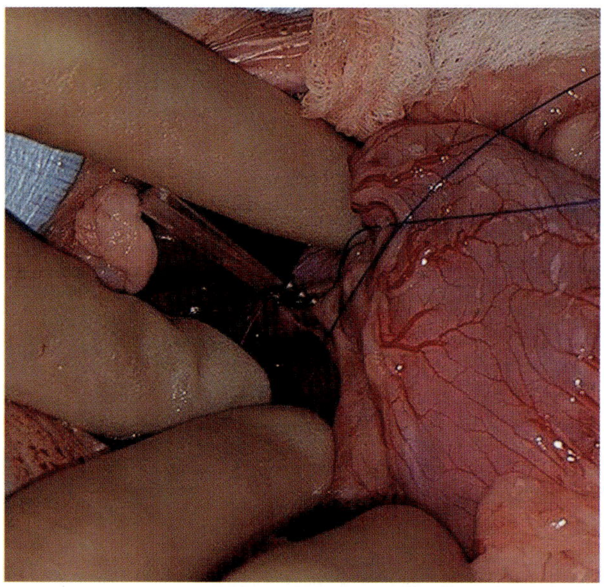

Figure 26.7. Intraoperative image of a cat with a left gastric vein extrahepatic congenital portosystemic shunt. A thin film band is placed around the shunt and secured with haemoclips. Note the length of loose polypropylene suture around the shunt; this will be left in situ and can be used to facilitate further attenuation at revision surgery if necessary.

has been described in a cat.[14] However, many cats with intrahepatic CPSSs may be too small for coil embolisation to be performed. A hybrid surgical approach in which the catheter is placed directly into the portal vein or a mesenteric vein via a small laparotomy has also been described in two cats.[15] Neither required a vena cava stent, but one had a coil anchor placed to prevent migration. The authors are uncertain whether this approach offers significant advantages over traditional open surgery performed by experienced surgeons, especially as most intrahepatic shunts in cats are left divisional, which offers a consistently accessible posthepatic location with predictable morphology for open surgical dissection around the shunt.[16]

Surgical complications and mortality

Shunt attenuation in cats has been associated with several complications, including haemorrhage, hypoglycaemia, PH, and post-attenuation neurological signs (PANS). Cats should be monitored carefully postoperatively for complications, particularly PANS.

Intraoperative haemorrhage from the shunt could occur during dissection but is rare, especially for extrahepatic CPSSs. Glucose should be measured perioperatively and supplemented as needed. PH can occur if attenuation of the CPSS has been overzealous or there is kinking of an AC. However, with the use of a gradual attenuation device and/or careful intraoperative assessment to ensure that any acute attenuation is appropriate, serious PH is a rare complication.

PANS are the most common perioperative complication in cats undergoing shunt surgery. PANS vary in form and severity and include mild tremors or ataxia, abnormal behaviour, central blindness, partial or generalised seizures, and status epilepticus (Fig. 26.8). Signs typically occur within the first 72 hours after surgery, and cats should be monitored very closely for signs to allow early treatment. The authors treat affected cats promptly and aggressively with anti-seizure medication including phenobarbitone, levetiracetam, propofol, and medetomidine.[12] The cause of PANS is unknown, but it is not directly related to hypoglycaemia or HE, as it can occur despite normal glucose or ammonia levels and does not respond to treatment for acute HE. It is speculated that PANS are related to changes in false neurotransmitters, although this remains unproven. Importantly, PANS do not seem to relate to the specific surgical technique and occur with similar frequency, even with gradual attenuation devices. PANS are more frequent in cats compared with dogs and are reported in 36.7%–62.0% of cats undergoing shunt surgery, with seizures in 22.0%–23.5%.[4,13,17] Unfortunately, PANS result in the death or euthanasia of a proportion of cats, and they are the most common cause of mortality in cats undergoing shunt surgery. In a recent study, the mortality rate for cats that suffered postoperative seizures was 45.5%.[4] This study found that serum osmolality at a median of 24 hours after surgery was significantly lower in cats that suffered PANS, suggesting a possible link.[4] The study did not find any benefit in the preoperative administration of anti-seizure medication. Despite suffering PANS, a proportion of cats can still make a full recovery. However, some do require ongoing medication for their neurological signs but can still have a good quality of life.

The overall mortality rate following shunt surgery in cats is variable. See Table 26.1 for more details.

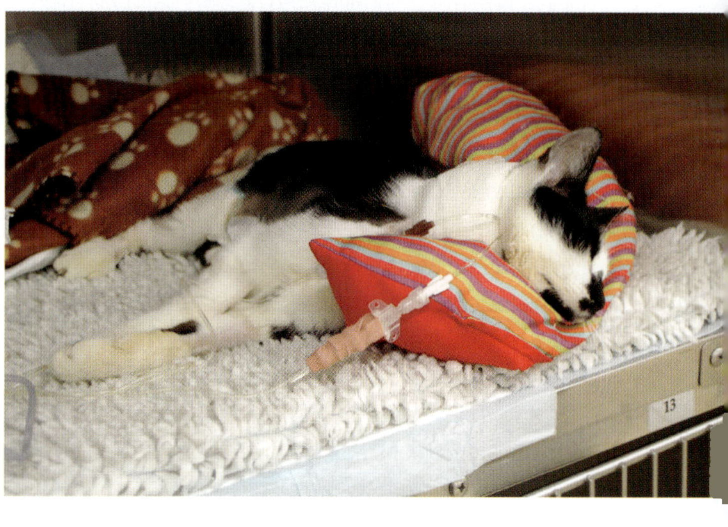

Figure 26.8. Image of a cat suffering from neurological complications following full suture ligation of a congenital portosystemic shunt. He initially recovered well from surgery; however, the following day he became increasingly uncoordinated and mentally depressed. These signs were consistent with post-attenuation neurological signs rather than hepatic encephalopathy. The cat was treated with phenobarbitone and levetiracetam. His neurological signs gradually improved, and he was discharged from the hospital on continued treatment.

Table 26.1. Mortality rates from studies of surgical treatment for congenital portosystemic shunts in cats.

Study	Number of cats and type of shunt	Surgical treatment	Mortality rate prior to discharge
Kyles et al. 2002[8]	23 extrahepatic	Ameroid constrictor	4.3% (1 cat)
Havig and Tobias 2002[19]	12 extrahepatic	Ameroid constrictor	0%
Lipscomb, Jones, and Brockman 2007[13]	49 total 36 extrahepatic 13 intrahepatic	Suture ligation	4.1% (2 cats)
Cabassu et al. 2011[18]	9 extrahepatic	Thin film band	22.2% (2 cats)
Valiente et al. 2020[17]	34 extrahepatic	Thin film band	11.8% (4 cats)
Strickland et al. 2020[4]	50 total 40 extrahepatic 10 intrahepatic	46 suture ligation 4 thin film band	12% (6 cats)

Prognosis and outcome

Successful shunt surgery should result in improvement in liver function and hence resolution of clinical signs. It has been shown that portal blood flow improves following partial attenuation, and it is presumed that liver regeneration occurs resulting in increased liver volume.[10] A good clinical response is normally mirrored by an improvement in BA levels. However, in some cats, BAs may be persistently mildly increased despite a good outcome.[13] This could be due to persistent subclinical shunting or concurrent primary PPVH. Some cats will have persistent shunting due to incomplete shunt attenuation or the development of MAS, and this can cause ongoing or recurrent clinical signs (Fig. 26.9). Cats with clinical signs should undergo further imaging to assess for persistent shunting and can be treated with further surgery or long-term medical management as appropriate. However, some cats can still have a good outcome despite persistent shunting. It remains unclear how much shunting can be associated with a good clinical outcome, and this may well vary between individuals. The authors perform complete acute suture ligation in cats whenever possible, so that no cat that can tolerate this procedure is denied the opportunity for complete shunt closure, as abolishing all shunting is a universally accepted excellent prognostic factor. The authors use a gradual attenuation method in cats that cannot tolerate complete acute ligation and always leave a loose polypropylene suture in situ around the shunt, regardless of the gradual attenuation method used (Figs. 26.6 and 26.7). This suture facilitates any further surgery if needed for cats that are demonstrating clinical signs associated with residual flow through their shunt.

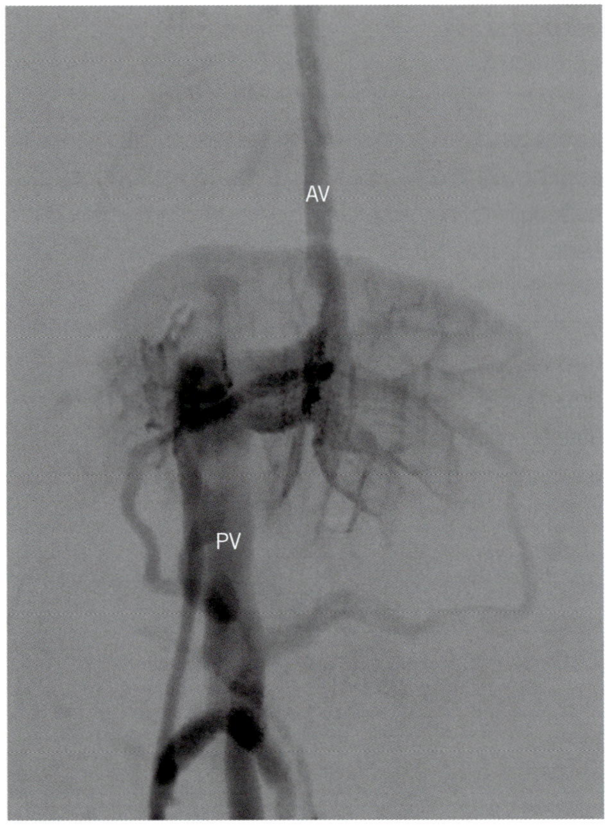

Figure 26.9. Intraoperative mesenteric portovenogram from revision surgery in a cat with an intrahepatic congenital portosystemic shunt. The cat is in dorsal recumbency, with cranial to the top of the image. Contrast has been injected through a catheter in a jejunal vein under fluoroscopic guidance with digital subtraction. The cat previously underwent placement of a thin film band for attenuation of a central divisional intrahepatic congenital portosystemic shunt. The portovenogram shows multiple acquired shunts within the liver, connecting to the azygous vein (AV). PV, portal vein.

There is limited long-term outcome data available in the literature and most relies on owner and veterinary assessment. Nevertheless, most cats are expected to have a good long-term outcome following surgery (Table 26.2). The long-term outcome for cats treated with suture ligation, AC, or TFB has been reported to be excellent or good in 75.0%–86.6% of cats.[8,13,17] However, smaller studies of AC and TFB placement have reflected a poorer outcome.[18,19] Further research is necessary to determine the best surgical treatment for CPSSs in cats.

HEPATIC ARTERIOVENOUS MALFORMATION

Epidemiology and aetiology

HAVM is an extremely rare congenital condition that has only been reported in a small number of cats in the literature.[20–22] The malformation represents a direct communication between the high-pressure arterial circulation and the low-pressure portal system via a vessel or vessels connecting a branch of the hepatic artery (or coeliac artery) with a branch of the portal vein. This results in hepatofugal flow (away from the liver) in the portal system and hence PH. The PH results in the development of MAS in order to relieve the pressure (Fig. 26.10).

History and physical examination

Limited information exists to describe typical history and physical examination findings. It is a congenital condition, and therefore cats are likely to be presented when immature. Clinical signs may include vomiting, diarrhoea, poor appetite, poor growth, heart murmur, cranial abdominal bruit, lethargy, ascites, and signs of HE.

Diagnostic investigation

Routine blood testing may show evidence of hepatic dysfunction, and increased ammonia levels have been reported.[20] HAVM can be readily diagnosed on abdominal ultrasonography, although CTA provides more detailed information about the precise nature of the abnormality to allow surgical planning. IOMP, alongside intraoperative portal pressure measurement, can be used during surgical treatment to confirm the morphology and to document treatment success during surgery.

Treatment and prognosis

Medical management of HE may not resolve the clinical signs.[20] In dogs, ligation of the artery supplying the malformation, surgical removal of the affected liver lobe, and glue embolisation using interventional radiology have been reported for the treatment of HAVM. Successful treatment of an arterioportal venous malformation

Table 26.2. Long-term outcome for cats surgically treated for congenital portosystemic shunts.

Study	Surgical treatment	Follow-up	Outcome			
			Excellent Clinically normal, no medication	**Good** Mild clinical signs and no treatment, or no clinical signs with ongoing treatment	**Fair** Ongoing or recurrent clinical signs and ongoing medication	**Poor** Euthanasia or death due to progression or recurrence of clinical signs
Kyles et al. 2002[8]	Ameroid constrictor	3–51 months (mean 27 months)	15/20 (75%)*	1/20 (5%)	1/20 (5%)	3/20 (15%)
Havig and Tobias 2002[19]	Ameroid constrictor	6–60 months	2/9 (22.2%)	1/9 (11.1%)	2/9 (22.2%)	4/9 (44.4%)
Lipscomb, Jones, and Brockman 2007[13]	Suture ligation	4–105 months (median 47 months)	20/36 (55.6%)	7/36 (19.4%)	7/36 (19.4%)	2/36 (5.6%)
Cabassu et al. 2011[18]	Thin film band	Median 240 days	4/7 (57.1%)	1/7 (14.3%)	1/7 (14.3%)	1/7 (14.3%)
Valiente et al. 2020[17]	Thin film band	0.5–84 months (median 8 months)	26/30 (86.6%)	0/30 (0%)	2/30 (6.7%)	2/30 (6.7%)

*Includes six cats on a low-protein diet.

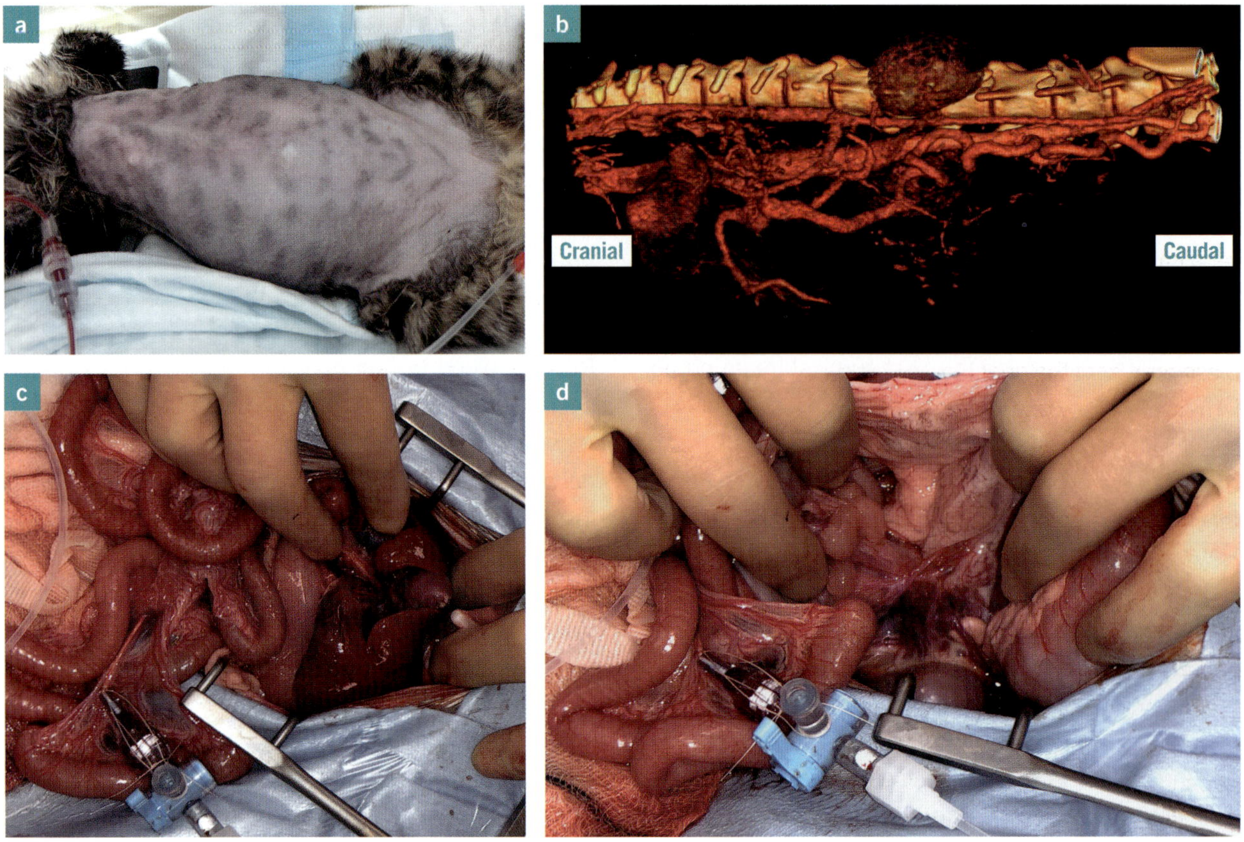

Figure 26.10. Images of a cat with a hepatic arteriovenous malformation (HAVM). Prior to surgery, abdominal distension due to ascites caused by the portal hypertension could be observed (a). Sagittal computed tomography angiogram of the cat's abdomen showing the HAVM (b). Exploratory laparotomy showing an extremely dilated left portal vein branch (c). Multiple acquired shunts can also be seen in the region of the left kidney (d). These have formed as a result of portal hypertension due to the HAVM.

in a cat described ligation of a single "feeder" arterial branch, identified on CTA, that supplied the abnormality.[23] Another case report describes the successful management of a cat with HAVM using coil embolisation via laparotomy.[20] However, surgical treatment was not successful in two other reports.[21,22] Due to the nature of the condition and the presence of MAS, ongoing medical treatment of HE may be necessary in some cats.

PRIMARY PORTAL VEIN HYPOPLASIA

PPVH is a congenital disorder which involves portosystemic shunting at the microvascular level. Histopathology is consistent with portal vein hypoperfusion, and the changes associated with CPSS and PPVH are indistinguishable. It has been suggested that some or all dogs with CPSSs have concurrent PPVH, and it is likely that the same may be true in cats. In dogs, a variation of PPVH can be associated with PH, typically with more marked fibrosis on histopathology, and this results in MAS and ascites.

PPVH appears to be extremely rare in cats, and although it is mentioned in several articles, very little specific information exists. Two reports have described cats with clinical signs consistent with a CPSS but no macroscopic shunt and liver histopathology consistent with PPVH.[24,25] Another report described a cat with signs of HE, MAS, and a splenosystemic shunt on CTA and liver histopathology consistent with PPVH.[26] Therefore, it seems that PPVH can exist in combination with or without PH, similar to what occurs in dogs. However, more cases are needed to establish this fully.

OTHER TYPES OF MACROSCOPIC SHUNTS

MAS occur as a result of PH due to chronic liver pathology. Classically they consist of a plexus of multiple small vessels connecting the portal system with the vena cava and are typically found in the retroperitoneum adjacent to either kidney, although they can also develop around the site of shunt attenuation. It is assumed that these represent the opening up of vestigial vessels or the formation of new ones as a response to PH. MAS seem to be much less common in cats compared to dogs, but there is limited information in the literature. In cats, they have been reported as a consequence of PH due to HAVM, excessive attenuation of a CPSS, PPVH, congenital hepatic fibrosis, portal vein thrombosis/obstruction, and other chronic liver diseases. History, clinical signs, and the results of diagnostic investigations may vary with the underlying cause. However, cats with significant liver disease and PH may show signs of HE and/or ascites, depending on the severity of their condition.

Another form of vascular anomaly reported in cats is a splenosystemic shunt.[27,28] This is a relatively large vessel that connects the splenic vein with the left gonadal or left renal vein. The aetiology of this abnormality is unclear, and it is uncertain whether it is congenital or acquired. It is diagnosed almost exclusively in older, neutered female cats (91%–100%), although it can occur in male cats.[27,28] Splenosystemic shunts can be identified as a well-defined, tortuous, tubular soft tissue structure in the left midabdominal cavity on plain digital radiography ("spaghetti sign") but are more likely to be diagnosed with ultrasonography or CTA.[27,28]

Importantly, the history, clinical signs, and biochemical abnormalities are quite variable, and it seems to be an incidental finding in many cats. Splenosystemic shunts can be associated with conditions predisposing the cat to PH and have been assumed to be a form of acquired shunt. Indeed, there is circumstantial evidence for this abnormality being an acquired condition with similar shunts forming as a response to experimental PH in cats. In addition, splenosystemic shunts can occur in tandem with MAS in cats with PH, and there is a report of spontaneous formation of a similar shunt due to PH following ligation of an intrahepatic CPSS.[26,29] Nevertheless, many cats do not seem to have any evidence of PH or liver disease, and this may suggest a congenital origin. Such cats, however, appear clinically unaffected and do not show the classic clinical signs associated with CPSSs. As these shunts drain the splenic circulation rather than the portal system, there may be effectively less shunting, and this may account for the apparent lack of clinical signs. It is also possible that cats with splenosystemic shunts had suffered a previous episode of PH due to an issue that has subsequently resolved. As most cats with splenosystemic shunts are neutered females, it has also been suggested that they could be an acquired shunt as a result of adhesions and neovascularisation following removal of the left ovary, although this is unproven.[27] Treatment of splenosystemic shunts has not been described, beyond management of any concurrent or apparently causative condition.

The cause and significance of splenosystemic shunts seems to vary between individuals, and it is possible that it might represent both a congenital and an acquired abnormality, depending on the presence or absence of PH. More research is needed to further elucidate this.

PELIOSIS HEPATIS

Epidemiology and aetiology

Peliosis hepatis is a very uncommon vasculoproliferative disorder in cats, although it is even less common in dogs. Affected cats have multiple, irregular, cystic blood-filled spaces randomly distributed throughout the liver. These are individually small (1–5 mm) but coalesce to cause enlargement of the liver and mass lesions.

The cause of peliosis hepatis remains unknown in cats. In people, it has been associated with a variety of inciting factors, including anabolic androgenic steroids, oestrogenic steroids, and infection with HIV or *Bartonella*. However, a postmortem study of the livers of 26 cats with peliosis hepatitis failed to detect evidence of *Bartonella henselae*, suggesting that this is not the underlying cause in this species.[30]

Peliosis hepatis can be divided into two types: parenchymal and phlebectatic (also referred to as telangiectasis). The parenchymal type is due to focal necrosis of hepatocytes as a result of an acute, severe ischaemic lesion. The phlebectatic type develops more slowly as a result of local obstruction of small portal vein branches, with associated hepatic atrophy and sinusoidal dilation. Both types can be seen concurrently in the same individual.

History and physical examination

Cats with peliosis hepatis can have clinical signs relating to abdominal haemorrhage due to rupture of one or more of the cysts. In one study, 69% (11/16) of cats had abdominal haemorrhage identified pre- or post-mortem.[31] Cats without haemorrhage may have signs of liver enlargement or have cystic liver masses identified. However, it is likely that in some cats peliosis hepatis may be an incidental finding, or it is possible that it may remain unidentified during their lifetime.

Diagnostic investigation

Liver enlargement or cystic lesions can be identified on abdominal imaging including ultrasonography or computed tomography. In cats with haemorrhage, peritoneal effusion will be present, and sampling will yield frank blood. In cats with intra-abdominal bleeding, a complete blood count will show evidence of acute and/or chronic haemorrhage.

Treatment and prognosis

There is very limited information regarding the treatment of peliosis hepatis in cats. Surgery can be performed to remove the affected liver lobe(s), but as the condition can be present in multiple lobes, the prognosis is typically guarded due to the potential for ongoing haemorrhage.

Take-home messages

- Most congenital portosystemic shunts in cats are extrahepatic, and the most common intrahepatic morphology is left divisional.
- Surgery to attenuate the shunt is the recommended treatment for congenital portosystemic shunts in cats. A cat that can tolerate complete acute ligation at surgery should benefit from this, whereas other cats require a gradual attenuation method.
- The most common perioperative complication and cause of mortality in cats undergoing congenital portosystemic shunt surgery is post-attenuation neurological signs, regardless of the method used.
- Other vascular disorders include primary portal vein hypoplasia and hepatic arteriovenous malformation, but these are very uncommon.

REFERENCES

[1] Levy JK, Bunch SE, Komtebedde J. Feline portosystemic vascular shunts. In: Bonagura JD, editor. *Kirk's Current Veterinary Therapy XII: Small Animal Practice*. Philadelphia, WB Saunders: 743, 1995.

[2] Bayton WA et al. Histopathological frequency of feline hepatobiliary disease in the UK. *J Small Anim Pract* 59:404, 2018.

[3] Swinbourne F et al. Histopathological findings in the livers of cats with a congenital portosystemic shunt before and after surgical attenuation. *Vet Rec* 172:362, 2013.

[4] Strickland R et al. Incidence and risk factors for neurological signs after attenuation of a single congenital portosystemic shunt in 50 cats. *Vet Surg*, 2020 [epub ahead of print].

[5] White RN, Shales C, Parry AT. New perspectives on the development of extrahepatic portosystemic shunts. *J Small Anim Pract* 58:669, 2017.

[6] Tivers M, Lipscomb V. Congenital portosystemic shunts in cats: investigation, diagnosis and stabilisation. *J Feline Med Surg* 13:173, 2011.

[7] Tzounos CE et al. Haematology and coagulation profiles in cats with congenital portosystemic shunts. *J Feline Med Surg* 19:1290, 2017.

[8] Kyles AE et al. Evaluation of ameroid ring constrictors for the management of single extrahepatic portosystemic shunts in cats: 23 cases (1996–2001). *J Am Vet Med Assoc* 220:1341, 2002.

[9] Ruland K, Fischer A, Hartmann K. Sensitivity and specificity of fasting ammonia and serum bile acids in the diagnosis of portosystemic shunts in dogs and cats. *Vet Clin Pathol* 39:57, 2010.

[10] Lipscomb VJ et al. Association of mesenteric portovenographic findings with outcome in cats receiving surgical treatment for single congenital portosystemic shunts. *J Am Vet Med Assoc* 234:221, 2009.

[11] Greenhalgh SN et al. Long-term survival and quality of life in dogs with clinical signs associated with a congenital portosystemic shunt after surgical or medical treatment. *J Am Vet Med Assoc* 245:527, 2014.

[12] Tivers M, Lipscomb V. Congenital portosystemic shunts in cats: surgical management and prognosis. *J Feline Med Surg* 13:185, 2011.

[13] Lipscomb VJ, Jones HJ, Brockman DJ. Complications and long-term outcomes of the ligation of congenital portosystemic shunts in 49 cats. *Vet Rec* 160:465, 2007.

[14] Weisse C et al. Transjugular coil embolization of an intrahepatic portosystemic shunt in a cat. *J Am Vet Med Assoc* 221:1287, 2002.

[15] Uemura A, Nakata TM, Tanaka R. Hybrid surgical treatment for 2 feline cases of intrahepatic shunt. *Can Vet J* 59:47, 2018.

[16] White RN, Burton CA. Anatomy of the patent ductus venosus in the cat. *J Feline Med Surg* 3:229, 2001.

[17] Valiente P et al. Complications and outcome of cats with congenital extrahepatic portosystemic shunts treated with thin film: thirty-four cases (2008–2017). *J Vet Intern Med* 34:117, 2020.

[18] Cabassu J et al. Outcomes of cats undergoing surgical attenuation of congenital extrahepatic portosystemic shunts through cellophane banding: 9 cases (2000–2007). *J Am Vet Med Assoc* 238:89, 2011.

[19] Havig M, Tobias KM. Outcome of ameroid constrictor occlusion of single congenital extrahepatic portosystemic shunts in cats: 12 cases (1993–2000). *J Am Vet Med Assoc* 220:337, 2002.

[20] Uemura A et al. Hybrid technique coil embolisation for intrahepatic arterioportal fistula in a cat: case report. *JFMS Open Rep* 2:2055116916642256, 2016.

[21] Legendre AM et al. Ascites associated with intrahepatic arteriovenous fistula in a cat. *J Am Vet Med Assoc* 168:589, 1976.

[22] McConnell JF et al. Ultrasonographic diagnosis of unusual portal vascular abnormalities in two cats. *J Small Anim Pract* 47:338, 2006.

[23] Phillips A et al. Surgical management of a cat with hepatic arterioportal fistula. *J Small Anim Pract* 60:126, 2019.

[24] Vandermeulen E et al. Transsplenic portal scintigraphy using ^{99m}Tc-pertechnetate for the diagnosis of portosystemic shunts in cats: a retrospective review of 12 patients. *J Feline Med Surg* 15:1123, 2013.

[25] d'Anjou MA et al. Ultrasonographic diagnosis of portosystemic shunting in dogs and cats. *Vet Radiol Ultrasound* 45:424, 2004.

[26] Sugimoto S et al. Multiple acquired portosystemic shunts secondary to primary hypoplasia of the portal vein in a cat. *J Vet Med Sci* 80:874, 2018.

[27] Palerme JS et al. Splenosystemic shunts in cats: a retrospective of 33 cases (2004–2011). *J Vet Intern Med* 27:1347, 2013.

[28] Specchi S et al. A "spaghetti sign" in feline abdominal radiographs predicts spleno-systemic collateral circulation. *Vet Radiol Ultrasound* 59:13, 2018.

[29] Zandvliet MM et al. Acquired portosystemic shunting in 2 cats secondary to congenital hepatic fibrosis. *J Vet Intern Med* 19:765, 2005.

[30] Buchmann AU et al. Peliosis hepatis in cats is not associated with *Bartonella henselae* infections. *Vet Pathol* 47:163, 2010.

[31] Brown PJ et al. Peliosis hepatis and telangiectasis in 18 cats. *J Small Anim Pract* 35:73, 1994.

CHAPTER 27

Hepatic lipidosis

Chiara Valtolina

Feline hepatic lipidosis (FHL) is a form of acquired liver disease in the cat. It presents as an acute critical syndrome that can result in the animal's death due to severe liver dysfunction and failure if therapeutic measures are not taken expeditiously. FHL is characterised by the accumulation of excessive triglycerides (TGs) in more than 50% of hepatocytes, resulting in hepatomegaly, intrahepatic cholestasis, and secondary impairment of liver function. It is believed to be a syndrome with multiple causative factors that is observed in anorexic cats.[1–4]

Cats have a propensity for hepatocellular lipid vacuolisation secondary to illness, which likely reflects unique aspects of feline metabolism. Their obligate carnivore status comes with several physiological and metabolic peculiarities in protein, carbon, and fatty acid (FA) metabolism that make them different from other animals that are not strict carnivores, like dogs, rats, mice, and humans.[1–3]

EPIDEMIOLOGY AND AETIOLOGY

The literature available on the epidemiology of FHL is scarce. A study performed in the United States of America in 1996 suggested that FHL was the most common liver disease in feline patients, with an overall prevalence of 49%, compared to other liver diseases.[5] More recent studies on the frequency and type of hepatobiliary liver diseases in cats performed in the United Kingdom and Japan revealed a much lower incidence of FHL (3.2% and 4.4%, respectively) when compared to other hepatobiliary diseases. Breed as well as dietary and other environmental differences have been proposed as the reasons for this discrepancy in the prevalence between the United States of America, United Kingdom, and Japan.[6,7]

Even though cats of any age and sex can be affected, FHL is mainly reported in middle-aged cats (median age 7 years).[3,4,8] Actual (body condition 4/5) or historical obesity seems to be a predisposing factor for the development of FHL.[2–4,8] A possible seasonality of the disease has been reported, with less cases being presented in spring, possibly due to seasonality-associated recorded stressful events, such as owners' vacation, and sudden introduction to outdoor access.[9] Furthermore, a significant proportion of cats with FHL, compared to a control group of cats presented to the hospital for other diseases, were indoor cats fed mainly dry food instead of a canned diet.[9]

Anorexia, and the resulting negative energy balance, is considered the trigger for FHL. Individual predisposition, however, cannot be excluded, as not every anorexic cat will develop FHL and not every sick cat with FHL will succumb to the disease. In a clinical setting, a period of anorexia of 2–14 days has been associated with the development of FHL.[1,3] Hepatic lipidosis has been divided into primary and secondary. In primary FHL, anorexia occurs in a healthy animal secondary to decreased food availability, administration of nonpalatable food, or decreased food intake secondary to a stressful event. Secondary FHL is considered the most common form of lipidosis, occurring in about 65%–95% of cases, in which anorexia develops as a consequence of an underlying disease. Most commonly reported underlying diseases include pancreatitis, diabetes mellitus, inflammatory hepatobiliary disease, gastrointestinal (GI) disease, renal failure, and neoplasia.[1,3,10] Secondary lipidosis can also occur in a hospitalised cat because of pain, nausea, vomiting, and critical illness interfering with adequate food intake for a period time. The development of FHL in an anorexic feline patient during hospitalisation can contribute to a worse outcome.

The pathophysiology of FHL is complex, multifactorial, and intertwined with the metabolic peculiarities of the cat as an obligate carnivore, which is considered an important cofounding factor for the development of FHL.[1,2] The unique lipid and protein metabolism of cats makes them dependent on indispensable essential fatty acids (EFAs), amino acids (especially arginine, taurine, methionine, and cobalamin), and vitamins (especially B vitamins), which easily become deficient after a period of prolonged anorexia.[1,2,11] Cats also possess limited ability to adapt their protein metabolic pathways to conserve nitrogen, and they rapidly develop severe protein malnutrition if anorexic. Carbohydrate metabolism in cats with FHL resembles that of critically ill cats, which is characterised by a high circulating concentration of insulin counter-regulatory hormones, such as glucagon, cortisol, and growth hormone. Furthermore, high circulating concentrations of glucose, lactate, and nonesterified fatty acids (NEFAs) and a low concentration of insulin have been found in critically ill cats.[12]

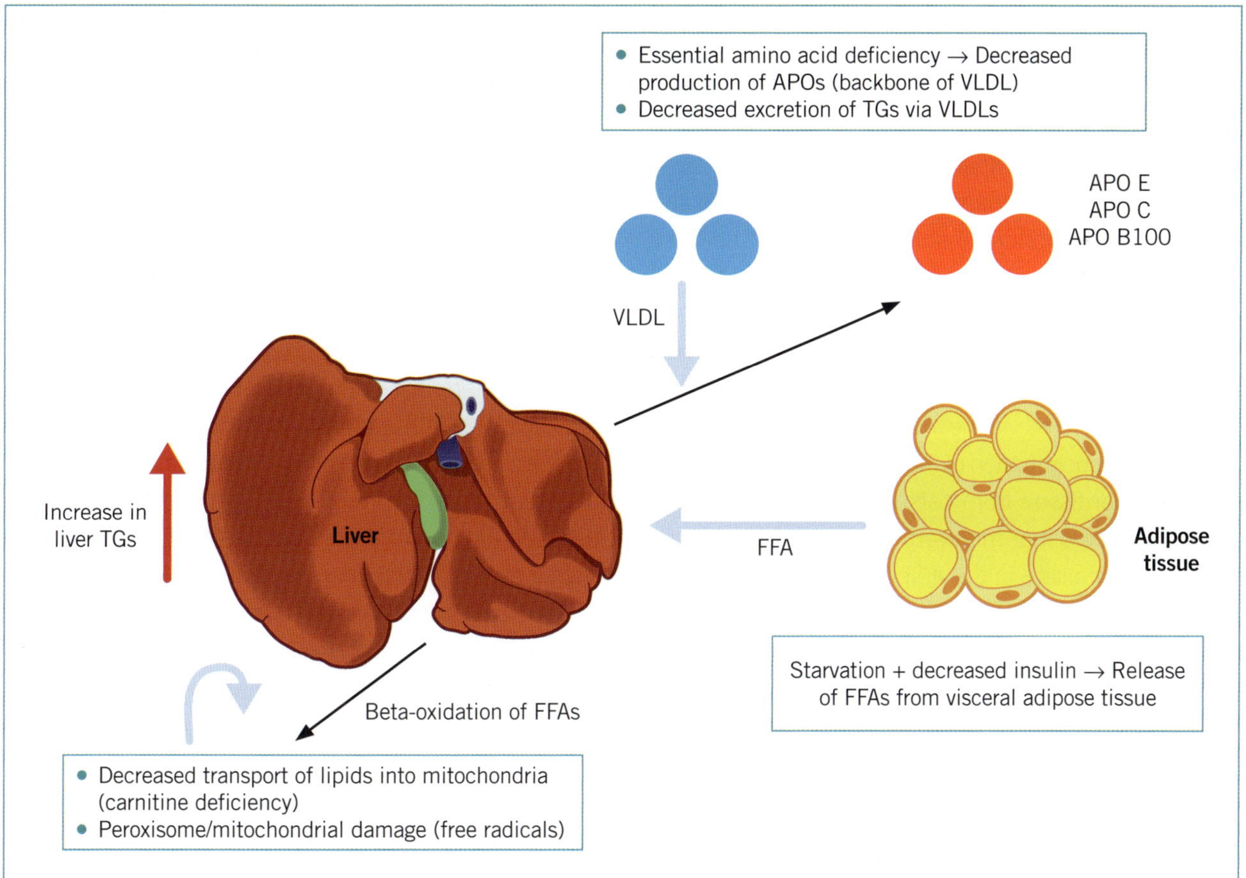

Figure 27.1. Pathogenesis of hepatic lipidosis in cats. Feline hepatic lipidosis (FHL) is usually a secondary disease that develops when a cat is ill from an underlying disease (often cholangiohepatitis or pancreatitis, but any disease can be the cause). The underlying disease causes anorexia, increased circulating concentrations of stress hormones, and decreased insulin concentration, which results in the release of large amounts of free fatty acids (FFAs) to the blood. The liver has two main mechanisms of dealing with increased FFAs. The first is beta-oxidation, the normal mechanism to produce energy in cells, which is dependent on carnitine—necessary to shuffle fatty acids into mitochondria to produce energy. This process is impaired in FHL because cats are protein-dependent and cannot produce carnitine themselves. Furthermore, a decreased number of mitochondria and mitochondrial damage has been described in FHL. The second mechanism involves esterification of fatty acids into triglycerides (TGs) by the liver and redistribution of TGs to other organs by packaging them into lipoproteins, mostly very-low-density lipoproteins (VLDLs). This process is also dependent on protein intake, as proteins are needed in the apolipoproteins (APO) to make the fat water-soluble for transportation in the blood. This process is thus also impaired in FHL and results in TG accumulation in the liver. This schematic makes it obvious that the single most important treatment of cats with FHL is tube feeding with sufficient protein and calories in order to reverse the negative energy balance, protein deficiency, and fat accumulation in the liver.

The primary metabolic abnormalities leading to the accumulation of TGs in the hepatocytes consist of disturbances in the pathways that regulate uptake, synthesis, degradation, and secretion of FAs. On the one hand, there is an imbalance between mobilisation of peripheral fat stores and de novo synthesis of FAs in the visceral adipose tissue, and on the other, the increase in the rate of hepatic FA beta-oxidation for energy production is insufficient. Furthermore, insufficient redistribution of hepatic TGs via very-low-density lipoprotein (VLDL) leads to accumulation of FAs in the liver (Fig. 27.1).[1–4]

The increased concentration of insulin counterregulatory hormones in FHL leads to an increased activity of hormone-sensitive lipase, which is associated with decreased circulating insulin, and promotes lipolysis and mobilisation of free fatty acids (FFAs) from the visceral adipose tissue while impairing lipogenesis and glucose tolerance. High concentrations of circulating FFAs also contribute to peripheral insulin resistance. The FFAs released from the adipose tissue are transported to the liver via the portal circulation. Once having reached the liver, FAs can enter two pathways: either they undergo beta-oxidation in the mitochondria, or they are esterified to TGs and secreted via the VLDL pathway (Fig. 27.1).

A higher concentration of the FA palmitate (16:0) was found in liver tissue from cats with FHL compared to control subjects that mirrored the increased concentrations of palmitate in the adipose tissue of the same animals.[13] The increased hepatic concentration of palmitate in cats with FHL supports the hypothesis that some de novo synthesis of FAs occurs in the visceral adipose tissue of cats with FHL, contributing to the FA overload in these subjects in FHL.[2,13–15] Obesity associated with increases in the visceral adipose tissue can predispose cats to FHL because of the quantity of FAs that can be rapidly released from peripheral fat stores and visceral adipose tissue, the release of inflammatory adipokines from the adipose tissue, and the insulin resistance associated with obesity.[3,4,16]

Mitochondrial beta-oxidation is the main oxidative pathway for the disposal of FAs from the liver under normal physiological conditions. Short-chain and medium-chain NEFAs freely enter the mitochondria, while the activity of the enzyme carnitine palmitoyltransferase 1 (CPT1) regulates the entry of long-chain FAs. L-carnitine is part of the two enzymes that regulate the transport of FAs from the circulation into the mitochondria and from the hepatic cytosol back into the plasma. In human medicine, abnormal beta-oxidation caused by mitochondrial dysfunction has been reported as a potential cause for lipid accumulation in hepatocytes during hepatic steatosis in nonalcoholic fatty liver disease.[17] A reduced number of mitochondria in FHL has been reported, suggesting that mitochondrial dysfunction could also occur in FHL and contribute to FA overload in the liver.[18] The occurrence of increased ketone body formation in cats with FHL, however, points more to an enhanced rate of beta-oxidation of FAs, and it is probably the result of the more complex catabolic state, increased insulin resistance, and decreased glucose tolerance that occurs in these patients.[1,3,10,19]

Once in the hepatocyte, FAs can be esterified to TGs, which usually accumulate in vacuoles within the hepatocytes or can be incorporated in VLDLs to be excreted into the peripheral circulation. Cats with FHL have always been considered to have increased levels of TGs in plasma, with the largest distribution in the VLDL fraction and increased plasma concentrations of VLDL.[20] This suggests that VLDL secretion in FHL is enhanced and not deficient, although it is insufficient to prevent the lipid overload of hepatocytes by the dramatic increase of FA uptake by the liver.[1,3,20] However, the relationship between FHL and VLDL is not straightforward, as conflicting results of both increased and decreased plasma TG or VLDL concentrations have been found in different studies on FHL.[9,20–22] Low VLDL concentrations in cats with FHL suggest that there may be a maximum capacity of the feline liver to secrete VLDLs.

In a recent article that evaluated lipid types and their distribution in the liver and plasma of cats with FHL, the concentration of sphingomyelin (SM) was significantly increased in the liver and plasma of cats with FHL when compared to healthy cats.[22] This phospholipid is a type of sphingolipid primarily present in the cell membrane, especially in the membranous myelin sheath that surrounds nerve cell axons. The availability of palmitic acid (16:0) is a rate-limiting step for SM synthesis, and cats with FHL have been shown to have an increased concentration of palmitic acid in their liver.[13,22] In human medicine, the increased synthesis of SM in livers affected by nonalcoholic fatty liver disease promotes hepatic insulin resistance, hepatocyte apoptosis, and increased release of inflammatory mediators, which ultimately worsens liver steatosis and predisposes the patient to the development of steatohepatitis.[23] The increased SM concentrations, both in the liver and in the plasma of cats with FHL, warrants further study in order to understand the potential role of SM in FHL and its correlation with cytokines, insulin resistance, and severity of the disease. Experimental studies targeting the enzymes involved in the pathway of ceramide synthesis have reported a decrease in the development of steatosis in a mouse model of obesity and nonalcoholic fatty liver disease, and these enzymes remain subject of research in human medicine.[23]

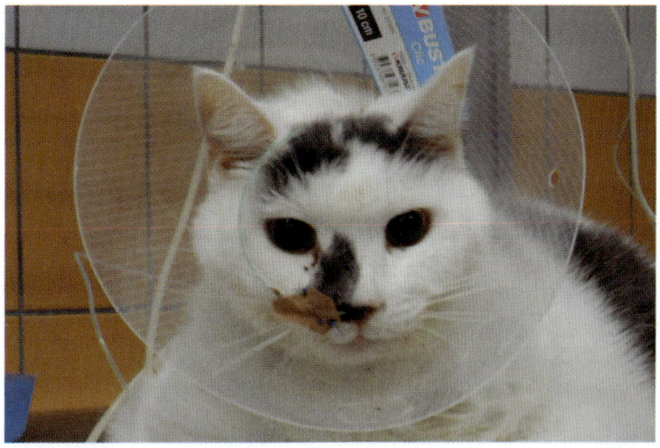

Figure 27.2. Cat with hepatic lipidosis. Note the icterus visible on the inner part of the pinnae.

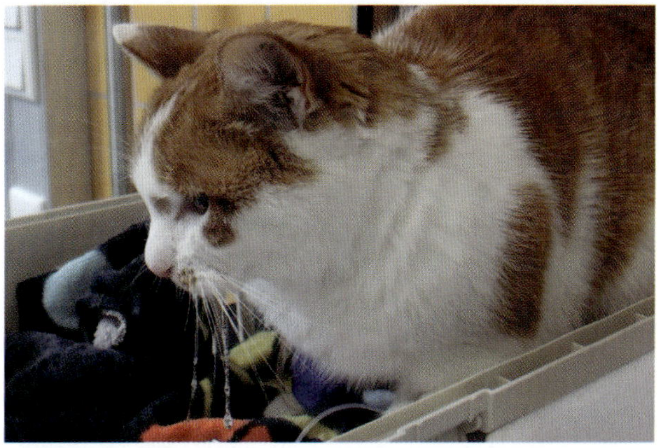

Figure 27.3. Cat with hepatic lipidosis displaying nausea and ptyalism.

HISTORY AND PHYSICAL EXAMINATION

Cats affected with FHL present with a history of anorexia and weight loss of different duration. If a cat develops FHL secondary to an underlying disease, the presenting clinical signs often overlap with those caused by the underlying primary disease process.

Icterus (Fig. 27.2) secondary to cholestasis is a common presentation in severe FHL (>70% of cases), and hepatomegaly can often be noted on abdominal palpation.[1,3,9] Other reported clinical signs include hypovolaemia, hypotension, and dehydration from decreased fluid intake and excessive fluid loss via diarrhoea or vomiting; nausea and ptyalism (Fig. 27.3) from concurrent GI disease, pancreatitis, or hepatic encephalopathy (HE); constipation or diarrhoea; and poor haircoat.[1,3] Lethargy and mental obtundation can be seen in cats with FHL and are often related to the presence of hypokalaemia and hyperammonaemia and secondary HE.[1,3,10] HE in cats with FHL is associated with decreased liver function and arginine deficiency and can be worsened by hypokalaemia.[1,24] Neck ventroflexion and severe muscle weakness can be secondary to severe hypokalaemia due to anorexia and vomiting.[1]

Cats with severe cholestasis have been reported to experience severe hypotension, often unresponsive to fluid therapy, especially if anaesthetised or if stressful procedures are being performed.[25] In the author's experience, this is also the case for some critically ill cats with FHL when general anaesthesia has been used for oesophagostomy tube placement or liver biopsy. In humans, the link between critical illness–related corticosteroid insufficiency and high circulating bile acid (BA) concentrations has been established.[26] High levels of circulating conjugated or unconjugated BAs in critical illness have been shown to inhibit glucocorticoid-metabolising enzymes and to inhibit the release of corticotropin-releasing hormone and adrenocorticotropic hormone (ACTH) from the hypothalamic–pituitary–adrenal (HPA) axis.[26] Critical illness–related corticosteroid insufficiency is characterised by haemodynamic instability and refractory hypotension despite fluid resuscitation and a concentration of corticosteroids that is insufficient for the severity of the underlying illness. In veterinary medicine, little is known about the effect of high serum BA concentrations on the function of the HPA axis. To date, only one study has been published investigating the relationship between delta cortisol (difference between basal cortisol and cortisol after ACTH stimulation) in cats with cholestatic liver disease and the survival or indicators of liver function. This study found that cats with cholestatic liver disease had high basal and stimulated cortisol levels, but a delta cortisol below 179 nmol/l defined a population with decreased survival at 30 days after discharge.[25] Critical illness–related corticosteroid insufficiency should be suspected in every patient with FHL that develops severe hypotension, and replacement therapy with corticosteroids should be considered.

DIAGNOSTIC INVESTIGATION

The presumptive diagnosis of FHL often begins as a clinical diagnosis based on the patient's history and clinical presentation. Clinicopathologic findings, ultrasonographic appearance of the liver, and liver fine needle aspiration (FNA) for cytological evaluation are often used to validate the initial clinical diagnosis and investigate for possible underlying and concomitant diseases.

Blood work

Haematology

Mild to moderate nonregenerative anaemia with poikilocytosis and Heinz bodies is common in FHL although considered a nonspecific finding.[1,3,10] Anaemia was recently considered a negative prognostic marker.[9] The leucogram can be influenced by the presence of an underlying inflammatory, infectious, or neoplastic disease. Thrombocytopenia does not occur frequently in cats with FHL, unless they are suffering from disseminated intravascular coagulation or concomitant liver failure.[1,10,27]

Biochemistry profile

Numerous biochemical abnormalities are present in cats with FHL. Bilirubin and BA concentrations and serum activities of alkaline phosphatase (ALP) and aspartate aminotransferase (AST) have been reported to be increased in cats with FHL compared to healthy cats and cats with other liver diseases (e.g. cholangitis).[3,8,10] Elevation in ALP activity and minimal elevation in gamma-glutamyltransferase (GGT) activity is considered by some authors to be a typical enzymatic pattern of FHL.[8,10] Mild hypoalbuminaemia secondary to anorexia and decreased hepatic function is also often reported in cats with FHL. Blood urea nitrogen was found to be decreased in 51% of cats as a consequence of chronic anorexia, concomitant GI diseases, and/or derangements in the urea cycle function.[1,3,10]

Anorexia, vomiting, diarrhoea, and dehydration, as well as fluid therapy to correct fluid disbalances, are responsible for the electrolyte abnormalities seen in FHL. Hypokalaemia, hypomagnesaemia, and hypophosphataemia are reported in almost 30% of cats with FHL.[1,3,8] Hypokalaemia and hypophosphataemia have been associated with increased morbidity and mortality in cats with FHL.[4,9] Hypocholesterolaemia, increased creatine kinase activity, and panhypoproteinaemia have been reported as significant risk factors for negative outcome.[9]

Cats with FHL often have higher serum concentration of beta-hydroxybutyric acid compared to healthy cats, which is likely a reflection of their negative energy balance.[19]

Evaluation of coagulation status

Coagulation abnormalities and clinical bleeding tendencies are frequently seen (45%–73%) in cats with FHL. Bleeding tendencies are recognisable even during small procedures like venepuncture and peripheral catheter placement, and they can become clinically relevant if invasive procedures like oesophageal tube placement and liver biopsy are performed.[10,27,28] The coagulopathy of patients with FHL is thought to be multifactorial: a combination of decreased production of coagulation factors and activation of haemostasis, with secondary increased consumption of coagulation factors likely contributing.[27]

Commonly reported alterations of haemostasis in cats with any liver disease are prolongation of prothrombin time (PT) as well as reduced factor II, VII, and X activities suggestive of vitamin K deficiency. Significant prolongation of activated partial thromboplastin time (aPTT) was also reported in 40% of cats with liver disease compared to healthy cats, and protein C was also decreased in 44% of cats with liver disease.[29] The most consistent abnormalities in cats with FHL were increased factor V activity and D-dimer concentration, with 54% of cats having values above the reference range for both parameters.[29] Furthermore, 31% of cats with FHL had severely reduced factor XIII (fibrin-stabilising factor) activity and fibrinogen concentration.[29]

Severe bleeding during liver biopsy procedures has been reported, with thrombocytopenia (<80000 platelets/ml) and an aPTT elevated more than 1.5 times the upper normal limit [30]

It is important to remember, however, that even a normal coagulation profile cannot predict with certainty if clinical bleeding will occur. It is crucial, especially in cats with FHL, to be extremely vigilant and to postpone any invasive procedure (e.g. oesophagostomy feeding tube placement, liver biopsy) until the cat has been appropriately stabilised and vitamin K_1 has been administered for a few days (see section "Management and treatment" in this chapter). A typed plasma transfusion might be necessary in patients with FHL that start to bleed after an invasive procedure or in coagulopathic cats when invasive procedures cannot be postponed.

Diagnostic imaging

Abdominal ultrasonography is usually the first diagnostic step performed in an icteric, anorexic cat to evaluate the size, echogenicity, and parenchyma of the liver and to highlight any changes in the gallbladder and bile duct. On ultrasound examination, the liver of cats with FHL appears enlarged and diffusely hyperechoic in comparison to the falciform fat. This finding is often used to diagnose FHL with an accuracy of 70%.[31] A study evaluating the use of computed tomography (CT) and X-ray attenuation in the liver for the diagnosis of FHL concluded that hepatic CT attenuation of the liver may be of limited value in detecting FHL in patients at risk for lipidosis and that values obtained for hepatic X-ray attenuation could vary between CT scanners.[32] For this reason, and since general anaesthesia is required before the procedure in these often clinically compromised patients, the routine use of CT to diagnose lipidosis cannot yet be recommended.[1]

Clinicopathologic findings

The definitive diagnosis of FHL is usually made by cytological evaluation of a liver sample obtained by FNA, which is considered a safe procedure with few minor complications when compared to liver histological biopsy. The cytological hallmark of lipidosis is the presence of cellular steatosis, which can be macro- or microvesicular (Fig. 27.4).[3,8,18] Cytological examination of samples obtained by FNA allows accurate detection of FHL and vacuolar hepatopathy in general; however, a study reported that only 51% of feline cases had overall agreement between cytological and histological diagnosis of FHL, and possible underlying liver diseases might be missed.[33] As previously mentioned, cats that are sick tend to accumulate lipid in their liver, often mimicking FHL; for this reason, a definitive diagnosis of FHL can only be made when at least 50% of the hepatocytes are affected.

Liver biopsy should not be routinely performed in cats suffering from FHL and should only be considered in subjects that fail to improve despite appropriate treatment. Other indications for liver biopsy are a history, clinical findings, or clinicopathologic findings suggestive of a possible underlying hepatic disease—neoplastic or inflammatory other than FHL.[1,3] Some authors have suggested that it might be safer to collect liver biopsy samples during an exploratory laparotomy or laparoscopy than using a Tru-Cut rapid-firing automatic biopsy needle.[1,10]

Histological examination of the liver of cats with FHL reveals diffuse lobular changes, with cytoplasmic lipid-containing vacuoles that fill more than 50% of hepatocytes. This disorder has always been described in the literature as an "acute disease that lacks a necroinflammatory component".[8,18] The liver contains parenchymal cells (i.e. hepatocytes) as well as nonparenchymal cells, including Kupffer cells (liver resident macrophages), hepatic stellate cells (involved in vitamin A metabolism),

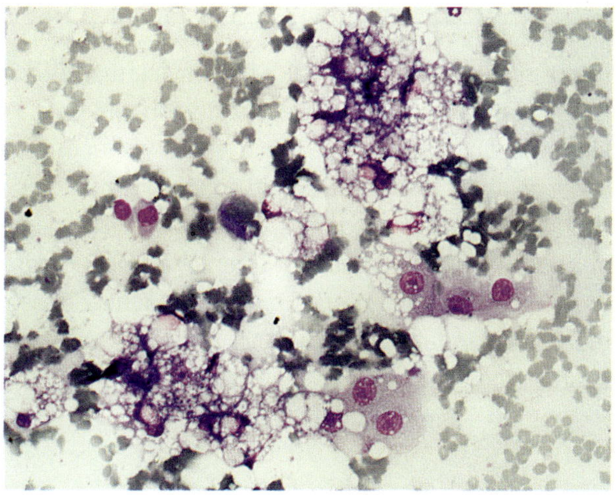

Figure 27.4. Liver cytology of a cat with hepatic lipidosis. Besides normal hepatocytes, numerous hepatic cells displaying severe (microvesicular) lipidosis can be seen.

and biliary epithelial cells (forming bile ducts), which contribute to maintain liver homoeostasis. When liver damage is severe enough to inhibit the replication capability of the hepatocytes (e.g. in steatosis), a quiescent population of pluripotent cells is activated: the hepatic progenitor cells (HPCs). In humans and animal models, the degree and niche activation of HPCs are directly related to disease severity, indicated by the amount of hepatocyte loss, the amount of inflammation, and the extent of fibrosis.[34] In a recent study, the HPCs and their niche was evaluated in cats with FHL.[35] A clear and definitive pattern between the histopathological changes and the activation of HPCs could not be established. In addition, a clear upregulation of niche factors was not shown in all cats with FHL, and no fibrosis or severe inflammatory changes were identified. Despite the presence of severe steatosis in all cats affected with FHL, the lack of a pattern of activation of HPCs could be explained by different factors. FHL is classified as an acute disease in which either the clinical condition of the cat improves and lipidosis resolves quickly or the cat dies or is euthanised. The acute nature of FHL may have limited the development of a clear relationship between HPC activation and hepatic lipidosis. Furthermore, the different results in HPC activation in FHL could also be caused by variations in the underlying disease that caused the anorexia and secondary lipidosis or by the effect of the therapeutic measures initiated by the clinician.

MANAGEMENT AND TREATMENT

Rapid assessment of all major body systems (neurological, cardiovascular, and respiratory) should be performed in any cat presented with a history of anorexia, lethargy, and icterus. Immediate supportive treatment should be directed to address any fluid and electrolyte abnormalities. Any other concurrent clinical findings, if present, (e.g. nausea and vomiting, abdominal pain, mental obtundation suggesting HE) should also be treated promptly.

Fluid therapy and electrolyte imbalance correction

Cats presenting with FHL can suffer from different degrees of hypoperfusion because of vomiting, anorexia, and adipsia. Hypoperfusion in cats is characterised by tachycardia (heart rate >220 bpm) or inappropriate bradycardia (heart rate <140 bpm), pale mucous membranes, prolonged capillary refill time, often hypothermia, and mild hypotension. Initial fluid therapy with a balanced isotonic crystalloid infusion (e.g. Ringer's lactate or acetate solution, Hartmann's solution, Plasma-Lyte) should be administered to correct hypoperfusion if present. Small volume resuscitation (5–10 ml/kg IV bolus given over 15–20 minutes) should be instituted in hypovolaemic cats, while slow rewarming should be implemented if hypothermia is present.[1] Once hypoperfusion has been addressed, fluid therapy to provide for maintenance requirements and to correct fluid deficits according to the estimated percentage of dehydration should be started, with the total volume administered over 24 hours.[1,10] The fluid therapy plan should be reevaluated and adjusted at least once daily based on the cat's requirements and clinical condition. The newly formulated fluid therapy plan should take into account the fluid balance and the body weight of the patient, the percentage of dehydration, and if ongoing losses (vomiting, diarrhoea) are still occurring.[1] If enteral or parenteral feeding is implemented, the amount of fluid administered with the nutritional plan should also be deducted from the calculated amount of fluid to avoid fluid overload, and the same should be done for any medications used.

There is a lot of debate on what is the best fluid to administer to patients with FHL. Due to poor hepatic function, lactate clearance may not be appropriate in cats with FHL. Therefore, the administration of lactate-based solutions might worsen hyperlactataemia in these patients.[3,4] However, this seems to only be a theoretical concern, as lactated Ringer's solution has been used without major complications in many of these patients.[1,3,4] Fluids containing glucose should not be used in cats with FHL to avoid worsening glucose intolerance and concurrent hyperglycaemia.

Correction of electrolyte abnormalities should take place in the initial phase of hospitalisation and before nutrition is started. Abnormalities of potassium and phosphate should be adequately corrected, and these electrolytes should be checked at least twice daily at the beginning of hospitalisation. The serum/plasma magnesium concentration should also be measured and supplemented, especially if hypokalaemia is difficult to correct, as hypomagnesaemia can worsen renal potassium wasting (Table 27.1).

Early enteral nutrition

Early enteral nutrition is the cornerstone of the treatment of FHL. Nutrition should be initiated as soon as the cat is cardiovascularly stable and electrolyte abnormalities have been corrected. Whenever possible, enteral feeding is preferred over parenteral nutrition because it helps to maintain intestinal structure and function.[36] However, in case of intractable vomiting or if there is minimal tolerance to enteral feeding, the parenteral route should be taken into consideration.[36] Partial parenteral nutrition can be easily administered via a peripheral catheter and does not require central venous access, which might initially not be advisable due to coagulation abnormalities.

The ideal diet for FHL should be high in protein (30%–40% of metabolisable energy), moderate in lipids (about 50% of metabolisable energy), and relatively poor in carbohydrates (about 20% of metabolisable energy).[1,3,4,10,36] In critically ill cats, 6 g of protein/100 kcal (or 25%–35% of their total energy requirements) is considered to be enough to support their unique metabolism.[36] The majority of the veterinary commercial diets formulated for recovery in cats meet these requirements.

Resting energy requirement (RER) in these patients can be estimated using the formula below. The use of an illness factor is no longer recommended, as feeding too much at once has been associated with hyperglycaemia, GI dysfunction, and hepatic dysfunction.[12,36,37]

$$\text{RER} = 70 \times (\text{body weight [kg]})^{0.75}$$

Forced enteral feeding should never be considered in a sick cat with FHL because of the risk of the development of food aversion and because this technique does not deliver enough nutrition to meet energy requirements. Feeding tubes (nasooesophageal, oesophageal) allow clinicians to reliably provide enteral nutrition without causing excessive stress to the patient. The author's initial feeding tube choice for cats with FHL is the nasooesophageal feeding tube (Fig. 27.5). The nasooesophageal feeding tube is ideal in an unstable and coagulopathic patient, as it does not require specialised techniques or general anaesthesia for placement, and it is noninvasive. Placing an oesophageal feeding tube should be delayed until fluid and coagulation abnormalities have been addressed and the cat is considered stable enough to undergo anaesthesia.

A commercial high-protein recovery food should be administered in increments: one-third of the calculated

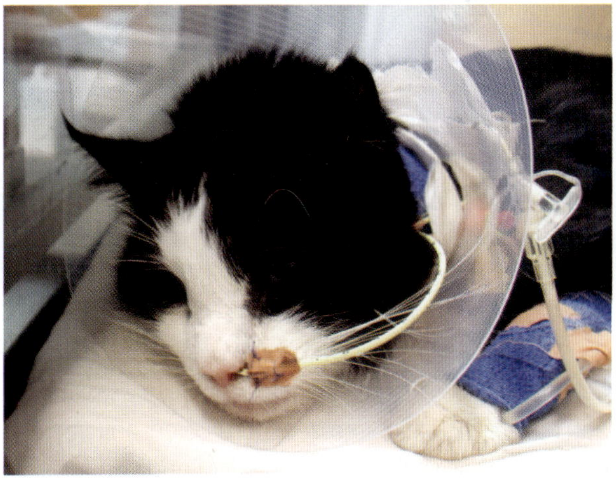

Figure 27.5. Cat with hepatic lipidosis being fed via a nasooesophageal tube.

Table 27.1. Guide to electrolyte imbalance correction.

Electrolyte	Dose	Route	Comments
Potassium	[4.5 – Potassium of the patient (mmol/l)] × 0.6 × body weight (kg) = mmol of potassium to administer to correct the patient's potassium deficit up to a potassium level of 4.5 mmol/l	IV	The amount in ml of the calculated potassium should be diluted 1:4 with NaCl 0.9% and administered with a dedicated syringe pump IV at a rate not faster than 0.5 mmol/kg/h Be careful not to administer the solution containing potassium as a bolus or rapid infusion
Phosphate	0.01–0.03 mEq/kg/h as a CRI for 6 h For severe deficits: 0.12 mEq/kg/h as a CRI	IV	–
Magnesium	0.75–1 mEq/kg/day for the first 24 h	IV	Diluted in 5% dextrose as a 20% solution

CRI, constant-rate infusion; IV, intravenous.

RER on the first day, followed by a slow increase over the next 2–3 days until the total RER is provided. The total volume of food required each day should initially be divided into six to eight portions or administered as a constant-rate infusion (CRI). Cats with FHL might have developed a smaller stomach volume because of the prolonged anorexia, and the amount of food they can tolerate per meal can be drastically reduced.[3] The author prefers to administer food initially as a trickle feeding because this method seems to reduce nausea, gastric discomfort, and vomiting associated with gastric distension after intermittent food administration. A regimen of 4 hours of food administration followed by 2 hours of no food is more physiological than CRI, as it offers the GI tract some rest between feedings and allows the clinician to evaluate any gastric residual volume. Food should always be administered lukewarm and, if intermittent administration is chosen, should be administered slowly over 15–20 minutes. If any signs of discomfort, retching, or vomiting occur, food administration should be interrupted for a few hours.

Other medical treatment

Antiemetics and gastroprotectants should be considered in cats that are nauseated and/or vomit and in order to enable enteral feeding as soon as possible. The different drugs act by diverse mechanisms, so they can be combined in the same patient. Metoclopramide (1 mg/kg/day IV as a CRI), ondansetron (0.1–0.5 mg/kg IV every 8–12 hours), and maropitant (1 mg/kg IV every 24 hours) can be used alone or in combination to decrease vomiting and nausea. Metoclopramide is not a potent antiemetic in cats, but it has some prokinetic effect and can facilitate gastric emptying, which makes it an attractive drug for use when enteral feeding is first initiated.[38] Omeprazole (1 mg/kg PO every 12 hours) can be used to prevent reflux oesophagitis in animals with frequent emesis.[38] The use of appetite stimulants has been discouraged in cats with FHL, especially during initial hospitalisation. Their effect in sick animals is unpredictable, and the reported side effects (e.g. agitation, tremors, depression. vomiting, hypersalivation) could worsen an already critical clinical situation.[1,10,36]

In cats with impaired coagulation and if invasive procedures (e.g. oesophageal tube placement) are planned, vitamin K_1 should be administered. Because the absorption of vitamin K_1 from the GI tract might be compromised by cholestasis, 0.5–1.5 mg/kg SC or IV (depending on the preparation) at 12-hour intervals for 3–4 doses has been recommended.[4]

Over the last years, L-carnitine supplementation (250–500 mg/cat/day) has received some interest as an important additional therapy for FHL.[3,4,39] In an experimental study in overweight cats undergoing rapid weight loss, dietary L-carnitine supplementation increased the rate of FFA beta-oxidation and decreased triacylglycerol accumulation in the liver.[40] These results seem to be in agreement with the clinical experience that exogenous L-carnitine supplementation can improve FA oxidation in cats with FHL, ameliorate their clinical signs, and increase the probability of survival.[4,39] Furthermore, in an organoid model for feline hepatic steatosis, L-carnitine supplementation to feline liver organoids attenuated lipid accumulation in high-fat conditions and improved cellular viability.[41]

Since cats with underlying pancreatitis or GI disease are also likely to be hypocobalaminaemic, vitamin B_{12} supplementation should be considered (250 µg SC injection once weekly for 6 weeks, then once monthly for 6 months).[4,10] Supplementation of taurine, vitamin E, and S-adenosylmethionine has been mentioned by some authors as supportive medical treatment in cats with FHL, but there is currently no evidence that supports their benefit in the available literature.[1,4,10]

PROGNOSIS AND OUTCOME

The prognosis does not seem to be related to the severity of FHL but more to the underlying disease and the early initiation of appropriate treatment. Cats with FHL have been reported to have a recovery rate of 80%–85% in the absence of a serious underlying disease and if they are rapidly treated with nutritional support.[1,4,8,40] The literature provides some prognostic factors relevant for patients with FHL. Reported positive prognostic factors are young age and higher serum potassium concentration and haematocrit at admission to the clinic.[4,8] Negative prognostic factors associated with increased mortality are older age, lethargy, mental depression, ptyalism, hypoproteinaemia, hypoalbuminaemia, increased serum creatine kinase activity, hypocholesterolaemia, and hepatic failure at presentation.[4,8,9]

Take-home messages

- Feline hepatic lipidosis should be considered a clinical diagnosis based on the patient's anamnesis and clinical presentation. Further tests should be used to confirm the diagnosis and concomitant diseases.
- Anorexia, weight loss, and icterus are the most common presenting clinical signs.
- Stabilisation of the cat's cardiovascular status and fluid and electrolyte imbalances should be rapidly instituted.
- Early enteral nutrition is the specific treatment for feline hepatic lipidosis and should not be delayed until a final diagnosis is reached.

REFERENCES

[1] Valtolina C, Favier RP. Feline hepatic lipidosis. *Vet Clin North Am Small Anim Pract* 47:683, 2017.

[2] Verbrugghe A, Bakovic M. Peculiarities of one-carbon metabolism in the strict carnivorous cat and the role in feline hepatic lipidosis. *Nutrients* 5:2811, 2013.

[3] Armstrong PJ, Blanchard G. Hepatic lipidosis in cats. *Vet Clin North Am Small Anim Pract* 39:599, 2009.

[4] Center SA. Feline hepatic lipidosis. *Vet Clin North Am Small Anim Pract* 35:225, 2005.

[5] Gagne JM et al. Clinical features of inflammatory liver disease in cats: 41 cases (1983–1993). *J Am Vet Med Assoc* 214:513, 1999.

[6] Bayton WA et al. Histopathological frequency of feline hepatobiliary disease in the UK. *J Small Anim Pract* 59:404, 2018.

[7] Hirose N et al. A retrospective histopathological survey on canine and feline liver diseases at the University of Tokyo between 2006 and 2012. *J Vet Med Sci* 76:1015, 2014.

[8] Center SA et al. A retrospective study of 77 cats with severe hepatic lipidosis: 1975–1990. *J Vet Intern Med* 7:349, 1993.

[9] Kuzi S et al. Prognostic markers in feline hepatic lipidosis: a retrospective study of 71 cats. *Vet Rec* 181:512, 2017.

[10] Webb CB. Hepatic lipidosis: clinical review drawn from collective effort. *J Feline Med Surg* 20:217, 2018.

[11] Trevizan L et al. Maintenance of arachidonic acid and evidence of $\Delta5$ desaturation in cats fed γ-linolenic and linoleic acid enriched diets. *Lipids* 47:413, 2012.

[12] Chan DL et al. Alterations in carbohydrate metabolism in critically ill cats. *J Vet Emerg Crit Care* 16:S7, 2006.

[13] Hall JA, Barstad LA, Connor WE. Lipid composition of hepatic and adipose tissues from normal cats and from cats with idiopathic hepatic lipidosis. *J Vet Intern Med* 11:238, 1997.

[14] Brown B et al. Metabolic and hormonal alterations in cats with hepatic lipidosis. *J Vet Intern Med* 14:20, 2000.

[15] Valtolina C et al. Gene expressions of de novo hepatic lipogenesis in feline hepatic lipidosis. *J Feline Med Surg* 22:500, 2020.

[16] Hoenig M et al. Insulin sensitivity, fat distribution, and adipocytokine response to different diets in lean and obese cats before and after weight loss. *Am J Physiol Regul Integr Comp Physiol* 292:R227, 2007.

[17] Wei Y et al. Nonalcoholic fatty liver disease and mitochondrial dysfunction. *World J Gastroenterol* 14:193, 2008.

[18] Center SA et al. Ultrastructural hepatocellular features associated with severe hepatic lipidosis in cats. *Am J Vet Res* 54:724, 1993.

[19] Aroch I, Shechter-Polak M, Segev G. A retrospective study of serum β-hydroxybutyric acid in 215 ill cats: clinical signs, laboratory findings and diagnoses. *Vet J* 191:240, 2012.

[20] Pazak HE et al. Characterization of serum lipoprotein profiles of healthy, adult cats and idiopathic feline hepatic lipidosis patients. *J Nutr* 128:2747S, 1998.

[21] Minamoto T et al. Altered lipoprotein profiles in cats with hepatic lipidosis. *J Feline Med Surg* 21:363, 2019.

[22] Valtolina C et al. Sex specific differences in hepatic and plasma lipid profiles in healthy cats pre and post spaying and neutering: relationship with feline hepatic lipidosis. *BMC Vet Res* 13:231, 2017.

[23] Bikman BT, Summers SA. Sphingolipids and hepatic steatosis. *Adv Exp Med Biol* 721:87, 2011.

[24] Lidbury JA, Cook AK, Steiner JM. Hepatic encephalopathy in dogs and cats. *J Vet Emerg Crit Care (San Antonio)* 26:471, 2016.

[25] Buckley FI, Mahony O, Webster CR. Adrenal function in cats with cholestatic liver disease. *J Vet Diagn Invest* 29:14, 2017.

[26] Petrescu AD et al. Hypothalamus-pituitary-adrenal dysfunction in cholestatic liver disease. *Front Endocrinol (Lausanne)* 9:660, 2018.

[27] Kavanagh C, Shaw S, Webster CR. Coagulation in hepatobiliary disease. *J Vet Emerg Crit Care (San Antonio)* 21:589, 2011.

[28] Center SA et al. Proteins invoked by vitamin K absence and clotting times in clinically ill cats. *J Vet Intern Med* 14:292, 2000.

[29] Dircks B, Nolte I, Mischke R. Haemostatic abnormalities in cats with naturally occurring liver diseases. *Vet J* 193:103, 2012.

[30] Bigge LA, Brown DJ, Penninck DG. Correlation between coagulation profile findings and bleeding complications after ultrasound-guided biopsies: 434 cases (1993–1996). *J Am Anim Hosp Assoc* 37:228, 2001.

[31] Feeney DA et al. Statistical relevance of ultrasonographic criteria in the assessment of diffuse liver disease in dogs and cats. *Am J Vet Res* 69:212, 2008.

[32] Lam R, Niessen SJ, Lamb CR. X-ray attenuation of the liver and kidney in cats considered at varying risk of hepatic lipidosis. *Vet Radiol Ultrasound* 55:141, 2014.

[33] Wang KY et al. Accuracy of ultrasound-guided fine-needle aspiration of the liver and cytologic findings in dogs and cats: 97 cases (1990–2000). *J Am Vet Med Assoc* 224:75, 2004.

[34] Roskams T, Katoonizadeh A, Komuta M. Hepatic progenitor cells: an update. *Clin Liver Dis* 14:705, 2010.

[35] Valtolina C et al. Immunohistochemical characterisation of the hepatic stem cell niche in feline hepatic lipidosis: a preliminary morphological study. *J Feline Med Surg* 21:165, 2019.

[36] Chan DL. The inappetent hospitalised cat: clinical approach to maximising nutritional support. *J Feline Med Surg* 11:925, 2009.

[37] Freeman LM, Chan DL. Total parenteral nutrition. In: DiBartola SP, editor. *Fluid, Electrolyte, and Acid-Base Disorders in Small Animal Practice*, 3rd ed. St Louis, Elsevier: 584, 2006.

[38] Trepanier L. Acute vomiting in cats: rational treatment selection. *J Feline Med Surg* 12:225, 2010.

[39] Center SA et al. Influence of dietary supplementation with (L)-carnitine on metabolic rate, fatty acid oxidation, body condition, and weight loss in overweight cats. *Am J Vet Res* 73:1002, 2012.

[40] Blanchard G et al. Dietary L-carnitine supplementation in obese cats alters carnitine metabolism and decreases ketosis during fasting and induced hepatic lipidosis. *J Nutr* 132:204, 2002.

[41] Kruitwagen HS et al. Long-term adult feline liver organoid cultures for disease modeling of hepatic steatosis. *Stem Cell Reports* 8:822, 2017.

CHAPTER 28

Hepatic encephalopathy

Adam G. Gow

Hepatic encephalopathy (HE) is defined as neurological dysfunction because of hepatic insufficiency or portosystemic shunting or both. This broad definition underlines the multifactorial nature of the syndrome and also encompasses more global effects of hepatic insufficiency such as hypoglycaemia as well as central nervous system (CNS) vascular events due to haemorrhage or clots as a result of disturbances in pro- and anticoagulant homoeostatic factors produced by the liver. However, it is more commonly thought of as a spectrum of clinical signs which can be intermittent and wax and wane in severity. Although it was previously considered to cause reversible pathology, long-term consequences are now recognised in humans.

EPIDEMIOLOGY AND AETIOLOGY

In the cat, the most common cause of HE is the presence of a congenital portosystemic shunt (CPSS). Although rare, acquired shunts as a result of portal hypertension have also been described (see Chapter 26). If blood draining from the gastrointestinal tract is diverted into the systemic circulation, this bypasses the filtering function of the hepatic sinusoids containing large numbers of macrophages as well as hepatocytes with their ability to metabolise and detoxify a vast array of endogenous and exogenous substances. Other causes of HE in the cat rather than vascular anomalies include acute liver failure as well as disruption of specific hepatic metabolic pathways due to a lack of substrate. Of particular mention is the syndrome of feline hepatic lipidosis (FHL), as it appears to be increasingly recognised worldwide (see Chapter 27). Encephalopathy is recognised as part of the constellation of signs seen in cats with FHL, although the vast majority of FHL cases do not present with HE signs.[1] It is important to be aware that HE may develop during institution of treatment of FHL due to feeding and also resulting electrolyte abnormalities (see Chapter 29).

As chronic hepatic diseases, and as a result HE, are becoming increasingly prevalent within the human population, there has been a sustained body of research to understand the pathogenesis. This has involved both clinical research with human patients and also experimental research with rodent models. More recently in veterinary medicine, much work has been done to unpick the potential mechanisms of HE in the dog. This has highlighted that the pathogenesis of HE appears similar between humans, dogs, and research animals. At present, there is little information on the triggers in the cat, aside from clinical reports and response to management. Although extrapolating disease pathogenesis between species (particularly dog and cat) must be done with caution, until further work is performed on feline HE, similar precipitating factors are thought to be likely triggers in feline HE. It is important to realise that in individual cats the likelihood of HE and its severity depends on multiple factors and the interplay/synergism between them (Fig. 28.1).

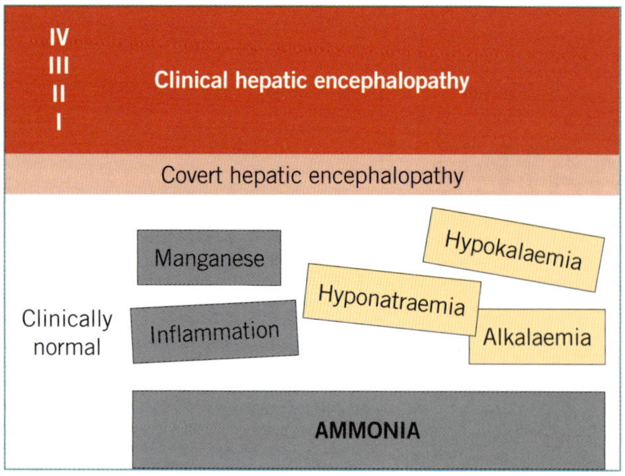

Figure 28.1. Building blocks of the pathogenesis of hepatic encephalopathy. Blocks in grey have the most evidence in veterinary medicine; however, there is evidence for all these factors playing a role from human and laboratory work. Many combinations can "build" upon each other to move an animal from being clinically normal to triggering clinical hepatic encephalopathy, but it is accepted that ammonia is a key driver.

Precipitating factors

Ammonia

Across all species examined, ammonia (NH_3) has been recognised as an important driver in HE pathogenesis. Portal blood, particularly postprandial, contains a high concentration of ammonia relative to the systemic circulation. Ammonia is potentially generated from a number of sources; however, enterocyte deamination of glutamine to provide energy likely plays a large role. Other sources of portal ammonia include bacterial degradation of protein (see dietary management below) and splitting of urea by urease-producing bacteria in the intestinal tract.

The liver is extremely efficient at removing ammonia before it is delivered into the systemic circulation. Hepatocytes have two mechanisms to detoxify ammonia. Periportal hepatocytes mainly remove ammonia to form urea via the urea cycle. This is a high-capacity, low-affinity system that removes the majority of delivered ammonia. As portal blood travels through the hepatic sinusoids, hepatocytes around the centrilobular vein use glutamine synthetase to remove ammonia, forming glutamine from glutamate. This is relatively high affinity but low capacity and captures residual ammonia within the blood.

High systemic concentrations of ammonia have long been recognised as causing neurotoxicity and contributing to the clinical signs of portosystemic shunting. Pavlov and Nencki demonstrated the role of the liver in ammonia metabolism and the CNS consequences of hyperammonaemia by experimentally creating portosystemic shunts in dogs between 1893 and 1896.[2] Since this time, further work has demonstrated that it is the astrocyte in the CNS that is mainly targeted by these high ammonia concentrations.[2] Astrocytes are the most numerous cells within the brain and act to buffer increasing CNS ammonia concentrations via the enzyme glutamine synthetase, which converts glutamate to glutamine consuming one molecule of ammonia. Both these compounds are neurotransmitters, and in the face of high ammonia the enzymatic reaction is shifted to reduced glutamate and increased glutamine, thus causing neurotransmitter disequilibrium. Glutamine is metabolised back to glutamate by mitochondria in the astrocyte, resulting in oxidative stress and disruption of mitochondrial function. Additionally, ammonia inhibits the tricarboxylic acid cycle, favouring anaerobic metabolism and increasing lactate concentrations in the astrocyte. The consequences of these effects are astrocyte dysfunction and cell swelling. Histologically, these swollen astrocytes are known as Alzheimer type II astrocytes and are almost pathognomonic for HE. As astrocytes contribute to a large percentage of CNS volume, this swelling, particularly in acute hepatic failure, can produce significant cerebral hypertension, leading to brain herniation. In the more usual scenarios of chronic HE seen in veterinary medicine, this swelling, although still present histologically, is less dramatic (at least in dogs and humans, although it has not been documented in cats).[3]

Skeletal muscle also contains the enzyme glutamine synthetase, and due to the large mass of muscles, when increased ammonia is delivered into the systemic circulation, this is thought to come into play as an important buffering system to mitigate the potential toxicity. This role of skeletal muscle would be decreased in cachectic patients with reduced muscle mass.

Infection and inflammation

Sepsis in its own right has been recognised as a cause of encephalopathy since the time of Hippocrates. It is now recognised as another key driver of HE in human patients and in experimental models, having a synergistic effect with ammonia. More recently, there is strong evidence of an association between inflammation and HE in canine patients with CPSSs.[4] This has important consequences for the management of HE, as it provides another therapeutic target. Systemic inflammation produces a neuroinflammatory state, with activation of microglial cells (specialised macrophages within the CNS). This pro-inflammatory state potentiates the effect of ammonia on astrocytes. There is evidence that hyperammonaemia reduces the effectiveness of the innate immune system, specifically neutrophil function, in humans and dogs;[5,6] therefore, high ammonia concentrations may predispose to a pro-inflammatory state, thereby potentiating HE. As yet, there have been no studies examining the role of inflammation in feline HE; however, as it has been shown to be important in all other species investigated so far, it should be considered as an important precipitating factor.

Manganese

Manganese (Mn), an essential trace element, is present in the portal vein in high concentrations due to high dietary intake. Hepatocytes clear almost all delivered Mn before blood reaches the systemic circulation. Cases with hepatic insufficiency or shunting vessels therefore have abnormally high systemic concentrations of this element. Mn toxicity results in neurological signs due to the presence of high-affinity Mn transporters in the membrane of astrocytes, and this transition element ultimately causes oxidative damage and inflammation. In human and rodent cases of Mn toxicity, identical astrocytic swelling (Alzheimer type II) to that seen in cases of hyperammonaemia is documented. In addition, astrocytic Mn accumulation results in production in pro-inflammatory cytokines from both astrocytes and microglial cells.[7] High systemic blood concentrations and Mn CNS deposition has been documented in humans and dogs with shunting vessels. There is one case report which documents hyperintense magnetic resonance imaging lesions suggestive of Mn deposition in a cat with a CPSS; therefore, this is likely to be a feature in cats with CPSSs.[8] Mn is present in almost all foodstuffs, making Mn dietary restriction difficult, and there is little information on Mn concentrations in pet foods. Chelation therapy to treat Mn toxicity is effective; however, this has not been explored in the management of HE in any species as yet.

Hypokalaemia

Hypokalaemia is recognised as a risk factor for HE in human medicine due to increased renal tubular cell ammoniagenesis. Two studies have investigated risk factors for HE in dogs with CPSSs and failed to implicate hypokalaemia. This is likely to be due to the low prevalence in this population rather than a species difference. As with previous triggers, this has not been examined in the cat; however, as cats appear to have an increased likelihood of hypokalaemia compared to dogs,[9] it may be relatively more important to be aware of this potential trigger in cats.

Additional precipitating factors

Other factors precipitating HE that are well recognised in human medicine are dehydration, alkalosis, hyponatraemia, constipation, and gastrointestinal bleeding, but these have not been implicated in dogs or cats, again likely due to the low prevalence in the studied population of dogs with CPSSs. As before, it is useful to be aware of these possible potentiators, as particularly in cats with FHL these metabolic derangements are more likely.

Of note is a condition termed bilirubin encephalopathy, in which high concentrations of free bilirubin result in CNS bilirubin deposition and encephalopathy. On histopathology, intraneuronal bilirubin accumulation is noted and CNS lesions are described.[10] This condition appears uncommon but could contribute to CNS signs if markedly high bilirubin concentrations are present.

HISTORY AND PHYSICAL EXAMINATION

Owner reports or main presenting complaints will depend on the underlying cause of HE, but the most dramatic signs are of neurological nature. Although an uncommon congenital abnormality compared to dogs, portosystemic shunting is the most common cause of HE in the cat. Neurological abnormalities vary in severity, and a clinical grading scale has been modified from human medicine for veterinary use (Table 28.1), which categorises the severity of HE from 0 (asymptomatic) to IV (comatose).[11] Video 28.1 demonstrates grade III HE and improvement after medical management in a cat. Clinical signs of HE can be further defined as episodic or persistent, with episodic signs being most common in veterinary medicine. In cats with CPSSs, more overt neurological signs are frequently seen; of note are aggression and seizures. However, with less overt signs, owners may be surprisingly unaware that their cat's behaviour is not normal, particularly if they have not had a kitten in the household before, ascribing any lethargy and dullness to having a very placid animal.

Table 28.1. West Haven grading scale modified for veterinary cases with hepatic encephalopathy.

Grade	Clinical signs
0	Asymptomatic
I	Mild decrease in mobility and/or apathy
II	Severe apathy and/or mild ataxia
III	Combination of hypersalivation, severe ataxia, head pressing, blindness, and circling
IV	Seizures and stupor or coma

Video 28.1. Sixteen-week-old Ragdoll cat demonstrating grade III hepatic encephalopathy. Note the evidence of prior hypersalivation. The second section of the video demonstrates resolution of clinical signs after institution of medical management.

In the cat, hypersalivation is another notable clinical sign which is not frequent in other species but reported in almost three-quarters of feline cases.[12] In cats with CPSSs, other clinical signs may be present or reported in the history to increase the index of suspicion and are further discussed in Chapter 26. Young animals may have reduced growth and have poor body condition. Golden-coloured irises are commonly reported in the literature, but it is important to note that this occurs in the minority of feline CPSS cases.[12] Polyuria/polydipsia and, due to ammonium urate cystoliths, lower urinary tract signs including dysuria, pollakiuria, and haematuria may be reported.

The age at which cats with CPSSs develop overt signs of HE varies between a few weeks of age to being mature animals, but the vast majority of affected cats are presented at a young age. This variation likely reflects a combination of shunt location, shunting fraction, owner awareness, and development of precipitating factors.

Cats with intrinsic liver dysfunction producing HE will have additional clinical signs related to the duration and severity of their hepatic disease, such as icterus or signs related to coagulopathy (see Chapter 27).

DIAGNOSTIC INVESTIGATION

Diagnosis of HE is primarily based on clinical suspicion of hepatic insufficiency and appropriate clinical signs of HE. As neurological signs are the most frequent presentation, other causes should be considered (Box 28.1).

Although ammonia is a key driver in the pathogenesis of HE, it is not a reliable indicator of the presence or severity of HE in individual humans or dogs. The majority of cats with CPSSs reported have high ammonia concentrations, potentially reflecting the higher animal protein content of feline diets. It is possible that high venous ammonia concentrations are a more reliable predictor of HE in the cat; however, the diagnosis should not be excluded based upon an ammonia concentration within the reference interval. Conversely, high ammonia concentrations have been reported in cats with severe azotaemia due to renal disease, and therefore high ammonia concentrations are not specific for HE.[13] Other clinicopathologic abnormalities will relate to the primary hepatic

Box 28.1. Differential diagnoses to be considered in cats presenting with signs compatible with hepatic encephalopathy.

Toxic
- Metaldehyde
- Ethylene glycol
- Lead
- Permethrin
- Organophosphates
- Nicotine (particularly, liquid from e-cigarettes)
- Human medication/illicit drugs

Metabolic
- Hypoglycaemia
- Severe hypokalaemia
- Hypocalcaemia
- Thiamine deficiency
- Uraemic encephalopathy
- Bilirubin encephalopathy
- Arginine deficiency

Infectious (CNS)
- Feline infectious peritonitis
- Toxoplasmosis
- Cryptococcosis
- Rabies

Congenital/acquired CNS disease

abnormality. For cats with CPSSs, a mild nonregenerative anaemia is most frequently reported, with hypoalbuminaemia, hypoglycaemia, and raised bile acids. Again, it is important to be aware that cases of feline CPSS have been reported with ammonia and fasting bile acids within reference intervals.[12] For cases with intrinsic hepatobiliary disease, raised hepatobiliary enzymes and bilirubin would also be expected.

MANAGEMENT AND TREATMENT

The ultimate aim of treatment is to remove the underlying cause; in the majority of cases this would be attenuation of the congenital shunt. Acquired shunts (rare in the cat) are a sign of portal hypertension most commonly due to hepatic disease, and attenuation of these is not an option. The level of medical intervention prior to shunt attenuation or as a sole treatment depends on the severity of the clinical signs at presentation. In addition, if intrinsic hepatic disease is present, there may be a wide spectrum of clinical and clinicopathologic abnormalities present which also require addressing. Cats that are suspected to have FHL as the cause of their HE should be further defined as to whether the hepatic lipidosis is thought to be primary (i.e. primarily due to decreased calorie intake) or secondary to another disease process resulting in anorexia (see Chapter 27).

At present, therapeutic strategies are aimed at lowering ammonia concentrations, although they may also have an effect on modulating the inflammatory state. Cases presenting with grade III–IV HE will require intensive supportive management appropriate for any stuporous or comatose patient.

Cats with primary portosystemic shunting should be stabilised prior to any surgical intervention to reduce perioperative risk. Medical management for ideally a minimum of 2 weeks is recommended; however, clinical signs of HE appear more difficult to control medically in the cat compared to the dog, and therefore surgery may have to be scheduled sooner. For cases with intrinsic liver disease, such as FHL, addressing the underlying cause and reversal of the metabolic abnormalities are important, along with medical HE management if required.

Lactulose/lactitol

Lactulose and lactitol are nonabsorbable disaccharides which are metabolised by colonic microflora into short-chain fatty acids (SCFAs). There are many potential beneficial effects of lactulose treatment. These SCFAs are utilised as a microbial energy source, which may favour a microbiome with less urease-producing bacteria. There is now evidence of the ability of lactulose to modulate the microbiome in dogs.[14] The acidification of the colon by the SCFAs will favour the formation of ammonium ions (NH_4^+) which become trapped in the lumen, as they cannot diffuse across cell membranes easily. Lactulose also acts as an osmotic laxative, removing trapped ammonium ions as well as nitrogen integrated into bacterial protein. All these mechanisms may contribute to lowering systemic ammonia concentrations. In both human and veterinary medicine, lactulose had become standard of care for HE treatment via clinical experience and anecdote. Despite many years of clinical experience suggesting a beneficial effect, there is no published data documenting that lactulose improves clinical signs, quality of life, or mortality rates in veterinary HE cases. Until very recently, a systematic review by the Cochrane group was "unable to find evidence to support the use of disaccharides" in human HE. However, possibly in response to this lack of evidence, further higher quality studies have now been performed. A meta-analysis of these studies concludes that there is sufficient evidence that lactulose improves mortality rate in humans and has a beneficial effect compared to a placebo.[15]

Lactulose appears to be very well tolerated in most patients, but adverse effects include nausea and diarrhoea, potentially causing dehydration and hypovolaemia. Lactulose is frequently recommended for feline HE, but compliance can be a problem because some cats do not tolerate the sweet syrup. Therefore, where available, powdered lactitol, although also sweet, may be accepted more readily mixed in food. If these are not accepted, as an alternative, lactose in the form of natural yogurt or milk may be trialled, relying on lactase deficiency; however, it is unclear how prevalent and severe lactase deficiency is in the adult cat and therefore how effective this may be.[16] Dosage of these medications is empirical and should be adjusted to produce two to three soft but formed faeces daily (Table 28.2).

Table 28.2. Medications commonly used to control hepatic encephalopathy signs in cats.

Treatment	Dosage and route of administration	Side effects and comments
Lactulose	Starting dose: 0.5–5 ml/cat PO every 8–12 h Titrated to produce 2–3 soft stools/day	Relative overdose causes diarrhoea and abdominal cramping
Lactulose enema	1 part lactulose to 3 parts warm water 10 ml/kg with Foley catheter, retain 30–60 minutes, and repeat as required	Consequent diarrhoea
Lactitol	Starting dose: 0.5–5 g/cat PO every 12 h Titrated to produce 2–3 soft stools/day	Relative overdose causes diarrhoea and abdominal cramping
Foods containing lactose (milk, yoghurt)	Empirical dosing to effect of 2–3 soft stools/day Protein content should be considered	Diarrhoea, dietary intolerance Prevalence and severity of lactase deficiency unknown in the cat

Antibiotics

Antibiotics will have an effect on the intestinal microbiome and also, if systemically absorbed, potentially treat any infectious focus as a source of inflammation (see Appendix for recommended dosages). Although enterically nonabsorbable antibiotics are attractive due to their more targeted effect, availability and concerns over potential toxicity have reduced their use. Neomycin was previously a widely used nonabsorbable choice for HE management and could be considered where still available. There is also experimental evidence that neomycin reduces ammonia production from hydrolysis of glutamine in the enterocytes. Rifaximin is a recent synthetic nonabsorbable antibiotic which has been shown to be effective in controlling HE in humans and has pharmacokinetic data in dogs. There is also one study demonstrating noninferiority to metronidazole for management of canine chronic enteropathy.[17] Anecdotally it has been used in cats; however, in many countries the lack of licensing and expense limits its veterinary use. Ampicillin, potentiated amoxycillin, and metronidazole are most commonly used in feline HE management.[11] Metronidazole is hepatically metabolised, and overdose causes neurological signs; therefore, if used, it should be at half the standard therapeutic dose.

There is justifiable increasing concern worldwide over nontargeted antibiotic use, and veterinary patients with HE fall into this category unless a bacterial inflammatory focus is identified. Therefore, antibiotic management of HE should only be instituted if thought required to control the clinical signs, and the need for their use should be reviewed regularly. Unfortunately, many cats with CPSSs continue to have significant HE despite medical management.

Diet

It is important to consider the underlying cause of hepatic encephalopathy when making diet choices: hepatic lipidosis cases require high-quality, high-protein diets fed early on to improve mortality, whilst some cases of congenital portosystemic shunting may require protein restriction.

Cats are obligate carnivores and have a higher protein requirement than dogs. Most cases of CPSS are diagnosed in young animals, which have a higher protein requirement than adults. Excess dietary protein will result in ammonia generation, as it is utilised as an energy source. Insufficient dietary protein will result in catabolism of body protein, leading to reduced muscle mass (potentially an important buffer of systemic ammonia) and risking deficiency of essential amino acids. Arginine, one such essential amino acid for cats, is required to convert ammonia to urea, and deficiency can produce hyperammonaemia in its own right.[18] It is important that enough protein is fed to meet the cat's life stage requirements. In addition, it should be recognised that total protein content is not the only important factor; it should also be usable protein (i.e. with high biological value) to prevent microbial digestion in the intestine and allow cellular protein incorporation without deamination and ammonia generation. There is evidence from dogs with CPSSs that using a vegetable protein source such as soya is preferable to meat-based diets. Although this is obviously more challenging in the cat, a commercial hydrolysed diet using soya protein is manufactured for adult cats and available in many parts of the world (Purina Pro Plan Veterinary Diets HA, Feline Dry) which is also suitable for growing animals. Otherwise, if possible, an appropriate high-quality diet for the patient's life stage should be used. If this is not possible with the additional therapies, careful protein restriction should be considered. Potentially, diets developed for hepatic and renal disease management are the next step towards this, generally being protein restricted and of high biological value, but ideally a veterinary nutritionist should be consulted before embarking on protein restriction in a growing cat.

For cats with HE as a consequence of FHL, ensuring early institution of feeding with a high protein content diet (35%–45% of metabolisable energy) is central to reversing the catabolic state. See Chapter 27 for further information on the management of FHL.

Seizure control

As previously noted, seizures are more commonly seen in cats with CPSSs than in other species. Phenobarbital has historically been used to manage these cases; however, more recently levetiracetam has been favoured due to its lack of hepatic metabolism (see Appendix for recommended dosages). A high percentage of cats that have seizures before surgery develop postattenuation seizures.[12] In the largest study to date of cats with CPSSs undergoing attenuation, postoperative seizures occurred in some cats with normal liver function tests and only in cats that had received anti-seizure medication (including cats which did not seizure before the procedure). Although the authors of the study noted that no conclusions could be drawn, they highlighted that levetiracetam has been reported to potentiate seizures in a proportion of human epileptics, particularly children.[19] Therefore, although it would appear prudent to continue medication in the immediate postoperative period, it is unknown if pre- and postattenuation treatment with levetiracetam improves outcome. Postoperative seizures are a significant complication in cats, with studies reporting prevalences of 14%–33%.[12] One large study of dogs with CPSSs which were pretreated with prophylactic levetiracetam did not demonstrate a reduction in postprocedural seizures.[20] Further research would be required to compare phenobarbital and levetiracetam protective effects compared to no treatment in cats with CPSSs undergoing attenuation.

Therapy of hepatic encephalopathy crisis (grade III–IV)

Cats that present with severe HE require triage, nonspecific life support management (beyond the scope of this chapter), and consideration of differential diagnoses (Box 28.1). Cats should be assessed for precipitating factors, hypoglycaemia, and electrolyte disturbances. Oral medication should be avoided in cases where reduced mentation makes them at risk for aspiration. For cases with status epilepticus, intravenous phenobarbital or levetiracetam is the treatment of choice. Many cases are dehydrated, and intravenous fluids will provide a dilutional effect for encephalopathic toxins as well as improve glomerular filtration rates and renal ammonia excretion. In cases which are due to hepatic failure, lactate-containing fluids should be avoided because this requires hepatic metabolism. Although not investigated in the cat, HE cases may be at risk of cobalamin deficiency, particularly if polyuria and reduced appetite are present. Cobalamin deficiency results in increased methylmalonic acid, which inhibits ammonia incorporation into the urea cycle. Therefore, until investigated, supplementation with cobalamin is recommended. Monitoring of potassium and glucose status during fluid therapy is important. Removal of colonic contents via a warm isotonic fluid enema and digital manipulation eliminates potential sources of ammonia. A lactulose retention enema has been shown to be helpful in human patients. Protocols vary, but 10 ml/kg of lactulose diluted 1:3 with warm water for 30–60 minutes and repeated as required may be useful after manual removal of faecal contents, although this has not been studied in veterinary patients. Close attention should be paid to body temperature, as encephalopathy, anaesthesia, and use of enemas can all precipitate hypothermia, prolonging recovery. Rarely, in acute cases of HE, most often due to acute hepatic failure, intracranial hypertension may occur necessitating specific standard treatment.

PROGNOSIS AND OUTCOME

Ultimately, prognosis depends on the underlying cause of HE and on the ability of the clinician to resolve or manage this. Many cats with CPSSs are reported to have continuing HE signs despite appropriate medical management, often necessitating scheduling earlier shunt occlusion. There is no data on long-term medical management of feline CPSS cases, but anecdotally quality of life is poorer than medically managed canine cases, often resulting in euthanasia. For cats with HE due to intrinsic hepatic failure, such as FHL, HE management will only be required until the predisposing factors are corrected and sufficient hepatic metabolism is restored.

Take-home messages

- Pathogenesis of hepatic encephalopathy is multifactorial.
- Blood ammonia concentrations within the reference interval do not completely exclude hepatic encephalopathy.
- Successful control depends on managing or resolving the underlying vascular or hepatocellular pathology.
- Cats with hepatic lipidosis may develop hepatic encephalopathy during treatment but should not be protein restricted.

REFERENCES

[1] Valtolina C, Favier RP. Feline hepatic lipidosis. *Vet Clin North Am Small Anim Pract* 47:683, 2017.

[2] Shawcross DL et al. Ammonia and hepatic encephalopathy: the more things change, the more they remain the same. *Metab Brain Dis* 20:169, 2005.

[3] Williams A et al. Astrocyte lesions in cerebral cortex and cerebellum of dogs with congenital ortosystemic shunting. *J Vet Sci* 21:e44, 2020.

[4] Tivers MS et al. Hyperammonemia and systemic inflammatory response syndrome predicts presence of hepatic encephalopathy in dogs with congenital portosystemic shunts. *PLoS One* 9:e82303, 2014.

[5] Breheny CR et al. The effect of ammonia on canine polymorphonuclear cells. *Vet Res Commun* 42:221, 2018.

[6] Shawcross DL et al. Ammonia impairs neutrophil phagocytic function in liver disease. *Hepatology* 48:1202, 2008.

[7] Sarkar S et al. Manganese exposure induces neuroinflammation by impairing mitochondrial dynamics in astrocytes. *Neurotoxicology* 64:204, 2018.

[8] Torisu S et al. Brain magnetic resonance imaging characteristics in dogs and cats with congenital portosystemic shunts. *Vet Radiol Ultrasound* 46:447, 2005.

[9] Hoehne SN, Hopper K, Epstein SE. Retrospective evaluation of the severity of and prognosis associated with potassium abnormalities in dogs and cats presenting to an emergency room (January 2014–August 2015): 2441 cases. *J Vet Emerg Crit Care (San Antonio)* 29:653, 2019.

[10] Saraiva LH et al. Bilirubin encephalopathy (kernicterus) in an adult cat. *JFMS Open Rep* 5:2055116919838874, 2019.

[11] Proot S et al. Soy protein isolate versus meat-based low-protein diet for dogs with congenital portosystemic shunts. *J Vet Intern Med* 23:794, 2009.

[12] Valiente P et al. Complications and outcome of cats with congenital extrahepatic portosystemic shunts treated with thin film: thirty-four cases (2008–2017). *J Vet Intern Med* 34:117, 2020.

[13] Adagra C, Foster DJ. Hyperammonaemia in four cats with renal azotaemia. *J Feline Med Surg* 17:168, 2015.

[14] Ferreira MDF et al. Lactulose drives a reversible reduction and qualitative modulation of the faecal microbiota diversity in healthy dogs. *Sci Rep* 9:13350, 2019.

[15] Gluud LL, Vilstrup H, Morgan MY. Non-absorbable disaccharides versus placebo/no intervention and lactulose versus lactitol for the prevention and treatment of hepatic encephalopathy in people with cirrhosis. *Cochrane Database Syst Rev* 2016:CD003044, 2016.

[16] Craig JM. Food intolerance in dogs and cats. *J Small Anim Pract* 60:77, 2019.

[17] Menozzi A et al. Rifaximin is an effective alternative to metronidazole for the treatment of chronic enteropathy in dogs: a randomised trial. *BMC Vet Res* 12:217, 2016.

[18] Morris JG, Rogers QR. Ammonia intoxication in the near-adult cat as a result of a dietary deficiency of arginine. *Science* 199:431, 1978.

[19] Nakken KO et al. A paradoxical effect of levetiracetam may be seen in both children and adults with refractory epilepsy. *Seizure* 12:42, 2003.

[20] Mullins RA et al. Effect of prophylactic treatment with levetiracetam on the incidence of postattenuation seizures in dogs undergoing surgical management of single congenital extrahepatic portosystemic shunts. *Vet Surg* 48:164, 2019.

CHAPTER 29

Refeeding syndrome

Daniel L. Chan

Refeeding syndrome is a rare but potentially life-threatening condition encountered when a patient with an extended period of complete anorexia is fed.[1,2] It is not simply any metabolic complication encountered when treating a starved animal, but rather a collection of specific metabolic derangements that follow feeding a severely and chronically debilitated malnourished patient. The metabolic complications most often encountered with refeeding syndrome include severe hypophosphataemia, hyperglycaemia, and vitamin deficiencies.[3] Less commonly, hypomagnesaemia, hypokalaemia, hyponatraemia, and hypocalcaemia can also be seen.[3] In addition to biochemical imbalances, other abnormalities that can develop related to refeeding syndrome include peripheral oedema, haemolytic anaemia, cardiac failure, neurological dysfunction, and respiratory failure. Many of these metabolic derangements are believed to be driven by the sudden release of insulin (stimulated by carbohydrate intake).[3–5] The electrolyte shifts caused by the surge in insulin are exacerbated by total body depletion of many nutrients. Successful management of patients at particularly high risk of developing refeeding syndrome involves careful use of intravenous fluids, frequent monitoring of electrolytes, and very conservative nutritional support.[5]

EPIDEMIOLOGY AND AETIOLOGY

An interesting observation is that refeeding syndrome is almost exclusively noted in cats but not in other domestic species. There are unfortunately too few reports of refeeding syndrome in cats to establish the epidemiology of this condition, other than to say that it is a rare complication.[4,6–8] Based on current understanding, this syndrome is believed to occur when nutrition (enteral or parenteral) is introduced too rapidly to severely malnourished patients.[3] In people, recent guidelines propose that the risk for developing refeeding syndrome is related to the presence of a reduction in phosphorus, potassium, or magnesium by more than 10% or if there is organ dysfunction as a result of any of these abnormalities or thiamine deficiency.[9] These guidelines also propose a classification scale of severity for refeeding syndrome based on the magnitude of the electrolyte abnormality such that refeeding syndrome should be classified as mild if electrolytes are reduced by 10%–20%, moderate if the abnormalities fall between 21% and 30%, or severe if the abnormalities are above 30%.[9] It is important to note that this broader scope for defining the risk for developing refeeding syndrome and severity scale has not been adopted in veterinary patients. In the cases reported in the veterinary literature, it would appear that these cats would be classified as having severe refeeding syndrome if these criteria were adopted.[4,6–9] The preponderance of electrolyte abnormalities stems from these patients often having intracellular depletion of electrolytes that are not readily identified at the initial evaluation. Upon refeeding, cells that have become metabolically dormant suddenly become active and increase their utilisation of phosphorus and magnesium to support glycolysis and production of adenosine triphosphate (ATP). The dramatic increase in intracellular phosphate utilisation, in conjunction with cotransport of potassium into cells via insulin-mediated glucose uptake, causes further depletion of these electrolytes. Typically, refeeding syndrome is observed within the first 2–5 days after feeding,[3] but clinical signs can be detected within hours of refeeding or delayed up to 10 days, at least in people.[4,8,10]

PATHOPHYSIOLOGY

During prolonged periods of anorexia, decreased dietary intake contributes to the depletion of electrolytes such as potassium and magnesium. Because of autoregulatory adjustments in renal electrolyte excretion, serum concentrations of electrolytes can be maintained, and clinical signs of electrolyte depletion may not be apparent. However, during refeeding, the carbohydrate content of the diet stimulates insulin release, resulting in conversion of the body from a catabolic to an anabolic state. It is this sudden increase in metabolic activity which increases the cellular demand for phosphorus, potassium, and water that results in the metabolic derangements observed. Newly synthesised cells require potassium for maintenance of electrical gradients and will translocate serum potassium and phosphorus intracellularly (thus contributing to hypokalaemia and hypophosphataemia). Activation of glycolysis and protein synthesis also require cellular uptake of phosphate and magnesium. Given that prolonged periods of poor food intake lead to whole-body depletion of these electrolytes, the ensuing cellular translocation further exacerbates serum electrolyte depletion and can result in life-threatening complications. Inorganic phosphate is required for generation of ATP and 2,3-diphosphoglycerate (2,3-DPG). Protein phosphorylation is also required for many intracellular enzymatic processes. With the onset of severe hypophosphataemia, there is a reduction in the capacity for ATP synthesis which leads to cellular energy deficits that then manifest as the various clinical signs associated with refeeding syndrome.

Changes observed in people with prolonged starvation include severe bradycardia, hypothermia, and hypoventilation. These changes reflect the reduction in metabolism that occurs within the first few days of anorexia. The reduction in apparent energy expenditure is related to the decrease in insulin activity, reduction of glucose utilisation, and loss of lean body mass.[1] Skeletal muscle wasting and the ensuing reduction in respiratory muscle function further compromise ventilation. Eventually, decreased myocardial mass and ventricular contractility occur, resulting in decreased cardiac output and heart failure. The reported incidence of cardiovascular-related complications in people with anorexia nervosa is high (up to 95%), and these include bradycardia, fluid overload, and cardiac arrhythmias, which are associated with a high mortality rate.[1,11]

HISTORY AND PHYSICAL EXAMINATION FINDINGS

The most pertinent aspect of the history in cats that go on to develop refeeding syndrome is inadequate food intake for weeks and sometimes months.[4–8] It is also important to recognise that refeeding syndrome is a specific set of complications that follow starvation, rather than a primary disease itself. Therefore, it is critical to have an acute awareness of cats that are at particularly high risk of developing refeeding syndrome and recognise those cats that are showing signs when affected by it. Physical examination findings of cats at high risk are not particularly specific but are marked in severity and include severe dehydration, hypothermia, bradycardia, and pronounced depletion of body fat and lean muscle tissue (Box 29.1). Cats are often very weak, debilitated, and obtunded (Fig. 29.1).

Box 29.1. Proposed list of risk factors associated with the development of refeeding syndrome in cats.

- History of significant period of inadequate food intake (>3 weeks)
- Significant weight loss (>20% of previous body weight)
- Poor body condition score (<3/9)
- Dehydration (>7%)
- Depletion of total body phosphorus, magnesium, potassium, and calcium
- Depletion of thiamine
- Premature and aggressive feeding (>20% of resting energy requirements) of calories rich in carbohydrates

Cats which go on to develop refeeding syndrome show additional clinical signs related to the metabolic changes that are triggered by refeeding. In particular, hypophosphataemia is the most common and consistent abnormality seen in refeeding syndrome and also results in many of the complications seen. Refeeding-associated hypophosphataemia has been reported previously in cats when it resulted in haemolytic anaemia, even though not all of the cases reported necessarily developed refeeding syndrome.[12] The ensuing depletion of phosphate results in neuromuscular, cardiovascular, and respiratory compromise (e.g. diaphragmatic muscle fatigue, respiratory failure). Arrhythmias could be induced by hypokalaemia in combination with hypocalcaemia and hypomagnesaemia. The sudden shift to

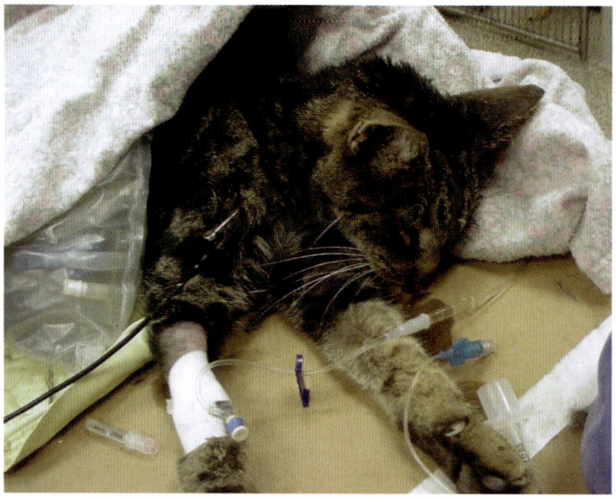

Figure 29.1. Severely malnourished cats (weight loss >20%) should be considered at high risk of developing refeeding syndrome and require special nutritional management strategies to ensure safe nutritional recovery.

carbohydrate metabolism may also explain the increased demand for magnesium and thiamine, which then leads to neurological and neuromuscular complications.[1–3] Signs of thiamine deficiency include ataxia, vestibular dysfunction, and visual disturbances. It is interesting to note that a high proportion of cats with refeeding syndrome also have blood glucose abnormalities (both hypo- and hyperglycaemia), which is not a reported feature of refeeding syndrome in people.[8,9]

DIAGNOSTIC INVESTIGATION

As this syndrome revolves around the metabolic changes that occur after refeeding, the most important aspect for recognising this condition is to perform serial assessments of electrolytes, in particular, potassium, calcium, magnesium, and phosphorus. In addition to electrolyte abnormalities,[5] there are derangements of glucose regulation. Whilst most cats affected by refeeding syndrome may develop hyperglycaemia, some develop hypoglycaemia.[6]

MANAGEMENT STRATEGIES

The general approach for the prevention of refeeding syndrome firstly contends that feeding should not be initiated prior to the correction of fluid, electrolyte, and vitamin imbalances (Table 29.1). Following stabilisation, nutrition should be administered gradually and in small increments. Recommendations for prevention of refeeding complications in people suggest that initial refeeding should not exceed 20 kcal/kg/day.[1] Refeeding syndrome has been reported to occur in cats fed only approximately 6 kcal/kg/day; it is therefore possible that refeeding complications in cats may be triggered at a lower level of caloric intake than is typically seen in people.[4,12] A loading dose of thiamine administered before initiation of feeding followed by daily injections until day 3 of nutritional therapy is recommended.[13–16]

Although there is insufficient information available from cats at risk for developing refeeding syndrome, protocols for reducing the risk of developing this disorder are available in people. According to a protocol adopted by the European Society for Clinical Nutrition and Metabolism (ESPEN), there should be careful patient assessment of patients at risk for developing refeeding syndrome; rehydration without overloading the cardiovascular system; empirical supplementation of phosphate, potassium, and magnesium (unless serum concentrations of these electrolytes are increased); and initiation of thiamine and other B vitamins and trace minerals with the exception of iron.[10] The caloric intake is gradually increased from 10 to 30 kcal/kg over the course of 10 days, with daily monitoring of potassium, phosphate, magnesium, and glucose.[5]

Extrapolating from recommendations in people, a sensible approach with cats at risk for developing refeeding syndrome would be to empirically supplement phosphate at 0.01–0.03 mmol/kg/h, potassium at 0.05 mEq/kg/h, and magnesium at 0.01–0.02 mEq/kg/h for the first 24 hours, provided that the patient does not have any of these electrolytes above the reference interval (Table 29.1).[5] Thiamine should be administered at a total dose of 25 mg/cat SC or IM every 24 hours until the neurological signs resolve. When nutritional support is instituted, no greater than 20% of resting energy requirement (RER) should be provided in the first day, and nutritional support should be increased gradually over 4–10 days. The estimation of RER is derived by the formula below.

$$\text{RER (kcal/day)} = 70 \times (\text{body weight [kg]})^{0.75}$$

Table 29.1. Proposed management strategies for managing cats at risk for refeeding syndrome.

Intervention	Dosing scheme
Phosphate supplementation	0.01–0.03 mmol/kg/h
Potassium supplementation	0.05 mEq/kg/h
Thiamine supplementation	25 mg/cat total dose SC or IM every 24 h
Nutritional support	Instituted at <20% of RER the first day, and increased gradually over 4–10 days to eventually reach 100% RER Feeding >100% RER can be instituted once patient is stable and recovery is progressing without complications

RER, resting energy requirement.

MONITORING

Patients considered at risk for developing refeeding syndrome require close monitoring of cardiovascular and neurological parameters and electrolytes. Body weight should be measured daily. At least twice a day, serum electrolytes (i.e. phosphorus, potassium, magnesium, calcium) electrocardiography, haematocrit, presence of haemolysis, and serum glucose should be monitored closely. Detection of metabolic abnormalities should prompt adjustments of nutritional therapy along with further correction of serum electrolyte concentrations.

PROGNOSIS AND OUTCOME

Given that many of the complications associated with this condition can be life-threatening, the best strategy for improving outcome is to prevent the triggering of this condition in the first place. With careful use of fluid therapy and early supplementation of electrolytes and vitamins before judicious use of nutritional support, cats can survive refeeding syndrome.[4–7] However, for a successful outcome, early recognition of patients at risk and careful nutritional planning are key.

Take-home messages

- The key clinical findings seen with refeeding syndrome include severe hypophosphataemia, hypomagnesaemia, hypokalaemia, hyperglycaemia, and thiamine deficiency.
- Additional complications seen include development of peripheral oedema, haemolytic anaemia, cardiac failure, neurological dysfunction, and respiratory failure, with neurological signs being most common.
- The main trigger for many of these changes is believed to relate to a sudden release of insulin (stimulated by carbohydrate intake).
- Thiamine should be administered prior to feeding at a total dose of 25 mg/cat SC or IM every 24 hours until the neurological signs resolve.
- Given the propensity for electrolyte imbalances, empirical supplementation of phosphate, potassium, and magnesium for the first 24 hours of therapy should be implemented, provided that the patient does not have any of these electrolytes above the reference interval.
- When nutritional support is instituted, no greater than 20% of RER (possibly only 10% RER) should be provided on the first day, and feeding should be gradually increased to eventually reach 100% RER over the subsequent 10 days or longer.

REFERENCES

[1] Crook MA, Hally V, Panteli JV. The importance of the refeeding syndrome. *Nutrition* 17:632, 2001.

[2] Kraft MD, Btaiche IF, Sacks GS. Review of the refeeding syndrome. *Nutr Clin Pract* 20:625, 2005.

[3] Skipper A. Refeeding syndrome or refeeding hypophosphatemia: a systematic review of cases. *Nutr Clin Pract* 27:34, 2012.

[4] Armitage-Chan EA, O'Toole T, Chan DL. Management of prolonged food deprivation, hypothermia, and refeeding syndrome in a cat. *J Vet Emerg Crit Care* 16:S34, 2006.

[5] Chan DL. Refeeding syndrome in small animals. In: Chan DL, editor. *Nutritional Management of the Hospitalized Small Animal Patient.* West Sussex, Wiley Blackwell: 159, 2015.

[6] DeAvilla MD, Leech EB. Hypoglycemia associated with refeeding syndrome in a cat. *J Vet Emerg Crit Care (San Antonio)* 26:798, 2016.

[7] Brenner K, KuKanich KS, Smee NM. Refeeding syndrome in a cat with hepatic lipidosis. *J Feline Med Surg* 13:614, 2011.

[8] Cook S et al. Retrospective evaluation of refeeding syndrome in cats: 11 cases (2013–2019). *J Feline Med Surg,* 2021 [epub ahead of print].

[9] da Silva JSV et al. ASPEN consensus recommendations for refeeding syndrome. *Nutr Clin Pract* 35:178, 2020.

[10] Hofer M et al. Safe refeeding management of anorexia nervosa inpatients: an evidence-based protocol. *Nutrition* 30:524, 2014.

[11] Mehler PS et al. Nutritional rehabilitation: practical guidelines for refeeding the anorectic patient. *J Nutr Metab* 2010:625782, 2010.

[12] Justin RB, Hohenhaus AE. Hypophosphatemia associated with enteral alimentation in cats. *J Vet Intern Med* 9:228, 1995.

[13] Solomon SM, Kirby DF. The refeeding syndrome: a review. *JPEN J Parenter Enteral Nutr* 14:90, 1990.

[14] Stanga Z et al. Nutrition in clinical practice—the refeeding syndrome: illustrative cases and guidelines for prevention and treatment. *Eur J Clin Nutr* 62:687, 2008.

[15] Boateng AA et al. Refeeding syndrome: treatment considerations based on collective analysis of literature case reports. *Nutrition* 26:156, 2010.

[16] Sriram K, Manzanares W, Joseph K. Thiamine in nutrition therapy. *Nutr Clin Pract* 27:41, 2012.

CHAPTER 30

Feline cholangitis and triaditis

Jonathan A. Lidbury

Feline cholangitis syndrome is one of the two most common liver disorders in cats (feline hepatic lipidosis being the other) and according to the World Small Animal Veterinary Association (WSAVA) Liver Standardization Group is histologically characterised by inflammation centred around the biliary tract with possible secondary extension into the hepatic parenchyma.[1] Cholangiohepatitis is another term that is usually used as a histomorphological diagnosis and that signifies that the inflammation extends beyond the limiting plate of hepatocytes into the hepatic parenchyma. However, it is preferable to call the clinical syndrome cholangitis, as the inflammation is centred around the bile ducts. Three forms of cholangitis are recognised in cats (in decreasing order of prevalence): neutrophilic cholangitis, lymphocytic cholangitis, and liver fluke–associated cholangitis. The terminology used to histologically describe inflammatory liver disease in cats is used inconsistently. For example, some older texts subdivide neutrophilic cholangitis into acute and chronic forms, and this distinction is still sometimes made by veterinary pathologists.

Cholangitis is an important cause of morbidity and mortality in cats. In one study, the 12-month mortality rate was reported to be 37%.[2] Additionally, this syndrome can present a diagnostic challenge for a number of reasons. Firstly, the clinical signs and laboratory abnormalities associated with cholangitis overlap with those of other conditions, such as feline hepatic lipidosis and pancreatitis. Furthermore, this syndrome cannot be definitively diagnosed by diagnostic imaging alone. Although cytological findings of hepatic fine needle aspirates and samples of bile can be helpful in diagnosing cholangitis, histological assessment of liver tissue is usually needed for definitive diagnosis and this invasive procedure may be contraindicated in unstable patients or may be declined by the client. Lastly, as discussed below, cats with cholangitis often have concurrent diseases.

In veterinary medicine, triaditis is the term used to describe concurrent inflammation of the liver, pancreas, and small intestine in cats. This somewhat poorly defined syndrome encompasses a spectrum of intestinal, pancreatic, and hepatobiliary diseases, including inflammatory bowel disease (IBD), alimentary small-cell lymphoma, cholangitis, and acute and chronic pancreatitis (Fig. 30.1). Some cats have involvement of two of these organs but not the third (e.g. cholangitis with concurrent pancreatitis in the absence of intestinal disease). Additionally, cats may present with disease of one organ predominating the clinical picture and histologically confirmed inflammation of other organs that may or may not be clinically important. The clinical signs and laboratory findings for the diseases comprising triaditis overlap creating a diagnostic challenge. Lastly, the presence of inflammation in other organs can complicate the treatment of each component (e.g. a cat with neutrophilic cholangitis with an active bacterial infection with concurrent IBD that requires immunomodulatory treatment). Although it has not been definitively proven, it is reasonable to speculate that disease in multiple organs may have prognostic implications.

This chapter reviews the epidemiology, aetiopathogenesis, diagnosis, and treatment of cholangitis and triaditis in cats. See Chapters 17 and 18 for an in-depth discussion of IBD. See Chapter 24 for an in-depth discussion of pancreatitis.

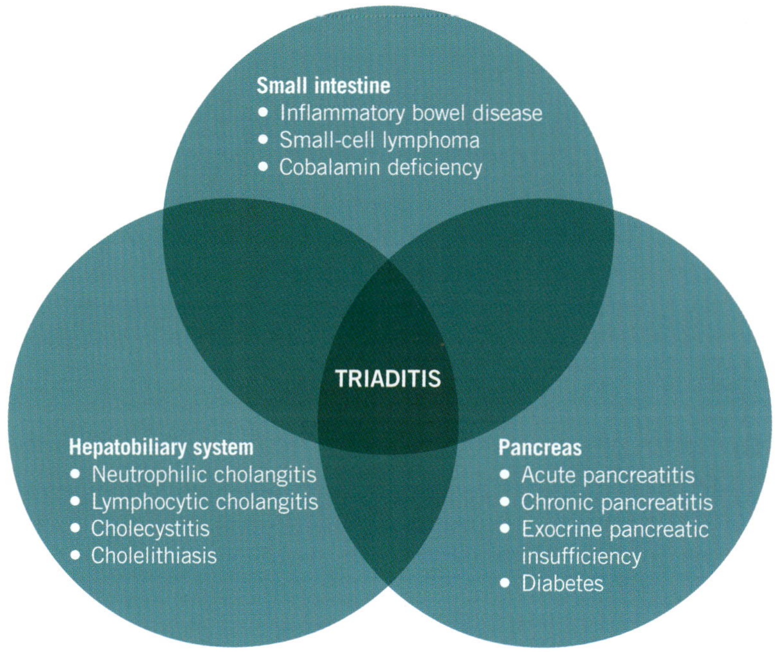

Figure 30.1. Components of the feline triaditis syndrome.

EPIDEMIOLOGY AND AETIOLOGY

Cholangitis

Cholangitis syndrome is one of the two most common liver diseases in cats, feline hepatic lipidosis being the other. These syndromes have a worldwide distribution, but there appears to be slight geographical variations in their relative prevalence.[3–6] For example, in a study of 1452 feline liver biopsies from the United Kingdom, neutrophilic cholangitis was the most common finding, reported in 20.5% of specimens, while lymphocytic cholangitis occurred in 6.8% and steatosis in only 3.5%.[3] Another study of 71 cat liver biopsy specimens from Japan found that neutrophilic cholangitis was the second most common finding (after parenchymal and interstitial hepatitis), present in 23.9% of specimens, while lymphocytic cholangitis was present in 14.1%.[5] However, in a study of 175 liver biopsy specimens from the United States of America, steatosis was the most common finding, recorded in 49% of specimens, and cholangitis was present in 26% of specimens.[6] Overall, neutrophilic cholangitis appears to be more common than lymphocytic cholangitis (Table 30.1).

The liver fluke species that can cause cholangitis in cats have a worldwide distribution, but their respective regional prevalence varies considerably and, in some areas, liver fluke–associated cholangitis is common.

Neutrophilic cholangitis

Most (but not all) cats with neutrophilic cholangitis have positive bile/liver cultures with single species of bacteria isolated. Additionally, many cats with this form of cholangitis respond favourably to antimicrobial therapy. *Escherichia coli* is the most commonly isolated bacteria from cat bile, but other frequently isolated species include *Enterococcus* sp., *Bacteroides* sp., *Clostridium* sp., *Staphylococcus* sp., and *Streptococcus* sp.[7–11] This strongly suggests that enteric bacteria are the aetiological agent in neutrophilic cholangitis. The mechanism by which these organisms reach the liver is somewhat controversial. It was previously assumed that they ascended the biliary tract. The common channel theory, whereby in approximately 80% of cats the common bile duct and pancreatic duct enter the duodenum together at the major duodenal papilla, is often purported to support this. However, a recent study that used fluorescence in situ hybridisation to look for bacteria in cats with inflammatory liver disease

Table 30.1. Most prevalent histopathological liver lesions/diseases described in cats.

1452 cat liver biopsy specimens from the UK[3]		152 cat liver biopsy specimens from New Zealand[4]		71 cat liver biopsy specimens from Japan[5]		175 cat liver biopsy specimens from the USA[6]	
Neutrophilic cholangitis	20.5%	Lymphocytic cholangitis	20.0%	Neutrophilic cholangitis	25.3%	Steatosis	49.1%
Reversible hepatitis	20.5%	Hepatitis	16.9%	Lymphocytic cholangitis	14.1%	Neutrophilic cholangitis	19.5%
Reversible hepatocellular injury	8.4%	Reversible hepatitis	16.4%	Hepatic degeneration	14.1%	Lymphocytic cholangitis	6.2%
Lymphocytic cholangitis	6.8%	Neutrophilic cholangitis	9.7%	Impaired hepatic perfusion	12.7%	Lymphoma	4.6%
Biliary cysts	5.7%	Haematopoietic neoplasia	9.7%	Chronic hepatitis	5.6%	Carcinoma	4.0%
Acute hepatitis	5.6%	Impaired hepatic perfusion	7.7%	Biliary cysts	5.6%	Vacuolar change	4.0%
Haematopoietic neoplasia	5.6%	Hepatocellular neoplasia	5.6%	Lymphoma	4.2%	Portal vascular anomalies	3.4%
Hepatocellular neoplasia	4.9%	Cholangiocellular neoplasia	4.1%	Hepatocellular neoplasia	4.2%	Other	2.9%
Congenital portosystemic shunt	3.8%	Metastatic neoplasia	3.1%	Other primary neoplasia	2.8%	Toxic hepatopathy	1.7%
Cholangiocellular neoplasia	3.1%	Biliary cystic disease	2.6%	Other neoplasia	2.8%	Hepatic cysts	1.1%

found that bacteria were more often localised to portal vessels, venous sinusoids, and parenchyma rather than to bile ducts.[12] This suggests that they may reach the liver by translocation across the intestinal wall or via the portal circulation rather than by ascending the biliary tract. This translocation could be caused by increased intestinal permeability and/or dysbiosis associated with intestinal disease.

Neutrophilic cholangitis in cats may be associated with concurrent cholecystitis and/or cholelithiasis. Additionally, as previously mentioned, concurrent pancreatitis and/or enteritis are common. Cats with neutrophilic cholangitis, especially those with septic bile, may develop systemic inflammation with resulting systemic inflammatory response syndrome or sepsis. A combination of intra- and extrahepatic cholestases (possibly due to pancreatitis, cholelithiasis, and obstruction of the common bile ducts with inflammatory debris) can contribute to the development of icterus.

Lymphocytic cholangitis

Lymphocytic cholangitis is thought to be caused by a loss of immune tolerance, resulting in the targeting of bile ducts by the adaptive immune response. An association between cholangitis, pancreatitis, and nephritis has been described in cats, possible due to a common autoimmune aetiology. Furthermore, cats with this form of cholangitis typically respond to immunomodulatory therapy. Although there is evidence that a loss of immune tolerance is responsible for the development of this form of cholangitis, the mechanisms behind this have not been determined. It is possible that a transient bacterial infection could lead to an aberrant and persistent immune response. Bacteria are not typically cultured from the liver or bile of cats with lymphocytic cholangitis, but sensitive molecular techniques have documented the presence of a variety of bacteria, including, *E. coli*, *Enterococcus*, and *Helicobacter* in the livers of these patients.[12–14] However, the significance of these organisms is not clear, as they were found in mixed populations and were also present in liver tissue from healthy cats. The other possibility is that bile duct-centric inflammation develops because of a loss of immune tolerance to members of the intestinal microbiota or dietary antigens, and the relatively high prevalence of enteropathy in cats with cholangitis supports this.

Lymphocytic cholangitis is not typically associated with systemic inflammatory response syndrome, sepsis, cholecystitis, or cholelithiasis. However, concurrent chronic pancreatitis is common. Therefore, combination of intra- and extrahepatic cholestases can contribute to the development of icterus.

Fluke-associated cholangitis

Species of liver fluke described to infect cats belong to the families Dicrocoeliidae (*Platynosomum* spp.) and Opisthorchiidae (*Opisthorchis* spp., *Clonorchis* spp., *Metorchis* spp., and *Amphimerus* spp.).[15–17] These trematodes have complex life cycles involving several hosts whereby cats (as well as dogs and humans) are definitive (reservoir) hosts. *Platynosomum* spp. is the best described in the literature, and cats acquire this parasite by ingesting lizards,[16] whereas cats acquire Opisthorchiidae infections by ingesting raw fish.[17] With either trematode family, the flukes migrate to the cat's liver and gallbladder, reproduce, and then eggs (ova) are shed in the faeces. *Platynosomum fastosum* is found in tropical and subtropical regions, and in endemic areas the prevalence rates are high in free-roaming cats. In the United States of America, this parasite is most common in the Southeast and Hawaii.[16]

The presence of flukes in the biliary tract leads to inflammation, fibrosis (with chronicity), and possibly biliary obstruction with resultant cholestasis and icterus. The severity of clinical signs is very variable and depends upon the parasite burden and chronicity of infection.

Triaditis

It is common for cats with inflammatory liver disease (including cholangitis) to have concurrent IBD and/or pancreatitis. For example, in one study of cats with neutrophilic cholangitis, 50% had pancreatitis, 83% had IBD, and 39% had triaditis.[18] In another study of cats with inflammatory liver disease, 62% had pancreatitis, 49% had IBD, and 32% had triaditis.[19] In a prospective study, IBD with cholangitis was noted to occur in 22% cats with gastrointestinal (GI) signs, IBD with pancreatitis in 4%, and triaditis in 30%, suggesting that triaditis or inflammation of two of these organs is relatively common. However, some combination of histopathological changes of two or more of these organs was also found in 11/20 (55%) asymptomatic cats undergoing ovariohysterectomy, although, interestingly, none of the cats in this group had histological inflammation in all three organs (Table 30.2).[20] This finding of histologically documented inflammation in cats without clinical signs may be because of limitations in our understanding of what constitutes histologically "normal" tissue or could be due to subclinical disease. Therefore, when evaluating cats with suspected triaditis (or its components), it is important to look at histopathological findings in conjunction with the patient's clinical signs, laboratory test results, and diagnostic imaging findings to help determine if inflammation in any organ is clinically relevant.

The aetiopathogeneses of IBD and pancreatitis in cats are reviewed in Chapters 17 and 24, respectively. The interplay between inflammation of the small intestine, pancreas, and biliary tract of cats has not been fully characterised. However, proposed mechanisms by which triaditis may occur are discussed below. Similar to the aetiopathogenesis of cholangitis in cats, bacterial infection and/or immune-mediated mechanisms are believed to play a role.

Two models have been proposed to explain the development of acute (suppurative) pancreatitis and neutrophilic cholangitis.[21] In the first, enteritis leads to dysbiosis and increased intestinal permeability. This leads to splanchnic bacteraemia and haematogenous seeding of bacteria in the liver and/or pancreas. A study of cats with inflammatory liver disease localising bacteria to be mainly around the portal vessels, venous sinusoids, and parenchyma supports this hypothesis.[12] Alternatively,

Table 30.2. Selected literature describing multi-organ (pancreas, liver, and/or intestines) histopathologically documented inflammation in cats.

Study	Study design	Number of cats	Pancreatitis	Cholangitis	IBD	Triaditis
Weiss et al. 1996[18]	Retrospective, necropsy	54 • NC: 18 • LC: 36	14/54 (26%) • NC: 9/18 (50%) • LC: 5/36 (14%)	54/54 (100%) • NC: 18/18 (100%) • LC: 36/36 (100%)	25/54 (46%) • NC: 15/18 (83%) • LC: 5/36 (28%)	9/54 (17%) • NC: 7/18 (39%) • LC: 2/36 (6%)
Callahan et al. 2011[19]	Retrospective, necropsy	43 • NC: 40 • LC: 3	21/34 (62%) • NC: 18/31 (58%) • LC: 3/3 (100%)	43/43 (100%) • NC: 40/40 (100%) • LC: 3/3 (100%)	17/35 (49%) • NC: 14/32 (44%) • LC: 3/3 (100%)	10/31 (32%) • NC: 7/28 (25%) • LC: 3/3 (100%)
Fragkou et al. 2016[20]	Prospective, biopsy, and necropsy	47 • Symptomatic: 27 • Asymptomatic: 20	12/47 (26%) • Symptomatic: 11/27 (41%) • Asymptomatic: 1/20 (5%)	30/47 (64%) • Symptomatic: 16/27 (59%) • Asymptomatic: 14/20 (70%)	40/47 (85%) • Symptomatic: 24/27 (89%) • Asymptomatic: 16/20 (80%)	8/47 (17%) • Symptomatic: 8/27 (30%) • Asymptomatic: 0/20 (0%)

IBD, inflammatory bowel disease; LC, lymphocytic cholangitis; NC, neutrophilic cholangitis.

reflux of duodenal contents into the pancreaticobiliary duct system could be the route by which enteric bacteria reach the liver and/or pancreas. In the other model, the development of acute pancreatitis is the initial event. This, in turn, leads to acute enteritis and/or cholangitis possibly due to the close anatomical relationship between the three organs. The enteritis then potentially leads to bacterial translocation to the pancreas and/or liver.

A third model could explain the development of chronic pancreatitis and lymphocytic cholangitis in cats with IBD. A combination of genetic and environmental factors in cats with IBD leads to a loss of immune tolerance to dietary components and/or the intestinal microbiota. The resulting enteritis is often associated with dysbiosis, and low-grade bacterial translocation could also occur. Activation of the innate/adaptive immune system then leads to immune-mediated injury in the pancreas and/or liver. One mechanism by which this may occur is by aberrant homing of T cells activated in the GI tract to the liver. This homing of T cells occurs in the human disease primary sclerosing cholangitis. Alternatively, gut- or host-derived molecules (pathogen-associated molecular patterns or bile acids) in the portal circulation may stimulate an immune response in the liver and/or pancreas. Lastly, IBD could be associated with the development of autoantibodies against hepatic and/or pancreatic proteins because of molecular mimicry.

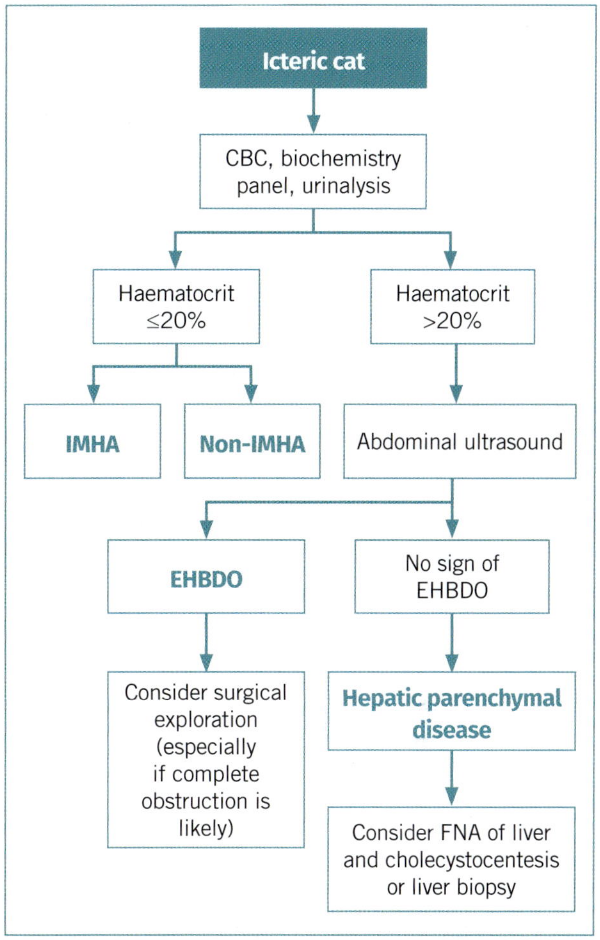

Figure 30.2. Diagnostic approach to icterus in cats. CBC, complete blood count; EHBDO, extrahepatic bile duct obstruction; FNA, fine needle aspiration, IMHA, immune-mediated haemolytic anaemia.

HISTORY AND PHYSICAL EXAMINATION

Cholangitis

Neutrophilic cholangitis

Cats of any age, breed, or sex can be affected by neutrophilic cholangitis. The median age of affected cats in one study was 8 years (range 1–20 years).[2] In general, cats with the neutrophilic form of cholangitis typically have an acute onset (<2 weeks).[15]

The most commonly reported historical findings are lethargy (in approximately 3/4 of cats), vomiting (in approximately 2/3), and dysrexia/anorexia (in approximately 1/2). Occasionally, owners may also notice obvious icterus. A diagnostic approach to icteric cats is outlined in Figure 30.2. Other signs related to concurrent illness may also be reported (e.g. diarrhoea).

The most common physical examination findings are icterus and pyrexia (both in approximately 1/3 of cats). Abdominal pain, hepatomegaly, and occasionally ptyalism may also be noted. It is important to note that cats with abdominal pain may show nonspecific clinical signs, such as decreased activity, withdrawal, or aggression.

Lymphocytic cholangitis

The signalment of cats with lymphocytic cholangitis described in the literature is very variable, and the only safe conclusion to draw is that cats of any age, breed, or sex can be affected by lymphocytic cholangitis. For example, the median age of affected cats in one study was 12.3 years,[22] whereas earlier studies reported that most cats were 4 years of age or younger.[23,24] In one study, Persian cats from the United Kingdom,[24] and, in another study, Norwegian Forest cats from the Netherlands[22] were reported to be predisposed. The former study also reported a predisposition for male cats, whereas other studies did not find this.

The lymphocytic form of cholangitis tends to be a more chronic condition in which clinical signs may wax and wane or can be slowly progressive. The most commonly reported historical findings are weight loss and lethargy, each occurring in about a third of cats. Other reported clinical findings include dysrexia/anorexia, polyphagia, and vomiting.

Commonly reported physical examination findings include icterus, hepatomegaly, and ascites (the prevalence of which is very variable between studies). Cats may also present with poor body condition/muscle wasting or, occasionally, neurological signs (presumably hepatic encephalopathy due to acquired portosystemic shunts). Pyrexia and abdominal pain are rarely reported. As for neutrophilic cholangitis, the clinical signs of concurrent diseases (e.g. diarrhoea due to IBD) may also be noted.

Fluke-associated cholangitis

Cats infected with low numbers of *P. fastosum* may have no clinical signs. Those with higher parasite burdens and more chronic infections may develop clinical signs ranging from transient inappetence, low-grade fever, or lethargy to more serious signs such as vomiting, icterus, or diarrhoea.

Triaditis

Sex and breed predilections for triaditis have not been demonstrated. Cats can present with triaditis at any age, but as IBD is more common in older cats, it reasonable to hypothesise that triaditis also becomes more likely with increasing age.

Because triaditis is a highly variable syndrome rather than a disease, cats can present with a wide array of clinical findings. Common historical observations include decreased appetite, lethargy, vomiting, diarrhoea, weight loss, and icterus. An increased appetite accompanied by weight loss is suggestive of exocrine pancreatic insufficiency or malassimilation due to IBD or small-cell GI lymphoma. There is considerable overlap in the clinical presentation of cats with pancreatitis, cholangitis, and IBD. This can create a diagnostic challenge for clinicians.

Possible physical examination findings include poor body condition, abdominal pain, ascites, icterus, or thickened intestinal loops.

DIAGNOSTIC INVESTIGATION

Laboratory testing

Biochemical changes consistent with cholangitis include hyperbilirubinaemia, increased alanine aminotransferase (ALT) activity, increased aspartate aminotransferase (AST) activity, increased alkaline phosphatase (ALP) activity, increased gamma-glutamyltransferase (GGT) activity, and hyperglobulinaemia. Hyperbilirubinaemia may be slightly less common and of lesser magnitude in lymphocytic cholangitis compared to neutrophilic cholangitis, whereas hyperglobulinaemia may be more common. Hypoalbuminaemia is an inconsistent finding and, when present, tends to be mild (>2.0 g/dl). Measuring serum pre- and postprandial total bile acid concentrations is a more sensitive test of liver dysfunction than bilirubin or other routinely measured biochemical parameters. However, there is generally little value in measuring total bile acid concentrations in hyperbilirubinaemic cats, unless haemolysis cannot be ruled out, as they are expected to be increased. Stress hyperglycaemia is common in hospitalised cats, and some patients may have concurrent diabetes mellitus. Electrolyte abnormalities may reflect dehydration (e.g. hypernatraemia) and increased losses because of vomiting (e.g. hypokalaemia) but are not consistent findings.

Cats with neutrophilic cholangitis often have an inflammatory leucogram, whereas this is less common with lymphocytic cholangitis. Mild to moderate normocytic normochromic anaemia consistent with anaemia of chronic disease may be noted with either form. Poikilocytosis has also been reported in cats with neutrophilic cholangitis and lymphocytic cholangitis. Severe anaemia in icteric cats should raise the suspicion for haemolysis.

The liver synthesises most coagulation and anticoagulant factors, and cats with cholestasis may have impaired vitamin K absorption. Cats with cholangitis may have prolonged coagulation times (prothrombin time [PT] and activated partial thromboplastin time [aPTT]). A prolonged PT was the most common abnormality recorded in 82% of cats with liver disease, and this was more common in cats with marked increases in ALP activity, suggesting the importance of cholestasis and impaired vitamin K absorption rather than hepatic synthetic failure.[25] However, vitamin K–replete cats with cholestatic liver disease were found to have a variety of haemostatic abnormalities on thromboelastography, including hypocoagulable states, hyperfibrinolysis, and hypercoagulable states.[26]

In ascitic patients, analysis of abdominal fluid usually reveals a modified transudate of relatively high protein content with increased globulin concentrations, small lymphocytes, and nondegenerate neutrophils.

Laboratory testing for pancreatic disease is described in Chapter 4. Traditional lipase and amylase activity assays have limited utility in cats and are not recommended. Measurement of feline pancreatic lipase immunoreactivity (fPLI) by Spec fPL or SNAP fPL is arguably the most useful laboratory test for helping to rule in or rule out pancreatitis. It is important to remember that positive SNAP fPL test results should be confirmed with the Spec fPL test, that false-positive and false-negative results can occur with either test, and that results should be integrated with other clinical and diagnostic imaging findings. 1,2-o-Dilauryl-rac-glycero-3-glutaric acid-(6'-methylresorufin) ester (DGGR) lipase activity assays are marketed as being more specific for pancreatic lipase than traditional activity assays. These assays mostly agree with pancreas-specific lipase assays, but they are not completely equivalent and discordant results can occur. Further studies are needed to fully determine their diagnostic performance. Cats with exocrine pancreatic insufficiency have reduced serum trypsin-like immunoreactivity (TLI) concentrations, and this test should be performed in cats with weight loss and soft stool.

Laboratory testing for chronic enteropathy is described in Chapter 3. Cats with chronic small intestinal disease often have serum cobalamin concentrations below the lower limit or in the lower part of the reference interval. They can also have serum folate concentrations below the lower limit of the reference interval. Increased serum folate concentrations may indicate dysbiosis, but this often occurs secondary to another disease process in cats and should not automatically lead to treatment aimed at modulating the GI microbiota (e.g. antimicrobial therapy). It is important to note that normal cobalamin and folate concentrations do not completely rule out chronic intestinal disease in cats.

Faecal analysis can identify trematode ova in cats suffering from liver fluke–associated cholangitis. However, negative results do not rule out infection. Possible reasons for false negatives include intermittent shedding of ova, low parasite burden, and technical issues with the faecal examination. Formalin–ether centrifugal sedimentation has been reported to be a more sensitive technique than centrifugal flotation in sugar solution, and its performance can be improved by serially analysing faecal samples collected over several days.

Diagnostic imaging

Diagnostic imaging of the GI tract and of the pancreas and hepatobiliary system is described in depth in Chapters 5 and 6, respectively. Abdominal radiographs are useful for ruling out other causes of vomiting, such as foreign bodies, or for detecting abdominal masses, but they often have limited utility for diagnosing cholangitis, pancreatitis, or IBD. Hepatomegaly or loss of serosal detail due to ascites may be appreciated in cats with cholangitis. Occasionally, mineralised cholecystoliths or choledocholiths may be appreciated in cats with cholangitis, but they can also be noted as incidental findings and may be nonmineralised and therefore not apparent on radiographs. A gas opacity in the region of the gallbladder suggests emphysematous cholecystitis (Fig. 30.3) Pancreatitis can lead to a focal loss of serosal detail in the right cranial abdomen, a soft tissue mass effect caudal to the stomach, increased soft tissue opacity in the cranial right abdomen, and a gas-distended descending duodenum. However, these findings can be subtle, are not completely specific for pancreatitis, and false-negative results are common. Radiography does not allow assessment of intestinal wall thickness and is not generally helpful for the diagnosis of IBD or other chronic enteropathies.

Abdominal ultrasonography is useful in the diagnosis of intestinal disease, pancreatitis, hepatobiliary disease, and combinations of the three. Changes to the hepatic parenchyma are variable in cats with cholangitis and include increased, decreased, or heterogeneous echotexture. The liver may be normal in size, or hepatomegaly may be appreciated. Abnormalities of the biliary tract are frequently observed and include gallbladder wall or

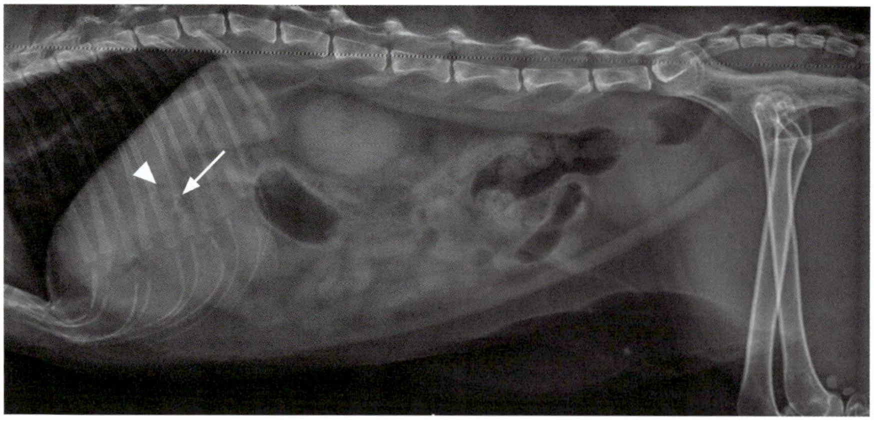

Figure 30.3. Lateral abdominal radiograph of a cat with cholecystoliths and emphysematous cholecystitis. A few mineralised opacities (arrow) represent cholecystoliths, and multiple gas opacities (arrowhead) within the liver in the region of the gallbladder represent gas bubbles within the gallbladder. Image courtesy of Dr John F. Griffin IV, Texas A&M University, USA.

common bile duct thickening, hyperechoic gallbladder contents, choleliths (Fig. 30.4), choledocholiths, and dilation of the common bile ducts (Fig. 30.5). The normal common bile duct should be less than or equal to 4 mm in width, and its wall should be less than or equal to 1 mm thick. Intra- and extrahepatic bile ducts are only visible on ultrasound if they are dilated. The finding of a gallbladder wall greater than 1 mm in thickness is a specific marker of disease (i.e. cholecystitis, oedema, or mucosal gland hyperplasia). It should be noted that the absence of ultrasonographic changes of the liver or biliary tract does not rule out cholangitis. Abdominal ultrasound also allows the collection of guided liver aspirates as well as percutaneous cholecystocentesis.

Ultrasonographic findings consistent with pancreatitis in cats include an enlarged pancreas, generalised hypoechogenicity (often seen with mild pancreatitis), hyperechogenicity of the surrounding mesentery, hyperechogenic areas of the pancreas (consistent with fibrosis), hypoechogenic areas of the pancreas (consistent with haemorrhage inflammation, haemorrhage, or necrosis), possibly cavitary lesions, or possibly dilation of the pancreatic duct. Occasionally, pancreatitis can lead to extrahepatic bile duct obstruction (EHBDO) in cats with resultant common bile duct dilation. It should be noted that the performance of this modality is operator dependent and that an unremarkable ultrasound examination does not rule out pancreatitis. Furthermore, it is not possible

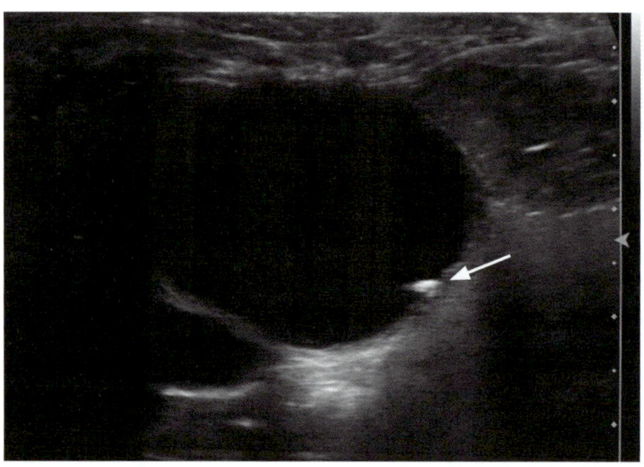

Figure 30.4. Ultrasonographic image of the gallbladder of a cat with cholelithiasis. A small hyperechoic calculus adherent to the gallbladder wall is apparent (arrow). Image courtesy of Dr Lindsey Gilmour, Texas A&M University, USA.

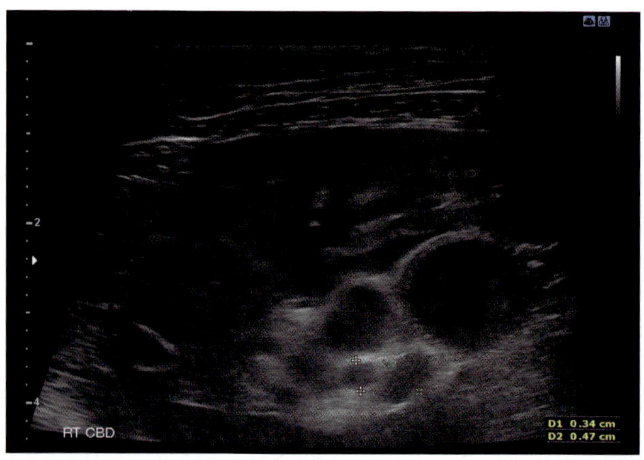

Figure 30.5. Ultrasonographic image of a dilated common bile duct in a cat with neutrophilic cholangitis. The measurement callipers show that the bile duct is 4.7 mm in width as it enters the duodenal papilla (>4.0 mm is considered to be dilated). Image courtesy of Dr Catherine Ruoff, Texas A&M University, USA.

to reliably differentiate acute and chronic pancreatitis sonographically.

In cats with IBD, the small intestinal wall thickness may be increased, while wall layering is maintained. However, this finding is insensitive, and normal wall thickness does not rule out IBD. Additionally, it is not possible to differentiate idiopathic IBD from other inflammatory enteropathies such as food-responsive enteropathy. The finding of muscularis thickening with preserved wall layers is suggestive of alimentary small-cell lymphoma. However, caution must be exercised, as muscularis thickening is only appreciated in about half of cats with this neoplasia and may also occasionally be seen in asymptomatic cats (Fig. 30.6).

Although they are generally less available and more costly than ultrasound, cross-sectional imaging modalities may be of use for the evaluation of cats with suspected cholangitis or triaditis. Ultrasonographic evaluation of the cranial abdomen is challenging because of superimposition of the stomach and gas in the adjacent intestinal loops. Computed tomography (CT) and magnetic resonance imaging (MRI) overcome these problems and are less operator dependent. These modalities are commonly used in people to image the pancreas, liver, and biliary tract. MRI and magnetic resonance cholangiopancreatography (MRCP) sequences were helpful for identifying lesions in 10 cats with cholangitis and/or pancreatitis.[27] CT and MRI may also allow the detection of cholecystoliths, choledocholiths, and EHBDO.

Cholecystocentesis

Percutaneous ultrasound-guided cholecystocentesis is typically performed in cats that are heavily sedated or anaesthetised. Either a right-sided transhepatic or right ventral abdominal approach can be used. Aspiration can be achieved with a 22- or 23-gauge 1.5-inch needle attached to a syringe with an extension set. Typically, as much bile is drained as possible to reduce leakage after aspiration. The procedure is cheaper and less invasive than liver biopsy and is generally well tolerated, but potential complications include gallbladder rupture with secondary bile peritonitis, haemorrhage, and increased vagal tone leading to bradycardia. Suspected emphysematous cholecystitis on ultrasound or severely increased bleeding risk are contraindications for percutaneous ultrasound-guided cholecystocentesis. In a retrospective study, postprocedural complications were recorded in 14/83 (17%) cats, of which 11 cats (13%) developed abdominal fluid following the procedure (all of which had concurrent procedures such as liver/splenic aspiration performed), one cat (1%) developed pneumoperitoneum, and no cats died or were euthanised due to complications of cholecystocentesis.[9] Bile can also be collected from the gallbladder during laparotomy or laparoscopy with direct visualisation.

Bacterial culture and cytological evaluation of bile revealed an abnormal result in one-third of cats with suspected hepatobiliary disease.[9] Cytologically confirmed septic suppurative inflammation (Fig. 30.7) and bacterial growth on bile culture are diagnostic for neutrophilic chol-

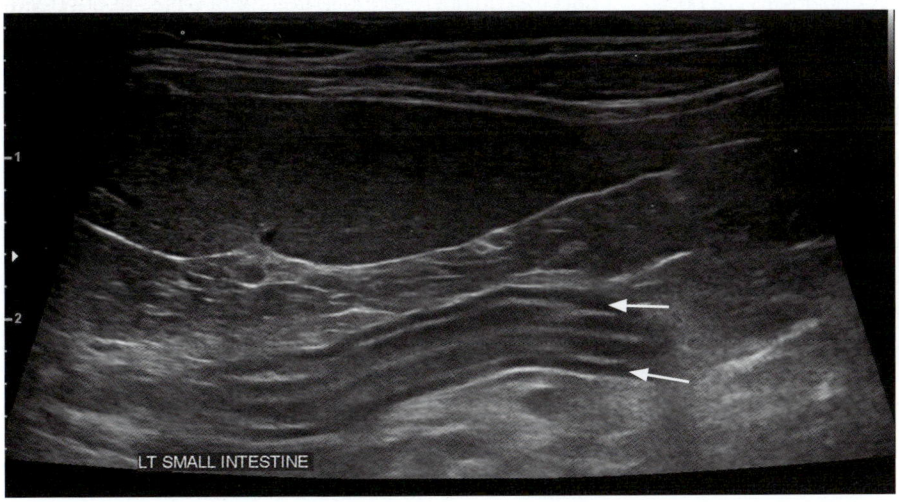

Figure 30.6. Ultrasonographic image of jejunal muscularis thickening in a cat. The thickened muscularis layer is highlighted by arrows. This change is suggestive of gastrointestinal small-cell lymphoma but may also be observed in healthy cats. Image courtesy of Dr Catherine Ruoff, Texas A&M University, USA.

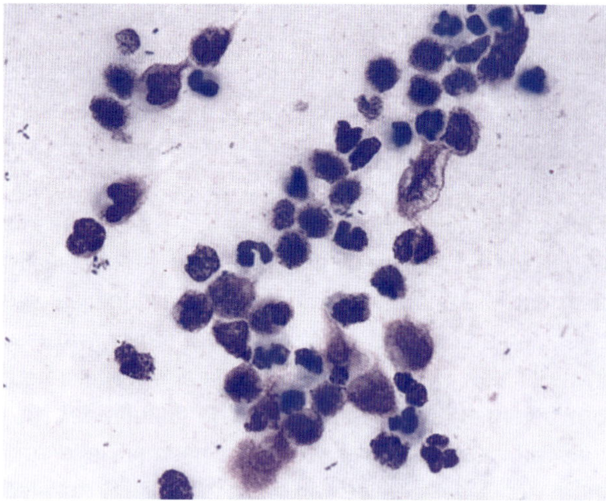

Figure 30.7. Microscopic image of bile from a cat with neutrophilic cholangitis. The neutrophils are severely degenerate, and some cells are difficult to identify (a common problem with bile cytological examination). Numerous extracellular and fewer intracellular bacteria are apparent. Image courtesy of Dr Mark C. Johnson, Texas A&M University, USA.

angitis. *E. coli* is the most frequently isolated bacterial species followed by *Enterococcus* spp. Other less frequently isolated bacteria include *Bacteroides* spp., *Clostridium* spp., *Streptococcus* spp., *Klebsiella pneumoniae*, *Pseudomonas aeruginosa*, *Enterobacter cloacae*, and *Bacillus* sp. (Table 30.3).[7–11] Bacteria are more commonly isolated from bile than from the liver. Of the cases with a positive bile culture, the cytological description of bacteria corresponded to the organism cultured in fewer than 50% of cases.[9] The sensitivity of bile culture for detecting bacterial infection has not been determined, and, for example, prior antibiotic administration could lead to false-negative results. In cats in which neutrophilic cholangitis is a possible differential diagnosis, percutaneous ultrasound-guided cholecystocentesis is a helpful diagnostic test to perform, but its diagnostic limitations must also be considered.

Platynosomum spp.–associated cholangitis can be diagnosed based on the visualisation of eggs in a bile sample. *Platynosomum* spp. egg counts in 27 cats were found to be higher in bile than in faeces. Therefore, percutaneous ultrasound-guided cholecystocentesis might be useful in cats in which this form of cholangitis is suspected but no eggs are found on faecal examination.[28]

Fine needle aspiration

Fine needle aspiration of the liver can easily be performed with ultrasound guidance in sedated or anaesthetised cats. This technique is generally well tolerated, but haemorrhage is a potential risk. Severe thrombocytopenia, coagulopathies, or anaemia are therefore potential contraindications.

The presence of increased numbers of nondegenerate or degenerate neutrophils on cytological evaluation of hepatic aspirates supports a diagnosis of neutrophilic cholangitis. However, the specificity of this finding is questionable, and it must be considered along with other clinical data. For example, blood contamination occurs with hepatic aspiration, and thus the peripheral neutrophil count must be considered when making this determination. The presence of increased numbers of predominantly small mature lymphocytes could support the presence of lymphocytic cholangitis (or small-cell lymphoma). With either form of cholangitis, variable degrees of intrahepatic cholestasis (characterised by bile plugs) and lipid-type vacuolar change may also be seen. Hepatic cytology has significant diagnostic limitations, and results should be cautiously interpreted. In cats that do not respond to treatment based upon a cytological diagnosis, hepatic biopsy should be considered. For example, in cats with hepatic lipidosis, cytological evaluation of hepatic aspirates can lead to a failure to

Table 30.3. Bacteria commonly isolated from the bile of cats with suspected hepatobiliary disease.

80 cats undergoing percutaneous ultrasound-guided cholecystocentesis[9]		78 cats undergoing cholecystocentesis[8]		70 cats undergoing percutaneous ultrasound-guided cholecystocentesis[11]	
Escherichia coli	8.8%	*Escherichia coli*	17.9%	*Escherichia coli*	35.7%
Streptococcus spp.	2.5%	*Enterococcus* spp.	5.1%	*Enterococcus* spp.	14.3%
Klebsiella pneumoniae	1.3%	*Clostridium* spp.	2.6%	*Streptococcus* spp.	2.9%
Pseudomonas aeruginosa	1.3%	*Proteus* spp.	1.3%	*Staphylococcus* sp.	1.4%
Enterococcus faecalis	1.3%	*Peptostreptococcus* spp.	1.3%	*Clostridium* spp.	1.4%
		Alpha-haemolytic *Streptococcus*	1.3%	*Bacillus* sp.	1.4%
				Enterobacter cloacae	1.4%

diagnose underlying cholangitis or neoplasia. In a study reviewing the agreement between cytological evaluation of hepatic fine needle aspiration samples and the histopathological diagnosis, only 51% of the cases had overall agreement.[29]

Liver biopsy

Definitive diagnosis of neutrophilic and lymphocytic cholangitis requires histological assessment of liver tissue. Liver biopsy is an invasive procedure; therefore, clinicians may opt to treat for this syndrome based on a presumptive diagnosis made after cytological assessment of the liver and bile as well as bacterial culture of bile. This approach is especially valid if neutrophilic cholangitis is suspected based on the findings of bacteribilia and/or bacteria growth in bile.

Liver biopsy may be performed percutaneously with a needle using ultrasound guidance, laparoscopically (Fig. 30.8), or via laparotomy. These techniques are discussed in detail in Chapter 8. Each method has advantages and disadvantages. The quality of samples collected with needle biopsy may be suboptimal, especially if an 18-gauge Tru-Cut biopsy needle is used instead of a 16-gauge needle. In cats suspected to have concurrent pancreatic or intestinal disease, the latter two techniques are preferable because these organs can be biopsied at the same time.

Liver biopsy is generally well tolerated, but the most common adverse event is haemorrhage. In a retrospective study of 30 cats undergoing percutaneous ultrasound-guided needle biopsy, minor bleeding (packed cell volume [PCV] decreased ≤6%) and major bleeding (PCV decreased >6%) occurred in 43% and 57% of cats, respectively. Major bleeding was more likely to occur in cats with feline hepatic lipidosis or in those with lower PCV before the procedure. However, physiological compromise necessitating an intervention or death were only recognised to occur in 17% of cats. Interestingly, clotting time (PT and aPTT) did not predict the occurrence of complication or magnitude of PCV decrease.[30] Automatic Tru-Cut biopsy devices should not be used in cats because they can cause fatal vagotonic shock.

Prior to liver biopsy, a bleeding risk assessment should be performed. This should include a platelet count, PT, aPTT, ideally measurement of plasma fibrinogen concentration, and a haematocrit. As mentioned above, the ability of these tests to predict haemorrhage is uncertain.

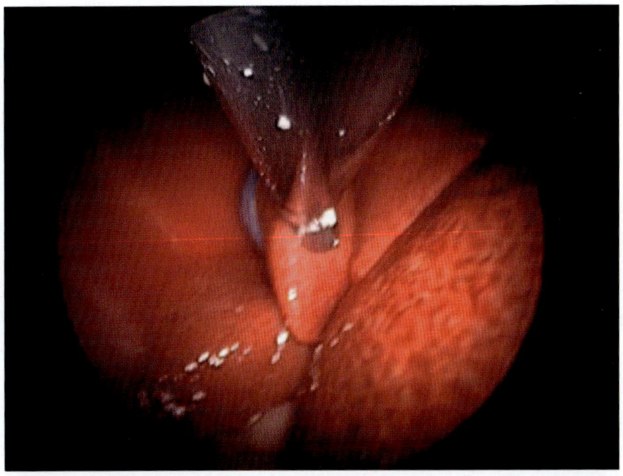

Figure 30.8. Laparoscopic view of a liver biopsy in a cat. The margin of the liver is being biopsied using oval closed cup forceps. Image courtesy of Dr Audrey K. Cook, Texas A&M University, USA.

If possible, several different liver lobes should be sampled to account for sampling variation, which is a concern with liver disease. In addition to placing several specimens in neutral buffered formalin for histopathological analysis, it is important to submit specimens of liver and bile for bacterial culture. It is also recommended to request that sections of liver are stained for copper, iron, and connective tissue.

Histopathology

Cholangitis

Acute neutrophilic cholangitis (formerly known as acute suppurative cholangitis/cholangiohepatitis) is characterised by an infiltrate of neutrophils and oedema centred around the bile ducts. As the disease progresses, the inflammatory infiltrate may cross the limiting plate of hepatocytes. When this occurs, the term cholangiohepatitis is used in the micromorphological diagnosis, but the initial injury was to the bile ducts. In chronic neutrophilic cholangitis (formerly known as chronic suppurative cholangitis/cholangiohepatitis), the inflammatory infiltrate is mixed with neutrophils, lymphocytes, and plasma cells, and there is also biliary hyperplasia, biliary epithelial degeneration, and varying degrees of periportal to bridging fibrosis. The most chronic phase of the disease may be represented by concentric periportal fibrosis (Fig. 30.9) and pseudolobule formation.[1]

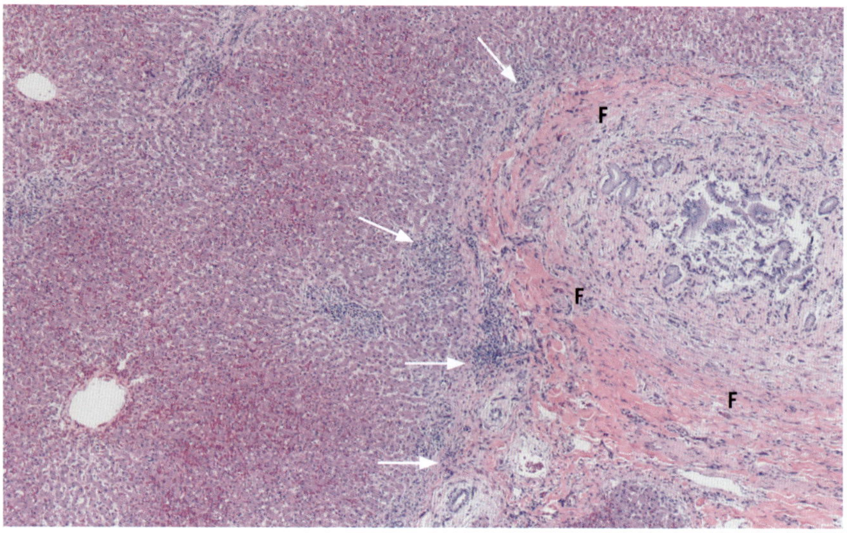

Figure 30.9. Microscopic image of the liver of a cat with (chronic) neutrophilic cholangitis. The image shows chronic, severe, multifocal to bridging, lymphoplasmacytic and neutrophilic cholangiohepatitis (arrows) and pericholangiolar concentric bands of fibrosis (F). Image courtesy of Dr Aline Rodrigues-Hoffmann, Texas A&M University, USA.

Lymphocytic cholangitis (formerly known as lymphocytic portal hepatitis or nonsuppurative cholangitis/cholangiohepatitis) is characterised by infiltration of lymphocytes in the portal region accompanied with bile duct proliferation, bile duct epithelial degeneration, bile duct loss, and varying degrees of fibrosis. When ductopenia is profound, the term sclerosing cholangitis is sometimes used. Although some authors suggest that this is a distinct disease entity (rather than a pattern of injury), it is not recognised as such in the WSAVA Standardization Guidelines.[1] Features of lymphocytic cholangitis that can help differentiate it from small-cell lymphoma include portal lipogranulomas, bile duct targeting, ductopenia, peribiliary fibrosis, and portal B-cell aggregates.[13] Immunophenotyping lymphocytic infiltrates and/or T-cell clonality can also help make this sometimes challenging determination (Fig. 30.10).

Platynosomum spp. lead to chronic cholangitis that is histologically characterised by marked periductal fibrosis, adenomatous proliferation of bile duct epithelium, dilation of intrahepatic bile ducts, and portal accumulations of inflammatory cells. Intraductal trematode fragments may or may not be appreciated (Fig. 30.11). Six out of 13 feline immunodeficiency virus (FIV)-positive cats with fluke-associated cholangitis also had bacterial cholangitis (*E. coli*).[28] Cases of fluke-associated cholangitis with concurrent cholangiocarcinoma have also been described in cats. It is possible that chronic inflammation due to the fluke can lead to neoplastic transformation of the biliary epithelium, but this has not been proven.

Triaditis

Histological confirmation of inflammation of the liver, pancreas, and small intestine is required before a definitive diagnosis of triaditis can be made. Many pathologists do not recognise triaditis as a syndrome in cats and therefore may not make this diagnosis or even mention it in their report. It is also important to note that the clinical importance of mild histopathological changes (e.g. minimal/mild lymphoplasmacytic enteritis) in these organs is uncertain and should be integrated with other clinical information.

Both neutrophilic and lymphocytic forms of cholangitis have been reported to occur in cats with triaditis. In a study of cats with cholangitis diagnosed after necropsy, 25% of those with neutrophilic cholangitis and 100% of those with lymphocytic cholangitis had triaditis.[19] The histopathological changes characteristic of cholangitis are described above.

The histopathological changes associated with pancreatitis are reviewed in Chapters 9 and 24. The most commonly type of pancreatitis observed in cats with triaditis is chronic interstitial pancreatitis whereby there is a monocytic infiltrate (lymphocytes, plasma cells, and occasional macrophages) and varying degrees of fibrosis. If the inflammatory infiltrate also contains neutrophils, the term chronic active pancreatitis may be used. However, acute pancreatitis, characterised by a neutrophilic infiltrate, pancreatic necrosis, and pancreatic oedema, can also occur in cats with triaditis.

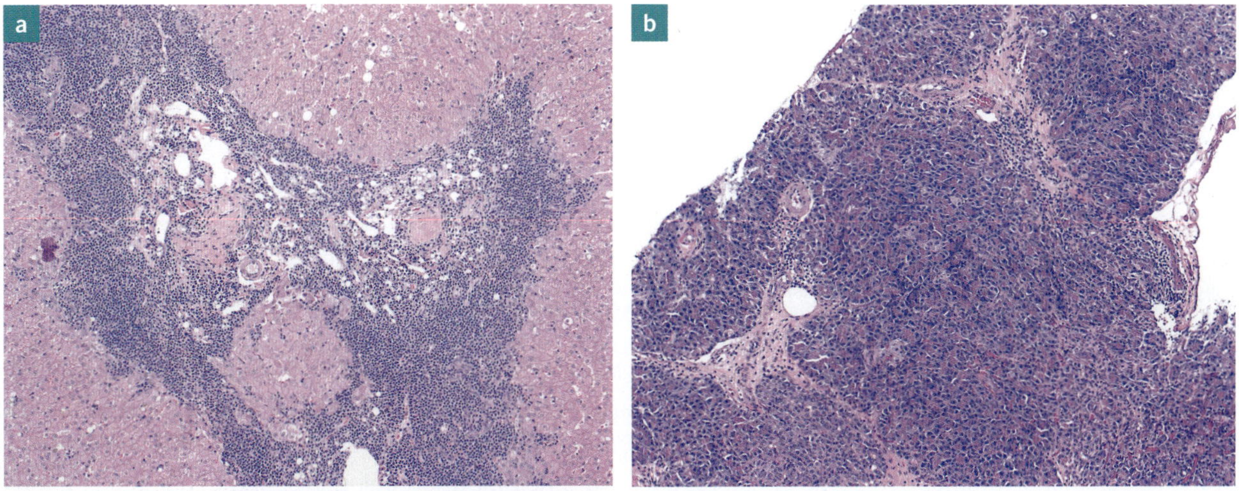

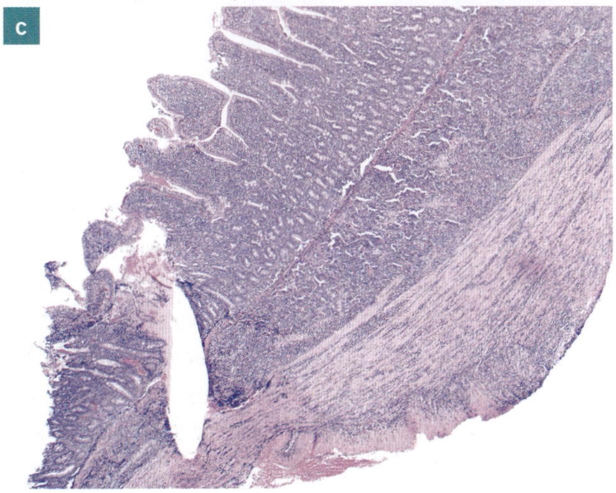

Figure 30.10. Microscopic images of the liver (a), pancreas (b), and duodenum (c) of a cat with severe lymphocytic cholangitis or hepatic small-cell lymphoma, mild chronic pancreatitis, and gastrointestinal small-cell lymphoma. In the liver, periportal tracts are markedly expanded, and often bridged, by a monomorphic population of small lymphocytes. The distinction of small-cell lymphoma and severe lymphocytic cholangitis can be challenging. In the pancreas, small to moderate numbers of small lymphocytes with rare plasma cells infiltrate along interlobular septae. In the duodenum, an infiltrative monomorphic population of neoplastic cells (small lymphocytes) is diffusely expanding and effacing the lamina propria and multifocally invading the mucosa and extending into the submucosa, tunica muscularis, and serosa. Images courtesy of Dr Maureen O'Brien, Texas A&M University, USA.

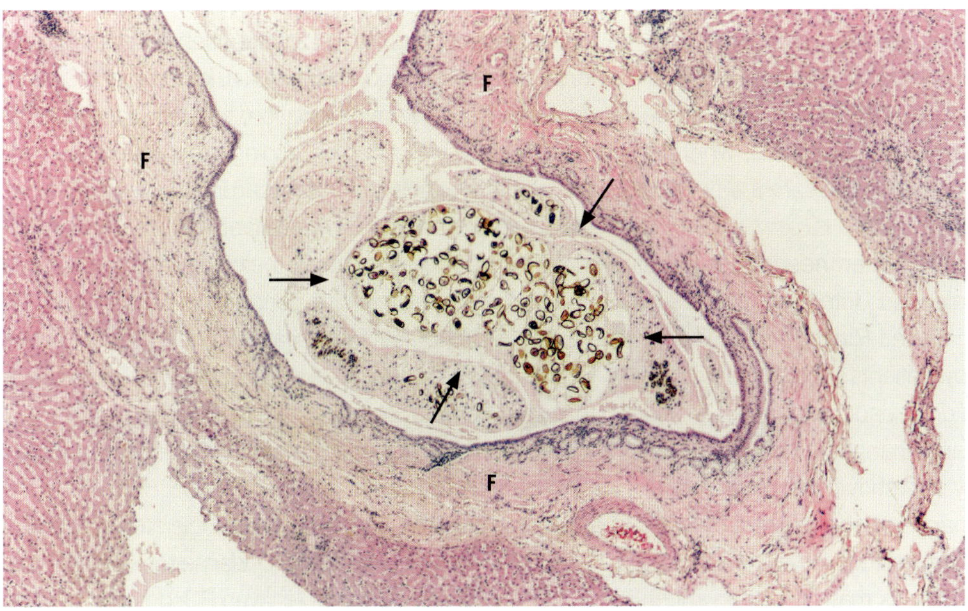

Figure 30.11. Microscopic image of the liver of a cat with fluke-associated cholangitis. Marked periductal fibrosis (F) and intraductal trematode fragments (arrows) are apparent. Image courtesy of Dr Randi M. Gold, Texas A&M Veterinary Medical Diagnostic Laboratory, USA.

The histopathological changes associated with IBD are reviewed in detail in Chapters 9 and 18. IBD is diagnosed in a cat with chronic GI signs by histologically documenting inflammation and ruling out other causes, including parasitism, infectious diseases, and food-responsive enteropathy. It is not possible to histologically distinguish IBD from other chronic enteropathies. However, the histological features of IBD include a variety of morphological (architectural) changes and inflammatory infiltrates. The morphological changes are more significant and include villous stunting, epithelial injury, crypt distension, lacteal dilation, and mucosal fibrosis. The inflammatory infiltrates are most commonly lymphoplasmacytic in nature, but eosinophilic and neutrophilic, or mixed, infiltrates can also occur. The clinical importance of low-grade inflammatory infiltrates, especially when they are lymphoplasmacytic, is questionable. There is a lack of interobserver agreement for diagnosing and grading these lesions even when using standardised diagnostic criteria. Furthermore, it can be difficult to distinguish lymphoplasmacytic enteritis from small-cell lymphoma.

MANAGEMENT AND TREATMENT

General supportive care and nutrition

Cats with cholangitis (especially, neutrophilic cholangitis) and triaditis may be critically ill. Severely affected patients may also be anorexic, which can have a variety of deleterious effects, including predisposing them to the development of feline hepatic lipidosis. Therefore, providing supportive care and nutritional support is essential to optimise outcome (see Appendix). Some cats can be managed effectively on an outpatient basis, whereas prolonged hospitalisation and intensive care are needed for others.

Intravenous fluid therapy is often needed for more severely affected cats. Balanced isotonic replacement crystalloid solutions (e.g. lactated Ringer's solution) are the mainstay of fluid therapy. Patients should be assessed for the three types of fluid disturbances: changes in volume, changes in content, and changes in distribution. An individualised fluid therapy plan should be made by considering the cat's maintenance needs, current deficits, ongoing losses, and its ability to tolerate intravenous fluids. Occasionally cats with cholangitis may present in shock (it should be remembered that cats with shock are often bradycardic rather than tachycardic) and may need to be given intravenous fluid boluses upon presentation. For cats that are refractory to boluses of isotonic replacement crystalloids, vasopressor therapy (if distributive shock is suspected) or administration of colloids (e.g. hydroxyethyl starch) should be considered. However, concerns about the safety of synthetic colloids in small animals require further investigation. It is also very important to promptly address potentially life-threatening electrolyte abnormalities such as hypokalaemia and hypophosphataemia. Standard intravenous potassium supplementation tables are helpful when doing this, and supplementation of potassium should not exceed 0.5 mEq/kg/h. It is essential to frequently reassess the cat's hydration status and serum biochemical parameters and then to adjust the fluid therapy plan accordingly.

In patients with cholestasis (intra- or extrahepatic) or prolonged clotting times, treatment with vitamin K_1 (0.5–1.5 mg/kg SC every 12 hours for three doses) is indicated, especially prior to performing invasive procedures such as hepatic aspiration/biopsy or feeding tube placement. Cats with clinically apparent coagulopathies may require treatment with fresh frozen plasma. Blood products are not typically recommended for patients with prolonged clotting times that are not haemorrhaging or at risk of bleeding due to a planned invasive procedure.

Some cats with cholangitis or triaditis may actively vomit or be nauseated, and thus antiemetics are frequently beneficial. Signs of nausea in cats are often nonspecific and include anorexia/hyporexia/dysrexia, lethargy, depression, restlessness, shivering, salivation, lip licking, frequent or exaggerated swallowing or gulping, abnormal body posture, food aversion, and tachycardia. The neurokinin-1 (NK_1) receptor antagonist maropitant is a potent antiemetic that also has analgesic effects; therefore, it is a good choice for cats with cholangitis or pancreatitis (1 mg/kg SC/IV/PO every 24 hours). Maropitant may be more effective in preventing emesis than in preventing nausea. Since this drug is metabolised in the liver by the cytochrome P450 enzyme CYP1A, the metabolism of this drug may be compromised in cats with liver disease. However, in the author's experience, maropitant is well tolerated in cats with liver disease at standard doses. Ondansetron (0.2–0.5 mg/kg IV/PO every 8–12 hours—if given PO, doses should be towards the high end of this range and should be given more frequently than when given IV or SC) is a potent 5-hydroxytryptamine (serotonin) 3 (5-HT_3) receptor antagonist antiemetic drug that is also reasonable to use. Since ondansetron is metabolised in the liver, it should be used cautiously in cats with liver disease. Combination therapy with maropitant and ondansetron is needed in some cats. Metoclopramide (0.2–0.5 mg/kg SC/PO every 6–8 hours, or 1–2 mg/kg/day IV as a CRI) is a dopamine 2 (D2) receptor and serotonin 4 (5-HT_4) receptor antagonist that is less effective than the previously mentioned drugs (cats have less D2 receptors in their chemoreceptor trigger zones than dogs) and, therefore, is not the author's first choice of antiemetic. It also has prokinetic effects and is sometimes used for this purpose. Metoclopramide interacts with the appetite stimulant mirtazapine, and some clinicians advise against its use in cats with pancreatitis because it may reduce pancreatic perfusion.

Cats with cholangitis and/or pancreatitis may experience abdominal pain and therefore require analgesia. Buprenorphine (0.01–0.03 mg/kg sublingual/IV/SC every 8–12 hours, or 0.24 mg/kg SC every 24 hours) is a partial mu-opioid receptor agonist that is a reasonable choice for hospitalised cats and can be given sublingually by owners. Full opioid receptor agonists such as fentanyl (1–6 μg/kg/h IV as a CRI) or methadone (0.1–0.2 mg/kg IV/IM every 4–6 hours) could also be used in hospitalised cats with severe pain. Nonsteroidal anti-inflammatory drugs may cause GI ulceration or nephrotoxicity and are contraindicated in cats with shock, dehydration, or preexisting GI signs.

Some cats with cholangitis (or triaditis) are hyporexic or anorexic. Therefore, nutritional support plays an essential role their management. Appetite stimulants such as mirtazapine (1.875–3.75 mg/cat PO every 24 hours, or 1.5 inches [≈2 mg] transdermally every 24 hours) can also be used as a short-term measure to help get cats to eat.[31] Potential side effects include vocalisation, increased affection, or sedation, and less commonly hypotension or tachycardia. Cats with liver disease may need less frequent mirtazapine administration than healthy cats. Forced syringe feeding of cats should be avoided, as it can lead to food aversion or aspiration. Enteral feeding is preferred to parenteral feeding, and placement of a feeding tube is often indicated. Feeding tubes can also make it easier for owners to medicate sick cats. Placement of nasogastric/nasooesophageal feeding tubes can be performed in conscious cats and is suitable for initial feeding of hospitalised cats, especially those that cannot immediately tolerate anaesthesia. However, they are not as well tolerated by patients as oesophageal feeding tubes, cats often remove them, and they are narrow bore, limiting the choice diets that can be fed. When feeding hospitalised cats through nasooesophageal/nasogastric tubes, high-caloric-density liquid recovery diets must be used in the short term only, as they are often not nutritionally balanced. Oesophageal feeding tubes are easy to place with readily available equipment, rarely have serious/life-threatening complications, and can be removed as soon as they are no longer needed. Gastrostomy tubes can be placed in anaesthetised cats percutaneously with endoscopic assistance or surgically. These tubes are suitable for long-term feeding but must be left in place for at least 2–3 weeks and occasionally result in serious/life-threatening complications. Cats that have been anorexic for more than a few days should be slowly reintroduced to food to reduce the chances of refeeding syndrome and gastric intolerance of larger volumes of food. Typically, in the first day of feeding, one-quarter to one-third of the cat's calculated resting energy requirement is fed, and if this is well tolerated, the amount is increased day by day. The choice of diet is not critical for cats with cholangitis, and the author typically feeds a high-quality maintenance diet or a low-residue highly digestible diet. Protein is arguably the most important macronutrient to prevent feline hepatic lipidosis; therefore, diets should have a protein content of ≈40% by metabolisable energy. For cats with concurrent chronic enteropathy, an elimination diet (novel protein source or hydrolysed protein) may be beneficial. The optimal diet to feed cats with pancreatitis is not currently known, but fat restriction has not been proven to be beneficial, and the author often feeds a commercial diet marketed for intestinal disease. Withholding food from cats with pancreatitis is no longer recommended, and early enteral nutrition is believed to be beneficial.

Deficient cats should be administered vitamin B_{12} (cobalamin). This can be done either parenterally (e.g. cyanocobalamin 250 μg/cat SC weekly for 6 weeks, then monthly until blood values are normal) or orally (250 μg/cat PO daily until blood values are normal).

Neutrophilic cholangitis

Antimicrobial agents are the primary treatment for cats with neutrophilic cholangitis (see Appendix). Ideally, these are selected based on the results of culture and sensitivity testing of bile and liver samples. Empirical antimicrobial therapy is usually started pending culture results or if there is no bacterial growth and neutrophilic cholangitis is histologically confirmed or suspected based on the cytological findings (see above). As previously mentioned, *E. coli.* is the most commonly isolated organism, followed by *Enterococcus* spp. The following antimicrobials are reasonable choices, as they are effective against most enteric bacteria (gram-positive and gram-negative aerobes and anaerobes) and have good biliary penetration: a potentiated penicillin alone, enrofloxacin (5 mg/kg PO every 24 hours) with concurrent potentiated penicillin or clindamycin, or pradofloxacin alone (7.5 mg/kg PO every 24 hours). Initial therapy with intravenous antimicrobials that provide broad-spectrum coverage should be started in critically ill cats. The coverage can then be narrowed once culture and sensitivity testing results are available. Treatment is switched to oral antimicrobials and typically continued for a total 4–6 weeks, as follow-up culture of bile and/or liver to confirm successful treatment is seldom performed. Clinical signs and biochemical changes are monitored closely during and after the cessation of treatment. In cases that have no bacterial growth and fail to respond to antimicrobial therapy, corticosteroids may be beneficial (see lymphocytic cholangitis below). If a cat has neutrophilic cholangitis and IBD, treatment with corticosteroids should be delayed until after (at least initial) treatment with antimicrobials.

Inflammatory liver disease, including neutrophilic cholangitis, is associated with depletion of hepatic glutathione in cats, suggesting oxidative stress. Therefore, there is justification for administering antioxidants. N-acetylcysteine (10% solution diluted 1:2 with saline as an IV bolus over 20 minutes through a 0.2 µm nonpyrogenic in-line filter at a dose of 140 mg/kg initially, followed by doses of 70 mg/kg every 8–12 hours) is a glutathione precursor that may be given intravenously in cats that cannot tolerate oral medications. When the cat can tolerate oral medications, combinations of S-adenosylmethionine (20 mg/kg PO every 24 hours on an empty stomach), silymarin (10 mg/kg of silymarin complexed with phosphatidylcholine PO every 24 hours), or vitamin E (alpha-tocopherol; 15 IU/kg PO every 24 hours) can be administered. Although there are few to no data documenting improved outcomes when these cytoprotective drugs are given, their use is unlikely to be detrimental to the patient. Ursodeoxycholic acid (10–15 mg/kg PO every 24 hours) may also be beneficial in cats with cholangitis, as in other species it has been shown to be a choleretic, to displace toxic bile acids, and to have potential antiapoptotic and immunomodulatory properties. However, it is important to prioritise medications that treat the underlying disease and essential supportive care over these cytoprotective agents and to be cognisant that giving multiple oral medications places a burden on the cat and its owner.

Cholecystectomy should be considered for cats with concurrent cholecystitis (especially if it is recurrent) or EHBDO. The management of these conditions is discussed in detail in Chapter 31.

Lymphocytic cholangitis

Immunomodulation with prednisolone (as opposed to prednisone) is the primary treatment for cats with lymphocytic cholangitis (see Appendix). An initial dose of 1–2 mg/kg PO every 24 hours is typically used followed by a gradual taper (e.g. a 25% dose decrease every 2–3 weeks) to the lowest effective dose, but long-term treatment is often needed. In a retrospective study, no difference in survival time was found between groups of cats treated with 1 mg/kg or 2 mg/kg PO of prednisolone every 24 hours.[22] Prednisolone-treated cats had a median survival time of more than 800 days,[22] and this drug has also been shown to result in an improvement in histologically documented hepatic inflammation but not in fibrosis.[32] Side effects of glucocorticoids are well described in cats and include polyphagia, polyuria/polydipsia, skin fragility, weight gain, and diabetes mellitus. In cats that fail to respond completely (or that have unacceptable glucocorticoid side effects), the addition of chlorambucil (2 mg/cat PO every 48–72 hours; several other protocols have also been described) may be needed, and the possibility of misdiagnosed or emergent small-cell lymphoma should be considered. As chlorambucil can cause myelosuppression, it is important to check complete blood counts during therapy.

Ursodeoxycholic acid may also be beneficial in cats with lymphocytic cholangitis and is a recognised treatment in humans with primary sclerosing cholangitis. This drug did not appear to be as effective as prednisolone for treating lymphocytic cholangitis in cats (median survival time <400 days vs. >800 days for prednisolone-treated cats).[22] However, it is not known whether or not the addition of this drug to prednisolone-treated cats is advantageous.

As repeat liver biopsy is seldom performed, response to treatment is assessed using clinical signs and improvement of biochemical parameters (liver enzymes activities and bilirubin concentration).

Fluke-associated cholangitis

Liver fluke infections can be successfully treated with praziquantel (10–25 mg/kg PO/SC for 3–5 days) (see Appendix).[16,17] Note that the dosage for this purpose is higher than for treating tapeworm infections. Praziquantel may cause injection-site reactions when given subcutaneously or GI side effects when given orally. It is important to identify and address concurrent bacterial cholangitis as described above for neutrophilic cholangitis.

Triaditis

The treatments of IBD and pancreatitis are discussed in detail in Chapters 18 and 24, respectively, and the treatment of cholangitis is described above.

Briefly, in addition to the supportive care described above, the treatment of IBD consists of immunomodulatory drugs and dietary intervention. In cats with chronic enteropathies a diet trial with a novel protein or hydrolysed antigen diet is usually performed at some point in the diagnostic process to rule out food-responsive enteropathy. Up to 50% of cats with mild chronic enteropathy respond to dietary intervention. The mainstay of treatment for feline IBD is prednisolone, which is normally started at a dose of 1–2 mg/kg PO every 24 hours and then gradually tapered (usually a 25% decrease every 2–3 weeks) to the lowest effective dose. Occasionally, chlorambucil is used as adjunctive treatment to allow the lowest effective dose of prednisolone to be decreased. Cats with serum cobalamin concentrations less than 400 ng/l should be supplemented as described above.

The treatment of acute pancreatitis is symptomatic in nature. As previously discussed, fluid therapy, analgesic drugs, and antiemetic drugs are often indicated. Antimicrobials are not routinely recommended for treating feline pancreatitis; however, they are indicated if the cat has concurrent documented or suspected neutrophilic cholangitis (see below), another source of bacterial infection is discovered, or there is a high suspicion of bacterial infection. Likewise, glucocorticoids and other immunomodulatory drugs are not currently recommended for cats with pancreatitis, especially acute pancreatitis. However, they are indicated in cats with concurrent IBD or lymphocytic cholangitis. Furthermore, in the author's experience, some cats with chronic pancreatitis appear to respond positively to treatment with corticosteroids or other immunomodulatory agents. Nevertheless, more information is needed before their use can be definitively recommended.

Treating cats with combinations of these conditions or triaditis can be challenging, but the principles of treating the individual components remain the same. In some cases, inflammation of all three organs may not have been histologically determined, and the diagnosis should be considered tentative based on clinical signs, laboratory testing, and diagnostic imaging. This can create uncertainty when making a therapeutic plan. It is essential to consider the patient's presenting clinical signs and the relative severity of the individual components, as often one of the three organ systems is more severely affected than the others and should be prioritised. Sometimes, histologically documented inflammation of one or more of these organs may be of questionable importance and may not require specific treatment. For example, in a cat with IBD that has an increased serum Spec fPL concentration and/or ultrasound changes consistent with chronic pancreatitis but no vomiting, hyporexia, or abdominal pain, treatment of IBD should be prioritised. One key principle is that treatments that could adversely affect another component or possible component of the cat's disease should be avoided or used with care. For example, in a cat with clinical histologically confirmed IBD that also has suspected but not histologically confirmed cholangitis, empiric antimicrobial therapy is often initiated before starting corticosteroids in case neutrophilic cholangitis with an active bacterial infection is present. In a cat with cholangitis, IBD, or pancreatitis that is not responding as expected to the treatment, the possibilities of concurrent inflammation in another organ, small-cell lymphoma, or exocrine pancreatic insufficiency should be considered.

PROGNOSIS AND OUTCOME

Neutrophilic cholangitis

The prognosis of cats with neutrophilic cholangitis is variable. This disease can be cured by appropriate antimicrobial treatment, but some critically ill cats may not survive initial hospitalisation and others develop chronic or recurrent disease. In one retrospective study of cats with neutrophilic cholangitis, 8/15 cats survived for more than 1 year. Of the cats that did not survive 1 year after diagnosis, 5/7 had a serious concurrent illness, such as chronic renal failure, diabetes mellitus, lymphoma, feline infectious peritonitis, or IBD that probably contributed to their death.[2] In another study of six cats with cholecystitis and neutrophilic cholangitis, one cat was euthanised within 3 weeks of diagnosis, one died of a motor vehicle trauma, one died of chronic kidney disease, and the other three survived for more than 1 year.[7]

Lymphocytic cholangitis

Although it is less common for cats with lymphocytic cholangitis to present in a critically ill condition compared to those with neutrophilic cholangitis, these cats may require long-term treatment. In a retrospective study, 16/25 cats with lymphocytic cholangitis survived for at least 1 year after diagnosis. Of the 7 cats that survived less than 1 year, all had a serious concurrent illness, such as peritonitis, IBD, systemic amyloidosis, or pneumonia, that likely contributed to their death.[2] In another retrospective study, the median survival time of cats treated with prednisolone was more than 800 days.[22]

Fluke-associated cholangitis

Many cases of fluke-associated cholangitis are asymptomatic or mildly symptomatic and respond readily to treatment with praziquantel. Cats with heavy fluke burdens or those with concurrent illness such as bacterial cholangitis might not respond as well and can even die, as can those with concurrent cholangiocarcinoma.

Triaditis

Although the prognosis has been described and some prognostic factors have been identified for pancreatitis, IBD, and cholangitis in cats, the outcome of cats with triaditis has not been well described in the literature. As triaditis is a complex and highly variable syndrome, the outcome of affected cats is also likely to be highly variable. Some cats are relatively mildly affected and respond well to treatment (e.g. a cat with IBD and suspected pancreatitis based on an increased feline-specific pancreatic lipase concentration). Other patients present in a critical condition and may or may not survive initial hospitalisation (e.g. a cat with acute suppurative pancreatitis and neutrophilic cholangitis). There is some evidence that cats with more than one of the constituent conditions have a worse prognosis. For example, cats with cholangitis and concurrent conditions (including IBD and pancreatitis) had a lower survival rate than those without,[2] and cats with triaditis had more severe histological inflammation than those with inflammation in only one or two organs.[20]

Take-home messages

- Combinations of inflammatory liver disease, inflammatory bowel disease, and pancreatitis are common in cats. Patients may present with disease of one organ predominating their clinical picture and histologically confirmed inflammation of other organs that may or may not be clinically important.
- Cytological evaluation of bile and liver aspirates is helpful for the diagnosis of feline cholangitis, but it is important to be aware of its diagnostic limitations.
- Cats with cholangitis or triaditis may be critically ill. Therefore, providing supportive care and nutritional support is essential to optimise the outcome.
- It is important to prioritise medications that treat the underlying disease and essential supportive care over cytoprotective agents, such as antioxidants and ursodeoxycholic acid.
- Treatments that could adversely affect another component or possible component of the cat's disease should be avoided or used with care. For example, in a cat with histologically confirmed inflammatory bowel disease that has concurrent neutrophilic cholangitis, empiric antimicrobial therapy is often initiated before starting corticosteroids.

REFERENCES

[1] van den Ingh TSGAM et al. Morphological classification of biliary disorders of the canine and feline liver. In: Rothuizen J et al., editors. *WSAVA Standards for Clinical and Histological Diagnosis of Canine and Feline Liver Diseases*. Edinburgh, W.B. Saunders: 61, 2006.

[2] Gagne JM et al. Clinical features of inflammatory liver disease in cats: 41 cases (1983–1993). *J Am Vet Med Assoc* 214:513, 1999.

[3] Bayton WA et al. Histopathological frequency of feline hepatobiliary disease in the UK. *J Small Anim Pract* 59:404, 2018.

[4] Fluen T et al. Retrospective study of the relative frequency of feline hepatobiliary disease in New Zealand based on 10 years of hepatic biopsy samples. *Vet Rec Open* 6:e000367, 2019.

[5] Hirose N et al. A retrospective histopathological survey on canine and feline liver diseases at the University of Tokyo between 2006 and 2012. *J Vet Med Sci* 76:1015, 2014.

[6] Gagne JM, Weiss DJ, Armstrong PJ. Histopathologic evaluation of feline inflammatory liver disease. *Vet Pathol* 33:521, 1996.

[7] Brain PH et al. Feline cholecystitis and acute neutrophilic cholangitis: clinical findings, bacterial isolates and response to treatment in six cases. *J Feline Med Surg* 8:91, 2006.

[8] Peters LM et al. Cytological findings of 140 bile samples from dogs and cats and associated clinical pathological data. *J Vet Intern Med* 30:123, 2016.

[9] Byfield VL et al. Percutaneous cholecystocentesis in cats with suspected hepatobiliary disease. *J Feline Med Surg* 19:1254, 2017.

[10] Schiborra F, McConnell JF, Maddox TW. Percutaneous ultrasound-guided cholecystocentesis: complications and association of ultrasonographic findings with bile culture results. *J Small Anim Pract* 58:389, 2017.

[11] Policelli Smith R et al. Association between gallbladder ultrasound findings and bacterial culture of bile in 70 cats and 202 dogs. *J Vet Intern Med* 31:1451, 2017.

[12] Twedt DC et al. Evaluation of fluorescence in situ hybridization for the detection of bacteria in feline inflammatory liver disease. *J Feline Med Surg* 16:109, 2014.

[13] Warren A et al. Histopathologic features, immunophenotyping, clonality, and eubacterial fluorescence in situ hybridization in cats with lymphocytic cholangitis/cholangiohepatitis. *Vet Pathol* 48:627, 2011.

[14] Otte CM et al. Detection of bacterial DNA in bile of cats with lymphocytic cholangitis. *Vet Microbiol* 156:217, 2012.

[15] Boland L, Beatty J. Feline cholangitis. *Vet Clin North Am Small Anim Pract* 47:703, 2017.

[16] Basu AK, Charles RA. A review of the cat liver fluke *Platynosomum fastosum* Kossack, 1910 (Trematoda: Dicrocoeliidae). *Vet Parasitol* 200:1, 2014.

[17] King S, Scholz T. Trematodes of the family Opisthorchiidae: a minireview. *Korean J Parasitol* 39:209, 2001.

[18] Weiss DJ, Gagne JM, Armstrong PJ. Relationship between inflammatory hepatic disease and inflammatory bowel disease, pancreatitis, and nephritis in cats. *J Am Vet Med Assoc* 209:1114, 1996.

[19] Callahan Clark JE et al. Feline cholangitis: a necropsy study of 44 cats (1986–2008). *J Feline Med Surg* 13:570, 2011.

[20] Fragkou FC et al. Prevalence and clinicopathological features of triaditis in a prospective case series of symptomatic and asymptomatic cats. *J Vet Intern Med* 30:1031, 2016.

[21] Simpson KW. Pancreatitis and triaditis in cats: causes and treatment. *J Small Anim Pract* 56:40, 2015.

[22] Otte CM et al. Retrospective comparison of prednisolone and ursodeoxycholic acid for the treatment of feline lymphocytic cholangitis. *Vet J* 195:205, 2013.

[23] Day MJ. Immunohistochemical characterization of the lesions of feline progressive lymphocytic cholangitis/cholangiohepatitis. *J Comp Pathol* 119:135, 1998.

[24] Lucke VM, Davies JD. Progressive lymphocytic cholangitis in the cat. *J Small Anim Pract* 25:249, 1984.

[25] Lisciandro SC, Hohenhaus A, Brooks M. Coagulation abnormalities in 22 cats with naturally occurring liver disease. *J Vet Intern Med* 12:71, 1998.

[26] Kakar N et al. Thromboelastography in cats with cholestatic liver disease. *J Feline Med Surg* 23:160, 2021.

[27] Marolf AJ et al. Magnetic resonance (MR) imaging and MR cholangiopancreatography findings in cats with cholangitis and pancreatitis. *J Feline Med Surg* 15:285, 2013.

[28] Köster L et al. Percutaneous ultrasound-guided cholecystocentesis and bile analysis for the detection of *Platynosomum* spp.-induced cholangitis in cats. *J Vet Intern Med* 30:787, 2016.

[29] Wang KY et al. Accuracy of ultrasound-guided fine-needle aspiration of the liver and cytologic findings in dogs and cats: 97 cases (1990–2000). *J Am Vet Med Assoc* 224:75, 2004.

[30] Pavlick M, Webster CR, Penninck DG. Bleeding risk and complications associated with percutaneous ultrasound-guided liver biopsy in cats. *J Feline Med Surg* 21:529, 2019.

[31] Benson KK et al. Drug exposure and clinical effect of transdermal mirtazapine in healthy young cats: a pilot study. *J Feline Med Surg* 19:998, 2017.

[32] Otte CM et al. A morphological and immunohistochemical study of the effects of prednisolone or ursodeoxycholic acid on liver histology in feline lymphocytic cholangitis. *J Feline Med Surg* 16:796, 2014.

CHAPTER 31

Extrahepatic bile duct obstruction and diseases of the gallbladder

Karla C. L. Lee

ANATOMY AND PHYSIOLOGY

Bile is synthesised and secreted by hepatocytes and modified by the bile duct epithelium. It contains bile salts, bilirubin, phospholipids, cholesterol, amino acids, steroids, enzymes, porphyrins, vitamins, heavy metals, drug metabolites, xenobiotics, and environmental toxins. Bile is an important excretory pathway for its constituents, which are potentially harmful if allowed to accumulate in the body. Bile also functions to facilitate absorption of fats, steroids, and lipid-soluble vitamins from the intestines, to maintain the immune function of the intestines, and to control the gut microbiota.[1]

Bile is secreted from hepatocytes into 1 μm diameter bile canaliculi, the space between adjacent hepatocytes. Bile passes from these canaliculi into the canals of Hering, which deliver bile to the finest branches of the biliary tree, the bile ducts within portal tracts. Bile ducts within the portal tracts merge to form ducts of increasing diameter as they pass through liver lobules and then between liver lobules, before eventually becoming the hepatic ducts that transport bile from each liver lobe to the common bile duct (CBD). The cystic duct of the gallbladder joins the CBD, proximal to the entry of the hepatic ducts. The gallbladder acts as a reservoir for bile and is partially encased by the right medial and quadrate liver lobes. The area of the liver that is adherent to the gallbladder is known as the hepatic fossa.[1]

The CBD enters the wall of the duodenum along its mesenteric surface and runs intramurally approximately 12 mm before entering the ampulla of Vater. The ampulla of Vater sits within the major duodenal papilla, which is located 2–3 cm distal to the pylorus, and opens into the duodenal lumen. The sphincter of Oddi is the muscle that surrounds the choledochoduodenal junction within the duodenal wall. It controls bile flow into the duodenum and prevents reflux of duodenal contents into the CBD. The pancreatic duct joins the CBD on entering the ampulla of Vater. Some cats also have an accessory pancreatic duct, which enters the duodenum at the minor duodenal papilla, 2 cm distal to the major duodenal papilla.[2]

DIAGNOSTIC INVESTIGATION

Clinical pathology

Blood sampling for clinical pathology tests, as for investigation of hepatic and pancreatic disorders, is indicated including, in particular, serum biochemistry, haematology, and coagulation profile.

Ultrasonography

Ultrasound is currently the most commonly used imaging modality for the extrahepatic biliary system in the cat. However, gas in the overlying intestine, patient discomfort, and operator experience can limit visualisation. The pear-shaped or ovoid-shaped gallbladder, located within the cranioventral abdomen to the right of the midline, is typically filled with an anechoic fluid. A normal variant of the gallbladder is a duplicated or septated gallbladder. The cystic duct can be followed from the gallbladder to the CBD. Alternatively, the CBD can be located immediately ventral to the portal vein. The CBD is an anechoic tubular structure surrounded by hyperechoic fat.

The median diameter of the CBD in healthy cats has been reported to be 2.7 mm (range 2–4 mm). The CBD ends at the duodenal papilla, which can be seen as an approximately 4 mm diameter elevation in the duodenal mucosa.[3]

Ultrasonographic gallbladder abnormalities reported in cats include a distended gallbladder, thickened wall, sludge, wall oedema, choleliths, mucosal hyperplasia, and gallbladder wall mass. Unlike in dogs, biliary mucoceles are rare in cats. These abnormalities are best interpreted in combination with other clinical data, as abnormalities can exist with or without other indications of clinical disease. In one study of 152 cats presenting for abdominal ultrasonographic examination, 14% of cats had gallbladder sludge and these cats had significantly higher serum concentrations of alanine aminotransferase (ALT), alkaline phosphatase (ALP), and total bilirubin compared to cats without gallbladder sludge.[4] In cats with a clinical indication for cholecystocentesis, positive bacterial culture has been associated with two or more abnormal gallbladder findings, including thickened wall and gallbladder sludge.[5] In cats with histopathological confirmed cholangitis, the gallbladder is more often normal, with a thickened wall and sludge reported in 8% and 38%, respectively, in one study.[6]

Ultrasound is the imaging technique of choice for diagnosis of extrahepatic bile duct obstruction (EHBDO). EHBDO results in dilation of the CBD to a diameter greater than 5 mm in over 97% of cases. Tortuosity of the CBD is also a common feature of severe EHBDO. In addition, dilation of the extrahepatic bile ducts and intrahepatic bile ducts has been reported in 67% and 85% of cases, respectively, but subjective dilation of the gallbladder is seen in less than 50% of cases. Ultrasound can also be used to identify the possible cause of EHBDO. Obstructing choleliths present as hyperechoic intraluminal structures with distal shadowing. In addition, intra- and extraluminal obstructing soft tissue masses, pancreatitis, and local abnormalities of the duodenal wall can be visualised. However, ultrasound cannot distinguish between inflammatory and neoplastic soft tissue masses.[3]

Ultrasound-guided fine needle aspiration (FNA) of liver, bile, pancreas, any free abdominal fluid, and abnormal local soft tissue masses is indicated for cytological examination, bacterial culture, and bile analysis.

Computed tomography and magnetic resonance imaging

The gallbladder is readily identified by computed tomography (CT), primarily due to its anechoic contents, but the CBD is not reliably seen due to its small size and lack of contrast enhancement.[7]

Drip infusion cholangiography with CT has been described in cats to highlight the extrahepatic biliary system and to rule in or out EHBDO. Meglumine iotroxate (105 mg meglumine iotroxate/ml) is the intravenous iodinated contrast agent used for these studies, as it is preferentially excreted via the biliary system. One report in cats describes giving 2 ml/kg meglumine iotroxate intravenously over 30 minutes, followed by CT in dorsal recumbency under general anaesthesia 1 hour after onset of infusion. Contrast was seen to highlight the gallbladder, cystic duct, hepatic duct, CBD, and duodenum, with an attenuation of 271 ± 37 HU, confirming a patent biliary system in three healthy cats. In two cats with obstructive cholelithiasis, contrast opacification of the extrahepatic biliary system was not seen and cholelith attenuation was noted to be 933 ± 119 HU. No complications were reported, but further validation of this technique in a greater number of cats is needed.[8]

Magnetic resonance imaging (MRI) cholangiography has been reported in cats. It permits visualisation of the fluid within the extrahepatic biliary system. Both CT and MRI can be used to identify choleliths, but further studies are required to determine the usefulness of CT and MRI over ultrasound.[7]

Cytology

Ultrasound-guided FNA of liver, bile, pancreas, any free abdominal fluid, and abnormal local soft tissue masses is indicated for cytological examination, bacterial culture, and bile analysis. A coagulation profile should be performed prior to sampling. Bleeding risk in cats presenting for ultrasound-guided liver biopsy has been reported to be greater if platelet counts are less than 80 000/μl or if activated partial thromboplastin time (aPTT) is greater than 1.5 times normal.[9]

Bile sampling

Ultrasound-guided percutaneous cholecystocentesis is indicated for cytology and bacterial culture of the bile. It has been recommended to use a 22-gauge, 3.81 cm (1.5 inch) needle attached to a 12 ml syringe. The needle is inserted into the cranial, right ventral abdomen. A transhepatic approach has been described to limit bile leak, but this may be associated with blood contamination of the sample and hepatic bleeding. Emptying the gallbladder during sampling is recommended, again to limit bile leak after the procedure. This procedure has been associated with a 2%–4% fall in packed cell volume and a 4000/µl increase in circulating neutrophils in healthy cats. The median total volume of bile obtained by cholecystocentesis from healthy cats is 0.9–3 ml. Healthy feline bile is acellular, containing an amorphous granular grey-green material and no bacteria.[10]

EXTRAHEPATIC BILE DUCT OBSTRUCTION

The aetiology of EHBDO in cats is commonly subdivided into neoplastic and inflammatory. Neoplasia has been reported in 32%–41% of cats presenting for surgical management of EHBDO. Inflammation has been reported in 59%–68% of cats presenting for surgical management of EHBDO and may include cholangiohepatitis, pancreatitis, cholecystitis, and/or cholelithiasis. In addition, EHBDO may be associated with bacterial infection: approximately 25% of cats in one case series of EHBDO were found to have positive bacterial cultures. Other reported primary causes of bile duct obstruction include biliary parasites, diaphragmatic rupture, grass awns within the CBD, duodenal foreign bodies, and pyloroduodenal adenomatous polyps.[11–16]

EHBDO leads to cholestasis, dilation of bile ducts proximal to the obstruction, and leak of bile into the portal areas of the liver parenchyma. Acutely, this results in portal oedema, neutrophilic inflammation, and a biliary reaction that is both degenerative and proliferative. Chronically this leads to portal fibrosis, bile duct proliferation, and a periductal inflammatory response characterised by pigment-laden macrophages, lymphocytes, plasma cells, and neutrophils.[17]

No breed predisposition has been clearly identified, with EHBDO commonly occurring in domestic longhair and shorthair cats. However, oriental breeds including the Siamese commonly appear to be overrepresented in reports of EHBDO. Cats of any age can be affected, but a median age of 8–10 years is reported.[11,12]

Clinical signs that occur almost consistently in EHBDO are icterus, anorexia, lethargy, weight loss, and intermittent vomiting. In addition, pyrexia, bleeding tendencies, acholic faeces, dehydration, hepatomegaly, and abdominal pain are seen. In experimental cats, icterus occurs 5.3 ± 0.4 days after complete ligation and transection of the CBD. In client-owned cats, the median time from onset of clinical signs to presentation for surgical intervention is 20–24 days.[11,12,18]

Common biochemical findings include marked elevations in aspartate aminotransferase (AST), ALT, ALP, cholesterol, and bilirubin. With complete acute EHBDO, these changes are seen within 7 days, peak at around 3 weeks, and decline thereafter. Other biochemical findings include hypoalbuminaemia and azotaemia. Haematologically, acute EHBDO is associated with progressive neutrophilia and regenerative anaemia. Abnormal clotting times, specifically prothrombin time (PT) and/or aPTT, have been reported in 46% of cats with EHBDO. Ultrasound is the most commonly used diagnostic tool for confirmation of a clinical suspicion of EHBDO.[11,12,18]

First-line therapy for EHBDO should be medical management of underlying disease, when possible, and is covered in other chapters in Section III. Surgical intervention for EHBDO is indicated when the cat is unresponsive to medical management of the underlying disease. The aims of surgery are:

- **Confirmation of the diagnosis of EHBDO,** by catheterisation of the CBD either via the duodenal papilla following duodenotomy or via the gallbladder following cholecystotomy.
- **Diagnosis of the cause of EHBDO,** by biopsy of any obstructing masses, pancreas, duodenum, and liver and sampling of bile.
- **Reestablishment of patency of the biliary system.** This may require removal of obstructing choleliths by retrograde flushing into the gallbladder, choledochotomy, or sphincterotomy. Alternatively, permanent biliary

diversion by cholecystoenterostomy or temporary biliary diversion by stenting of the CBD may be indicated.

- **Placement of a feeding tube as appropriate.** Many cats have anorexia, hyporexia, and/or vomiting both before and after surgery, making provision for feeding postoperatively a priority. Gastrostomy and jejunostomy tubes are preferred. These tubes may be more appropriate than nasooesophagostomy or oesophagostomy tubes in the presence of vomiting.

Prognosis for cats requiring surgery for EHBDO is poor. In one report by Mayhew et al. in 2002, cats with neoplasia as a primary cause died or were euthanised within 72 hours of presentation to a referral hospital.[11] In another study by Buote et al. in 2006, the median survival time of cats with neoplasia was 2 weeks.[12] In Mayhew et al.'s study, amongst cats with nonneoplastic disease, 40% died within 1 week of surgery and only 5% survived over 2 years without clinical signs.[11] In Buote et al.'s study, the median survival time of cats with nonneoplastic disease was 255 days, with less than 50% surviving more than 6 months.[12] For further discussion, see section "General complications of biliary surgery" in this chapter.

Cholelithiasis

Cholelithiasis is infrequently reported in cats, with veterinary reports including predominantly cats with cholelithiasis plus EHBDO (Fig. 31.1). Cats can present with multiple or single choleliths of varying sizes, with reports up to 12 mm. Choleliths can be located in the CBD, cystic duct, or gallbladder. Case presentation and diagnosis are as described for EHBDO.[19–21]

Feline cholelith composition includes 100% calcium carbonate, 100% bilirubin, and choleliths of a mixed composition, including—in addition to the aforementioned bile components—cholesterol, calcium bilirubinate, and unspecified bile pigments. This variation in composition likely reflects a varying pathogenesis.[19–21]

Choleliths composed entirely of bilirubin form in the presence of excess unconjugated bilirubin. They occur predominantly in the bile ducts, rather than in the cystic duct or gallbladder. Cats with 100% bilirubin choleliths tend to present with EHBDO at a young age, typically around 2 years of age. 100% bilirubin stones have been reported in Somali cats with haemolytic anaemia secondary to pyruvate kinase deficiency. EHBDO secondary to bilirubin cholelithiasis is therefore an important differential diagnosis for icteric cats with haemolytic anaemia. Excess unconjugated bilirubin can also result from ileal dysfunction or resection. The ileum normally absorbs 90% of bile salts. If these bile salts pass into the colon, they are solubilised into unconjugated bilirubin and reabsorbed into the enterohepatic circulation.[19–21]

Choleliths composed entirely of calcium carbonate are believed to form in the gallbladder as a result of chronic intermittent cystic duct obstruction, which stimulates gallbladder mucin secretion and thereby an increase in acid buffering capacity and calcium carbonate precipitation. This hypothesis is supported by case reports of cats with cholelithiasis that have a duplex gallbladder, in which one gallbladder either has a nonpatent cystic duct or contains a mucocele.[21] Cats with 100% calcium carbonate choleliths are more often middle-aged to older cats.

Choleliths of a mixed composition are associated with bacterial infection in human medicine.[22] Bacterial beta-glucuronidase results in hydrolysis of glucuronic acid from bilirubin, leading to a reduction in solubility of deconjugated bilirubin and the formation of choleliths composed of calcium salts of unconjugated bilirubin, deconjugated bile salts, and cholesterol. The finding of positive bacterial cultures in five out of nine cats in one case series of obstructive cholelithiasis supports a role for bacterial infection in feline cholelithiasis. Cats with

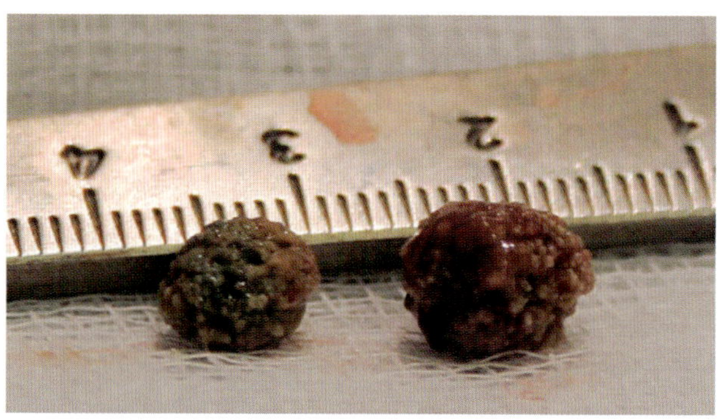

Figure 31.1. Mixed-composition choleliths found in the common bile duct and gallbladder of a cat with marked necrosuppurative cholangiohepatitis and cholecystitis, associated with bacterial infection. Analysis revealed 85% calcium carbonate and 15% mixed bile pigments.

mixed-composition choleliths are more often middle-aged to older cats (5–18 years).[20]

Choleliths consisting primarily of cholesterol crystals are the most common type of gallbladder stone in humans and result from a combination of excess secretion of cholesterol into the bile, gallbladder hypomotility, and a relative reduction in bile salt and phospholipid secretion into the bile.[22] These are rarely reported in cats.[20]

Surgical treatment for EHBDO secondary to cholelithiasis is indicated as for other causes of EHBDO. Choleliths are retrieved through the duodenal papilla following sphincterotomy, by choledochotomy, or by cholecystectomy and retrograde saline flushing. Choledochotomy has not been associated with obstructive stricture in cats unlike in humans. Cholecystectomy is indicated as a prophylactic measure, especially in the presence of a chronically diseased gallbladder, to reduce recurrence of, in particular, calcium carbonate choleliths.[11,19,20,23]

Whilst the prognosis for cats requiring surgical management of EHBDO is generally poor, the long-term prognosis for cats with EHBDO secondary to cholelithiasis that survive the immediate postoperative period can be good. In a study of seven cats with obstructive cholelithiasis that survived the immediate postoperative period, the median survival time was 24 months (range 13–27 months).[20]

Neoplasia

Hepatobiliary neoplasia represents 1.5%–2.3% of feline neoplasms. Of these, neoplasms arising from the biliary tract predominate in most studies (excluding lymphoma). Reported feline biliary neoplasms include bile duct carcinomas, bile duct adenomas, biliary cystadenomas, and biliary neuroendocrine tumours. They can be intrahepatic or extrahepatic. Intrahepatic biliary neoplasms can present as solitary mass lesions (massive), multiple mass lesions (nodular), multiple coalescing nodules (diffuse), or diffuse parenchymal change (diffuse). Extrahepatic biliary neoplasms can present as strictures of the bile ducts or mass lesions within the bile ducts, cystic duct, or gallbladder. Neoplasia of the ampulla of Vater has also been described in cats in single case reports, as has lymphoma of the gallbladder.[12,24–27]

Veterinary reports of biliary tumours in cats are sparse, making it difficult to accurately describe the clinical presentation of each specific tumour type distinct from the other. Cats with intrahepatic biliary tumours may present simply with abdominal enlargement or a range of nonspecific clinical signs including lethargy, anorexia, vomiting, and weight loss. Complete surgical resection of massive tumours can be associated with a cure for benign lesions. There is no reported effective treatment for nodular or diffuse disease. Cats with extrahepatic biliary tumours commonly present with clinical signs as for EHBDO. Surgical resection, if possible, is the treatment of choice. However, prognosis is extremely poor. Median survival times of 2 weeks after diagnosis have been reported, with the majority of cats not surviving to discharge from the hospital.[12,24–27]

Bile duct adenocarcinomas are the most commonly reported hepatobiliary tumours in cats (Fig. 31.2). Parasites may play a role in pathogenesis. They are highly malignant, with carcinomatosis or diffuse peritoneal metastasis being present in 67%–80% of cases at the time of diagnosis. Histopathological analysis suggests the potential for malignant transformation of bile duct adenomas, with 13% of bile duct adenomas demonstrating anaplastic or precancerous stages and 58% of bile duct adenocarcinomas demonstrating residual benign components.[24,28]

Biliary neuroendocrine tumours arise from neuroectodermal cells. In a case series of 17 cats with hepatobiliary neuroendocrine tumours, 9 cats had tumours arising from the extrahepatic biliary system. They had a mean age of 9 years (range 3–17 years). The tumours appeared as a stricture or mass lesion affecting the bile ducts, cystic duct, or gallbladder, and the clinical presentation was the same as for EHBDO. Two out of nine cats lived at least 1 year, the remainder were euthanised or died soon after surgery. Metastasis to lymph nodes, lungs, and intestines was seen at necropsy and emphasises the poor prognosis associated with neuroendocrine tumours.[27]

Biliary cystadenomas are benign neoplasms of the intrahepatic biliary epithelium and are composed of multilocular thin-walled cysts lined with normal biliary epithelium. The cystic fluid is clear and watery to slightly viscous. These neoplasms replace and compress the normal parenchyma, and examination of the adjacent liver may reveal bile duct hyperplasia, cholangiohepatitis, hepatic lipidosis, periportal fibrosis, and/or nodular

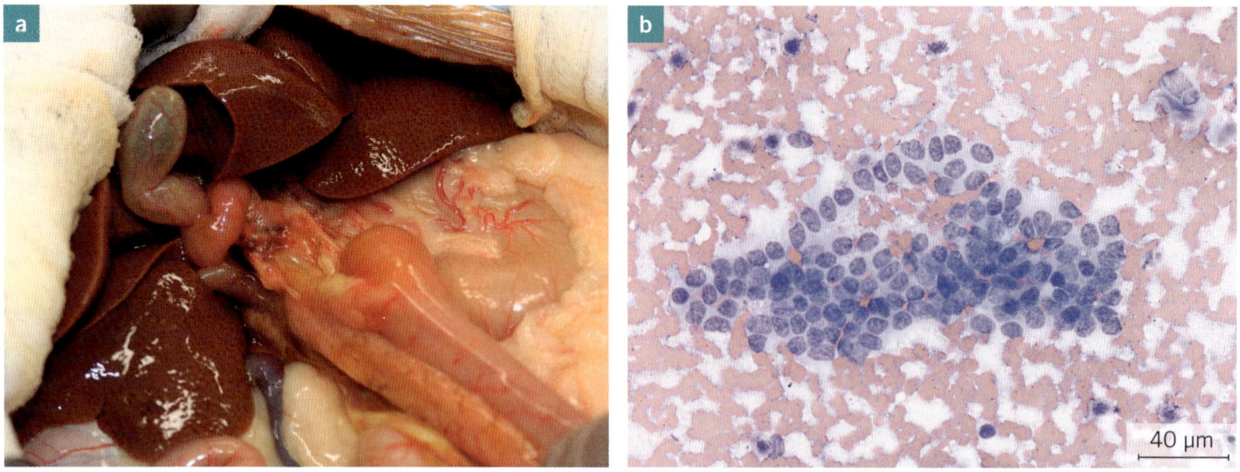

Figure 31.2. Intraoperative image of a cat with biliary carcinoma of the extrahepatic biliary tree (a). The main site of the neoplasm is central in the photo and is associated with haemorrhage from previous fine needle aspirations. The neoplasm could be palpated within the hepatic duct seen adjacent to the gallbladder: the infiltrated hepatic duct is creamy pink in colour compared to the more translucent wall of the gallbladder, through which green bile can be appreciated. Cytological examination of a biliary carcinoma (b). The neoplastic cells are arranged in cohesive clusters. They are cuboidal with a round to oval nucleus, smooth to finely stippled chromatin, an inapparent nucleolus, and a small amount of pale blue/grey cytoplasm. Image courtesy of Emma J. Holmes.

hyperplasia. They are seen predominantly in older cats, with reported mean ages of 13–14 years. They present as solitary focal lesions or multifocal lesions. They are most often associated with no clinical signs apart from abdominal enlargement. However, icterus related to hepatocellular disease or obstructive cholelithiasis has been reported. Ultrasonographic appearance is varied and includes multilocular thin-walled cysts, hyperechoic masses with cystic components, and mixed-echogenicity masses with cystic components. Surgical resection is recommended to avoid complications associated with the physical presence of a large abdominal mass and the possibility of neoplastic transformation. Prognosis is good following complete surgical resection.[26]

Pancreatitis and extrahepatic bile duct obstruction

There are few reports of EHBDO secondary to acute pancreatitis in cats. In one study, 5 out of 203 (2.5%) cats diagnosed with acute pancreatitis presented with severe EHBDO that warranted targeted intervention. No age, breed, or sex predispositions have been reported. Diagnosis of EHBDO secondary to pancreatitis is based on the abdominal ultrasonographic findings of gallbladder distension, bile duct dilation, and/or bile duct tortuosity. In addition, a mass-like lesion or thickening at the major duodenal papilla may be a frequent specific indicator of EHBDO secondary to pancreatitis. Subjective pancreatic duct distension, up to 5 mm in diameter, may also be a specific indicator of EHBDO secondary to pancreatitis, but it is not a consistent finding.[29,30]

The decision to pursue targeted therapy for EHBDO in cats with pancreatitis, in combination with therapy for pancreatitis, is based on worsening serial ultrasonographic findings, pancreas cytology consistent with necrosuppurative septic inflammation or necrosis, lack of clinical improvement, or worsening clinical signs. Cats meeting these criteria most often have elevations in liver enzymes and bilirubin. They may also demonstrate hypercholesterolaemia, hypoalbuminaemia, and azotaemia.[29,30]

Relief of EHBDO secondary to pancreatitis may require bile duct flushing alone or in combination with cholecystoenterostomy or choledochal stenting. A feeding tube should be considered in all of these cases; gastrostomy and gastrojejunostomy tubes are preferred. There is insufficient data to recommend one biliary intervention over the other. In one report of seven cats undergoing choledochal stenting, five cats survived beyond the immediate postoperative period and were either alive at the end of the study period, 14–15 months postoperatively, or had died of unrelated causes 7–24 months postoperatively.[29] For the five survivors, the stent passed in the faeces 3–4 months postoperatively in two cats, was removed endoscopically 6 months postoperatively in one cat, and one cat was lost to follow-up. The fifth survivor had recurrent EHBDO, and the stent was removed at a second surgery, in which cholecystoenterostomy was performed. In another report of three cats undergoing cholecystoenterostomy for relief of pancreatitis associated with EHBDO, two survived the immediate postoperative period and were alive at 5 months and 5.3 years postoperatively.[30]

Choledochal cysts

Choledochal cysts are congenital cystic dilations of the biliary tract not associated with EHBDO. They therefore represent an important but rare differential diagnosis for EHBDO. In humans, they have been associated with an anomalous pancreaticobiliary duct union, whereby this union occurs outside the duodenal wall. It has been hypothesised that this anomaly results in reflux of pancreatic enzymes into the biliary tree and subsequent cyst formation. Choledochal cysts can present as a fusiform dilation of the CBD (type I), a diverticulum of the CBD (type II), dilation of the intraduodenal component of the CBD (type III), and multiple extrahepatic (type IV) or intrahepatic (type V) dilations. Biliary stasis within the choledochal cysts may predispose to cholangitis, cholecystitis, and cholelithiasis, which may exacerbate preexisting pancreatitis. Resection is the recommended treatment in humans.[31]

Type I and type IV choledochal cysts have been reported in case reports of six cats with a median age of 8.5 years (range 5–11 years). Cats typically present with weight loss, hyporexia, lethargy, and vomiting. In addition, abdominal enlargement, diarrhoea, and inappropriate urination have been reported. Biochemistry may be normal in some cats, but in others varying degrees of liver enzyme and bilirubin elevations are seen. Mild normocytic, normochromic anaemia and neutrophilia are noted in at least 50% of case reports. Diagnosis is based on ultrasound. Biliary tract dilations range in size up to 52 mm in diameter and contain sludge or sediment. In addition, hepatomegaly may be seen. Mild chronic active cholangitis is a common histopathological feature, and positive bacterial cultures are also seen. Reported treatments and outcomes vary. Medical treatment for cholangitis with one or more of antibiotics, antacids, antiemetics, ursodeoxycholic acid, and S-adenosylmethionine for a period of 3–4 weeks has been reported in two cats: one made a full recovery and the other was euthanised after 1 month. Surgical treatment with choledochoduodenostomy or cholecystojejunostomy has been reported in two cats: one was normal postoperatively, whilst the other had recurrent cholangitis for 3 years.[31]

Liver fluke/hepatic trematode infection

Cats are the final host of the liver fluke *Platynosomum* spp. These hepatic trematodes are present in tropical and subtropical regions, where the intermediate hosts—terrestrial snails, terrestrial isopods, and lizards—reside. In cats, liver fluke infection is commonly known as "lizard poisoning", as lizards are the obligatory third intermediate host. In cats, the liver fluke lives in the bile ducts and gallbladder. Trematode infection may be asymptomatic, but severe infection can lead to EHBDO and the associated clinical, biochemical, haematologic, and ultrasonographic changes. Diagnosis of liver fluke is normally made by faecal analysis, but in severe cases the liver flukes are easily seen in bile samples. Praziquantel is an effective treatment, but surgery is indicated for severe infection associated with EHBDO. Surgical management to flush out the liver flukes from the biliary tract and to achieve biliary patency or diversion resulted in 100% mortality in one report of three cats.[13]

Traumatic injury to the extrahepatic biliary tract, bile peritonitis, and bilothorax

Traumatic injury to the extrahepatic biliary tract has been reported in single case reports in cats. Trauma due to gunshots are most common, but penetrating trauma of unknown cause and iatrogenic injury during placement of a thoracostomy tube have also been reported. Reported biliary tract injuries include perforation of the gallbladder and cystic duct, avulsion of the CBD from the duodenum, and stricture of the CBD. Concurrent injury to the diaphragm has been reported to result in adhesion of the biliary tract to the diaphragm and subsequent fistula formation and bilothorax. Wounds which result in bile leak tend to present 2–6 days after trauma, whilst those that result in CBD stricture present 7 days after trauma.[32–34]

Clinical signs of biliary tract trauma include vomiting, anorexia, and abdominal effusion in cats with bile peritonitis, and dyspnoea, depression, lethargy, pyrexia, dehydration, anorexia, icterus, and pleural effusion in cats with bilothorax. Diagnosis is based on bilirubin concentrations of body cavity effusions of more than twice serum concentrations. However, body fluid bilirubin concentrations up to 28 times normal have been reported. Cytological examination may reveal bacteria in the absence of positive bacterial cultures; this may be due to concurrent antibiotic treatment. Cats with traumatic stricture of the CBD may present with icterus, as well as other signs of trauma and sepsis including abdominal discomfort, abdominal wall bruising, abdominal effusion, and external wounds.[32–34]

Treatment aims to repair biliary tract rupture or stricture, to flush bilirubin and any associated bacteria out of the pleural/abdominal cavity, and to provide appropriate antibiotic therapy for bacterial infection when present. Successful primary repair of the gallbladder and cystic duct have been reported. Primary repair of CBD avulsion may not be possible, requiring choledochal jejunostomy or cholecystoenterostomy. Choledochal jejunostomy has been reported in one cat, with fatal outcome due to dehiscence of enterotomy wound and septic peritonitis. Stricture should be treated with appropriate biliary diversion if possible.[32–34]

SURGERY

Catheterisation of the common bile duct

Catheterisation of the CBD is indicated to check its patency (Fig. 31.3).[29,35] Gentle pressure on the gallbladder will result in expulsion of bile into the duodenum in a cat with a patent biliary tree. If this is unsuccessful, catheterisation can be performed via an incision in the antimesenteric surface of the proximal duodenum or via an incision made in the gallbladder. A small fine catheter, such as a 3–5 Fr silicone urinary cat catheter or latex red rubber catheter, can be used. Lubrication with an aqueous gel is advised. If the catheter does not pass easily, it may be possible to pass a lubricated stiff monofilament suture, which can be used like a guide wire to pass the catheter into the CBD. The CBD should be flushed through with sterile 0.9% saline solution in cases of EHBDO.

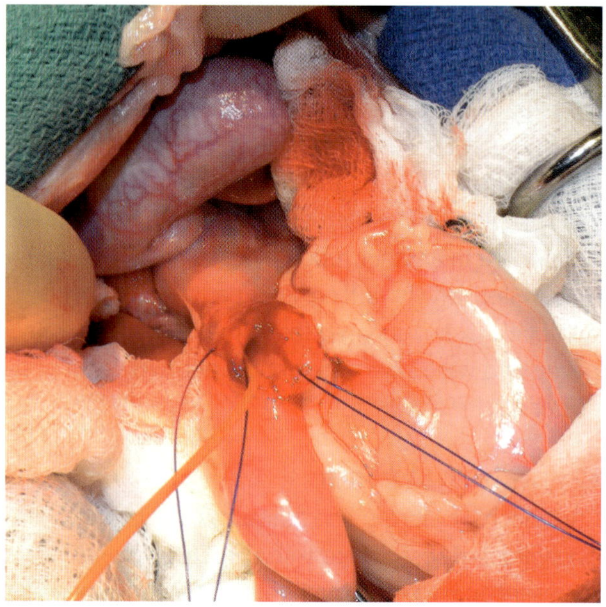

Figure 31.3. Intraoperative image of an antimesenteric duodenotomy and catheterisation of the common bile duct with a 3.5 Fr latex red rubber catheter in a cat with extrahepatic bile duct obstruction secondary to acute neutrophilic cholangiohepatitis. Note the distension of the gallbladder, cystic duct, common bile duct, and hepatic ducts.

Sphincterotomy of the sphincter of Oddi

Sphincterotomy is the creation of a 2–3 mm longitudinal incision in the ampulla of Vater.[2,36] This incision is made from within the duodenum and therefore requires an initial antimesenteric duodenotomy. Sphincterotomy begins at the natural opening of the ampulla and extends cranially along the normal pathway of the CBD in the duodenum. The effect is to increase the size of the choledochoduodenal junction, to decrease the pressure gradient between the CBD and the duodenum, and therefore to reduce resistance to bile flow. Sphincterotomy is indicated to permit catheterisation or stenting of the CBD, to remove choleliths within the distal CBD, and to relieve inflammatory or neoplastic stenosis of the ampulla. Bleeding is the major complication of this procedure; therefore, use of electrocautery using coagulation/blended (rather than cutting) settings is recommended. In an experimental setting, this procedure resulted in positive bile cultures in five out of six cats within 6 weeks but no evidence of active cholangiohepatitis.[36] In a clinical setting, sphincterotomy has been described in six cats with obstructive lesions of the choledochoduodenal junction: two had bile plugs, two cholelithiasis, one inflammatory bowel disease, and one bile duct carcinoma. Sphincterotomy successfully achieved intraoperative relief from obstruction in five cats, but was unsuccessful in the cat with bile duct carcinoma.[2]

Choledochal stenting

Choledochal stenting[29,36,37] is indicated for temporary management of EHBDO when it is hoped that the primary cause for EHBDO will respond to medical management or pending biopsy results and a definitive long-term plan.

Custom-made stents have been reported in cats. These are made from 3.5 or 5 Fr latex red rubber catheters, cut to an appropriate length. A 22-gauge IV catheter has also been reported in a single cat. Stent length within the CBD and duodenum should be the shortest possible. In humans, polyethylene stents with side flaps to prevent migration are most commonly used. In humans, entry of stents into the cystic duct is associated with increased morbidity, and a long stent section in the duodenum may increase the risk of duodenal ulceration and perforation. Recommended lengths in humans are 10–20 mm beyond the biliary obstruction and 10 mm within the duodenum.

An antimesenteric longitudinal duodenotomy is made to expose the major duodenal papilla extending approximately 2 cm aboral to the major duodenal papilla. The CBD should be catheterised and the CBD and gallbladder flushed thoroughly with sterile 0.9% saline solution. The stent should be passed through the major duodenal papilla into the CBD just beyond the site of obstruction, and a short section should extend aborally into the duodenum. The stent should be secured to the internal duodenal wall with two circumferential sutures placed partial thickness through the duodenal wall to include the submucosa. Monofilament absorbable sutures would be advised (e.g. polydioxanone, poliglecaprone). Ultrasound can be used to monitor the presence of the stent in the CBD (Fig. 31.4).

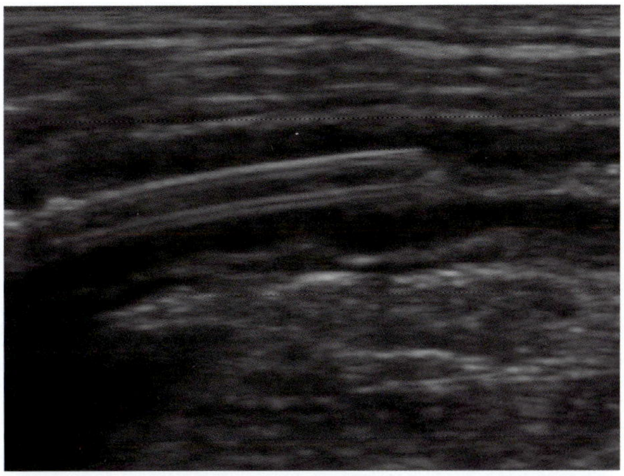

Figure 31.4. Ultrasonographic image of a 3.5 Fr latex red rubber choledochal stent in the common bile duct of a cat with extrahepatic bile duct obstruction secondary to acute bacterial cholangiohepatitis.

The effectiveness of choledochal stenting in cats for relief of EHBDO and the clinical implications of the risk of ascending infection have not been clearly determined. In an experimental study of six healthy cats undergoing choledochal stenting with a polyethylene tube, a bacterial biofilm on the stent and positive bile cultures were evident by 2 weeks. In addition, four out of six cats developed bile duct dilation, and complete stent occlusion was evident by 6 weeks.[36] Due to the risk of ascending infection, thorough flushing of the extrahepatic biliary system prior to stent placement should be performed. In addition, there may be a rationale for prophylactic as well as ongoing antibiotics. Moreover, stent removal should be a planned procedure if the stent does not pass naturally in the faeces.

Cholecystotomy

Cholecystotomy[35] is indicated for antegrade catheterisation of the CBD and retrieval of choleliths from a gallbladder with a healthy wall. The gallbladder may be handled with stay sutures: fine loops of suture passed through the gallbladder wall. Repair of the cholecystotomy can be achieved with a fine, monofilament, absorbable suture. Nonabsorbable suture may act as a nidus for cholelith formation. Use of a simple continuous or a continuous inverting pattern has been reported.

Choledochotomy

Choledochotomy[23] has been reported in cats for removal of choleliths from obstructed dilated CBDs. A longitudinal incision is made in the CBD, which is then closed in a longitudinal or transverse orientation. A transverse closure is performed if excessive luminal narrowing is a concern. A simple interrupted pattern may be preferable to a simple continuous pattern. The use of polydioxanone, polypropylene, and nylon have been reported, but there is a lack of evidence to support the use of one suture material over another. Suture material size and choice should be based on bile duct size and tissue friability.

Cholecystectomy

Cholecystectomy[35] is indicated for removal of a diseased or traumatised gallbladder in the presence of a patent CBD and for the prevention of recurrent cholelithiasis (Fig. 31.5). The gallbladder is adherent to the quadrate and right medial liver lobes. The area of adherence is known as the hepatic fossa. Sharp dissection is required to release the peritoneal attachments at the margins of the hepatic fossa. Blunt dissection with moist cotton tip applicators, swabs, or a fine Poole suction tip are then used to release the remainder of the gallbladder wall from the hepatic fossa. If a Poole suction tip is used, care should be taken to monitor carefully for blood loss, as this can be underestimated if blood is continuously suctioned from the surgical site. Haemostasis of the hepatic fossa can be achieved using electrocautery and topical haemostatic materials. Release of the gallbladder from the liver should be complete, resulting in circumferential access to the cystic duct. Dissection should not be extended into the CBD to avoid damage to the hepatic ducts. The cystic artery runs alongside the cystic duct; this artery is often transected before it is noticed. Suture ligation or electrocautery of the cystic artery is advised to minimise blood loss. The cystic duct is clamped and circumferentially ligated. The use of permanent and absorbable suture material has been described (e.g. polypropylene, polyglactin 910, polydioxanone). The transected cystic duct should be examined carefully for leak and double ligated if appropriate. A transfixing suture may be appropriate if the cystic duct is thickened or dilated and ligature slip is a concern. The specific complication of cholecystectomy is bile leak leading to bile peritonitis.

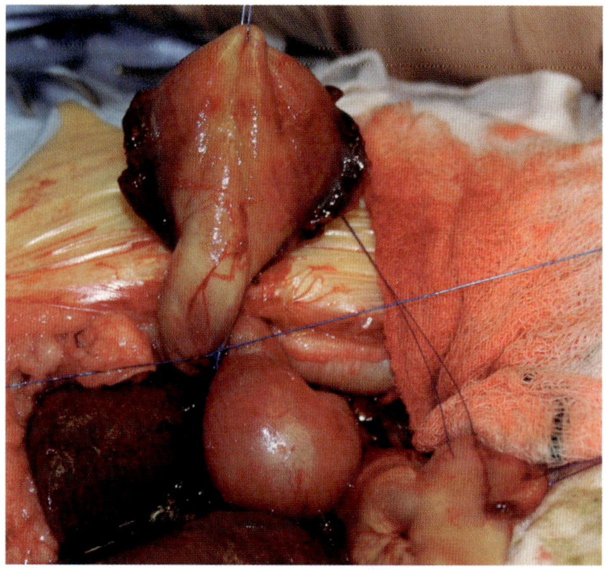

Figure 31.5. Intraoperative image of the ligation of the cystic duct with polypropylene (blue suture) in a cat undergoing cholecystectomy for management of extrahepatic bile duct obstruction secondary to severe obstructive cholelithiasis. The gallbladder has an opaque, thickened wall and has been dissected out of the hepatic fossa: it is being held with a single stay suture. Marked dilation of the common bile duct can be seen below the gallbladder. The liver is also swollen, dark in colour, and friable. This cat had marked acute necrosuppurative cholangiohepatitis and cholecystitis associated with bacterial infection.

Cholecystoenterostomy

Cholecystoenterostotomy[12,35] is indicated for the management of permanent obstruction of the CBD (Fig. 31.6). The gallbladder is released from its hepatic fossa as for cholecystectomy. The gallbladder wall is then sutured to the seromuscular layer of the antimesenteric surface of the duodenum for cholecystoduodenostomy or to a section of jejunum for cholecystojejunostomy. Corresponding incisions are then made in the gallbladder and duodenum parallel to this suture line. These incisions are sutured to each other to create a new stoma. Finally, another suture line is placed between the gallbladder and the duodenum to seal the stoma site. The use of a single suture line for each side of the stoma is also reported. Simple continuous or interrupted suture patterns and 3-0 or 4-0 monofilament delayed absorbable suture materials are appropriate. The stoma is expected to contract down to 50% of its original size, so stoma size should be maximised.

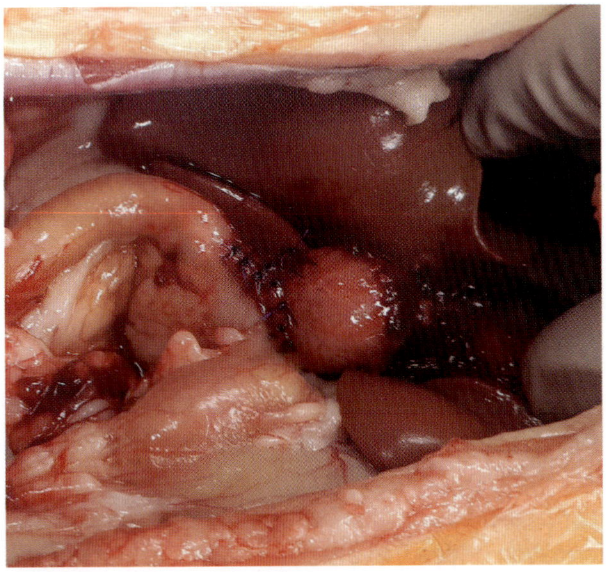

Figure 31.6. Intraoperative image of a cholecystoduodenostomy in a cat with extrahepatic bile duct obstruction that failed catheterisation of the common bile duct via the duodenum. The cat was eventually diagnosed with neoplasia of the ampulla of Vater.

The use of a 30 mm endoscopic gastrointestinal anastomosis stapler for cholecystoduodenostomy has been described in four cats.[38] Follow-up was limited to 2 weeks and no comparison was made with the sutured technique, so no conclusions can be made about the success of this technique.

Specific complications of this surgery include recurrent bacterial cholangiohepatitis characterised by pyrexia, anorexia, and lethargy; chronic diarrhoea secondary to exocrine pancreatic insufficiency; chronic vomiting; chronic weight loss; and stricture requiring revision surgery. Long-term medical treatments are frequently indicated including antibiotics, pancreatic enzyme supplements, and low-fat prescription diets. These chronic, recurrent problems frequently lead to euthanasia or death. In one study of cats undergoing cholecystoenterostomy, in the absence of neoplasia, the median survival time was 255 days (range 4–2196 days), with less than 50% surviving more than 6 months.[12]

GENERAL COMPLICATIONS OF BILIARY SURGERY

Hypotension

Persistent and frequently unresponsive hypotension is a commonly reported anaesthetic complication of biliary surgery seen in most, if not all, cats. Unresponsiveness to treatment results in persistent hypotension into the postoperative period and can progress to fatal cardiorespiratory arrest.[39]

A number of hypotheses have been suggested for refractory hypotension in cats undergoing biliary surgery including the following. First, endotoxaemia and hyperbilirubinaemia may result in a decrease in the responsiveness or functional activation of α_1-adrenergic receptors, resulting in inappropriate vasodilation. Second, obstructive jaundice has been associated with the release of nitric oxide, which is a potent vasodilator. Third, a reduction in hepatic angiotensinogen synthesis may lead to failure of the renin–angiotensin–aldosterone system to maintain normotension.[39]

Treatment of intraoperative hypotension with intravenous fluid boluses, constant-rate infusions of positive inotropes and/or vasopressors, dosed to effect, and reduction in inhalant anaesthetic agents has been described. Intravenous fluids used for bolus therapy include crystalloids and colloids, such as tetrastarch and haemoglobin-based volume expanders. Haemoglobin-based volume expanders have the added benefit of being an endothelial nitric oxide scavenger, which may stimulate vasoconstriction, as well as contributing to plasma volume expansion. Positive inotropes used include dopamine, which activates myocardial β_1-adrenergic receptors to increase systolic blood pressure and heart rate, and ephedrine, which increases cardiac output by activation of β_1-adrenergic receptors and at higher doses stimulates vasoconstriction by activation of α-adrenergic receptors. Vasopressors include norepinephrine, which activates α_1- and β_1-adrenergic receptors to induce vasoconstriction. Reduction in inhalant anaesthetic agents, which appear to have a greater cardiovascular depressant effect in cats than in other species, and replacement with intravenous alternatives can also improve mean arterial pressure intraoperatively. Reduction in inhalant anaesthetic agents can also be achieved by careful consideration of analgesia with the incorporation of epidural opioids, local anaesthetics, and constant-rate intravenous infusions of analgesics into anaesthetic plans.[39]

Acute kidney injury

Acute kidney injury characterised by elevation in serum creatinine concentrations is also commonly reported.[39]

This may result from preoperative dehydration and intraoperative kidney hypoperfusion secondary to unresponsive hypotension. Careful preoperative rehydration and management of intraoperative hypotension are indicated in an attempt to decrease incidence of acute kidney injury.

Hypothermia

Hypothermia is reported in up to 100% of cats undergoing biliary surgery.[39] This may result from the duration of surgery and be exacerbated by poor body condition, emphasising the need for preoperative planning and active warming.

Pancreatitis

Pancreatitis is a commonly reported postoperative complication of biliary surgery.[39] It may be preexisting. This emphasises the need to consider postoperative nutrition intraoperatively by placement of a feeding tube.

Anaemia

Anaemia is frequently seen in cats presenting for biliary surgery and is also a reported complication of biliary surgery. Anaemia has been reported preoperatively in 36%–60% of cats presenting with complete EHBDO and postoperatively in 82% of cats undergoing cholecystoenterostomy. Preoperatively, blood loss may occur as a result of gastrointestinal bleeding, resulting in a regenerative anaemia.[11,12]

Cats presenting with biliary disease may have underlying coagulopathy. In studies of cats presenting for surgical intervention of EHBDO, 45%–46% of cats had abnormal clotting times.[11,12] This may be due to an associated decrease in liver function, leading to reduction in hepatic synthesis of multiple procoagulants, anticoagulants, and proteins involved in fibrinolysis. In addition, vitamin K is required for hepatic activation of a number of procoagulants (factors II, VII, XI, and X) and anticoagulants (protein C and protein S), and as a fat-soluble vitamin, vitamin K is dependent on the normal release of bile salts into the intestine for its absorption. In cats, cholangitis has been associated with vitamin K deficiency, decrease in the procoagulant factor XIII, increase in fibrinogen, and elevations in PT and aPTT.

However, control of haemostasis is complex and dependent not only on synthesis and activation of protein factors but also on their interplay with the vascular endothelium and platelets. A decrease in liver function may be associated with proportional decline in the procoagulants and anticoagulants produced by the liver, enhanced endothelial production and activation of factor VIII and von Willebrand factor, release of procoagulant microparticles from monocytes, platelets and endothelium, and dampened fibrinolytic capacity. Further, endotoxins are known to activate coagulation and fibrinolysis. The coagulopathy of feline biliary disease may therefore include a spectrum of abnormalities including both an increase in bleeding tendency and an increase in clot formation. Indeed, in a report of portal vein thrombosis in cats, all six cats had hepatobiliary disease,[40] and elevations in clotting times are seen in less than 50% of cats presenting for biliary surgery.[11,12] Further studies in cats with biliary disease, including global evaluations of coagulation (e.g. thromboelastography), are needed.

Cats presenting with necrotising pancreatitis may have anaemia secondary to bleeding within the pancreas and peripancreatic tissues due to enzymatic degradation of blood vessels. In one histopathological study of severe acute necrotising pancreatitis and acute suppurative pancreatitis in 40 cats, 26% of cats were anaemic on presentation and 55% of cats were anaemic terminally.[41] Anaemia was normochromic, normocytic. At postmortem examination, petechiation and gastrointestinal haemorrhage were seen in 15% of cats, serosanguineous fluid in body cavities in 47%, and thrombosis in 20%. This study suggests that anaemia in cats with pancreatitis may be due to intravenous fluid therapy, acute blood loss, and coagulopathy.

Bleeding risk in cats presenting for ultrasound-guided liver biopsy has been reported to be greater if platelet counts are less than 80000/μl or if aPTT is greater than 1.5 times normal.[9] Pretreatment with vitamin K has been shown to normalise clotting times in over 80% of cats with abnormal clotting times due to vitamin K deficiency within 3–5 days, so it is recommended in all cats prior to biliary surgery. Recommended treatment of spontaneous or iatrogenic bleeding includes packed red blood cells but also fresh frozen plasma due to coagulation factor content.

Take-home messages

- Extrahepatic bile duct obstruction (EHBDO) may be due to one or a combination of neoplastic and inflammatory causes, as well as bacterial infection, parasitic infection, trauma, and foreign bodies.
- Irrespective of cause, EHBDO always results in cholestasis and a clinical picture characterised by icterus, anorexia, lethargy, weight loss, and vomiting.
- Initial diagnostic investigation of EHBDO should include serum biochemistry, haematology, coagulation profile, abdominal ultrasound, and noninvasive fine needle aspiration of bile, pancreas, and liver.
- Medical management of inflammatory causes of EHBDO should be initiated prior to surgical management due to frequent complications associated with biliary surgery in cats.
- The aims of surgery in cats with EHBDO are to confirm the disease, diagnose its cause, establish patency of the biliary system, and place a feeding tube.
- Complications of biliary surgery are frequently life-threatening and include hypotension, hypothermia, acute kidney injury, pancreatitis and anaemia, as well as complications associated with the specific surgery performed, including ascending bacterial cholangiohepatitis.

REFERENCES

[1] Boyer JL. Bile formation and secretion. *Compr Physiol* 3:1035, 2013.

[2] Furneaux RW. A series of six cases of sphincter of Oddi pathology in the cat (2008–2009). *J Feline Med Surg* 12:794, 2010.

[3] Larson MM. Ultrasound imaging of the hepatobiliary system and pancreas. *Vet Clin North Am Small Anim Pract* 46:453, 2016.

[4] Harran N et al. Gallbladder sludge on ultrasound is predictive of increased liver enzymes and total bilirubin in cats. *Can Vet J* 52:999, 2011.

[5] Policelli Smith R et al. Association between gallbladder ultrasound findings and bacterial culture of bile in 70 cats and 202 dogs. *J Vet Intern Med* 31:1451, 2017.

[6] Marolf AJ et al. Ultrasonographic findings of feline cholangitis. *J Am Anim Hosp Assoc* 48:36, 2012.

[7] Marolf AJ. Computed tomography and MRI of the hepatobiliary system and pancreas. *Vet Clin North Am Small Anim Pract* 46:481, 2016.

[8] Tanaka T et al. Drip infusion cholangiography with CT in cats. *J Feline Med Surg* 20:1173, 2018.

[9] Bigge LA, Brown DJ, Penninck DG. Correlation between coagulation profile findings and bleeding complications after ultrasound-guided biopsies: 434 cases (1993–1996). *J Am Anim Hosp Assoc* 37:228, 2001.

[10] Savary-Bataille KC et al. Percutaneous ultrasound-guided cholecystocentesis in healthy cats. *J Vet Intern Med* 17:298, 2003.

[11] Mayhew PD et al. Pathogenesis and outcome of extrahepatic biliary obstruction in cats. *J Small Anim Pract* 43:247, 2002.

[12] Buote NJ et al. Cholecystoenterostomy for treatment of extrahepatic biliary tract obstruction in cats: 22 cases (1994–2003). *J Am Vet Med Assoc* 228:1376, 2006.

[13] Haney DR, Christiansen JS, Toll J. Severe cholestatic liver disease secondary to liver fluke (*Platynosomum concinnum*) infection in three cats. *J Am Anim Hosp Assoc* 42:234, 2006.

[14] Della Santa D et al. Imaging diagnosis—extrahepatic biliary tract obstruction secondary to a duodenal foreign body in a cat. *Vet Radiol Ultrasound* 48:448, 2007.

[15] Brioschi V, Rousset N, Ladlow JF. Imaging diagnosis—extrahepatic biliary tract obstruction secondary to a biliary foreign body in a cat. *Vet Radiol Ultrasound* 55:628, 2014. Daure E et al. Ultrasonographic and clinicopathological features of pyloroduodenal adenomatous polyps in cats. *J Feline Med Surg* 19:141, 2017.

[16] van den Ingh TSGAM et al. Morphological classification of biliary disorders of the canine and feline liver. In: WSAVA Liver Standardization Group. *WSAVA Standards for Clinical and Histological Diagnosis of Canine and Feline Liver Diseases.* Philadelphia, Elsevier: 61, 2006.

[17] Center SA et al. Hematologic and biochemical abnormalities associated with induced extrahepatic bile duct obstruction in the cat. *Am J Vet Res* 44:1822, 1983.

[18] Harvey AM et al. Treatment and long-term follow-up of extrahepatic biliary obstruction with bilirubin cholelithiasis in a Somali cat with pyruvate kinase deficiency. *J Feline Med Surg* 9:424, 2007.

[19] Eich CS, Ludwig LL. The surgical treatment of cholelithiasis in cats: a study of nine cases. *J Am Anim Hosp Assoc* 38:290, 2002.

[20] Woods KS et al. Congenital duplex gallbladder and biliary mucocele associated with partial hepatic cholestasis and cholelithiasis in a cat. *Can Vet J* 53:269, 2012.

[21] Grünhage F, Lammert F. Gallstone disease. Pathogenesis of gallstones: a genetic perspective. *Best Pract Res Clin Gastroenterol* 20:997, 2006.

[22] Baker SG, Mayhew PD, Mehler SJ. Choledochotomy and primary repair of extrahepatic biliary duct rupture in seven dogs and two cats. *J Small Anim Pract* 52:32, 2011.

[23] Patnaik AK. A morphologic and immunocytochemical study of hepatic neoplasms in cats. *Vet Pathol* 29:405, 1992.

[24] Haines VL et al. Adenocarcinoma of the hepatopancreatic ampulla in a domestic cat. *Vet Pathol* 33:439, 1996.

[25] Trout NJ. Surgical treatment of hepatobiliary cystadenomas in cats. *Semin Vet Med Surg Small Anim* 12:51, 1997.

[26] Patnaik AK et al. Hepatobiliary neuroendocrine carcinoma in cats: a clinicopathologic, immunohistochemical, and ultrastructural study of 17 cases. *Vet Pathol* 42:331, 2005.

[27] Basu AK, Charles RA. A review of the cat liver fluke *Platynosomum fastosum* Kossack, 1910 (Trematoda: Dicrocoeliidae). *Vet Parasitol* 200:1, 2014.

[28] Mayhew PD, Weisse CW. Treatment of pancreatitis-associated extrahepatic biliary tract obstruction by choledochal stenting in seven cats. *J Small Anim Pract* 49:133, 2008.

[29] Son TT et al. Surgical intervention in the management of severe acute pancreatitis in cats: 8 cases (2003–2007). *J Vet Emerg Crit Care (San Antonio)* 20:426, 2010.

[30] Spain HN et al. Ultrasonographic and clinicopathologic features of segmental dilatations of the common bile duct in four cats. *JFMS Open Rep* 3:2055116917716881, 2017.

[31] Ludwig LL et al. Surgical treatment of bile peritonitis in 24 dogs and 2 cats: a retrospective study (1987–1994). *Vet Surg* 26:90, 1997.

[32] Murgia D. A case of combined bilothorax and bile peritonitis secondary to gunshot wounds in a cat. *J Feline Med Surg* 15:513, 2013.

[33] Linton M et al. Extrahepatic biliary duct obstruction as a result of involuntary transcavitary implantation of hair in a cat. *JFMS Open Rep* 1:2055116915610359, 2015.

[34] Mayhew PD, Weisse C. Liver and biliary system. In: Tobias K, Johnston S, editors. *Veterinary Surgery: Small Animal*, 2nd ed. Missouri, Saunders: 1828, 2017.

[35] Sung JY et al. Ascending infection of the biliary tract after surgical sphincterotomy and biliary stenting. *J Gastroenterol Hepatol* 7:240, 1992.

[36] Dumonceau JM et al. Endoscopic biliary stenting: indications, choice of stents, and results: European Society of Gastrointestinal Endoscopy (ESGE) clinical guideline—updated October 2017. *Endoscopy* 50:910, 2018.

[37] Morrison S, Prostredny J, Roa D. Retrospective study of 28 cases of cholecystoduodenostomy performed using endoscopic gastrointestinal anastomosis stapling equipment. *J Am Anim Hosp Assoc* 44:10, 2008.

[38] Monticelli P et al. Life-threatening perianaesthetic complications in five cats undergoing biliary tract surgery: case series and literature review. *J Feline Med Surg* 19:717, 2017.

[39] Rogers CL et al. Portal vein thrombosis in cats: 6 cases (2001–2006). *J Vet Intern Med* 22:282, 2008.

[40] Hill RC, Van Winkle TJ. Acute necrotizing pancreatitis and acute suppurative pancreatitis in the cat. A retrospective study of 40 cases (1976–1989). *J Vet Intern Med* 7:25, 1993.

CHAPTER 32

Pancreatic and hepatobiliary neoplasia

Davide Berlato

PANCREATIC NEOPLASIA AND PARANEOPLASTIC ALOPECIA

The pancreas is a multilobular organ of exocrine secretory units that produces digestive enzymes. Isles of endocrine cells are scattered throughout the lobules.

Primary pancreatic tumours are divided into exocrine and endocrine. Tumours of the exocrine pancreas are uncommon and can be benign (pancreatic adenoma) or malignant (pancreatic carcinoma). Tumours of the endocrine pancreas are rare in cats, the most common being insulinoma. Other reported tumours of the feline pancreas are lymphoma, sarcoma, undifferentiated tumours, and metastatic neoplasia.[1]

Epidemiology and aetiology

Tumours of the pancreas are rare in cats. The estimated incidence of primary pancreatic carcinoma, which is the most common pancreatic tumour, is 12.6 per 10000 cats.[2] In a recent study that included 540 feline pancreatic samples,[1] there were 54 (10%) exocrine carcinomas, 21 (4%) exocrine adenomas, 17 (3%) non-epithelial tumours, and 2 (<0.5%) endocrine tumours.

Experimentally, N-ethyl-N'-nitro-N-nitrosoguanidine has been shown to induce pancreatic duct adenocarcinoma when administered intraductally in dogs,[3] but there is no documented causative evidence in cats.

History and physical examination

Pancreatic tumours tend to occur in middle-aged to older cats, with a median age of 11–12 years.[4,5] Typical presenting clinical signs are similar to those of other pancreatic diseases, such as pancreatitis, and include weight loss, vomiting, diarrhoea, anorexia, abdominal pain, abdominal enlargement, and icterus.[4–6] The presence of a midabdominal mass is also frequent in the late stage of the disease.[3] Rare clinical presentations include diabetes mellitus and pleural effusion.[5]

Cats with insulinoma present with clinical signs related to the hypoglycaemia (e.g. weakness, seizure, visual impairment) or with clinical signs related to the secondary catecholamine release (e.g. tremor, anxiety).[7]

Paraneoplastic alopecia

Another clinical presentation of pancreatic or biliary tract tumours is paraneoplastic alopecia (Fig. 32.1). The main clinical feature is acute, progressive, and symmetric alopecia affecting the ventrum and then extending to the head and medial aspect of the limbs.[8] Hair epilates easily, and alopecic skin is shiny, inelastic, and thin, but not fragile. Involvement of the pads is common. Some cats might also present excessive grooming, even though pruritus is not a typical feature of this disorder. Pruritus can be present with concurrent complications, such as *Malassezia* spp. infection or flea infestation.

Histopathological evaluation of alopecic skin biopsy samples reveals a nonscarring alopecia, with characteristic marked follicular telogenisation, miniaturisation, and atrophy.[8] These features are nonspecific and might also be present in endocrinopathies, dermatophytosis, self-induced alopecia, telogen defluxion, feline symmetrical alopecia, and alopecia areata. The alopecia can be reversible after resection of the tumour.[9]

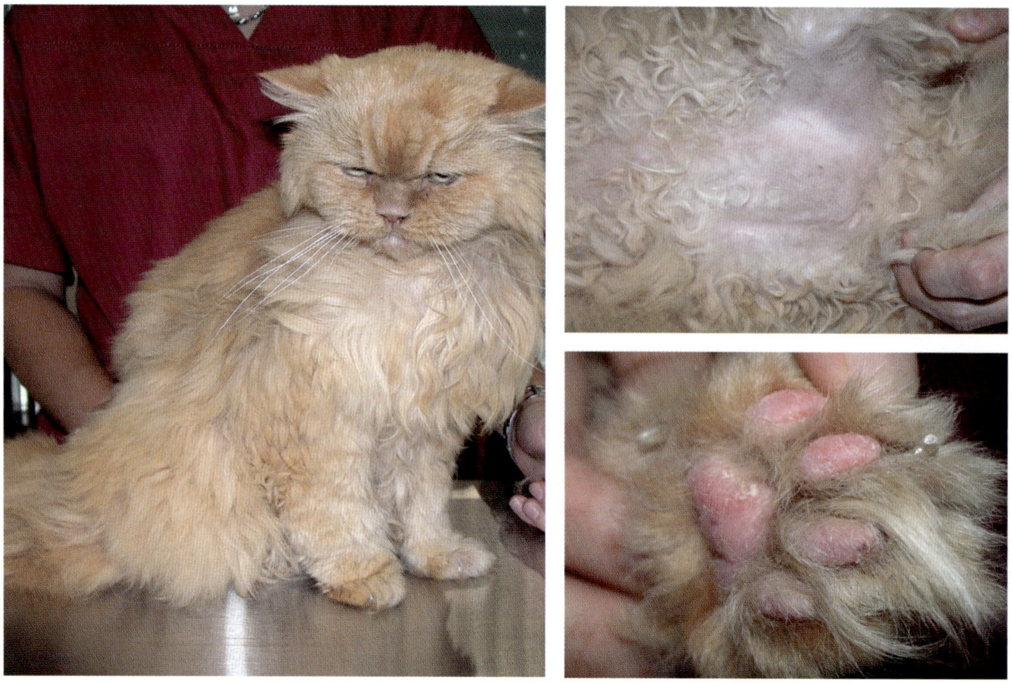

Figure 32.1. Persian cat with a pancreatic carcinoma presented with paraneoplastic alopecia characterised by bilateral symmetrical nonpruritic alopecia, with glossy and slightly oedematous skin and involvement of the footpads. Images courtesy of Claudia Nett, Ennet-SeeKlinik, Hünenberg, Switzerland.

Diagnostic investigation

Common alterations seen in routine blood analysis of cats with pancreatic tumours are nonspecific and include neutrophilia, mild anaemia, hyperglycaemia, increased liver enzyme activities, and bilirubinaemia.[5,10] A recent study described the association between histopathology and feline pancreatic lipase immunoreactivity (fPLI) in cats with a normal pancreas and cats with hyperplastic, inflammatory, and neoplastic pancreatic diseases.[6] Cats with pancreatitis and pancreatic exocrine carcinoma had a significantly higher fPLI compared to cats with a normal pancreas, but the degree of fPLI increase did not allow differentiation between pancreatitis and exocrine pancreatic carcinoma.

Standard diagnostic criteria for the diagnosis of insulinoma are not available in cats, but the concomitant documentation of hypoglycaemia and a normal or high (inappropriate) insulin blood concentration should be considered a good indicator for the diagnosis.[7] The final diagnosis should be confirmed by histopathology and immunohistochemistry.

Imaging modalities can be helpful in the diagnosis of pancreatic disease, including pancreatic cancer. Abdominal radiographs are not sensible for the detection of pancreatic masses, but nonspecific findings (e.g. loss of abdominal serosal detail, cranial abdominal organomegaly) are commonly reported.[4,5] Thoracic radiographs are an important part of staging, as they can allow the diagnosis of lung metastatic disease, mediastinal lymphadenomegaly, and pleural effusion.

Ultrasound can be a valuable tool in the diagnosis of pancreatic disease, but it cannot reliably differentiate neoplasia from pancreatitis, pseudocysts, abscesses, or nodular hyperplasia.[10] Pancreatic tumours can be focal, multifocal, or diffuse, and also cystic or solid. In a study describing the ultrasonographic features of 19 cats with pancreatic neoplasia,[11] the only imaging feature able to discriminate neoplasia from other pancreatic diseases was the presence of a single focal mass larger than 2 cm (Table 32.1, Fig. 32.2). Cystic pancreatic tumours are more likely to be benign (70%), whereas solid pancreatic tumours are more likely to be malignant (90%).[12] Another feature that can indicate the presence of a malignant pancreatic tumour is the infiltration of the surrounding mesentery or abdominal fat (carcinomatosis), which occurs in approximately 50% of the cases and can cause secondary peritoneal effusion.[12] Metastases can also be found in up to 80% of exocrine pancreatic carcinomas at diagnosis, and common sites include the abdominal lymph nodes but also the intestine, spleen, kidneys, liver, and lungs.[4,5,12]

Table 32.1. Ultrasonographic features suggestive of benign vs. malignant pancreatic neoplasia.

Pancreatic neoplasia	Ultrasonographic features
Benign	Dimension <2 cm Cystic
Malignant	Dimension >2 cm Solid Carcinomatosis (abdominal effusion, nodules/ infiltration of mesentery or abdominal fat) Metastasis in regional lymph nodes: confirmed by FNA Metastasis in distant abdominal sites (intestine, spleen, kidneys, liver): confirmed by FNA

FNA, fine needle aspiration.

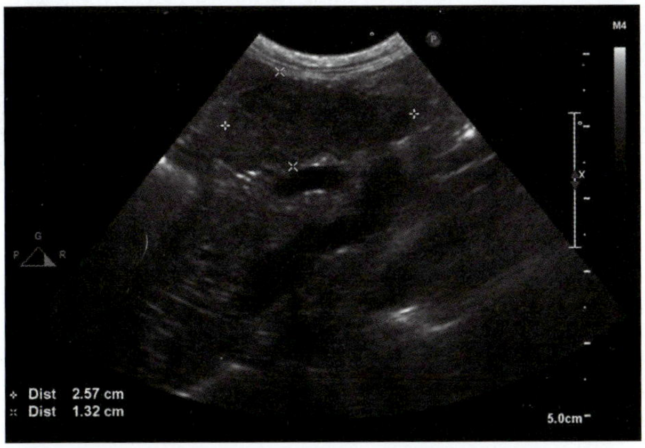

Figure 32.2. Parasagittal B-mode ultrasonographic image showing a heterogeneous, slightly hypoechogenic mass (between callipers) with irregular contour in the left pancreatic limb. The normal pancreatic tissue is almost isoechoic to the surrounding mesentery. The splenic vein is noted deep to the pancreatic tissue. The mass was confirmed to be a pancreatic carcinoma on cytological examination.

Most cats with insulinoma have an ultrasonographically detectable mass;[7] this is in contrast with dogs, in which the mass is frequently missed.[10]

The use of computed tomography (CT) or magnetic resonance imaging (MRI) in the diagnosis and staging of pancreatic tumours in cats has not been described in the literature. In dogs, CT angiography is commonly used to visualise insulinomas for surgical planning and staging, but in cats this imaging modality has not yet been investigated.[13]

The final diagnosis of pancreatic neoplasia relies on cytology or histopathology. Ultrasound-guided fine needle aspiration (FNA) is a safe procedure in cats with pancreatic disease. In a case-control study,[14] cats with pancreatic disease undergoing FNA of the pancreas had a similar risk (10%–15%) of developing complications during hospitalisation than matched cats with pancreatic disease that did not have the pancreas aspirated. The diagnostic yield of pancreatic aspirates in this study was approximately 70%, with a good correlation with histopathology (Fig. 32.3). Similar results were also obtained in a study evaluating aspiration of pancreatic lesions in dogs.[15]

When a cytological diagnosis cannot be obtained, the next diagnostic step is surgical or laparoscopic biopsy.[16,17] Both these techniques are relatively safe, but they carry a low risk of inducing acute pancreatitis. Before performing the procedure, it is important to discuss with the owner that collecting a representative sample is not always possible and that obtaining a nonrepresentative sample occurs in as many as half of the cases.[16] The reason why this happens is that most pancreatic lesions are focal, and when the mass lesion cannot be identified, the sample is collected from a randomly selected area of the pancreas (usually the distal end of the right pancreatic limb).

Management and treatment

At the time of this writing, there is no standard of care for the treatment of pancreatic neoplasia in cats.

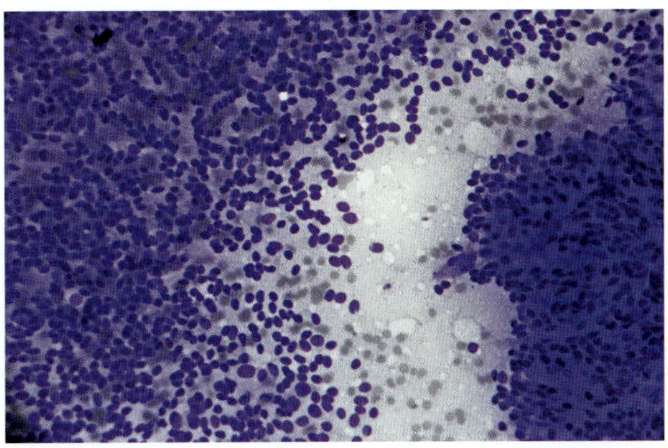

Figure 32.3. Endocrine (islet cell) pancreatic tumour in a cat. The neoplastic cells appear as naked nuclei, haphazardly to more linearly arranged, within a pale basophilic background of cytoplasmic material. The nuclei display moderate anisokaryosis and are round with indistinct nucleoli. The exfoliation of bare nuclei is typically associated with neuroendocrine/endocrine tumours. Diff-Quik, ×500. Image courtesy of Roger Powell, DragonVet Consulting, Hitchin, UK.

Marginal excision should be recommended for localised pancreatic masses if staging does not show infiltration of the surrounding tissues or spread to the regional lymph nodes or to distant sites. In these cases, the use of adjuvant chemotherapy after surgery is probably beneficial, but currently there is no supportive evidence.

For locally advanced pancreatic neoplasia or in presence of distant metastases, palliative chemotherapy should be considered only in cats that respond favourably to symptomatic and supportive treatment. Common chemotherapy agents that have been prescribed include gemcitabine, carboplatin, and mitoxantrone. The efficacy of tyrosine kinase inhibitors is currently unknown.

Supportive treatment should be considered for cats with pancreatic neoplasia because all of them also suffer from concurrent pancreatitis, which can be moderate or severe.[6] The use of nonsteroidal anti-inflammatory drugs has been associated with a negative outcome, but this finding was probably related to selection bias.[4]

Prognosis and outcome

The prognosis of pancreatic cancer is in general guarded to poor because the most common tumour is exocrine carcinoma. Most cats are euthanised shortly after admission or at the time of surgical biopsy. In a case series,[12] the intraoperative mortality rate for pancreatic exocrine carcinoma was 65% (32/50). Cats with a focal pancreatic mass without metastatic disease are an exception; in a study describing the long-term outcome of nine cats undergoing marginal resection, followed by adjuvant chemotherapy in six cases, the median survival time was 10 months (range 1–32).[18] The survival time for cats with a more advanced disease that received chemotherapy or underwent surgery is in the order of 6 months.[4] The presence of abdominal effusion is a negative prognostic factor, with a median survival time of 1 month.[4]

The outcome of cats with pancreatic adenoma is variable. In the nine cats reported in a case series, the mean and median survival times were, respectively, 16 and 4 months (range 0.5–60).[12]

HEPATOBILIARY NEOPLASIA

Feline hepatic neoplasms are classified as hepatocellular adenomas and carcinomas, cholangiocellular adenomas and carcinomas, mixed hepatocellular and cholangiocellular carcinomas, and hepatic carcinoids.[19–23] A single feline hepatoblastoma has been described in the literature.[24]

Epidemiology and aetiology

Primary liver tumours represent 1.0%–2.9% of all tumours in cats.[25] The classification of primary liver tumours was updated in 2006, challenging the diagnosis of many older manuscripts.[21,22] Cholangiocellular carcinomas are reported to be the most frequent primary hepatic malignancy.[20,23] In a recent study,[23] 61 feline primary liver tumours were classified as nodular hyperplasia (10%), hepatocellular tumours (34%), cholangiocellular tumours (41%), hepatic carcinoids (13%), and squamous cell carcinoma (2%). The incidence of hepatocellular and cholangiocellular tumours in cats is similar, but while hepatocellular tumours are mostly benign (85% adenoma, 15% carcinoma), almost all cholangiocellular tumours are malignant (100% carcinoma).[21–23] Cholangiocellular adenomas are thought to be extremely rare, and probably all feline cholangiocellular adenomas (or cystadenomas) described in the veterinary literature[19,26–28] are likely to represent nonneoplastic adult-type cystic liver disease.[21]

Primary hepatic carcinoids (neuroendocrine carcinoma) are also rare. They can arise from the liver parenchyma or from the biliary tract and can be intrahepatic or extrahepatic.

Currently, the aetiology of primary liver tumours in cats is unknown.

History and physical examination

The age of cats with cholangiocellular carcinomas, hepatocellular carcinomas, or hepatic carcinoids is usually greater than 9 years, and there is no sex or breed predisposition.[20,26,27,29] In a series of cats with hepatocellular carcinoma, most cats had one or more coexistent or preexistent health disorders, the most common being hyperthyroidism.[30]

The clinical signs associated with primary hepatic neoplasia are nonspecific, such as weight loss, anorexia, vomiting, and lethargy. Other less common clinical signs include icterus, diarrhoea, and abdominal effusion. During physical examination, documenting hepatomegaly causing abdominal enlargement and a palpable mass in the cranial abdomen is common.[20,26,27,30]

A rare clinical presentation of biliary tract tumours is paraneoplastic alopecia (see section “Paraneoplastic alopecia” in this chapter for more details).[8] Hypoglycaemia has also been reported as a rare paraneoplastic effect of hepatocellular carcinomas and hepatic carcinoids and appears to be secondary to the aberrant secretion of the insulin-like growth factor 2 (IGF-2) precursors.[31]

Diagnostic investigation

There is no pattern of clinical chemistry abnormalities that suggests hepatocellular neoplasia over any other diseases of the liver. Common clinicopathologic abnormalities in a series of cats with hepatocellular carcinoma included increased activities of liver enzymes (aspartate aminotransferase [AST] in 90%; alanine aminotransferase [ALT] and alkaline phosphatase [ALP] in 71%) and hyperbilirubinaemia in 38%. Prolonged prothrombin time (PT) and activated partial thromboplastin time (aPTT) was found in 37%.[30] The abnormalities present in other primary liver tumours are not well documented in the literature but are likely to be similar to the ones just described.

In cats with primary liver neoplasia, radiographs can be obtained for staging purposes to evaluate the presence of distant metastasis to the lungs or to the sternal lymph node, but it is uncommon to be able to visualise the hepatic tumour (Fig. 32.4).[30]

Abdominal ultrasound is the most common imaging modality used to investigate the liver and provide information on its size, contour, and echogenicity. Primary tumours can appear ultrasonographically as solitary/multifocal masses, diffuse coalescing nodular lesions, or diffuse hypo- or hyperechogenicity (Fig. 32.5).[32] Nodular hyperplasia is a differential diagnosis for every focal hepatic disease. A variable amount of free abdominal fluid can also be identified in approximately 20% of the cats with primary liver neoplasia.[30]

The most common feline hepatic mass lesion is what was incorrectly called “cystadenoma” in the old literature.[28] These lesions are now thought to be non-neoplastic adult-type cystic liver disease, and they appear ultrasonographically as a multilocular mass with numerous thin-walled cysts that can vary in diameter from 1 mm to 8 cm or as a hyperechoic or mixed-echogenicity mass with a cystic element.[32] The second most common hepatic mass lesion is cholangiocarcinoma, but there is no description of its ultrasonographic appearance in the veterinary literature. In human medicine, the differentiation between biliary carcinoma and adenoma relies on histopathology because their ultrasonographic appearance is similar.[32] The ultrasonographic characterisation of hepatocellular neoplasia is also poorly described in the veterinary literature, but these tumours appear most commonly as a solitary hepatic mass with heterogeneous echogenicity and multiple hypoechoic fluid-filled nodules.[30] Ultrasound should also be used in these cases to assess regional lymph nodes and guide FNA.

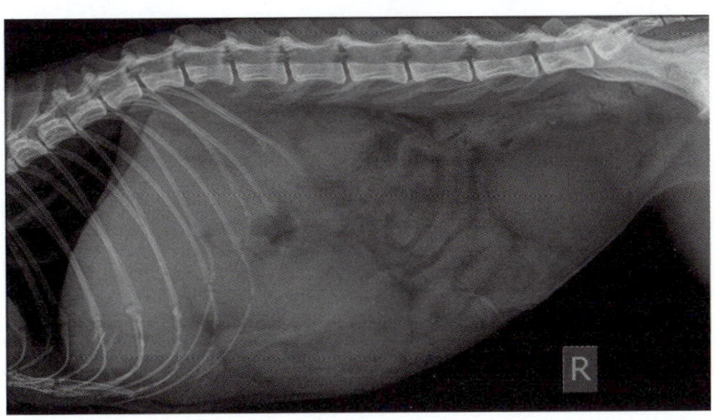

Figure 32.4. Right lateral abdominal radiograph of a domestic shorthair cat with cholangiocellular carcinoma affecting the right liver and with multiple intrahepatic metastases. A large soft tissue mass effacing the liver and causing dorsal displacement of the stomach can be seen.

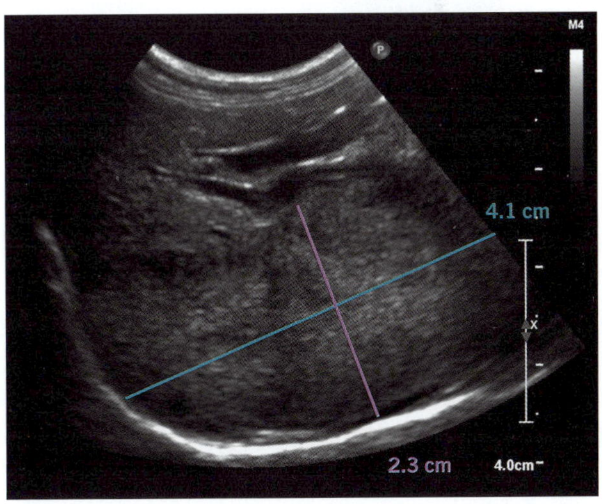

Figure 32.5. Parasagittal B-mode ultrasonographic image of the same patient as in Figure 32.2 showing a large, slightly hyperechogenic, heterogeneous mass in the right liver.

The use of CT or MRI in the diagnosis and staging of hepatic tumours in cats is not described in the literature. In dogs, CT is commonly used to plan surgical resection and for staging purposes, but in cats this imaging modality has not yet been investigated.[13]

In general, there is no individual imaging feature that allows distinction between benign hepatic mass lesions (e.g. nodular hepatic hyperplasia, adult-like cystic liver disease) and neoplasia, benign or malignant. As always, the final diagnosis of neoplasia relies on cytology and/or histopathology (Figs. 32.6 and 32.7).[33] Cystic lesions should never be aspirated because of the risk of causing bleeding, and biopsy specimens should be obtained only during laparotomy. Ultrasound-guided FNA is safe, and the cytological interpretation correlates with the histological diagnosis in 50%–80% of the cases.[34] Samples for histopathology can be obtained with Tru-Cut needle biopsy, laparoscopy, or surgery. The correlation between Tru-Cut needle biopsy and surgical wedge biopsy is 55%–65%,[35] and the risk of major complications, mainly bleeding, is around 5%.[36] Liver biopsy specimens should not be obtained in cats with an automatic Tru-Cut biopsy gun device because these devices have been associated with a high risk of death caused by severe vagal shock.[37]

In cats with cholangiocellular carcinoma, metastasis should be expected in almost all cases; the most common metastatic sites include the liver itself, regional lymph nodes, abdominal serosa, and lungs.[20,23] The coexistence of cholangiocellular carcinoma and adult-type congenital cystic liver disease has also been reported in 10%–15% of the cases, making it difficult to predict whether multifocal liver disease represents intrahepatic metastases or not.[23] Interestingly, carcinomatosis is not a feature of cholangiocellular carcinoma.[20]

In a recent large case series of hepatocellular carcinoma,[30] metastasis was not recognised in any cat, but, in older reports, metastases were reported to occur in 30% of the cases, with regional lymph nodes as the most common location—and rarely the lungs and spleen.[20]

Management and treatment

The treatment of choice for liver tumours is surgery; the efficacy of radiotherapy and chemotherapy is minimal. Surgery should be attempted in cats with solitary hepatic masses, but it is not advisable when multifocal masses or metastatic disease is present. Often, benign lesions (e.g. benign nodular hyperplasia, adult-type cystic liver disease) coexist with malignant tumours in the same patient,

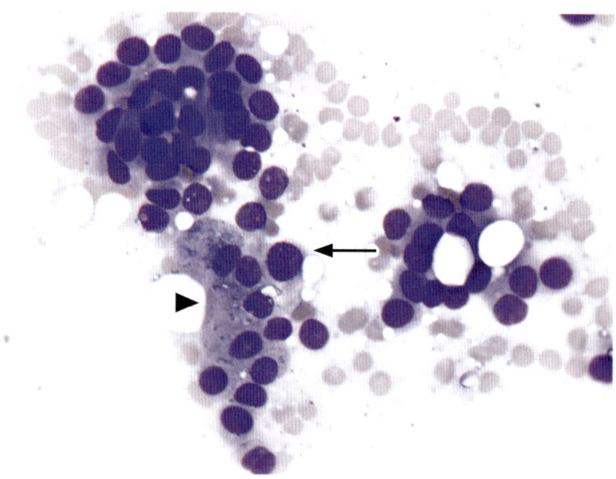

Figure 32.6. Cholangiocellular carcinoma in a cat. The neoplastic biliary epithelial cells have exfoliated in cohesive, crowded, and more irregular clusters. They are cuboidal to columnar and display mild anisokaryosis and anisocytosis. They have round nuclei with indistinct nucleoli, nuclear moulding, and a small to moderate amount of pale basophilic cytoplasm. Low numbers of hepatocytes are also present (arrowhead), with a single mitotic figure (arrow) and background blood. Modified Wright–Giemsa, ×1000. Image courtesy of Roger Powell, DragonVet Consulting, Hitchin, UK.

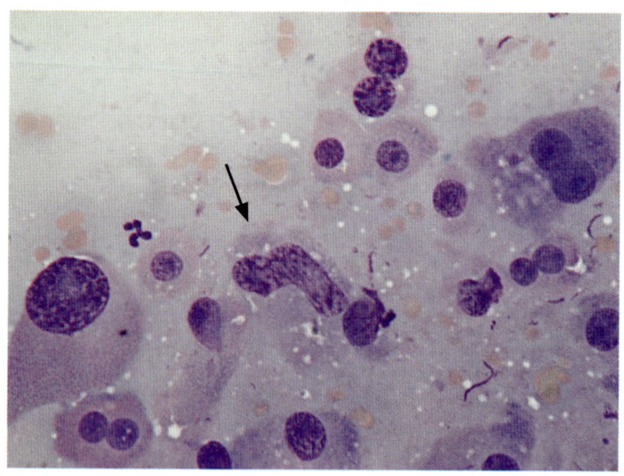

Figure 32.7. Hepatocellular carcinoma in a cat. The hepatocytes display prominent features of atypia and pleomorphism. They show marked anisokaryosis and anisocytosis, karyomegaly, frequent binucleation, and dyscohesion. Their nuclear chromatin is variably coarse and stippled to more irregular, with variably prominent and often irregular nucleoli. A hepatocyte with a large and irregularly shaped nucleus is seen (arrow). Modified Wright–Giemsa, ×1000. Image courtesy of Roger Powell, DragonVet Consulting, Hitchin, UK.

making it difficult to recommend surgery for veterinary clinicians. Performing cytology of all accessible noncystic lesions is always a good initial step, but it is important to keep in mind that malignant neoplasia can never be entirely ruled out in this way. After explaining all these limitations, if the cat owner still elects to pursue surgery, it is essential to ensure that all the accessible suspicious lesions are biopsied at the time of surgery. This will allow the veterinary clinician to provide accurate staging and associated prognosis and plan follow-up appointments.

Prognosis and outcome

The prognosis for benign hepatic mass lesions is good, even without any intervention. Reaching the diagnosis can, however, be difficult and require surgical intervention.

The prognosis of cholangiocellular carcinomas and primary hepatic carcinoids is poor. Most cats show clinical signs at the time of diagnosis, and the neoplasia is already at an advanced stage, with intrahepatic, nodal, and distant metastases. When surgery is attempted, perioperative mortality is common.

The prognosis of hepatocellular carcinoma is fair. At the time of diagnosis, metastases are rarely found, but they might develop later in the course of the disease in some cases. The tumour-associated morbidity most commonly results from the tumour growth, which leads to local compression, necrosis, and haemorrhage.[20] In a recent case series,[30] the median survival time of eight cats diagnosed with hepatocellular carcinoma was 1.4 years (range 0.6–6.5). The six cats that underwent complete tumour resection had a median survival time of 2.4 years (range 1.0–6.5).

Take-home messages

Pancreatic neoplasia

- Clinical signs of pancreatic neoplasia are similar to those of other pancreatic diseases.
- Most cats with pancreatic neoplasia suffer from concurrent pancreatitis.
- Abdominal ultrasound, thoracic radiographs, and fine needle aspiration are helpful in obtaining a final diagnosis and for staging purposes.
- Metastatic disease is present in 80% of cats with pancreatic carcinoma at presentation.
- Surgery should be considered for the few cats with focal nonmetastatic pancreatic neoplasia. The prognosis for cats that survive the perioperative period is guarded for carcinomas and fair for adenomas.

Hepatobiliary neoplasia

- Presenting clinical signs of hepatic neoplasia are nonspecific.
- Physical examination often reveals a cranial abdominal mass.
- The radiological distinction between benign hepatic mass lesions and neoplasia is not possible. For diagnosis, solid lesions should be aspirated, while cystic lesions should be biopsied surgically.
- In all cases, abdominal ultrasound and thoracic radiographs should be obtained for staging before performing any invasive procedure. Most cats with cholangiocellular carcinoma have detectable metastasis at presentation.
- Surgery should be attempted in cats with solitary hepatic masses, but it is not advisable when multifocal masses or metastatic disease is present.
- The prognosis for cholangiocellular carcinoma is poor, while hepatocellular tumours carry a fair prognosis.

REFERENCES

[1] Törner K et al. Clinical and pathological data of 17 non-epithelial pancreatic tumors in cats. *Vet Sci* 7:55, 2020.

[2] Priester WA. Data from eleven United States and Canadian colleges of veterinary medicine on pancreatic carcinoma in domestic animals. *Cancer Res* 34:1372, 1974.

[3] Selmic LE. Exocrine pancreatic cancer. In: Vail DM, Thamm DH, Liptak JM, editors. *Withrow and MacEwen's Small Animal Clinical Oncology*, 6th ed. St Louis, Elsevier Saunders: 451, 2020.

[4] Linderman MJ et al. Feline exocrine pancreatic carcinoma: a retrospective study of 34 cases. *Vet Comp Oncol* 11:208, 2013.

[5] Seaman RL. Exocrine pancreatic neoplasia in the cat: a case series. *J Am Anim Hosp Assoc* 40:238, 2004.

[6] Törner K et al. Histopathology and feline pancreatic lipase immunoreactivity in inflammatory, hyperplastic and neoplastic pancreatic diseases in cats. *J Comp Pathol* 174:63, 2020.

[7] Gifford CH et al. Diagnosis of insulinoma in a Maine Coon cat. *JFMS Open Rep* 6:2055116919894782, 2020.

[8] Turek MM. Cutaneous paraneoplastic syndromes in dogs and cats: a review of the literature. *Vet Dermatol* 14:279, 2003.

[9] Tasker S et al. Resolution of paraneoplastic alopecia following surgical removal of a pancreatic carcinoma in a cat. *J Small Anim Pract* 40:16, 1999.

[10] Larson MM. Ultrasound imaging of the hepatobiliary system and pancreas. *Vet Clin North Am Small Anim Pract* 46:453, 2016.

[11] Hecht S, Penninck DG, Keating JH. Imaging findings in pancreatic neoplasia and nodular hyperplasia in 19 cats. *Vet Radiol Ultrasound* 48:45, 2007.

[12] Törner K et al. Primary solid and cystic tumours of the exocrine pancreas in cats. *J Comp Pathol* 169:5, 2019.

[13] Marolf AJ. Computed tomography and MRI of the hepatobiliary system and pancreas. *Vet Clin North Am Small Anim Pract* 46:481, 2016.

[14] Crain SK et al. Safety of ultrasound-guided fine-needle aspiration of the feline pancreas: a case-control study. *J Feline Med Surg* 17:858, 2015.

[15] Cordner AP et al. Cytologic findings and diagnostic yield in 92 dogs undergoing fine-needle aspiration of the pancreas. *J Vet Diagn Invest* 27:236, 2015.

[16] Pratschke KM et al. Pancreatic surgical biopsy in 24 dogs and 19 cats: postoperative complications and clinical relevance of histological findings. *J Small Anim Pract* 56:60, 2015.

[17] Webb CB, Trott C. Laparoscopic diagnosis of pancreatic disease in dogs and cats. *J Vet Intern Med* 22:1263, 2008.

[18] Nicoletti R et al. Postsurgical outcome in cats with exocrine pancreatic carcinoma: nine cases (2007–2016). *J Am Anim Hosp Assoc* 54:291, 2018.

[19] Patnaik AK. A morphologic and immunocytochemical study of hepatic neoplasms in cats. *Vet Pathol* 29:405, 1992.

[20] Cullen JM. Tumors of the liver and gallbladder. In: Meuten DJ, editor. *Tumors in Domestic Animals*, 5th ed. Ames, John Wiley & Sons: 602, 2017.

[21] Charles JA et al. Morphological classification of neoplastic disorders of the canine and feline liver. In: WSAVA Liver Standardization Group. *WSAVA Standards for Clinical and Histological Diagnosis of Canine and Feline Liver Diseases*. Edinburgh, WB Saunders: 117, 2006.

[22] van den Ingh TSGAM et al. Morphological classification of biliary disorders of the canine and feline liver. In: WSAVA Liver Standardization Group. *WSAVA Standards for Clinical and Histological Diagnosis of Canine and Feline Liver Diseases*. Edinburgh, WB Saunders: 61, 2006.

[23] van Sprundel RG et al. Classification of primary hepatic tumours in the cat. *Vet J* 202:255, 2014.

[24] Ano N et al. Hepatoblastoma in a cat. *Vet Pathol* 48:1020, 2011.

[25] Liptak JM. Hepatobiliary tumors. In: Vail DM, Thamm DH, Liptak JM, editors. *Withrow and MacEwen's Small Animal Clinical Oncology*, 6th ed. St Louis, WB Saunders: 432, 2020.

[26] Post G, Patnaik AK. Nonhematopoietic hepatic neoplasms in cats: 21 cases (1983–1988). *J Am Vet Med Assoc* 201:1080, 1992.

[27] Lawrence HJ, Erb HN, Harvey HJ. Nonlymphomatous hepatobiliary masses in cats: 41 cases (1972 to 1991). *Vet Surg* 23:365, 1994.

[28] Nyland TG, Koblik PD, Tellyer SE. Ultrasonographic evaluation of biliary cystadenomas in cats. *Vet Radiol Ultrasound* 40:300, 1999.

[29] Patnaik AK et al. Hepatobiliary neuroendocrine carcinoma in cats: a clinicopathologic, immunohistochemical, and ultrastructural study of 17 cases. *Vet Pathol* 42:331, 2005.

[30] Goussev SA et al. Clinical characteristics of hepatocellular carcinoma in 19 cats from a single institution (1980–2013). *J Am Anim Hosp Assoc* 52:36, 2016.

[31] Guillen A et al. Non-islet-cell tumour hypoglycaemia in a cat with hepatocellular carcinoma. *JFMS Open Rep* 5:2055116919856129, 2019.

[32] Griffin S. Feline abdominal ultrasonography: what's normal? What's abnormal? The liver. *J Feline Med Surg* 21:12, 2019.

[33] Warren-Smith CM et al. Lack of associations between ultrasonographic appearance of parenchymal lesions of the canine liver and histological diagnosis. *J Small Anim Pract* 53:168, 2012.

[34] Wang KY et al. Accuracy of ultrasound-guided fine-needle aspiration of the liver and cytologic findings in dogs and cats: 97 cases (1990–2000). *J Am Vet Med Assoc* 224:75, 2004.

[35] Cole TL et al. Diagnostic comparison of needle and wedge biopsy specimens of the liver in dogs and cats. *J Am Vet Med Assoc* 220:1483, 2002.

[36] Bigge LA, Brown DJ, Penninck DG. Correlation between coagulation profile findings and bleeding complications after ultrasound-guided biopsies: 434 cases (1993–1996). *J Am Anim Hosp Assoc* 37:228, 2001.

[37] Proot SJ, Rothuizen J. High complication rate of an automatic Tru-Cut biopsy gun device for liver biopsy in cats. *J Vet Intern Med* 20:1327, 2006.

CHAPTER 33

Antiemetic and gastroprotective agents

M. Katherine Tolbert

ANTIEMETIC DRUGS

Vomiting and nausea, often resulting from systemic illness or gastrointestinal (GI) disease, are common in hospitalised and sick cats. Consequently, feline practitioners are faced with managing the resulting sequelae (e.g. aspiration pneumonia, dehydration, electrolyte derangements, hepatic lipidosis) and their effect on morbidity and mortality. For this reason, antiemetics and anti-nausea drugs are amongst the most commonly prescribed medications in veterinary medicine. Uncontrolled vomiting and nausea can contribute to weakness and lethargy, two of the leading reasons for euthanasia of cats. Thus, the selection of antiemetic and anti-nausea therapy can have a profound impact on the cat's outcome. See Appendix for recommended dosages.

Pathophysiology of vomiting

The vomiting reflex involves a complex circuit in which the vomiting centre can be stimulated by pathways from the abdominal viscera, chemoreceptor trigger zone (CRTZ), vestibular apparatus, and central nervous system. The receptors and the signalling pathways into the vomiting centre differ between dogs and cats. Additionally, administering medications to a cat, especially one that is sick, can be challenging for owners. Thus, the choice of antiemetic drug is dictated by three considerations: the likely stimulus of vomiting (i.e. peripheral vs. CRTZ), the recognition that cats do not always pharmacologically behave like small dogs, and the need to reduce frequency of administration and optimise route of administration for the owner in order to enhance medication compliance.

Antiemetics should not be prescribed unless the practitioner is confident that a mechanical obstruction is not the cause of vomiting. Caution is also advised when using antiemetics prior to achieving a diagnosis, as antiemetic therapy can mask an otherwise lack of response to direct therapy.

Commercially available antiemetics commonly used in veterinary medicine include maropitant, serotonin antagonists, and metoclopramide and are discussed below along with other less commonly used medications with antiemetic potential, including mirtazapine, glucocorticoids, and cannabinoids.

Antiemetic agents

Maropitant citrate

The neurokinin-1 (NK_1) inhibitor maropitant citrate (hereafter referred to as maropitant) has largely replaced many of the older antiemetic drugs for the treatment of vomiting in dogs and cats. NK_1 receptors are expressed in many locations throughout the body, and for this reason, maropitant is an effective antiemetic for cats with GI and systemic causes of vomiting as well as for motion sickness.[1,2]

Maropitant is available as a Food and Drug Administration (FDA)–approved injectable drug for the treatment of acute vomiting in cats 16 weeks of age or older. The time at which the maximum blood concentrations (T_{max}) are observed after subcutaneous injection (1 mg/kg) in cats is between 30 minutes and 2 hours.[2] The terminal half-life is 13–17 hours, regardless of the method of administration, providing antiemetic activity for up to 24 hours.[2] A longer interval between maropitant and administration of proemetic substances (≈18 hours) has been recommended to promote greater antiemetic effects. However, the same antiemetic effects are observed when maropitant is administered 2 hours prior to the emetogen.[3,4] Oral maropitant administration is extralabel in cats but is also an effective treatment for feline vomiting due to a wide variety of causes including vomiting secondary to administration of proemetic substances.[2–4] The T_{max} following oral maropitant administration at 1 mg/kg in the cat is similar to that in the dog at 2–3 hours, and bioavailability is 50%.[2]

Because of its effects on blockade of the inflammatory neuropeptide substance P at the NK_1 receptor, maropitant also exhibits efficacy against painful visceral stimuli and might alleviate pain in cats undergoing surgical procedures, as exhibited by a reduction in their overall sevoflurane requirement during ovarian ligament stimulation.[5]

Although maropitant is an effective antiemetic, it—and most other antiemetic therapies—may not alleviate nausea for all conditions.[1,3,4,6] Thus, alternative (e.g. ondansetron for chemotherapy-induced nausea) and additional therapies (e.g. mirtazapine for chronic kidney disease [CKD] in cats)[1,7] or higher doses of maropitant may be needed to help control nausea, depending on the underlying disease.

Although once-daily subcutaneous maropitant injections were determined to be safe up to 15 days in 6-month-old cats,[2] bone marrow hypocellularity was observed in puppies younger than 11 weeks receiving injectable maropitant; therefore, repeated administration in kittens younger than 16 weeks is discouraged. Pain at the injection site is a commonly reported adverse effect of subcutaneous injection in cats. Injection of the drug immediately following its removal from refrigeration might help alleviate pain associated with the injection. The reported side effects from the FDA prescribing information, in order of frequency, were depression/lethargy, anorexia, hypersalivation, pain/vocalisation upon injection, dyspnoea, ataxia, fever, recumbency, vomiting, panting, convulsion, and muscle tremor.

Maropitant is metabolised by the cytochrome P450 (CYP450) system; therefore, administration in cats with liver dysfunction is not recommended. Close monitoring is also advised with concurrent administration of drugs that are CYP450 inhibitors (e.g. omeprazole, ketoconazole). Maropitant is highly protein bound (≈99%) and therefore caution is recommended with concurrent administration of other highly protein-bound drugs (e.g. nonsteroidal anti-inflammatory drugs [NSAIDs], anticonvulsants). There may be an age-related effect on the pharmacokinetics of maropitant, with higher clearance in kittens compared to adult cats. Safety data for administration of maropitant in pregnant or lactating animals is not available.

Adverse effects reported following repeated oral administration of maropitant in dogs over a 28-day period included lymphadenomegaly, corneal oedema, lethargy, vomiting, and decreased appetite. Similar adverse effects may be observed in cats following repeated exposure to oral maropitant; however, this data, beyond the aforementioned 15-day study, is not available for the cat.

Serotonin antagonists

A major cause of chemotherapy-induced vomiting is induction of 5-hydroxytryptamine (serotonin) 3 ($5\text{-}HT_3$) release, which stimulates the vomiting centre. Serotonin antagonists, such as ondansetron or dolasetron, block peripheral serotonin $5\text{-}HT_3$ receptors[8] and therefore are often considered to be frontline antiemetics and antinausea drugs for cats receiving chemotherapy. Ondansetron, however, has poor oral bioavailability (32%), with wide interindividual variation (range 11%–50%), and a short half-life (≈75 minutes) in cats. Subcutaneous administration results in an improved bioavailability (75%) and a longer half-life (≈3 hours) when compared to oral or intravenous administration (≈1.5 hours).[9] Therefore, subcutaneous administration and thrice-daily dosing, in cats without liver or renal dysfunction, are recommended. Unlike with maropitant, ondansetron must be administered simultaneously with emetogens such as α_2-agonists rather than as a premedication to be effective for preventing nausea and vomiting associated with these drugs.[10] Ondansetron is not effective against opioid-induced vomiting. For cats with opioid-induced vomiting, maropitant may be a better option.

Ondansetron is metabolised predominantly by the liver, with a small fraction metabolised by the kidney. Twice-daily dosing is recommended for cats with liver dysfunction.[11] Frequency reduction of ondansetron in cats with compromised glomerular filtration may also be recommended if the renal impairment is severe. Transdermal application of 4 mg ondansetron did not result in clinically relevant blood concentrations in cats and is not recommended.[12] Dolasetron also exhibits a short half-life in the blood of cats and was ineffective in preventing xylazine-induced emesis in cats. Therefore, dolasetron is not recommended as a sole antiemetic for cats.

Metoclopramide

Metoclopramide is a dopamine 2 receptor (low doses) and 5-HT_3 (high doses) antagonist. Metoclopramide is a less effective antiemetic in cats because of the reduced dopaminergic receptors in the feline CRTZ. However, metoclopramide can help to reduce the frequency of vomiting episodes in cats sedated with α_2-agonists.[13] It also may be a helpful adjunctive, but not sole, therapy in cats with GI dysmotility, as it has been demonstrated to enhance gastric emptying of a liquid meal[14] and improve the antral motility index in healthy cats.[15] Metoclopramide is touted to inhibit gastric relaxation and enhance intestinal motility; however, studies in healthy awake or anaesthetised dogs suggest that these effects are weak or absent. Oral metoclopramide has no effect on lower oesophageal sphincter tone in cats.[14]

Mirtazapine

Mirtazapine antagonises presynaptic α_2-adrenergic receptors and serotonin and histamine type 1 receptors and stimulates appetite through 5-HT_2 receptor antagonism. Antagonism of 5-HT_3 receptors provides its antiemetic and anti-nausea effects. Mirtazapine decreases nausea and vomiting and stimulates appetite in cancer-bearing human patients undergoing chemotherapy. In a placebo-controlled, masked crossover clinical trial, mirtazapine administration resulted in a significant decrease in vomiting episodes and an increase in appetite and body weight in cats with CKD.[7] Compliance with administration of oral medications is an important concern for cat owners, especially those with cats displaying nausea or vomiting. Thus, transdermal medications are a desirable route of administration. Unfortunately, the majority of transdermal products are compounded and suffer from stability and safety concerns. However, mirtazapine is commercially available as an FDA-approved transdermal mirtazapine ointment and labelled for the promotion of weight gain in cats. In cats with unintended weight loss from a variety of underlying diseases which may be associated with chronic vomiting, application of the transdermal product resulted in a 3.9% increase of body weight following 14 days of daily topical treatment. Mirtazapine might also promote GI motility, as it improved gastric emptying, normalised rectal distension-induced delay in gastric emptying, and accelerated colonic transit in healthy purpose-bred research dogs. No such studies are available in the cat.

Mirtazapine is largely metabolised by the liver and eliminated by the kidneys. In a study of cats with liver disease, the half-life of mirtazapine was prolonged when compared to aged-matched control cats.[16] The T_{max} was also unexplainably prolonged. The half-life and clearance were also prolonged in cats with CKD.[17] Thus, frequency reductions are recommended in cats with liver or kidney disease.

Side effects of mirtazapine tend to be dose-dependent and observed with doses greater than or equal to 3.75 mg/cat. Common adverse effects can include vocalisation, excitability, and hypersalivation.[18] Rarely, mirtazapine may induce vomiting. There is a single report of increased liver enzyme activity in a cat following mirtazapine administration, thus careful monitoring of liver enzyme activity, especially in cats with underlying liver disease, is recommended when using the drug long-term.[7]

Chlorpromazine/prochlorperazine

Chlorpromazine and prochlorperazine inhibit vomiting at both the CRTZ and vomiting centre through antagonism of dopamine, histamine type 1, α_2-adrenergic, and muscarinic receptors. The requirements for frequent dosing (0.1–0.5 mg/kg every 8 hours) and parenteral administration limit the use of the drug to hospitalised patients. Adverse effects include sedation and hypotension, and therefore these drugs should not be used in patients prior to stabilisation or as outpatient treatments. These drugs should not be combined with metoclopramide because of the concern for extrapyramidal effects via dopamine antagonism.

Corticosteroids

Corticosteroids, specifically the glucocorticoid dexamethasone, have been demonstrated to have central antiemetic effects targeted at the vomiting centre in cats. Glucocorticoids are effective antiemetics, especially in the context of chemotherapy-induced vomiting, and also have appetite stimulant properties.[19] Other uses without additional indications for steroid therapy are avoided because of the multitude of adverse effects associated with long-term steroid use, including increased risk for diabetes mellitus, infections, proteinuria, and thromboembolic disease.

Additional antiemetic therapies

Cannabinoids, active compounds derived from the cannabis plant, are both marketed and under development for their antiemetic and anti-nausea properties in cats. Cannabinoids, which include psychoactive (e.g. tetrahydrocannabinol [THC]) and nonpsychoactive compounds (e.g. cannabidiol, cannabigerol), exert their antiemetic effects largely through agonism of the central presynaptic cannabinoid type 1 (CB_1) receptor.[20] Cannabinoids have demonstrated antiemetic, antianxiety, antinociceptive, and antineuropathic properties in humans. For this reason, cannabinoid-containing products targeting pet owners are already sold at many licensed medical marijuana dispensaries. However, these products are neither FDA-approved nor undergo any regulatory oversight at this time. Post-production product quality assurance from independent labs, including the assurance of being free from contaminants such as herbicides and pesticides and 100% THC-free (or minimally less than 0.1%), is largely lacking in most commercial products. Moreover, there are no placebo-controlled clinical trials investigating the efficacy of cannabinoids in cats. Finally, at the time of this writing, with the exception of California, veterinary practitioners in the United States of America are prohibited from recommending the use of cannabinoids for the treatment of any clinical sign or disease in animals. Thus, more studies, quality testing, and regulatory approval are needed prior to the recommendation for the use of cannabinoids as an antiemetic in cats.

In animals with chronic disease states where the underlying cause of vomiting cannot be removed (e.g. CKD, neoplasia), placement of an oesophageal or gastric feeding tube may help to reverse the deficit in water and nutritional status and optimise medication compliance.

GASTROPROTECTIVE AGENTS

Gastroprotective agents such as gastric acid suppressants and cytoprotective agents are most commonly administered to the cat for the treatment of oesophagitis and gastroduodenal ulceration. Gastroduodenal ulceration is relatively uncommon in the cat but, when observed, is most commonly caused by gastroduodenal or pancreatic neoplasia or feline GI eosinophilic sclerosing fibroplasia. Although sporadic cases are reported, cats appear to be less susceptible than dogs to develop NSAID-induced ulceration. Other causes of ulceration in the cat include high-dose corticosteroid administration, inflammatory bowel disease, parasitic disease, foreign bodies, trichobezoars, and severe stress (e.g. critical illness).

The efficacy of gastroprotective agents for the treatment of oesophagitis and gastroduodenal ulceration is highly dependent on the underlying cause and its ability to be removed. The medical treatment of oesophagitis and upper GI ulceration can be directed towards neutralising or decreasing the production of gastric acid (see Figure 33.1 for an illustration on gastric acid production), promoting prostaglandin production or action, and coating and protecting denuded epithelium.

The commercially available gastroprotective agents commonly used in veterinary medicine, including acid suppressant drugs, antacids, and coating agents, are discussed below. See Appendix for recommended dosages. For more details on the indications and rationale for the use of gastroprotective therapy in cats, please refer to the American College of Veterinary Internal Medicine (ACVIM) consensus statement.[21]

Histamine type 2 receptor antagonists

Gastric acid secretion is triggered by hormonal and neural stimulation of parietal cells, the acid-producing cells of the stomach. Acid suppressant drugs, which take aim at these physiological targets on the parietal cell surface, have largely supplanted antacids (acid-neutralising drugs) as the drugs of choice for acid-related diseases. Healing of acid-related disorders was determined to be partially dependent on gastric acid suppression. The histamine type 2 receptor antagonists (H_2RAs; e.g. famotidine, ranitidine, cimetidine hydrochloride) are competitive

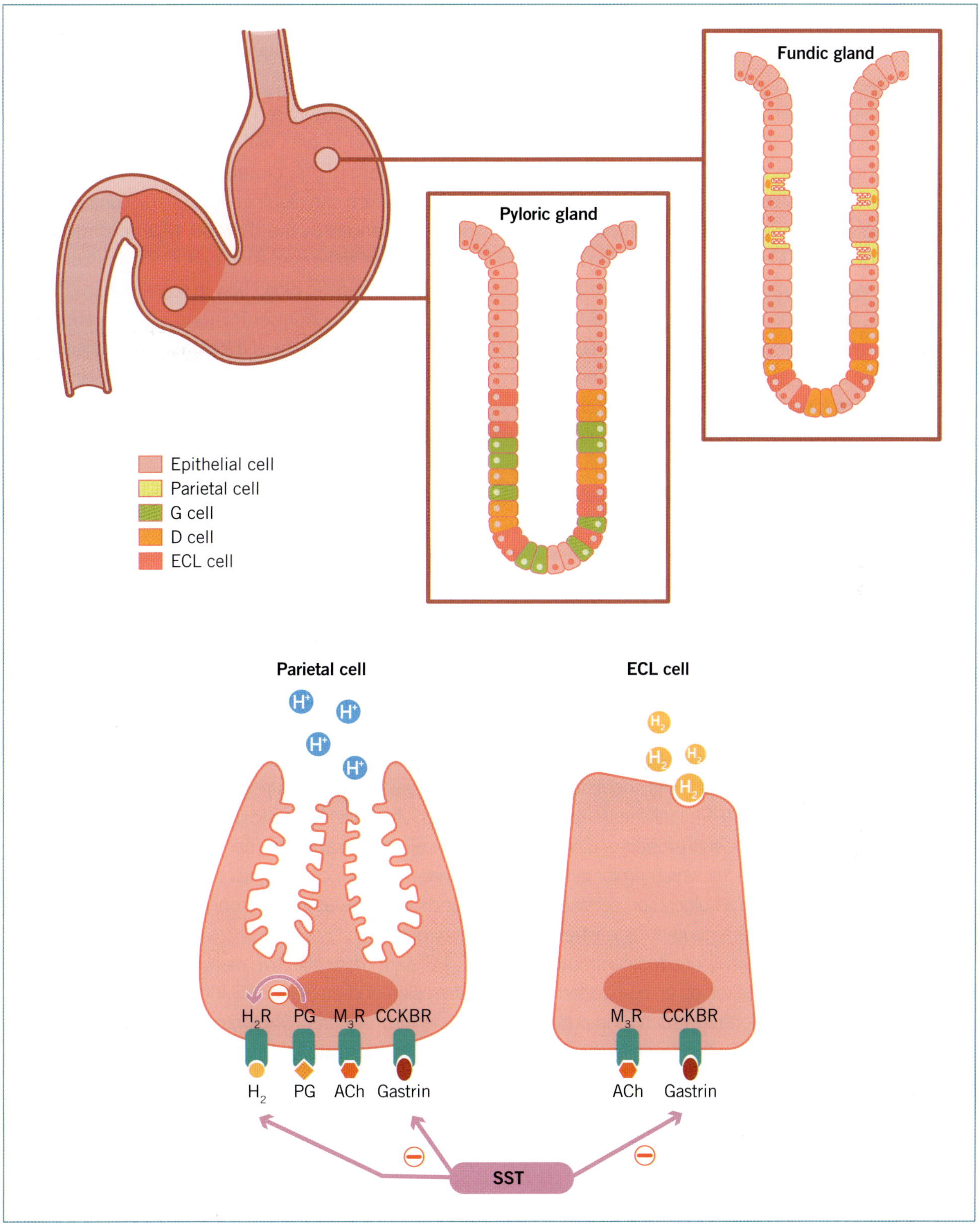

Figure 33.1. Gastric acid secretion in the cat. The gastric acid–secreting parietal cells, located in the gastric fundus and body (shaded light pink), are stimulated by histamine (H_2) secreted by enterochromaffin-like (ECL) cells, gastrin secreted by gastrin (G) cells (predominantly in the pyloric antrum), and vagal inputs (acetylcholine [ACh]) and inhibited by somatostatin (SST) secreted by delta (D) cells and prostaglandins (PG). Vasoactive intestinal peptide potentiates meal-induced acid secretion in the cat, unlike in dogs. CCKBR, cholecystokinin type B receptor; H_2R, histamine type 2 receptor; M_3R, muscarinic type 3 receptor.

inhibitors of the interaction of histamine with the parietal cell histamine type 2 receptors. They have a good safety profile and are not affected by the presence of a meal.

Cimetidine was the first H_2RA to be used experimentally or clinically in cats. It is thought to be less potent as a gastric acid inhibitor compared to famotidine and ranitidine and has rapidly fallen out of favour for clinical use.

Ranitidine has poor acid-suppressing activity, as determined by studies in healthy cats in which it was no better than placebo in raising gastric pH when administered orally at approximately 2 mg/kg every 12 hours.[22] Ranitidine is more commonly used to promote GI motility, although to the author's knowledge, there are no studies evaluating the prokinetic effect of ranitidine in the cat.

Famotidine has fair to good acid-suppressing activity during the first few days of oral administration, has a good safety profile, and is more effective as a gastric acid suppressant than ranitidine in cats.[23–25] Repeated daily oral administration of famotidine, and likely the other H_2RAs, results in a diminished effect over time.[24] In humans, tolerance to the drug occurs regardless of the type of H_2RA used or dosage or frequency administered as long as the drug is given daily. Intravenous famotidine administration also results in tolerance in humans, but this effect has not been demonstrated in cats.

Because of their relatively weak acid-suppressing activity after several days of use, H_2RAs should not supplant proton pump inhibitors (PPIs) for the treatment of moderate to severe gastroduodenal erosion or ulceration, especially in those conditions for which prolonged treatment may be required such as ulceration secondary to gastric tumours. H_2RAs are a good choice when only weak acid-suppressing activity is needed, for immediate relief of clinical signs when taken on an as-needed basis (e.g. bilious vomiting), or short-term such as in preventative therapy for oesophageal reflux under anaesthesia. H_2RAs are also effective against basal acid secretion and, as a result, have efficacy against nocturnal gastric acidity. Therefore, although combination therapy is not recommended for treatment of gastric or duodenal ulceration, there might be some benefit in the combination of a PPI with night-time famotidine for the treatment of gastrooesophageal reflux in susceptible individuals such as brachycephalic cats or for the medical treatment of hiatal hernia. H_2RAs might also have local protective oesophageal effects and reduce acid-induced oesophageal injury, although this has only been demonstrated with cimetidine.[26]

H_2RAs are largely renally excreted and should be dose-reduced in cats with severe renal impairment. Unlike other H_2RAs, cimetidine is a known CYP450 inhibitor, which can result in drug interactions with other drugs influenced by the CYP450 system, although this effect has yet to be proven in cats.[27–29] Cimetidine may also reduce hepatic blood flow in some species.[30]

Recently, low concentrations of the carcinogen N-nitrosodimethylamine (NDMA) were identified in prescription and over-the-counter generic and brand-name ranitidine preparations. In the United States of America, the FDA has requested the withdrawal of all ranitidine drugs from the market as of April 1, 2020. The European Medicines Agency is reviewing the problem but has not made a decision at the time of this writing.

Intravenously administered famotidine was anecdotally reported to cause haemolysis in cats; however, this effect has not been documented when the drug is intravenously administered as a slow bolus over 5 minutes.[31]

Proton pump inhibitors

PPIs (e.g. omeprazole, esomeprazole, pantoprazole) target the final common pathway of acid production and inhibit gastric secretion regardless of the stimulus. PPIs are lipophilic, weakly basic drugs that permeate the parietal cell membrane and become trapped in its acidic environment. Once trapped, the drug forms disulphide bonds with the active proton-pumping H^+/K^+-ATPase enzymes.

PPIs are more effective than H_2RAs in healing upper GI erosion and ulceration.[32] Indeed, a variety of omeprazole formulations (whole and divided enteric-coated tablet, encapsulated, reformulated paste, suspension) have been evaluated and demonstrated to be superior in increasing the gastric pH in cats when compared to H_2RAs.[22,23,33] Although peak concentrations of H_2RAs occur within hours of oral administration and the PPIs can take up to 4 days to reach peak effect, PPIs are likely as effective as H_2RAs on day 1 of administration.[34] Meal-induced gastric acid secretion has the most potent effect on gastric pH. Therefore, orally administered PPIs should be given on an empty stomach immediately (30–

60 minutes) prior to offering a full meal or with a small treat prior to the full meal to improve efficacy.[22] Although keeping the enteric-coated tablet intact is desired if possible, the tablet can be divided to optimise dosing for cats.[23] The degree of acid suppression is likely not as good on day 1 compared to an intact tablet, but provides good acid suppression over time, as any drug that escapes premature gastric degradation begins to provide its own "enteric coating" by raising the gastric pH.

For most causes of upper GI ulceration or bleeding, cats should be treated twice-daily with a PPI.[22,35,36] If once-daily administration is necessary or compliance is a concern, orally administered esomeprazole may be an effective option although likely less effective than twice-daily administration.[37] In published and preliminary studies, both twice-daily administered omeprazole and esomeprazole appear to be effective in raising feline gastric pH. However, caution is recommended when opting for newer acid suppressants such as lansoprazole and dexlansoprazole in cats, as these might not be as effective as esomeprazole and omeprazole.

Adverse effects of PPI administration in cats can include a transient induction of faecal dysbiosis,[38] hypergastrinaemia, and drug withdrawal–induced rebound gastric acid hypersecretion.[39] Serum gastrin concentrations should normalise within 7 days following PPI cessation.[40] PPIs are inhibitors of the hepatic CYP450 system. Thus, interactions due to concurrent PPI administration are possible with drugs that are affected by increased gastric pH or CYP450 inhibition. Chronic use of PPIs and H_2RAs or prophylactic administration for diseases in which a benefit has not been demonstrated is discouraged due to reports of an association with a wide variety of adverse effects in people following long-term PPI use, including CKD, osteoporosis and pathological fractures, community-acquired pneumonia, *Clostridioides difficile*–associated diarrhoea, and spontaneous bacterial peritonitis. However, the quality of evidence for causation of PPIs for most of these adverse effects is low.

Antacids

Antacids (e.g. calcium carbonate, aluminium hydroxide, magnesium hydroxide) neutralise local gastric acid but do not effectively inhibit gastric acid secretion and are therefore less effective than acid suppressants in treating gastric ulceration. Moreover, they likely need to be administered frequently when used as a monotherapy to maintain their effect on gastric acid neutralisation, which can lead to poor compliance in cats. Therefore, antacids are not recommended as a sole therapy for the treatment of gastric ulceration.

Antacids can have a beneficial effect in cats with painful erosive or ulcerative lesions such as oral mucositis or erosive oesophagitis. They may also promote local prostaglandin production.

Side effects of antacid administration include constipation (aluminium preparations), diarrhoea (magnesium preparations), and electrolyte derangements. Antacids have been observed to cause a minor increase in urinary pH in people. This effect has not been evaluated in cats, but long-term use in cats with a predisposition towards struvite stones is not advised.

Coating agents

Sucralfate

Sucralfate is the basic aluminium hydroxide salt of sucrose octasulphate and is divided into sucrose sulphate and aluminium salts in the presence of gastric acid. The negatively charged sulphate groups protect the ulcerated tissue from additional injury by binding electrostatically to positively charged proteins exposed in ulcerated areas. Sucralfate's affinity for abnormal, injured tissue is five times greater than that for normal mucosa. Sucralfate also reduces pepsin activity and stimulates the release of protective prostaglandins, which in turn increases mucosal blood flow and increases mucus production and viscosity.[41] Sucralfate is particularly beneficial when pain is an anticipated sequela, such as with reflux oesophagitis. In an experimental model of acid-induced feline oesophagitis, high-dose (1 g) orally administered sucralfate was more effective in preventing lesions as compared to high-dose (40–100 mg/kg) topical and intraperitoneal injections of cimetidine[26] or misoprostol (5–100 µg/kg).[42] Sucralfate is not effective when administered as a whole or divided tablet and should be orally administered as a suspension or slurry.

Sucralfate is associated with very few adverse effects, aside from constipation and drug interactions. However, its use, especially at high doses, is discouraged in cats with CKD.[43] Sucralfate does change the pH of the stomach and therefore can interfere with the metabolism of drugs that are dependent on an acidic gastric pH (e.g. PPIs). It also interferes with drugs affected by the aluminium component of sucralfate (e.g. tetracyclines, ciprofloxacin).[44,45] Therefore, these drugs should be administered at least 2 hours before or after sucralfate administration.

Barium

Barium, like sucralfate, is proposed to have mucosal protecting effects and haemostatic properties. However, to the author's knowledge, there are no published studies evaluating the efficacy of barium for gastric injury or bleeding in cats. Barium enemas are effective for treatment of lower GI bleeding in humans. The dose recommended for mucosal haemostasis (1–2 ml/kg) can be challenging to administer in cats, especially in those displaying dysrexia or vomiting. Although barium is inert, aspiration of barium with gastric fluid contents can be fatal. Barium should be discontinued for at least 24 hours prior to GI endoscopy, and it should not be used if GI perforation is suspected.

Take-home messages

- Drug dissolution, absorption, and metabolism in cats can be distinctly different from those in humans and dogs. The ability to administer medications into a moribund cat is also a concern. Therefore, drug choice, route, and frequency of administration should be considered on a patient-by-patient basis and specifically tailored for the cat.
- Maropitant and mirtazapine are available in Food and Drug Administration–approved formulations for the treatment of vomiting and unintended weight loss, respectively, in the cat.
- Proton pump inhibitors are the most effective drug for the medical treatment of gastric ulceration. However, they are not effective for all causes of gastrointestinal ulceration. The choice of gastroprotective drug should be guided by the cause and location of gastrointestinal injury and the potential for adverse effects.

REFERENCES

[1] Quimby JM et al. Chronic use of maropitant for the management of vomiting and inappetence in cats with chronic kidney disease: a blinded, placebo-controlled clinical trial. *J Feline Med Surg* 17:692, 2015.

[2] Hickman MA et al. Safety, pharmacokinetics and use of the novel NK-1 receptor antagonist maropitant (Cerenia) for the prevention of emesis and motion sickness in cats. *J Vet Pharmacol Ther* 31:220, 2008.

[3] Martin-Flores M et al. Maropitant administered orally 2–2.5 h prior to morphine and dexmedetomidine reduces the incidence of emesis in cats. *J Feline Med Surg* 19:876, 2017.

[4] Kanda T et al. Antiemetic effect of oral maropitant treatment before the administration of brimonidine ophthalmic solution in healthy cats. *J Feline Med Surg* 22:557, 2020.

[5] Niyom S et al. Effect of maropitant, a neurokinin-1 receptor antagonist, on the minimum alveolar concentration of sevoflurane during stimulation of the ovarian ligament in cats. *Vet Anaesth Analg* 40:425, 2013.

[6] Martin-Flores M et al. Effects of maropitant in cats receiving dexmedetomidine and morphine. *J Am Vet Med Assoc* 248:1257, 2016.

[7] Quimby JM, Lunn KF. Mirtazapine as an appetite stimulant and anti-emetic in cats with chronic kidney disease: a masked placebo-controlled crossover clinical trial. *Vet J* 197:651, 2013.

[8] Milano S et al. Vagal-induced vomiting in decerebrate cat is not suppressed by specific 5-HT3 receptor antagonists. *J Auton Nerv Syst* 31:109, 1990.

[9] Quimby JM et al. Oral, subcutaneous, and intravenous pharmacokinetics of ondansetron in healthy cats. *J Vet Pharmacol Ther* 37:348, 2014.

[10] Santos LC et al. A randomized, blinded, controlled trial of the antiemetic effect of ondansetron on dexmedetomidine-induced emesis in cats. *Vet Anaesth Analg* 38:320, 2011.

[11] Fitzpatrick RL et al. Limited sampling pharmacokinetics of subcutaneous ondansetron in healthy geriatric cats, cats with chronic kidney disease, and cats with liver disease. *J Vet Pharmacol Ther* 39:350, 2016.

[12] Zajic LB et al. Assessment of absorption of transdermal ondansetron in normal research cats. *J Feline Med Surg* 19:1245, 2017.

[13] Kolahian S, Jarolmasjed S. Effects of metoclopramide on emesis in cats sedated with xylazine hydrochloride. *J Feline Med Surg* 12:899, 2010.

[14] Hillemeier C et al. Effect of bethanechol and metoclopramide on upper gastrointestinal motility in the kitten. *J Pediatr Gastroenterol Nutr* 5:134, 1986.

[15] Mangel AW, Stavorski JR, Pendleton RG. Effects of bethanechol, metoclopramide, and domperidone on antral contractions in cats and dogs. *Digestion* 28:205, 1983.

[16] Fitzpatrick RL et al. In vivo and in vitro assessment of mirtazapine pharmacokinetics in cats with liver disease. *J Vet Intern Med* 32:1951, 2018.

[17] Quimby JM, Gustafson DL, Lunn KF. The pharmacokinetics of mirtazapine in cats with chronic kidney disease and in age-matched control cats. *J Vet Intern Med* 25:985, 2011.

[18] Ferguson LE et al. Mirtazapine toxicity in cats: retrospective study of 84 cases (2006–2011). *J Feline Med Surg* 18:868, 2016.

[19] Ho CM et al. Dexamethasone has a central antiemetic mechanism in decerebrated cats. *Anesth Analg* 99:734, table of contents, 2004.

[20] Darmani NA, Belkacemi L, Zhong W. Δ^9-THC and related cannabinoids suppress substance P-induced neurokinin NK_1-receptor-mediated vomiting via activation of cannabinoid CB_1 receptor. *Eur J Pharmacol* 865:172806, 2019.

[21] Marks SL et al. ACVIM consensus statement: support for rational administration of gastrointestinal protectants to dogs and cats. *J Vet Intern Med* 32:1823, 2018.

[22] Šutalo S et al. The effect of orally administered ranitidine and once-daily or twice-daily orally administered omeprazole on intragastric pH in cats. *J Vet Intern Med* 29:840, 2015.

[23] Parkinson S et al. Evaluation of the effect of orally administered acid suppressants on intragastric pH in cats. *J Vet Intern Med* 29:104, 2015.

[24] Golly E et al. The frequency of oral famotidine administration influences its effect on gastric pH in cats over time. *J Vet Intern Med* 33:544, 2019.

[25] Coruzzi G et al. Inhibitory effect of famotidine on cat gastric secretion. *Agents Actions* 19:188, 1986.

[26] Clark S et al. Comparison of potential cytoprotective action of sucralfate and cimetidine. Studies with experimental feline esophagitis. *Am J Med* 83:56, 1987.

[27] Johnson LM, Lankford SM, Bai SA. The influence of cimetidine on the pharmacokinetics of the enantiomers of verapamil in the dog during multiple oral dosing. *J Vet Pharmacol Ther* 18:117, 1995.

[28] Maskasame C, Lankford S, Bai SA. The effects of chronic oral diltiazem and cimetidine dosing on the pharmacokinetics and negative dromotropic action of intravenous and oral diltiazem in the dog. *Biopharm Drug Dispos* 13:521, 1992.

[29] Shah SS et al. Inhibitory effects of ketoconazole, cimetidine and erythromycin on hepatic CYP3A activities in cats. *J Vet Med Sci* 71:1151, 2009.

[30] Sako J, Yasuda Y. The effect of intravenous cimetidine and histamine on splanchnic circulation in the dogs. [In Japanese]. *Nihon Shokakibyo Gakkai Zasshi* 90:1405, 1993.

[31] de Brito Galvao JF, Trepanier LA. Risk of hemolytic anemia with intravenous administration of famotidine to hospitalized cats. *J Vet Intern Med* 22:325, 2008.

[32] Williamson KK et al. Efficacy of omeprazole versus high-dose famotidine for prevention of exercise-induced gastritis in racing Alaskan sled dogs. *J Vet Intern Med* 24:285, 2010.

[33] Lane M et al. Medical management of gastrinoma in a cat. *JFMS Open Rep* 2:2055116916646389, 2016.

[34] Garcia RS et al. Prevalence of gastroesophageal reflux in cats during anesthesia and effect of omeprazole on gastric pH. *J Vet Intern Med* 31:734, 2017.

[35] Tolbert K et al. Efficacy of oral famotidine and 2 omeprazole formulations for the control of intragastric pH in dogs. *J Vet Intern Med* 25:47, 2011.

[36] Bersenas AM et al. Effects of ranitidine, famotidine, pantoprazole, and omeprazole on intragastric pH in dogs. *Am J Vet Res* 66:425, 2005.

[37] Hwang JH et al. Pharmacokinetics and acid suppressant efficacy of esomeprazole after intravenous, oral, and subcutaneous administration to healthy Beagle dogs. *J Vet Intern Med* 31:743, 2017.

[38] Schmid SM et al. Omeprazole minimally alters the fecal microbial community in six cats: a pilot study. *Front Vet Sci* 5:79, 2018.

[39] Gould E et al. A prospective, placebo-controlled pilot evaluation of the effect of omeprazole on serum calcium, magnesium, cobalamin, gastrin concentrations, and bone in cats. *J Vet Intern Med* 30:779, 2016.

[40] Parente NL et al. Serum concentrations of gastrin after famotidine and omeprazole administration to dogs. *J Vet Intern Med* 28:1465, 2014.

[41] Shorrock CJ, Rees WD. Effect of sucralfate on human gastric bicarbonate secretion and local prostaglandin E2 metabolism. *Am J Med* 86:2, 1989.

[42] Katz PO et al. Acid-induced esophagitis in cats is prevented by sucralfate but not synthetic prostaglandin E. *Dig Dis Sci* 33:217, 1988.

[43] Quimby J, Lappin M. Evaluating sucralfate as a phosphate binder in normal cats and cats with chronic kidney disease. *J Am Anim Hosp Assoc* 52:8, 2016.

[44] KuKanich K, KuKanich B. The effect of sucralfate tablets vs. suspension on oral doxycycline absorption in dogs. *J Vet Pharmacol Ther* 38:169, 2015.

[45] KuKanich K et al. Effect of sucralfate on the relative bioavailability of enrofloxacin and ciprofloxacin in healthy fed dogs. *J Vet Intern Med* 30:108, 2016.

CHAPTER 34

Antibiotics

Thomas Spillmann, Thomas Grönthal, Susanne Kilpinen

Originally, the term "antibiotics" referred to compounds naturally produced by microorganisms, but it stands increasingly as a synonym also for synthetic and semi-synthetic antimicrobials.

The overuse of antibiotics in human and veterinary medicine has led to the development of a wide range of bacteria resistant to one or multiple antibiotics. Drug resistance amongst protozoa is also of growing concern, but data on the prevalence of resistance amongst protozoa isolated from cats is scarce, and testing resistance in protozoa has not yet become a part of routine faecal examination.

Facing increasing amounts of multidrug-resistant bacteria with the potential of life-threatening infections led to the requirement of redefining the principles of antibiotic usage. State authorities and scientific societies are continuously updating guidelines that aim at a reduced use of antibiotics.

Optimal antimicrobial treatment in veterinary practice should include:

- reducing the overall antimicrobial usage;
- increasing the use of diagnostic testing (bacterial culture, antimicrobial susceptibility testing, polymerase chain reaction, fluorescence in situ hybridisation [FISH], molecular methods of faecal microbiota analysis such as dysbiosis index, etc.);
- limiting the empiric use of second-line critical important agents (e.g. fluoroquinolones, extended-spectrum cephalosporins);
- banning last-resort antibiotics from use in animals (e.g. carbapenems, vancomycin);
- optimising dosage regimens.

The current lack of scientific evidence and clinical data limits possibilities for informed decisions about the use of antibiotics in clinical practice. Cheap and reliable point-of-care tests are missing that discriminate viral and bacterial infections or detect bacterial or protozoal resistance to first-line antimicrobials. There is an increasing demand to find and introduce so-called green antimicrobials that are not chemically related to medically important antibiotics in humans and intended for veterinary use only.[1]

MODES OF RESISTANCE DEVELOPMENT

Resistance to an antibiotic emerges de novo (i.e. anew) through natural selection. Due to the diversity of any bacterial community, including intestinal microbiota, some of the bacteria will be less sensitive to the applied antibiotic than others are. As antibiotic treatment continues, only the strongest of each bacterial generation survive, and haphazard mutations (e.g. to the target of the antibiotic) will be favoured, giving access to more space and nutrients for those bacteria. This, combined with the ability of bacteria to transfer genes horizontally (from one strain to another), via for example plasmids, can lead to the development of multidrug resistance. De novo evolution of resistance is not required for infection; simple exposure to multidrug-resistant bacteria is enough. If an animal is an asymptomatic carrier of multidrug-resistant bacteria, any favourable selective pressure (e.g. antibiotic treatment) will likely increase the number of these organisms and thus the likelihood of prolonged carriage and possible spread.

The four major mechanisms of antimicrobial resistance in bacteria are reduced cell wall permeability, antimicrobial agent modification, active efflux, and target modification.[2] The rise of extended-spectrum beta-lactamase (ESBL)-producing bacteria has become a growing concern. These enzymes are produced primarily by *Escherichia coli* and other *Enterobacterales* species and can inactivate most beta-lactam antibiotics. The plasmids carrying genes that code for the diverse group of ESBL enzymes may also carry several other resistance genes. Antibiotic treatment increases the rate of transfer of ESBL plasmids between bacterial species, and likely increases the number of these bacteria in an animal carrier.

BACTERIA AND PROTOZOA ASSOCIATED WITH FELINE GASTROINTESTINAL DISEASES AND THEIR REPORTED RESISTANCES

Bacteria and protozoa associated with diseases of the feline gastrointestinal (GI) tract are listed in alphabetical order in Table 34.1. The only report about resistance of protozoa in cats concerns the in vitro and in vivo resistance of *Tritrichomonas blagburni* (former feline *T. foetus*) to ronidazole, which is the current drug of choice to treat feline tritrichomoniasis (Table 34.4). The main pathogenic or suspected pathogenic bacteria of the feline GI tract are *Campylobacter* spp., *Clostridioides difficile* (*C. diff*), *Clostridium perfringens*, *E. coli*, and *Salmonella* spp.[3] Bacterial resistance profiles differ between studies and regions, and local resistance data should be taken into account whenever empirical therapy is initiated.

One recent study from Italy revealed a high frequency of multidrug resistance (31% of the isolates) and presence of ESBL/plasmid-mediated AmpC (pAmpC)-type beta-lactamase-producing *Enterobacterales* in samples taken from cats (including their GI tract). The percentage of resistant isolates was 61.3% for amoxicillin–clavulanate, 33.6% for trimethoprim–sulphamethoxazole, and 36% for third-generation cephalosporins. Nine isolates had pAmpC beta-lactamases.[4] Another study tested the resistance profile of anaerobes in dogs, cats, and horses. Most samples from cats originated from abdominal fluid followed by liver, gallbladder, bile, GI tract, and faeces. Only specimens from abdominal fluid yielded obligate anaerobes, with the most common isolated species being *C. perfringens* followed by *Bacteroides fragilis*. Resistance against amoxicillin–clavulanate, ampicillin, chloramphenicol, clindamycin, metronidazole, and penicillin was rare, implying that anaerobes are generally sensitive to antimicrobial drugs in vitro. The results suggest an empirical choice of antimicrobial drugs based on animal species and location of infection remains a reasonable clinical decision for treatment of suspected anaerobic infections.[5]

Campylobacter spp.–positive faecal cultures have been reported for healthy and diseased cats. There is limited information on the sensitivity of feline *Campylobacter* spp. isolates to antibiotics, with some evidence for regional differences. An Iranian study reported that the largest proportion of *C. jejuni* and *C. coli* was resistant to tetracycline followed by erythromycin. *C. jejuni* was also highly resistant to nalidixic acid, fluoroquinolones, amoxicillin, cefazolin, and lincomycin. In contrast, an Irish study found that the majority of *C. jejuni* isolates expressed no resistance at all. Ciprofloxacin resistance was 20%, while resistance to tetracycline (14%) and erythromycin (12%) was less common. No resistance to erythromycin was detected in a Norwegian study on *Campylobacter* spp. in pets. The results of a case control study suggest an association of mucosal invasion by *C. coli* with feline neutrophilic but not with lymphoplasmacytic chronic enteropathy (CE).

C. diff is rarely reported in cats and there is limited information on antimicrobial susceptibility. According to reports 0%–21% of cats in the general population are colonised with *C. diff*, but a recent study showed a very low prevalence (2%) in Brazil and all reported 16 isolates were sensitive to metronidazole but resistant to ciprofloxacin.

C. perfringens has an unclear role as a pathogen, and there is a lack of evidence for benefits of antimicrobial treatment of *C. perfringens*–associated diarrhoea in cats.

E. coli is part of the normal intestinal microbiome in cats. However, cats have also been described as carriers of diarrhoeagenic *E. coli* (DEC), such as enterohaemorrhagic *E. coli*, Shiga toxin–producing *E. coli*, and verotoxigenic *E. coli*. Sensitivity to antibiotics amongst isolates varies significantly, from completely sensitive to multidrug-resistant, but resistance to ampicillin may be high in certain regions.[6]

Table 34.1. Bacteria and protozoa associated with diarrhoea in cats.

Organism	Comments	Antibiotics of choice (see Appendix for recommended dosages)
Bacteria		
***Campylobacter* spp.**	Commonly asymptomatic, but young animals may show signs of mild to moderate enteritis. Molecular methods superior to bacterial culture for rapid and accurate diagnosis. *C. coli* possibly associated with feline neutrophilic chronic enteropathy.	Erythromycin (drug of choice), cefazolin, clindamycin
Clostridioides difficile	No clear association with clinical disease in cats. Prevalence in faecal samples of cats in Germany = 2.5%, but no parallel occurrence of *C. diff* in cats and owners of the same household.	No recommendations
Clostridium perfringens	Studies have failed to show an association with clinical disease in cats.	No recommendations
Escherichia coli	• Toxigenic: no clear association with clinical disease in cats. • Intracellular: one case report of *E. coli*–induced granulomatous colitis diagnosed with fluorescence in situ hybridisation.	Toxigenic: no recommendations Intracellular: enrofloxacin (14 days); use with caution and at recommended dose—overdose can cause retina degeneration
***Mycobacterium* spp.**	Intestinal disease, weight loss, anaemia, vomiting, and diarrhoea may be present as well as enlarged mesentery lymph nodes. *M. tuberculosis* is a zoonosis.	Rapidly growing mycobacteria: high-dose doxycycline or a fluoroquinolone Tuberculosis: clarithromycin, rifampin, and a fluoroquinolone; euthanasia may be preferred
***Salmonella* spp.**	Prevalence in feline faecal samples sent to US laboratories <1%, diarrhoeic and nondiarrhoeic cats can shed *Salmonella* spp. May cause sepsis in individuals. Important zoonosis.	Diarrhoea: no treatment Severe cases: treatment based on susceptibility testing Sepsis: ampicillin + enrofloxacin (avoid dose >5 mg/kg every 24 h)
***Yersinia* spp.**	*Y. enterocolitica* and *Y. pseudotuberculosis* can both be detected in faeces of healthy cats. • *Y. enterocolitica*: prevalence in feline faecal samples sent to a European laboratory = 0.03%. Cats with and without diarrhoea can shed *Y. enterocolitica* 4/O:3 especially when being fed raw pork. • *Y. pseudotuberculosis*: single case reports of infectious hepatitis in cats. One cat responded to potentiated amoxicillin and marbofloxacin.	Fluoroquinolones or aminoglycosides are indicated in systemic illness
Protozoa	All enteric protozoal infections may cause abdominal discomfort, increased gas or fluid in the intestinal tract, and thickened intestinal loops.	
***Cryptosporidium* spp.**	Commonly asymptomatic; immunocompromised cats can have small intestinal diarrhoea. *C. felis* can cause disease in immunocompetent and immunocompromised humans.	Azithromycin, paromomycin, tylosin tartrate
Cystoisospora felis* *Cystoisospora rivolta	Commonly asymptomatic; immunocompromised kittens and cats can have large or mixed intestinal diarrhoea (mucoid diarrhoea, haematochezia, weight loss).	Sulphadimethoxine, trimethoprim–sulphamethoxazole, trimethoprim–sulphadiazine
Entamoeba histolytica	Commonly large or mixed intestinal diarrhoea.	Metronidazole and diiodohydroxyquin
***Giardia* spp.**	Commonly small intestinal diarrhoea; can be asymptomatic or cause chronic continuous or intermittent diarrhoea and weight loss. Clinical illness most commonly seen in young animals.	Metronidazole, fenbendazole (preferred due to higher efficacy)
Toxoplasma gondii	Commonly subclinical; intestinal form once in a lifetime and brief (3 weeks), with possible small intestinal diarrhoea. Kittens shed much higher numbers of oocysts than adult cats. Systemic form in young or immunocompromised cats with ocular, respiratory, and neurological signs.	Clindamycin
Tritrichomonas blagburni* *Pentatrichomonas hominis	Commonly large or mixed intestinal diarrhoea in young animals. Feline *T. blagburni* biologically different from *T. foetus* of cattle, no transmission to humans reported. *P. hominis* is zoonotic.	Ronidazole

Salmonella spp. can be multidrug-resistant and have shown to spread between cats in the same animal shelter or cattery and infect humans. It is important, however, to note that the overall prevalence of *Salmonella* spp. in cats is low (0%–6%).

PLANNING ANTIBIOTIC TREATMENT IN CATS WITH CLINICAL SIGNS OF A GASTROINTESTINAL TRACT DISEASE

To decide for or against the use of an antibiotic, it is helpful to follow a flow chart (Fig. 34.1) and to consider the patient's clinical conditions and findings that may raise the suspicion of a bacterial or protozoal infection (Table 34.2). Once the decision is in favour of an antibiotic, its selection should be based on its antimicrobial spectrum and pharmacokinetics. In addition, considerations whether the bacterial or protozoal infection is local or generalised should influence the decision about the use of single or combined antibiotics and the route of administration.

Important pharmacokinetics of antibiotics

When designing the antibiotic treatment regime for a patient, it is important to differentiate between time- and concentration-dependent antibiotics. The three main

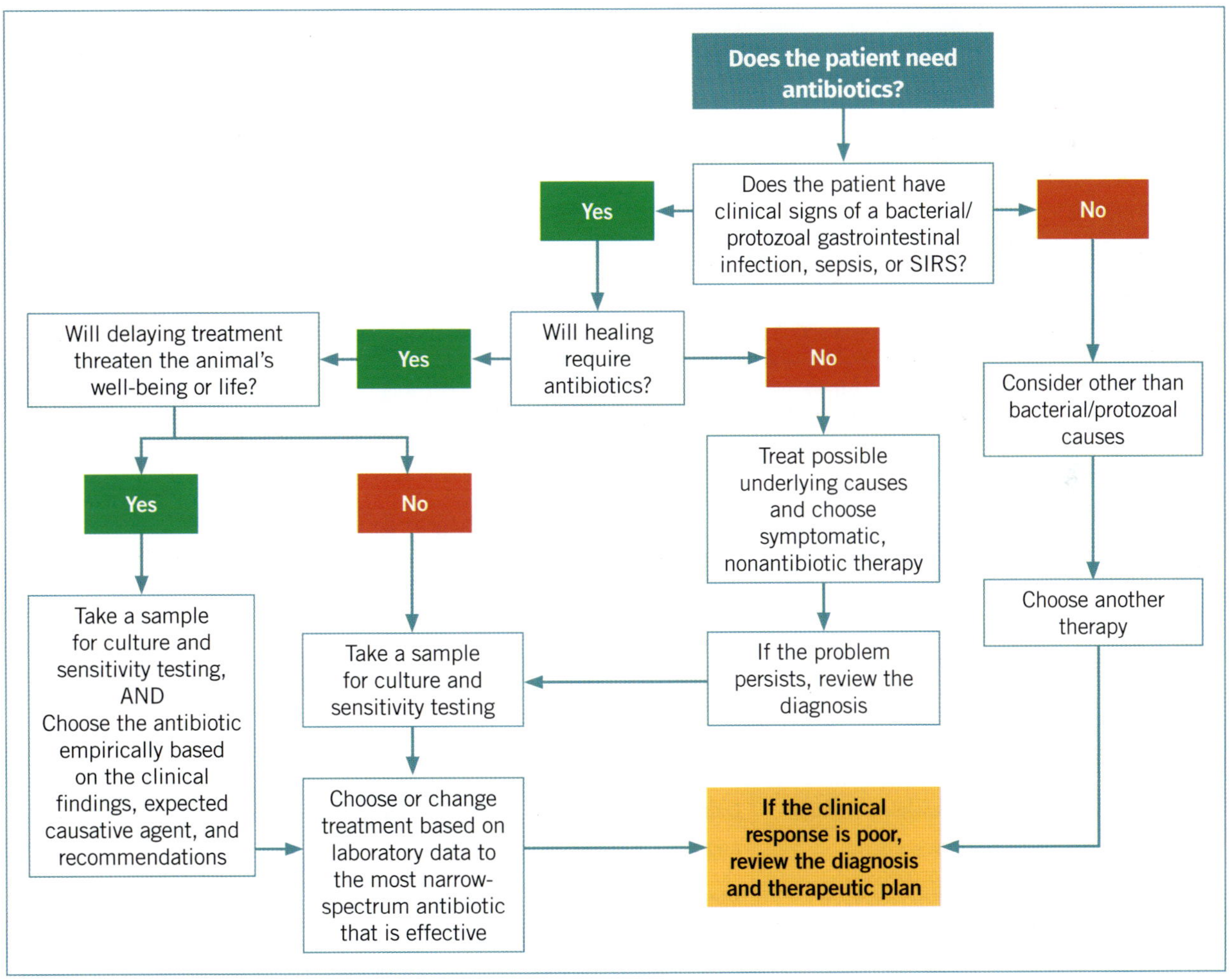

Figure 34.1. Flow chart about deciding for or against the use of antibiotics in cats with alimentary tract diseases. SIRS, systemic inflammatory response syndrome. Based on the Federation of European Companion Animal Veterinary Associations (FECAVA) Advice on Responsible Use of Antimicrobials, 2018. Available from: https://www.fecava.org/wp-content/uploads/2020/01/FECAVA-Advice-on-Responsible-use-of-Antimicrobials-ENGLISH.pdf.

pharmacokinetic parameters of interest are T>MIC, C_{max}/MIC, and AUC/MIC (T, time; C_{max}, maximum plasma concentration; AUC, area under the curve; MIC, minimum inhibitory concentration—the concentration that inhibits the growth of the bacteria causing the infection) (Table 34.3).[2,7]

- **T>MIC.** Time-dependent antibiotics rely on the prolonged exposure of the bacterium to the antibiotic. An increase of the dosage will not significantly improve their efficacy and may even hamper antimicrobial potency. Antibiotics with very short half-lives (e.g. beta-lactams) are more effective when given in shorter

Table 34.2. Patient status, conditions, signs, and laboratory findings increasing the suspicion of a bacterial infection as cause of diarrhoea in cats.

Patient status, condition, or findings	Detailed information
Signalment	Young, old, debilitated
Housing	Overcrowded, breeding facility, shelter, hospitalisation, clinical signs in contact animals or humans
Husbandry	Feeding raw or undercooked food
Medical history	Vaccination, receiving antibiotics or immunosuppressive drugs, comorbidities (e.g. diabetes mellitus)
Clinical signs	Haematochezia (predisposition for bacterial translocation) Sepsis/systemic inflammatory response syndrome (SIRS) • Pale mucous membranes • Prolonged capillary refill time • Poor to absent pulses SIRS criteria (without evidence for infection) • Rectal temperature: ≤37.8°C or ≥39.7°C (≤100°F or ≥103.5°F) • Heart frequency: <140 or >225 beats/minute • Respiratory rate: ≥40 breaths/minute

Laboratory findings	Blood
	• Leucopenia/leucocytosis with clinical signs of sepsis
	  • <5000/µl or
	  • >19500/µl or
	  • >5% band neutrophil percentage
	• Hypoglycaemia (in sepsis)
	• Hypoalbuminaemia (in sepsis)
	• Serological evidence of infection
	Faeces
	• Negative virology and parasitology
	• Positive faecal culture or PCR for potentially pathogenic bacteria
	• Presence of bacterial toxins
	Rectal scrape cytology
	• Leucocytosis
	Biopsy samples of intestinal mucosa
	• Fluorescence in situ hybridisation detects intracellular bacteria

Table 34.3. Pharmacodynamic/pharmacokinetic parameters for antibiotics.

	Time-dependent (T>MIC)	Concentration-dependent (C_{max}/MIC)	Concentration- and time-dependent (AUC/MIC)
Bactericidal	Penicillins Cephalosporins Sulpha–trimethoprim	Aminoglycosides Fluoroquinolones* Metronidazole	Fluoroquinolones*
Bacteriostatic	Chloramphenicol Erythromycin Tylosin		Azithromycin Clindamycin Tetracycline

AUC, area under the curve; C_{max}, maximum concentration; T, time; MIC, minimum inhibitory concentration.
*In some cases, the AUC/MIC parameter is better at predicting clinical outcome in severely ill patients.

dosing intervals than by increasing the dose. In contrast, doubling the dose only adds one half-life to the effective time (approximately 1 hour with ampicillin).

- **C_{max}/MIC.** Concentration-dependent antibiotics need to be administered only once or twice daily. The higher the concentrations of the antibiotic, the more effective the treatment will be (i.e. higher concentrations kill bacteria faster). The main limitation for treatment or dosing are potential adverse drug reactions. Concentration-dependent antibiotics commonly have a postantibiotic effect (bacterial killing continues after the concentration has fallen below the MIC).[7]
- **AUC/MIC.** The AUC measures the total area of a concentration–time curve. The higher the concentration and the longer this high concentration is maintained, the better the treatment results. A sufficiently high AUC/MIC is also important for preventing development of antimicrobial resistance. The route of administration can also significantly affect the AUC. As an example, the AUC of enrofloxacin for kittens is 16.7 (μg × h/ml) when given IV at the recommended dose of 5 mg/kg, but only 5.7 when given PO at the same dose.

Clinical indications of antibiotics

Several authorities and scientific organisations have published guidelines on the empiric use of antibiotics, for example, the consensus statement of the American College of Veterinary Internal Medicine (ACVIM) on the treatment of enteropathogenic bacteria.[5] Regardless of regional differences, it should be the primary goal to use culture and sensitivity results for treatment decision whenever possible.

Oral diseases

The normal feline gingival margin hosts mostly anaerobic bacteria (71%–77%) that are very similar in composition to those found in catfight abscesses and feline pyothorax. Next generation sequencing revealed that the oral microbiota is largely conserved between healthy cats. Eight bacterial phyla comprise 98% of all sequences and include *Proteobacteria*, *Bacteroidetes*, *Firmicutes*, uncultured Bacteria candidate division Sulphur River 1 (SR1), *Spirochaetes*, *Fusobacteria*, and *Actinobacteria*.[8] The most commonly isolated aerobic/facultative anaerobic species is *Pasteurella multocida* followed by different *Actinomyces* spp. and *Propionibacterium terium*.[9]

Anaerobic bacteria associated with severity of gingivitis consist of *Bacteroides* spp., *Eubacterium aerofaciens*, and *Peptostreptococcus anaerobius*. Aerobe gingival bacteria include *Pasteurella multocida*, *Streptococcus* spp., *Enterococcus* spp., *Staphylococcus* spp., *Bacillus cereus*, *E. coli*, and *Pseudomonas aeruginosa*.

Since the primary aetiology of feline oral and dental diseases is mostly nonbacterial and their treatment rather local or surgical, national and international guidelines prioritise the removal of dental tartar, followed by local treatment with chlorhexidine or other antiseptic preparations. The American Veterinary Dental College (AVDC) recommends the use of systemically administered antibiotics only for animals that are immunocompromised, have underlying systemic disease (e.g. clinically evident cardiac, hepatic, and renal disease), and/or severe oral infections. The use of antibiotics for monotherapy or preventive management of oral conditions is discouraged.[10,11] In addition, the wide variety of drugs used (7 antibiotics in 28 cats in one study) and the lack of standardised treatment protocols do often not allow for useful conclusions. For more detailed information see Chapter 10.

Oesophageal diseases

The feline oesophageal mucosa is sensitive to a large variety of drugs including certain antibiotics. Tetracycline, doxycycline, and clindamycin can cause ulcers and strictures when given orally to cats without being accompanied by swallowing either water or food. For doxycycline, there is some evidence that its monohydrate salt has less ulcerogenic effects on the oesophageal mucosa than the hydrochloride salt. It seems likely that a recently introduced liquid formulation might produce less oesophageal irritation than doxycycline tablets.

Feline oesophageal diseases rarely require antibiotic treatment (see Chapter 11). Some clinicians have used antibiotics after endoscopic treatment procedures such as foreign body removal, stricture balloon dilation or bougienage, and stent placement. However, cats often improved after such procedures without antibiotics, putting their regular use after endoscopic interventions in question.

Oesophageal perforation as well as caudal mediastinal paraoesophageal abscesses (CMPA) with pneumomediastinitis and/or thoracic effusion in cats generally require surgical management and antibiotic treatment. The bacteria most commonly associated with CMPA have been *Nocardia* spp. and *Actinomyces* spp.

Aspiration pneumonia can occur in cats with oesophageal disorders but also in a plethora of other conditions. The antibiotic treatment of suspected bacterial pneumonia is often empirical. It should follow, however, the recommendations of the Antimicrobial Guidelines Working Group of the International Society for Companion Animal Infectious Diseases. It is advised to reevaluate animals 10–14 days after starting the antibiotics to decide whether to extend their use or not.[12]

Gastric diseases

The use of antibiotics in feline gastric diseases is very limited. There are no reports about acute bacterial gastric infections in cats, making the use of antibiotics in acute gastritis obsolete. Chronic bacterial infections of the feline stomach include the controversial *Helicobacter*-associated gastritis and the rather rare gastric actinomycosis. The prevalence of *Helicobacter* spp. in cats is high but their presence does not correlate with clinical signs or histological severity of gastritis, probably since most *Helicobacter* spp. belong to the normal gastric microbiota. However, there is some evidence that *Helicobacter* spp. induce lymphoid follicular hyperplasia and mild gastritis and can possibly be associated with gastric lymphoma. Some consensus exists that *Helicobacter* spp. infection should only be treated in cats with massive gastric pit or intracellular colonisation in connection with marked inflammation. Treatment regimens include the combination of three to four drugs. Triple therapy (metronidazole, amoxicillin, omeprazole or bismuth subsalicylate) does not lead to full eradication. *Helicobacter* spp. can persist in extragastric sites like plaque, saliva, and gastric fluid. Quadruple therapy (amoxicillin, metronidazole, clarithromycin, omeprazole) of asymptomatic cats did also not succeed in an eradication.

Gastric actinomycosis was successfully treated in one cat with partial gastric resection and cefovecin for 4 months.[13]

Intestinal diseases

Primary bacterial infections of the intestine are rare in cats (see Chapter 14). In addition, the detection of potentially pathogenic bacteria in faeces of cats does not always establish a causality since healthy cats can shed such bacteria as often as cats with diarrhoea.

Acute intestinal disorders are mostly self-limiting, do not require antibiotics, and respond to symptomatic treatment. Primary bacterial infections of the intestine are considered likely in cats with acute diarrhoea under conditions listed in Table 34.2 when other infections and non-infective intra- or extraintestinal disorders are excluded.

Feline parvovirus infection with panleucopenia poses a risk for sepsis and requires coverage with a broad-spectrum antibiotic effective against gram-negative and anaerobic bacteria.

Salmonella infections in asymptomatic cats or cats with signs of mild enteritis should rather not be treated with antibiotics. It has been suggested that signs of digestive tract disease persist longer, and antibiotic treatment may prolong the excretion of *Salmonella* in faeces. In severe cases of intestinal disease, antibiotics effective against enteric gram-negative bacteria should be used such as amoxicillin, ampicillin, trimethoprim–sulphonamide, or fluoroquinolones. Septic patients should be treated with a beta-lactam (e.g. ampicillin or amoxicillin–clavulanic acid) combined with a fluoroquinolone.

Protozoal infections with *Giardia duodenalis*, *Tritrichomonas blagburni*, or *Pentatrichomonas hominis* can also be treated with antibiotics. Table 34.1 lists bacteria and protozoa next to the antibiotics of choice, if there is sufficient evidence to indicate their empirical or targeted use. Recommended dosages of antibiotics are provided in Appendix.

Feline CE is treated based on far less robust evidence than canine CE (see Chapters 17 and 18). In contrast to dogs, antibiotic-responsive diarrhoea or enteropathy has never been definitively identified in cats (see Chapter 18). Even though there is some low-level evidence in support of metronidazole as adjunctive treatment for CE, the actual effect of metronidazole in a multimodal treatment regimen remains questionable. Some review articles and textbooks recommend the use of tylosin in cats to treat possible antibiotic-responsive CE or colitis, but they refer to studies performed in dogs or other species. There have been no pharmacokinetic or clinical studies on tylosin in healthy cats or cats with CE. Feline neutrophilic CE has been associated with invasive *Campylobacter coli*. Whether an antibiotic treatment against *Campylobacter* spp. results in clinical improvement remains to be studied.

A case report suggests that feline granulomatous colitis involving enteroinvasive *E. coli* occurs, albeit more rarely than in dogs. The cat responded to a 14-day treatment course with enrofloxacin.[14]

Intestinal actinomycetomas are rarely reported. They resemble tumours and are treated with a combination of surgery and antibiotics such as clindamycin or cefovecin.

Pancreatic diseases

Studies in feline pancreatitis models have shown that *E. coli* can spread into the pancreas from the blood stream, small intestine, gallbladder (reflux into the pancreatic duct), or colon (transmural). Translocation of enteric bacteria was regarded the most likely source of infection in a clinical study evaluating pancreatic tissue sections of cats with and without acute or chronic pancreatitis by FISH. 35% of cats with moderate to severe pancreatitis were positive for *E. coli*, with the infection being most prevalent in cats with necrotising or suppurative severe acute pancreatitis and poor outcome.[15] A recent retrospective study in 157 cats with pancreatitis revealed that withholding antibiotic treatment was associated with an increased odd of death.[16] However, review articles on feline pancreatitis recommend that antibiotics should be reserved for cats presenting with shock, fever, marked leucocytosis, evidence of GI barrier breakdown, or pancreatic abscesses (see also Chapter 24). Prospective studies allowing an assessment of the necessity for prophylactic antibiotics in feline pancreatitis are lacking.

Pancreatic abscesses have been reported sporadically and bacterial infection with *E. coli* or *Staphylococcus aureus* has been documented. Infected pancreatic abscesses can be treated with antibiotics (based on antibiotic susceptibility testing) in combination with nonsurgical drainage or surgical intervention with omentalisation.

Biliary diseases

The World Small Animal Veterinary Association (WSAVA) Liver Standardization Group recognises three forms of feline cholangitis: neutrophilic (acute and chronic), lymphocytic, and chronic, liver fluke–associated (see Chapters 30 and 31). Neutrophilic cholangitis is the most commonly reported form and often accompanied by cholecystitis.[17] Bile analysis and/or liver biopsy for cytology/histology and bacterial culture are necessary for definitive diagnosis, and antimicrobial treatment should be selected according to in vitro susceptibility testing.

However, empirical antibiotic treatments may be indicated in clinically unstable cats with suspected neutrophilic cholangitis, when invasive procedures are a risk or declined by the owners. The most common organisms identified in bacterial cultures of bile and liver tissue are *E. coli*, *Enterococcus* spp., *Bacteroides* spp., and *Clostridium* spp. Numerous isolates of *E. coli* are reportedly resistant to amoxicillin–clavulanate and first-generation cephalosporins. Anaerobic gram-negative rods (primarily *Bacteroides* spp.) were reported as beta-lactamase positive. Thus, empirical antimicrobial therapy should include extended coverage for aerobic gram-positive and gram-negative bacteria and anaerobes, and may require more than one antimicrobial agent. Antibiotics chosen for cholangitis treatment should be excreted into the bile in their active form. Several reports show multidrug-resistant bacteria in cats with cholangitis, such as *Providencia rettgeri* (treated with pradofloxacin) or *Enterococcus faecium* (persistent infection despite treatment with vancomycin). It is of importance to be aware of the resistance patterns of the own region since it might not be the same as in published articles.

The optimal duration of antimicrobial therapy in feline cholangitis and cholecystitis is unknown and treatment success is often monitored by resolution of clinical signs. In most cases, a 4- to 6-week course has been recommended, but the lack of references indicates that such recommendations are based on anecdotal clinical experience. In people, a duration of antimicrobial treatment of 4–7 days is recommended.[18] Whether repeated deter-

Table 34.4. Antibiotics used in cats (alphabetical order): main indication, comments, and precautions. See Appendix for recommended dosages.

Drug	Main indications in diseases of the feline GI tract, liver, and pancreas	Comments and precautions
All		Any antibiotic given orally will cause changes in the intestinal microbiome and may lead to GI upset (i.e. vomiting and diarrhoea) (see Chapter 16). Any condition affecting drug metabolism or elimination (e.g. decreased function of liver or kidney) increases the risk of adverse effects and may warrant dose adjustment or change of drug. Susceptibility test results should be used whenever possible to guide treatment.
Amikacin	Rarely indicated. Use only in severe cases of multidrug-resistant organisms or when fluoroquinolones are contraindicated.	Broad spectrum against many aerobic bacteria. Less vestibular toxicity than gentamicin, potentially nephrotoxic, avoid in dehydrated animals and animals with renal disease, pregnant animals, and neonates.
Amoxicillin	Enteric infections caused by sensitive organisms.	Extended-spectrum penicillin. Very safe, only rare side effects. Aminopenicillins have a rather low volume of distribution and short half-life. Effective against many gram-positive bacteria. Many enteric bacteria are resistant such as *Bacteroides fragilis*, *Klebsiella* spp., *Enterobacter* spp., and *Yersinia enterocolitica* as well as beta-lactamase-producing staphylococci.
Amoxicillin–clavulanate	Numerous. May be of particular benefit in peritonitis and sepsis/bacteraemia (when combined with aminoglycoside or fluoroquinolone).	Like amoxicillin alone but has a broader spectrum, including beta-lactamase-producing staphylococci. Also effective against most anaerobes. Ineffective against MRSP/A and AmpC-producing bacteria. Uncertain effect against ESBL-producing bacteria. Repeated SC injection is not recommended due to the possibility of abscess formation.
Ampicillin sodium	See amoxicillin.	See amoxicillin.
Azithromycin	*Cryptosporidium felis* infection. May be used as a second choice for toxoplasmosis (see clindamycin). Also used in combination therapy in cases of mycobacterial infection.	Advanced-generation macrolide. More active against gram-negative bacteria than erythromycin and generally effective against *Mycoplasma* spp., variable effect against anaerobes. Fewer GI adverse effects than erythromycin and longer half-life. Bioavailability in cats is approximately 50%. Tissue concentration is generally 10–100x higher than in serum. Wide range of dose recommendations, no efficacy studies for feline cryptosporidiosis.
Cefoxitin	Severe mixed infections, including peritonitis.	Second-generation cephalosporin with a medium spectrum. Less effective than cefazolin against gram-positive bacteria, but broader gram-negative spectrum (*Serratia* spp. and *Enterobacter* spp.). Hypothrombinaemia has been described in humans. Pain when injected IM (avoid).
Cefovecin	Not often indicated.	Third-generation cephalosporin with a broad spectrum, similar to that of amoxicillin–clavulanate. MRSP/A and ESBL/AmpC producers are resistant. Strong binding to proteins leads to a long-lasting effect as well as a long period of sub-MIC levels. Very low volume of distribution (<0.1 l/kg). Vomiting and diarrhoea, as well as neurological signs and local reactions have been described in very rare cases.
Clindamycin	Periodontal disease and osteomyelitis (see Chapter 10). *Toxoplasma gondii.*	Activity against many aerobic gram-positive bacteria, anaerobic bacteria as well as *Campylobacter jejuni* and the protozoa *Toxoplasma gondii.* Most aerobic gram-negative bacteria are resistant. It has peripheral neuromuscular blocking and cardiac depressive effects—do not give with anaesthetics or by rapid IV injection. Generally safe in cats. However, oesophagitis and oesophageal ulceration/stricture have been reported. Use with caution in patients with liver failure.
Doxycycline	Chlamydial and mycoplasmal disease (as well as tick-borne diseases).	Broad spectrum, including *Mycoplasma* spp. and *Chlamydia* spp. Relatively safe but oral application may cause oesophageal ulceration and stricture in cats when not given with water or a small amount of food. Can be used in kittens >4 weeks of age without enamel discolouration. Give IV slowly. Also has anti-inflammatory effects. Avoid use in pregnant animals.
Enrofloxacin	Severe systemic illness (sepsis/bacteraemia) or peritonitis in combination with a beta-lactam.	Good tissue penetration and broad spectrum but not effective against anaerobes. Generally safe. Dose shall not exceed 5 mg/kg every 24 h. Side effects: • Most commonly nausea, vomiting, and diarrhoea. • Overdose >5 mg/kg/day can cause retinal degeneration. • Chronic, high-dose therapy may be harmful to cartilage formation in young animals <8 months of age. • Neurotoxic effects have been described. • Use with caution in patients with renal failure and pregnant animals.

Drug	Main indications in diseases of the feline GI tract, liver, and pancreas	Comments and precautions
Erythromycin	Drug of choice in treating *Campylobacter jejuni* enteritis.	Good spectrum against gram-positive aerobes and many anaerobes. Has effect against *Clostridium* spp. and *Campylobacter* spp. but is ineffective against all *Enterobacterales*. Relatively safe. Food interferes with absorption. Use with caution in patients with liver failure.
	Effect in upper GI tract (motilin agonist, serotonergic antagonist).	The use of an antibiotic as a prokinetic should be considered only when other prokinetics such as ranitidine/nizatidine, metoclopramide, or cisapride have failed.
Gentamicin	With sepsis or peritonitis in combination with a beta-lactam.	Requires parenteral dosing. Can be used as a substitute for fluoroquinolones in severe infections. Highly effective against aerobic gram-negative bacteria. Intracellular *Salmonella* are often resistant. Moderate otic and renal toxicity.
Marbofloxacin	See enrofloxacin.	See enrofloxacin. Reports about cases of retinal degeneration.
Metronidazole	Anaerobic (including clostridial) infections, giardiasis.	Very good activity against most anaerobes but ineffective against aerobic bacteria and *Actinomyces* spp. Neurotoxicity possible, with forebrain signs of seizures, altered mental status, behavioural changes, and visual deficits (acute with dose >60 mg/kg/day, delayed onset with dose >30 mg/kg/day). Reduce dose by 50% in animals with hepatic insufficiency. May cause chromosomal damage—do not give to pregnant queens and avoid use in neonates. Cats accept metronidazole benzoate better, when using recommended metronidazole dose, the benzoate concentration is nontoxic.
Pradofloxacin	In combination with other antibiotics in infections caused by rapidly growing mycobacteria.	Also see enrofloxacin. Broader spectrum than enrofloxacin, effective against gram-positive and some anaerobic bacteria. Effect against rapidly growing mycobacteria in vitro, but only few case reports regarding in vivo efficacy. Higher retinal safety in comparison to enrofloxacin (no retinal toxic effects at 6× and 10× the recommended dose). Only available in oral formulation.
Ronidazole	*Tritrichomonas blagburni* (formerly feline *T. foetus*).	Neurotoxicity in cats (lethargy, inappetance, ataxia, seizures). Side effects generally resolve, but drug needs to be discontinued immediately and signs may worsen for the next few days. Close monitoring is needed. Do not reinstitute or repeat treatment when toxicity occurred. Low doses (10 mg/kg) are prone to relapse, and treatment failure to higher dose should raise concern of resistance.
Sulphadimethoxine	*Cystoisospora* spp.	Sulphonamide antibiotic, see trimethoprim–sulphamethoxazole for main side effects.
Trimethoprim–sulphamethoxazole Trimethoprim–sulphadiazine	A wide variety of infections caused by sensitive bacteria. *Cystoisospora* spp.	Broad spectrum against aerobic gram-positive and gram-negative bacteria. Ineffective against anaerobes. Diverse set of adverse effect, which are usually reversible; crystalluria (followed by haematuria and even obstruction), haematopoietic disorders (thrombocytopenia, anaemia, leucopenia), and skin irritation. Significant reactions are rare when treatment lasts <2 weeks. Drooling may be apparent. Use with caution in patients with renal failure (combination) or liver failure (sulphonamides). Avoid use in pregnant animals and neonates.
Tylosin tartrate	*Cryptosporidium felis.*	See erythromycin. Only anecdotic use for feline cryptosporidiosis. Beneficial effects in dogs with CE, but no data on effect in cats with CE. Very few data on use in respiratory disorders. Use with caution in patients with liver failure.

CE, chronic enteropathy; ESBL, extended-spectrum beta-lactamase; GI, gastrointesinal; IM, intramuscular; IV, intravenous; MIC, minimum inhibitory concentration; MRSP/A, methicillin-resistant *Staphylococcus pseudintermedius/aureus*; SC, subcutaneous.

mination of feline serum amyloid A may help to assess antibiotic effects and to reduce the duration of antibiotic treatments still needs to be studied.

Feline extrahepatic bile duct obstruction (EHBDO) is reported in connection with extramural, intramural, or intraluminal biliary pathologies, and treatment aims at achieving patency of the common bile duct (CBD) and antibiotic treatment of bacterial infections (see Chapter 31). A bacterial cholangitis due to *E. coli* was reported in one icteric cat with a CBD cyst causing an intramural EHBDO. The cat was treated, with very good long-term outcome (7 months follow up), by performing surgical CBD stenting and intravenous application of metronidazole and cephalexin around the time of surgery. Based on sensitivity testing, cephalexin was continued orally for another 6 weeks. Intraluminal CBD blockage was described in one cat with bilirubin cholelithiasis and concurrent cholecystitis. Bacterial culture of the gallbladder contents at cholecystectomy yielded a pure growth of *Actinomyces* spp. The cat was successfully treated according to the susceptibility profile using oral cephalexin 15 mg/kg every 12 hours and metronidazole 10 mg/kg every 12 hours for 4 weeks. Minimally invasive endoscopic EHBDO treatment such as cholelith removal, papillary sphincterotomy, or stent placement is performed in humans, and there have been first attempts to establish such techniques also for cats.[19] However, experimental studies in cats revealed that sphincterotomy and CBD stenting can lead to ascending infections of the biliary tract and stent blockage, which can be partly addressed by prophylactic ciprofloxacin (25 mg every 12 hours PO for 16 weeks). When using endoscopic treatment options of EHBDO in cats, the result of those experimental studies should be taken into consideration in the attempt to prevent possible secondary bacterial cholangitis with recurrence of the CBD blockage.

Hepatic encephalopathy

The indication for antibiotics in cats depends on the hepatic encephalopathy (HE) type (see Chapter 28). In general, antibiotics should only be given short-term and during clinical exacerbations of HE. In human medicine, the nonabsorbable antibiotic rifaximin is widely used, but missing safety and efficacy data for cats prohibit its use in this species. Antibiotics used in feline HE include metronidazole, ampicillin, potentiated amoxicillin, and neomycin. Metronidazole is recommended to be given orally at a reduced dose of 7.5 mg/kg every 8–12 hours due to its hepatic metabolisation and possible neurological effects when being overdosed. Ampicillin can be given intravenously to cats that cannot receive oral medication. Neomycin is rather poorly absorbed by the intestine and has been used in conjunction with lactulose to treat feline HE. However, substantial systemic absorption can lead to ototoxicity and nephrotoxicity, and it is therefore not anymore used in people to treat HE.[20]

Take-home messages

- Growing resistance of bacteria and protozoa against antibiotics is of major concern.
- It is strongly advised that treatment decisions should be based on clinical and laboratory findings and the results of bacteriologic and parasitological examinations for pathogens (culture and sensitivity, PCR, fluorescence in situ hybridisation).
- Regional differences of antimicrobial resistance should be considered.
- Empiric antibiotic treatment can be started based on clinical suspicion if significant clinical deterioration or threat to life would otherwise occur, and while waiting for results of bacterial culture and sensitivity.
- Antibiotic treatments should be adjusted if necessary when test results of bacteria become available.
- Antibiotic treatment failure should always raise the suspicion for suboptimal dosing, immunosuppression, multidrug resistance, reinfection, or persistent infection due to sequestration in a "protected niche" from the immune system or the antibiotic.

REFERENCES

[1] Guardabassi L et al. Optimization of antimicrobial treatment to minimize resistance selection. *Microbiol Spectr* 6, 2018.

[2] Giguère S, Prescott JF, Dowling PM, editors. *Antimicrobial Therapy in Veterinary Medicine*, 5th ed. John Wiley & Sons, 2013.

[3] Marks SL et al. Enteropathogenic bacteria in dogs and cats: diagnosis, epidemiology, treatment, and control. *J Vet Intern Med* 25:1195, 2011.

[4] Piccolo FL et al. Detection of multidrug resistance and extended-spectrum/plasmid-mediated AmpC beta-lactamase genes in Enterobacteriaceae isolates from diseased cats in Italy. *J Feline Med Surg* 22:613, 2020.

[5] Lawhon SD, Taylor A, Fajt VR. Frequency of resistance in obligate anaerobic bacteria isolated from dogs, cats, and horses to antimicrobial agents. *J Clin Microbiol* 51:3804, 2013.

[6] Joosten P et al. Antimicrobial usage and resistance in companion animals: a cross-sectional study in three European countries. *Antibiotics (Basel)* 9: 87, 2020.

[7] Jessen LR et al. *Antibiotic Use Guidelines for Companion Animal Practice*, 2nd ed. Frederiksberg, Danish Small Animal Veterinary Association SvHKS, 2019.

[8] Sturgeon A et al. Characterization of the oral microbiota of healthy cats using next-generation sequencing. *Vet J* 201:223, 2014.

[9] Love DN, Vekselstein R, Collings S. The obligate and facultatively anaerobic bacterial flora of the normal feline gingival margin. *Vet Microbiol* 22:267, 1990.

[10] American Veterinary Dental College. *Position Statement: the Use of Antibiotics in Veterinary Dentistry*, 2019. Available from: https://avdc.org/wp-content/uploads/2019/AVDC-pos-stmts/Antibiotic_Use_April_2019.pdf.

[11] Sarkiala E. Use of antibiotics and antiseptics. In: Verstraete FJM, Lommer MJ, Arzi B. *Oral and Maxillofacial Surgery in Dogs and Cats*, 2nd ed. St Louis, Elsevier: 14, 2020.

[12] Lappin MR et al. Antimicrobial use guidelines for treatment of respiratory tract disease in dogs and cats: Antimicrobial Guidelines Working Group of the International Society for Companion Animal Infectious Diseases. *J Vet Intern Med* 31:279, 2017.

[13] Pietra M et al. Gastric inflammatory pseudotumour secondary to *Actinomyces hordeovulneris* infection in a cat. *Ir Vet J* 69:12, 2016.

[14] Matsumoto I et al. *Escherichia coli*-induced granulomatous colitis in a cat. *JFMS Open Rep* 5:2055116919836537, 2019.

[15] Simpson KW et al. Culture-independent detection of bacteria in feline pancreatitis. *Proceeding from the ACVIM Forum*, Denver (CO), USA, June 15–18, 2011.

[16] Nivy R et al. A retrospective study of 157 hospitalized cats with pancreatitis in a tertiary care center: clinical, imaging and laboratory findings, potential prognostic markers and outcome. *J Vet Intern Med* 32:1874, 2018.

[17] Boland L, Beatty J. Feline cholangitis. *Vet Clin North Am Small Anim Pract* 47:703, 2017.

[18] Gomi H et al. Tokyo Guidelines 2018: antimicrobial therapy for acute cholangitis and cholecystitis. *J Hepatobiliary Pancreat Sci* 25:3, 2018.

[19] Spillmann T et al. Feasibility of endoscopic retrograde cholangiopancreatography in healthy cats. *Vet Radiol Ultrasound* 55:85, 2014.

[20] Gow AG. Hepatic encephalopathy. *Vet Clin North Am Small Anim Pract* 47:585, 2017.

CHAPTER 35

Anti-inflammatories and immunosuppressants

Lauren Lacorcia, Julien R. S. Dandrieux

This chapter reviews the main drugs in current or emergent use for anti-inflammatory and immunosuppressant effect in feline gastroenterology. Some immunosuppressant drugs, such as prednisolone, have anti-inflammatory properties at lower doses. Pure anti-inflammatory drugs such as nonsteroidal anti-inflammatory drugs will not be discussed, as they do not play a significant role in the management of most diseases covered in this book.

Information on the pharmacological action, pharmacokinetics, pharmacodynamics, clinical use, and adverse effects for each drug will be summarised. For advice on treatment of specific conditions, please refer to the corresponding chapters.

GLUCOCORTICOIDS

Glucocorticoids (GCs) are steroid hormones naturally synthesised in the adrenal cortex that have major metabolic, anti-inflammatory, and immunosuppressive effects. Synthetic versions are frequently used in the management of inflammatory and immune-mediated feline gastrointestinal (GI) and hepatobiliary diseases, including chronic gingivostomatitis, idiopathic inflammatory bowel disease (IBD), and lymphocytic cholangitis, and for cytotoxic effect in round cell neoplasia.

Pharmacological effects

The effect of GCs is predominantly exerted by passive diffusion into the cell to bind to cytosolic GC receptors, forming activated complexes which then translocate into the cell nucleus and bind to genomic GC response elements.[1] This interaction then modulates expression of multiple genes, resulting in wide-ranging effects on virtually every cell type and system in the body (Table 35.1).[2] Nongenomic effects also occur by direct interactions with cell membranes to modulate cell signalling pathways and may account for some of the more rapid effects of GCs, particularly when used at high doses.

One of the major desirable clinical effects of GCs is to potently reduce inflammation of any cause, at all phases of the process.[4] Natural amounts of GCs caused by physiological stress sensitise the innate immune system to respond to harmful stimuli by increasing the expression of pattern recognition receptors, cytokine receptors, and complement factors, promoting a normal inflammatory response. In allergic and immune-mediated diseases, inflammation becomes excessive, prolonged, and causes tissue damage. In this situation, pharmacological use of synthetic GCs can dampen the inflammatory response.

In the initial phase of inflammation, GCs inhibit the release of biogenic amines and production of eicosanoids from tissue mast cells and macrophages, reducing vascular dilation and permeability. Both the production of and endothelial response to vasodilators and vasoconstrictors are altered, reducing blood flow to inflammatory sites. The barrier function of the endothelium is preserved to further reduce fluid leakage into tissues. Production of many pro-inflammatory cytokines is inhibited, including interleukin (IL)-1α, IL-1β, IL-2, IL-6, interferon gamma (IFN-γ), and tumour necrosis factor (TNF). Cell responses to these cytokines are attenuated. Reduced expression of adhesion molecules, chemokines, and chemoattractants prevents leucocyte migration into the tissues. As this is normally important for clearing pathogens and cell debris, suppressing this function can be detrimental in undiagnosed cases of infection.

In the natural resolution phase of inflammation, GCs have a physiological role in stimulating monocytes and macrophages to phagocytise apoptotic cells and debris before levels subside so that tissue healing can occur. Pharmacological use of GCs inhibits multiple important aspects of normal wound healing, including collagen deposition, angiogenesis, and reepithelialisation.

Table 35.1. Major pharmacological and adverse effects of glucocorticoids.

System	Major pharmacological effects across species	Adverse effects reported in cats
Immune	Inhibition of neutrophil, macrophage, and monocyte migration Inhibition of phagocytosis and chemotaxis Inhibition of lymphocytes (T to a greater extent than B) Reduced antigen processing and cell-mediated killing	Secondary infections
Haematopoietic	Increased circulating platelets, neutrophils, and erythrocytes Reduced circulating lymphocytes, monocytes, and eosinophils	
Metabolic and miscellaneous	Increased hepatic gluconeogenesis Mobilisation of fatty acids, increased plasma cholesterol and triglycerides, increased central fat deposition Increased protein catabolism Insulin resistance Inhibition of fibroblast proliferation and wound healing	Onset of diabetes mellitus Steroid hepatopathy
Cardiovascular	Positive inotropic effect Reduced capillary permeability Increased blood pressure (vasoconstriction and increased blood volume)	Onset of congestive heart failure
Renal, fluid, and electrolyte balance	Increased sodium, chloride, and water retention Increased potassium and calcium excretion Diuresis Proteinuria	Polyuria and polydipsia
Endocrine	Suppression of adrenocorticotropic hormone production Suppression of thyroid stimulating hormone and thyroid hormone production Suppression of reproductive hormones Reduced renal antidiuretic hormone activity	
Musculoskeletal	Muscular weakness and atrophy Osteoporosis Inhibition of bone and fibrocartilage growth	Muscle wasting*
Gastrointestinal and hepatobiliary	Increased secretion of gastric acid, pepsin, and trypsin Altered mucin structure Decreased gastrointestinal mucosal cell proliferation Reduced iron and calcium absorption Increased fat absorption Increased hepatocellular glycogen and fat deposition Increased serum liver enzymes	Gastrointestinal ulceration
Cutaneous	Dermal atrophy Alopecia	Skin fragility syndrome Poor hair regrowth or alopecia Medial curling of the ears (rare)
Nervous	Altered mood and behaviour (humans) Stimulation of appetite Lowered seizure threshold (humans) Reduced response to pyrogens Maintenance of normal adrenergic sensitivity	Polyphagia (and weight gain)
Eye	Increased intraocular pressure Glaucoma Cataracts	

*Muscle wasting has been reported in other species, but not specifically in cats. In a study in which cats were treated with 4.4 mg/kg/day of prednisolone for 56 days, no muscle atrophy was noted clinically, although there was a significant decrease in creatinine.[3] It is unclear if this decrease was due to increased glomerular filtration rate or subclinical muscle wastage. It is also unclear if longer treatment at high doses is a risk factor for muscle wasting.

The spectrum of activity of GCs extends from anti-inflammatory to immunosuppressive, and these cannot be completely separated. With high doses and prolonged use, overt immunosuppression becomes clinically apparent. The extensive anti-inflammatory effects of GCs dampen the innate immune response to tissue injury and pathogens, flowing on to dampen the adaptive immune response. GCs are also potent lympholytic agents, especially of T cells, and interfere with their function, directly supressing cell-mediated immunity.[4] They suppress function of dendritic antigen-presenting cells, and B-cell function is both directly and indirectly reduced due to the lack of effective costimulation from T cells.

This extensive range of actions makes GCs effective in many immune-mediated diseases regardless of pathogenesis. Much of the damage in immune-mediated diseases also occurs through inflammation, adding to the efficacy of GCs.[5] Figure 35.1 demonstrates the extensive cellular targeting of GCs (represented by prednisolone), in addition to the targets of some of the other immunosuppressive drugs discussed in this chapter. The low cost, established efficacy, rapid onset of action, and familiarity of veterinary practitioners with both the beneficial and adverse effects of these GCs make them popular first-line immunosuppressive agents.

Synthetic GCs have been developed to reduce the relative mineralocorticoid activity and to increase the bioavailability and duration of action of these compounds relative to endogenous GCs.[2] The type of GC used, dose, frequency, and duration of therapy determine both the efficacy and adverse effects of treatment. The holy grail of safe steroid therapy is the development of a GC that has all the desired effects without significant adverse effects. This has not yet been achieved in human medicine despite ongoing work in development of selective glucocorticoid receptor agonists and modulators (SEGRAMs). These drugs are not yet routinely available for clinical use in veterinary medicine.

Clinical use

The recommended dosages of the common GCs used for anti-inflammatory and immunosuppressive therapy for GI and hepatobiliary diseases in cats is provided in Appendix. Much of the pharmacological information about these drugs is derived from humans and dogs. Prednisone is not advised for use in cats due to poor hepatic methylation to

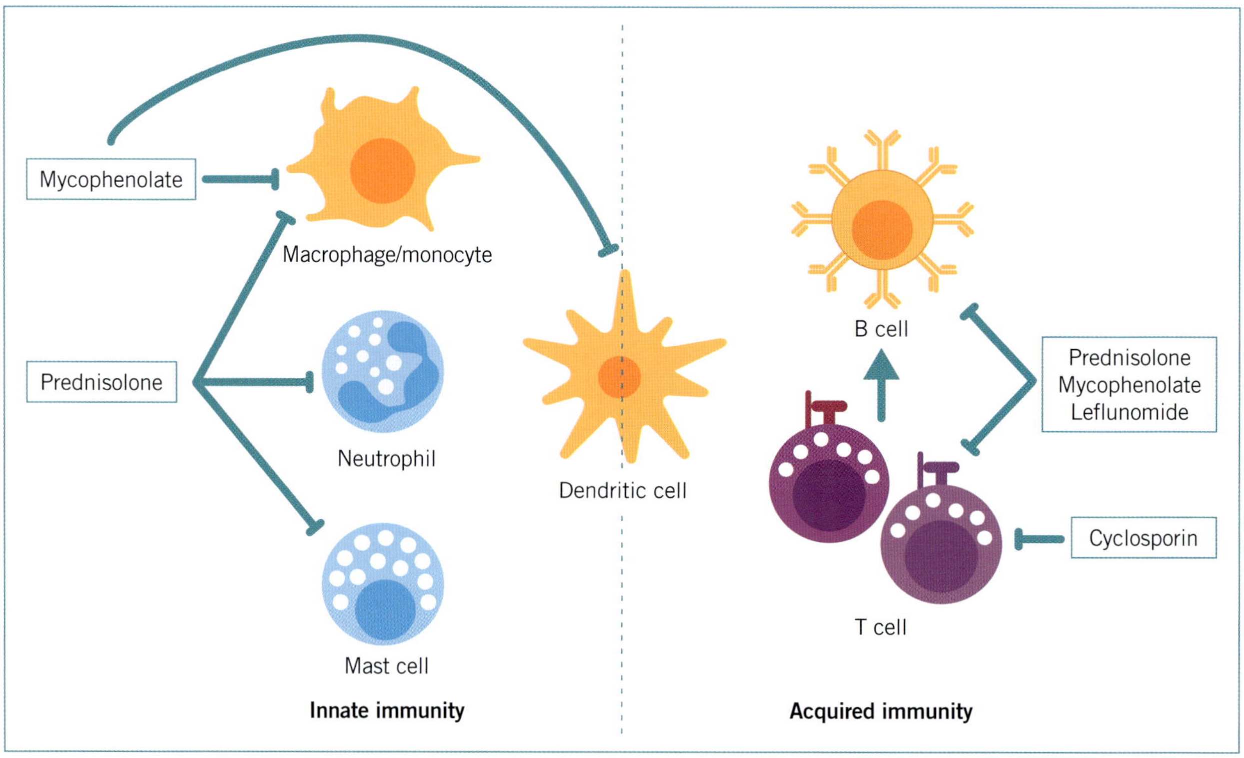

Figure 35.1. Main targets of the different immunosuppressive drugs described in this chapter.

active prednisolone when compared with other species. Prednisolone achieves significantly higher and more reliable plasma drug levels and is the oral drug of choice.

Recommended doses of GCs for cats have traditionally been based on anecdotal observations, which indicate that cats often require higher doses than dogs do to achieve a clinical response, and on the relative tolerance of cats to GCs. This has led to published dose ranges that double those recommended for dogs, commonly 1–2 mg/kg/day prednisolone or equivalent for anti-inflammatory effect and ranges as wide as 2–8 mg/kg/day for immunosuppression. However, this is partially based on historic use of prednisone in cats, which is not bioequivalent to prednisolone in this species. Cats are also predisposed to the more serious adverse effects of GCs (Table 35.1), and it is likely that doses at the higher end of the range simply increase adverse effects without increasing efficacy. There is little evidence to support any particular dose regimen, but for a small number of cats treated with prednisolone for lymphocytic cholangitis there was no difference in outcome between cats receiving 1 mg/kg/day vs. 2 mg/kg/day.[6] The 2 mg/kg/day dose has also been documented to be immunosuppressive in cats,[7] and doses in the 1–2 mg/kg/day range are clinically effective for immune-mediated diseases.[8,9]

The diabetogenic effect of prednisolone is mild in the 1–2 mg/kg/day oral dose range but moderate at the 4.4 mg/kg/day dose, further supporting conservative dosing.[10] In a tertiary referral centre, 9.7% of cats treated with a dose of prednisolone greater than 1.9 mg/kg/day for a minimum of 3 weeks developed diabetes mellitus (DM), the majority within 3 months of starting therapy.[11] In comparison, the prevalence of spontaneous DM in first opinion practice in the same country is less than 0.5%. Although the median starting dose of prednisolone was slightly higher in cats developing DM (3.5 mg/kg) vs. those that did not (2.9 mg/kg), this did not reach statistical significance. There were also no significant differences between the groups in age, breed, sex, or weight, but the small number of cats affected (14/143) limits the assessment. Two of these cats had been managed with prednisolone for over 2 years before requiring a dose increase due to relapsing primary disease. Onset of DM followed the dose increase.

For these reasons, the authors consider a dose of 0.5–1 mg/kg anti-inflammatory and 1–2 mg/kg immunosuppressant. If a higher dose is required to manage the primary disease, a second-line immunosuppressant should be considered.

Overweight cats dosed for body weight achieve higher plasma prednisolone levels compared with cats in normal body condition and may be at higher risk of adverse metabolic effects.[12] Dosing based on ideal body weight has not been well investigated but may reduce this risk.

Oral formulations of GCs are recommended over long-acting injectable formulations whenever possible, as the latter are more commonly associated with serious adverse effects such as DM and congestive heart failure[10,13] and cannot be withdrawn once given. Therapy with GCs can cause congestive heart failure and structural cardiac changes in cats without preexisting signs of heart disease. It is known that significant plasma volume expansion occurs with intramuscular GC administration in cats, but even short oral courses can expand plasma volume.[14,15] Oral dexamethasone may be less likely to promote fluid retention but may also be more diabetogenic in cats, and a prolonged biologic effect makes it poorly suited to daily or alternate day use.[2,16]

Anecdotally, off-label "topical" treatment of idiopathic IBD in cats with oral budesonide has been used to limit systemic drug absorption and adverse effects. In humans, the drug has a high local potency and undergoes extensive first-pass hepatic metabolism after absorption from the intestine. The pharmacokinetics have been studied in dogs but not in cats, but enough drug is still absorbed to cause suppression of the hypothalamic–pituitary–adrenal (HPA) axis in dogs. In cats, inhaled budesonide has shown HPA axis suppression in 3 out of 15 cats, suggesting similarly systemic absorption, although no studies have been done with oral budesonide.[2] When using budesonide in cats, compounding is required to reformulate commercial enteric-coated capsules to the appropriate dose, and monitoring for clinical adverse effects is still recommended. See section "Drug compounding" in this chapter for considerations when using compounding pharmacies.

The following considerations can help guide clinicians when formulating an individual treatment plan (Fig. 35.2):

Do I have a definitive diagnosis?

- Has there been an extensive investigation to exclude other causes of clinical signs?
- Do I have a biopsy-confirmed diagnosis in which histopathology is most consistent with sterile inflammatory, allergic, or immune-mediated disease?
- Have infectious causes been excluded?
- Have other appropriate treatment trials been carried out prior to considering GCs?
- Can I start at an anti-inflammatory dose, or am I likely to need a higher dose to control the disease?

These questions can help assess the likely risks and benefits of proceeding with GC treatment and help to decide on the starting dose. If a high dose is not effective, the clinician needs to review the diagnosis. If immunosuppression is required and a dosage of 2 mg/kg is ineffective, addition of a second-line agent should be considered.

How severe is the disease?

For severe or life-threatening conditions that are likely immune-mediated, starting at the higher end of the dose range is appropriate. If malabsorption or emesis is a concern, initial parenteral therapy may be most appropriate.

Are there contraindications to glucocorticoid therapy?

The presence of DM (active or in remission) suggests that an alternative first-line immunosuppressive agent should be used, particularly if effectiveness has been demonstrated for that disease.

A prior diagnosis of cardiac disease may prompt consideration of whether to use steroids, or whether to consider oral anti-inflammatory GC therapy but not use higher doses or depot formulations. Budesonide has been used anecdotally for chronic enteropathy (CE) in these situations, but some systemic absorption may occur. One cat treated with oral budesonide (0.2 mg/kg PO every 24 hours) had an increase in N-terminal pro–B-type natriuretic peptide consistent with plasma volume expansion.[15]

GI ulceration or bleeding is a relative contraindication; in some cases, the primary disease is corticosteroid-responsive, and GCs are necessary to control the disease. Concurrent gastroprotectant and/or antacid secretory therapy may assist with management. If surgical full-thickness biopsy samples have been collected, a general guide is to allow 2 weeks for healing before starting corticosteroid therapy.

How long do I need to treat?

In feline gastroenterology, GCs are most often used for conditions such as steroid-responsive CE and lymphocytic cholangitis, in which the long-term goal is management rather than cure. GCs are used to induce remission and for chronic maintenance therapy, and the starting dose depends on the disease process and severity and any relative contraindications to treatment. Oral formulations are preferable because their dose can be rapidly adjusted to limit adverse effects, and prednisolone is typically the drug of choice. Once-daily therapy rather than divided dosages should be effective and easier for cat owners to comply with. Time of day does not matter, as diurnal variation in cortisol secretion does not appear to occur in cats; however, the drug should be given at approximately the same time each day.[1]

The rate of drug tapering depends on how good the clinical response to therapy is and how well the cat is tolerating treatment. Generally, the aim is to taper the dose by 25% every 2–4 weeks, aiming to reduce to alternate-day therapy relatively rapidly as this theoretically causes less suppression of the HPA axis and fewer adverse effects. It can take months to reach a maintenance dose that effectively controls the disease, and over time the drug may or may not be able to be further tapered to the point that it can be withdrawn. The goal should always be to use the lowest dose of corticosteroid that controls the disease, whilst tapering slowly enough to reduce the risk of relapse. If adverse effects are excessive or relapse occurs during tapering, an additional or alternative immunosuppressant should be considered so that the steroid can be reduced or withdrawn. Other concurrent therapies (e.g. a novel protein diet for CE) should also be implemented in an attempt to reduce the amount of GC needed to manage the disease.

How am I going to monitor?

Knowledge of the disease being treated determines whether the expectation is cure or chronic clinical remission, and whether the treatment course is likely to be short or protracted. Establishing realistic expectations regarding whether complete resolution of clinical signs vs. a significant reduction in clinical signs is expected is also important. There may be clinicopathologic parameters that can easily be monitored to assess response to therapy, but when objective monitoring may be invasive or expensive, clinical response to therapy using scoring systems and parameters such as body weight and faecal scoring may be more practical. For severe disease or when using high doses of GCs, assessing regularly for both treatment response and adverse effects prior to each dose taper is ideal.

A baseline consisting of haematology, biochemistry, and urinalysis should be considered. For cats requiring chronic maintenance therapy, laboratory work should be considered every 3–4 months to assess for adverse effects and to decide whether a dose reduction has become possible. At a minimum, a urinalysis should be performed monthly for the first 3 months of therapy with immunosuppressive doses, as most cats developing diabetes will do so within this time frame. Repeat haematology and biochemistry can be considered every 6 months for stable cats on chronic treatment.

Can I vaccinate?

At anti-inflammatory doses, immune responses to vaccination are not impaired.[17] With immunosuppressive therapy with any drug, immune responses are more likely to be impaired, and, for safety, modified live vaccines should be avoided.

SECOND-LINE OR ALTERNATIVE IMMUNOSUPPRESSIVE AGENTS

Second-line immunosuppressive agents are typically added when the inflammatory or immune-mediated disease being treated is poorly controlled with GCs, or to allow a more rapid or greater reduction in GC dose when adverse effects are marked. Combination immunosuppressive therapy holds a greater risk for adverse complications such as opportunistic infection. The goal when the disease is in remission is always stepwise tapering of both agents. Often, depending on clinical response to therapy, the dose of GC can be tapered by 25% every 2–4 weeks until a low anti-inflammatory dose every other day is reached. Tapering of the second-line immunosuppressant may begin at this point, or the GC may be discontinued before the second-line agent is tapered. Ultimately discontinuation of both drugs is the aim, but if this is not possible, the lowest effective maintenance dose of one agent should be selected for ongoing use.

Cyclosporin is effective as a single first-line agent for some diseases and may be chosen if GCs are contraindicated or relatively contraindicated, such as for cats with DM or preexisting heart disease. Cats may also be transitioned to cyclosporin if complications develop during GC therapy. For other agents, use alongside a GC is usually required to achieve disease remission, but they may be suitable as single agents for chronic maintenance therapy for some animals or with certain diseases.

CYCLOSPORIN

Cyclosporin has been registered for the treatment of chronic allergic dermatitis in cats and has been used off-label for diseases such as CE, feline stomatitis, other immune-mediated skin diseases, pure red cell aplasia, and in renal transplant recipients.[2] Cyclosporin has also been used as a single agent in diabetic cats or in cats that develop DM with prednisolone treatment, but it can cause disturbances in glucose homoeostasis in some dogs. Cyclosporin has the advantage of a rapid onset of effect compared with some other second-line agents, although the clinical response in conditions such as CE is still expected to take 2–4 weeks.

Pharmacological effects

Cyclosporin is a cyclic polypeptide extracted from the fungus *Tolypocladium inflatum* and a potent immunosuppressant. It binds to cyclophilin within the cell cytosol, preventing the activation of calcineurin and subsequent nuclear transcription of multiple genes coding for important cytokines including IL-2, the key cytokine for activation and proliferation of T cells.[18] Cyclophilin is present in high concentration in the cytoplasm of T cells, and for this reason cyclosporin has a targeted effect on their activation, causing potent downregulation of cell-mediated immunity and a lesser effect on humoral immunity due to the reduced T-helper cell support of this response.

Cyclosporin decreases the expression of several other inflammatory cytokines including IL-4, IL-5, IL-6, IL-8,

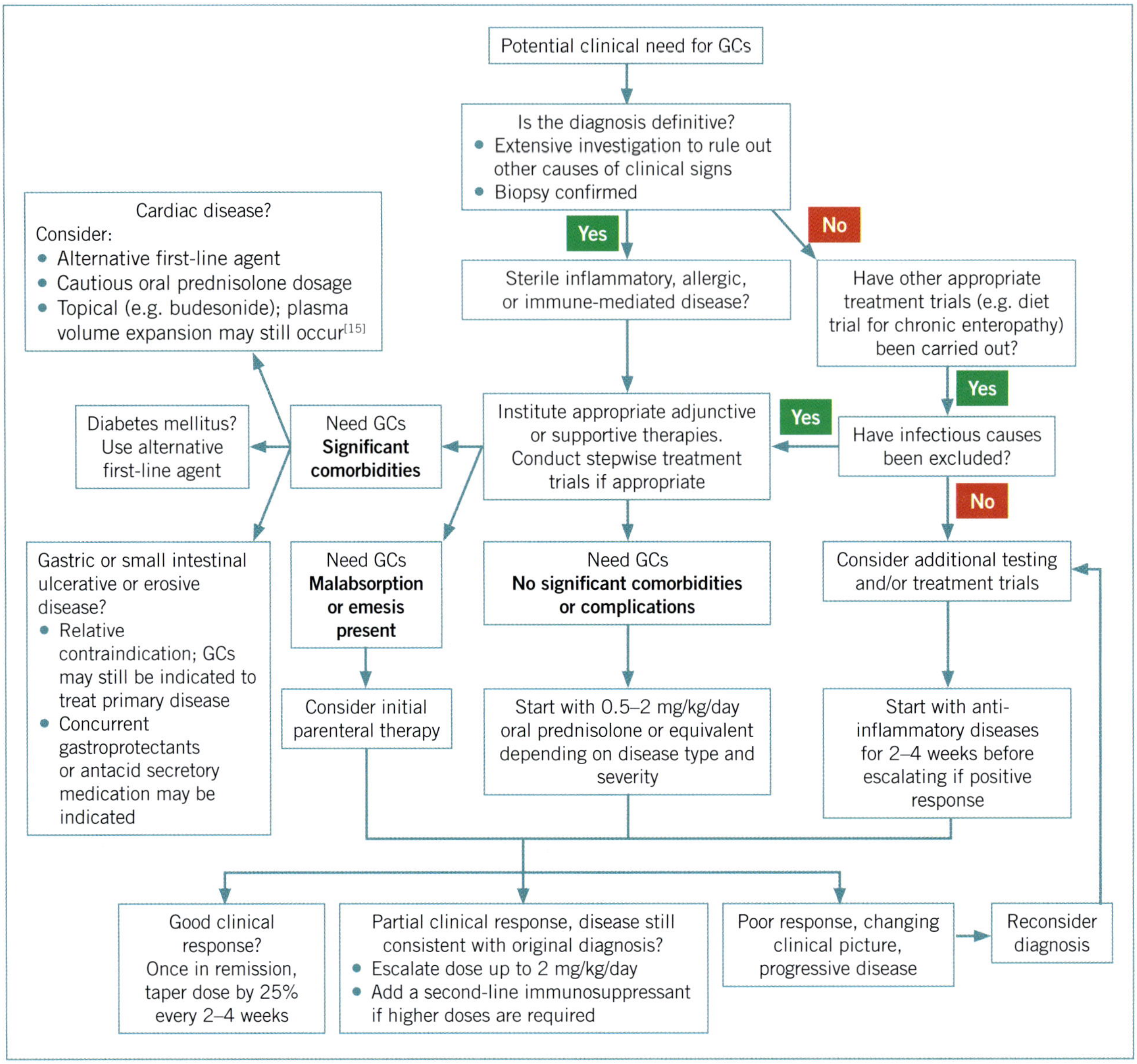

Figure 35.2. Therapeutic considerations in the use of glucocorticoids (GCs).

IL-13, IFN-γ, TNF-α, and granulocyte–macrophage colony-stimulating factor (GM-CSF) in cats.[18] This inhibition suppresses the activity of other immune cells such as macrophages, granulocytes, and mast cells. Proliferative activity of keratinocytes is reduced, endothelial cells express fewer adhesion molecules, and antigen-presenting cells are suppressed. There are few studies specific to cats, but reduction in lymphocyte proliferation after activation with concanavalin A and induction of apoptotic changes in peripheral blood mononuclear cells have both been demonstrated in vitro.

Pharmacokinetics

As in other species, oral cyclosporin absorption is highly variable between individual cats for a given dose.[18] Cyclosporin can be given with or without food in cats, with minimal effect on absorption, which is overall poor (<30%) and limited by P-glycoprotein drug efflux pumps in the enterocytes. Only use of microemulsified cyclosporin is recommended to improve intestinal absorption, as reported in other species. With this formulation in cats, peak plasma concentrations are reached after 1–2 hours, with a half-life of around 8 hours. Trough levels are still highly variable. Transdermal absorption is too poor to reach effective blood concentrations. Subcutaneous administration is associated with local reactions.

Cyclosporin is widely distributed in the body but also highly lipophilic and therefore accumulates in the skin and adipose tissue. Cyclosporin is mainly metabolised in the liver via the cytochrome P450 complex, and excretion is mostly via the bile, with limited excretion in the urine. Drugs that inhibit or induce the cytochrome P450 complex will affect cyclosporin blood concentration, and this should be considered when using cyclosporin (Table 35.2). In cats the effects of ketoconazole, itraconazole, and clarithromycin have been specifically studied, and all significantly increase blood cyclosporin concentration.

Clinical use

Dosage and therapeutic drug monitoring

Challenges with the clinical use of cyclosporin include pharmacokinetic variability and lack of correlation between blood concentrations and clinical efficacy. Measuring blood concentrations (therapeutic drug monitoring, TDM) from 3–5 days into therapy is advised in life-threatening situations that require heavy immunosuppression (e.g. avoidance of graft rejection, severe immune-mediated disease). TDM is particularly recommended if there is concurrent drug therapy that can increase cyclosporin concentrations, as the effect of the combination is not predictable. One such situation is the intentional use of ketoconazole to lower dose requirements and cost of cyclosporin therapy. This is practically less useful in cats than in large dogs, and cost of monitoring offsets any savings.

Adjusting the dose to target a therapeutic blood concentration should ensure a therapeutic effect while limiting adverse effects. However, therapeutic ranges differ between species and diseases in humans and dogs and do not seem to correlate reliably with treatment response. Similar challenges are expected in cats. Pharmacodynamic studies correlate better with clinical effect in dogs but are not established yet for cats.

Microemulsified human and canine labelled cyclosporin in gelatine capsules has previously been used off-label in cats. The registered feline liquid product has a labelled dose of 7 mg/kg every 24 hours for treatment of allergic dermatitis in cats. For this disease, TDM is not recommended unless adverse effects are seen, as cyclosporin is expected to accumulate in the skin (hence blood concentration does not reflect target tissue concentration) and the clinical effect is easily observed.

For systemic immunosuppression, as the required dose is expected to be higher, cyclosporin is usually given every 12 hours (see Appendix). TDM has been used in feline renal transplant recipients with an initial

Table 35.2. Main known drug interactions that can affect plasma concentration of immunosuppressants.*

Drug	Increased blood concentration	Reduced blood concentration
Cyclosporin	**Azole antifungals** Calcium channel blockers (e.g. amlodipine) Corticosteroids Fatty acids (essential/omega) Fluoroquinolones **Macrolide antibiotics** Metronidazole Omeprazole Cisapride	Clindamycin Famotidine Phenobarbital Sulphasalazine Terbinafine Griseofulvin
Mycophenolate mofetil		Amoxicillin–clavulanic acid Antacids (aluminium and magnesium containing)† Ciprofloxacin Cyclosporin Iron† Lanthanum carbonate Proton pump inhibitors Telmisartan

*Drug interactions reported in cats are indicated in bold type, and drug interactions reported in humans in plain type.
†Affects absorption. Separate dosing by at least 2 hours.

target trough (just before the next pill is due) blood concentration of ≈300–500 ng/ml[18] and a maintenance therapy trough target level of ≈250 ng/ml. Peak concentration targets are not well established in cats. Chronic refractory feline gingivostomatitis in cats has been successfully managed with cyclosporin at 2.5 mg PO every 12 hours.[19] Whole-blood cyclosporin concentrations above 300 ng/ml were associated with significant improvement in oral inflammation in cats with chronic stomatitis that had previously undergone premolar/molar or full-mouth extraction. If TDM is performed, a whole-blood assay using high-performance liquid chromatography (HPLC) is recommended, as cyclosporin concentrates in erythrocytes. Reference intervals and monitoring guidelines are specific to each laboratory. The utility of TDM when cyclosporin is used for other indications in cats is currently unknown. Cyclosporin at the 5 mg/kg PO once-daily "atopy" dose is effective for steroid-refractory IBD in dogs, but blood cyclosporin concentrations do not correlate with clinical efficacy.[20] TDM is therefore not routinely used, and 2–4 weeks should be allowed for clinical effect. The use of cyclosporin for the management of CE in cats is anecdotal.

Regardless of dose, administering at a consistent time of day, and consistently with or without food, is recommended to maintain relatively consistent drug absorption and blood concentrations. For the liquid formulation, mixing it with food or placing it in a capsule can be beneficial to hide the bitter taste. Other strategies reported to reduce adverse GI effects include concurrent administration of maropitant or freezing the capsule for 30–60 minutes prior to administration.

Adverse effects

The most common adverse effects reported with cyclosporin treatment at standard doses (up to 7 mg/kg every 24 hours) are GI (reduced appetite, hypersalivation, vomiting, and diarrhoea).[18] These are usually self-limiting, resolving within the first few weeks of treatment.

Hyporexia and weight loss usually resolve with dose reduction or cessation of the treatment. Hepatic lipidosis is a rare outcome of significant weight loss. Other rare adverse effects reported include gingival hyperplasia, acute bullous keratopathy, polyphagia, polydipsia, lethargy, hyperactivity, and hypertrichosis.

Mild decreases in some cell lines (lymphocytes, neutrophils, eosinophils) have been reported as well as mild increases in some biochemistry values (bilirubin, glucose, urea), but all values remain within the reference interval, and the significance of these findings is unclear.

A significantly increased risk of malignant neoplasia has been reported in feline transplant recipients immunosuppressed with cyclosporin and prednisolone in multiple studies. Reports of neoplasia in cats treated with standard cyclosporin doses are rare.

Risk of infection with the use of cyclosporin

As previously mentioned, cyclosporin is a very potent immunosuppressant, and an increased risk of opportunistic infection has been reported with its use.[2,18] No increase in risk for subclinical bacteriuria was noted in cats treated with cyclosporin for at least 3 months for dermatologic disease. Relapse of latent feline herpesvirus infection has been reported (usually mild), and fatal toxoplasmosis has also been reported, with some cats suspected to have a newly acquired infection and others possible reactivation of a previous infection.

A prospective study of experimental *Toxoplasma gondii* infection using oral cyclosporin at 7.5 mg/kg/day found that there was no reactivation of toxoplasmosis in previously infected cats but that cats newly infected with *T. gondii* during treatment had a more severe infection.[22] Out of the ten cats in this group, one died of toxoplasmosis and had a markedly high blood cyclosporin trough concentration (1690 ng/ml) compared to the other cats in the group (626 ± 259 ng/ml). Fortunately, oocyst shedding was not increased in either group of cats, indicating that there is not an increased zoonotic risk to humans with cyclosporin treatment. Although this study suggests that the risk is highest for naïve cats that are newly infected during treatment with cyclosporin, it may not completely exclude the possibility of reactivation of prior infection. Firstly, the cats were all young adults, and none had comorbidities as is usually the case for cats treated with cyclosporin. Secondly, the duration of cyclosporin treatment of previously infected cats was relatively short (40 days), whereas longer treatment periods are more likely for chronic therapy of immune-mediated diseases.

For anti-*Toxoplasma* IgG positive (previously infected) cats, the prophylactic use of antibiotics has been suggested for renal transplant recipients undergoing heavy immunosuppression, although prospective studies to recommend this approach are missing. For other uses, as recrudescence of infection is not likely, prophylactic treatment is not indicated. Reducing the risk of new infections is achieved by housing indoors to limit hunting behaviour and avoiding feeding raw meat.[22] This is especially important for seronegative cats. TDM might be useful to identify cats with a higher risk of opportunistic infections, although a cutoff cyclosporin blood concentration above which risk is increased is not currently available.

Baseline screening and monitoring of therapy

Ideally, a full baseline screening should be obtained prior to initiating cyclosporin therapy, including haematology, biochemistry panel, urinalysis, urine culture, feline leukaemia virus (FeLV) antigen, feline immunodeficiency virus (FIV) antibody, and *Toxoplasma* IgG and IgM serology. Treatment of FIV- or FeLV-infected cats with cyclosporin is not recommended. For other treatable active infections, appropriate treatment should be implemented prior to using cyclosporin. New infections that develop during cyclosporin therapy may require discontinuation of cyclosporin in addition to specific treatment.

Cyclosporin should be used cautiously in cats with liver dysfunction, as it is highly metabolised by the liver and mostly excreted in the bile. Closer monitoring of cats with preexisting renal disease or DM is also advised. For cats with normal major organ function, monitoring haematology, biochemistry, and urinalysis every 6 months is advised, although more frequent monitoring may be indicated depending on the primary disease process. Otherwise, monitoring is primarily based on physical examination findings including body weight, assessing clinical response to treatment, and watching for adverse effects.

Vaccination during cyclosporin therapy

Experimentally, booster vaccinations for feline calicivirus, feline herpesvirus 1, feline parvovirus, FeLV, and rabies have provoked an adequate humoral immune response during treatment with very high doses of cyclosporin.[18] A novel vaccination for FIV was not effective, and it is expected that any primary vaccination response may be impaired. Live vaccinations are not recommended during immunosuppressive therapy with any drug.

CHLORAMBUCIL

Chlorambucil has been widely used in cats to treat immune-mediated skin and haematologic diseases, CEs, and small-cell GI lymphoma. It is also used in some antineoplastic chemotherapy protocols.

Pharmacological effects

Chlorambucil is a nitrogen mustard derivative that is metabolised in the liver to its active metabolite, phenylacetic acid mustard.[2] Phenylacetic acid mustard is further metabolised in the liver to other inactive metabolites that are excreted in the urine and faeces. The cytotoxic effect of the active metabolite is due to cell cycle–nonspecific alkylation of DNA strands that results in their cross-linking, inhibiting replication and promoting cellular apoptosis. Toxicity occurs to both resting and dividing cells, with dividing lymphocytes being particularly sensitive. Both humoral and cell-mediated immunity are affected, but the onset of drug action is slow, with an immunosuppressive effect expected 2–4 weeks after starting treatment.

Adverse effects

Chlorambucil is a cytotoxic agent and has the potential for teratogenic effects.[2] Risks should be discussed with the owners prior to dispensing the drug, and recommendations to reduce exposure should be provided (e.g. use of gloves, no splitting of the tablets). Any local legal requirements should be adhered to.

Chlorambucil is myelosuppressive and, for this reason, should be used cautiously in cats with preexisting bone marrow suppression or when used in conjunction with other drugs likely to cause myelosuppression (e.g. other chemotherapeutic drugs). In a large study of 56 cats treated for small-cell lymphoma with prednisolone and chlorambucil, adverse events were reported in 19 cats.[23] Myelosuppression, including anaemia, leucopenia, and thrombocytopenia, was the most frequently reported adverse effect (11/19 cats). Myelosuppression is usually mild, generally occurs 7–14 days after the start of the therapy, and resolves 7–14 days after treatment cessation. However, marked thrombocytopenia can be seen after months of treatment and might take months to resolve. For this reason, platelet count should be monitored with chronic treatment. GI adverse effects (inappetence, vomiting, and diarrhoea) and hepatotoxicity are also common, with seven events of each reported in the aforementioned study. GI signs are usually mild and self-limiting. The severity of hepatotoxicity described in case reports is more variable, but contribution of an underlying disease process is not always excluded. In the case series described above, the drug was withdrawn in 5/6 cats with hepatotoxicity, and alanine aminotransferase (ALT) improved in all cats in an average of 76 days (range 6–228 days).

Reversible neurological signs (agitation, facial twitching, myoclonus, and tonic–clonic seizures) have been reported in one cat following a drug overdose.[2] Acquired Fanconi syndrome was reported in four cats within 2–26 months of starting chlorambucil treatment.[2] Improvement or resolution occurred in 3/4 cats within 3 months of discontinuing treatment.

Clinical use

Combination of chlorambucil and prednisolone is the chemotherapy protocol of choice for cats diagnosed with low-grade alimentary lymphoma or poorly responsive CE (idiopathic IBD). Either continuous or pulse dosing has been described. There is no randomised prospective study to compare the protocols, but different studies report similar median survival times of 2 years or longer. For this reason, there is no strong reason to support one protocol in favour of the other. A typical continuous dosage protocol is 2 mg/cat PO every 48 hours for cats weighing over 4 kg or every 72 hours for cats weighing less than 4 kg.[2] Pulse treatment varies from 15 mg/m^2 (rounded to the nearest 2 mg) PO every 24 hours for 4 days every 3 weeks, to 20 mg/m^2 PO once every 2 weeks.[2] Treatment once every 2 weeks with chlorambucil rather than every second or third day has the potential benefit of reduced exposure for the owner and less handling of the patient.

Varying doses of prednisolone have been used concomitantly, ranging from 1–2 mg/kg PO every 24 hours or 5 mg/cat every 12–24 hours up to 3 mg/kg PO every 24 hours (tapering to 1–2 mg/kg once in remission). There is no study available to determine optimal treatment duration or tapering strategies. The preferred strategy of the authors is to start treatment at a prednisolone dose of 1–2 mg/kg PO every 24 hours with reduction over several weeks to 0.5 mg/kg every other day in order to reduce the risk of adverse effects of long-term GC treatment.

Monitoring

There is no strict consensus on laboratory monitoring for chlorambucil adverse effects. A baseline haematology, biochemistry, and urinalysis are recommended. For continuous dosing, repeat haematology should be considered 1 month after starting treatment and every 2–3 months thereafter. For pulse treatment, haematology should be repeated 1 week after treatment. Treatment should be discontinued if the platelet count is lower than 75000/μl, the haematocrit drops below 20%, or the neutrophil count is lower than 1.5×10^9/l. The frequency of rechecks should be increased if one or more values are trending towards these cutoffs. Resolution of cytopenias is expected following discontinuation of therapy but may be slow. If resolution is not occurring, other causes should be investigated.

Biochemistry should be repeated after 1 month and, if normal, every 3 months thereafter. Urinalysis, and especially monitoring of glycosuria, should be considered at the same time intervals as biochemistry.

MYCOPHENOLATE MOFETIL

Mycophenolate mofetil (MMF) is an immunosuppressive agent used in people as an alternative to azathioprine, primarily alongside cyclosporin and GCs, to prevent transplant rejection.[17] There is some literature on its use in dogs in transplantation, immune-mediated haematologic diseases, meningoencephalitis of unknown origin, immune-mediated dermatologic disease, and myasthenia gravis.[2] Clinical use reported in cats has been limited to immune-mediated haemolytic anaemia (IMHA).[24] Like chlorambucil, onset of effect is slow, and clinical immunosuppression is expected after 2–4 weeks of therapy.

Pharmacological effects

MMF is a prodrug that is metabolised to mycophenolic acid (MPA), the active immunosuppressive agent.[2] MPA is a selective, reversible inhibitor of inosine-5'-monophosphate dehydrogenase, particularly the type II isoform found in activated lymphocytes. This protease is rate-limiting for the de novo synthesis of guanosine nucleotides required for cell proliferation. As T and B cells lack alternative synthesis pathways, their differentiation and proliferation are inhibited, as is B cell immunoglobulin production. This impairs both cell-mediated and humoral immunity. Additional effects include suppression of dendritic cell maturation and prevention of monocyte and lymphocyte recruitment into tissue sites of chronic inflammation.

Safety

Reported adverse effects in dogs include GI signs (inappetence, vomiting, diarrhoea, GI bleeding), lethargy, weight loss, papillomatosis, allergic reactions, and lymphopenia. More severe myelosuppression or hepatotoxicity have not yet been reported. A hepatopathy and pancreatopathy have been associated with MMF treatment in one cat.[25]

Short-term safety of intravenous and oral MMF has been evaluated in 24 healthy cats.[21] Intravenous doses ranged from 5 mg/kg once up to 20 mg/kg every 12 hours for 1 day, with a 10 mg/kg twice-daily dose given for either 1 or 3 days. Oral MMF was given at a low (10 mg/kg every 12 hours), intermediate (15 mg/kg every 12 hours), or high dose (15 mg/kg every 8 hours) for 7 days. Adverse effects reported included mild weight loss in 11/24 cats (median 0.2 kg, range 0.1–0.4 kg), which stabilised or improved within 7–10 days of treatment cessation. One cat given oral MMF became hyporexic. Self-limiting diarrhoea was reported in 4/14 cats treated with intravenous MMF within 48 hours and in 4/10 cats treated with oral MMF. As reported in people and dogs, this appeared to be dose-dependent, affecting 4/4 cats receiving the high oral dose and 1/4 receiving the intermediate oral dose. Diarrhoea resolved in all cats within 24 hours of discontinuing MMF. Clinicopathologic changes reported included variably lower packed cell volume in 19/24 cats and variable thrombocytopenia in 19/24 cats from baseline by the end of the study. Many cats had large platelets or aggregates, and none had clinical bleeding. The reason for thrombocytopenia was not further assessed, but iatrogenic blood loss from repeat sampling or consumption in the GI tract were not excluded. White blood cell counts and ALT were not affected.

Overall, intravenous MMF at 10 mg/kg every 12 hours for 3 days and oral MMF at a dose of up to 15 mg/kg every 12 hours for up to 1 week appears to be well tolerated in healthy cats.

Pharmacokinetics and pharmacodynamics

In dogs, peak MPA blood concentrations occur 1–2 hours after oral MMF administration.[2] Hepatic glucuronidation to form an inactive metabolite (mycophenolic acid glucuronide, MPAG) follows, some of which is excreted into the biliary system and undergoes enterohepatic circulation, causing a second peak in MPA 4–12 hours after MMF ingestion. The majority of MMF is excreted in urine, primarily as MPAG. Cats also biotransform MMF to MPA. Although cats typically do not glucuronidate medications well, they metabolise MPA adequately by glucosidation, and it appears to also undergo some enterohepatic circulation.[2] As in humans, after both intravenous and oral MMF administration, there is high intercat variability in plasma concentrations, which could lead to unpredictable drug responses.

One concern arising from studies in cats is that total MPA drug exposure did not reach concentrations known to be effective for immunosuppression in humans, even at the 15 mg/kg PO every-8-hour dose for 7 days, which resulted in GI toxicity.[26] There were also no measurable effects on peripheral blood mononuclear counts or the $CD4^+$:$CD8^+$ ratio after treatment. In dogs, these changes may take 2 weeks or more to be seen. It is uncertain whether longer treatment duration is needed to achieve an effect or whether toxicity will prevent achievement of an effective dose in cats. Further studies would be required to establish whether there is an effective dose for cats, the time to effect, and the ideal TDM.

Some drug interactions have been reported in humans that might be relevant in cats and are listed in Table 35.2. Drugs that reduce enterohepatic circulation might reduce MMF serum concentration. These include cholestyramine, ciprofloxacin, and cyclosporin.[2]

Clinical use

There is currently very limited information regarding the use of MMF in cats. Two cats were treated with MMF at 10 mg/kg PO every 12 hours alongside prednisolone 4 mg/kg/day for IMHA, and the drug was well tolerated.[24] In a third cat treated similarly, a hepatopathy and suspected pancreatitis developed 2 months into therapy.[25] These adverse effects have been reported in humans, and they resolved in this cat following drug withdrawal and supportive care.

Given the lack of proven efficacy in cats and the frequency of adverse GI side effects, the authors do not currently recommend considering MMF as a second-line agent for cats with inflammatory or immune-mediated GI, hepatic, or pancreatic disease.

LEFLUNOMIDE

Leflunomide is an isoxazole immunosuppressive drug. There is very limited information on the use of leflunomide in cats, and this is restricted to treatment of rheumatoid arthritis—the main indication for the drug in humans. Small numbers of dogs are reported in the literature treated with leflunomide either as an adjunctive therapy for various refractory immune diseases or, in some cases, as a single agent where GCs were poorly tolerated or contraindicated. Uses include transplant recipients, immune-mediated haematologic and histiocytic diseases, immune-mediated polyarthritis, granulomatous meningoencephalitis, IBD, and inflammatory colorectal polyps.[27]

Pharmacological effects

Leflunomide is the prodrug of teriflunomide, a pyrimidine synthesis inhibitor.[2] After ingestion, leflunomide is converted to its active metabolite teriflunomide (A77 1726) in the plasma and intestinal tract mucosa. Teriflunomide inhibits the enzyme dihydroorotate dehydrogenase, which is important for de novo pyrimidine synthesis. Reduced DNA and RNA synthesis reduce cell proliferation, causing a cytostatic effect. Activated T and B cells are dependent on this pathway for pyrimidine synthesis, and therefore leflunomide acts relatively specifically on these cells, with less effect on other rapidly dividing cells. Both cell-mediated and humoral immunity are affected. The drug also causes some tyrosine kinase inhibition and has antiviral effects.

Pharmacokinetics and pharmacodynamics

In an experimental setting, healthy cats were treated orally with 2 mg/kg of leflunomide every 24 hours for 2 days followed by 2 mg/kg every 48 hours for six treatments.[28] Bioavailability was 100%, and the half-life of the active metabolite was 60 hours. The mean plasma teriflunomide concentration that achieved 50% inhibition of lymphocytes was 16 µg/ml. Targets for TDM have otherwise not been established. One day after receiving the last dose of leflunomide, the mean lymphocyte proliferation was still inhibited by 51 ± 9.5%, supporting a prolonged biological effect. The half-life of this drug in cats is of note, as it is quite different to that in dogs (21 hours) and people (7–10 days);[17] consequently, doses cannot be extrapolated between species.

Elimination mechanisms are not known in cats. Renal excretion is the main mechanism in humans, and dose adjustment may be required if renal function is impaired.

Adverse effects

Self-limiting intermittent vomiting was reported in 2/6 cats treated experimentally with oral leflunomide following multiple doses, and mild sedation occurred in 2 cats after intravenous administration. There is report of only mild significant adverse effects in 12 cats treated for rheumatoid arthritis, including a mild transient increase in liver enzymes and increased defecation in one cat.[29]

In a large retrospective study of 92 dogs treated with leflunomide for various conditions, possible adverse events reported in 11/92 dogs included lethargy, reduced appetite, vomiting, diarrhoea, unexplained haemorrhage (including haematochezia in all three cases), mild thrombocytopenia, and mild increases in liver values.[27] The clinicopathologic abnormalities responded to a reduction of the leflunomide dose by 50%. Nonspecific signs resolved with drug reduction or withdrawal. Bleeding resolved within days in both dogs treated by drug withdrawal.

Clinical use

To date, there is only one study that reports the use of a combination of methotrexate and leflunomide (at 10 mg/cat PO every 24 hours until remission, twice a week thereafter) for feline rheumatoid arthritis with good success.[29]

The study in healthy cats suggests that a dose of 2 mg/kg PO every 24 hours for 2 days followed by 2 mg/kg every 48 hours is effective to inhibit lymphocyte proliferation.

With reported efficacy in some canine enteropathies and in Crohn's disease in people, leflunomide may have a place in feline gastroenterology in the future, but more research is needed in this area.

AZATHIOPRINE AND CYCLOPHOSPHAMIDE

Azathioprine is a thiopurine that has been used widely in dogs. The mechanism of immunosuppression is not fully understood, but the enzyme thiopurine methyltransferase (TPMT) plays a central role in azathioprine metabolism. Cats have extremely low concentrations of TMPT and, for this reason, produce large amounts of 6-thioguanine nucleotides that are myelotoxic.[2]

Though treatment of cats with low doses of azathioprine has been reported in the literature, because of the myelotoxic risk and the array of other safer drugs available as second-line immunosuppressants in cats, azathioprine should be avoided in this species.

Similarly, cyclophosphamide is a potent nitrogen mustard cytotoxic and immunosuppressive drug, with a high risk of myelosuppression and other adverse effects in both cats and dogs. It is best reserved for use as an antineoplastic agent.

DRUG COMPOUNDING

Drug compounding has been widely used in veterinary medicine, but concerns have been raised regarding stability, purity, strength, and absorption of the compounded drugs.[17] Some reasons to compound drugs include inadequate strength of manufactured drugs on the market, need for another type of formulation (e.g. liquid form for cats that cannot be given tablets), and cost.

Although compounding is very attractive, the clinician needs to keep in mind that the final product will be dependent on the compounding pharmacy used and significant differences can be present when compared with the licensed formulations, which may affect efficacy and safety. This has been demonstrated in a recent study assessing the strength and stability of compounded chlorambucil.[30] The authors of the study used four different compounding pharmacies to compound chlorambucil at a strength of 1 mg. One of the products had a strength of less than 90% of the intended strength on the day of arrival and two products less than 80% by day 42.

Similarly, inadequate strength has been reported in compounded liquid cyclosporin from five different compounding pharmacies.[2] The additional difficulty with cyclosporin is the lack of certainty around bioavailability of the product, as the equivalence of various human generic microemulsified forms to the original human or veterinary commercial products has not been studied in veterinary species.[17] There are anecdotal reports of loss of disease control in cats after changing cyclosporin product. Hence, the risk of compounding needs to be discussed with the owners.

Take-home messages

- Prednisolone is the preferred oral glucocorticoid for cats, as this species metabolises prednisone to active prednisolone poorly.
- Traditional published doses for oral glucocorticoids are probably excessive. Dosing with prednisolone at the higher end of the range likely increases adverse effects without increasing clinical efficacy.
- The risk of severe clinical toxoplasmosis in cats treated with cyclosporin is greatest in seronegative cats. It is recommended that they be housed indoors and not be fed raw meat during treatment.
- Compounding is popular in feline medicine for accurate dosing or to help with compliance by changing formulation. However, compounding can significantly alter drug stability, purity, strength, and absorption.

REFERENCES

[1] Ferguson DC, Hoenig M. Glucocorticoids, mineralocorticoids, and adrenolytic drugs. In: Riviere JE, Papich MG, editors. *Veterinary Pharmacology and Therapeutics*, 10th ed. Newark, John Wiley & Sons: 729, 2018.

[2] Plumb DC. *Plumb's Veterinary Drug Handbook*, 9th ed. Stockholm (Wisconsin), PharmaVet, 2018.

[3] Lowe AD et al. Clinical, clinicopathological and histological changes observed in 14 cats treated with glucocorticoids. *Vet Rec* 162:777, 2008.

[4] Cain DW, Cidlowski JA. Immune regulation by glucocorticoids. *Nat Rev Immunol* 17:233, 2017.

[5] Flammer JR, Rogatsky I. Minireview: glucocorticoids in autoimmunity: unexpected targets and mechanisms. *Mol Endocrinol* 25:1075, 2011.

[6] Otte CM et al. Retrospective comparison of prednisolone and ursodeoxycholic acid for the treatment of feline lymphocytic cholangitis. *Vet J* 195:205, 2013.

[7] Miller C et al. Immunopathologic effects of prednisolone and cyclosporine A on feline immunodeficiency virus replication and persistence. *Viruses* 11:805, 2019.

[8] Simpson DL, Burton GG. Use of prednisolone as monotherapy in the treatment of feline pemphigus foliaceus: a retrospective study of 37 cats. *Vet Dermatol* 24:598, 2013.

[9] Kohn B et al. Primary immune-mediated hemolytic anemia in 19 cats: diagnosis, therapy, and outcome (1998–2004). *J Vet Intern Med* 20:159, 2006.

[10] Khelik IA et al. Clinicopathologic, hemodynamic, and echocardiographic effects of short-term oral administration of anti-inflammatory doses of prednisolone to systemically normal cats. *Am J Vet Res* 80:743, 2019.

[11] Nerhagen S et al. Prednisolone-induced diabetes mellitus in the cat: a historical cohort. *J Feline Med Surg* 1098612X20943522, 2020 [epub ahead of print].

[12] Center SA et al. Influence of body condition on plasma prednisolone and prednisone concentrations in clinically healthy cats after single oral dose administration. *Res Vet Sci* 95:225, 2013.

[13] Smith SA et al. Corticosteroid-associated congestive heart failure in 12 cats. *Int J Appl Res Vet Med* 2:159, 2004.

[14] Ployngam T et al. Hemodynamic effects of methylprednisolone acetate administration in cats. *Am J Vet Res* 67:583, 2006.

[15] Block CL, Oyama MA. Echocardiographic and biomarker evidence of plasma volume expansion after short-term steroids administered orally in cats. *J Vet Intern Med* 34:29, 2020.

[16] Lowe AD et al. A pilot study comparing the diabetogenic effects of dexamethasone and prednisolone in cats. *J Am Anim Hosp Assoc* 45:215, 2009.

[17] Papich MG. Immunosuppressive drugs. In: Riviere JE, Papich MG, editors. *Veterinary Pharmacology and Therapeutics*, 10th ed. Newark, John Wiley & Sons: 1226, 2018.

[18] Colombo S, Sartori R. Ciclosporin and the cat: current understanding and review of clinical use. *J Feline Med Surg* 20:244, 2018.

[19] Lommer MJ. Efficacy of cyclosporine for chronic, refractory stomatitis in cats: a randomized, placebo-controlled, double-blinded clinical study. *J Vet Dent* 30:8, 2013.

[20] Allenspach K et al. Pharmacokinetics and clinical efficacy of cyclosporine treatment of dogs with steroid-refractory inflammatory bowel disease. *J Vet Intern Med* 20:239, 2006.

[21] Slovak JE, Villarino NF. Safety of oral and intravenous mycophenolate mofetil in healthy cats. *J Feline Med Surg* 20:184, 2018.

[22] Lappin MR et al. Effect of oral administration of cyclosporine on *Toxoplasma gondii* infection status of cats. *Am J Vet Res* 76:351, 2015.

[23] Pope KV et al. Outcome and toxicity assessment of feline small cell lymphoma: 56 cases (2000–2010). *Vet Med Sci* 1:51, 2015.

[24] Bacek LM, Macintire DK. Treatment of primary immune-mediated hemolytic anemia with mycophenolate mofetil in two cats. *J Vet Emerg Crit Care (San Antonio)* 21:45, 2011.

[25] Kopke MA, Galloway PEJ. Suspected hepatopathy and pancreatitis associated with mycophenolate mofetil use in a cat with immune-mediated haemolytic anaemia. *JFMS Open Rep* 6:2055116920905038, 2020.

[26] Slovak JE et al. Pharmacokinetics of mycophenolic acid and its effect on $CD4^+$ and $CD8^+$ T cells after oral administration of mycophenolate mofetil to healthy cats. *J Vet Intern Med* 33:2020, 2019.

[27] Sato M et al. A retrospective study on the safety and efficacy of leflunomide in dogs. *J Vet Intern Med* 31:1502, 2017.

[28] Mehl ML et al. Pharmacokinetics and pharmacodynamics of A77 1726 and leflunomide in domestic cats. *J Vet Pharmacol Ther* 35:139, 2012.

[29] Hanna FY. Disease modifying treatment for feline rheumatoid arthritis. *Vet Comp Orthop Traumatol* 18:94, 2005.

[30] Burton JH et al. Potency and stability of compounded formulations of chlorambucil, melphalan and cyclophosphamide. *Vet Comp Oncol* 15:1558, 2017.

CHAPTER 36

Prebiotics, probiotics, synbiotics, and postbiotics

Silke Salavati Schmitz

Probiotics are gaining increasing interest as alternative or ancillary treatment options for a number of gastrointestinal (GI) conditions in small animals. This is due to the fact that antibiotic stewardship is gaining traction in veterinary medicine around the world, and alternatives to antibiotics are sought for many diseases. In addition, increased understanding of the relevance of the intestinal microbiota in a number of conditions inside and outside the GI tract allows more targeted interventions to modify it.

Unfortunately, the label "probiotic" is often misused as an umbrella term and applied to products that do not meet the definition of a "true" probiotic.[1] Worldwide, there is insufficient regulation to scrutinise if a product can be defined as a probiotic, as legislation varies from including them as foods for human consumption to animal feeds, nutritional supplements, or drugs. To uphold principles of evidence-based veterinary medicine, it seems prudent that sufficient scientific scrutiny is applied to assess if a suspected probiotic achieves desired outcomes in the disease of interest and, crucially, in the target species.

So far, even though many studies examining probiotic effects on a number of organ systems are available, these were mostly conducted in laboratory animals, cell cultures, or other ex vivo systems. Human clinical trials often examine small numbers of patients, are not controlled, or do not include sufficiently specific information about the probiotics used. The number of high-quality probiotic trials in cats (and dogs) is even more limited. In small studies, the bacterial strains used were often isolated specifically for the study purpose, making it nearly impossible to reproduce any reported findings. This chapter reviews the supposed or demonstrated mechanisms of action of probiotics and examines the evidence for their use in clinical conditions of the GI tract in cats. In addition, it explores the connection between probiotics, prebiotics, and dietary fibre, and briefly discusses the relatively novel concept of postbiotics.

DEFINITION OF PROBIOTICS, PREBIOTICS, SYNBIOTICS, AND POSTBIOTICS

The definition of probiotics as used today was established by the Food and Agriculture Organization of the United Nations and World Health Organization (FAO/WHO) in 2001/2002 and amended by the International Scientific Association for Probiotics and Prebiotics in 2014, as "live microorganisms which when administered in adequate amounts confer a health benefit on the host". In a further attempt to clarify what constitutes a probiotic, a newly created "probiotic framework" separates live microbes used as processing aids or those in naturally fermented foods from those administered primarily for their health benefits (Fig. 36.1). It also dictates that until any microorganisms or gut commensals are isolated, characterised, and their health effects sufficiently demonstrated, they cannot be called probiotics.

In contrast, prebiotics are defined as "nondigestible food ingredients that beneficially affect the host by selectively stimulating the growth and/or activity of one or a limited number of bacterial species already established in the colon, and thus in effect improve host health", as outlined originally by Gibson and Roberfroid in 1995.[2]

In some cases, prebiotics may be directly beneficial for a probiotic, providing a synbiotic concept. Synbiotics are

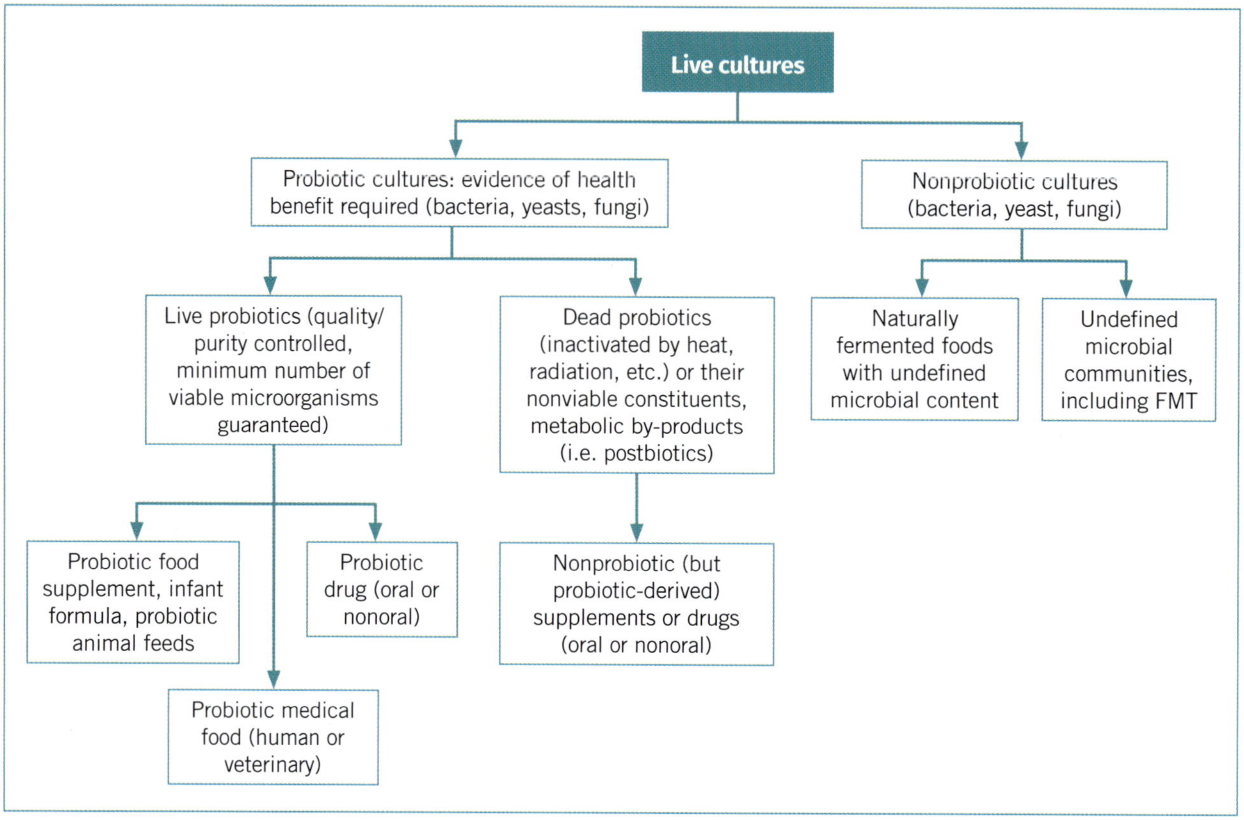

Figure 36.1. The probiotic framework and its regulation. The definition of probiotics currently includes live cultures with a proven health benefit to the host. FMT, faecal microbiota transplantation. Adapted from DE SIMONE C. The unregulated probiotic market. *Clin Gastroenterol Hepatol* 17:809, 2019.[1]

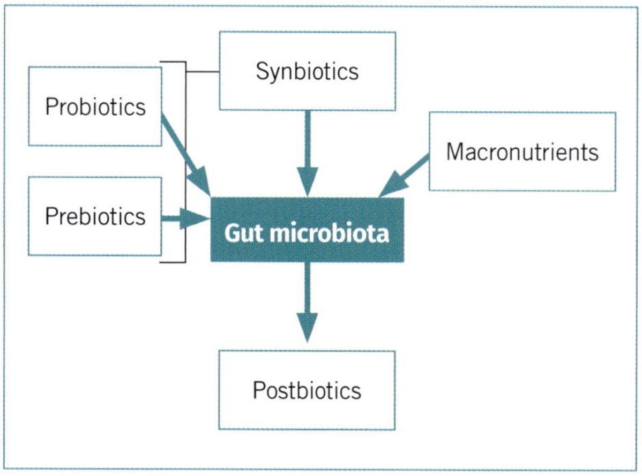

Figure 36.2. Schematic metabolism of pre-, pro-, or synbiotics alongside macronutrients by the gut microbiota to postbiotic products. Pro- or prebiotics (or their combination, i.e. synbiotics), as well as the composition of macronutrients, have a modifying effect on the composition and function of the gut microbiota. Metabolic products from the microbiota are collectively termed postbiotics and can be derived mainly from carbohydrate and fibre fermentation, plant polyphenols, protein putrefaction, microbial gas postbiotics, or vitamin postbiotics. Adapted from https://www.myhillsvet.com.au/blog/gut-feeling-on-postbiotics/.

hence defined as "mixtures of probiotics and prebiotics that beneficially affect the host by improving the survival and implantation of live microbial dietary supplements in the gastrointestinal tract of the host".[3]

Postbiotics is a relatively new term that has been created to refer to the nonviable metabolic (by)products of live commensal or probiotic microorganisms that have biological activity in the host (Fig. 36.2). These include short-chain fatty acids (SCFA), indol, indoxyl sulphate, phenolic metabolites, vitamins, and others, as well as enzymes, peptides, polysaccharides, cell surface proteins, and organic acids released after bacterial lysis. Even though most of them are largely unexplored, some researchers believe that they are responsible for many of the beneficial effects of probiotics.[4]

MECHANISMS OF PROBIOTIC ACTION IN THE GASTROINTESTINAL TRACT

Several mechanisms of action within the GI tract and the gut-associated immune system have been proposed for probiotics (Fig. 36.3), but very few of them have been confirmed specifically in small animals. These include displacement of intestinal pathogens (e.g. by interfering with their adherence to the intestinal epithelial cells [IECs] or by inducing mucus/mucin production), production of antimicrobial substances (e.g. organic acids, defensins, specific toxins aimed at pathogens, proteases that in turn can deactivate toxins), enhancement of innate and adaptive immune responses within IECs or the lamina propria immune cells, and upregulation of various nonspecific cellular defence mechanisms (e.g. heat shock proteins, inflammasomes).[5]

Many of these actions are strain-specific; even bacterial strains of the same species can alter cellular responses differentially. For example, *Lactobacillus reuteri* ATCC PTA 6475 can inhibit lipopolysaccharide-induced tumour necrosis factor alpha (TNF-α) production from myeloid cells in vitro through suppression of the activator protein-1 pathway, while another *L. reuteri* strain, DSM 17938, does not exhibit this behaviour.[6] Details on cellular interactions of specific probiotic strains have been summarised in several reviews,[5,7,8] but it is overall believed that key biological signalling pathways, for example for the transcription of cytokines, cell survival, and apoptosis are common targets for probiotics or their products both in vitro and in vivo,[7] particularly in innate immune cells like macrophages and IECs (Fig. 36.3). Probiotics also regulate adaptive local immunity by influencing T-cell maturation and proliferation towards a more

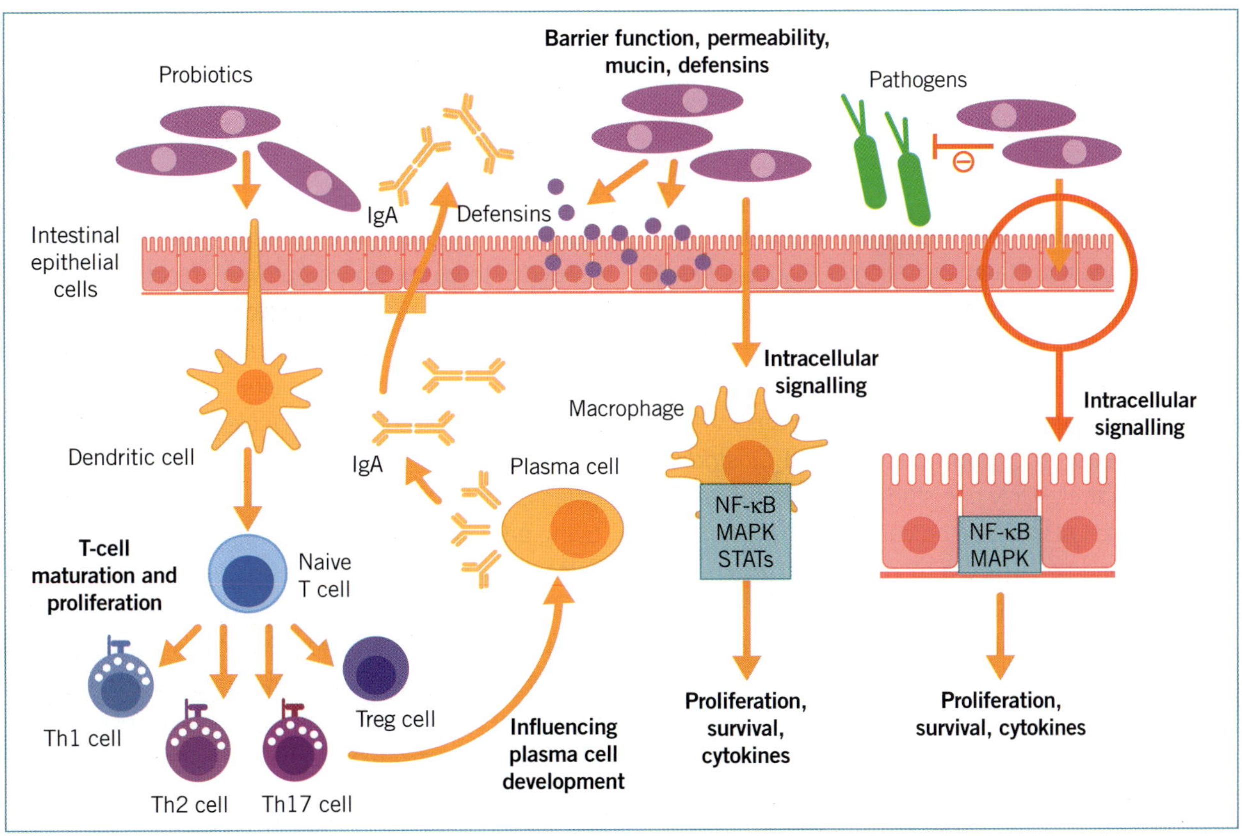

Figure 36.3. Proposed mechanisms of action of probiotics on the intestinal mucosa and the associated local immune system. Yellow arrows indicate direct promoting effects. The red T-shaped arrow indicates an inhibitory effect. IgA, immunoglobulin A; MAPK, mitogen-activated protein kinase; NF-κB, nuclear factor kappa B; STAT, signal transducer and activator of transcription; Th cell, T-helper cell; Treg cell, regulatory T cell. Adapted from Thomas CM, Versalovic J. Probiotics-host communication: modulation of signaling pathways in the intestine. *Gut Microbes* 1:148, 2010.[7]

tolerogenic environment (shift to regulatory T cells), and plasma cell development/class switching to specific IgA production (Fig. 36.3).[7]

THE EFFECT OF PRO- OR SYNBIOTICS ON FELINE HEALTH

Enterococcus faecium (EF) is one of the most widely used "probiotics" in small animals, but no studies have focused on its effects when administered to healthy cats. Most information stems from administering EF to healthy dogs. For example, when EF 10415 SF68 was given to healthy puppies for a year, they had significantly higher total faecal and serum IgA levels compared to the control animals.[9]

In healthy cats, three studies investigated the effect of potential probiotic lactic acid bacteria (LAB) on faecal characteristics like visual scores, volatile compounds, pH, and selected bacteria based on culture methods, as well as assessment of physical examination and routine clinicopathologic data findings (Table 36.1). Changes in these latter parameters were generally not observed, while faecal scores also either remained the same or improved slightly.[10–12] Faecal pH decreased, while volatile compounds remained unchanged in one study (with administration of *Lactobacillus acidophilus*),[10] but in another study (administration of *Bifidobacterium pseudocatenulatum*) a reduction of faecal ammonia and lactic, n-valeric and isovaleric acids in combination with an increase in acetic acid was reported.[12] Faecal culture results generally showed an increase in LAB and a decrease in coliform bacteria and *Clostridium* spp., respectively. Only one study assessed the effects of a synbiotic LAB mixture on cats beyond faecal characteristics and performed a more in-depth analysis on faecal microbiota composition (Table 36.1).[13] They also observed a significant increase in *Lactobacillus* spp. during synbiotic supplementation, while major bacterial phyla as assessed by 454-pyrosequencing were not altered. Reduction in microbiota species diversity was observed during synbiotic supplementation, but overall, the functional significance of any of these observed changes remains unclear.

In the majority of studies in healthy animals, "probiotic" bacterial strains were undetectable immediately or shortly after administration ceased, and described effects were transient. However, as most of these studies did not use commercially available "probiotic" products, but commensal bacterial strains isolated from individual animals, this makes them difficult to reproduce or translate into practice.

USE OF PRO- OR SYNBIOTICS IN FELINE GASTROINTESTINAL DISEASES

Peer-reviewed studies investigating in vivo use of pro- or synbiotics in the prevention or treatment of disease in cats are sparse. Only five clinical trials report the use of pro- or synbiotics in feline GI diseases. One of them is a randomised controlled trial,[14] three are experimental[15,16] or in vitro[17] studies, and one is a conference abstract that has so far not been published in a peer-reviewed journal.[18] A variety of different pro- and synbiotics from different sources have been assessed, making comparison of individual studies difficult (Tables 36.2 and 36.3).

Probiotics in acute gastrointestinal conditions

Acute GI diseases in which the merit of pro- or synbiotic treatment has been investigated in cats can be roughly divided in three categories: "proven" infectious diseases (viral, bacterial, parasitic/protozoal), "idiopathic" or otherwise ill-defined gastroenteritis (in which an infectious component might or might not be present), and antibiotic-induced diarrhoea (Table 36.2).

In acute uncomplicated diarrhoea ("idiopathic" gastroenteritis not further classified, or due to kennelling stress/being admitted to a shelter), only one study included cats as well as dogs, and no effect on the prevalence or duration of shelter-associated diarrhoea was found.[14] It might, however, be noteworthy that this study included animals regardless of their parasitic burden at the time of diarrhoea, and that the overall incidence of diarrhoea was low, which might have influenced the results.

For acute viral enteritis, no study in cats is available. However, as one study reports a significant clinical improvement with a commercially available LAB mixture added to standard treatment in canine parvovirosis, with an improved survival rate of 90% (vs. 70% in stand-

Table 36.1. Suspected pro- or synbiotics tested for health-promoting effects in healthy cats.

Microorganism used (source)	Dose and duration	Test animals (n)	Control group	Measured outcomes	Reference
***Bifidobacterium pseudocatenulatum* (BP-B82) (isolated from a healthy cat) + galacto-oligosaccharides**	10^{10} CFU/day for 15 days	10 client-owned healthy cats	No	Faecal volatile compounds: reduced faecal ammonia concentration; higher faecal acetic acid concentration; lower faecal lactic, n-valeric, and isovaleric acids concentration; no change in faecal polyamines. Faecal cultures: faecal bifidobacteria increased, while counts of *C. perfringens*, coliforms, and enterococci were unchanged.	Biagi et al. 2013[12]
LAB mixture: *E. faecium* *S. salivarius* subsp. *thermophilus* *B. longum* *L. acidophilus* *L. casei* subsp. *rhamnosus* *L. plantarum* *L. delbrueckii* subsp. *bulgaricus* + FOS, arabinogalactans (Proviable-DC, Nutramax Laboratories)	5×10^9 CFU/day (exact proportions are proprietary) for 3 weeks	12 privately-owned healthy cats (mostly domestic shorthair cats) & 12 privately-owned healthy dogs (various breeds)	No	Faecal scores: normal with the exception of 2 cats and 2 dogs (pulpy faeces for 2 days). CBC & serum biochemistry, serum cobalamin/folate, f/cTLI, and f/cPLI (day 0, 21 [last day of supplementation], and day 42 [3 weeks after cessation of supplementation]): decrease in lymphocytes (cats) and neutrophils (dogs) during supplementation. Other parameters unchanged. Faecal total IgA (day 0, 21, and 42): no change. Canine/feline faecal alpha$_1$-proteinase inhibitor (day 0, 21, and 42): no change. 16S rRNA PCR followed by DGGE (day 0, 21, and 38 [2 weeks after cessation of supplementation]): 11/12 (92%) of cats and 5/11 (45%) of dogs specific DGGE bands observed during supplementation that were absent at baseline or after supplementation. Sequencing identified *Enterococcus faecium*. 16S rRNA gene clone libraries for *Lactobacillus* spp. and *Bifidobacterium* spp. (days 14–17 [last week of supplementation] and 2 weeks after cessation of supplementation): at least one LAB was detected during supplementation in 8/11 (73%) of cats and 9/11 (82%) of dogs, but were undetectable before or after supplementation. qPCR for bacterial targets of interest: *Bifidobacterium* spp., *Enterococcus* spp., *Lactobacillus* spp., *Streptococcus* spp. (day 1, 8, and 17 in cats, and days 3, 5, and 17 in dogs): abundances of *Enterococcus* spp. and *Streptococcus* spp. increased in at least 1 time point during supplementation in both cats and dogs. In cats, *Lactobacillus* spp. increased significantly on day 17 of supplementation. Massive parallel 16S rRNA 454-pyrosequencing (day 0, 5, and 23): no changes in major bacterial phyla, no clustering on PCoA, no differences in diversity indices in dogs. Cats had higher Shannon–Weaver diversity index before supplementation when compared to during or after supplementation.	Garcia-Mazcorro et al. 2011[13]
***Lactobacillus acidophilus* D2/CSL (CECT 4529) (commercial culture)**	5×10^9 CFU/kg feed over 5 weeks	10 adult cats (5 each in control and probiotic group)	Yes (feed alone)	Body weight and BCS: no change. Faecal characteristics: less faecal moisture and better faecal scores on probiotics. Faecal culture: increase in lactobacilli and decrease in *E. coli*.	Fusi et al. 2019[11]
***Lactobacillus acidophilus* DSM13241**	2×10^8 CFU/day for 4.5 weeks	15 adult cats	No	Assessments before, after 4.5 weeks of supplementation, and after additional 4 weeks without supplementation. Physical exam findings, haematology, biochemistry, food intake, and body weight: no change Faecal scores: no change Faecal volatile compounds (hydrogen sulphide, ammonia): no change Faecal pH decreased Faecal culture: clostridia reduced during probiotic feeding and increased after cessation; coliform and *Enterococcus* spp. decreased during the study	Marshall-Jones et al. 2006[10]

BCS, body condition score; CBC, complete blood count; CFU, colony-forming unit; cPLI, canine pancreatic lipase immunoreactivity; cTLI, canine trypsin-like immunoreactivity; DGGE, denaturing gradient gel electrophoresis; FOS, fructooligosaccharides; fPLI, feline pancreatic lipase immunoreactivity; fTLI, feline trypsin-like immunoreactivity; Ig, immunoglobulin; LAB, lactic acid bacteria; PCoA, principal coordinate analysis; qPCR, quantitative polymerase chain reaction.

ard treatment only), this might or might not be a viable adjunctive treatment in feline panleucopenia. It should be considered that no causal relationship between probiotic administration and shortening of treatment duration, improvement in disease evolution, antibody production, or faecal virus excretion was established, and the mechanism by which probiotics improved clinical outcomes remain unclear. For potential future use, it should also be noted that the LAB mixture used was originally marketed under the trade name of VSL#3. However, the currently available product VSL#3 does no longer contain the same strains. The originally used "de Simone" formulation of the LAB mixture is currently available as Visbiome (in the United States of America and Canada) and as VivoMixx (in Europe). As strain specificity is important, only the original mixture should be used.

In acute parasitic disease, pro- or synbiotics have not been assessed in cats so far. In dogs, they had limited to no effects. *Giardia* cyst shedding was not altered by the administration of EF, while subclinical *Ancylostoma* egg shedding was significantly, but only transiently, suppressed using a LAB mixture.

Antibiotic-induced diarrhoea was assessed in two experimental studies. Healthy cats were either given potentiated amoxicillin[15] or clindamycin,[16] and different probiotics were used to counter their effects on the GI tract (EF[15] and a LAB mixture[16], respectively). No statistical difference was noted in faecal scores, faecal dysbiosis index, or faecal microbiota characteristics. In one of the studies, complex metabolic changes of the microbiota were described, but these were more likely associated with the administration of antibiotics than with the administration of probiotics.[16]

Probiotics in chronic gastrointestinal conditions

Probiotics have been assessed in the context of chronic *Tritrichomonas blagburni* (*foetus*) infection and chronic constipation in cats (Table 36.3). Evidence for the adjunctive use of EF in feline *T. blagburni* infection is based on

Table 36.2. Pro- or synbiotics assessed for their effect in acute gastrointestinal conditions in cats.

Pro- or synbiotic used (trade name, manufacturer)	Dose	Target species	Animals (n)	Disorder	Observed outcomes	Reference
***E. faecium* SF68 NCIMB 10415 (Fortiflora, Nestle Purina)**	2.1×10^9 CFU/day	Dog, cat	Dogs: 182 (102 treatment, 80 placebo) Cats: 217 (130 treatment, 87 placebo)	Shelter-associated diarrhoea (some animals also positive for various parasites)	Dogs: no difference in number of dogs having diarrhoea (9.8% treatment, 12.5% placebo) Cats: no difference in prevalence or duration of diarrhoea (26% treatment, 32% placebo)	Bybee, Scorza, and Lappin 2011[14]
***E. faecium* SF68 NCIMB 10415 (commercial product not specified)**	Not disclosed	Cat	27 (13 treatment, 14 placebo)	Antibiotic-induced diarrhoea (potentiated amoxicillin)	No statistical difference in faecal scores between treatment groups No difference in number of observed species of the faecal microbiota between treatment groups	Torres-Henderson et al. 2017[15]
LAB mixture: *B. bifidum* *E. faecium* *E. thermophilus* *L. acidophilus* *L. bulgaricus* *L. casei* *L. plantarum* + FOS and arabinogalactan (Proviable-DC, Nutramax)	1×10^{10} CFU/day	Cat	16 (8 treatment, 8 placebo)	Antibiotic-induced diarrhoea (clindamycin)	Higher abundance of faecal *Ruminococcaceae* in probiotic-treated group No difference of dysbiosis index, microbiota richness, or diversity indices between treatment groups Some complex metabolomic changes were observed, but most likely due to antibiotics rather than probiotics	Whittemore et al. 2019[16]

CFU, colony-forming unit; FOS, fructooligosaccharides; LAB, lactic acid bacteria.

a small clinical trial, in which it did not accelerate time to clinical improvement compared to ronidazole alone but significantly reduced relapse,[18] and on a study investigating the effects of different enterococci on *T. blagburni* growth and cytotoxicity in an IEC culture model. The enterococci (one of them sourced from a commercial product) were able to completely inhibit *T. blagburni* growth both prophylactically (before cell infection) and therapeutically (after log-phase growth had been achieved).[17] However, it is yet unclear if this translates into similar efficacy in vivo.

There is some preliminary evidence that a probiotic blend called SLAB51 could be beneficial in feline chronic constipation or idiopathic megacolon.[19] This is based on a small study including 10 cats. Only three of these cats had been diagnosed with idiopathic megacolon; in the others, the cause of the constipation—that had to be present at least twice within a month—was ill-defined, and it remained unclear if all cats had investigations allowing the diagnosis of "idiopathic" constipation. There was also no alternative treatment group included (and it is unclear how many cats had subtotal colectomy performed as part of the treatment), only tissue samples obtained from an ill-defined control group. In all constipated cats, clinical severity significantly reduced at the end of the probiotic treatment, and the number of interstitial cells of Cajal within colonic tissue increased. There were also some changes of faecal bacterial species of unclear significance.[19] There are no studies assessing the use of pro- or synbiotics in chronic noninfectious

Table 36.3. Pro- or synbiotics assessed for their effect in chronic gastrointestinal conditions in cats.

Pro- or synbiotic used (trade name, manufacturer)	Dose	Animals (n)	Disorder	Observed outcomes	Reference
***E. faecium* (isolated from commercial product containing *E. faecium* SF68 NCIMB10415—Fortiflora, Nestle Purina) or *E. hirae* (isolated from a healthy kitten) vs. placebo**	1×10^5–10^8 CFU/cell culture well	N/A (no clinical trial)	*Tritrichomonas blagburni* (*foetus*) infection of IECs in vitro: coculture experiment using enterococci with *T. blagburni* infecting porcine intestinal epithelial cells (IPEC-J2)	When enterococci and *T. blagburni* were added simultaneously, enterococci completely inhibited *T. blagburni* growth When enterococci were added after *T. blagburni* had achieved early log-phase growth (18 h), enterococci significantly inhibited growth Viable enterococci were needed for this effect, as direct interaction and colonisation of the IECs was necessary; this effect was also shown to be partially pH dependent	Dickson et al. 2019[17]
***E. faecium* DSM 10663 NCIMB 10415 4b/E1707 + FOS and gum arabic, kaolin, montmorillonite, pectin, alpha-glucan butyrogenic, patented mucopolysaccharide starch (Pro-Kolin paste, Protexin)**	Dose not disclosed	26 (13 ronidazole 10–30 mg/kg every 24 h & placebo; 13 ronidazole 10–30 mg/kg every 24 h & synbiotic)	Natural *Tritrichomonas blagburni* (*foetus*) infection	In both groups, faecal scores and body weight improved Cats on synbiotic had significantly less relapses (2/13) compared to placebo-treated cats (8/13)	Lalor and Gunn-Moore 2012 (congress abstract)[18]
SLAB51 blend: *Scc. thermophilus* DSM32245 *L. acidophilus* DSM32241 *L. plantarum* DSM32244 *L. casei* DSM32243 *L. helveticus*, DSM32242 *L. brevis* DSM27961 *B. lactis* DSM32246 *B. lactis* DSM32247 (Sivoy/SivoMixx, Mendes/Omendes)	2×10^{11} CFU lyophilised bacteria per 5 kg body weight	10 with naturally occurring disease (10 healthy cats used as controls for tissue, but not treated with probiotic)	Chronic constipation (7/10) & idiopathic megacolon (3/10)	Clinical severity score significantly reduced at end of probiotic treatment Number of ICCs increased significantly Significant increase in faecal streptococci and lactobacilli after treatment (of total of 9 analysed taxa)	Rossi et al. 2018[19]

CFU, colony-forming unit; FOS, fructooligosaccharides; ICC, interstitial cell of Cajal; IEC, intestinal epithelial cell.

diarrhoea or inflammatory bowel disease (IBD) in cats, even though there is some evidence that the de Simone probiotic blend is as effective as treatment with a metronidazole–prednisolone combination in dogs with IBD, and also in prevention of recurrence in human IBD.

PREBIOTICS, DIETARY FIBRE, AND POSTBIOTICS IN FELINE GASTROENTEROLOGY

The supplementation of plant fibre to feline diets has been associated with beneficial effects on the general health of the GI tract.[20,21] Despite a short colon, the lack of a functional caecum, and other adaptations to a strict carnivorous diet, fermentation of a broad range of dietary fibres takes place in the feline large intestine.[20,22] Concentrations of postbiotics like volatile fatty acids in the colon of healthy cats is comparable to those of other monogastric mammals,[20] and one study shows that the metabolic capacities of the feline microbiota are comparable to those of the microbiota of other omnivores.[23] Regardless, species differences should be taken into account, and studies on dietary fibre should ideally be done in the target species. Besides plant fibres, the importance of animal fibre for wild carnivorous species has been demonstrated.[21] In domestic cats, however, little research has been done on animal fibre, despite the fact that animal meal is the main fibre and protein source in the majority of commercially available cat foods, and despite the growing popularity of raw meat-based diets.[21]

Most studies assessing the effect of prebiotics on cats are feeding trials investigating nutrient digestibility or changes in fermentation properties or composition of the intestinal microbiota. This includes fructooligosaccharides (FOS), galactooligosaccharides (GOS),[12,24] pectin, inulin, and yeast-wall extracts. In most early culture-based studies, an increase in faecal *Bifidobacterium* spp. was observed.[21,23] Especially, FOS were described as a useful fibre source for promotion of feline GI health based on changes in the faecal microbiota.[23] A lack of significant effects in follow-up studies might be due to a lower dose of FOS. When GOS or a FOS–GOS combination was supplemented, the increase in *Bifidobacterium* spp. counts was higher. However, in more recent studies, even with relatively high doses of prebiotics, changes seen in the microbiota composition or richness when assessed by modern sequencing techniques were not sufficient to separate bacterial communities or predicted metabolic profiles according to administration of prebiotics.[25]

The direct influence of fibre fermentation and concomitant SCFA production on colonic morphology has been assessed in healthy lean cats[26] and in overweight cats.[27] Beneficial effects on morphology (colonic weight, mucosal cell density, crypt structure), function (mucosal tissue energetics, transport of SCFA), and microbiota composition within the colon (reduced pathogenic bacteria) were observed.[26,28] According to the authors, the supplementation of a moderately fermentable fibre source to diets for lean felines generated the best combination of beneficial effects. In contrast, in overweight cats, the supplementation of fibre did not affect the histological findings in colonic biopsies.[27]

Oligofructose and inulin have also been assessed for their effect on glucose and amino acid metabolism in healthy domestic cats: they did not modulate fasting blood glucose, insulin concentrations, or responses to glucose administration.[29,30] In contrast, in another study, decreases in mean blood glucose concentration and area under the curve were achieved by supplementing sugarcane fibre to diets of overweight cats.[27]

Despite the availability of some studies into the role of fibres in the nutritional management of extra-GI diseases in cats (chronic renal disease, hepatobiliary and pancreatic diseases, obesity), there are no studies investigating the effect of specific dietary fibres or prebiotics alone (i.e. not as a synbiotic) in cats with GI conditions apart from one exception: a psyllium-enriched extruded dry diet was found to be efficient in the management of recurrent feline constipation in an uncontrolled study.[31] No follow-up controlled clinical trials in constipation or other feline GI conditions like IBD are available.

Production of postbiotics might be modified by selectively increasing specific pre-, pro-, or synbiotics in the diet (Fig. 36.2). Overall, studies suggest that postbiotics from carbohydrate fermentation (e.g. SCFAs) or polyphenol metabolism result in beneficial effects, whereas postbiotics from excessive protein putrefaction (e.g. ammonia, phenols, p-cresol, certain amines, hydrogen sulphide) may be detrimental by increasing intestinal barrier permeability, inflammation, DNA damage, and cancer progression.[4,32]

For example, the SCFA acetate is produced by many bacteria, but propionate and butyrate tend to be produced by specific bacteria only. Postbiotics are proposed to act locally in the colon or be taken up by the host into the systemic circulation. The most important factor that determines which postbiotics are being formed in the intestine is the amount and type of substrate available for microbial digestion. Providing primarily carbohydrates to the gut microbiota results in a saccharolytic type of fermentation. In the colon, this primarily involves resistant starch, oligosaccharides, or fibre. The major postbiotics generated by feline intestinal microbiota are straight SCFAs (acetate, propionate, butyrate),[20] which are products of saccharolytic fermentation. SCFAs reduce inflammation via receptors on immune cells and alter gene expression. A number of experimental studies show that they maintain mucosal integrity and growth. Particularly, butyrate is an important energy source for colonocytes and has the capacity to modify cell growth. SCFAs also stimulate feline colonic smooth muscle contractions.[33] The main beneficial effects of SCFAs are summarised in Figure 36.4.

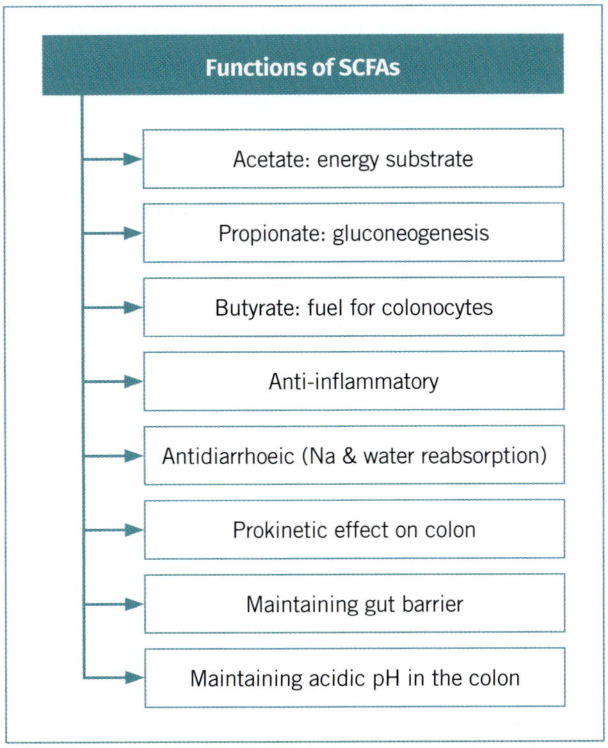

Figure 36.4. Physiological functions of short-chain fatty acids (SCFAs) as examples of postbiotics. Adapted from https://www.myhillsvet.com.au/blog/gut-feeling-on-postbiotics/.

Other postbiotics are not as well investigated as SCFAs and some of them only recently recognised as important (Fig. 36.5).

Polyphenols are a diverse class of plant metabolites, synthesised as a protection against UV light and pathogens, classed broadly into flavonoids, phenolic acids, lignans, and stilbenes (Fig. 36.6).[34] They can often be found in skin, flesh, and fibre of fruits and grains and are associated with their colour and taste. The colon does not only receive unmodified dietary polyphenols, but

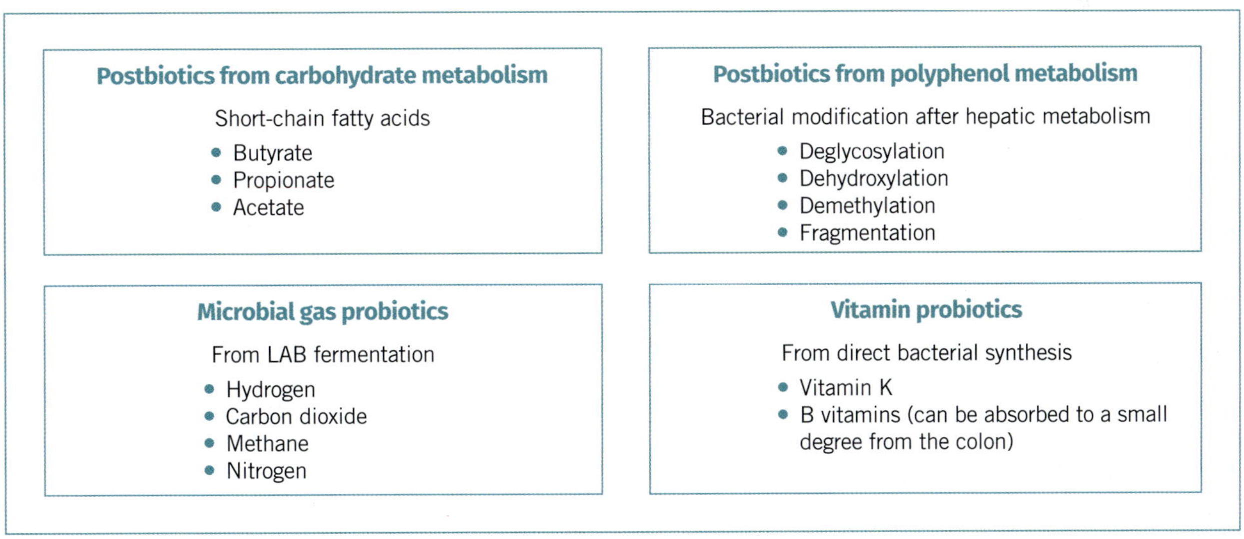

Figure 36.5. The four main sources of beneficial postbiotics. LAB, lactic acid bacteria.

a mixture of their metabolites, as they undergo excessive hepatic metabolism and enterohepatic recycling. Polyphenols and their metabolites have been reported to have antioxidant, anti-inflammatory, antimicrobial, and disease-modulating properties.[34] They likely retain their bioactive roles after ingestion, either in their native form or as metabolites. A recent review of health outcomes in people concluded that a critical mass of data strongly suggests a protective effect of a polyphenol-rich diet, even if further well-targeted studies are needed to define specific recommendations.[34]

The effect of polyphenols in cats has not been fully investigated, but a conference abstract suggests a "health-promoting" effect: polyphenols in the diet modulated feline gut microbiota by increasing the relative abundance of beneficial bacteria. Food containing pea

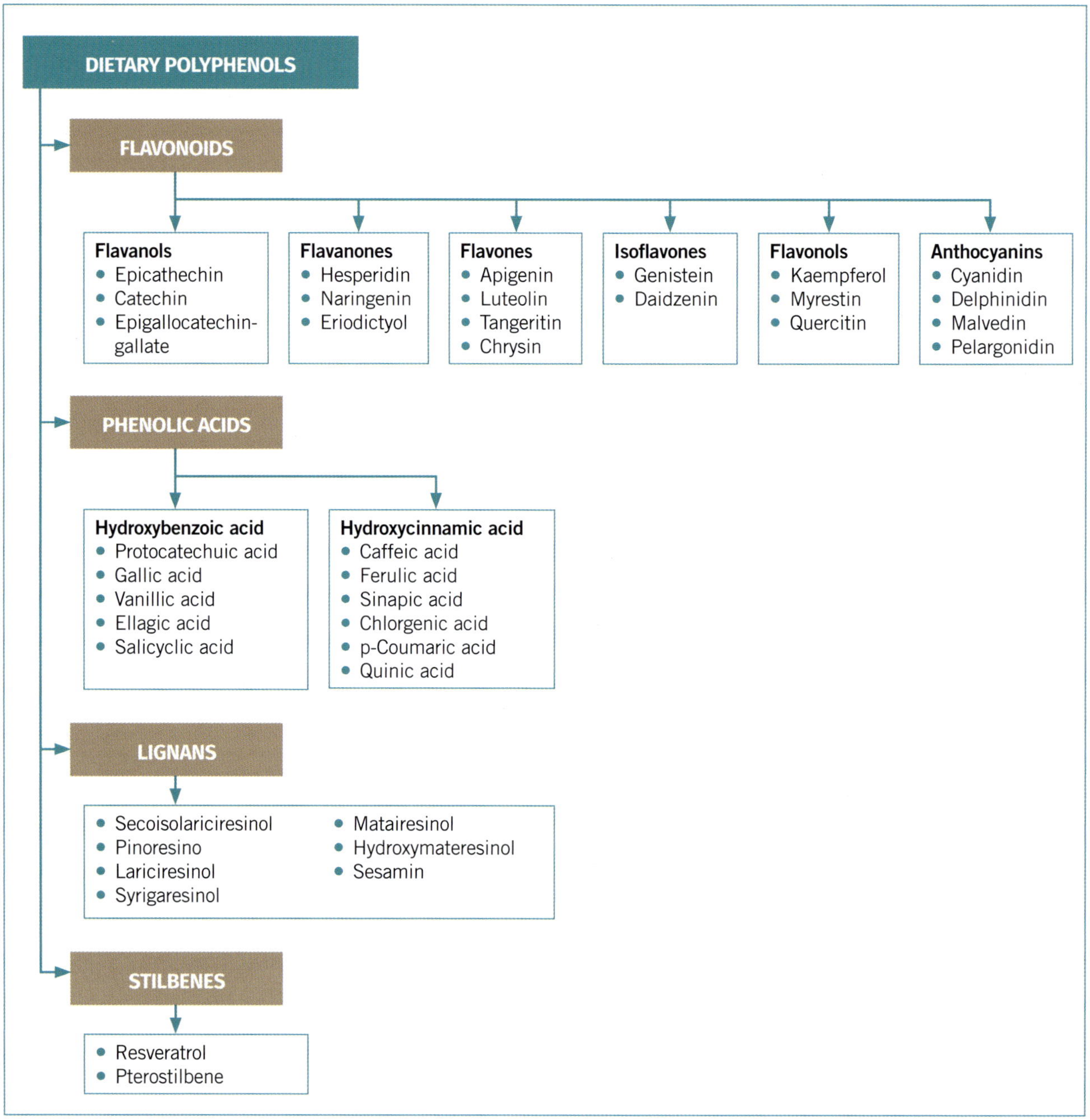

Figure 36.6. Classes of dietary polyphenols grouped by their chemical structure. Examples for each type are given.

powder, tomato pomace, and broccoli powder led to a significant increase in *Bifidobacterium* spp. and reduction in *Clostridium* spp. and *Eubacterium* spp., and influenced markers of aging in senior dogs and cats, but only the data of dogs have been published in a peer-reviewed journal so far.[35] A citrus polyphenol-supplemented diet reduced plasma acute phase proteins in obese cats.[36] Studies on rice bran might assess the effect of polyphenols indirectly, as it contains the polyphenols ferulic acid and α-lipoic acid: it was found to reduce plasma taurine and increase the faecal excretion of conjugated bile acids. This, by proxy, might improve gut health, as bile acids have only recently been considered in the pathogenesis of canine (but not feline) chronic enteropathies.

CONCLUSIONS

Many products or strains marketed or tested as probiotics or synbiotics in small animals do not strictly fulfil the criteria to be defined as a probiotic, as this is based on a proven beneficial effect on the host. Whilst there are only a few clinical trials in the correct "target species" allowing a direct inference of results to feline clinical practice, studies investigating mechanisms of action of potential probiotics in cats are even more sparse. The studies available in both acute and chronic GI conditions suffer from a number of problems. In several clinical trials, there was no control group, animals with ill-defined diseases were included, or inappropriate and nonspecific inclusion criteria were applied. Most studies in which inclusion criteria are better defined, and hence examined conditions more convincingly stratified, have been conducted using small numbers (Tables 36.2 and 36.3), with statistical power either not assessed or likely insufficient. In addition, a wide range of different potential probiotics has been used at different dosages and in various conditions. This is problematic, as there is evidence that molecular effects of probiotics are not only specific to the genus of the bacteria used, but even species- or strain-specific. This, together with a huge discrepancy in measured outcomes (ranging from assessment of nonspecific routine clinicopathologic parameters and purely observational assessments like faecal scores to complex faecal microbiota sequencing and metabolic profiles), makes it difficult to compare studies. Especially when assessing faecal microbial diversity and function, very few studies have applied modern molecular techniques that allow a more realistic assessment of the microbiota composition and diversity compared to culture-based techniques. Microbiota function or metagenomics have hardly been employed using feline samples.

There is preliminary evidence that certain pro- or synbiotic preparations could be beneficial in some infectious GI conditions, namely parvovirosis in dogs and *T. blagburni* infection in cats, while results in undefined or "idiopathic" acute enteritis are mixed. The effect on well-defined chronic noninfectious GI conditions has only been investigated in dogs, in which little benefit was observed with adjunctive administration of probiotics. A relatively new blend of probiotics (SLAB51) might be beneficial in cats with constipation, but further studies are needed. This blend is currently also used by many gastroenterologists (including the author) in IBD, especially if the de Simone (formerly VSL#3, now Visbiome or VivoMixx) formulation is not available. The composition of the de Simone formulation and SLAB51 is very similar, but neither of them have been investigated for their use in IBD in cats, and there are no studies comparing these two blends for their efficacy in any feline condition.

Recent studies suggest that the feline gut microbiota produce many different postbiotics. Even for cats, postbiotics from carbohydrate fermentation likely result in beneficial effects, whereas postbiotics from excessive protein putrefaction may be detrimental. However, research into finding the best nutritional strategies to maintain and activate the gut microbiota using prebiotics and dietary fibre to assess long-term health benefits or use in GI disease is still lacking. The relationship between gut health, microbiota composition and function, carbohydrate fermentation, and protein putrefaction, and the associated connection between pro-, pre-, and postbiotics in cats, will require more research to derive specific recommendations for optimal gut microbial function in health and disease.

In summary, more well-designed studies into the potential benefit of probiotics in feline GI conditions are needed; and they should be designed to have sufficient statistical power to detect meaningful effects. Studies should focus on assessing functional outcomes that can further the understanding of probiotic-specific mechanisms of action and can inform and drive rational and evidence-based clinical use of pro-, pre-, syn-, and postbiotics.

Take-home messages

- Probiotics need stricter regulation in the veterinary market, and products should be tested to exert the health benefits claimed.
- Probiotics are likely useful in acute gastrointestinal conditions, and their effect is likely strain-specific.
- The type of probiotics beneficial in chronic gastrointestinal disease needs further investigation, but mixtures are likely preferred over single-strain preparations.

REFERENCES

[1] de Simone C. The unregulated probiotic market. *Clin Gastroenterol Hepatol* 17:809, 2019.

[2] Gibson GR, Roberfroid MB. Dietary modulation of the human colonic microbiota: introducing the concept of prebiotics. *J Nutr* 125:1401, 1995.

[3] Andersson H et al. Health effects of probiotics and prebiotics. A literature review on human studies. *Näringsforskning* 45:58, 2001.

[4] Oliphant K, Allen-Vercoe E. Macronutrient metabolism by the human gut microbiome: major fermentation by-products and their impact on host health. *Microbiome* 7:91, 2019.

[5] Oelschlaeger TA. Mechanisms of probiotic actions—A review. *Int J Med Microbiol* 300:57, 2010.

[6] Lin PW et al. *Lactobacillus rhamnosus* blocks inflammatory signaling in vivo via reactive oxygen species generation. *Free Radic Biol Med* 47:1205, 2009.

[7] Thomas CM, Versalovic J. Probiotics-host communication: modulation of signaling pathways in the intestine. *Gut Microbes* 1:148, 2010.

[8] Schmitz S, Suchodolski J. Understanding the canine intestinal microbiota and its modification by pro-, pre- and synbiotics—what is the evidence? *Vet Med Sci* 2:71, 2016.

[9] Benyacoub J et al. Supplementation of food with *Enterococcus faecium* (SF68) stimulates immune functions in young dogs. *J Nutr* 133:1158, 2003.

[10] Marshall-Jones ZV et al. Effects of *Lactobacillus acidophilus* DSM13241 as a probiotic in healthy adult cats. *Am J Vet Res* 67:1005, 2006.

[11] Fusi E et al. Effects of *Lactobacillus acidophilus* D2/CSL (CECT 4529) supplementation on healthy cat performance. *Vet Rec Open* 6:e000368, 2019.

[12] Biagi G et al. Effect of feeding a selected combination of galacto-oligosaccharides and a strain of *Bifidobacterium pseudocatenulatum* on the intestinal microbiota of cats. *Am J Vet Res* 74:90, 2013.

[13] Garcia-Mazcorro JF et al. Effect of a multi-species synbiotic formulation on fecal bacterial microbiota of healthy cats and dogs as evaluated by pyrosequencing. *FEMS Microbiol Ecol* 78:542, 2011.

[14] Bybee SN, Scorza AV, Lappin MR. Effect of the probiotic *Enterococcus faecium* SF68 on presence of diarrhea in cats and dogs housed in an animal shelter. *J Vet Intern Med* 25:856, 2011.

[15] Torres-Henderson C et al. Effect of *Enterococcus faecium* strain SF68 on gastrointestinal signs and fecal microbiome in cats administered amoxicillin–clavulanate. *Top Companion Anim Med* 32:104, 2017.

[16] Whittemore JC et al. Effects of a synbiotic on the fecal microbiome and metabolomic profiles of healthy research cats administered clindamycin: a randomized, controlled trial. *Gut Microbes* 10:521, 2019.

[17] Dickson R et al. The effect of enterococci on feline *Tritrichomonas foetus* infection in vitro. *Vet Parasitol* 273:90, 2019.

[18] Lalor S, Gunn-Moore D. Effects of concurrent ronidazole and probiotic therapy in cats with *Tritrichomonas foetus*-associated diarrhoea. Abstract. *J Feline Med Surg* 14:650, 2012.

[19] Rossi G et al. Effects of a probiotic (SLAB51™) on clinical and histologic variables and microbiota of cats with chronic constipation/megacolon: a pilot study. *Benef Microbes* 9:101, 2018.

[20] Brosey BP, Hill RC, Scott KC. Gastrointestinal volatile fatty acid concentrations and pH in cats. *Am J Vet Res* 61:359, 2000.

[21] Rochus K, Janssens GP, Hesta M. Dietary fibre and the importance of the gut microbiota in feline nutrition: a review. *Nutr Res Rev* 27:295, 2014.

[22] Sunvold GD et al. In vitro fermentation of selected fibrous substrates by dog and cat fecal inoculum: influence of diet composition on substrate organic matter disappearance and short-chain fatty acid production. *J Anim Sci* 73:1110, 1995.

[23] Barry KA et al. Effects of dietary fiber on the feline gastrointestinal metagenome. *J Proteome Res* 11:5924, 2012.

[24] Kanakupt K et al. Effects of short-chain fructooligosaccharides and galactooligosaccharides, individually and in combination, on nutrient digestibility, fecal fermentative metabolite concentrations, and large bowel microbial ecology of healthy adults cats. *J Anim Sci* 89:1376, 2011.

[25] Garcia-Mazcorro JF et al. Molecular assessment of the fecal microbiota in healthy cats and dogs before and during supplementation with fructo-oligosaccharides (FOS) and inulin using high-throughput 454-pyrosequencing. *PeerJ* 5:e3184, 2017.

[26] Bueno AR et al. Feline colonic microbes and fatty acid transport: effects of feeding cellulose, beet pulp and pectin/gum arabic fibers. *Nutr Res* 20:1319, 2000.

[27] Fischer MM et al. Fiber fermentability effects on energy and macronutrient digestibility, fecal traits, postprandial metabolite responses, and colon histology of overweight cats. *J Anim Sci* 90:2233, 2012.

[28] Bueno AR et al. Feline colonic morphology and mucosal tissue energetics as influenced via the source of dietary fiber. *Nutr Res* 20:985, 2000.

[29] Verbrugghe A et al. Oligofructose and inulin modulate glucose and amino acid metabolism through propionate production in normal-weight and obese cats. *Br J Nutr* 102:694, 2009.

[30] Verbrugghe A et al. Intestinal fermentation modulates postprandial acylcarnitine profile and nitrogen metabolism in a true carnivore: the domestic cat (*Felis catus*). *Br J Nutr* 104:972, 2010.

[31] Freiche V et al. Uncontrolled study assessing the impact of a psyllium-enriched extruded dry diet on faecal consistency in cats with constipation. *J Feline Med Surg* 13:903, 2011.

[32] Wilson AS et al. Diet and the human gut microbiome: an international review. *Dig Dis Sci* 65:723, 2020.

[33] Rondeau MP et al. Short chain fatty acids stimulate feline colonic smooth muscle contraction. *J Feline Med Surg* 5:167, 2003.

[34] Del Bo' C et al. Systematic review on polyphenol intake and health outcomes: is there sufficient evidence to define a health-promoting polyphenol-rich dietary pattern? *Nutrients* 11:1355, 2019.

[35] Gebreselassie EE et al. Anti-aging food that improves markers of health in senior dogs by modulating gut microbiota and metabolite profiles. Preprint. *bioRxiv* 324327, 2018.

[36] Leray V et al. Effect of citrus polyphenol- and curcumin-supplemented diet on inflammatory state in obese cats. *Br J Nutr* 106:S198, 2011.

CHAPTER 37

Faecal microbiota transplantation

Frédéric P. Gaschen

The gastrointestinal (GI) microbiota consists of trillions of microorganisms including bacteria, archaea, fungi, and protozoa. These microorganisms contribute to the health of the host in several ways: they ensure development and support of the immune system, they produce metabolites with nutritional value or signalling function, they maintain homoeostasis (e.g. by maintaining the intestinal barrier), and they provide resistance to colonisation by pathogenic bacteria. Altogether, these effects ultimately exert an essential and positive influence on the host's general health.[1–3] More information on the feline GI microbiome and its importance in health and disease can be found in Chapter 16.

Faecal microbiota transplantation (FMT) describes the transfer of faeces from a healthy donor into the gut of a diseased recipient with the goal of modulating the recipient's intestinal microbiome. It can be performed via enema, upper or lower GI endoscopy, nasogastric or nasojejunal feeding tube, or by ingestion of capsules.[4,5] In human medicine, the first reports describing the use of various forms of FMT to treat patients date back to ancient China. The procedure was first investigated in North America more than 60 years ago to treat patients with pseudomembranous colitis. In recent years, the technique has gained great popularity and approval for use in patients with *Clostridioides difficile* (*C. diff*) infection,[4,6] and its potential for the treatment of other GI and non-GI disorders is under continued exploration.[6,7] In veterinary medicine, transfer of GI microbiota has been used in ruminants for centuries. More recently, FMT has gained notoriety in small animal gastroenterology following its regain of popularity in human medicine. Commercial FMT products are now available for use in dogs and cats in the United States of America and elsewhere. However, there are only few peer-reviewed scientific publications that establish the value of FMT in the treatment of GI diseases in small animals and only one case report about its use in cats.[5,8,9]

MODE OF ACTION

As is the case in people and in dogs, GI inflammation severely impacts the intestinal microbiome of cats.[3,10,11] Changes in the intestinal microbiota might be at the origin of events leading to chronic enteropathies such as inflammatory bowel disease (IBD) and alimentary lymphoma, or alternately the microbiota may merely be an innocent bystander in the pathogenesis of these diseases. Nevertheless, the resulting dysbiosis has measurable repercussions on the metabolome that may exert a negative impact on the host's health. Interestingly, the intestinal microbiome is also profoundly altered after oral administration of antibiotics to cats.[12,13] See Chapter 16 for more details on intestinal microbiota and dysbiosis.

The beneficial effects of FMT on the intestinal microbiota and the host have not been definitely identified yet and are the topic of ongoing investigations. It is probable that multiple changes associated with faecal transfer are ultimately beneficial to the host. A recent review listed several factors that underpin the positive response observed following FMT in animal models and in clinical studies performed in people with intestinal inflammation.[14] They include an increase in richness and diversity in the microbiome and a shift of recipient microbial profiles towards those of the healthy donor. Additionally, more butyrate-producing bacteria are observed in the microbiota profiles of FMT responders, increasing the production of short-chain fatty acids known to induce regulatory

T cells and promote interleukin (IL)-10 production, which ultimately result in a decrease of underlying inflammatory processes. In addition, increases in the production of specific antimicrobial peptides, secretory immunoglobulin A, and mucin help minimise pathogen invasion. Moreover, increased mucin production also restores the integrity of the intestinal barrier by strengthening the mucus layer separating the epithelial cells from the gut lumen.[14] This list is not comprehensive, and it is likely that many other yet unidentified factors contribute to the beneficial effects of FMT in GI diseases. Importantly, other microorganisms from the donor faeces such as yeasts and bacteriophages may also exert positive effects on the host.

USE IN HUMAN AND CANINE MEDICINE

Faecal microbiota transplantation in people

FMT is now recognised as the treatment of choice for recurrent *C. diff* infection.[6] Its effects have also been investigated in patients with other intestinal diseases such as Crohn's disease, ulcerative colitis, irritable bowel syndrome, and colorectal cancer, with a promising outlook in some instances.[6] Interestingly, there is also preliminary evidence about the benefits of FMT in non-GI diseases that are associated with intestinal dysbiosis, such as hepatic encephalopathy, psoriasis, some neurological disorders, metabolic syndrome, and cancer.[7] For example, FMT increased insulin sensitivity in people with metabolic syndrome. This preliminary evidence needs to be confirmed, and the mechanisms through which FMT exerts beneficial effects in these disorders need to be further elucidated. However, these studies underscore the very broad potential of FMT as an adjunctive treatment in human medicine.

Complications of FMT in human patients appear to be generally minimal and limited to abdominal discomfort, bloating, cramping, diarrhoea/constipation, nausea/vomiting, and low-grade fever.[4,15] However, rarely, more serious infectious complications have been reported, such as high-grade fever and bacteraemia with multidrug-resistant bacteria and death.[15] This highlights the central importance of diligent donor screening, including faecal multidrug-resistant bacteria, in human medicine.

Faecal microbiota transplantation in dogs

The currently available clinical data on FMT in dogs was recently reviewed.[5] The positive effects of FMT are best documented in acute gastroenteritis: repeat FMT treatments shortened the time to return of normal faeces and the duration of hospital stay in puppies with parvovirus infection. In addition, in dogs with uncomplicated acute gastroenteritis, a single FMT treatment improved faecal consistency and was associated with recovery of the faecal microbiota (based on the faecal dysbiosis index) at days 7 and 28 after the procedure, while treatment with metronidazole improved faecal consistency at day 7 but was not associated with normalisation of the faecal microbiota at any time point. In contrast, the effects of FMT in chronic canine GI disorders are much less well documented. Based on a few case reports and small case series, the technique may be beneficial in some instances; however, well-designed prospective studies are needed to better define the chronic GI diseases for which FMT may be a reliably successful therapeutic option.

FAECAL MICROBIOTA TRANSPLANTATION IN CATS

Currently, there is only very limited and anecdotal evidence available about the use of FMT in cats. This may be due, at least in part, to the fact that diarrhoea is a less common presenting complaint in cats than it is in dogs. In fact, cats with IBD or small-cell intestinal lymphoma typically show fairly nonspecific signs such as hyporexia or anorexia, lethargy, weight loss, and chronic vomiting without concurrent diarrhoea, particularly if their disease is limited to the small intestine (see Chapters 18 and 20).

The only published case report to date described the use of FMT in a 10-year-old spayed female Abyssinian cat with chronic large bowel diarrhoea that was refractory to symptomatic and immunosuppressive treatments. The cat was ultimately diagnosed with ulcerative colitis. The consistency and appearance of the cat's faeces normalised within 4 days of the first FMT treatment, but diarrhoea returned progressively. The improvement in faecal appearance and consistency occurred more slowly after the second FMT treatment; however, the faeces were still normal 3 and 11 months after the procedure.[9]

Indications

Based on the published case report, additional anecdotal data obtained from several members of the Comparative Gastroenterology Society (CGS), and the author's own experience, FMT has been used either to treat young shelter cats with acute diarrhoea and young cats with persistent *Tritrichomonas blagburni* (*foetus*) infection, or as an add-on treatment for middle-aged to older cats with IBD or low-grade alimentary lymphoma. Half of the veterinary practitioners gave one dose of FMT once, while the other half used between two and five sequential administrations in their patients. FMT was often used after other more traditional treatments had failed, and success rate ranged from poor to excellent.

Patient (recipient) selection

FMT may be beneficial in any cat with diarrhoea. However, a proper diagnostic workup is recommended to identify the cause of the problem, as diarrhoea is likely to recur if underlying causes are not addressed. Therefore, parasitic infections, hyperthyroidism, food-responsive enteropathy, antibiotic-associated diarrhoea, and other causes of diarrhoea should be identified and appropriately treated before considering FMT. It was shown in people with *C. diff* infection that antibiotics negatively impact the microbiome and limit the beneficial effects of FMT. Therefore, it is not generally recommended to give FMT to patients that are simultaneously receiving antibiotics. Based on the sparse anecdotal evidence cited above, it appears that FMT can be safely given to cats with uncontrolled IBD treated with high doses of steroids and/or other immunosuppressants. Nevertheless, immunosuppressed patients should receive FMT from carefully screened donors and be monitored closely following FMT to ensure they do not develop infectious complications.

Donor selection

The selection of a faecal donor needs to include a rigorous screening process for infectious diseases that could jeopardise the health of the recipient. In human medicine, faecal donors undergo very strict screening procedures aimed at preventing transmission of infections or other diseases and ensuring transplantation of a desirable faecal microbiome and metabolome. Potential donors are screened for dietary habits, recent use of medication (e.g. antibiotics, immunosuppressants, chemotherapy drugs, proton pump inhibitors), and for any history of chronic diseases, including GI diseases, diabetes, obesity, and psychiatric disorders. Candidates with risk behaviours for infections (e.g. travel to other countries, illegal drug use) are generally not accepted. A complete blood count, biochemistry panel, and protein C concentration are obtained as well as titres for common infectious agents, such as hepatitis viruses and human immunodeficiency virus (HIV). Parasitic diseases need to be ruled out, as does the presence of enteric pathogens and multidrug-resistant bacteria in the faeces.[4,16]

In canine medicine, screening protocols vary amongst published studies. General screening criteria were proposed in a recent review with the goals to ensure the safety of FMT and to optimise the quality of the transplanted faeces.[5]

The screening protocol for feline faecal donors shown in Box 37.1 has comparable goals to protocols recommended for human and canine donor candidates. Strictly indoor cats are preferred, as they live in a more controlled environment with less potential exposure to infectious agents. A comparable approach is used by a commercial feline faecal bank* that states that they collect faeces from "indoor cats that have no current or prior health issues, no antibiotic treatment in the prior 6 months, have diverse and species-rich microbiomes, healthy body weight, good temperament, and good faecal consistency". In addition, faeces are screened for feline coronavirus, feline parvovirus, *Cryptosporidium* spp., *Giardia* spp., *Salmonella* spp., *Toxoplasma gondii*, and *Tritrichomonas blagburni*. Ultimately, the desired depth of screening depends on the general condition of the recipient and on the personal preference of the veterinary practitioner in charge. Intestinal function tests (serum cobalamin concentration), pancreatic enzymatic immunoassays (pancreatic lipase immunoreactivity and trypsin-like immunoreactivity), and endocrine tests (serum thyroxine in cats older than 5 years) could be performed to more definitely rule out abnormal intestinal function, pancreatitis, exocrine pancreatic insufficiency, and hyperthyroidism. Unfortunately, there is currently no simple test to assess the diversity and composition of the faecal microbiome in cats that is comparable to the faecal dysbiosis index established in dogs. While this information

*https://www.animalbiome.com/fecal-microbiota-transplant-capsules-aka-poo-pills/

would be valuable for the identification of desirable faecal donors, it is currently impossible to obtain without access to a research laboratory able to evaluate specific bacterial taxa using quantitative PCR assays.

Preparation of the faecal solution

Based on recommendations used in human medicine, preparation of the faecal solution should be done rapidly in order to protect anaerobic bacteria. However, obtaining faeces from a feline donor in a noninvasive manner may be challenging, as the delay between spontaneous defecation and collection and processing of faeces may be prolonged. Fortunately, refrigerated storage (4°C) of feline faeces for up to 14 days had only minimal repercussions on the microbiota,[17] and keeping feline faeces at room temperature for up to 4 days did not cause any changes in composition or richness of the microbiota.[18] In addition, a study in dogs showed that the viability of faecal bacteria was maintained in homogenised faecal samples for 1 week in a refrigerator (4°C), although this has not been tested with feline faeces.[19] Altogether, this information suggests that processing of faeces could be delayed without jeopardising the beneficial properties of the faeces for FMT.

The technique for preparation of faecal solution used in the author's laboratory is described in Box 37.2 and illustrated in Fig. 37.1. It is comparable to the technique used in the published case report mentioned above.[9]

Administration of the faecal solution

In human medicine, a randomised clinical trial showed high efficacy of FMT administered as an enema without colonic lavage and demonstrated that both fresh and frozen faecal solutions were equally effective.[20] There are no corresponding studies for FMT in small animals, and the outcome could be different considering FMT is often used to treat diseases affecting the small intestine. However, administration via enema can easily be applied to veterinary clinical settings and is often preferred because it does not require general anaesthesia or

Box 37.1. Recommended selection criteria for feline faecal donors.

History and physical examination

- Preferably of 1–10 years of age
- Indoor cat
- No recent stay in a shelter or boarding facility, no travel history
- No health issues in the last 6–12 months
- No history of chronic gastrointestinal diseases, allergies, or immune-mediated diseases
- Has not received any antibiotics in the last 12 months
- Regularly vaccinated according to existing guidelines
- Fed a balanced diet, raw diets excluded
- Not overweight or underweight (body condition score of 4–6/9)
- Normal faecal consistency
- Deemed healthy on physical examination

Laboratory screening

- Normal complete blood count and serum biochemistry; consider testing for hyperthyroidism (>5 years old), hypocobalaminaemia, exocrine pancreatic insufficiency, etc.
- Negative retrovirus panel (FeLV antigen, FIV antibodies)*
- Negative for feline coronavirus in the faeces*
- Negative for parasite ova on faecal flotation; consider empirical deworming with a broad-spectrum anthelmintic drug*
- Negative for *Giardia* cysts on faecal flotation and ELISA faecal test; see above for empirical deworming*
- Consider testing for other faecal parasites and pathogens (e.g. *Cryptosporidium felis*, *Salmonella* spp., *Campylobacter* spp., etc.)*

FeLV, feline leukaemia virus; FIV, feline immunodeficiency virus.
*The extent of infectious disease screening should be based on a risk assessment taking into account the likelihood of exposure of each individual donor candidate to infectious agents.

Box 37.2. Preparation of faecal solution for use in faecal microbiota transplantation.

Preparation for immediate use or short-term storage (Fig. 37.1)

1. Weigh faeces from the donor on a gram scale.
2. Add nonbacteriostatic 0.9% NaCl solution in a volume (ml) equivalent to 4 times the faecal weight, creating a 20% faecal solution (e.g. if 10 g faeces, add 40 ml 0.9% NaCl).
3. Mix the solution by hand in a sealed plastic bag or in a blender.
4. Filter the solution through a fine mesh strainer to remove large particles.
5. Collect the filtered solution in a 60 ml catheter tip syringe.
6. If not used immediately, store in a refrigerated environment (4°C) for up to 1 week.

A more concentrated solution could also be prepared by diluting faeces with 2–3 volumes of 0.9% NaCl to decrease the total volume of faecal solution to be administered to the recipient.

Preparation for long-term storage (to preserve viability of faecal microbiota)

Steps 1–6 as described above.

7. Add glycerol to the faecal solution (1/9 of the faecal solution volume obtained after step 6, resulting in a 10% glycerol solution)
8. Store the faecal solution with added glycerol at –20°C for up to 3 months or at –80°C for up to 6 months; do not refreeze the faecal solution after it has been thawed

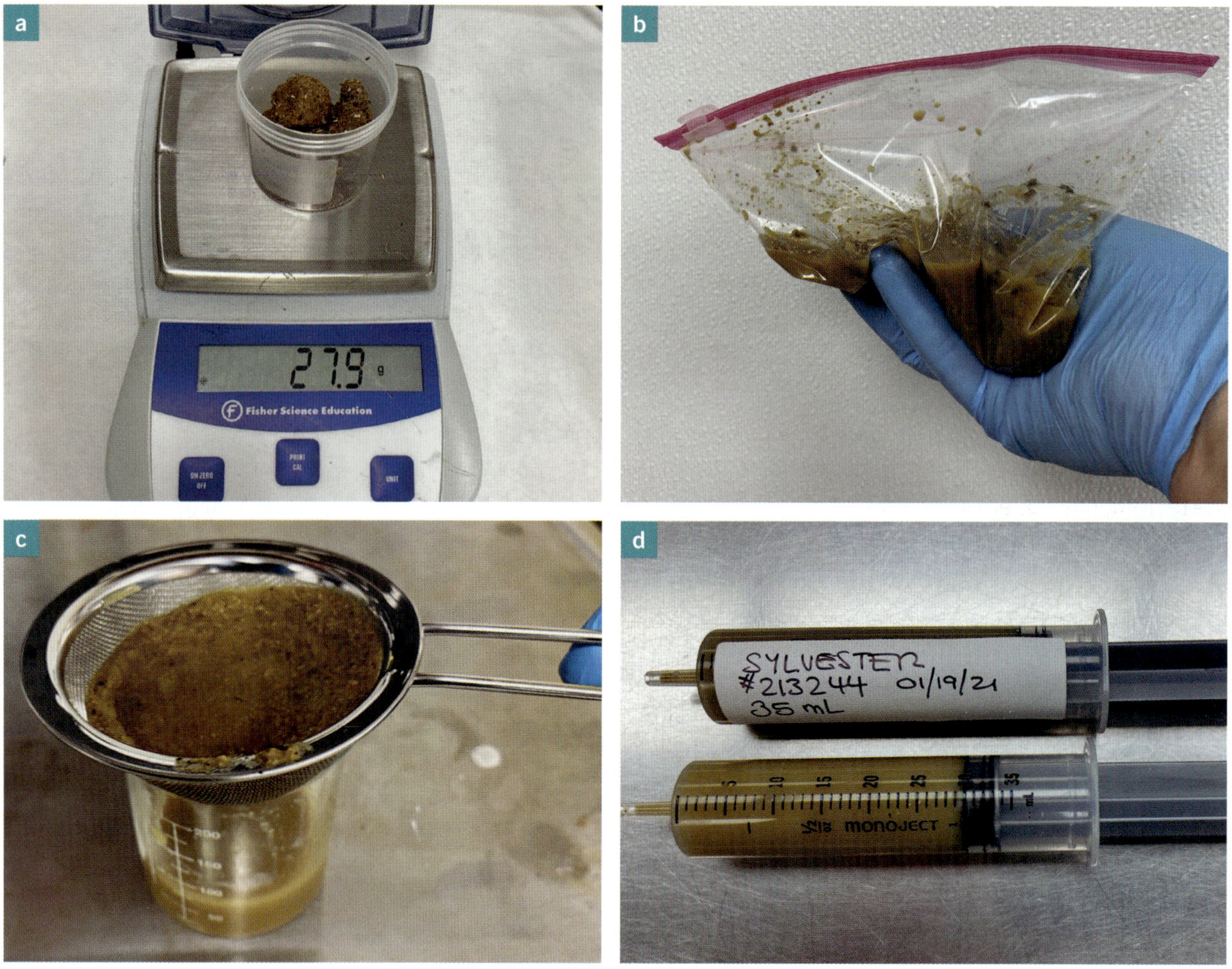

Figure 37.1. Preparation of faecal solution for faecal microbiota transplantation. The faeces from the donor are weighed (a). The faeces are placed in a sealable plastic bag, and nonbacteriostatic 0.9% NaCl is added (total volume [ml] = 4 × faecal weight [g]; in this instance, 4 × 27.9 g = 111.6 ml). The air is expressed out of the bag, and the bag is sealed. The solution is mixed by hand for a few minutes until the faeces are dissolved (b). The solution is filtered through a fine mesh strainer into another container to filter out particles that could obstruct the catheter during administration (c). The filtered faecal solution is ready for use after being transferred to properly labelled syringes (d).

special equipment. Some veterinary practitioners administer FMT through an endoscope while performing upper or lower GI endoscopy. Finally, FMT could also be given orally through syringe feeding or nasooesophageal tube or using capsules with frozen faecal solution or lyophilised faeces that may be available commercially.

Based on studies in people and in dogs, the recommended dose of faeces for feline FMT was determined to be between 1.5 and 5 g of donor faeces per kg body weight of recipient. Using the faecal solution recipe in Box 37.2, this would approximately equate to a volume of 7.5–20 ml/kg. The author usually administers at least 2 g/kg faeces or 10 ml/kg faecal solution. Ultimately, the final volume should be tolerated by the recipient without triggering rapid spontaneous evacuation. While a warm water enema can be administered to cleanse the colon prior to FMT,[9] many veterinary practitioners administer FMT without specific preparation of the recipient. However, it is recommended to administer sedation to the recipient to ensure feasibility of the FMT procedure, including the additional dwell time of 20–30 minutes during which the anus can be maintained closed to prevent the cat from expelling the faecal solution. It is noteworthy that some docile or debilitated cats may tolerate the procedure without sedatives. Sedation protocols should be adapted to the age and health status of the cat. In middle-aged cats without significant comorbidities, the author uses dexmedetomidine and buprenorphine at conventional doses and reverses the sedation with atipamezole at the very end of the procedure. The FMT procedure is illustrated in Video 37.1. The cat is placed in right lateral recumbency with the hind end elevated with a rolled towel. A large-bore catheter (e.g. 18–20 Fr red rubber catheter) is used, and its dead space is determined prior to the procedure and added to the required volume of faecal solution. After being warmed up in a water bath at body temperature, the syringe containing the faecal solution is attached to the catheter. The catheter is prefilled with faecal solution to avoid injecting air in the recipient's colon. It is coated with water-soluble lubricant and slowly introduced in the rectum, then carefully advanced through the rectum and descending colon to the level of the colonic flexure. The faecal solution is then slowly injected into the colon over a period of 10 or more minutes depending on the final volume administered, followed by withdrawal of the catheter. Based on the fact that people receiving FMT are requested to remain on their back for approximately 30 minutes after completion of the procedure to limit the urge to defecate,[4] the author recommends maintaining the cat in right lateral recumbency for an additional 20–30 minutes. In order to ensure proper distribution of the faecal solution, some veterinary practitioners prefer moving the cat from right lateral to ventral, left lateral, and dorsal recumbency during the instillation and/or the post-FMT period.

Video 37.1. Faecal microbiota transplantation procedure in a cat.

CONCLUSION AND OUTLOOK

There is currently very little data available about the benefits of FMT in cats, and this chapter is based solely on comparative data obtained from other species and anecdotal evidence from veterinary practitioners who have used the technique in their own patients. This void of scientific evidence underscores the urgent need for well-designed studies of FMT in cats so that the benefits of the technique can be applied in the approach to feline diseases. Given the wide impact of the GI microbiome on health and disease, it is conceivable that the benefits of FMT may range beyond the GI tract in cats as well.

Take-home messages

- The gastrointestinal microbiota consists of bacteria, archaea, fungi, and bacteriophages and plays a central role in health and disease of cats.
- Faecal microbiota transplantation aims at restoring a healthy gastrointestinal microbiota in sick cats with suspected gastrointestinal dysbiosis and holds promise in the treatment of feline digestive, metabolic, and other diseases.
- The technique is simple and easy to use in practice, including preparation of the faecal solution and colonic administration via enema or other methods.
- Special attention must be given to donor selection to prevent disease transmission and ensure that the donor has a desirable faecal microbiome.
- There is currently almost no data on faecal microbiota transplantation in cats. Anecdotally, the technique has been used with some success both in acute and chronic feline gastrointestinal diseases.

REFERENCES

[1] Pilla R, Suchodolski JS. The role of the canine gut microbiome and metabolome in health and gastrointestinal disease. *Front Vet Sci* 6:498, 2020.

[2] Lyu Y et al. Past, present, and future of gastrointestinal microbiota research in cats. *Front Microbiol* 11:1661, 2020.

[3] Minamoto Y et al. Feline gastrointestinal microbiota. *Anim Health Res Rev* 13:64, 2012.

[4] Cammarota G et al. European consensus conference on faecal microbiota transplantation in clinical practice. *Gut* 66:569, 2017.

[5] Chaitman J, Gaschen F. Fecal microbiota transplantation in dogs. *Vet Clin North Am Small Anim Pract* 51:219, 2021.

[6] Borody TJ, Eslick GD, Clancy RL. Fecal microbiota transplantation as a new therapy: from *Clostridioides difficile* infection to inflammatory bowel disease, irritable bowel syndrome, and colon cancer. *Curr Opin Pharmacol* 49:43, 2019.

[7] D'Haens GR, Jobin C. Fecal microbial transplantation for diseases beyond recurrent *Clostridium difficile* infection. *Gastroenterology* 157:624, 2019.

[8] Chaitman J et al. Commentary on key aspects of fecal microbiota transplantation in small animal practice. *Vet Med (Auckl)* 7:71, 2016.

[9] Furmanski S, Mor T. First case report of fecal microbiota transplantation in a cat in Israel. *Isr J Vet Med* 72:35, 2017.

[10] Suchodolski JS et al. The fecal microbiome in cats with diarrhea. *PLoS One* 10:e0127378, 2015.

[11] Marsilio S et al. Characterization of the fecal microbiome in cats with inflammatory bowel disease or alimentary small cell lymphoma. *Sci Rep* 9:19208, 2019.

[12] Whittemore JC et al. Effects of a synbiotic on the fecal microbiome and metabolomic profiles of healthy research cats administered clindamycin: a randomized, controlled trial. *Gut Microbes* 10:521, 2019.

[13] Torres-Henderson C et al. Effect of *Enterococcus faecium* strain SF68 on gastrointestinal signs and fecal microbiome in cats administered amoxicillin–clavulanate. *Top Companion Anim Med* 32:104, 2017.

[14] Quraishi MN et al. Immunological mechanisms underpinning faecal microbiota transplantation for the treatment of inflammatory bowel disease. *Clin Exp Immunol* 199:24, 2020.

[15] Dailey FE et al. The dirty aspects of fecal microbiota transplantation: a review of its adverse effects and complications. *Curr Opin Pharmacol* 49:29, 2019.

[16] Bibbò S et al. Fecal microbiota transplantation: screening and selection to choose the optimal donor. *J Clin Med* 9:1757, 2020.

[17] Weese JS, Jalali M. Evaluation of the impact of refrigeration on next generation sequencing-based assessment of the canine and feline fecal microbiota. *BMC Vet Res* 10:230, 2014.

[18] Tal M et al. The effect of storage at ambient temperature on the feline fecal microbiota. *BMC Vet Res* 13:256, 2017.

[19] Rodriguez E et al. Bacteria viability in stored canine feces for use in fecal microbiota transplantation. ACVIM Forum, 2020.

[20] Lee CH et al. Frozen vs fresh fecal microbiota transplantation and clinical resolution of diarrhea in patients with recurrent *Clostridium difficile* infection: a randomized clinical trial. *JAMA* 315:142, 2016.

CHAPTER 38

Nutritional assessment

Aarti Kathrani

Nutritional status of cats is considered the fifth vital sign to assess after body temperature, pulse, respiration, and pain. The purpose of nutritional assessment is to determine the cat's nutritional status and identify malnutrition, as well as to allow for monitoring of any changes to this status (Fig. 38.1). Malnutrition is defined by the World Health Organization as a deficiency, excess, or imbalance in a person's intake of energy and/or nutrients. Malnutrition can develop quickly even in adequately nourished cats. In cats with gastrointestinal (GI) disease, the severity and duration of disease, impaired digestion and absorption of nutrients, comorbidities, complications of disease, adverse effects from treatment, and an unbalanced diet are all risk factors for malnutrition.

Malnutrition is linked to adverse outcomes in humans with inflammatory bowel disease (IBD) and is associated with in-hospital death and increased hospital stay,[1] as well as increased risk for infection and nonelective surgery. Adequate nutritional support can preserve lean body mass, reverse the maladaptive metabolic response to injury, maintain organ function, and decrease morbidity. Therefore, nutritional assessment should be performed in all cats to ensure that any deficiencies are adequately addressed. Nutritional assessment involves assessment of the cat, the diet, the feeding strategy, and the environment.[2]

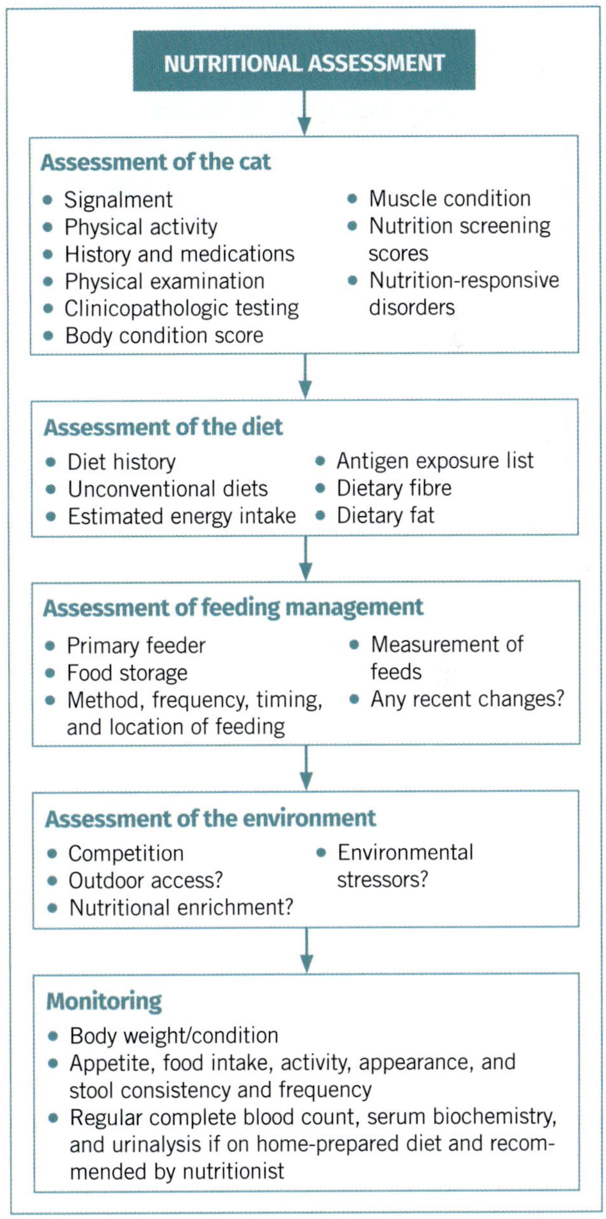

Figure 38.1. Nutritional assessment of cats with gastrointestinal disease.

ASSESSMENT OF THE CAT

Signalment

The age of the cat greatly affects its daily energy and nutrient requirements. Kittens have higher energy and nutrient requirements than adult cats; thus, ensuring that any therapeutic diet intended for kittens meets the recommendations for growth is important. Twelve months of age is generally considered to be a safe time to transition most kittens to adult cat food.[3]

The nutritional requirements of geriatric cats are also different from those of adult cats. Approximately 30% and 20% of cats older than 12 years of age have decreased fat absorption and decreased protein digestibility, respectively.[4] Hence, in some geriatric cats, reduced digestion and absorption may lead to deficiencies in essential nutrients. Consequently, older cats that are losing weight despite presumed adequate intake should be fed increased amounts or transitioned to an energy-dense diet that is higher in fat and protein.

Sex and neuter status, as well as pregnancy and lactation, can also affect the energy and nutrient requirements of cats. Neutering cats can lower their energy needs, whereas pregnancy and lactation substantially increase their needs. All cats should be monitored closely via body weight, body condition scoring, assessment of muscle and dermatologic condition, and general physical examination (see the corresponding sections in this chapter) to ensure that adequate nutrition and calories are being provided.

Physical activity

The outdoor status of the cat and the level of activity should be ascertained, as this will directly impact the energy needs. It is also important to note that activity may decrease as cats get older due to comorbidities such as arthritis.

History and medications

The collection of a thorough history regarding the current GI condition should include information pertaining to the cat's appetite, weight loss, and activity as well as to the frequency, duration, and character of any regurgitation, vomiting, or diarrhoea. The past medical history and any comorbidities such as chronic kidney disease, pancreatitis, or diabetes mellitus should also be ascertained, as this will help in the selection of an appropriate therapeutic diet for the GI condition that also meets dietary strategies for the comorbidities. If the cat is receiving laxatives or medication for hyperthyroidism, ensuring that any dose changes do not coincide with the onset of weight loss is important. Similarly, ensuring that any weight loss did not start with the withdrawal of certain therapies such as mirtazapine or pancreatic enzymes is valuable.

Physical examination

Body weight should be measured, on a scale that is regularly calibrated, and recorded at each visit. This should then be compared to body weight histories to determine if there have been any significant changes. If any weight loss is present, the degree should be quantified as mild (<5% of body weight loss), moderate (5%–10% of body weight loss), or severe (>10% of body weight loss), as this will help to guide the severity of undernutrition present. Assessing body weight, as well as trends, is not only important for nutritional assessment but may also provide prognostic information (Box 38.1).

Box 38.1. Calculation and characterisation of the severity of body weight loss in cats.

Calculation of percentage body weight loss in cats		
$\frac{\text{historical body weight} - \text{current body weight}}{\text{historical body weight}} \times 100$		
Mild weight loss: <5%	Moderate weight loss: 5%–10%	Severe weight loss: >10%
In the following example, the weight loss of a cat that has gone from 5.2 to 4.8 kg is considered moderate: $\frac{5.2\text{ kg} - 4.8\text{ kg}}{5.2\text{ kg}} \times 100 = 8\%$		

There are many aspects of the physical examination that may be impacted by a nutrient deficiency (Table 38.1). A deficiency in the number of daily calories can result in a body condition score (BCS) that is less than ideal (ideal BCS for a cat is 5/9; see section "Body condition score" in this chapter). Protein deficiency can lead to muscle atrophy and low muscle condition. Protein deficiency may also impact the quality of the haircoat, and, depending on the individual amino acid involved, may impact coat colour (e.g. phenylalanine/tyrosine deficiency can cause a coat colour change from black to red) or result in footpad lesions. Taurine deficiency can result in dilated cardiomyopathy, which may result in abnormalities when assessing the cardiovascular system or cause retinal changes that can be assessed by fundic examination. Omega-6 fatty acid and zinc deficiencies could result in dermatologic abnormalities. Vitamin A and E deficiency could result in dermatologic and retinal changes. Vitamin D or calcium deficiency may result in skeletal changes. Potassium and thiamine deficiency can lead

Table 38.1. Examples of nutrient deficiency and their possible effects on the physical examination findings of cats.*

Nutrient deficiency	Possible abnormalities
Proteins	Reduced body, muscle, and coat condition Poor wound healing
Amino acids	Phenylalanine/tyrosine: coat colour change from black to red Taurine: dilated cardiomyopathy, retinal changes
Essential fatty acids (e.g. linoleic acid)	Dermatologic abnormalities
Vitamins	Vitamin D: skeletal abnormalities Thiamine: neck ventroflexion, neurological abnormalities
Macrominerals	Calcium: tetany, seizures, skeletal abnormalities Potassium: muscle weakness, neck ventroflexion
Micronutrients	Zinc: dermatologic abnormalities

*Not an exhaustive list.

to neck ventroflexion. Additionally, thiamine deficiency can cause central nervous system signs. Hypocalcaemia can lead to tetany and seizures. Therefore, assessing the cat's stature, body condition and musculature, haircoat, footpads, eyes, and cardiovascular, nervous, and skeletal systems is important to assess overall nutritional health. In addition, dental examination should be performed to assess for any periodontal and dental disease.

Additionally, the presence of poor wound healing on physical examination may be an indication of inadequate nutritional intake. Assessment of petechia, ecchymosis, bruising, or bleeding on physical examination, which may be evidence of a coagulopathy, is important, as this could be a contraindication to the placement of an enteral feeding tube. Similarly, ensuring adequate mentation and the presence of a gag reflex is important if enteral assisted feeding is being considered.

Clinicopathologic testing

Unfortunately, no definitive clinicopathologic tests are available for establishing a cat's nutritional status. Increased serum creatine kinase activity has been found to be associated with anorexia in feline patients.[5] A minimum database consisting of complete blood count, serum biochemistry with electrolytes and total thyroxine concentration if the cat is over 6 years of age, and urinalysis should be performed. Although the packed cell volume, total solids, and some electrolytes such as potassium can be an indication of the nutritional status, they may be poor markers as these parameters can also be influenced by confounding factors such as the disease process itself or increased losses.

Body condition score

BCS is a reliable and repeatable measure of the body fat percentage, with strong correlation with dual-energy X-ray absorptiometry, and is therefore one of the measures used to assess nutritional status. Assessment of BCS should be performed using a standardised scoring system. The World Small Animal Veterinary Association (WSAVA) Global Nutrition Committee recommends the use of a 9-point scale* for assessment of BCS, which is based on characterisation of body silhouette and palpation of body fat.

Ideal body fat composition in cats ranges from 15% to 24%.[6] Using the 9-point BCS scale, each unit of increase in BCS above the ideal of 5/9 is approximately equivalent to 10%–15% over the ideal body weight. Whenever possible, owners should be taught to score body condition, as they will then be able to assess it regularly at home. It is important to note that BCS is informative of peripheral fat status in cats, but this score does not take into account intra-abdominal fat, muscle condition, or bone density, all of which can be affected by malnutrition and are therefore important in its assessment.

*https://wsava.org/wp-content/uploads/2020/02/Body-Condition-Score-Cat.pdf

Muscle condition

Cachexia is defined as a complex metabolic syndrome associated with underlying illness and characterised by loss of muscle with or without loss of fat mass, whereas sarcopenia is an age-related disease characterised by low muscle mass, loss of muscle strength, and decreased physical performance. Although sarcopenia refers to the loss of muscle mass, it differs from cachexia, as it is a syndrome associated with ageing in the absence of disease.

Assessment of muscle condition is important to identify cachexia and sarcopenia. However, there is currently no standardised scoring system for muscle mass in cats. Therefore, assessment of muscle condition can be performed subjectively by using the 4-point scale* recommended by the WSAVA Global Nutrition Committee or by assessing the muscle mass as adequate or mildly, moderately, or severely atrophied together with its symmetry and distribution. Muscle mass should be evaluated both by visual assessment and palpation of the head, scapulae, epaxial muscles over the thoracic and lumbar vertebrae, and pelvic bones. It is important to note that to ensure accuracy for both BCS and muscle condition, this should be assessed not just visually but also by palpation, especially in cats with medium- or long-haired coats.

Nutrition screening scores

Scores assessing nutrition risk screening are important in the nutritional assessment of human IBD patients. Earlier identification of malnourished patients may allow for earlier intervention and impact on clinical outcomes. Unfortunately, there have been no studies published to date utilising nutrition scores in feline GI disease or evaluating the impact of nutritional support on the clinical outcome in malnourished cats with GI disease.

Nutrition-responsive disorders

The documentation of any comorbidities that are nutrition responsive (e.g. liver disease, pancreatitis, kidney disease) is important, as nutritional strategies for these diseases may also need to be incorporated into any dietary recommendations for the GI disease.

ASSESSMENT OF THE DIET

Diet history

A complete and thorough diet history is paramount in determining sufficient nutrient intake and the need for immediate nutritional intervention. Collection of the diet history should encompass all foods that the cat is eating, including all commercial pet food, commercial treats, human food, dietary supplements, and food used to administer medications, with specification of the manufacturer, brand, dry or tinned formula, and flavour if applicable. The ability to scavenge and hunt, as well as access to additional food outdoors, should also be ascertained.

An assessment of the diet that the cat is consuming just prior to or at the onset of GI signs is important, as this may help to determine if there could be a dietary trigger for the signs. The diet should be assessed to ensure it is appropriate for long-term feeding (i.e. it is complete and balanced). This is especially important in cases with GI signs to prevent exacerbation of malnutrition, to which the cat may already be susceptible. In addition to the diet being complete and balanced, it should also meet the recommendations† outlined by the WSAVA Global Nutrition Committee. This involves contacting the pet food manufacturer directly to ask a series of eight questions, which help to ascertain the credentials of the person formulating their diet, whether the diet meets nutrient requirements via formulation or animal feeding tests, where the foods are produced and manufactured, what specific quality control measures are taken to assure quality and consistency of their ingredients and end products, their willingness to provide full nutrient profiles including caloric density for their products, and what product research has been done and whether this has been published in peer-reviewed journals. Manufacturers that employ individuals with a doctorate degree or board certification in small animal nutrition, that have good quality control and safety measures, that are willing to provide full nutrient profiles of their products when requested, and that publish research on their products in peer-reviewed journals should be recommended.[3]

*https://wsava.org/wp-content/uploads/2020/01/Muscle-Condition-Score-Chart-for-Cats.pdf
†https://wsava.org/wp-content/uploads/2020/01/Selecting-the-Best-Food-for-your-Pet.pdf

One study assessed early-life risk factors, including diet, in cats presenting to veterinary practices specifically for GI signs on at least two occasions between 6 and 30 months of age.[7] Of the 1212 cats enrolled in the study, cats reported with vomiting or diarrhoea, or both, and/or those not exclusively fed a commercial diet that met the WSAVA Global Nutrition Committee guidelines before 16 weeks of age were more likely to visit veterinary practices specifically for GI signs on at least two occasions between 6 and 30 months of age. Therefore, feeding a diet that does not comply with the WSAVA Global Nutrition Committee guidelines may raise concerns regarding the source of ingredients, nutritional composition, and quality control of the diet—factors that may impact the GI mucosal immune system, microbiota, and intestinal permeability. However, further studies are needed to determine if any attributes of these diets are specifically implicated in disease pathogenesis in cats with chronic GI signs. Nevertheless, all cats should be assessed to ensure that they are exclusively consuming diets that meet the recommendations outlined by the WSAVA Global Nutrition Committee.

Unconventional diets

It is important to determine if the cat is consuming an unconventional diet, such as a home-prepared diet not formulated by a board-certified veterinary nutritionist, a diet consisting of raw meat, a vegetarian or vegan diet (either home-prepared or commercially bought), or a boutique, exotic, or grain-free diet.

Home-prepared diets for cats, if not formulated by a board-certified veterinary nutritionist, are often deficient in essential nutrients, with the following nutrients most frequently below recommended allowances: choline, iron, thiamine, zinc, manganese, vitamin E, and copper.[8] Therefore, if a home-prepared diet is fed, a board-certified veterinary nutritionist, a list of which can be found on the American and European nutrition specialty websites, must be consulted for guidance.

Diets consisting of raw meat are not currently recommended for cats. Firstly, due to concerns regarding bacterial contamination, which can pose a threat to both the cat and the people in contact with the cat and its environment, and secondly because of potential nutritional inadequacy of these diets. Therefore, at the time of this writing, any documented benefits of feeding raw meat do not outweigh its potential adverse health risks, and consequently these diets should be avoided. It is important to note that methods such as dehydration and freeze-drying are not effective at killing all pathogenic bacteria.

Cats are obligate carnivores and, as such, should not be fed vegetarian or vegan diets, mainly due to concerns regarding taurine deficiency—but also other nutrients such as preformed vitamin A and arachidonic acid. One study demonstrated that most commercial vegetarian diets formulated for dogs and cats were not compliant with the Association of American Feed Control Officials (AAFCO) labelling regulations, and there were concerns regarding adequacy of amino acid content.[9] Thus, cat owners should be cautioned against feeding these diets.

Finally, boutique, exotic, and grain-free diets have been associated with dilated cardiomyopathy in companion animals; therefore, cat owners should be questioned with regard to feeding these diets.

Estimating energy intake

Once the diet and any additional foods that are being fed have been ascertained, the next step involves estimating the daily number of calories that the cat consumes. In the United States of America, the number of calories is listed on the pet food label. Unfortunately, this is not a requirement in Europe, and therefore either reading the product guide, if a therapeutic diet is being fed, calling the pet food manufacturer, or visiting their website is required to determine the calorie content of the diet. Once the total number of daily calories being consumed has been estimated, it can be compared to calculations of daily maintenance energy requirement (MER) to determine if the cat is consuming enough. To estimate the MER, firstly the resting energy requirement (RER) is calculated using the equation: $70 \times \text{body weight (kg)}^{0.75}$, which is then multiplied by a factor to determine the MER. This factor depends on the neuter status, activity, and body condition of the cat. As an example, a factor of 1.2 may be used for a neutered female cat with ideal body condition and moderate activity. However, it is important to note that the calculated MER provides a ballpark and therefore may under- or overestimate the actual energy requirement by up to 50% in individual cats. Accordingly, if the calculated MER is chosen as a starting point, the cat's body weight and BCS should be regularly monitored and adjustments to caloric intake made as necessary to ensure an ideal body condition.

Ensuring that the cat is not consuming table food or unbalanced treats in excess of 10% of the total daily energy intake is important to ensure that the diet does not become unbalanced overall.

Compiling an antigen exposure list

Once the total number of daily calories consumed has been estimated, the next step involves assessing the ingredients in past and currently fed diets. Listing the ingredients will firstly allow an antigen exposure list, which can then be used to determine what would be novel for the cat. Secondly, determining the ingredients of diets that helped or exacerbated the GI signs can aid in prioritising ingredients for a home-prepared diet or choosing a commercial therapeutic diet containing or avoiding those ingredients, respectively. The most commonly identified dietary antigens in cats are beef, dairy products, and fish.

Assessing dietary fibre

Once an antigen exposure list and a list of ingredients that are tolerated or exacerbate the GI signs have been compiled, the fibre and fat content of the diet can be estimated to determine their effects on the GI signs. Unfortunately, the fibre content of a diet is not as easily obtained from the pet food label. Crude fibre is listed on the label; it measures most but not all of the insoluble fibre and none of the soluble fibre. One study demonstrated that crude fibre concentration was not a reliable indicator of total dietary fibre (TDF) concentration or dietary fibre composition.[10] Therefore, TDF is a better measure of dietary fibre, however this is often unavailable from the manufacturers. Ascertaining which diets the owner has previously tried for the GI signs and the fibre content of these diets will help to determine whether a high- or low-fibre diet should be trialled next.

Assessing dietary fat

The fat content of the diet can be assessed to determine the amount the cat is consuming and the impact of different amounts from previous diets on the GI signs. However, dietary fat does not seem to affect the outcome of cats with chronic diarrhoea.[11] Hence, dietary fat may be less of a nutrient of concern in cats with GI signs. Nevertheless, the fat content of diets should be compared on a metabolisable energy basis to remove confounding factors of moisture content and energy density between the diets. This can be done on a percentage or gram per 100 or 1000 kcal basis.

ASSESSMENT OF FEEDING MANAGEMENT

Nutritional assessment of feeding management should ascertain the primary feeder of the cat and include which other family members are actively involved in feeding. Determining how the food is stored and the method, frequency, timing, and location of feeding is also important. Confirming how the owner measures the daily allocation of food (using a gram scale or a measuring device) will help to determine how accurately this is performed. It is important to confirm whether any changes in feeding management have occurred. If the cat has an ideal body condition and is fed ad libitum, then this feeding method is acceptable and can be continued. For those cats that are overweight or obese, meal feeding should be encouraged. Frequent feeding of small meals is likely advantageous in cats with GI disease. Ensuring that cats on exclusion diets do not have access to other sources of food is important to determine success of the diet in controlling the GI signs.

ASSESSMENT OF THE ENVIRONMENT

Cat owners should be questioned with regard to the current household and any potential issues with competition of food from other pets. Outdoor access should also be ascertained to determine if there could be additional food providers or sources. The extent of environmental enrichment should be determined, such as access to toys or food delivery devices. In order to improve environmental enrichment, daily meals can be provided via puzzle or food dispensing toys rather than traditional bowls. In addition, owners can enrich their cat's nutritional experience by interacting with them during mealtime or providing food toys or playing with them. Therapeutic diets intended for long-term feeding should not be fed during hospitalisation to avoid the development of a food aversion.

Environmental stressors, such as any recent changes that have occurred in the environment (the introduction or death of an animal or family member, any changes in routine, house moves, or new cats in the neighbourhood), should be questioned. The role of the environment has been demonstrated in certain nutrient-sensitive disorders in cats (e.g. feline lower urinary tract disease, type 2 diabetes mellitus); however, further studies are needed to ascertain the role of the environment in feline GI diseases.

MONITORING

The cat should be reassessed regularly after any new diet changes to determine whether the recommendations are being adhered to or whether any problems with diet acceptance and tolerance or feeding methods have been seen. Dietary changes in cats should be performed very slowly, preferably over 2 weeks, to help with acceptance of the new diet. It is also important to ascertain if the desired outcomes (e.g. reduction in frequency of vomiting) have been achieved or if any adverse effects associated with the new diet (e.g. exacerbation of diarrhoea) have occurred. As a minimum, body weight and BCS should be regularly assessed to ensure that the cat is maintaining, or achieving and then maintaining, an ideal body condition. The owner should also ideally monitor the cat's appetite, food intake, overall appearance, activity, and stool quality, consistency, and frequency. For those cats receiving a complete and balanced home-prepared diet formulated by a board-certified veterinary nutritionist, regular complete blood count, serum biochemistry, and urinalysis should be performed as recommended by the nutritionist due to the potential unknown bioavailability of these diets.

Take-home messages

- Nutritional status of cats is considered the fifth vital sign to assess, after body temperature, pulse, respiration, and pain.
- The purpose of nutritional assessment is to determine the cat's nutritional status and identify malnutrition, as well as to allow for monitoring of any changes to this status.
- In cats with gastrointestinal disease, the severity and duration of disease, impaired digestion and absorption of nutrients, comorbidities, complications of disease, adverse effects from treatment, and an unbalanced diet are all risk factors for malnutrition.
- Nutritional assessment involves assessment of the cat, the diet, the feeding strategy, and the environment.
- Assessment of the cat includes consideration of the signalment, physical activity, history and medications, physical examination, clinicopathologic testing, body condition score, muscle condition, nutrition screening score, and the presence of nutrition-responsive disorders.
- Assessment of the diet for cats with gastrointestinal disease involves collecting a thorough diet history, ascertaining if unconventional diets are fed, estimating energy intake, compiling an antigen exposure list, and determining dietary fibre and fat.
- Assessment of the feeding management and the environment, as well as monitoring, are also important in the nutritional assessment of cats with gastrointestinal disease.

REFERENCES

[1] Nguyen GC, Munsell M, Harris ML. Nationwide prevalence and prognostic significance of clinically diagnosable protein-calorie malnutrition in hospitalized inflammatory bowel disease patients. *Inflamm Bowel Dis* 14:1105, 2008.

[2] Baldwin K et al. AAHA nutritional assessment guidelines for dogs and cats. *J Am Anim Hosp Assoc* 46:285, 2010.

[3] Rollins AW, Murphy M. Nutritional assessment in the cat: practical recommendations for better medical care. *J Feline Med Surg* 21:442, 2019.

[4] Laflamme DP. Nutrition for aging cats and dogs and the importance of body condition. *Vet Clin North Am Small Anim Pract* 35:713, 2005.

[5] Fascetti AJ, Mauldin GE, Mauldin GN. Correlation between serum creatine kinase activities and anorexia in cats. *J Vet Intern Med* 11:9, 1997.

[6] Cline MG et al. Body composition of lean outdoor intact cats vs lean indoor neutered cats using dual-energy x-ray absorptiometry. *J Feline Med Surg* 21:459, 2019.

[7] Kathrani A et al. Exploring early life events including diet in cats presenting for gastrointestinal signs in later life. *Vet Rec* 185:144, 2019.

[8] Wilson SA et al. Evaluation of the nutritional adequacy of recipes for home-prepared maintenance diets for cats. *J Am Vet Med Assoc* 254:1172, 2019.

[9] Kanakubo K, Fascetti AJ, Larsen JA. Assessment of protein and amino acid concentrations and labeling adequacy of commercial vegetarian diets formulated for dogs and cats. *J Am Vet Med Assoc* 247:385, 2015.

[10] Owens TJ et al. Total dietary fiber composition of diets used for management of obesity and diabetes mellitus in cats. *J Am Vet Med Assoc* 245:99, 2014.

[11] Laflamme DP, Xu H, Long GM. Effect of diets differing in fat content on chronic diarrhea in cats. *J Vet Intern Med* 25:230, 2011.

CHAPTER 39

Nutritional strategies

Aarti Kathrani

NUTRITIONAL STRATEGIES IN GASTROINTESTINAL DISEASE

Nutrition has many direct beneficial effects on the components and function of the gastrointestinal (GI) tract and is therefore important in the management of various feline GI diseases. This section of the chapter discusses specific nutritional strategies for the management of acute gastroenteritis, GI adverse food reaction (AFR), food-responsive enteropathy (FRE), and constipation.

Acute gastroenteritis

Vomiting and diarrhoea due to acute gastroenteritis are a familiar presentation in veterinary practice. There are many causative factors, such as infectious, inflammatory, toxic, and dietary indiscretion, although the underlying cause is frequently not determined. Treatment focuses on the underlying cause if identified, symptomatic care, and dietary management once the cat is appropriately rehydrated and stabilised.

The absence of nutrients within the GI tract can result in small intestinal villous atrophy within days. The absence of luminal nutrition also results in suppressed crypt cell proliferation, marked decrease in GI-associated lymphoid tissue and function, increased intestinal permeability and risk of bacterial translocation, and enhanced pro-inflammatory cytokine production, whereas nutrients within the intestinal lumen stimulate intestinal mass and function and are an important stimulus for intestinal mucosal growth, repair, and integrity. Enteral feeding with as little as 10% of resting energy requirement (RER) to piglets resulted in significantly greater jejunal lactase and sucrase activities and taller villi and deeper crypts vs. findings in animals fed *nil per os*.[1] Similarly, significantly higher survival rates were achieved in cats receiving enteral nutrition with parenteral nutrition (PN), as compared to PN alone.[2] Therefore, enteral nutrition should be prioritised over starvation or total PN whenever possible. The former is particularly important for the prevention of hepatic lipidosis in cats.

Nutrients of focus

Energy

As discussed before, cats presenting with acute gastroenteritis, once stabilised and rehydrated, should not have food withheld and instead small amounts of food should be offered as soon as possible. Food intake should be initiated with 25% of the calculated RER [70 × body weight (kg)$^{0.75}$] divided into multiple meals to aid gastric emptying and intestinal motility. If the cat does not tolerate enteral feeding initially, food should be withheld for as short a time as possible and then offered again at a reduced amount of 10%–15% of RER. If 25% of RER is well tolerated, this can be increased slowly by 25% increments every 24 hours until full RER is reached on day 4. A slow increase over 4 days will help to prevent GI tract overload and exacerbation of clinical signs, as well as allow for assessment of tolerance. Feeding above RER should not be performed in hospital due to complications associated with overfeeding.

Digestibility

Unfortunately, studies are lacking to determine the ideal dietary composition for cats with acute gastroenteritis. However, commercial therapeutic GI diets are commonly selected for management of these cases, as these diets typically have higher digestibility compared to over-the-counter diets. Cats with acute gastroenteritis likely have compromise of their digestion and absorption of nutrients and, consequently, diets with high digestibility should be prioritised. In addition, diets with high digestibility help to provide fewer osmotic residues in the GI tract.

Fat

A reduction in dietary fat can help to hasten gastric transit and may help those cats with vomiting or nausea. GI disease may reduce fat digestion and cause excess dietary fat to pass into the colon. Increased fat in the colon can potentially result in dysbiosis as well as induce epithelial cell damage and fluid secretion into the colon. However, dietary fat did not seem to affect the outcome of cats with chronic diarrhoea.[3] Thus, dietary fat may be less of a nutrient of concern in cats with acute gastroenteritis. Nevertheless, as older cats can have impaired fat digestion, lower-fat diets may be a consideration for these cases depending on their initial response to therapeutic GI diets with moderate levels of fat.

Fibre

Dietary fibre can have many beneficial effects within the GI tract, such as modification of gastric emptying, normalisation of intestinal motility, buffering of toxins, binding of excess water, support of the growth of beneficial bacteria, and alteration of the viscosity of the ingesta. In cats with colitis, one study showed response to diets high in fibre or supplemented with fibre.[4] However, an increase in dietary fibre can reduce the digestibility of the food. Therefore, this strategy is usually trialled if the cat's clinical signs do not respond to a highly digestible diet or if the clinical signs are predominantly large intestinal in origin.

Probiotics

Cats with acute diarrhoea in an animal rescue centre were shown to benefit from *Enterococcus faecium* SF68 probiotic by having fewer episodes of diarrhoea for two or more days when compared to controls.[5] Hence, probiotics may be beneficial in reducing the duration of signs in cats with acute gastroenteritis. However, further studies, particularly in immunocompromised cats, are needed to definitively define the role of probiotics in the treatment protocol of cats with acute gastroenteritis.

Feeding plan

Cats with acute gastroenteritis should be fed small, frequent meals throughout the day to ensure their daily requirements are met without overloading the GI tract. Food for kittens should also meet their requirements for growth. Once clinical signs have resolved, the regular diet can be slowly introduced over 10–14 days. If the cat is at an ideal body condition score (BCS) of 5/9, then the number of daily calories previously fed can be continued.

Reassessment

The prognosis for recovery in most cases of acute gastroenteritis is very good. Body weight and hydration status as well as monitoring of GI signs should be performed at least daily during hospitalisation. Further diagnostic investigations should be pursued if vomiting or diarrhoea persists, or if signs become chronic.

Gastrointestinal adverse food reaction

Many conditions are included under the term GI AFR and can be grouped depending on their underlying aetiology (Fig. 39.1). The first classification of GI AFR is toxic (e.g. aflatoxin ingestion) or nontoxic. Nontoxic causes are then subclassified further into nonimmune-mediated or immune-mediated. Nonimmune-mediated causes include pharmacological (e.g. ingestion of vasoactive amines) or enzymatic (e.g. brush border enzyme deficiency). Immune-mediated causes are subclassified depending on whether the innate immune system or the adaptive immune system is implicated. The majority of studies in humans and animal models have focused on the role of the adaptive immune system in GI AFR, with three further subdivisions including IgE-mediated, non-IgE-mediated, and mixed IgE- and non-IgE-mediated. Dietary intolerance comprises the nontoxic, nonimmune-mediated causes of GI AFR (i.e. pharmacological and enzymatic), whereas the term food allergy or food hypersensitivity is used to describe the immune-mediated causes (i.e. innate and adaptive immune systems).[6] Therefore, GI AFR in cats can have many underlying causes.

A complete and thorough diet history will help to diagnose toxic and nontoxic, nonimmune-mediated causes of GI AFR in cats. However, the diagnosis of immune-mediated causes (food hypersensitivity or

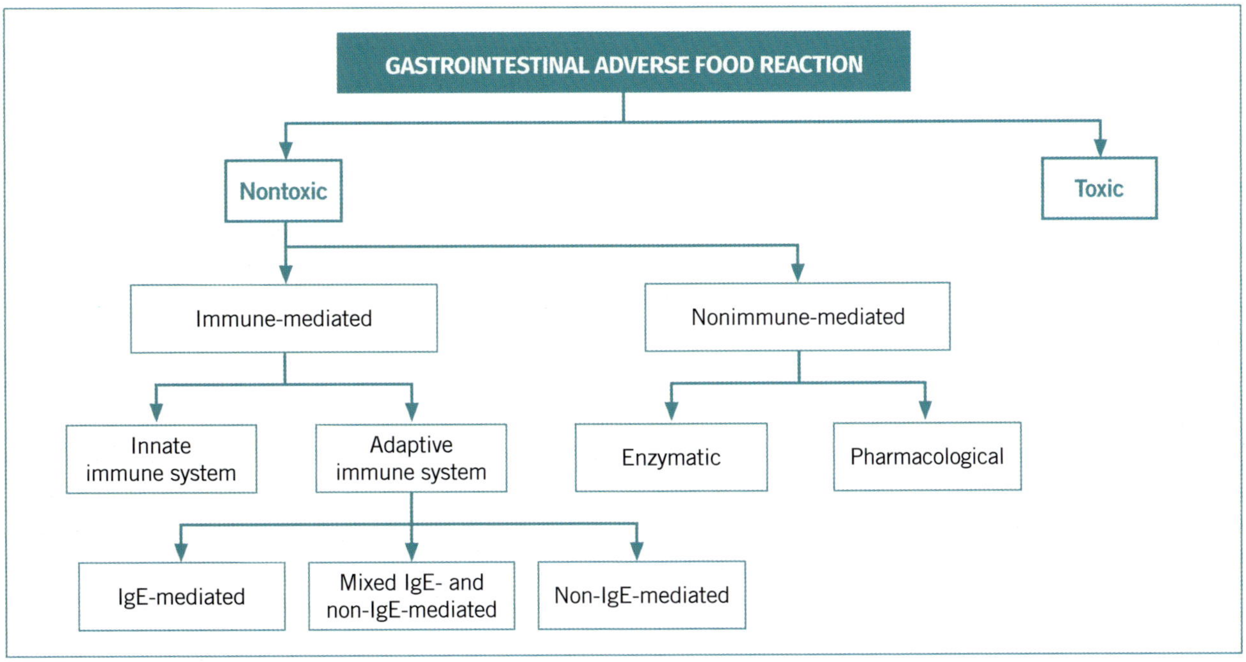

Figure 39.1. Classification system used in humans with gastrointestinal adverse food reaction.

allergy) is currently more challenging. This is because there is currently no laboratory test commercially available that allows for a definitive diagnosis. Testing for serum food-specific IgE and IgG showed low accuracy in cats. Therefore, this test should be avoided for the diagnosis of food allergy in cats. Similarly, patch, gastroscopic, and colonoscopic testing with food is not useful, and neither is food-specific faecal IgE measurement or hair and saliva testing, and these tests should not be used for the diagnosis of food allergy in cats. Although lymphocyte proliferation tests have been shown to be more accurate for the diagnosis of food allergy in cats, they are not available commercially due to the difficulty in performing the tests, as samples need to be processed immediately in a laboratory. Thus, the gold standard diagnostic test for food allergy in cats remains an exclusion diet trial with provocation testing. However, provocation testing is commonly not carried out due to low owner compliance, and hence a definitive diagnosis of food allergy in cats is frequently not reached.

Commercial therapeutic diets

Hydrolysed diets are effective in cases of food allergy, as they contain proteins that are considered small enough to theoretically avoid a type 1 IgE-mediated hypersensitivity. They avoid this immune response by preventing cross-linking of two IgE antibody receptors on a mast cell. Although the exact type of aberrant immune response is unknown in cats with GI food allergy, hydrolysed diets are used to diagnose and treat this condition. However, one study showed that a significant proportion (21%) of dogs sensitised to the intact protein still reacted adversely to the hydrolysed diet.[7] In consequence, persistent signs may be anticipated with hydrolysed diets, particularly in cats with a non-IgE-mediated aetiology for their food allergy. Accordingly, if the GI signs fail to respond to a hydrolysed diet, then a commercial therapeutic diet or a home-prepared, limited-ingredient, novel protein diet should be trialled.

Home-prepared diets

In some cases, cats may be allergic to an antigen that developed or was unmasked during the commercialisation process of the diet and may be unable to tolerate any commercial cat food. In these cases, a positive response to a home-prepared diet can be used to diagnose and manage these cats.

Feeding plan and reassessment

A strict exclusion diet trial should be performed for at least 6 to 8 weeks. After this time, a provocation challenge with the original diet or single ingredients would be needed to confirm the diagnosis of food allergy. However, this is not frequently performed, and the diagnosis remains tentative in these cats.

Food-responsive enteropathy

The term FRE is defined as those cases of chronic enteropathy (CE) that are responsive to dietary therapy alone. Studies have demonstrated that FRE encompasses approximately two thirds of dogs presenting with CE in a secondary to tertiary referral population. Although information is unavailable for the feline population, it is similarly thought to involve approximately two thirds of cats presenting with CE. Unfortunately, the exact aetiology of CE in cats is unknown; however, it is hypothesised to involve the variable interplay of four key components: genetic susceptibility, environmental risk factors, intestinal dysbiosis, and altered GI mucosal immune response.[8] Thus, cats with CE may be able to attain remission with dietary therapy alone due to the advantageous effects of diet on intestinal microbiota, mucosal immune response, GI permeability and motility, mucosal healing, and gene expression. In addition, diet may act as a significant environmental trigger for the disease in some cats, and removal of this inciting cause may resolve clinical signs.

Dietary therapy for inflammatory bowel disease (IBD) in humans is considered a personalised approach, as responses to different dietary strategies likely depend on the underlying genetic susceptibility and are thus not the same for all IBD patients. Similarly, an advantageous response to specific dietary strategies in cats with CE is likely dependent on the underlying genetic susceptibility as well as environmental risk factors. Therefore, nutrition should also be individualised in cats with CE to ensure that the most effective dietary strategy that will allow control of the clinical signs is employed. Unfortunately, at this time, dietary management remains trial and error in cats with CE to determine which strategy is the most effective. Although owners may find it frustrating to trial different dietary strategies, one study demonstrated that most cats with chronic idiopathic GI problems that respond to dietary therapy alone respond quickly, within 2–3 days, suggesting that these diets do not need to be fed long-term to determine clinical response.[9] Therefore, if the cat shows no response to a trial with a therapeutic diet after 2 weeks of exclusive feeding, a different diet or pharmacological treatment should be considered.

Nutrients of focus

Protein

Studies in cats have demonstrated that diets containing either hydrolysed protein, protein from novel sources, or highly digestible protein can be successfully used in the management of FRE in cats. Hydrolysed protein diets are likely effective in the management of CE in cats due to their effect on the immune system, which is known to be dysregulated in this disease. The hydrolysed protein strategy may evade the immune system, and one study demonstrated less systemic cytokine response to these diets in cats compared to intact protein.[10] Novel protein diets may escape detection by the immune system, as they have not previously been fed and therefore may not be recognised. Highly digestible proteins are likely to be more completely digested before presenting to the immune system. However, further studies are needed to determine the exact mechanism for the effectiveness of these diets in feline chronic enteropathy (FCE).

Nearly 50% of cats with chronic GI signs respond to a novel protein diet.[9] Deciding which specific novel protein formula to use will depend on the cat's previous antigen exposure list. One study demonstrated the presence of other common food antigens in over-the-counter novel protein diets; thus, these diets should be avoided in cats for the treatment of suspected FRE.[11]

Digestibility

Highly digestible diets have been used successfully in the management of FCE. The efficacy of these diets is likely due to less protein presenting intact to the immune system because of the higher digestibility, as well as less digestion required by the already compromised GI tract. However, digestibility alone may be unlikely to maintain remission, as one study in dogs with CE showed that although a highly digestible therapeutic GI diet was able to induce remission, these dogs were less likely to remain asymptomatic at subsequent rechecks when compared to dogs managed with a hydrolysed diet.[12] However, further studies comparing highly digestible therapeutic GI diets with hydrolysed diets are needed in FCE to determine if the same is also true in cats.

Fat

High-fat diets can have adverse effects on the GI microbiota, permeability, and mucosal immune response in individuals with a relevant genetic susceptibility. Therefore, although dietary fat has been shown to be generally well tolerated in cats with chronic diarrhoea, further studies are needed to determine if individual cats are likely to benefit from low-fat diets due to the underlying pathophysiology of their CE.

Omega-3 fatty acids and soy are immunomodulatory and may be beneficial in some cats with CE. Commercial hydrolysed diets for cats are known to contain these ingredients, which may explain why these diets are effective in the management of FCE. Further studies are needed to determine the optimal dose of omega-3 fatty acids in the management of cats with CE.

Vitamin B_{12}

Several studies have documented low vitamin B_{12} in FCE. Hence, measuring serum vitamin B_{12} concentrations to determine if supplementation is warranted is important, as this may help to improve not only clinical signs and gut health but also the response to other treatments such as glucocorticoids. One study showing the effects of oral cobalamin supplementation at normalising serum vitamin B_{12} concentrations in cats has been reported.[13]

Fibre

Dietary fibres are plant-based carbohydrates, which cannot be digested by mammalian enzymes. Fibre has numerous advantageous effects and is hypothesised to exert an anti-inflammatory effect via fermentation to short-chain fatty acids by intestinal microbiota, thereby playing a role in maintaining intestinal barrier function. Unfortunately, there have been limited studies assessing the efficacy of dietary fibre in FCE. One study demonstrated response to diets high in fibre or supplemented with fibre in cats with colitis.[4] Therefore, selecting formulas within the hydrolysed or novel protein category that have higher total dietary fibre may also help to encompass this dietary strategy in those cases with signs attributable to the large intestine.

Feeding plan

A slow transition to the new diet should be performed over 2 weeks to increase the chances of acceptance, and in some cases 3–4 weeks may be needed. It is important to ensure that the cat does not get access to other foods when outdoors to increase the chances of success. Feeding multiple small meals throughout the day will help digestion and absorption and prevent overloading of the GI tract. If the cat has an ideal BCS of 5/9, then the number of daily calories that were previously fed can be continued. If the cat's BCS is low, then the quantity fed should be increased by 10% increments to account for any malassimilation from the CE until an ideal BCS is reached.

Reassessment

Regularly assessing the cat's appetite, activity, body weight, BCS, and GI signs will help to determine the effectiveness of the therapeutic diet. Return to normal appetite, activity, body weight, and BCS and absence of GI signs indicate success of dietary management. Serial measurement of the clinical CE activity index offers a more objective measure of assessing response to treatment. Assessing serum vitamin B_{12} concentrations is important in those cases that were deficient to ensure adequate dose and frequency of supplementation. Transition to an over-the-counter diet could be considered after the 6-week diet trial if the cat's clinical signs are in remission; however, most owners elect to continue to feed the therapeutic diet lifelong.

Failure to respond to the therapeutic diet may require a different dietary strategy or immunosuppressive drugs (e.g. glucocorticoids) in addition to diet to control clinical signs or may suggest owner noncompliance with feeding, intercurrent diseases (e.g. triaditis, exocrine pancreatic insufficiency [EPI]), or misdiagnosis (e.g. small-cell alimentary lymphoma).

Constipation

Constipation is a common clinical problem in cats presenting to veterinary practice. Constipation may lead to obstipation, which necessitates medical intervention.

Dietary management forms an important component in the treatment of feline constipation, with recommendations varying depending on the level of colonic motility remaining.

Nutrients of focus

Fibre

For those cats presenting with constipation that still have some level of colonic motility, insoluble or a mix of insoluble and soluble fibre may help. Insoluble fibres are less fermentable in the large intestine and provide bulk to the faeces, which can then help to improve colonic motility by causing distension of the colon. On the other hand, soluble fibres are generally fermentable in the large intestine resulting in the production of short-chain fatty acids, which have numerous beneficial effects on the colonocytes and colonic motility and increase the moisture content of the faeces. As soluble fibres increase the moisture of faeces, an excess of these fibres can lead to diarrhoea.

Psyllium is a soluble fibre with low fermentability; however, its ability to produce a gel when mixed with water helps to provide bulk to the faeces. One uncontrolled trial in cats with constipation showed that a commercial psyllium-enriched dry diet was able to improve stool quality and clinical outcome in over 80% of cats within a week of starting the diet.[14] However, the long-term use and effects of this diet in decreasing the risk of megacolon have not been studied.

Digestibility

In cats presenting with obstipation, the motility patterns of the large intestine are completely abolished. Therefore, in these cats, diets with increased fibre content and supplements containing fibre should be avoided, as they may worsen clinical signs. Instead, a highly digestible, low-residue diet with a high caloric density should be fed to markedly reduce faecal content.

Feeding plan

Constipated cats should be well hydrated before a diet high in fibre is introduced. This will help to maximise the therapeutic effect of dietary fibre, as well as minimise any potential for impaction of fibre in the large intestine. Similarly, in obstipated cats, multiple cleansing enemas with or without mechanical removal of impacted faeces should be performed before dietary changes are introduced. Feeding smaller and more frequent meals may help to improve colonic motility patterns and reduce the amount of ingesta entering the colon at one time. If the cat is overweight, a weight reduction programme should be initiated. Ensuring adequate water intake is important, and active encouragement with the use of water fountains and running taps should be used to ensure adequate hydration.

Reassessment

Body weight, BCS, appetite, and faecal frequency and consistency should be monitored at least daily during hospitalisation. Return of normal activity and appetite, weight stability or intentional weight loss or gain, and absence of clinical signs at home are all indicators of successful dietary management.

NUTRITIONAL STRATEGIES IN PANCREATIC DISEASE

Dietary therapy is an important adjunctive treatment for two of the pancreatic diseases diagnosed in cats: pancreatitis and EPI. Different dietary strategies and nutrients of focus are prioritised for each of these conditions; therefore, selecting the right diet and feeding strategy will help to optimise treatment.

Pancreatitis

Voluntary enteral nutrition

If the cat is able to eat enough food to meet its daily energy requirements, voluntary enteral nutrition should be prioritised. *Nil per os*, which was historically recommended for these cases, should no longer be advocated if the cat is not actively vomiting. Inflammation and necrosis of the pancreas are exacerbated when exocrine activity is suppressed, and food should not be deliberately withheld. In addition, withholding food can have detrimental effects on intestinal function, such as the promotion of mucosal atrophy, increased rate of apoptosis of the enterocytes, decreased transport of glutamine and arginine, increased permeability of the intestinal tract, and adverse effects on renal, respiratory, immune, cardiovascular, muscular, and skeletal systems, which could exacerbate concurrent illness in cats with pancreatitis. *Nil per os* can also increase morbidity and mortality. Therefore, enteral feeding is crucial in these cases.

Unfortunately, dietary management of feline pancreatitis has not been well studied or described. The diet chosen should be highly digestible. The role of dietary fat is less certain in cats compared to dogs. Nevertheless, some internists have anecdotally seen pancreatitis in cats initiated by a high-fat diet. Thus, although dietary fat restriction is unlikely to be a major strategy in cats with pancreatitis, high-fat diets should be avoided. Dietary protein is more likely to be a stimulant for pancreatic secretion than dietary fat, so diets high in protein should also be avoided. Commercial therapeutic GI diets should be offered due to their high digestibility.

Assisted enteral nutrition

For those cats unable to meet their daily energy requirements voluntarily, an assisted enteral feeding tube should be considered. Three to five days of anorexia, either prior to or during hospitalisation, is an indication to intervene nutritionally. One study documented that 69% of cats with pancreatitis were anorexic at presentation, and 96% hyporexic.[15] Nutritional intervention should be started sooner in cats younger than 6 months, older and debilitated, severely cachectic, or if the anticipated period of anorexia will be protracted due to the underlying disease. Nutritional intervention should also be considered sooner in obese cats due to their increased risk for hepatic lipidosis. In one study with 55 cats with pancreatitis, feeding could occur early in the course of hospitalisation (<72 hours after admission) with nasogastric tube feeding, and this study reported a survival rate of 91%.[15]

Assisted enteral feeding consists of either feeding directly into the oral cavity using a syringe or placing a feeding tube. The author does not recommend assisted oral feeding with a syringe due to difficulty achieving daily caloric requirements, as well as the risk of aspiration and food aversion. Appetite stimulants, such as mirtazapine or cyproheptadine, can also be tried to help support caloric intake and may reduce the need for feeding tube placement. However, this can have varied individual effects and may not increase voluntary intake enough to meet daily requirements, necessitating an enteral feeding tube. There are four common types of enteral assisted feeding tubes used in cats: nasoenteral, oesophagostomy, gastrostomy, and jejunostomy. See Chapter 40 for further details on enteral nutrition and feeding tubes.

Unfortunately, certain conditions preclude enteral feeding, such as intractable vomiting and diarrhoea, dull mentation, absent gag reflex, and the inability to place an enteral feeding tube due to coagulopathy or contraindications to sedation or anaesthesia. Therefore, in such cats, PN is indicated for assisted feeding.

Parenteral nutrition

This type of nutrition is recommended for those cats that are not consuming enough of their daily energy and nutrient requirements and placement of an enteral feeding tube is contraindicated. PN is made up of three main constituents: a dextrose solution, an amino acid solution, and a lipid solution. Light-sensitive B complex vitamins are frequently included into the PN solution because of their important role in metabolism. As PN is not intended to be administered long-term, it does not contain all of the cat's daily nutrient requirements. However, if administration is likely to exceed 5 days, some veterinary nutritionists may include certain minerals to the PN solution.

Administration of PN can be made via central (single- or multi-lumen central intravenous catheter into the jugular vein or the lateral or medial saphenous veins) or peripheral venous access (catheter into the cephalic vein). Catheter placement should occur aseptically, and the port should be new and not have been used for any purpose before the PN administration. The osmolarity of the resultant PN formulation determines whether it can be administered centrally or peripherally. For central administration, the osmolarity of the final formulation should not exceed 1400 mOsm/l, whereas for peripheral administration the osmolarity is typically 600–750 mOsm/l to help prevent thrombophlebitis. Because of this restriction on osmolarity, providing the cat's full daily energy requirement by peripheral PN can be restrictive. However, because the lipid constituent of the PN solution has the lowest osmolarity and highest caloric density, a solution with a high amount of lipid could provide the cat's full daily energy requirement via peripheral administration. However, some veterinary nutritionists advise not to exceed 2 grams of lipid per kilogram of body weight per day because of the concern for immunosuppression.

In addition, if the cat is hyperlipidaemic, high-fat PN solutions should be avoided.

A PN solution containing more than 50% dextrose and an excess of 4 mg/kg/minute of dextrose infusion should be avoided due to potential complications associated with hyperglycaemia, which is also a poor prognostic indicator in cats.[16] If the cat has concurrent kidney or liver dysfunction, the protein content of the PN solution should be reduced. Pancreatitis is not an indication to reduce the fat content in the PN solution, as parenteral fat does not stimulate the pancreas. However, if the cat has hyperlipidaemia, the amount of lipid in the PN solution should be reduced.

Parenteral feeding should be complemented with enteral feeding whenever possible, even if the latter makes up no more than 10% of the daily RER, as some enteral nutrition will help to maintain the integrity of the GI lining. In humans, the addition of the amino acid glutamine was shown to reduce hospital stay and decrease overall complications in those patients with acute pancreatitis given PN. However, this has not been investigated in cats with pancreatitis. One study, which evaluated the risk of PN in cats with pancreatitis amongst other diseases, reported a mortality rate of 19%, with more cats surviving when PN was administered with enteral nutrition.[2] Another study reported a 46% mortality rate in 35 cats with pancreatitis fed parenterally.[16]

If PN is to be used, the solution can be compounded under a laminar flow hood with a closed, semiautomated system or manually using an all-in-one system. However, strict adherence to asepsis is paramount in both techniques. Another option is the use of three-in-one solutions, which are also available commercially. A board-certified veterinary nutritionist can be consulted for further recommendations with regard to PN formulation.

Cats should be monitored closely for complications throughout PN administration and should ideally be hospitalised in an intensive care unit with 24-hour supervision. Parenteral feeding can be associated with mechanical, metabolic, and septic complications. Further information regarding these complications are beyond the scope of this chapter and therefore the reader is encouraged to examine more in-depth reviews of PN in cats or consult with a board-certified veterinary nutritionist for more guidance before use.

Nutrients of focus

Water

Cats with pancreatitis are particularly susceptible to dehydration due to vomiting and anorexia. It is important to ensure that the cat is adequately hydrated so that perfusion to the pancreas is not compromised. Intravenous fluids should be initiated if the cat is moderately to severely dehydrated. It is important to delay nutritional support until fluid, electrolyte, and acid–base abnormalities have been corrected.

Energy

Ensuring that cats meet their daily energy requirements is paramount to avoid negative energy balance, which can have deleterious effects on the GI tract as well as other organs. Feeding, whether via enteral or parenteral nutrition, should be initiated at 25% of the RER, with daily increases of 25% until 100% RER is reached on day 4 if the cat is tolerating the feeds. In-hospital feeding should not exceed 100% RER to prevent complications associated with overfeeding.

Once the cat is discharged home and recovering, the number of calories should be increased to ensure that an ideal body weight is achieved or maintained for underconditioned or ideal-conditioned cats, respectively. Overweight and obese cats should be started on a weight loss plan when they have recovered from the pancreatitis episode.

Dietary fat

Although dietary fat is less of a concern in cats than in dogs, excessively high-fat diets should be avoided due to their anecdotal association with pancreatitis. However, if hyperlipidaemia is present, dietary fat should be decreased. Unfortunately, unlike in dogs, there are few commercial therapeutic diets available for cats that are low in fat. Some commercial therapeutic weight loss diets that are low in caloric density or senior diets may be low in fat. However, these diets may not be sufficiently energy-dense to ensure sufficient calories for an ill cat. Thus, if these diets are used, the cat should be closely monitored to ensure adequate intake.

Obesity has been associated with canine pancreatitis, likely due to the inflammatory effects of adipose tissue. Although the effect of obesity on feline pancreatitis is not definitively known, overconditioned cats should be started on a weight loss plan once recovered from the current bout of pancreatitis, as this may help to prevent reoccurrence.

Dietary protein

Dietary protein is a strong stimulus for pancreatic secretion in cats.[17] Hence, excess dietary protein should be avoided in cats with pancreatitis while still providing adequate amounts for tissue repair and recovery.

Vitamin B_{12}

In cats, intrinsic factor, which helps to promote vitamin B_{12} absorption in the ileum, is produced solely in the pancreas. Therefore, many cats with pancreatitis may be deficient in vitamin B_{12}. If a deficiency is documented, parenteral or oral cobalamin supplementation should be initiated.

Omega-3 polyunsaturated fatty acids

Studies in humans have demonstrated the benefit of omega-3 polyunsaturated fatty acids in pancreatitis. Omega-3 polyunsaturated fatty acids helped to decrease hospital stay and complications in people with acute pancreatitis. The mechanism for their efficacy is likely due to their anti-inflammatory effects. Further studies are needed in cats to demonstrate efficacy before a dose for supplemental use can be recommended. However, omega-3 polyunsaturated fatty acids have been shown to be beneficial in the treatment of hypertriglyceridaemia and so they could be considered for these cats.

Antioxidants

Studies in humans have proven the beneficial effects of antioxidants in pancreatitis. A combination of antioxidants involving selenium, beta-carotene, vitamin C, and vitamin E helped to reduce abdominal pain, disease recurrence, chronicity, and hospital stay in people. Although studies of experimental pancreatitis in dogs demonstrated an increased generation of free oxygen radicals, a study assessing the effects of superoxide dismutase showed no improvement in laboratory parameters or survival rates.[18] However, further studies are needed, particularly in cats, to prove any efficacy before supplemental use can be recommended.

Probiotics

Studies in humans showed equivocal results with regard to the use of probiotics in pancreatitis. Some studies have cited the beneficial effects of probiotics to be due to their ability to maintain the integrity of the intestinal barrier and consequently minimise bacterial translocation, as well as promote the production of antimicrobial factors. However, it is important to note that some human studies have shown that probiotics do not make a difference, and others have even shown a worsening effect. In consequence, studies are needed in cats before a recommendation can be made on the use of probiotics for pancreatitis in this species.

Cats with comorbidities

Cats presenting with pancreatitis may have additional comorbidities that are dietary responsive. In one study, 84% of cats with acute pancreatitis were suspected to have concurrent diseases.[15] The most common comorbidities included concurrent CE and cholangitis (i.e. triaditis), diabetes mellitus, kidney disease, and hepatic lipidosis. Hepatic lipidosis can occur within 72 hours of anorexia and has been reported as an exacerbating illness in 59% of cats with pancreatitis, increasing mortality up to 80%.[19] Hence, diets will need to be selected and dietary strategies employed to ensure that they also meet the recommendations of these additional diseases if present.

Feeding strategy

Cats with pancreatitis should be fed smaller amounts more frequently to prevent GI tract overloading. A slow transition to the new diet should be performed over 1–2 weeks. However, some cats may require a slower transition—over a month—until full acceptance is achieved. Ensuring that access to other foods is not available during a therapeutic diet trial is important to avoid interfering with the required dietary strategies.

Reassessment

Assessment of the body weight and condition are important to ensure adequate hydration and caloric intake. Haematocrit and potassium, phosphorus, and glucose concentrations should be monitored regularly in cats receiving nutrition after a period of prolonged anorexia to ensure that refeeding does not develop. If PN is used, daily monitoring of electrolytes, glucose, and triglycerides is needed to determine if any adjustments are required in the composition of the PN solution. The cat should be monitored closely for any GI signs, including new onset or worsening regurgitation, vomiting, inappetence, weight loss, or diarrhoea. The return to normal activity and appetite and maintenance of body weight in the absence of clinical signs are measures of successful dietary management. Laboratory parameters including feline pancreatic lipase immunoreactivity should be regularly monitored.

Exocrine pancreatic insufficiency

Chronic pancreatitis is likely the most common cause of feline EPI. Feline EPI is associated with severe nutrient malassimilation due to failure of intraluminal digestion from a deficiency in pancreatic enzymes. Also, the deficiency of other pancreatic secretory products, such as bicarbonate, GI trophic factors, intrinsic factor to help with vitamin B_{12} absorption, and antimicrobial factors, can lead to impaired intestinal function and nutrient malassimilation. The lack of GI trophic factors and concurrent small intestinal bacterial overgrowth may lead to impaired mucosal enzyme activity, resulting in reduced absorption of amino acids, fatty acids, and sugars. Although oral pancreatic enzyme supplementation is the foundation of treatment, enteral nutrition is also extremely important in the management.

Enteral nutrition

Nutrients of focus

Energy

If the cat is underweight, the daily caloric intake should be increased until an ideal body condition is reached. For those cats that are already at or have reached an ideal body condition, it will be necessary to offer above the average amount of food that would be needed for a healthy cat to compensate for the malabsorption present.

Digestibility

Diets with high digestibility should be prioritised to help with nutrient digestion and absorption.

Dietary fat

Cats with EPI can present with steatorrhoea. However, reducing dietary fat in dogs with EPI can lead to worsening of clinical signs, so moderate fat content is recommended.[20,21] This will also help to ensure that enough calories are provided to help with achieving and then maintaining an adequate body condition. However, the effect of dietary fat in feline EPI has not been specifically reported. Accordingly, different levels of dietary fat may need to be tried to find the optimal level for each individual cat.

Dietary fibre

Diets for cats with EPI should contain very little fibre in order to maximise the digestibility of the food. Dietary fibre has also been shown to hinder pancreatic enzyme activity in vitro.

Medium-chain triglycerides

Although medium-chain triglycerides have been suggested as a source of fat in cats with EPI, one study suggested that their addition did not improve clinical signs in dogs with EPI.[22] In addition, medium-chain triglycerides are associated with poor palatability in cats and may reduce overall food intake.

Cobalamin and folate

Cobalamin deficiency has been associated with EPI and has been reported in 77% of cats.[23] Several mechanisms are likely to explain this deficiency: the lack of bicarbonate secretion from the pancreas, which may reduce intestinal pH and the affinity of cobalamin for intrinsic factor; a deficiency in intrinsic factor, which is primarily secreted from the pancreas in cats; and concurrent small intestinal bacterial overgrowth, which may consume cobalamin before it is able to be absorbed. Thus, supplementation should be initiated either parenterally or orally in these cases. Furthermore, supplementation of cobalamin to cats with EPI improves overall outcome.[23] If folate concentrations are low, supplementation should also be considered. Interestingly, folate deficiency has been shown to inhibit pancreatic exocrine function in rats.

Fat-soluble vitamins

As EPI can cause fat malassimilation, fat-soluble vitamins (A, D, E, and K) may be deficient in these cats. Clinically, vitamin K deficiency has been reported in a cat with EPI. Accordingly, if a coagulopathy is documented, subcutaneous vitamin K therapy should be initiated at 0.5–1 mg/kg subcutaneously every 12 hours for 2–4 doses. Empirical supplementation of vitamin A and D should be avoided unless these can be documented to be deficient, as excess levels may be harmful. Supplementation with vitamin E is considered to be safe and can be dosed orally at 10 IU/kg every 24 hours.

Minerals

Although there is no information with regard to whether macro- and micromineral deficiencies exist in cats with EPI, one study in dogs with experimental EPI found lower serum and tissue concentrations of zinc and copper compared to control dogs.[24] However, this was not replicated in spontaneous cases of canine EPI.[25] Hence, empirical supplementation of these minerals is not currently recommended in cats with EPI until further research in the feline disease is available.

Feeding strategy

Cats with EPI should be fed multiple small meals per day with pancreatic enzyme supplementation to maximise digestion and prevent intestinal overload and resultant osmotic diarrhoea.

Reassessment

Regular assessment of food intake, body weight, body condition, coat condition, and faecal consistency and frequency should be undertaken. It is crucial to remember that these cats are likely to require more food than expected to ensure that they maintain an optimal body weight and condition. It is also important to assess serum cobalamin concentrations to ensure that supplementation is adequate.

Indicators of successful dietary management of cats with EPI include achieving or maintaining an optimal body weight and body condition, normal activity and appetite, good coat condition, and absence of clinical signs.

NUTRITIONAL STRATEGIES IN HEPATOBILIARY DISEASE

The liver plays a central role in nutrient digestion and metabolism. It is involved in bile salt production for fat digestion and absorption and is essential in the metabolism of proteins, fat, and carbohydrates. Therefore, nutrition helps provide a supportive role in the management of feline hepatobiliary diseases, although it is the cornerstone of treatment for hepatic lipidosis and hepatic encephalopathy (HE).

Feline hepatic lipidosis

Pathophysiology

The pathophysiology of feline hepatic lipidosis involves the excessive accumulation of triglycerides in the hepatocytes, which leads to intrahepatic cholestasis and hepatic dysfunction. A negative energy state caused by anorexia is considered the inciting cause of hepatic lipidosis. Cats presenting with this syndrome are usually obese, with a history of anorexia and weight loss following a stressful episode or due to an underlying disease. Feline hepatic lipidosis can be categorised as either primary, when no inciting underlying disease for anorexia is identified, or more commonly secondary, when anorexia is a consequence of an underlying disease (e.g. diabetes mellitus, pancreatitis, inflammatory hepatobiliary disease, CE, kidney disease, neoplasia). Unfortunately, the exact pathophysiology of this syndrome is still unknown. Possible underlying aetiologies include protein deficiency, excess of peripheral lipolysis, increased lipogenesis, inhibition of oxidation of lipids, and inhibition of very-low-density lipoprotein synthesis.[26]

Treatment should initially be directed towards addressing any cardiovascular, fluid, or electrolyte abnormalities and HE if present. Treatment should also focus on identifying and treating any underlying cause for the hepatic lipidosis, such as cholangitis, pancreatitis, CE, chronic kidney disease, or neoplasia. The cornerstone of treatment is early, long-term assisted enteral feeding with oesophagostomy or gastrostomy tubes, which has helped to increase the prognosis of this potentially life-threatening condition. If general anaesthesia cannot be safely performed for placement of an oesophagostomy or gastrostomy feeding tube, a nasoenteral feeding tube should be initially placed instead and a liquid diet administered (Table 39.1) until the cat is stable for the placement of a more permanent and longer-lasting enteral feeding tube.

Nutrients of focus

Energy

Ensuring that cats with hepatic lipidosis meet their daily energy requirement is paramount to the successful management of these cases. A sufficient supply of energy will help to prevent catabolism of amino acids for use as energy and inhibit peripheral lipolysis and hepatic triglyceride accumulation. Nutrition should be started on the day of admission to ensure reversal of the negative energy state, unless the cat is cardiovascularly unstable or has severe electrolyte derangements. Caloric intake in hospital should meet the RER, and this can be increased to 1.2 times the RER when the cat is discharged for at-home management. Feeding should be via an assisted enteral feeding tube. Forced feeding should not be attempted, as this can result in food aversion and increase the risk of aspiration. Although appetite stimulants such as mirtazapine or cyproheptadine can be tried, they rarely result in the achievement of an oral intake of 100% RER. Oral diazepam should be avoided as an appetite stimulant in cats due to its association with fulminant hepatic failure.[27]

The use of oesophagostomy and gastrostomy feeding tubes will help to ensure the daily RER is met long-term and are well tolerated by cats. If the cat is unstable for general anaesthesia, a nasoenteral feeding tube will need to be placed initially to ensure that the cat meets some of its energy and nutrient requirements. The small diameter of these tubes (5–8 Fr) requires the feeding of a liquid diet to prevent clogging. Commercial therapeutic veterinary liquid diets that are designed for nasoenteral feeding are available, with caloric density varying from 1.0 to 2.0 kcal/ml to allow full daily energy requirements to be met. Diets can be fed continuously via pump infusion or using bolus feeding schedules. Feeding should be started at 25% of RER on day 1 and increased by 25% increments daily if the cat tolerates the feedings and electrolytes and phosphorus concentrations remain stable. Gradually increasing to 100% RER over at least 4 days may help to prevent refeeding syndrome, which has been reported in a cat with hepatic lipidosis.[28] Refeeding syndrome is characterised by hypophosphataemia, hypokalaemia, and hypomagnesaemia and is the consequence of rapid caloric administration in a previously starved patient that was in a chronic negative catabolic state, causing a surge in insulin release and resulting in electrolyte deficiencies.

Complications associated with the use of nasoenteral feeding tubes include intubation into the respiratory tract and associated pneumonia, epistaxis, rhinitis, dacryocystitis, vomiting, diarrhoea, tube removal or displacement by the cat, and tube clogging. Once the cat is stable for

Table 39.1. Nutritional supplements and nutraceuticals for feline hepatic lipidosis.

Supplement/nutraceutical	Route of administration	Dose
L-carnitine	PO	250–500 mg every 24 h
Taurine	PO	250–500 mg every 24 h
Vitamin K	SC	0.5–1 mg/kg every 12 h for 2–4 doses
Thiamine	PO	50–100 mg every 24 h
Cyanocobalamin	SC	0.25 mg every week
	PO	0.25 mg every 24 h
Vitamin E	PO	10 IU/kg every 24 h
Potassium	PO	2–6 mEq every 24 h
	IV crystalloid fluids	Not to exceed 0.5 mEq/kg/h
B complex vitamins	IV crystalloid fluids	1–2 ml per litre of crystalloid fluids
Lactulose	PO	0.25–0.5 mg/kg every 8–12 h
S-adenosylmethionine	PO	20 mg/kg every 24 h

IV, intravenous; PO, per os; SC, subcutaneous.

general anaesthesia, placement of an oesophagostomy or gastrostomy tube should be pursued to enable long-term assisted feeding. Commercial dry or tinned diets should be blenderised with water to provide a slurry for gastrostomy or oesophagostomy tube feeding. Gastrostomy tubes should be placed under percutaneous endoscopic guidance rather than via laparotomy, as the latter is associated with high risk of postoperative morbidity and stomach displacement.[29] Gastrostomy tubes have the advantage of allowing greater movement of the head and neck of the cat, since these are not bandaged as they would be for an oesophagostomy tube, and consequently would allow the cat to self-groom. If enteral assisted nutrition is not possible (e.g. intractable vomiting, coagulopathy, comatose patient, inability to swallow), PN should be considered. See Chapters 40 and 41 for further details on enteral and parenteral nutrition, respectively.

Protein

Cats with hepatobiliary disease may require higher amounts of protein to maintain positive nitrogen balance compared to healthy cats. Hence, protein restriction in these cats may result in protein–calorie malnutrition and may worsen clinical signs associated with their disease. Thus, cats with hepatic lipidosis that do not have evidence of HE should not have dietary protein restricted. Commercial therapeutic diets containing 25%–30% protein on a metabolisable energy (ME) basis have been well tolerated in most cats with hepatic lipidosis without evidence of HE. Although a diet with 25% protein on a ME basis was shown to attenuate but not ameliorate hepatic lipidosis, a diet with 35%–45% protein on a ME basis was shown to reverse the catabolic state and improve clinical signs in cats.[30,31] Commercial therapeutic feline recovery diets generally provide protein in the latter range and are suited for cats without signs of HE. Commercial therapeutic hepatic diets are moderately reduced in protein and should be prioritised in those cats with HE that will not tolerate diets with higher protein contents. Therefore, commercial therapeutic hepatic diets should not be fed universally to all cats with hepatic lipidosis and instead should be reserved for those cats that are not able to tolerate higher amounts of protein. Ultimately, the goal is to provide sufficient dietary protein to avoid catabolism and support hepatic regeneration while avoiding excess dietary protein that might contribute to or exacerbate HE.

Potassium

Hypokalaemia is relatively common in cats with hepatic lipidosis and likely develops due to anorexia reducing oral intake, vomiting, polydipsia and polyuria, magnesium depletion, and in cats with concurrent kidney disease. Hypokalaemia has been shown to be a negative prognostic indicator in cats with hepatic lipidosis and can exacerbate HE, as well as cause muscle weakness, ileus, and anorexia.[32] Hence, hypokalaemia should be actively corrected, and diets selected for cats with hepatic lipidosis should be potassium replete. Alternatively, potassium can be supplemented orally at 2–6 mEq potassium gluconate per day or via intravenous fluids. The rate of intravenous potassium supplementation should not exceed 0.5 mEq/kg/h.

L-carnitine

Carnitine is involved in the beta-oxidation of long-chain fatty acids by serving as a cofactor for the transport of these fatty acids across the inner mitochondrial membrane into the mitochondrial matrix. Cats meet their carnitine requirements through the diet and via biosynthesis in the liver. Mean concentrations of carnitine have been shown to be significantly higher in the plasma, liver, and skeletal muscle of cats with hepatic lipidosis compared to controls.[33] However, studies have shown that feline diets supplemented with L-carnitine helped to facilitate fatty acid oxidation in obese cats undergoing rapid weight loss and also protected obese cats from hepatic lipid accumulation during calorie restriction and rapid weight loss.[34,35] One study also showed that diets supplemented with L-carnitine can safely facilitate rapid weight loss in privately owned obese cats.[36] Based on the results of these studies, L-carnitine is recommended in the treatment of cats with hepatic lipidosis at an oral dose of 250–500 mg of L-carnitine per cat per day. Although rigorous placebo-controlled clinical trials evaluating the benefits of L-carnitine in cats with hepatic lipidosis are lacking, anecdotally, supplementation is considered to result in faster recovery and higher survival rates.

Vitamin B_{12}

Cats with hepatic lipidosis can have concurrent diseases that may reduce their vitamin B_{12} concentrations, such as CE or kidney disease. Therefore, serum vitamin B_{12} concentrations should be measured and either parenteral or oral cyanocobalamin supplementation started if concentrations are found to be low.

Vitamin K

Significant increases in plasma concentrations of proteins induced by vitamin K antagonism (PIVKA) have been demonstrated in cats with hepatic lipidosis.[37] Vitamin K deficiency in these cats may develop due to prolonged anorexia, oral antibiotic treatment which may destroy intestinal microbiota that normally synthesise vitamin K, or fat malabsorption. Thus, vitamin K should be supplemented via subcutaneous vitamin K_1 injection (0.5–1.0 mg/kg every 12 hours for 2–4 doses) prior to fine needle aspiration of the liver or placement of an oesophagostomy or gastrostomy tube.

Taurine

Taurine is a nutritionally essential amino acid in cats, as they are unable to synthesise it in sufficient amounts to meet their daily requirement. In cats, bile acids are exclusively conjugated with taurine. Intestinal bacteria can deconjugate bile acids, resulting in an increased loss of taurine in the faeces, thereby increasing requirements. In addition, food-induced bile salt excretion into the intestinal tract and interruption of the normal enterohepatic recirculation can result in significant loss of taurine. Consequently, cats with hepatic disease may be at risk of taurine deficiency. A deficiency in taurine has been associated with secondary accumulation of nonesterified fatty acids in the liver.[38] So, providing additional taurine via oral supplementation at 250–500 mg/day PO may help to reduce total liver lipid content, as well as help to prevent mobilisation of muscle protein to meet taurine requirements. Taurine supplementation is particularly important if home-prepared diets or human enteral foods are fed to cats.

Arginine

Arginine is an important substrate in the urea cycle. Deficiency of this amino acid has been associated with the development of hyperammonaemia and HE in cats with hepatic lipidosis. Adult cats fed diets devoid of arginine develop hyperammonaemia and HE;[39] thus, food for cats should contain adequate arginine levels. Home-prepared vegetable-based diets and human enteral foods may be devoid of sufficient arginine to meet daily requirements in cats and should be supplemented if used.

Thiamine

Cats with hepatic lipidosis may have many vitamin and mineral deficiencies due to anorexia, fat malabsorption, reduced GI function, and loss of hepatic reserves. Thiamine is a vital cofactor in enzymatic pathways carried out in hepatic cells, and its deficiency can cause neurological signs and may mimic signs of HE. Thiamine should be supplemented at 50–100 mg/day PO. Parenteral administration should be avoided due to possible adverse effects.

Additional water-soluble vitamins

Many cats with hepatic lipidosis likely have water-soluble vitamin deficiencies due to prolonged anorexia, impaired nutrient digestion and absorption, impaired hepatic metabolism and storage, and increased requirements. Hence, these can be supplemented by adding a complex of B vitamins to the intravenous fluid bag. The bag and line containing this vitamin complex should be protected from light.

Antioxidants

Vitamin E deficiency can result in a reduction of cellular defences against prooxidant damage. Antioxidants should be provided as vitamin E (D-α-tocopherol acetate at 10–15 IU/kg/day PO) and S-adenosylmethionine (SAMe, 20 mg/kg/day PO). SAMe is needed for the synthesis and reduction of glutathione, which is an important hepatic antioxidant.

Feeding strategy

Assisted enteral feeding should continue long-term until the cat resumes eating voluntarily. Initially, feedings should be provided in small amounts, at least in six to eight portions per day, or as a constant-rate infusion to improve digestibility, prevent release of free fatty acids from adipose tissue, and reduce the amount of ingesta entering the colon where bacterial fermentation occurs. All food should be administered lukewarm, and bolus feeding should be administered over 20–30 minutes while assessing for any signs of discomfort, retching, or vomiting. Food can be offered to determine if the cat will eat voluntarily, but if the cat shows any signs of nausea, food should be removed immediately and not persisted with.

Reassessment

Although the prognosis for hepatic lipidosis depends on the underlying cause, it is also dependent on the ability of the veterinary surgeon and owner to vigorously meet the cat's energy requirements via assisted enteral feeding. A decrease in serum beta-hydroxybutyrate during hospitalisation in cats with hepatic lipidosis was associated with higher survival rates,[40] which likely indicates an improvement in the catabolic state. Assessment of appetite, body weight, body condition, frequency and severity of any GI signs, and neurological function should be performed at least daily during hospitalisation. At home, an improvement in the cat's attitude, activity, and appetite and regular monitoring of body weight and body condition will help to determine response to dietary management. The assisted enteral feeding tube can be removed once the cat is eating 100% of its daily requirement consistently over at least 3–4 days. Once the assisted enteral feeding tube has been removed and any comorbidities have resolved, adult maintenance over-the-counter diets can be introduced. If nutritional support is rapidly and sufficiently provided and no serious underlying disease is present, cats with hepatic lipidosis have a reported recovery rate of 80%–85%.[26]

Hepatic encephalopathy

Pathophysiology

This syndrome is defined as "a brain dysfunction caused by liver insufficiency and/or portosystemic shunt; it manifests as a wide spectrum of neurological or psychiatric abnormalities ranging from subclinical alterations to coma".[41] In cats, it is most often associated with congenital or acquired portosystemic shunts and end-stage liver failure.

There are three main objectives of treatment in cats with HE:

- ensuring early recognition of encephalopathy and its predisposing factors, such as GI bleeding or hypokalaemia, to allow for correction;
- reducing the production and absorption of toxins within the GI tract, which includes reducing or modifying dietary protein, altering the intestinal microbiota, and decreasing intestinal transit time;
- providing optimal supportive care, which includes correcting any dehydration, hypovolaemia, or electrolytes and acid base abnormalities.

Nutrients of focus

Energy

Cats should be fed 1.0 × RER in hospital, unless they are growing animals (2–3 × RER). The use of illness factors can lead to overfeeding, which has been associated with hyperglycaemia and GI and hepatic dysfunction. Once discharged home, they can be fed 1.2 × RER or their historical daily caloric intake if this maintains their body weight at an ideal condition.

Protein

Cats with a portosystemic shunt and no evidence of HE should not have dietary protein restricted, and instead these cats should be fed as much protein as they will tolerate without becoming clinically encephalopathic. A failure to feed adequate amounts of protein can cause catabolism with a decrease in muscle mass, resulting in the release of ammonia and reducing the cat's ability to buffer through glutamine synthetase in skeletal muscle. Similarly, for those cats that have undergone surgical repair of the portosystemic shunt, slowly weaning onto a maintenance over-the-counter diet should be attempted over a 4- to 6-week period following surgery. If there is any evidence that the level of dietary protein in the maintenance diet is not tolerated, a moderately reduced protein diet, such as a commercial therapeutic hepatic diet, should be fed. It is important that dietary protein needs for growth are also met for kittens.

Consumption of a high-protein meat-based diet, GI bleeding, and azotaemia are the most common causes of HE in animals with end-stage liver disease or portosystemic shunt.[42] The source of dietary protein is important in the management of HE; for example, dogs with experimentally created portosystemic shunts had significantly prolonged survival and fewer signs of encephalopathy when fed a milk-based diet as opposed to a meat-based diet.[43] It is hypothesised that haem,

RNA, and other nitrogenous bases in the meat-based diet led to the exacerbation of HE and shortened survival times, whereas milk-based diets may be beneficial due to their lack of porphyrins, haem, and other nitrogenous bases as well as the elicitation of a short intestinal transit time and low colonic pH, which decrease nitrogen absorption. Although casein-based diets have been fed to cats with liver disease, they may be low in arginine, warranting supplementation of this essential amino acid if these diets are administered to cats. Dietary arginine deficiency in otherwise healthy cats can cause hyperammonaemia and encephalopathy signs within 30 minutes of consumption of a high-protein, arginine-deficient diet.[44] Care should also be taken to ensure that diets are adequately supplemented with taurine. Commercial therapeutic hepatic diets for cats meet these requirements and commonly contain animal- and vegetable-derived proteins, which are of high digestibility and biologic value.

Dietary formulas designed for parenteral or enteral use containing lower aromatic amino acids and higher branched-chain amino acids have been studied in various clinical trials in humans with HE. A recent review showed that branched-chain amino acids had a beneficial effect on signs of HE in humans but no effect on mortality. Unfortunately, supplementation of diets with branched-chain amino acids can be expensive and may decrease palatability.

Although commercial therapeutic renal diets are lower in protein, their protein source is mainly meat-based compared to hepatic diets, which are both animal and vegetable in origin. Therefore, commercial therapeutic renal diets may not be optimal for the management of HE in cats. Home-prepared diets formulated by a board-certified veterinary nutritionist with a combination of meat-based and vegetable protein sources can be used as effective alternatives to commercial therapeutic hepatic diets in cats.

Fat and carbohydrates

Cats with HE should receive adequate quantities of fat and carbohydrates to spare the use of protein as an energy source and decrease ammonia production.

Nonabsorbable disaccharides

Oral administration of lactulose is fundamental to the treatment of HE. Lactulose is a synthetic disaccharide that is hydrolysed by colonic bacteria to lactic acid and acetic acid. Lactulose has many roles in reducing the degree of HE. Firstly, it reduces the pH of the colon, which results in trapping of ammonium ions, thereby decreasing their absorption. Secondly, it inhibits ammonia generation by bacteria in the colon via a process known as catabolite repression. Thirdly, it decreases the intestinal transit time, as it is able to act as a cathartic. Lastly, it can suppress bacterial and intestinal ammonia generation by providing an alternative carbohydrate source. Although there is individual variation with regard to the dose needed, most cats can be managed with a dose of 0.25–0.5 mg/kg PO every 8–12 hours. The dose should be optimised to yield faeces that are soft-serve ice cream consistency.

Dietary fibre

Dietary fibre helps to reduce the production and availability of nitrogenous waste in the GI tract. Dietary fibre is also able to bind noxious bile acids and other toxins and alter the pH of the colon to help with ammonia trapping.

Zinc

Zinc has direct hepatoprotective effects via inhibition of lipid peroxidation and destabilisation of lysosomal membranes. Depletion of zinc has been suggested as a precipitant of HE in humans with liver failure. Commercial therapeutic hepatic diets are suitably supplemented with zinc.

Vitamin E

Vitamin E serves as a cellular membrane-bound antioxidant, which protects membrane-associated phospholipids from oxidative damage. Therefore, vitamin E is important for protection against oxidative damage in hepatocytes and is supplemented in commercial therapeutic hepatic diets.

Feeding strategy

Ensuring that owners feed several small meals throughout the day will help cats with HE, as this will likely help to reduce the total ammonia load associated with each meal.

Reassessment

Assessment of appetite, body weight, body condition, frequency and severity of any GI signs, and neurological function should be performed at least daily during hospitalisation. At home, an improvement in the cat's attitude, activity, and appetite and regular monitoring of body weight and body condition will help to determine response to dietary management. Assessment of serum albumin is recommended to ensure that protein and calorie requirements are being met. If there are any concerns with feeding a cat with HE, a board-certified veterinary nutritionist should be consulted. If the shunt has been successfully ligated, an over-the-counter maintenance diet can be slowly introduced to assess tolerance to the diet and protein content.

Cholangitis

Cholangitis is the most common feline inflammatory liver disease, with the two most common forms being neutrophilic and lymphocytic. Cats with cholangitis commonly have concurrent diseases, such as CE and pancreatitis. Therefore, dietary management of these cases should focus on the nutritional strategies for CE and pancreatitis, as discussed previously in this chapter. In addition, serum cobalamin concentrations should be assessed and supplemented if found to be low. Cats with cholangitis rarely need a commercial therapeutic hepatic diet, unless they are showing signs of HE, and so these diets should not be fed due to their lower protein content.

Bile duct obstruction

Cats presenting with bile duct obstruction are commonly candidates for corrective surgery. Assisted enteral feeding is usually used prior to and after surgery in these cases. Standard adult maintenance diets are usually indicated during the recovery process. However, in cats with concurrent CE, EPI, or pancreatitis, diets that meet the different nutritional strategies for each of these conditions should be fed. Cats with complete bile duct obstruction are at risk of vitamin K deficiency, and for this reason this should be supplemented subcutaneously, as described previously.

Take-home messages

Nutritional strategies in gastrointestinal disease

- Nutrition has many direct beneficial effects on the components and function of the gastrointestinal tract and is therefore important in the management of various feline gastrointestinal diseases.
- Nutritional management of acute gastroenteritis in cats includes consideration of the digestibility, fat, and fibre of the diet, as well as the use of probiotics.
- Commercial therapeutic hydrolysed diets, commercial therapeutic limited-ingredient novel protein diets, and complete and balanced limited-ingredient novel protein home-prepared diets can all be used for the diagnosis and management of food hypersensitivity in cats.
- Dietary management of food-responsive enteropathy in cats involves trial and error to determine the most effective nutritional strategy. Categories of diets commonly used include commercial therapeutic gastrointestinal diets, commercial therapeutic hydrolysed diets, commercial therapeutic limited-ingredient novel protein diets, and complete and balanced home-prepared diets. Different amounts of dietary fat and fibre within these categories of diets can be trialled to determine the most effective for individual cats.
- Dietary management forms an important component in the treatment of feline constipation, with recommendations varying depending on the level of colonic motility remaining. For those cats presenting with constipation that still have some level of colonic motility, insoluble or a mix of insoluble and soluble fibre may help. In cats presenting with obstipation, a highly digestible, low-residue diet with a high caloric density should be fed to markedly reduce faecal content.

Nutritional strategies in pancreatic disease

- Dietary therapy is an important adjunctive treatment for pancreatitis and exocrine pancreatic insufficiency.
- *Nil per os*, which was historically recommended for pancreatitis, should no longer be the case if the cat is not actively vomiting. If the cat is able to eat enough food to meet its daily energy requirements, voluntary enteral nutrition should be prioritised. For those cats that are unable to meet their daily energy requirements voluntarily, an assisted enteral feeding tube should be considered. Parenteral nutrition is recommended for those cats that are not consuming enough of their daily energy and nutrient requirements and placement of an enteral feeding tube is contraindicated.
- Nutrients of focus in cats with pancreatitis include water, energy, dietary fat, dietary protein, vitamin B_{12}, omega-3 polyunsaturated fatty acids, antioxidants, and probiotics.
- Although oral pancreatic enzyme supplementation is the foundation for the treatment of exocrine pancreatic insufficiency, enteral nutrition is also extremely important in the management.
- Nutrients of focus in cats with exocrine pancreatic insufficiency include energy, digestibility, dietary fat, dietary fibre, medium-chain triglycerides, cobalamin, folate, fat-soluble vitamins, and minerals.
- In cats with exocrine pancreatic insufficiency, highly digestible diets should be prioritised to help with nutrient digestion and absorption.
- It is very important to remember that cats with exocrine pancreatic insufficiency are likely to require more food than expected to ensure that they maintain an optimal body weight and condition.

Nutritional strategies in hepatobiliary disease

- Nutrition helps to provide a supportive role in the management of feline hepatic diseases, although it is the cornerstone of treatment for hepatic lipidosis and hepatic encephalopathy.
- The cornerstone of treatment of feline hepatic lipidosis is with early, long-term assisted enteral feeding with oesophagostomy or gastrostomy tubes, which has helped to increase the prognosis of this potentially life-threatening condition. If general anaesthesia cannot be safely performed for placement of an oesophagostomy or gastrostomy feeding tube, a nasoenteral feeding tube should instead be initially placed and a liquid diet administered until the cat is stable for placement of a more permanent enteral feeding tube.
- Nutrients of focus in feline hepatic lipidosis include energy, protein, potassium, L-carnitine, vitamin B_{12}, vitamin K, taurine, arginine, thiamine, additional water-soluble vitamins, and antioxidants.
- Cats with a portosystemic shunt and no evidence of hepatic encephalopathy should not have dietary protein restricted. Instead, these cats should be fed as much protein as they will tolerate without becoming clinically encephalopathic.
- Nutrients of focus in cats with portosystemic shunt—with or without hepatic encephalopathy—include energy, protein, carbohydrate, fat, nonabsorbable disaccharides, dietary fibre, zinc, and vitamin E.

REFERENCES

[1] Remillard RL et al. Intravenous glutamine or limited enteral feedings in piglets: amelioration of small intestinal disuse atrophy. *J Nutr* 128:2723S, 1998.

[2] Chan DL et al. Retrospective evaluation of partial parenteral nutrition in dogs and cats. *J Vet Intern Med* 16:440, 2002.

[3] Laflamme DP, Xu H, Long GM. Effect of diets differing in fat content on chronic diarrhea in cats. *J Vet Intern Med* 25:230, 2011.

[4] Dennis JS, Kruger JM, Mullaney TP. Lymphocytic/plasmacytic colitis in cats: 14 cases (1985–1990). *J Am Vet Med Assoc* 202:313, 1993.

[5] Bybee SN, Scorza AV, Lappin MR. Effect of the probiotic *Enterococcus faecium* SF68 on presence of diarrhea in cats and dogs housed in an animal shelter. *J Vet Intern Med* 25:856, 2011.

[6] Anvari S et al. IgE-mediated food allergy. *Clin Rev Allergy Immunol* 57:244, 2019.

[7] Jackson HA et al. Evaluation of the clinical and allergen specific serum immunoglobulin E responses to oral challenge with cornstarch, corn, soy and a soy hydrolysate diet in dogs with spontaneous food allergy. *Vet Dermatol* 14:181, 2003.

[8] Jergens AE. Feline idiopathic inflammatory bowel disease: what we know and what remains to be unraveled. *J Feline Med Surg* 14:445, 2012.

[9] Guilford WG et al. Food sensitivity in cats with chronic idiopathic gastrointestinal problems. *J Vet Intern Med* 15:7, 2001.

[10] Kathrani A et al. A descriptive pilot study of cytokine production following stimulation of ex-vivo whole blood with commercial therapeutic feline hydrolyzed diets in individual healthy immunotolerant cats. *BMC Vet Res* 13:297, 2017.

[11] Raditic DM, Remillard RL, Tater KC. ELISA testing for common food antigens in four dry dog foods used in dietary elimination trials. *J Anim Physiol Anim Nutr (Berl)* 95:90, 2011.

[12] Mandigers PJ et al. A randomized, open-label, positively-controlled field trial of a hydrolyzed protein diet in dogs with chronic small bowel enteropathy. *J Vet Intern Med* 24:1350, 2010.

[13] Toresson L et al. Oral cobalamin supplementation in cats with hypocobalaminaemia: a retrospective study. *J Feline Med Surg* 19:1302, 2017.

[14] Freiche V et al. Uncontrolled study assessing the impact of a psyllium-enriched extruded dry diet on faecal consistency in cats with constipation. *J Feline Med Surg* 13:903, 2011.

[15] Klaus JA, Rudloff E, Kirby R. Nasogastric tube feeding in cats with suspected acute pancreatitis: 55 cases (2001–2006). *J Vet Emerg Crit Care (San Antonio)* 19:337, 2009.

[16] Pyle SC, Marks SL, Kass PH. Evaluation of complications and prognostic factors associated with administration of total parenteral nutrition in cats: 75 cases (1994–2001). *J Am Vet Med Assoc* 225:242, 2004.

[17] Backus RC et al. Elevation of plasma cholecystokinin (CCK) immunoreactivity by fat, protein, and amino acids in the cat, a carnivore. *Regul Pept* 57:123, 1995.

[18] Sato T. Role of free radicals on canine bile-induced pancreatitis and effect of superoxide dismutase. [In Japanese]. *Nihon Geka Gakkai Zasshi* 96:388, 1995.

[19] Akol KG et al. Acute pancreatitis in cats with hepatic lipidosis. *J Vet Intern Med* 7:205, 1993.

[20] Suzuki A et al. Effect of bacterial or porcine lipase with low- or high-fat diets on nutrient absorption in pancreatic-insufficient dogs. *Gastroenterology* 116:431, 1999.

[21] Biourge VC, Fontaine J. Exocrine pancreatic insufficiency and adverse reaction to food in dogs: a positive response to a high-fat, soy isolate hydrolysate-based diet. *J Nutr* 134:2166S, 2004.

[22] Rutz GM et al. Effects of exchange of dietary medium chain triglycerides for long-chain triglycerides on serum biochemical variables and subjectively assessed well-being of dogs with exocrine pancreatic insufficiency. *Am J Vet Res* 65:1293, 2004.

[23] Xenoulis PG et al. Feline exocrine pancreatic insufficiency: a retrospective study of 150 cases. *J Vet Intern Med* 30:1790, 2016.

[24] Adamama-Moraitou K et al. Iron, zinc, and copper concentration in serum, various organs, and hair of dogs with experimentally induced exocrine pancreatic insufficiency. *Dig Dis Sci* 46:1444, 2001.

[25] Williams DA. Exocrine pancreatic insufficiency. In: Anderson NV, editor. *Veterinary Gastroenterology*, 2nd ed. Philadelphia, Lea & Febiger: 283, 1992.

[26] Valtolina C, Favier RP. Feline hepatic lipidosis. *Vet Clin North Am Small Anim Pract* 47:683, 2017.

[27] Center SA et al. Fulminant hepatic failure associated with oral administration of diazepam in 11 cats. *J Am Vet Med Assoc* 209:618, 1996.

[28] Brenner K, KuKanich KS, Smee NM. Refeeding syndrome in a cat with hepatic lipidosis. *J Feline Med Surg* 13:614, 2011.

[29] Center SA. Feline hepatic lipidosis. *Vet Clin North Am Small Anim Pract* 35:225, 2005.

[30] Biourge V et al. Nitrogen balance, plasma free amino acid concentrations and urinary orotic acid excretion during long-term fasting in cats. *J Nutr* 124:1094, 1994.

[31] Biourge VC et al. Effects of protein, lipid, or carbohydrate supplementation on hepatic lipid accumulation during rapid weight loss in obese cats. *Am J Vet Res* 55:1406, 1994.

[32] Center SA et al. A retrospective study of 77 cats with severe hepatic lipidosis: 1975–1990. *J Vet Intern Med* 7:349, 1993.

[33] Jacobs G et al. Comparison of plasma, liver, and skeletal muscle carnitine concentrations in cats with idiopathic hepatic lipidosis and in healthy cats. *Am J Vet Res* 51:1349, 1990.

[34] Blanchard G et al. Dietary L-carnitine supplementation in obese cats alters carnitine metabolism and decreases ketosis during fasting and induced hepatic lipidosis. *J Nutr* 132:204, 2002.

[35] Ibrahim WH et al. Effects of carnitine and taurine on fatty acid metabolism and lipid accumulation in the liver of cats during weight gain and weight loss. *Am J Vet Res* 64:1265, 2003.

[36] Center SA et al. The clinical and metabolic effects of rapid weight loss in obese pet cats and the influence of supplemental oral L-carnitine. *J Vet Intern Med* 14:598, 2000.

[37] Center SA et al. Proteins invoked by vitamin K absence and clotting times in clinically ill cats. *J Vet Intern Med* 14:292, 2000.

[38] Cantafora A et al. Dietary taurine content changes liver lipids in cats. *J Nutr* 121:1522, 1991.

[39] Morris JG, Rogers QR. Ammonia intoxication in the near-adult cat as a result of a dietary deficiency of arginine. *Science* 199:431, 1978.

[40] Kuzi S et al. Prognostic markers in feline hepatic lipidosis: a retrospective study of 71 cats. *Vet Rec* 181:512, 2017.

[41] Vilstrup H et al. Hepatic encephalopathy in chronic liver disease: 2014 Practice Guideline by the American Association for the Study of Liver Diseases and the European Association for the Study of the Liver. *Hepatology* 60:715, 2014.

[42] Center SA. Chronic hepatitis, cirrhosis, breed-specific hepatopathies, copper storage hepatopathy, suppurative hepatitis, granulomatous hepatitis and idiopathic hepatic fibrosis. In: Guilford WG et al., editors. *Strombeck's Small Animal Gastroenterology*, 3rd ed. Philadelphia, WB Saunders: 705, 1996.

[43] Condon RE. Effect of dietary protein on symptoms and survival in dogs with an Eck fistula. *Am J Surg* 121:107, 1971.

[44] Morris JG. Nutritional and metabolic responses to arginine deficiency in carnivores. *J Nutr* 115:524, 1985.

CHAPTER 40

Enteral nutritional support

Craig Breheny, Silke Salavati Schmitz

In recent years, the appreciation and understanding of the necessity of nutritional support in a patient's management continues to grow, and body condition score is considered "the fifth vital sign" in cats (see Chapter 38). Enteral nutrition is the process by which nutrition is supplied to the gastrointestinal (GI) tract. In the absence of enteral nutrition, there are several local and systemic consequences that are encountered as a result. A study in humans identified that the relative risk of dying is more than double for those eating less than 25% of their recommended calorie intake and increased to triple for those that were completely anorexic.[1] These patients have also been shown to have a reduced diversity of their intestinal microbiota, which improves upon renourishment.[2] As the microbiota have roles in metabolising nutrients and vitamins, outcompeting enteropathogens, bestowing immunomodulatory effects, and influencing intestinal permeability, any alterations in their composition, richness, or function can have far reaching consequences (see Chapter 16).

The enterocytes themselves are another key component of GI function. These highly metabolically active cells, supported by a large number of enzymes, are a key site of absorption of many essential biochemical components such as iron.[3] Together, with tight junctions and desmosomes, they are also a crucial component of GI integrity. Almost 70% of the nutrition required for enterocyte survival is obtained from the lumen, primarily as glutamine and ketone bodies. The remaining 30% is derived from the intestinal blood flow. With periods of hyporexia, these cells are then more reliant upon the mesenteric blood supply.[4,5] As many patients are presented with systemic disease, the combination of catecholamines and increased sympathetic tone results in vasoconstriction of the splanchnic circulation, further diminishing enterocyte nutrition. With the high metabolic activity of these cells, consequent inadequate ATP generation results in cellular death, manifesting as blunting and atrophy of the villi, with subsequent diminished function.[6]

In recent years, with the above consequences in mind, there has been a shift to instituting early enteral nutrition as soon as feasible and safe for the patient. This can be achieved by encouraging voluntary intake or, if this is not possible, by the use of feeding tubes. For cats, this is particularly important in the light of this species propensity to develop hepatic lipidosis (see Chapter 27). Due to the alterations of influx and efflux of fatty acids in response to insufficient dietary intake of energy, this can have consequences which are more severe than the originating cause of anorexia. However, considering the right amount and type of food while not being overzealous is equally crucial, as metabolic derangements known as refeeding syndrome can otherwise occur (see Chapter 29). Specific nutritional strategies for GI, pancreatic, and biliary conditions are covered in Chapter 39.

STIMULATION OF VOLUNTARY FOOD INTAKE

Anorexia as a clinical sign can often be relatively vague with a large number of potential differential diagnoses (see Chapter 1).

In the early stages of anorexia, up to 72 hours since last food intake, supportive care and medical therapy can be attempted. Beyond this, the risk of hepatic lipidosis increases and a more definitive approach to addressing the nutritional requirements should be pursued. In some patients, hepatic lipidosis may occur at an earlier point in time, or be of greater consequence, such as in those with preexisting liver disease, diabetes mellitus, hyperadrenocorticism, and obesity. In these patients, earlier more invasive interventions may be necessary (see Chapter 27). Figure 40.1 summarises some of the key questions in deciding whether to manage a patient medically or whether tube placement is necessary.

Symptomatic treatment of anorexia can consist of:

- anti-nausea/antiemetic and gastroprotective treatment (see Chapter 33)
- appetite stimulants (e.g. mirtazapine, cyproheptadine, capromorelin; see below)
- assisted nutrition (tube feeding).

In cases where anti-nausea medication (and treatment of the identified underlying cause) does not lead to a swift improvement, anorexia can be managed with appetite stimulants (Table 40.1). However, at this point, a renewed effort should be undertaken to identify an underlying cause if not already addressed simultaneously.

CONSIDERATIONS WHEN COMMENCING NUTRITIONAL SUPPORT

Patient factors

Although it is important that patients receive nutrition as early as possible to negate the consequences associated with malnutrition, it is also important that they can tolerate enteral nutrition. If patients are presenting in a critical condition with any degree of shock, compensated or otherwise, there is a concern that stimulation of the alimentary tract could have a negative impact.

As a compensatory mechanism to decreased tissue perfusion, there will be a release of catecholamines and stimulation of the sympathetic component of the autonomic nervous system. A consequence of this is shunting of blood from the GI tract via splanchnic vasoconstriction. If patients are fed during this state, there are two possible and equally deleterious consequences. One is that the hypoperfused GI tract will have decreased motility, with the potential secondary ileus which can lead to discomfort and poses a risk for regurgitation and subsequent aspiration. The other potential consequence is that the presence of food instilled within the stomach after feeding will elicit an increase in GI metabolism, motility, and blood flow, all of which would be diverted from the crucial organs in more critical need. Therefore, it is essential to evaluate the patient prior to each feed, and ideally measure blood pressure before administration.

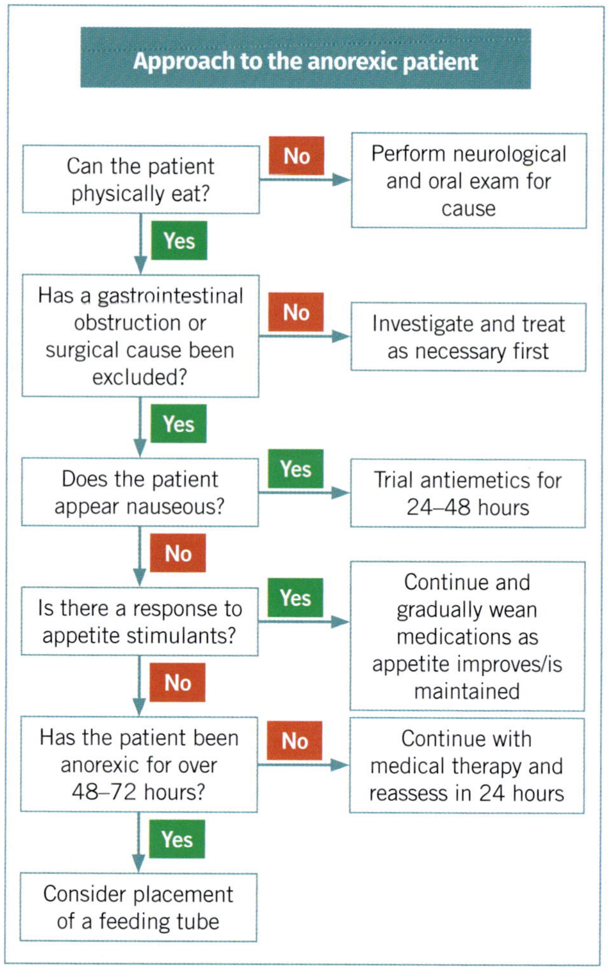

Figure 40.1. Flow chart demonstrating key questions and factors to be considered when deciding whether to manage an anorexic cat medically or with a feeding tube.

Delivery and type of tube feed

There are two main methods of delivery of enteral nutrition. This consists of either bolus feeding or constant infusions (trickle feeding). Bolus feeding consists of administering an equal portion of the daily nutritional volume over the course of the day, typically with feeds every 4–6 hours depending on the practicalities involved. This is often administered over a 15–30-minute time period, depending on how well the patient copes with the procedure.

Table 40.1. Relevant details of the medications most commonly used in anorexic patients.

	Mirtazapine	Cyproheptadine	Capromorelin
Mechanism of action	Presynaptic α_2-adrenergic receptors, 5-HT_3 antagonist and H_1 antagonist	H_1 and potentially serotonin antagonist	Ghrelin receptor agonist
Site of action	Centrally	Centrally	Centrally
Metabolism	Hepatic	Hepatic	Hepatic
Elimination	Hepatic and renal	Renal	Renal (37%) and faecal (63%)
Protein binding	Moderate to high	Unknown	Not highly protein bound
Contraindications	Consider dose reducing in patients with hepatic or renal disease	Pyloric outflow obstruction, bladder neck obstruction, cardiac failure, glaucoma	Hepatic or renal dysfunction (consider liver and kidney function)
Side effects	Potential for serotonin syndrome (hypersalivation, tachycardia, hypotension, behavioural changes)	Dry mucous membranes (xerostomia), sedation, or paradoxical agitation	Increased salivation can be seen following dosing Diarrhoea, vomiting, and polydipsia have also been reported
Dosage	3–4 mg/cat PO every 72 h	2–4 mg/cat PO every 12–24 h	3 mg/kg PO every 24 h
Comments	May have some antiemetic properties		Wide safety margin and has been dosed at 17.5 times the therapeutic dose for 1 year without clinical consequence*

*Zollers B et al. Evaluation of the safety in dogs of long-term, daily oral administration of capromorelin, a novel drug for stimulation of appetite. *J Vet Pharmacol Ther* 40:248, 2017.[16]

Continuous feeding is usually only possible with commercial liquid diets, and most often utilised with nasogastric and oesophageal feeding tubes. Syringe drivers can be used, setting them at a constant rate avoiding the delivery of larger volumes of food, with a resultant decrease in stomach distension. This approach has the benefit that it is less personnel intense, but also means that the patient may not be as intensively monitored whilst the food is delivered.

While several studies, in both the veterinary and human fields, have investigated which of the above approaches is most effective and efficient, to date there has been no consensus, and therefore either is appropriate to use depending on the patient and their associated circumstances.[7,8]

The volume delivered will depend on the caloric requirement as well as the capacity of the stomach to receive this. Stomach volume, in that which has not received consistent meals, is often quoted as 5–10 ml/kg. Assessing the gastric residual volume can be extremely useful in deciding upon the best approach for an individual cat, as well as having diagnostic and patient welfare implications. The gastric residual volume is the amount of fluid obtained prior to the next feed being delivered. A noninvasive method of evaluating the residual volume of material within the stomach is via the use of abdominal ultrasound. With the cranial abdomen scanned with a standard abdominal probe, the degree of stomach distension can be evaluated. This is however subjective, with no standard formulas or measurements to correlate this to specific volumes. Despite this, ultrasound can be a useful tool for making clinical decisions such as whether to feed at that point in time or not. It can also aid in the decision of which type of tube should be placed, with a nasogastric tube (NG tube) having the benefit of allowing suction of stomach contents.

A more invasive approach is the utilisation of a feeding tube to remove any residual volume within the stomach immediately prior to the next meal. This could be achieved with an NG tube placed solely for this purpose, or other techniques such as using a gastrostomy tube that is already in situ or placing an NG tube through an oesophageal feeding tube into the stomach. This allows a more objective measurement of whether the residual volume is static or progressing. It can also deliver diagnostic information, such as if there is evidence of gastric bleeding. An additional benefit is simultaneous decompression of the stomach, minimising the risk of regurgitation and assisting with any discomfort associated with the ileus that is often present in critical patients.

Feeding volumes for tube feeding

In order to ensure that an adequate amount of calories is administered, the resting energy requirement (RER) should be calculated as follows:

$$\text{RER} = 70 \times (\text{body weight [kg]})^{0.75}$$

Previously described illness factors, which the RER was multiplied by, are no longer used. Instead the focus is to meet the RER initially. However, RER is increased in kittens due to higher energy requirements to support basal metabolic processes and the additional energy required for appropriate growth. The kitten factor is often (but anecdotally) quoted as 2–3 times the RER, although the origin of these factors is unclear.

Refeeding syndrome is a concern in feline patients with prolonged anorexia when nutritional delivery is reestablished. This arises as a result of severe electrolyte imbalances and fluctuations, particularly decreases in phosphate, magnesium, and potassium (see Chapter 29). Measures which can be taken to minimise the risk of refeeding syndrome include feeding an aliquot of the calculated RER initially and increasing this incrementally over several days. It is also recommended to check electrolytes (including phosphate and magnesium) and basic blood work daily whilst nutrition is increased.

TYPES OF FEEDING TUBES

There are several options for tube placement, each with their own advantages, limitations, and complications. The different tubes and their relative merits are summarised in Table 40.2, and the appropriate decision-making for the type of feeding tube used is illustrated in Figure 40.2.

Nasooesophageal and nasogastric feeding tubes

Nasooesophageal tubes (NO tubes) and NG tubes are some of the most commonly employed feeding tubes. These tubes are placed into the nares and terminate either in the last third of the oesophagus or in the stomach.[9] The main use of NO/NG tubes is to facilitate feeding of liquid diets for short periods of time. NG tubes can have the additional advantage of being used to retrieve the contents of the stomach, particularly effective with a wider gauged tube (see comments above). NG tubes can be used to empty the stomach as completely as possible in a conscious patient, for example prior to anaesthesia being induced when the risk of regurgitation and aspiration is deemed high (e.g. in cases with proximal GI obstruction).

As mentioned above, gastric residual volume can act as a surrogate marker for stomach motility and guide further feeding as well as fluid planning. Gastric residual volume is usually evaluated at 4–8 hourly intervals.

Table 40.2. Key features of commonly placed tubes used to provide enteral nutrition.

	Nasooesophageal/ nasogastric tube	Oesophagostomy tube	Percutaneous endoscopic gastrostomy (PEG) tube	Jejunostomy tube
Cost	Inexpensive	Moderately expensive	Expensive	Expensive
Ease of placement	Easy	Relatively easy	More difficult	Difficult
Need for general anaesthesia	No	Yes	Yes	Yes
Length of time in place	Short-term	Short- to mid-term	Long-term	Mid-term
Contraindications	Nasal disease Facial trauma/fractures Coagulopathy Raised intracranial pressure Fractious patients	Skin infection of surgical site Coagulopathy Oesophageal disease Neck pain/trauma	Primary gastric ulceration Intractable vomiting Splenomegaly Coagulopathy Exogenous steroids (consideration rather than contraindication)	Primary intestinal disease such as ulceration Coagulopathy
Complications	Rhinitis/epistaxis Tube obstruction Perforation of oesophagus or stomach (rare) Tube dislodgement	Stoma site infection/abscess Haemorrhage Tube dislodgement Oesophageal trauma Nervous structure damage	Dehiscence and septic peritonitis Organ perforation Stoma site infection Haemorrhage Patient dislodgement	Dehiscence and septic peritonitis Stoma site infection Haemorrhage Patient dislodgement

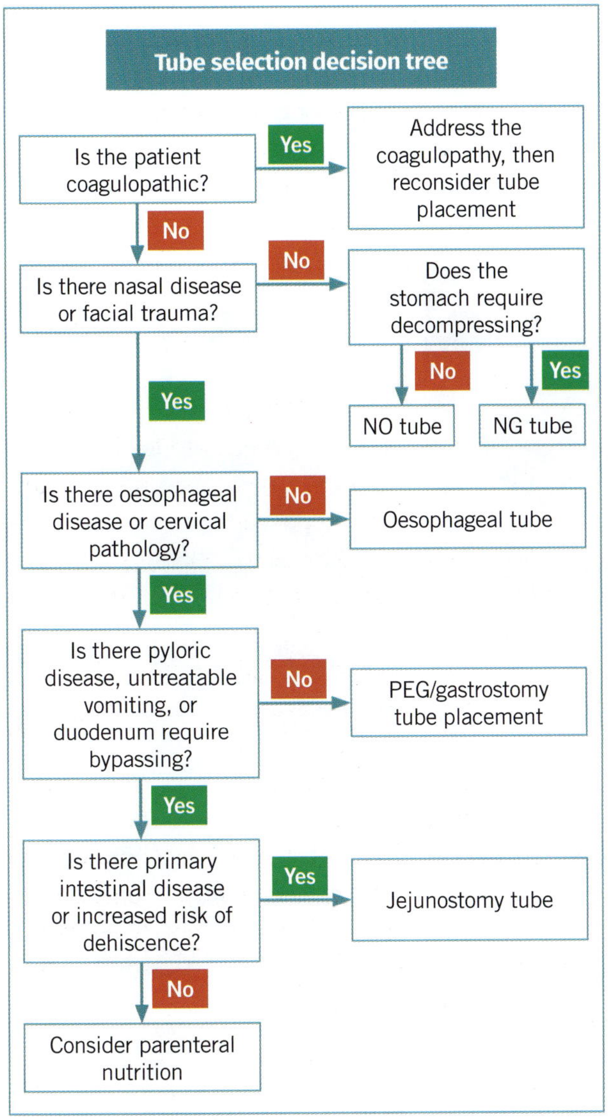

Figure 40.2. Flow chart depicting the key decisions when selecting the most appropriate feeding tube for a patient. NG, nasogastric; NO, nasooesophageal; PEG, percutaneous endoscopic gastrostomy.

NG or NO tubes can also be used for administering medications that cats may not take voluntarily, whilst avoiding the need for general anaesthesia. This is of particular use for administering laxatives like polyethylene glycol either to prepare feline patients for endoscopic procedures or to treat cats with constipation or obstipation (see Chapter 23). Lactulose may be best avoided, as given the smaller gauge, the risk of it obstructing the tube is higher.

Benefits, disadvantages, contraindications, and complications of NO and NG tubes are listed in Table 40.2, but briefly, these tubes can be placed in conscious animals, augmented with topical anaesthesia, which is often beneficial when general anaesthesia can have a negative impact, such as in those patients that are cardiovascularly unstable or unable to tolerate the potentially resultant hypotension.

They are relatively well tolerated by most patients but can result in some irritation during and the initial period after placement. A buster collar is an essential whilst these tubes are in place to avoid accidental removal, and they can be left in place for several days provided the patient remains comfortable. On the other hand, they can be removed immediately with ease and no requirement for sedation or anaesthesia when no longer required.

One of the major limitations of NO and NG tubes is their small gauge. This means that these tubes can be exclusively used for liquid diets or water-like medications. As such, grinding tablets or opening capsules and administering through the tubes should be avoided, as they can readily obstruct the tube, necessitating its removal. For the same reason, the infusion of liquid food should be constant, or the tube flushed adequately with water afterwards to prevent concretion of the food material within the tube.

Contraindications to NO or NG tube placement include primary nasal disease, where the placement of the tube could be hindered by the nasal disease, or in which the placement can cause further trauma and discomfort. There is also the possibility that the cribriform plate could be fragile or eroded. Additional contraindications include facial trauma or facial fractures, coagulopathic patients, patients with raised intracranial pressure (restraint necessary or sneezing can exacerbate this), and fractious or aggressive patients in which utilising the tube could be met with difficulty.

The procedure is not always pleasant, and anxious patients may require sedation. It should be borne in mind that if a patient has required sedatives to facilitate placement, their normal swallow and gag reflexes may be diminished and placement of the tube into the trachea or airways is a possibility and should be evaluated for.

Main complications of NO or NG tube placement include epistaxis (often self-limiting), development of rhinitis, and tube displacement (regurgitation or vomiting can cause the tube to project into the mouth, which can then become damaged if bitten). If the tube is dislodged into the airways, the main concern is aspiration pneumonia or worse when feeding. For this reason, these tubes are typically only used in hospitalised patients as a temporary solution to address the nutritional need. Each tube feeding should be slow and the patient monitored carefully whilst administering the food. Rare complications include oesophageal or gastric perforation, possibly due to preexisting defects or disease, but this is based on speculation rather than strong evidence.

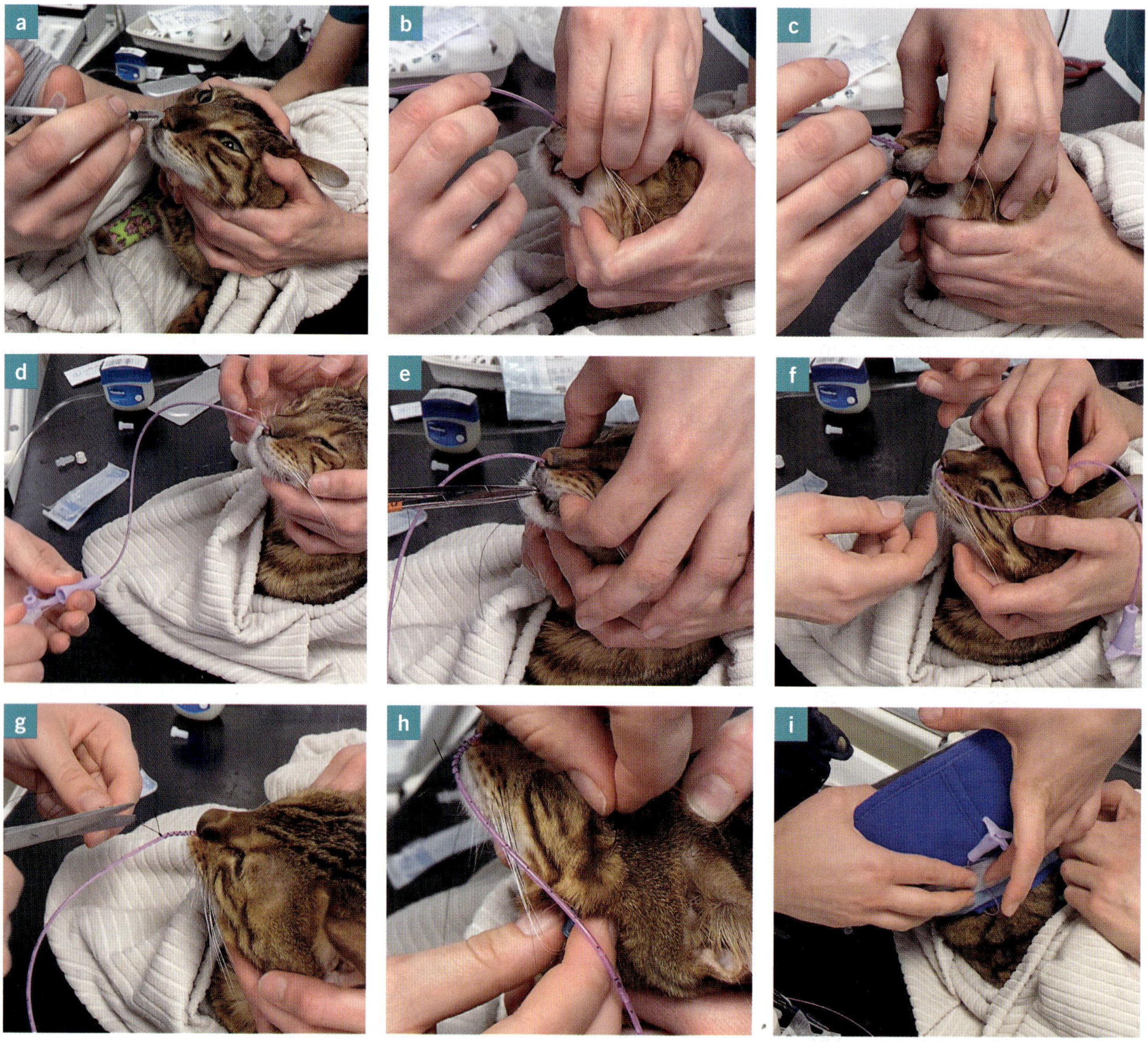

Figure 40.3. Placement of a nasooesophageal or nasogastric tube (NO/NG tube) in a cat. Instill a local anaesthetic (e.g. proxymetacaine or lidocaine, approx. 0.5 ml) into the nares and *planum nasale* (a). A drop can also be placed into each lower conjunctiva to assist anaesthesia of the caudal nasopharynx. Allow 15–20 minutes to take effect. Fill and lubricate the tube. Lubricate the stylet if present. Premeasure the tube (NO tube: 7th–8th intercostal space; NG tube: 13th rib), extend the cat's neck, and insert the tip of the tube, aiming ventromedially (b). To help direct the tube, deviate the *planum nasale* and lips dorsally to form a "pig snout" (c). After advancing the tube in short gentle bursts, release it (d). If resistance is met, gently retract and readvance the tube or twist along long axis. Stimulate the patient to swallow once the tube reaches the pharynx. To confirm the tube is in the correct position, attach an empty syringe (remove stylet if present) and apply negative pressure in pulses. An NO tube should maintain the negative pressure, while with an NG tube gastric content can be aspirated. Secure the tube by a single suture at the ventrolateral corner of the nares, either with a swaged needle/needle holder (e) or by using a 23-gauge injection needle to guide the suture (f). Secure the tube with a Roman sandal suture (g). The knots should be tight enough to allow grip, but not causing narrowing of the tube. Secure the tube at a further point on the patient—typically centre of head or lateral aspect of face, but avoid whiskers or vision (h). Place buster collar and tape the tube to it (i). Confirm position of the tube (e.g. radiographs).

Figure 40.3 and Box 40.1 give some practical guidance for placing an NO or NG tube in a cat. Video 40.1 also demonstrates this.

Video 40.1. Nasogastric feeding tube placement in a cat. Video courtesy of Dr Efa Llewellyn.

Box 40.1. Equipment needed for nasooesophageal or nasogastric tube (NO/NG tube) placement in cats.

- 3-0 nonabsorbable suture material (e.g. nylon)
- 5 ml and 10 ml syringes
- 23-gauge needle
- 100 ml 0.9% saline
- Appropriate type of tube for NO/NG placement
- Local anaesthetic (lidocaine or proxymetacaine)
- Needle holders, if preferred over hand ties
- Permanent marker pen
- Water-soluble medical lubricant

Oesophagostomy feeding tube

One of the major benefits of an oesophagostomy tube (O-tube) in comparison to NO or NG tubes is that a wider gauge can be used, as the nasal passages are bypassed. This is particularly useful when a specific diet is desired that does not come in a liquid form (e.g. hydrolysed or low-fat food). The wider tube can accommodate blended food, provided enough water is added and the food is suitably liquidised. Equally, ground or powdered medications can be mixed with food or water and administered with a lower risk of tube obstruction.

As the tubes does not interfere with the cat's face and whiskers, it is usually very well tolerated. With a relatively light dressing or a Kitty Kollar, cats can carry on with normal functions without impedance. With anorexia often being one of the clinical signs of illness in cats that is slower to abate, the use of these tubes can decrease hospitalisation time, as owners can be instructed how to use and care for these tubes. In patients that require medication for a longer period but are difficult for owners to tablet, they could have placement of this feeding tube considered solely for this purpose.

An additional benefit is that O-tubes can be in place for a longer time than NO/NG tubes. A median time of 11 days was reported in a recent survey, but long-term use (>90 days) has also been described.[10] Premature dislodgement or removal of O-tubes by the patient, whilst frustrating, is unlikely to carry any negative complications, especially in comparison with early removal of percutaneous endoscopic gastrostomy (PEG) tubes, which can have catastrophic consequences. Equally, O-tubes are very easy to remove conscious when no longer required, by removing the suture and pulling the tube. The O-tube stoma site will heal by secondary intention, usually within 24–48 hours.

As mentioned above, O-tubes can also be utilised as a guide to place a smaller tube to access the stomach and allow decompression, either for therapeutic or diagnostic sampling. This, however, only works if the distal end has been cut, as most tubes are not manufactured open-ended but rather have several side openings (Fig. 40.4a). Along these lines, O-tubes can be altered with additional side holes, creating fenestrations that allow suctioning of oesophageal material (Figs. 40.4b and 40.4c). This has been reported in the context of O-tubes being used in animals with megaoesophagus.[11] These case studies suggest that intermittent suction can reduce the occurrence of regurgitation and episodes of aspiration pneumonia. However, this use has been reported in a relatively small patient number, all of which were dogs.

In that context it should also be noted that in O-tubes with premanufactured side openings, care should be taken to place the tube in a way that the first opening does not end up being located too high up in the cervical part of the oesophagus. This can easily happen particularly in cats due to their small size. To prevent this, the authors often cut off the lower part of the O-tube before placement (Fig. 40.4a), as this will simultaneously allow creation of a large-bore open end of the tube.

Another potential use of these tubes would be to provide an inexpensive alternative to maintain a functional oesophagus akin to an oesophageal stent in patients with risk of recurrence of oesophageal strictures. The placement of O-tubes with integrated balloon dilators has been described in a small case series of nine dogs and three cats, where overall tube management was reported to be well tolerated and effective in maintaining dilation of benign oesophageal strictures while reducing anaesthetic time and cost.[12]

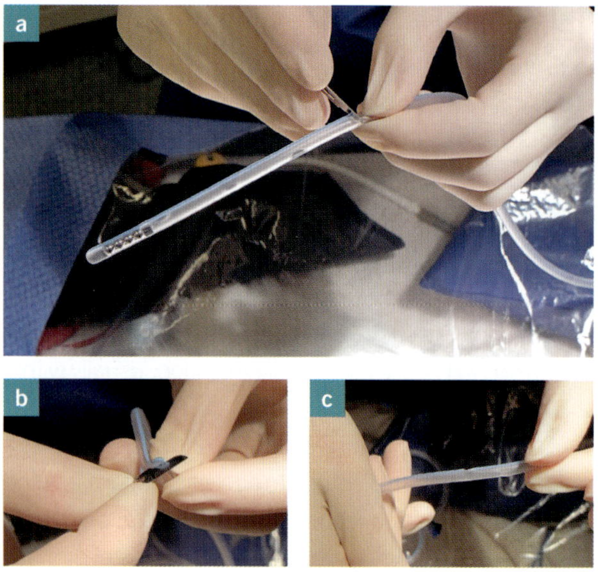

Figure 40.4. Suggested manipulations of commercial oesophagostomy tubes when placed in cats. To create an open-ended oesophagostomy tube as well as to avoid having the most oral side opening too close to the larynx, the tip has to often be cut off (a). If additional suctioning of the oesophagus via the tube is required, additional openings can be cut before placement (maximum 40% of the circumference to avoid tearing) (b,c).

One of the major drawbacks to the use of O-tubes is the necessity for general anaesthesia for placement. There are also a number of potential contraindications, most of which are related to any underlying conditions. Patients with superficial skin disease within the surgical field, such as atopic skin disease or pyoderma, will be at a higher risk of secondary infection of the stoma site. Given the risk of abscessation, an alternative tube or approach should be considered. Patients with coagulopathies are another relative contraindication. Whilst the incision into the skin and oesophagus is relatively small with minimal trauma, this could still lead to substantial bleeding if the patient is unable to coagulate effectively. There is also the potential for trauma from the other actions necessary for placement, such as the right-angled forceps insertion. In those with oesophageal disease (possibly with the exception of megaoesophagus as mentioned above), the use of O-tubes should also be avoided. In oesophagitis or oesophageal ulceration, there is the risk of oesophageal tear or rupture. There are reports of oesophageal rupture or leakage following placement. Patients with neck pain or trauma are also not ideal candidates for O-tube placement. To facilitate placement, the neck is heavily manipulated including flexion and extension as the tube is placed. If there are unstable vertebral fractures or intervertebral disc disease, the necessary manipulations could risk worsening these comorbidities.

There are two recent studies evaluating the complications associated with oesophageal feeding tubes. Complications are reported to occur in 35%–44% of cases.[10,13] Complications at the time of placement are relatively rare and can include haemorrhage (often minor, but the jugular vein should be carefully identified before making the initial incision) or damage to the sympathetic trunk (during placement or associated with local inflammation). If this happens, Horner's syndrome can develop. However, this is unlikely to be clinically relevant and will likely resolve with time.

The most common complication is tube dislodgement (14.5%), either by the patient or otherwise. For this reason, the patient's demeanour and their environment, such as other cats or dogs in the household that may be inquisitive and could assist with removal, should be taken into account before placing. Owners should be informed of how to manage the stoma site following premature removal and how to remove the tube, if necessary, in an emergency. If the patient were to vomit, this can force the tube out of the oesophagus and into the mouth or potentially into the pharynx. In patients with intractable vomiting, an alternative option should be considered.

Tube stoma site infection is also common (12.1%), which is not entirely surprising, as the tube acts as a foreign body and micromovements can cause ongoing irritation. Bacteria isolated from infected stoma sites are mostly oral or skin commensals. Many patients with O-tubes will also receive systemic antibiotics to manage or treat their underlying conditions, which can promote the development of multidrug-resistant infections. The use of chemotherapy or immunosuppressive dosages of steroids is associated with a greater odds ratio of infection occurring.[10,13] The duration of tube being in place was, however, not associated with infection rate. Topical therapy is often enough to help resolve the infection, but removing the tube may be necessary to facilitate management.

Obstruction of an O-tube is mostly associated with incomplete flushing at the end of usage. This can be worsened if the cats are grooming excessively, as the hair can accumulate in the distal portion of the oesophagus, obstructing the tube openings and causing a blockage. Changing to a smaller gauge NG tube down the O-tube can be attempted to dislodge a small plug, or alternatively synthetic pancreatic enzyme can be placed into the tube to digest the materials.

Box 40.2 lists equipment needed for placing an O-tube in a cat, while Figures 40.5 and 40.6 give some practical guidance for placing and securing the tube. The whole process can be watched in Video 40.2.

Box 40.2. Equipment needed for oesophagostomy tube placement in cats.

- Clippers
- Dressing materials
- Oesophageal feeding tube (12- or 14-gauge in cats)
- Permanent marker pen
- Radiography facilities
- Right-angled forceps
- Scalpel blade
- Surgical drape
- Surgical gloves
- Surgical preparation solutions/swabs

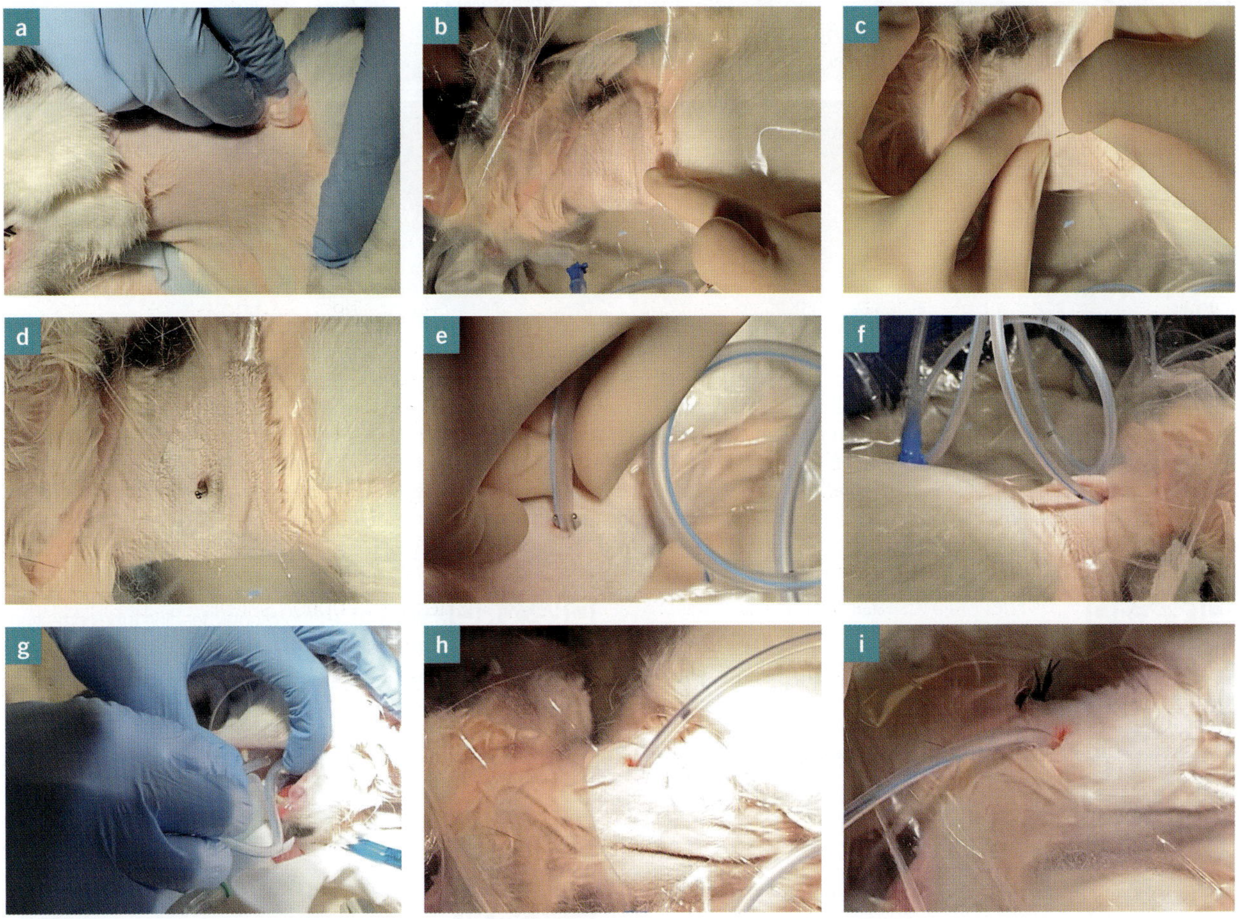

Figure 40.5. Placement of an oesophagostomy tube in a cat. With the patient in right lateral recumbency, the area from the caudal mandible to the thoracic inlet is clipped and aseptically prepared (a). While the neck is maximally extended, the right-angled forceps is inserted into the cat's mouth, aiming for the two o'clock position to enter the oesophagus, advanced, and then pushed upwards to tent the tissues from underneath, so that it can be palpated easily through the skin (b). The jugular vein should be raised to ensure the proposed incision site is at a suitable distance. A short (≈1 cm) incision is made through the skin until the forceps is reached (c). The forceps is then advanced through the incision and opened to the size of the tube diameter (d). The tube is placed in the centre between the jaws of the forceps (on occasion, the edges need to be trimmed slightly to allow smooth movement), clamped tightly, and pulled gently out through the mouth, while being pushed from the skin side (e). A loop is formed and the tube advanced back into the mouth and oesophagus (f,g); the loop should be long enough to avoid kinking, but tangling should be avoided. Once the loop is no longer palpable from the mouth, the tube has to be slowly pulled from the incision site. There is often a characteristic "flip" in the tube direction from pointing cranial (h) to caudal (i), confirming it is now facing in the correct direction (towards the stomach). This can be confirmed by gently moving the tube, which should move aborally without resistance. In addition, no part of the tube should be visible or palpable from the oral cavity (use laryngoscope if necessary). Once comfortable that the tube is facing the correct direction, it should be retracted until the marker previously determined is visible at the level of the skin incision. Correct position of the tube tip should be confirmed via radiograph or fluoroscopy (tip in last third of oesophagus) before suturing.

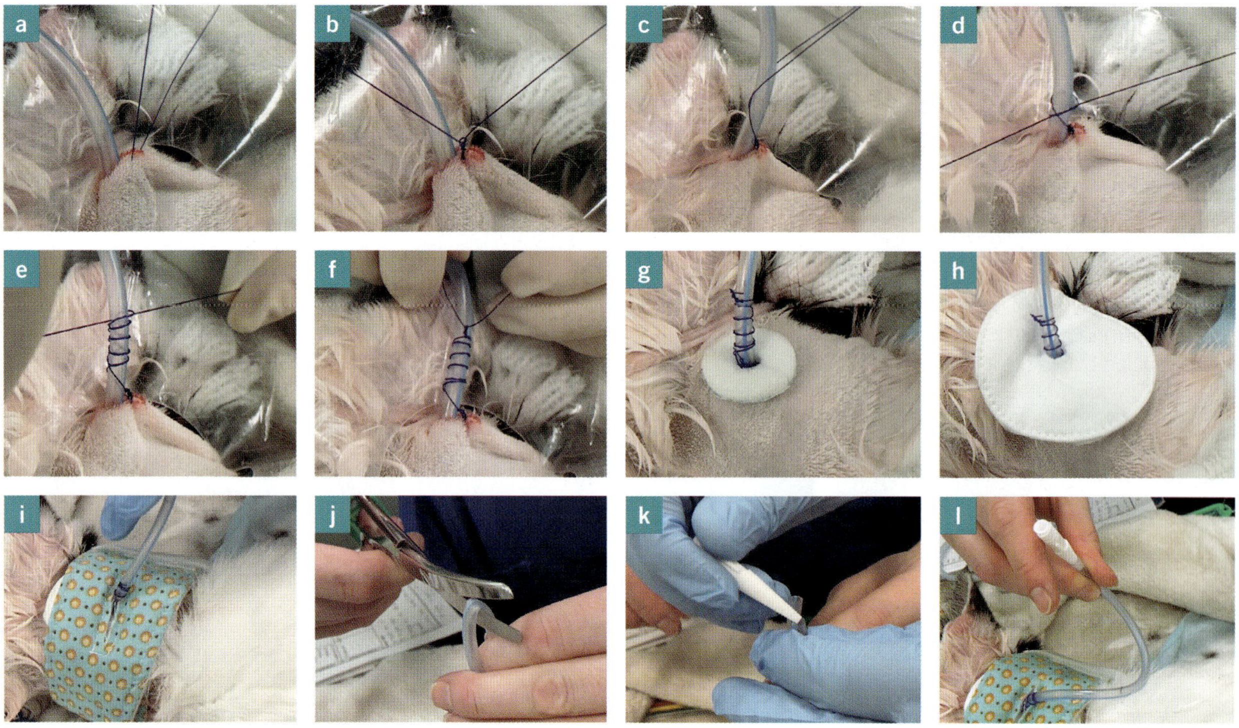

Figure 40.6. Securing and dressing of an oesophagostomy tube in a cat. A purse-string suture is placed around the tube insertion point (a). The two ends of the suture should be pulled until equal in length. A knot is tied, bearing in mind some level of post-placement swelling. A Roman sandal suture is used to prevent the tube from slipping (b–f): the suture ends are passed behind the tube and crossed over before pulling them back (c). A surgeon's knot is tied tight enough to grip the tube without causing the lumen to narrow (d). A total of at least six of these manoeuvres including knots should be tied (e) and finished with six throws (f). The tube can then be covered (g–i), for example, with biopatches, which are circular pieces of material impregnated with chlorhexidine, followed by a loose-fitting bandage or Kitty Kollar (i). The tube might require shortening to reduce the dead space volume (j). Depending on the type of tube used, a Christmas tree connector (k,l) can be placed to allow fitting of a bung as well as the attaching of syringes.

Video 40.2. Oesophageal feeding tube placement in a cat. Video courtesy of Dr Petra Cerna.

Video 40.3. Fluoroscopic feeding tube correction. Videos 40.3–40.5 demonstrate oesophageal feeding tubes having kinks corrected under fluoroscopic guidance by applying gentle traction to the tube until it is corrected.

One of the most commonly encountered difficulties in placing O-tubes is that a kink develops in the tube whilst being placed. This often occurs close to the incision site within the oesophagus. If manual manipulation as described above is unsuccessful in rectifying this, additional imaging procedures like endoscopic assessment of the tube (Fig. 40.7) or—depending on availability—fluoroscopy can be used (Videos 40.3–40.5).

If an animal is discharged with an O-tube in place, care should be taken to give correct instructions for aftercare to the owner. For an example of this, see Online Supplement 40.1.

Video 40.4. Fluoroscopic feeding tube correction.

Video 40.5. Fluoroscopic feeding tube correction.

Online Supplement 40.1. Instructions for oesophageal feeding tube use and care in cats.

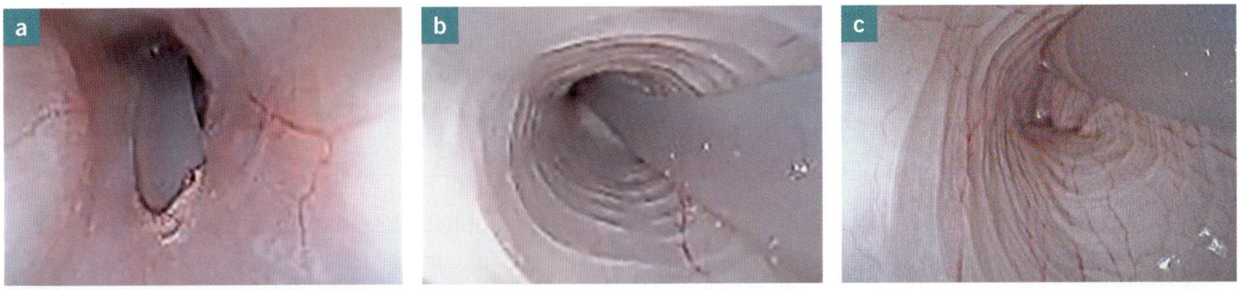

Figure 40.7. Assessment of correct oesophagostomy tube positioning via videoendoscopy. Assessment of the tube insertion site; the tube has no kinks and is fully pointing aborally (a). The tip of the tube is seen to cross the lower oesophageal sphincter, hence the tube needs to be retracted before suturing (b). The tip of the tube from image b is now in the correct position (c): lower third of the oesophagus, not traversing the lower oesophageal sphincter.

Percutaneous endoscopic gastrostomy tube

In some patients, it might be desirable to bypass the upper GI tract (e.g. severe oesophageal disease), or a more permanent enteral feeding solution is required. Gastrostomy tubes can either be placed surgically or endoscopically, with the latter being preferred due to reduced invasiveness (no need for larger incisions) and a reduced amount of time required in experienced hands. However, surgical placement should be considered as part of another necessary procedure (diagnostic or therapeutic laparotomy) in the rare situation that an O-tube is considered inappropriate. In this chapter, PEG tubes will be discussed; however, the use, care, removal, and complications of surgically placed gastrostomy tubes are similar.

Compared to O-tubes, PEG tubes often are of even wider gauge (possibly less relevant in cats compared to dogs), which facilitates feeding, and obstruction (from food or medication) is less likely to occur. In patients in which potentially long-term or lifelong assisted feeding is anticipated, standard paediatric PEG tubes can—once a stoma has formed—be replaced with low-profile gastrostomy tubes, which facilitate daily use, have cosmetic benefits (hardly visible under long fur, do not require a bandage), and can easily be replaced if necessary.

Contraindications to PEG tube placement are gastric diseases (gastritis, ulceration, neoplasia). Conditions giving rise to splenomegaly should be considered relative contraindications. If the spleen is greater in size, the risk of it becoming punctured or lacerated during the placement procedure is potentially higher. Ultrasound guidance can help identify a safe passage for the needle during placement if still considered necessary. In addition, gastrostomy tubes should be avoided in patients treated with immunosuppressive dosages of steroids, as this was found to increase complication rates to 43%, compared to 18% in the control group, in one study.[14]

As with O-tubes, general anaesthesia is required for placement of a PEG tube. Contrary to the other tubes described above, gastrostomy tubes have to be in place for a minimum of 12–14 days to allow formation of a secure stoma. If removed prematurely, either by the patient or iatrogenic, there is the risk of detachment of the gastric wall from the abdominal wall, resulting in leakage of gastric content into the abdominal cavity and septic peritonitis. For the same reason, feeding cannot be started for 24–48 hours following placement, which is the main downside in comparison to NO, NG, or O-tubes.

Haemorrhage from either the stomach or the spleen can occur during or soon after placement (splenic puncture during the initial stages of the procedure), with the potential that an occult haemoabdomen could occur. As stated above, ultrasound can provide some guidance if the position of the spleen is unclear during the procedure.

Long-term usage of a PEG tube requires the owner's acceptance of the tube and accompanied lifestyle changes. For some, this is not feasible, which is why it is important that this is discussed at the outset to ensure informed consent. A limiting factor rather than a true disadvantage of PEG tubes is the specialised equipment and skills needed for placement. Whilst theoretically easy to place, practice and proficiency as well as availability of endoscopic equipment is essential (see Box 40.3, Video 40.6, and Online Supplement 40.2).

Box 40.3. Equipment needed for percutaneous endoscopic gastrostomy tube placement in cats.

- 3-0 and 2-0 nonabsorbable suture material
- Biopsy/rat tooth forceps compatible with the endoscope used
- Commercial percutaneous endoscopic gastrostomy tube kit (often paediatric)
- Gastrointestinal-compatible flexible (video)endoscope of appropriate length
- Scalpel blade
- Surgical preparation equipment
- Ultrasonography availability is also useful

Video 40.6. Endoscopic component of percutaneous endoscopic gastrostomy tube placement.

Online Supplement 40.2. Step-by-step instructions for percutaneous endoscopic gastrostomy tube placement.

After placement, owners must be warned of the severity of the consequences of dislodgement or premature removal. Even longer-term, damage or loss of parts of the PEG tube can be an issue. If the tube is partially chewed, components can serve as an obstructive foreign body. PEG tubes can be dislodged or displaced if not properly used. If the tube is not clamped securely or were to migrate, there is the risk that the side holes within the tube move out the stomach and into the abdominal cavity. If the patient were to be fed whilst the tube is in an incorrect position, the food would be instilled into the abdominal cavity, giving rise to a septic peritonitis. To prevent this, the number on the tube at the position it inserts at the skin should be recorded both in clinical records and the patient's hospitalisation sheet. Prior to any food being administered, the tube measurements should be checked to ensure that they corroborate with the clinical record and therefore the risk of tube migration is less likely.

Stoma site infection can also be seen, as both skin and GI commensals can take advantage of the continually open stoma, while the tube acts as a foreign body and can contribute to biofilm formation. If the infection is severe, local extension can risk septic peritonitis or may necessitate removal of the tube to allow healing while minimising the risk of abscess formation.

Removal of PEG tubes, provided they were in place for a minimum of 12–14 days, can be achieved without the need for general anaesthesia (sedation only, or even awake depending on the cat's temperament). The tube needs to be straightened (depending on the model used) and should be pulled with consistent traction (sometimes needed to be "aided" with a sharp tuck), which will pull the button portion through the stoma. This might not be possible if a PEG tube with a large button on the gastric side is used. In these cases, removal under general anaesthesia with endoscopic guidance to grasp the intragastric part once cut off from the outside is advised. If a patient removes a PEG tube once a stoma site has formed, but it is still required, a new tube can often be replaced (using the same procedure as for initial placement) into the previous stoma site. However, this should be done ideally on the same day, as the longer the interval

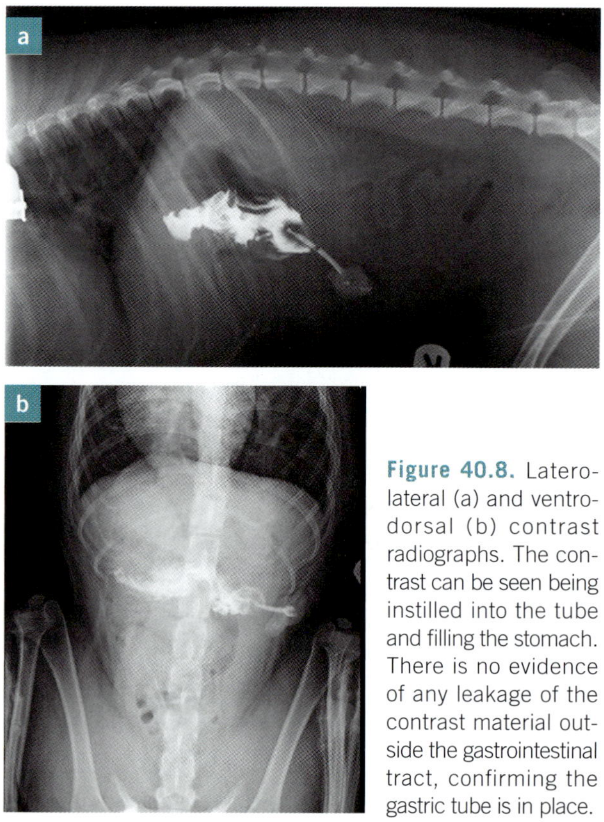

Figure 40.8. Latero-lateral (a) and ventrodorsal (b) contrast radiographs. The contrast can be seen being instilled into the tube and filling the stomach. There is no evidence of any leakage of the contrast material outside the gastrointestinal tract, confirming the gastric tube is in place.

between removal and replacement, the more difficult it will be, as the stoma site often narrows relatively quickly. Low-profile PEG tubes can also be used long-term once a stoma has formed, as they are easier to maintain by owners (often considered more aesthetic) and easier to change if needed.

The paramount concern following placement of gastrostomy tubes is the premature removal or leakage around the tube. If leakage is suspected, contrast radiography can be employed (Fig. 40.8). Abdominal ultrasound can also be useful in identifying free abdominal fluid, which should then be sampled.

Jejunostomy tubes

Jejunostomy tubes (J-tubes) are the least commonly used in veterinary medicine, and indications are narrow and relatively rare, particularly in the cat. They could be useful in cases with functional gastric obstructions, compromised gastric outflow anatomy, or patients not tolerating gastric nutrition for another reason. There is no indication that in small animals—contrary to humans—bypassing the duodenum and hence the pancreatic outflow (e.g. in severe pancreatitis) is beneficial. Hence, even though jejunal feeding is likely to decrease pancreatic stimulation and secretion, pancreatitis is not a primary indication for J-tube placement.

J-tubes can be placed surgically or through existing tubes, for example as nasojejunal tubes needing endoscopy-assisted placement, or through gastrostomy tubes to allow slightly larger tubes to be used. Interventional radiography might be needed to place these tubes with a noninvasive procedure.[15] As with gastrostomy tubes, the main risk with J-tubes is their premature removal or leakage resulting in septic peritonitis. Additional complications include haemorrhage, tube occlusion, and intestinal obstruction.

WHEN TO REMOVE THE TUBES

In some circumstances, the decision on when to remove a feeding tube is clear-cut, such as when the patient can prehend food normally following a facial fracture. Other times it is more challenging, such as medical patients where nausea has been the main driver.

Once the patient has received and tolerated their full RER for 3–4 days in a row, the authors will often reduce the frequency of the meals to evaluate whether this can help stimulate appetite. Even if this does not immediately stimulate appetite, the animal will also have had time to adjust to being tube-fed and should tolerate larger gastric volumes. This is of particular relevance when considering discharging the patient back into the care of the owner, when the number of feeds should be reduced to the minimum necessary to assist with compliance and preventing home care becoming onerous for the owner.

With the patient at home, the authors would suggest that if the patient has eaten voluntarily for 3 days consistently, then O-tubes can be removed. However, the ease of medicating the patient and owner compliance with tube care should also be a factor in making this decision.

Take-home messages

- Providing adequate nutrition to critical patients is crucial in terms of patient welfare, owner interpretation of quality of life, and prognosis.
- Whilst there is a slight learning curve associated with feeding tube placement, this is relatively shallow with nasogastric and oesophageal feeding tubes, both of which are suitable for the majority of patients in need of nutrition.
- Each tube has its own relative merits and issues, which can be considered to pick the best option. This chapter helps with this decision-making.

REFERENCES

[1] Hiesmayr M et al. Decreased food intake is a risk factor for mortality in hospitalised patients: the NutritionDay survey 2006. *Clin Nutr* 28:484, 2009.

[2] Kleiman SC et al. The intestinal microbiota in acute anorexia nervosa and during renourishment: relationship to depression, anxiety, and eating disorder psychopathology. *Psychosom Med* 77:969, 2015.

[3] Barton JC, Acton RT. Hepcidin, iron, and bacterial infection. *Vitam Horm* 110:223, 2019.

[4] Chen S et al. Glutamine supplementation improves intestinal cell proliferation and stem cell differentiation in weanling mice. *Food Nutr Res* 62, 2018.

[5] Kim MH, Kim H. The roles of glutamine in the intestine and its implication in intestinal diseases. *Int J Mol Sci* 18:1051, 2017.

[6] Wang ZE et al. Effects of glutamine on intestinal mucus barrier after burn injury. *Am J Transl Res* 10:3833, 2018.

[7] Holahan M et al. Intermittent and continuous enteral nutrition in critically ill dogs: a prospective randomized trial. *J Vet Intern Med* 24:520, 2010.

[8] Nasiri M et al. Comparison of intermittent and bolus enteral feeding methods on enteral feeding intolerance of patients with sepsis: a triple-blind controlled trial in intensive care units. *Middle East J Dig Dis* 9:218, 2017.

[9] Yu MK et al. Comparison of complication rates in dogs with nasoesophageal versus nasogastric feeding tubes. *J Vet Emerg Crit Care (San Antonio)* 23:300, 2013.

[10] Breheny CR et al. Esophageal feeding tube placement and the associated complications in 248 cats. *J Vet Intern Med* 33:1306, 2019.

[11] Manning K et al. Intermittent at-home suctioning of esophageal content for prevention of recurrent aspiration pneumonia in 4 dogs with megaesophagus. *J Vet Intern Med* 30:1715, 2016.

[12] Tan DK et al. Prospective evaluation of an indwelling esophageal balloon dilation feeding tube for treatment of benign esophageal strictures in dogs and cats. *J Vet Intern Med* 32:693, 2018.

[13] Nathanson O et al. Esophagostomy tube complications in dogs and cats: retrospective review of 225 cases. *J Vet Intern Med* 33:2014, 2019.

[14] Aguiar J, Chang YM, Garden OA. Complications of percutaneous endoscopic gastrostomy in dogs and cats receiving corticosteroid treatment. *J Vet Intern Med* 30:1008, 2016.

[15] Beal MW, Brown AJ. Clinical experience utilizing a novel fluoroscopic technique for wire-guided nasojejunal tube placement in the dog: 26 cases (2006–2010). *J Vet Emerg Crit Care (San Antonio)* 21:151, 2011.

CHAPTER 41

Parenteral nutritional support

Daniel L. Chan

In most cases, the preferred route of providing nutrition to hospitalised patients is enterally, and feeding tubes have become the modality of choice in critically ill cats. However, an often overlooked therapeutic modality for hospitalised animals that cannot tolerate enteral nutrition is to feed parenterally. Feeding animals with parenteral nutrition (PN) allows effective provision of calories, protein, and other nutrients. However, as with all interventions, there are a number of possible complications that can be seen with its use. For this reason, careful patient selection, appropriate formulation, and safe and effective administration practices are critical if one chooses to administer PN to patients. Therefore, whilst enteral nutrition should continue to be the mainstay of nutritional support in most cases, clinicians need to be aware of cases that can benefit from PN and how to implement it safely and effectively.[1–4]

Part of the reason that PN is often overlooked as a treatment modality relates to the perception that this technique is fraught with complications, too difficult to implement, and that clinicians often feel inadequately trained in this technique. However, with greater understanding of how this technique can be managed in practice, it could give clinicians another important option for critically ill patients, particularly those with significant gastrointestinal dysfunction. In this chapter, the following will be discussed: proper identification of patients most likely to benefit from this treatment modality, the considerations for formulation of PN, how it can be implemented, and how these patients should be monitored.

DEFINITIONS

In discussing PN, it is worth noting that the terms used in veterinary medicine have changed to better reflect the different modes of PN. The previously commonly used term of "total parenteral nutrition" was coined with the assumption that it could meet "all" of the patient's protein, calorie, and micronutrient requirements intravenously, whereas "partial parenteral nutrition" was thought to meet a proportion of this requirement (typically 40%–70% of the energy requirement).[5] As the true full energy and nutrient requirements of critically ill animals remain largely unknown, recent recommendations emphasise describing PN by the mode of delivery such that PN administered via a central vein is termed "central parenteral nutrition" and when administered via a peripheral vein is called "peripheral parenteral nutrition".[6,7]

INDICATIONS

Much of the reason that PN has gained a notorious reputation as a technique that should be avoided stems from studies in people that indicated that some populations treated with PN had higher complications and worse outcome compared with populations treated with enteral nutrition.[1,3,4] Even the timing of initiating PN has been associated with greater complications in people when PN was initiated within the first 48 hours of intensive care unit (ICU) admission compared with delayed initiation of PN until after a week in the ICU.[8] On closer analysis, the increase in the complication rate may have been more related to selecting inappropriate patients (e.g. those that were too well-nourished ICU patients who would have done better on enteral nutrition rather than PN).[9] However, the use of PN in critically ill patients is not without controversy. One large prospective controlled study demonstrated that the implementation of early PN in critically ill patients was not associated with higher mortality, and in fact these patients had lower morbidity.[10] A more recent study compared the timing of initiating enteral nutrition or PN within 36 hours of ICU admission and also found fewer complications when using PN.[11] When considering these findings, patient selection appears to be an important first step, and therefore a nutritional assessment should be carried out (Table 41.1). What nutritional assessment allows is a stepwise process that will help to select which patients need more urgent feeding as well as the most appropriate route of feeding. The primary indication for considering PN is when animals cannot voluntarily or safely consume (i.e. animals unable to protect their airways) sufficient food to meet their needs. Persistent anorexia itself is not a sufficient justification to initiate PN out of convenience, and this would constitute inappropriate patient selection and use of PN. The use of PN could be justified in patients that have contraindications for placement of feeding tubes (e.g. coagulopathic, unstable patients for general anaesthesia).

ROUTES OF ADMINISTRATION

One of the important complications that can occur with PN is the development of thrombophlebitis. The factors that impact the incidence of this complication include the catheter placement technique and the pH and osmolarity of the solution used. A study evaluating the peripheral use of PN in paediatric human patients found greater incidence of phlebitis when PN solutions had an osmolarity greater than 1000 mOsm/l.[12] However, a study evaluating PN (osmolarity 1350 mOsm/l) use in dogs did not find high rates of phlebitis occurrence.[13] Most of the dogs (two-thirds) received a high-osmolarity solution peripherally, and thrombophlebitis was only found in one dog.[13] Some published protocols state that PN solutions should have osmolarities below 950 mOsm/l to be safely administered peripherally. To lower the osmolarity of these solution below 1000 mOsm/l, one would need to dilute the solutions or decrease the amino acids and dextrose content, which would also decrease the caloric density of the solutions. If adjusted as such, the PN would only meet a proportion of the calculated resting energy requirement (RER), and therefore, ideally, it should be used short-term.

In order to reduce the risk of septic complications, the administration of PN requires a newly placed catheter using strict aseptic technique. Such a catheter should be used solely for PN administration. Catheters made of silicone or polyurethane are recommended, as they further reduce the risk of phlebitis. In cats, multilumen jugular catheters are often recommended for PN administration.

Table 41.1. Identification of patients in need of nutritional support via nutritional assessment. A patient with two or more high-risk factors present should receive nutritional support as soon as they are stabilised. Patients with fewer than two high risk factors should be closely monitored and reassessed every few days.

Parameter		Low risk	Moderate risk	High risk
Food intake <80% RER	<3 days	✓		
	3–5 days		✓	
	>3 days			✓
Presence of weight loss			✓	
Severe vomiting/diarrhoea				✓
Body condition score <4/9				✓
Muscle mass score <2				✓
Hypoalbuminaemia			✓	
Expected course of illness	<3 days	✓		
	2–3 days		✓	
	>3 days			✓

RER, resting energy requirement.

COMPONENTS OF PARENTERAL NUTRITION

Amino acids

In cats, perhaps the most important nutrient requirement is protein, and in parenteral solutions this will be met by amino acid solutions. The most commonly used amino acid solution concentration in veterinary patients is 8.5%, and this solution has an energy density of 0.34 kcal/ml. In most cases, it is easier to use amino acid solutions with added electrolytes, but in cats with very abnormal serum electrolyte concentrations it may be preferable to use amino acids without electrolytes and address these imbalances with fluid therapy. As these formulations are designed to meet essential amino acid requirements for people, they are not considered complete for cats. However, these solutions can be used for short-term support, as they are unlikely to result in clinically relevant deficiencies.

As the protein requirement for critically ill cats has not been established, a common recommendation for protein is to provide 6–8 g/100 kcal for cats.[5,14,15] This is higher than maintenance requirements, and the presumed increase in requirements in ill animals relate to factors such as increased protein losses and altered metabolic and inflammatory pathways.[16,17]

It is worth noting that the goal of nutritional support is to provide sufficient amino acids to minimise lean muscle catabolism. During health, animals deprived of food can alter their metabolism to conserve lean body mass and rely on stored fat for energy (simple starvation). However, critically ill cats tend to have accelerated muscle breakdown (stressed starvation) to generate amino acids used for other metabolic pathways such as gluconeogenesis and the generation of acute phase proteins.[17,18] However, there are cats with protein intolerance (e.g. hepatic encephalopathy, severe kidney failure) that should be fed reduced levels of protein (i.e. 3 g protein/100 kcal).

Carbohydrates

Cats do not have a carbohydrate requirement; however, dextrose solutions, ranging from 5% to 50%, provide a readily available source of calories (a 5% solution provides 0.17 kcal/ml; a 50% solution provides 1.7 kcal/ml). Given the high osmolarity of 50% dextrose solutions (>2500 mOsm/l), they are only suitable for central PN. When formulating PN solutions, the different components (e.g. amino acids, dextrose, and lipids) will make up different proportions of the total calories provided. Therefore, the carbohydrate component will depend somewhat on the patient's individual circumstances, and it typically translates to 50% of the nonprotein calories. The overall ratio of calories provided by lipids and carbohydrates are adjusted as required by the patient's needs. One general parameter is to limit dextrose infusion to no more than 4 mg/kg/minute; otherwise, persistent hyperglycaemia can be seen with infusions exceeding that limit.[19] When considering managing diabetic patients on PN, a greater proportion of calories should be provided from lipids and amino acids rather than glucose. Insulin therapy may also be necessary to manage hyperglycaemia.

Lipids

The lipid portion of PN provides a source of essential fatty acids and energy. Most PN solutions employ a 20% solution of lipid emulsion, providing 2 kcal/ml. Lipid emulsions used for PN are primarily composed of omega-6 fatty acids. Although omega-6 fatty acids can reportedly have deleterious effects on the inflammatory response, this fact has not translated into major changes of the way that PN is formulated. In some in vivo studies, an exaggerated inflammatory response has been noted following long-chain triglyceride infusion (mostly omega-6 derived) in people.[20] Other concerns relate to the effects of omega-6 fatty acid on host immune function, oxidative stress, and haemodynamics. Other known complications include an increased risk for hyperlipidaemia and lipid embolisation.[21–22] To address these issues, alternative lipid emulsions containing omega-3 fatty acids, omega-9 fatty acids, medium-chain triglycerides, or structured lipids have been developed but are not widely available at this time.[23,24] When using the typical omega-6-based lipid emulsion, the author usually limits the dosage in cats to 2 g/kg/day (30%–40% of total calories provided) to decrease risk of development of lipaemia. Cats with preexisting lipaemia may also require lower rates of lipid infusion. It is possible to formulate PN without lipids, but this approach is uncommon.

Electrolytes and trace minerals

Given that critically ill patients often have electrolyte imbalances, it is often necessary to adjust the electrolyte composition of PN. Most formulations of PN contain 20–30 mmol/l (20–30 mEq/l) of potassium, as is common in maintenance fluid solutions. For management of hypokalaemic patients, potassium chloride or potassium phosphate can be used. If patients require additional phosphorus (e.g. severe hypophosphataemia), phosphate can be provided as a separate infusion. As a general approach, it is easier to adjust electrolytes separately from PN solutions, which allows greater flexibility and avoids frequent reformulation.

Trace minerals are not necessary in most veterinary patients requiring PN, as the majority of cases only receive short-term PN (<7 days). However, patients that require prolonged PN support (>10 days) or are severely malnourished could benefit from the addition of zinc, copper, manganese, and chromium, although there are no studies confirming the importance of these trace minerals in veterinary patients.

Vitamins

As critically ill patients deemed in need for nutritional support may already be malnourished, supplementation with B vitamins may be of benefit. It is important to note that some B vitamins (e.g. riboflavin) are light sensitive, and as such it may be best to add B vitamins to the PN solution immediately before administration. The dosage regimen for B vitamins in PN (per 1000 kcal of PN solution) is 0.29 mg thiamine, 0.63 mg riboflavin, 3.3 mg niacin, 2.9 mg pantothenic acid, 0.29 mg pyridoxine, and 6 μg cyanocobalamin.[7]

FORMULATION OF PARENTERAL NUTRITION SOLUTIONS

The most practical way to provide PN is to use admixtures of amino acids, dextrose, and lipids in a single bag. A stepwise method of calculating the PN formulation can be found in Box 41.1. The calculation of the animal's caloric requirements is the first step. Most hospitalised animals should have their RER calculated. Illness energy factors are no longer recommended, as they lead to overfeeding and its associated complications. Given that compounding of PN solutions requires very specialised equipment, it is more practical for veterinary practices to obtain PN solutions from human hospitals using the formulations outlined below.

ALTERNATIVES TO COMPOUNDING PARENTERAL NUTRITION ADMIXTURES

As an alternative to compounding PN solutions, there are a number of combination products commercially available that could be used in practice. A very convenient product is a multichambered sealed bag that keeps the components separate until the seals are broken by squeezing the bag. (Fig. 41.1). The advantage of these ready-to-use products is that they are widely available, and veterinary practices can avoid having to compound solutions themselves. The major disadvantage of these ready-to-use products is that their composition cannot be adjusted to suit the needs of the patient (e.g. reducing the lipid content for patients with lipaemia, reducing the amino acid content for encephalopathic patients).

Box 41.1. Worksheet for calculating parenteral nutrition for cats using commonly available components.

1) Resting energy requirement (RER)

70 × (current body weight in kilograms)$^{0.75}$ = kcal/day

Or for animals 3–25 kg, can also use:

[30 × (current body weight in kilograms)] + 70 = kcal/day

RER = _____kcal/day

This caloric target can be adjusted down (e.g. 70% RER) if necessary

2) Protein requirement

Recommended values (use the most appropriate in the formula):

- Standard: 6 g/100 kcal
- Decreased requirement (hepatic/renal failure): 4–5 g/100 kcal
- Increased requirement (protein-losing conditions): 6–8 g/100 kcal

$\frac{\text{RER}}{100}$ × _____g/100 kcal = _____g protein required/day

3) Volumes of nutrient solutions required each day

a) 8.5% amino acid solution = 0.085 g protein/ml

$\frac{\text{\_\_\_\_\_ g protein required/day}}{0.085 \text{ g/ml}}$ = _____ml of amino acids/day

b) Nonprotein calories: the calories supplied by protein (4 kcal/g) are subtracted from the RER to get total nonprotein calories needed

_____g protein required/day × 4 kcal/g = _____kcal provided by protein

RER – kcal provided by protein = _____nonprotein kcal needed/day

c) Nonprotein calories are usually provided as a 50:50 mixture of lipid and dextrose. However, if the patient has a preexisting condition (e.g. diabetes, hypertriglyceridaemia), this ratio may need to be adjusted

20% lipid solution = 2 kcal/ml

To supply 50% of nonprotein kcal:

$\frac{\text{\_\_\_\_\_ lipid kcal required}}{2 \text{ kcal/ml}}$ = _____ml of lipid

50% dextrose solution = 1.7 kcal/ml

To supply 50% of nonprotein kcal:

$\frac{\text{\_\_\_\_\_ dextrose kcal required}}{1.7 \text{ kcal/ml}}$ = _____ml dextrose

4) Total daily requirements

_____ml 8.5% amino acid solution

_____ml 20% lipid solution

_____ml 50% dextrose solution

_____ml total volume of parenteral nutrition solution

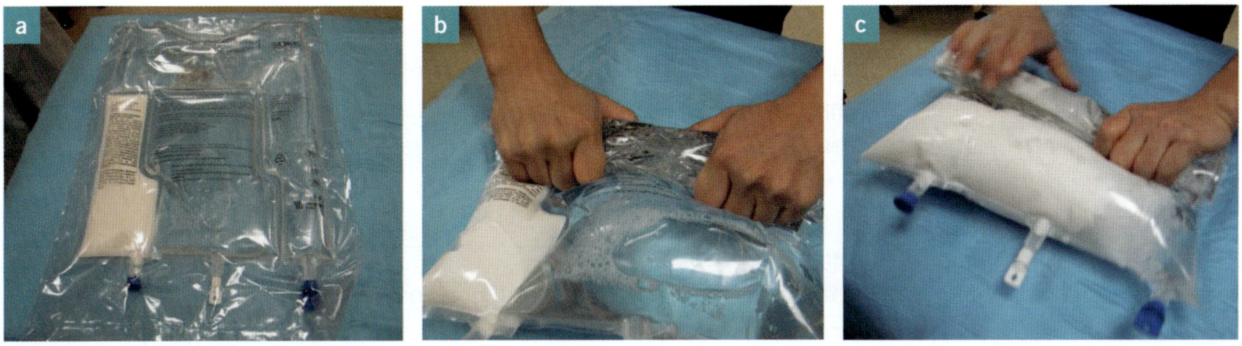

Figure 41.1. Commercially available three-in-one parenteral nutrition products are available, which allow fixed-formulation admixtures to be used in veterinary practices unable to compound parenteral nutrition. Components (dextrose, amino acids, lipids) are held in separate compartments until the solution is prepared for administration (a). For mixing the various components, the bag is rolled from the top and the pressure opens the internal seals, first between the dextrose and amino acids (b) and then of the lipid compartment (c). After all the internal seals are opened, the bag is gently inverted to ensure complete mixing. The bag is then ready for set up and administration.

ADMINISTRATION OF PARENTERAL NUTRITION

As with enteral nutrition, PN administration should be introduced gradually over 48–72 hours. Most animals can be administered 50% of total target energy provision on the first day, and this can increase to 100% of total energy target on the second day. Animals that are debilitated or anorexic for long periods may require slower introduction (e.g. 33% on the first day, 66% on the second day, and 100% on the third day). It is important to adjust the animal's other intravenous fluids when initiating PN support to avoid fluid volume overload.

Once PN is connected to a patient, the infusion lines should not be disconnected until the infusion is complete (i.e. it should remain a closed system). The PN solution must be connected to a catheter that is used solely for PN administration. Infusions should be administered through a 1.2 µm in-line filter.

MONITORING

Since critically ill patients are at risk of various complications, close monitoring is required during PN administration. Catheters must be checked daily for signs of phlebitis or cellulitis. In addition to vital signs, general attitude, body weight, body temperature, packed cell volume, and concentrations of total plasma protein (also checking the serum for presence of gross lipaemia or haemolysis), blood glucose, and electrolytes should be assessed at least daily. Should a patient develop a metabolic complication, discontinuation of PN is not usually required but reformulation may be warranted (e.g. a reduction of dextrose content for patients that develop hyperglycaemia). The overall nutritional plan should be reevaluated on a regular basis so that adjustments can be made based on the response to treatment.

COMPLICATIONS

Metabolic complications

There are three main metabolic complications associated with PN: hyperglycaemia, lipaemia, and electrolyte imbalances.[6,25,26] Although common, the development of hyperglycaemia following PN administration may not necessarily negatively impact outcome; however, it may still be prudent to avoid this complication. Using energy targets that only meet the RER may reduce the frequency and severity of hyperglycaemia. Hyperlipidaemia is also commonly reported in cats receiving PN and can be managed by using more conservative energy targets and a lower proportion of lipids.[25,27–29]

Electrolyte imbalances can develop following institution of PN or may worsen in animals with preexisting abnormalities. Hyponatraemia, hypokalaemia, hypocalcaemia, hypophosphataemia, and hypochloraemia have been reported but not associated with worse survival.[6,25,27–29]

Septic complications

Septic complications are uncommon in animals receiving PN. In all reports to date, fewer than 7% of all animals described had septic complications noted.[6,13,25–29] Catheter-related infection is the most commonly reported complication, and most patients were simply dealt with by removal of the intravenous catheter. The overall low rates of septic complications may be the result of strict adherence to aseptic techniques during catheter placement and handling of PN bags and infusing sets.

TRANSITION TO ENTERAL FEEDING

Given the benefits of enteral feeding, animals receiving PN should be transitioned to enteral feeding as soon as possible. In the absence of clear contraindications, animals receiving PN should be offered food enterally. The use of antiemetic and prokinetic therapies may improve tolerance to enteral feeding.

SUMMARY

Despite the various considerations required to safely administer PN, this form of nutritional support remains an important technique in patients unable to tolerate enteral feeding. Proper patient selection (i.e. those most likely to benefit from PN) along with proper formulation are critical for successful management of these cases. Despite some challenges associated with the use of PN in animals, it can be successfully adopted in many practice settings.

Take-home messages

- Parenteral nutrition is the mode of choice for nutritional support in patients intolerant of enteral nutrition.
- Before initiation of parenteral nutrition support, it is important to carry out a full nutritional assessment so that complicating factors can be identified and appropriate plans can be made.
- Potential complications associated with parenteral nutrition include hyperglycaemia, lipaemia, and electrolyte imbalances.
- Transitioning to enteral nutrition should occur as soon as it is feasible.

REFERENCES

[1] Braunschweig CL et al. Enteral compared with parenteral nutrition: a meta-analysis. *Am J Clin Nutr* 74:534, 2001.

[2] Biffl WL, Moore EE, Haenel JB. Nutrition support of the trauma patient. *Nutrition* 18:960, 2002.

[3] Gramlich L et al. Does enteral nutrition compared to parenteral nutrition result in better outcomes in critically ill adult patients? A systematic review of the literature. *Nutrition* 20:843, 2004.

[4] Simpson F, Doig GS. Parenteral vs. enteral nutrition in the critically ill patient: a meta-analysis of trials using the intention to treat principle. *Intensive Care Med* 31:12, 2005.

[5] Chan DL, Freeman LM. Parenteral nutrition. In: DiBartola SP, editor. *Fluid, Electrolyte, and Acid-Base Disorders in Small Animal Practice*, 4th ed. St Louis, Saunders Elsevier: 605, 2012.

[6] Queau Y et al. Factors associated with adverse outcomes during parenteral nutrition administration in dogs and cats. *J Vet Intern Med* 25:446, 2011.

[7] Perea SC. Parenteral nutrition. In: Fascetti AJ, Delaney SJ, editors. *Applied Veterinary Clinical Nutrition*, 1st ed. St Louis, Saunders Elsevier: 353, 2002.

[8] Casaer MP et al. Early versus late parenteral nutrition in critically ill adults. *N Engl J Med* 365:506, 2011.

[9] Lee H et al. Relationship of delayed parenteral nutrition protocol with the clinical outcomes in a medical intensive care unit. *Clin Nutr Res* 3:33, 2014.

[10] Doig GS et al. Early parenteral nutrition in critically ill patients with short-term relative contraindications to early enteral nutrition: a randomized controlled trial. *JAMA* 309:2130, 2013.

[11] Harvey SE et al. Trial of the route of early nutritional support in critically ill adults. *N Engl J Med* 371:1673, 2014.

[12] Dugan S, Le J, Jew RK. Maximum tolerated osmolarity for peripheral administration of parenteral nutrition in pediatric patients. *JPEN J Parenter Enteral Nutr* 38:847, 2014.

[13] Gajanayake I, Wylie CE, Chan DL. Clinical experience with a lipid-free, ready-made parenteral nutrition solution in dogs: 70 cases (2006–2012). *J Vet Emerg Crit Care (San Antonio)* 23:305, 2013.

[14] Michel KE, Eirmann L. Parenteral nutrition. In: Silverstein DC, Hopper K, editors. *Small Animal Critical Care Medicine*, 2nd ed. St Louis, Saunders Elsevier: 687, 2014.

[15] Chan DL. Nutrition in critical care. In: Bonagura JD, Twedt DC, editors. *Kirk's Current Veterinary Therapy*, 15th ed. St Louis, Saunders Elsevier: 38, 2002.

[16] Michel KE, King LG, Ostro E. Measurement of urinary urea nitrogen content as an estimate of the amount of total urinary nitrogen loss in dogs in intensive care units. *J Am Vet Med Assoc* 210:356, 1997.

[17] Chan DL. Nutritional requirements of the critically ill patient. *Clin Tech Small Anim Pract* 19:1, 2004.

[18] Biolo G et al. Metabolic response to injury and sepsis: changes in protein metabolism. *Nutrition* 13:52S, 1997.

[19] Rosmarin DK, Wardlaw GM, Mirtallo J. Hyperglycemia associated with high, continuous infusion rates of total parenteral nutrition dextrose. *Nutr Clin Pract* 11:151, 1996.

[20] Krogh-Madsen R et al. Effect of short-term intralipid infusion on the immune response during low-dose endotoxemia in humans. *Am J Physiol Endocrinol Metab* 294:E371, 2008.

[21] Grimes JB, Abel RM. Acute hemodynamic effects of intravenous fat emulsion in dogs. *JPEN J Parenter Enteral Nutr* 3:40, 1979.

[22] Mirtallo J et al. Safe practices for parenteral nutrition. *JPEN J Parenter Enteral Nutr* 28:S39, 2004.

[23] Wanten GJ, Calder PC. Immune modulation by parenteral lipid emulsions. *Am J Clin Nutr* 85:1171, 2007.

[24] Sala-Vila A, Barbosa VM, Calder PC. Olive oil in parenteral nutrition. *Curr Opin Clin Nutr Metab Care* 10:165, 2007.

[25] Lippert AC, Fulton RB Jr, Parr AM. A retrospective study of the use of total parenteral nutrition in dogs and cats. *J Vet Intern Med* 7:52, 1993.

[26] Crabb SE et al. Retrospective evaluation of total parenteral nutrition in cats: 40 cases (1991–2003). *J Vet Emerg Crit Care* 16:S21, 2006.

[27] Reuter JD et al. Use of total parenteral nutrition in dogs: 209 cases (1988–1995). *J Vet Emerg Crit Care* 8:201, 1998.

[28] Chan DL et al. Retrospective evaluation of partial parenteral nutrition in dogs and cats. *J Vet Intern Med* 16:440, 2002.

[29] Pyle SC, Marks SL, Kass PH. Evaluation of complications and prognostic factors associated with administration of total parenteral nutrition in cats: 75 cases (1994–2001). *J Am Vet Med Assoc* 225:242, 2004.

Appendix:
Recommended drugs and dosages

Recommended drugs for the management of digestive disorders in cats.

Drug	Indications	Dosage and route of administration	Comments
Alpha-tocopherol (see vitamin E)			
Amoxicillin	Hepatic encephalopathy	10–20 mg/kg SC/IM/PO every 8–12 h	Time-dependent bactericidal antibiotic Active against gram-positive and gram-negative aerobes and many anaerobes Ineffective against *Pseudomonas* spp., *Mycoplasma* spp., and *Enterobacter* spp., amongst others Ineffective against beta-lactamase-producing bacteria
Amoxicillin–clavulanate	Neutrophilic cholangitis Hepatic encephalopathy	10–20 mg/kg PO every 8–12 h 62.5 mg/cat PO every 12 h	Aminopenicillin + beta-lactamase inhibitor which extends spectrum of action Active against gram-positive and gram-negative aerobes and many anaerobes Ineffective against *Pseudomonas* spp. and *Enterobacter* spp. Reasonable choice for at-home empiric therapy or pending C&S testing
Ampicillin	Neutrophilic cholangitis Hepatic encephalopathy	10–20 mg/kg PO	Time-dependent bactericidal antibiotic Active against gram-positive and gram-negative aerobes and many anaerobes Ineffective against *Pseudomonas* spp., *Mycoplasma* spp., and *Enterobacter* spp., amongst others Ineffective against beta-lactamase-producing bacteria
Ampicillin–sulbactam	Neutrophilic cholangitis	20–40 mg/kg (of ampicillin) IV/IM every 6–8 h	Aminopenicillin + beta-lactamase inhibitor which extends spectrum of action Active against gram-positive and gram-negative aerobes and many anaerobes Ineffective against *Pseudomonas* spp. and *Enterobacter* spp. Reasonable choice for empiric therapy of hospitalised cats or pending C&S testing
Azithromycin	*Cryptosporidium* spp.	7–15 mg/kg PO every 12–24 h for 5–14 days (might require several weeks)	Optimal duration of treatment is unknown Potential for liver toxicity
Barium	GI mucosal bleeding/ulceration	1–2 ml/kg PO or per rectum (colorectal bleeding) every 8–12 h	Coating agent Can cause severe pneumonitis if inhaled or aspirated
Bisacodyl	Long-term management of constipation/obstipation	5 mg/cat PO every 24 h, short-term use only	Stimulant laxative (oral tablets)
Budesonide	Lymphocytic cholangitis, IBD, +/– chronic pancreatitis GI small-cell lymphoma	0.5–1 mg/cat PO every 24 h	Off-label use for IBD High topical activity, but systemic absorption and HPA axis suppression still occur in humans and dogs
Buprenorphine	Visceral pain associated with pancreatitis	0.01–0.03 mg/kg sublingual (off-label)/ IV/IM/SC every 6–8 h	Partial mu-opioid receptor agonist Effective analgesic agent in cats Provides moderate analgesia Can cause mydriasis, behavioural changes, and rarely respiratory depression Controlled drug, with potential for abuse
Butorphanol	Visceral pain associated with pancreatitis	0.2–0.4 mg/kg IV/SC every 2–6 h	Provides only mild to moderate analgesia
Capromorelin	Anorexia	3 mg/kg PO every 24 h	Ghrelin receptor agonist Not available in Europe

Chlorambucil	Lymphocytic cholangitis or IBD that does not respond adequately to prednisolone only GI small-cell lymphoma (in combination with prednisolone)	2 mg/cat PO every 48 h (every 72 h if <4 kg body weight) 15 mg/m^2 PO every 24 h for 4 days every 3 weeks 20 mg/m^2 PO every 2 weeks	Use gloves and do not split or crush the tablets* Can cause anaemia, leucopenia, thrombocytopenia, vomiting, and diarrhoea; can rarely cause neurotoxicity and Fanconi syndrome Increased risk of myelosuppression if used with additional myelosuppressive agents Monitoring: • Baseline CBC, biochemistry, urinalysis (including UPC ratio) • Repeat CBC after 1 month, thereafter every 2–3 months • Biochemistry and urinalysis (including UPC ratio) every 3 months
Chlorpromazine	Vomiting	0.5 mg/kg IM/SC every 6–8 h	Phenothiazine antiemetic
Cisapride	Gastrooesophageal reflux Gastric hypomotility Long-term management of constipation/obstipation	2.5-5 mg/cat PO every 8–12 h	Prokinetic agent Serotonin 4 agonist Stimulates smooth muscle Multiple known drug interactions with cisapride due to hepatic cytochrome P450 enzyme metabolism Geographical differences in availability or from compounding pharmacies
Cobalamin (see vitamin B_{12})			
Cyclosporin	Chronic gingivostomatitis Immunosuppression	Chronic gingivostomatitis: 2.5 mg/kg PO every 12 h Immunosuppressant: 3–4 mg/kg PO every 12 h 5–7 mg/kg PO every 24 h	Can cause GI signs (vomiting, diarrhoea, hypersalivation, hyporexia/anorexia); can rarely cause lethargy, malaise, behavioural changes, hirsutism, acute bullous keratopathy, gingival hyperplasia, recurrence of latent infections (viral, systemic toxoplasmosis), anaphylaxis, nephrotoxicity, and hepatotoxicity Absorption not significantly altered when administered with or without food, but highly variable between cats Half-life is very variable between cats Contraindications: hypersensitivity, neoplastic disease, known persistent infection (FeLV, FIV), possible insulin resistance Monitoring: • CBC and biochemistry at baseline, every 1 month for 3 months, then every 3–6 months • Blood glucose in diabetic cats • Body weight • Consider therapeutic drug monitoring
Dexamethasone (sodium phosphate)	Lymphocytic cholangitis, IBD, +/– chronic pancreatitis GI small-cell lymphoma	1/7th the calculated prednisolone dose IV/IM every 24 h	May be used during induction phase for 1–5 days if PO therapy is not possible
Docusate sodium or calcium	Long-term management of constipation/obstipation	50 mg/cat (mix with food or administer with syringe)	Emollient laxative (powder or liquid)

This table is intended only as a reference. The reader is referred to a pharmacology textbook or an approved drug formulary for comprehensive review of pharmacokinetics, pharmacodynamics, and known interactions and adverse effects of each drug.

CBC, complete blood count; C&S, culture and sensitivity; FeLV, feline leukaemia virus; FIV, feline immunodeficiency virus; GI, gastrointestinal; HPA, hypothalamic–pituitary–adrenal; IBD, inflammatory bowel disease; IM, intramuscular; IV, intravenous; PO, per os; SC, subcutaneous; UPC, urine protein:creatinine.

*Recommendations for the use of chemotherapy and safety guidelines are country dependent. The reader should be familiar with the requirements or seek advice prior to using chlorambucil.

Drug	Indications	Dosage and route of administration	Comments
Dolasetron	Vomiting, nausea	0.6–1.0 mg/kg PO/IV every 24 h	PO administration is not recommended for sole or long-term use due to poor bioavailability
Enrofloxacin	Neutrophilic cholangitis Granulomatous colitis caused by adherent–invasive *Escherichia coli* (AIEC) strains	5 mg/kg SC/PO every 24 h or divided in two doses every 12 h	Second-generation fluoroquinolone Bactericidal agent Active against gram-negative aerobes including *Pseudomonas* spp. Ineffective against anaerobes Prescribe only based on C&S results Can cause anorexia, vomiting, diarrhoea, retinal blindness, and cartilage abnormalities in young animals IV use is not recommended for cats **Other fluoquinolones represent a safer alternative in cats, as enrofloxacin has been associated with retinal blindness in this species.**
Epsiprantel	Tapeworms	2.75 mg/kg PO single dose	
Esomeprazole (see omeprazole)			
Famotidine	Oesophagitis	1 mg/kg PO/SC/IV every 12 h	Histamine type 2 receptor antagonist Inferior to proton pump inhibitors in inducing lasting increase in gastric pH
Fenbendazole	*Giardia* spp., roundworms, hookworms, *Physaloptera* spp., *Ollulanus tricuspis*	50 mg/kg PO every 24 h for 3–7 days	Able to eliminate *Giardia* in about 2/3 of cases
Fentanyl	Visceral pain associated with pancreatitis	0.005–0.01 mg/kg IV/IM/SC every 2 h 0.001–0.006 mg/kg/h CRI	Full mu-opioid receptor agonist Provides excellent analgesia Can cause dose-related CNS, respiratory, and circulatory depression Controlled drug, with potential for abuse Fentanyl patches may also be used
Lactulose	Long-term management of constipation/obstipation	0.5 ml/kg PO every 8–12 h (mix with food or administer with syringe)	Osmotic laxative (liquid)
Leflunomide	Immunosuppression	2 mg/kg PO every 24 h for 2 days, then 2 mg/kg PO every 48 h	Metabolised in plasma and intestinal tract Can rarely cause vomiting, and sedation (when given parenterally); other adverse effects reported in dogs: diarrhoea, lethargy, unexplained haemorrhage, thrombocytopenia, and increased liver enzymes Very limited information in cats Monitoring: CBC and biochemistry (hepatic enzymes) at baseline, every 1 month for 3 months, then every 3–6 months
Levetiracetam	Control of seizures associated with hepatic encephalopathy	20 mg/kg IV/PO every 8 h	Can cause sedation, hypersalivation, and inappetence
Marbofloxacin	Neutrophilic cholangitis Granulomatous colitis caused by adherent–invasive *Escherichia coli* (AIEC) strains	2 mg/kg PO every 24 h	Second-generation fluoroquinolone Bactericidal agent Active against gram-negative aerobes including *Pseudomonas* spp. Ineffective against anaerobes Prescribe only based on C&S results

Maropitant	Vomiting, nausea	1 mg/kg SC/IV (off-label) every 24 h 2 mg/kg PO (extralabel)	Neurokinin-1 receptor antagonist More effective in controlling vomiting than nausea Also has an analgesic effect Can cause injection-site pain, rarely depression, anorexia, and hypersalivation
Meperidine	Visceral pain associated with pancreatitis	2–5 mg/kg IM/SC every 2–4 h	
Methadone	Visceral pain associated with pancreatitis	0.1–0.2 mg/kg IV/IM every 4–6 h	Full mu-opioid receptor agonist and NMDA receptor competitive inhibitor Effective analgesic agent in hospitalised cats Can cause dose-related CNS, respiratory, and circulatory depression, as well as dysphoria and vomiting Controlled drug, with potential for abuse
Methylprednisolone	Same as prednisolone	2–4 mg/cat PO every 24 h or divided in two doses every 12 h, then taper gradually	Chronic use at any dose for more than 1–2 weeks will cause HPA axis suppression, and tapering therapy is advised
Methylprednisolone acetate	Same as prednisolone	10–20 mg/cat IM every 1–3 weeks	
Metoclopramide	Gastrooesophageal reflux Gastric hypomotility Vomiting, nausea	0.2–0.5 mg/kg IV/IM/SC/PO every 6–8 h 1–2 mg/kg/day CRI	Dopamine 2 receptor and serotonin 4 receptor antagonist Not effective antiemetic in cats Weak prokinetic (stimulates gastric antral contractions) CRI might be more effective Can cause frenzied behaviour, ataxia, and constipation
Mirtazapine	Inappetence	2 mg transdermally every 24 h 1.875–3.75 mg/cat PO every 24 h	Tricyclic antidepressant, serotonin 3 receptor antagonist Can interact with other drugs, including tramadol Can cause application-site reactions, vocalisation, increased affection, hyperactivity, and vomiting, and less commonly hypotension or tachycardia (PO route)
Mosapride	Long-term management of constipation/obstipation	5 mg/cat PO every 12 h	Serotonin 4 agonist Colonic prokinetic Available in select Asian countries
Mycophenolate mofetil	Immunosuppression	10 mg/kg PO every 12 h 10 mg/kg IV every 12 h	Very limited information in cats Can cause diarrhoea (dose dependent) and hyporexia Monitoring: • CBC, renal and hepatic function at baseline • Monitor periodically
Neomycin	Hepatic encephalopathy	20 mg/kg PO every 12 h	Allergies reported in some cats Can cause oto- and nephrotoxicity if systemically absorbed

This table is intended only as a reference. The reader is referred to a pharmacology textbook or an approved drug formulary for comprehensive review of pharmacokinetics, pharmacodynamics, and known interactions and adverse effects of each drug.

CBC, complete blood count; CNS, central nervous system; CRI, constant-rate infusion; C&S, culture and sensitivity; HPA, hypothalamic–pituitary–adrenal; IM, intramuscular; IV, intravenous; NMDA, N-methyl-D-aspartate; PO, per os; SC, subcutaneous.

Drug	Indications	Dosage and route of administration	Comments
Nitazoxanide	*Cryptosporidium* spp.	10–25 mg/kg PO every 12 h for 4 weeks	Used in humans; large data regarding use in cats is lacking Might cause vomiting and diarrhoea
Omeprazole **Pantoprazole** **Esomeprazole**	Oesophagitis Gastrooesophageal reflux	1 mg/kg PO every 12 h	Proton pump inhibitors Increase gastric pH Based on comparative studies in healthy cats, oral esomeprazole might be superior to pantoprazole in suppressing gastric pH Can be used depending on the formulation available in respective countries
Ondansetron	Vomiting, nausea	0.1–2 mg/kg slow IV every 6–12 h 0.2–0.5 mg/kg PO every 12 h	Serotonin 3 receptor antagonist PO administration is not recommended for sole or long-term use due to poor bioavailability If PO doses are given, should be towards the high end of the range and should be given more frequently
Pantoprazole (see omeprazole)			
Paromomycin	*Cryptosporidium* spp.	125–165 mg/kg PO every 12 h for 5–7 days	Likely low efficacy Potentially toxic (nephrotoxicity, ototoxicity)
Petrolatum	Prevention of hairballs	Use according to manufacturers' instructions	Lubricant laxative used mostly for hairball prevention
Phenobarbital	Control of seizures associated with hepatic encephalopathy	Status epilepticus: 6–12 mg/kg IV, repeat at lower dose after 20 minutes if required 1.5–2 mg/kg PO every 12 h	Can cause sedation Metabolised in the liver; hence, avoid high dose
Phytomenadione (see vitamin K_1)			
Piroxicam	Palliative therapy for squamous cell carcinoma	0.3 mg/kg PO every 24–72 h	NSAID Antitumour, anti-inflammatory
Polyethylene glycol 3350 (macrogol)	Long-term management of constipation/obstipation	1/8–1/4 tsp/cat PO every 12 h (mix with canned food)	Osmotic laxative (powder)
Ponazuril	*Isospora* spp.	30–50 mg/kg PO every 24 h for 2–6 days	
Pradofloxacin	Neutrophilic cholangitis Granulomatous colitis caused by adherent–invasive *Escherichia coli* (AIEC) strains	5 (extralabel)–7.5 mg/kg PO every 24 h	Third-generation fluoroquinolone Bactericidal agent Compared to second-generation fluoroquinolones, it has activity against gram-positive aerobes and some anaerobes May interact with other drugs, including cyclosporin and NSAIDs Can cause anorexia, vomiting, diarrhoea, and leucopenia
Praziquantel	Tapeworms Liver fluke–associated cholangitis	5–20 mg/kg PO single dose 10–25 mg/kg SC/PO every 24 h for 3–5 days	Anticestodal Can cause GI signs, injection-site pain

Prednisolone	Lymphocytic cholangitis, IBD, +/– chronic pancreatitis GI small-cell lymphoma Feline GI eosinophilic sclerosing fibroplasia Acquired myasthenia gravis Chronic gingivostomatitis	Immunosuppressive: 1–2 (–4) mg/kg every 24 h or divided every 12 h then gradually tapered Anti-inflammatory: 0.5–1 (–2) mg/kg every 24 h then gradually tapered	Glucocorticoid Can cause polyuria, polydipsia, polyphagia, weight gain, and diabetes Avoid with untreated bacterial cholangitis or other infections Chronic use at any dose for more than 1–2 weeks will cause HPA axis suppression, and tapering therapy is advised
Prochlorperazine	Vomiting	0.1–0.5 mg/kg IM/SC every 6–8 h	Phenothiazine antiemetic
Prucalopride	Same as cisapride	1 mg/cat PO every 8–24 h	Serotonin 4 agonist Gastric and colonic prokinetic At 0.64 mg/kg PO given to healthy cats, it induced defecation within 1 hour whilst it had no efficacy at 0.32 mg/kg
Psyllium husk	Long-term management of constipation/obstipation	1 tsp PO every 12–24 h (mix with canned food)	Bulk laxative (powder)
Pumpkin (canned)	Long-term management of constipation/obstipation	1 tsp PO every 12–24 h (mix with food)	Bulk laxative
Pyrantel pamoate	Roundworms, hookworms, *Physaloptera* spp., *Ollulanus tricuspis*	5–20 mg/kg PO single dose	Safe and effective Ideal for very young kittens (2–3 weeks)
Pyridostigmine	Acquired myasthenia gravis	0.2–2 mg/kg PO every 8–12 h (extrapolated from dogs)	Acetylcholine esterase inhibitor
Ranitidine	Oesophagitis Long-term management of constipation/obstipation (mild cases)	2.0–3.5 mg/kg PO/SC/IV every 12 h	Histamine type 2 receptor antagonist Mildly increases gastric pH (inferior efficacy compared to famotidine and proton pump inhibitors) Some prokinetics effects on colon
Rifaximin	Hepatic encephalopathy	5 mg/kg PO every 12–24 h	Expense restricts use Limited anecdotal use for hepatic encephalopathy
Ronidazole	*Tritrichomonas blagburni* (*foetus*)	30 mg/kg PO every 24 h for 14 days	Only drug that works for *T. blagburni* Relatively safe and effective Higher doses might be associated with neurological signs
S-adenosylmethionine	Cholangitis Hepatic lipidosis	20 mg/kg or 90 mg/cat PO every 24 h on an empty stomach	Antioxidant (glutathione precursor), possible anti-inflammatory and choleretic effects Well tolerated
Silymarin	Cholangitis Hepatic lipidosis	5–10 mg/kg/day (silybin–phosphatidylcholine complex) 20–50 mg/kg/day PO divided every 8 h (less bioavailable forms)	Reduces lipid peroxidation, purported anti-inflammatory and antifibrotic effects Well tolerated Essential medications should be prioritised

This table is intended only as a reference. The reader is referred to a pharmacology textbook or an approved drug formulary for comprehensive review of pharmacokinetics, pharmacodynamics, and known interactions and adverse effects of each drug.

GI, gastrointestinal; HPA, hypothalamic–pituitary–adrenal; IBD, inflammatory bowel disease; IM, intramuscular; IV, intravenous; NSAID, nonsteroidal anti-inflammatory drug; PO, per os; SC, subcutaneous; tsp, teaspoon.

Drug	Indications	Dosage and route of administration	Comments
Sucralfate	Oesophagitis Gastrooesophageal reflux	250–500 mg/cat PO every 6–8 h, dissolve in water to form slurry	Mucosal cytoprotectant Provides diffusion barrier Slurry (tab crushed and dissolved in water) or suspension
Sulphadimethoxine	*Isospora* spp.	50–60 mg/kg PO every 24 h for 5–20 days	Safe and effective
Toltrazuril	*Isospora* spp.	30 mg/kg PO every 24 h for 2–6 days	Safe and effective
Triamcinolone	Oesophageal stricture	1 mg intramucosal/intralesional injection (applied circumferentially, dose divided between four locations, after stricture balloon dilation, using a sclerotherapy injection needle)	Glucocorticoid Inhibits fibrosis
Trimethoprim–sulphadiazine	*Isospora* spp.	30 mg/kg PO every 24 h (or 15 mg/kg PO every 12 h) for 10 days	Safe and effective
Ursodeoxycholic acid	Hepatic lipidosis, +/– cholangitis	10–15 mg/kg PO every 24 h	Displaces hydrophobic bile acids, choleretic, and possibly reduces hepatocellular apoptosis Can rarely cause diarrhoea Essential medications should be prioritised
Vitamin B_{12} (cobalamin)	Cobalamin deficiency associated with IBD, EPI, and other causes	EPI: 250–500 µg SC/IM weekly for 6 weeks, then monthly until blood values are in high end of reference range Causes other than EPI: 250 µg/cat SC/IM weekly for 6 weeks, then monthly until blood values are in high end of reference range 250 µg/cat PO daily for 12 weeks (until blood values are in high end of reference range)	Measure serum cobalamin concentrations every 3–6 months after initial supplementation, and treat as necessary with additional supplementation every 14–30 days
Vitamin E (alpha-tocopherol)	Cholangitis Hepatic lipidosis	10–15 IU/kg/day PO	Reduced lipid peroxidation Well tolerated when given PO Essential medications should be prioritised
Vitamin K_1 (phytomenadione)	Cholestasis, hepatic lipidosis	0.5–1.5 mg/kg SC/PO every 12 h for three doses	Cofactor for vitamin K–dependent coagulation factors Best absorbed PO when given with a meal Can rarely cause anaphylactoid reactions when given SC

This table is intended only as a reference. The reader is referred to a pharmacology textbook or an approved drug formulary for comprehensive review of pharmacokinetics, pharmacodynamics, and known interactions and adverse effects of each drug.

EPI, exocrine pancreatic insufficiency; IBD, inflammatory bowel disease; IM, intramuscular; PO, per os; SC, subcutaneous.

Subject index

A

B

C

F

G

H

N

O

P

R